ORAL RADIOLOGY

Principles and Interpretation

ORAL RADIOLOGY

Principles and Interpretation

EDITION 7

Stuart C. White, DDS, PhD
Distinguished Professor
Oral and Maxillofacial Radiology
School of Dentistry
University of California, Los Angeles
Los Angeles, California

Michael J. Pharoah, DDS, MSc, FRCD(C)
Professor, Department of Radiology
Faculty of Dentistry
University of Toronto
Toronto, Ontario
Canada

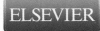

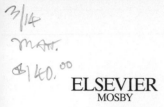

ELSEVIER
MOSBY

3251 Riverport Lane
St. Louis, Missouri 63043

ORAL RADIOLOGY PRINCIPLES AND INTERPRETATION,   ISBN: 978-0-323-09633-1
SEVENTH EDITION
Copyright © 2014, 2009, 2004, 2000, 1994, 1987, 1982 by Mosby, an imprint of Elsevier Inc.

Notices

Knowledge and best practice in this field are constantly changing. As new research and experience broaden our understanding, changes in research methods, professional practices, or medical treatment may become necessary.

Practitioners and researchers must always rely on their own experience and knowledge in evaluating and using any information, methods, compounds, or experiments described herein. In using such information or methods they should be mindful of their own safety and the safety of others, including parties for whom they have a professional responsibility.

With respect to any drug or pharmaceutical products identified, readers are advised to check the most current information provided (i) on procedures featured or (ii) by the manufacturer of each product to be administered, to verify the recommended dose or formula, the method and duration of administration, and contraindications. It is the responsibility of practitioners, relying on their own experience and knowledge of their patients, to make diagnoses, to determine dosages and the best treatment for each individual patient, and to take all appropriate safety precautions.

To the fullest extent of the law, neither the Publisher nor the authors, contributors, or editors, assume any liability for any injury and/or damage to persons or property as a matter of products liability, negligence or otherwise, or from any use or operation of any methods, products, instructions, or ideas contained in the material herein.

ISBN: 978-0-323-09633-1

Vice President and Publisher: Linda Duncan
Executive Content Strategist: Kathy Falk
Senior Content Development Specialist: Brian Loehr
Publishing Services Manager: Julie Eddy
Project Manager: Jan Waters
Design Direction: Maggie Reid

Printed in Canada

Last digit is the print number: 9   8   7   6   5   4   3   2   1

Contributors

Mariam Baghdady, BDS, MSc, PhD, FRCD(C), Dip ABOMR
University of Toronto
Faculty of Dentistry
Toronto, Ontario
Canada

Byron W. Benson, DDS, MS
Professor and Vice Chair
Department of Diagnostic Sciences
Texas A&M University
Baylor College of Dentistry
Dallas, Texas

Sharon L. Brooks, DDS, MS
Professor Emerita
Periodontics and Oral Medicine
University of Michigan
School of Dentistry
Ann Arbor, Michigan

Laurie C. Carter, DDS, PhD
Professor and Director
Oral and Maxillofacial Radiology
Director of Advanced Dental Education
Virginia Commonwealth University
School of Dentistry
Richmond, Virginia

Allan G. Farman, BDS, PhD (Odont), DSc (Odont)
Professor, Radiology and Imaging Science
Surgical and Hospital Dentistry
Clinical Professor, Department of Diagnostic Radiology School
   of Medicine
Adjunct Professor, Department of Anatomical Sciences and
   Neurobiology
University of Louisville
Louisville, Kentucky

Fatima Jadu, BDS, MSc, PhD, FRCD(C), Dipl ABOMR
Assistant Professor
Oral and Maxillofacial Radiology
King Abdulaziz University
Faculty of Dentistry
Jeddah, Saudi Arabia

Mel L. Kantor, DDS, MPH, PhD
Professor and Chief
Oral Diagnosis, Oral Medicine & Oral Radiology
Department of Oral Health Practice
University of Kentucky
College of Dentistry
Lexington, Kentucky

Ernest W. N. Lam, DMD, PhD, FRCD(C)
Dr. Lloyd & Mrs. Kay Chapman Chair in Clinical Sciences
Professor and Head of Oral and Maxillofacial Radiology
University of Toronto
Toronto, Ontario
Canada

Linda Lee, DDS, MSc, Dipl ABOP, FRCD(C)
Oral Medicine and Pathology
Princess Margaret Hospital
University Health Network
Associate Professor
University of Toronto
Toronto, Ontario
Canada

John B. Ludlow, DDS, MS, FDS, RCSEd
Professor
Oral and Maxillofacial Radiology
University of North Carolina at Chapel Hill
School of Dentistry
Chapel Hill, North Carolina

Alan G. Lurie, DDS, PhD
Professor and Chair
Oral and Maxillofacial Radiology
University of Connecticut
School of Dental Medicine
Farmington, Connecticut

Sanjay M. Mallya, BDS, MDS, PhD
Assistant Professor
Oral and Maxillofacial Radiology
UCLA School of Dentistry
Los Angeles, California

André Mol, DDS, MS, PhD
Clinical Associate Professor
Department of Diagnostic Sciences
University of North Carolina at Chapel Hill
School of Dentistry
Chapel Hill, North Carolina

Carol Anne Murdoch-Kinch, DDS, PhD
Clinical Professor
Associate Dean for Academic Affairs
University of Michigan School of Dentistry
Ann Arbor, Michigan

Susanne Perschbacher, DDS, MSc, FRCD(C), Dipl ABOMR
Assistant Professor
Oral and Maxillofacial Radiology
University of Toronto
Toronto, Ontario
Canada

Axel Ruprecht, DDS, MScD, FRCD(C)
Gilbert E. Lilly Professor of Diagnostic Sciences
Professor and Director of Oral and Maxillofacial Radiology
Professor of Radiology
Professor of Anatomy and Cell Biology
The University of Iowa
Iowa City, Iowa

William C. Scarfe, BDS, MS, FRACDS
Professor
Radiology and Imaging Sciences
University of Louisville
School of Dentistry
Louisville, Kentucky

Vivek Shetty, DDS, Dr Med Dent
Professor
Oral and Maxillofacial Surgery
UCLA School of Dentistry
Los Angeles, California

Sotirios Tetradis, DDS, PhD
Professor and Chair
Oral and Maxillofacial Radiology
UCLA School of Dentistry
Los Angeles, California

Ann Wenzel, PhD, Dr Odont
Professor and Head
Department of Oral Radiology
School of Dentistry
University of Aarhus
Aarhus, Denmark

Robert E. Wood, DDS, PhD, FRCD(C), DABFO
Head, Department of Dental Oncology
Princess Margaret Hospital
Associate Professor
University of Toronto
Toronto, Ontario
Canada

Preface

Oral radiology is a vibrant field of study. The discovery of x rays by Wilhelm Röntgen in December 1895 forever changed the practice of dentistry and medicine. During the next year, the first dental radiographs were made by Dr. Otto Walkhoff in Germany, Dr. C. Edmund Kells in New Orleans, and Dr. W. H. Rollins in Boston. Dr. Rollins was also a pioneer in the field of radiation safety, and we follow his basic principles to this day. We dedicate this edition to Dr. Harry M. Worth, who devoted his life study to the radiographic appearances of diseases of the jaws. His textbook, issued 50 years ago in 1963, set the standard for radiographic interpretation. He was an inspiration to us both.

Dentists today have ready access to a variety of excellent imaging modalities to assist in the care of their patients. To best use dental radiography in the practice of dentistry, it is important to understand the basic principles of imaging. To this end, this book includes chapters describing the means of producing x rays, the mechanisms by which radiation interacts with living systems, and the safe operation of dental x-ray machines. Other chapters focus on how to make intraoral images and on the imaging principles underlying panoramic and cone-beam computed tomographic (CBCT) machines, multidetector computed tomographic (CT) scanners, and magnetic resonance imaging scanners. We describe how images are captured on film and, increasingly often, with digital sensors.

Of course, the primary purpose of oral radiology is to produce images that may be interpreted for the detection of disease or other abnormalities. The second half of this book is dedicated to the systematic description of the radiographic manifestation of diseases and other conditions in the oral cavity and associated structures, including the paranasal sinuses and temporomandibular joints. Emphasis is placed on the role of understanding the underlying mechanisms of various disease processes to enhance the interpretation of abnormalities as they can appear in various imaging modalities. To be a good diagnostician, it is helpful to be curious, observant, systematic, and thorough. This applies not only to interpreting diagnostic images but also to obtaining a patient's history, conducting the physical examination, and combining this information to arrive at a proper differential diagnosis. Successful treatment critically depends on accurate diagnosis.

In general, dentists interpret most of the images they prescribe and produce. This responsibility places a special burden on dentists to be well versed in the means of acquiring optimal images as well as in their interpretation. Interpretation of images may be especially challenging for dentists who rarely see abnormalities such as cysts, inflammatory diseases, tumors, or other forms of disease. Also challenging is the unfamiliar presentation of images in a new format, such as a sequence of image slices of an image volume or three-dimensional representations as in advanced imaging modalities, such as cone-beam CT imaging or other types of scanners. This situation is largely remedied by a cadre of trained and experienced oral and maxillofacial radiologists. These individuals assist general dentists and other medical and dental specialists by helping to interpret the images of unusual cases or by suggesting appropriate advanced imaging to investigate an unknown condition more thoroughly. General dentists and their patients benefit by calling on the services of these individuals whenever they come across an image that they are not confident interpreting.

Each new edition of this textbook provides the opportunity to describe recent progress in our rapidly changing field of diagnostic imaging. Every chapter has been revised in light of new knowledge, technology, and techniques. In this edition, two new chapters dealing with the image acquisition and image processing involved with cone-beam CT technology have been added. It is the continuing goal of our textbook to present the underlying science of diagnostic imaging, including the core principles of image production and interpretation for the dental student. We also offer supplemental resources to both instructors and students at a companion Evolve website (http://evolve.elsevier.com) for the seventh edition. For instructors, a test bank and image collection will save time in preparing for lectures and examinations.

It is our hope that the reader will find the study of oral radiology as exciting and fulfilling as we have.

Stuart C. White
Michael J. Pharoah

Acknowledgments

We are sincerely appreciative of all authors for sharing their expertise with the reader. Their rich body of knowledge and experience have contributed substantively to this edition. We thank all for sharing their expertise and skills.

This edition welcomes three new authors: Drs. Mariam Baghdady and Fatima Jadu, both from the University of Toronto, and Dr. Sanjay Mallya from UCLA. Dr. Baghdady has extended the chapter on the principles of interpretation, bringing more emphasis on the science behind diagnostic reasoning and image interpretation. Dr. Jadu rewrote the chapter on systemic diseases, with special emphasis on the underlying disease mechanisms. Dr. Mallya rewrote the chapter on panoramic imaging, extending the coverage of the principles underlying image formation as well as novel features available on new panoramic machines. Drs. William Scarfe and Allan Farman extended their coverage of cone-beam CT imaging from one chapter to two, the first on image acquisition and the second on image preparation for interpretation. A new chapter by Drs. Mallya and Sotirios Tetradis describes the radiographic anatomy seen on sagittal, coronal, and axial cone-beam CT images. Finally, Dr. Robert Wood has prepared a new chapter on forensics in dentistry focusing on the role of dental radiography in identifying human remains. And we are most appreciative of authors who continue to contribute their expertise in updating their chapters for the current edition. Lastly, we wish to remember the outstanding contributions of two deceased gentlemen, Drs. A. Peter Fortier and S. Julian Gibbs. Each of these men wrote insightful chapters in the early editions of this book and contributed to the advancement of our field.

We are particularly grateful to our colleagues and students whose sharp eyes and minds uncover errors and suggest ways for us to improve each edition. Among these individuals are Drs. Mansur Ahmad, Mohamed Khaled Alashiry, Ali Bagherpour, Silvina Friedlander-Barenboim, Mohammed Hussain, Marc Levitan, Gang Li, Brian Lozano, Peter Mah, Matheus Oliveira, Colin Price, Elham Radan, Greg Smith, Susan White, Lisa Yi, Eugene Yu, and Ed Zinman. Also, from the world of industry, we appreciate the assistance of Drs. Kim Brown and Adam Chen, Herb Clay, Betsy Guffey, Gary Piper, Jacqueline Sacrey, Christopher Warren, and Douglas Yoon. We apologize for any individuals inadvertently overlooked on these lists.

Finally, we are also grateful to the staff at Elsevier for their generous support and energy and creativity in the presentation of the content of this book. In particular, we thank Brian Loehr for his calm persistence in keeping us ever moving forward, as well as Ellen Thomas and Jan Waters for their close review and improvements to the text. We also thank Ms. Jeanne Robertson for her many new skillful illustrations, as well as Joe Robertson for his insightful contributions to the test bank review questions.

Stuart C. White
Michael J. Pharoah

"Man erblickt nur, was man schon weiss und versteht."

Johann Wolfgang von Goethe

Gespräche mit F.V. Müller

24.4.1819

One recognizes only what one already knows and understands.

Contents

CHAPTER

1

Physics

OUTLINE

One atom says to a friend, "I think I lost an electron." The friend replies, "Are you sure?" "Yes," says the first atom, "I'm positive."

Dentists make radiographic images of patients when they seek additional information beyond that available from a clinical examination or their patient's history. Dentists combine the information from these images with their findings from the clinical examination and history to form a diagnosis. When a diagnosis is established, treatment can be provided. This chapter considers the initial steps in making radiographic images including the operation of an x-ray machine and the interactions of radiation with matter.

COMPOSITION OF MATTER

Matter is anything that has mass and occupies space. All visible matter in the universe (all stable matter) is made of up quarks, down quarks, and electrons. These particles are fundamental because they have no inner structure and cannot be divided. Up quarks and down quarks combine to form neutrons and protons in atomic nuclei. Electrons are located in orbitals outside the nuclei. Historically, the atom has been viewed as a miniature solar system with a nucleus at the center and revolving electrons. This

classic view of the atom has been replaced by the Standard Model, which describes the subatomic particles (Table 1-1), and the Quantum Mechanical Model, which describes the arrangement of electrons in an atom. In addition to matter particles, the Standard Model also describes force carrier particles—particles that mediate interactions between matter particles (Table 1-2).

ATOMIC STRUCTURE

Nucleus

In all atoms except hydrogen, the nucleus consists of positively charged protons and neutral neutrons. A hydrogen nucleus contains a single proton. Protons and neutrons are made of quarks (Fig. 1-1). Protons consist of two up quarks and one down quark and thus have a charge of +1. Neutrons are made of one up quark and two down quarks and thus are neutral. Although the positively charged protons repel each other, the nucleus is held together by the strong nuclear force, the rapid exchange of gluons. The strong nuclear force overwhelms the repulsive electromagnetic effect at the incredibly short distances inside an atomic nucleus.

The number of protons in the nucleus determines the identity of an element. This is its atomic number (Z), the nuclear charge. A change in the number of protons in an atom changes it to another element. Each of the more than 100 elements has a unique atomic number, a corresponding number of orbital electrons in the ground state, and unique chemical and physical properties. The

TABLE 1-1   Fundamental Particles

	Charge	FAMILIES OF PARTICLES					
		I		II		III	
Quarks	$+\frac{2}{3}$	Up	u	Charm	c	Top	t
	$-\frac{1}{3}$	Down	d	Strange	s	Bottom	b
Leptons	-1	Electron	e	Muon	μ	Tau	τ
	0	Electron neutrino	ν_e	Muon neutrino	ν_μ	Tau neutrino	ν_τ

Stable particles

TABLE 1-2   Force-Carrier Particles

Particle	Symbol	Action
Photon	γ	Make up x-ray beams and mediate electromagnetic interactions
Gluon	g	Mediate strong nuclear force that binds quarks into protons and neutrons and bind nuclei together
W boson	W	Mediate weak interactions; associated with beta decay
Z boson	Z	Mediate weak interactions; associated with neutrino scatter

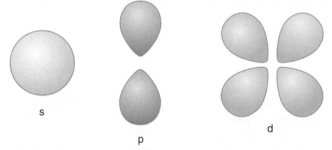

s

p

d

FIGURE 1-2 Electron orbitals are clouds of varying density, probability plots of the location of the electron. The s-type electron orbital is spherical and centered around the nucleus. The p-type electron orbitals are bilobed and centered around the nucleus. Four of the five d-type electron orbitals are made up of four lobes, centered on the nucleus. The fifth d-type orbital is bilobed with an encircling ring (not shown).

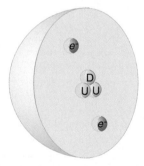

FIGURE 1-1 Schematic view of a hydrogen atom showing a nucleus with one proton, composed of two up quarks (U) and one down quark (D) and two surrounding electrons (e^-) within a 1s spherical orbital. Compared with the scale of the 1s orbital, the nucleus and electrons are much smaller than shown.

total number of protons and neutrons in the nucleus of an atom is its **atomic mass** (A). A change in the number of neutrons in an atom changes the stability of the element. Nearly the entire mass of the atom consists of the protons and neutrons in the nucleus.

Electron Orbitals

Electrons exhibit both particle-like properties (e.g., they have mass) and wavelike properties (e.g., they generate interference patterns). Electrons exist within three-dimensional volumes called **orbitals**. Orbitals represent the probability locations of the electron in space at any instant in time—the regions in which the electron is most likely to exist. The letters s, p, d, f, g, and h are used to describe orbital shapes (Fig. 1-2). These letters replace the K, L, M, N, O, and P designations previously used. Only two electrons may occupy an orbital. The s-type orbital is spherical. The s-type

orbitals are the first to be filled in every element. Next are the p-type orbitals, which are bilobed and centered on the nucleus. Next are the d-type orbitals, which consist of four lobes arranged around the nucleus—they are bilobed with a ring. In an atom with many electrons, the electron clouds of one orbital are superimposed with the electron clouds of other orbitals. No known atom has more than seven orbitals. Electrons occupy the lowest energy available orbitals—those not already occupied by other electrons. A change in the number of electrons of an atom changes the charge of an atom.

IONIZATION

When the number of electrons in an atom is equal to the number of protons in its nucleus, the atom is electrically neutral. If a neutral atom loses an electron, it becomes a positive ion, and the free electron becomes a negative ion. This process of forming an ion pair is termed **ionization**. Ionizing an atom requires sufficient energy to overcome the **electron binding energy**, the electrostatic force binding the electrons to the nucleus. The binding energy of an electron is related to the atomic number of the atom and the orbital type. Elements with a large atomic number (high Z) have more protons in their nucleus and thus bind electrons in any given orbital more tightly than smaller Z elements. Within a given atom, electrons in the inner orbitals are more tightly bound than the more distant outer orbitals. Tightly bound electrons require the energy of x rays or high-energy particles to remove them, whereas loosely bound outer electrons can be displaced by ultraviolet radiation. However, nonionizing types of radiation, such as visible light, infrared, and microwave radiation, and radio waves do not have sufficient energy to remove bound electrons from their orbitals.

NATURE OF RADIATION

Radiation is the transmission of energy through space and matter. It may occur in two forms: (1) particulate (Table 1-3) and (2) electromagnetic. Natural radioactivity and radiation therapy may involve both particulate and electromagnetic radiation. Oral and maxillofacial radiology involves only electromagnetic radiation.

PARTICULATE RADIATION

Small atoms have roughly equal numbers of protons and neutrons, whereas larger atoms tend to have more neutrons than protons. Larger atoms are unstable because of the unequal distribution of protons and neutrons, and they may break up, releasing α (alpha) or β (beta) particles or γ (gamma) rays. This process is called radioactivity. When a radioactive atom releases an α or a β particle, the atom is transmuted into another element. α particles are helium nuclei consisting of two protons and two neutrons. They result from the radioactive decay of many large atomic number elements. Because of their double positive charge and heavy mass, α particles densely ionize matter through which they pass. They quickly give up their energy and penetrate only a few micrometers of body tissue. (An ordinary sheet of paper absorbs them.) After stopping, α particles acquire two electrons and become neutral helium atoms.

An unstable atom with an excess of neutrons may decay by converting a neutron into a proton, a β⁻ particle, and a neutrino. β⁻ particles are identical to electrons. High-speed β⁻ particles are not densely ionizing; they are able to penetrate matter to a greater depth than α particles can—up to 1.5 cm in tissue. This deeper penetration occurs because β⁻ particles are smaller and lighter and carry a single negative charge; they have a much lower probability of interacting with matter than α particles. β⁻ particles from radioactive iodine-131 are used for treatment of some thyroid cancers. An unstable atom with an excess of protons may decay by converting a proton into a neutron, a β⁺ particle (positron), and a neutrino. Positrons quickly annihilate with electrons to form two γ rays. This reaction is the basis for positron emission tomography scanning (see Chapter 14).

The capacity of particulate radiation to ionize atoms depends on its mass, velocity, and charge. The rate of loss of energy from a particle as it moves along its track through matter (tissue) is its linear energy transfer (LET). A particle loses kinetic energy each time it ionizes adjacent matter. The greater the physical size of the particle, the higher its charge, and the lower its velocity, the greater its LET. For example, α particles, with their high mass compared with an electron, high charge, and low velocity, are densely ionizing, lose their kinetic energy rapidly, and have a high LET. β⁻ particles are much less densely ionizing because of their lighter mass and lower charge; they have a lower LET. High LET radiations concentrate their ionization along a short path, whereas low LET radiations produce ion pairs much more sparsely over a longer path length.

Another type of radioactivity is γ decay. γ rays are photons, a form of electromagnetic radiation (see next section). They result as part of a decay chain where a nucleus converts from an excited state to a lower level ground state; this often happens after a nucleus emits an α or β particle or after nuclear fission or fusion.

ELECTROMAGNETIC RADIATION

Electromagnetic radiation is the movement of energy through space as a combination of electric and magnetic fields. It is generated when the velocity of an electrically charged particle is altered. γ rays, x rays, ultraviolet rays, visible light, infrared radiation (heat), microwaves, and radio waves all are examples of electromagnetic radiation (Fig. 1-3). γ rays originate in the nuclei of radioactive atoms. They typically have greater energy than x rays. In contrast, x rays are produced outside the nucleus and result from the interaction of electrons with large atomic nuclei in x-ray machines. The higher energy types of radiation in the electromagnetic spectrum—ultraviolet rays, x rays, and γ rays—are capable of ionizing matter. Some properties of electromagnetic radiation are best explained by quantum theory, whereas others are most successfully described by wave theory.

Quantum theory considers electromagnetic radiation as small discrete bundles of energy called photons. Each photon travels at the speed of light and contains a specific amount of energy. The unit of photon energy is the electron volt (eV), the amount of energy acquired by one electron accelerating through a potential difference of one volt. The relationship between wavelength and photon energy is as follows:

$$E = h \times c / \lambda$$

where E is energy in kiloelectron volts (keV), h is Planck's constant (6.626×10^{-34} joule-seconds or 4.13×10^{-15} eV-seconds), c is the

TABLE 1-3		Particulate Radiation	
Particle	Symbol	Elementary Charge*	Rest Mass (amu)
Alpha	α	+2	4.00154
Beta⁺ (positron)	β⁺	+1	0.000549
Beta⁻ (electron)	β⁻	−1	0.000549
Electron	e⁻	−1	0.000549
Neutron	n⁰	0	1.008665
Proton	p	+1	1.007276

amu, Atomic mass units, where 1 amu = 1/12 the mass of a neutral carbon-12 atom.
*Elementary charge of 1 equals that the charge of a proton or the opposite of an electron.

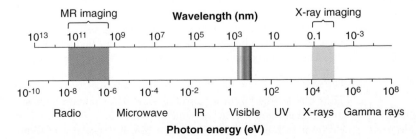

FIGURE 1-3 Electromagnetic spectrum showing the relationship between photon wavelength and energy and the physical properties of various portions of the spectrum. Photons with shorter wavelengths have higher energy. Photons used in dental radiography (blue) have energies of 10 to 120 keV. Magnetic resonance (MR) imaging uses radio waves (orange).

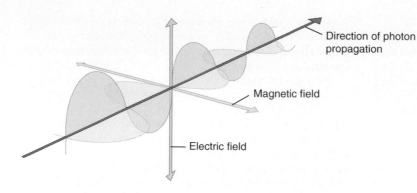

FIGURE 1-4 Electric and magnetic fields associated with electromagnetic radiation.

velocity of light, and λ is wavelength in nanometers. This expression may be simplified to:

$$E = 1.24/\lambda$$

Quantum theory has been successful in correlating experimental data on the interaction of radiation with atoms, the photoelectric effect, and the production of x rays. The wave theory of electromagnetic radiation maintains that radiation is propagated in the form of waves, similar to the waves resulting from a disturbance in water. Such waves consist of electric and magnetic fields oriented in planes at right angles to one another that oscillate perpendicular to the direction of motion (Fig. 1-4). All electromagnetic waves travel at the velocity of light ($c = 3.0 \times 10^8$ m/s) in a vacuum. Waves of all kinds exhibit the properties of wavelength (λ) and frequency (ν) and are related as follows:

$$\lambda \times \nu = c = 3 \times 10^8 \text{ m/s}$$

where λ is in meters and ν is in cycles per second (hertz). Wave theory is more useful for considering radiation in bulk when millions of quanta are being examined, as in experiments dealing with refraction, reflection, diffraction, interference, and polarization.

High-energy photons such as x rays and γ rays are typically characterized by their energy (electron volts), medium-energy photons (e.g., visible light and ultraviolet waves) are typically characterized by their wavelength (nanometers), and low-energy photons (e.g., AM and FM radio waves) are typically characterized by their frequency (KHz and MHz).

X-RAY MACHINE

X-ray machines produce x rays that pass through a patient's tissues and strike a digital receptor or film to make a radiographic image. The primary components of an x-ray machine are the x-ray tube and its power supply. The x-ray tube is positioned within the tube head, along with some components of the power supply (Fig. 1-5). An electrical insulating material, usually oil, surrounds the tube and transformers. Often, the tube is recessed within the tube head to improve the quality of the radiographic image (see Chapter 6). The tube head is typically supported by an arm that is usually mounted on a wall. A control panel allows the operator to adjust the duration of the exposure, and often the energy and exposure rate, of the x-ray beam.

X-RAY TUBE

An x-ray tube is composed of a cathode and an anode situated within an evacuated glass envelope or tube (Fig. 1-6). Electrons

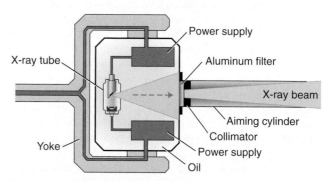

FIGURE 1-5 Tube head showing a recessed x-ray tube, components of the power supply, and oil that conducts heat away from the x-ray tube. Path of useful x-ray beam (blue) from the anode, through the glass wall of the x-ray tube, oil, and finally an aluminum filter. The beam size is restricted by the metal tube housing and collimator. Low-energy photons are preferentially removed by the filter.

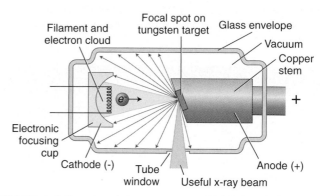

FIGURE 1-6 X-ray tube with the major components labeled. The path of the electron beam is shown in yellow. X rays produced at the target travel in all directions. The useful x-ray beam is shown in blue.

stream from the filament in the cathode to the target in the anode, where the energy from some of the electrons is converted into x rays. For the x-ray tube to function, a power supply is necessary to:
- Heat the cathode filament to generate electrons.
- Establish a high-voltage potential between the anode and cathode to accelerate the electrons toward the anode.

Cathode

The cathode (Fig. 1-7, *B*; see also Fig. 1-6) in an x-ray tube consists of a filament and a focusing cup. The filament is the source of electrons within the x-ray tube. It is a coil of tungsten wire about

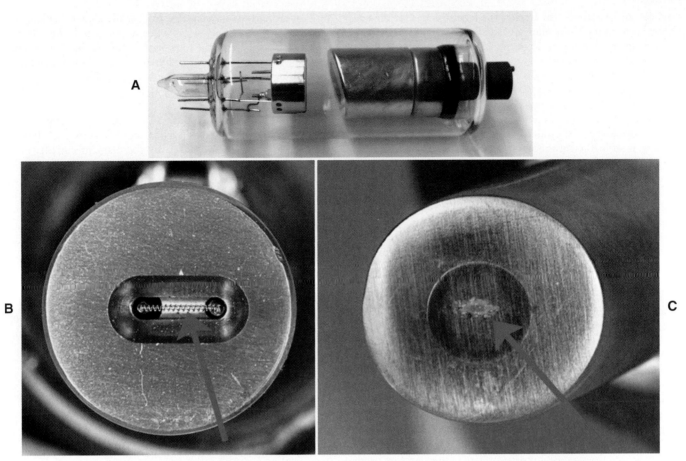

FIGURE 1-7 **A,** Dental stationary x-ray tube with cathode on left and copper anode on right. **B,** Focusing cup containing a filament *(arrow)* in the cathode. **C,** Copper anode with tungsten inset. Note the elongated actual focal spot area *(arrow)* on the tungsten target of the anode. (**B** and **C,** Courtesy John DeArmond, Tellico Plains, TN.)

2 mm in diameter and 1 cm or less in length. Filaments typically contain about 1% thorium, which greatly increases the release of electrons from the heated wire. The filament is mounted between two stiff support wires that carry an electrical current. These two mounting wires lead through the glass envelope and connect to both the high-voltage and the low-voltage electrical sources. The filament is heated to incandescence by the flow of current from the low-voltage source and emits electrons at a rate proportional to the temperature of the filament.

The filament lies in a focusing cup (Fig. 1-7, *B;* see also Fig. 1-6), a negatively charged concave reflector made of molybdenum. The parabolic shape of the focusing cup electrostatically focuses the electrons emitted by the filament into a narrow beam directed at a small rectangular area on the anode called the focal spot (Fig. 1-7, *C,* and Fig. 1-8). The electrons move to the focal spot because they are both repelled by the negatively charged cathode and attracted to the positively charged anode. The x-ray tube is evacuated to prevent collision of the fast-moving electrons with gas molecules, which would significantly reduce their speed. The vacuum also prevents oxidation, or "burnout," of the filament.

Anode

The anode in an x-ray tube consists of a tungsten target embedded in a copper stem (see Figs. 1-6 and 1-7, *C*). The purpose of the

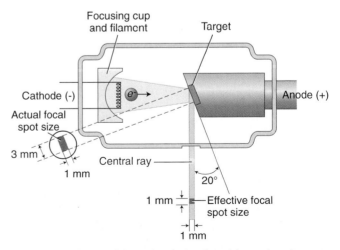

FIGURE 1-8 The angle of the target to the central ray of the x-ray beam has a strong influence on the apparent size of the focal spot. The projected effective focal spot (seen below the target) is much smaller than the actual focal spot size (projected to the left). This provides a beam that has a small effective focal spot size to produce images with high resolution, while allowing for heat generated at the anode to be dissipated over the larger area.

target in an x-ray tube is to convert the kinetic energy of the colliding electrons into x-ray photons. The target is made of tungsten, an element that has several characteristics of an ideal target material, including the following:
- High atomic number (74)
- High melting point (3422°C)
- High thermal conductivity (173 W · m⁻¹ · K⁻¹)
- Low vapor pressure at the working temperatures of an x-ray tube

The conversion of the kinetic energy of the electrons into x-ray photons is an inefficient process with more than 99% of the electron kinetic energy converted to heat. A target made of a high atomic number material is most efficient in producing x rays. Because heat is generated at the anode, the requirement for a target with a high melting point is clear. Tungsten also has high thermal conductivity, readily dissipating its heat into the copper stem. Finally, the low vapor pressure of tungsten at high temperatures helps maintain the vacuum in the tube at high operating temperatures. The tungsten target is typically embedded in a large block of copper. Copper, also a good thermal conductor, removes heat from the tungsten, reducing the risk of the target melting. Additionally, the insulating oil between the glass envelope and the housing of the tube head carries heat away from the copper stem.

The focal spot is the area on the target to which the focusing cup directs the electrons and from which x rays are produced. The sharpness of a radiographic image increases as the size of the focal spot decreases (see Chapter 6). However, the heat generated per unit target area becomes greater as the focal spot decreases in size. To take advantage of a small focal spot while distributing the electrons over a larger area of the target, the target is placed at an angle to the electron beam (see Fig. 1-8). The apparent size of the focal spot seen from a position perpendicular to the electron beam (the effective focal spot) is smaller than the actual focal spot size. Typically, the target is inclined about 20 degrees to the central ray of the x-ray beam; this causes the effective focal spot to be approximately 1 mm × 1 mm, as opposed to the actual focal spot, which is about 1 mm × 3 mm. This smaller effective focal spot results in a small apparent source of x rays and an increase in the sharpness of the image (see Fig. 5-2), with a larger actual focal spot size to improve heat dissipation. This type of anode is a stationary anode because it has no moving parts.

Another method of dissipating the heat from a small focal spot is to use a rotating anode. In this design, the tungsten target is in the form of a beveled disk that rotates when the tube is in operation (Fig. 1-9). As a result, the electrons strike successive areas of the target, widening the focal spot by an amount corresponding to the circumference of the beveled disk, distributing the heat over this extended area. The focal spot of a stationary tube is now a focal track in rotating anode machines. Narrow focal tracks in rotating anode tubes can be used with tube currents of 100 to 500 milliamperes (mA), which is 10 to 50 times that possible with stationary targets. The target and rotor (armature) of the motor lie within the x-ray tube, and the stator coils (which drive the rotor at about 3000 revolutions per minute) lie outside the tube. Such rotating anodes are not used in intraoral dental x-ray machines but are occasionally used in cephalometric units; are usually used in cone-beam machines; and are always used in medical computed tomography x-ray machines, which require high radiation output for longer, sustained exposures.

POWER SUPPLY

The primary functions of the power supply of an x-ray machine are to:

- Provide a low-voltage current to heat the x-ray tube filament.
- Generate a high potential difference to accelerate electrons from the cathode to the focal spot on the anode. The x-ray tube and two transformers lie within an electrically grounded metal housing called the head of the x-ray machine.

Tube Current

The filament transformer (Fig. 1-10) reduces the voltage of the incoming alternating current (AC) to about 10 volts in the filament circuit. This voltage is regulated by the filament current control (mA selector), which adjusts the resistance and the current flow through the filament; this regulates the filament temperature and the number of electrons emitted by the cathode. The *tube current* is the flow of electrons through the tube—that is, from the cathode filament across the tube to the anode. Beyond the anode, this current is carried through the power supply back to the cathode. The numerical mA setting on the filament current control refers

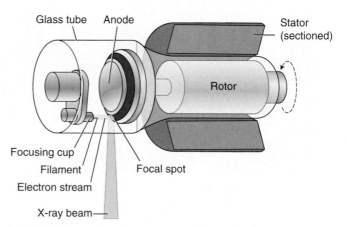

FIGURE 1-9 X-ray tube with a rotating anode allows heat at the focal spot to spread out over a large surface area (dark band). Current applied to the stator induces rapid rotation of the rotor and the anode. The path of the electron beam is shown in yellow, and the useful x-ray beam is shown in blue.

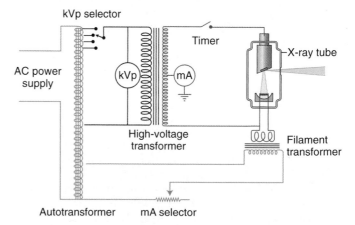

FIGURE 1-10 Schematic of dental x-ray machine circuitry and x-ray tube with the major components labeled. The operator selects the desired kVp from the autotransformer. The voltage is greatly increased by the high-voltage step-up transformer and applied to the x-ray tube. The kVp dial measures the voltage on the low-voltage side of the transformer but is scaled to display the corresponding voltage in the tube circuit. The timer closes the tube circuit for the desired exposure time interval. The mA dial measures the current flowing through the tube circuit. The filament circuit heats the cathode filament and is regulated by the mA selector.

to this tube current, typically about 10 mA, which is measured by the milliammeter. This current is not the same as the current flowing through the filament to heat it.

Tube Voltage

A high voltage is required between the anode and cathode to give electrons sufficient energy to generate x rays. The actual voltage used on an x-ray machine is adjusted with the autotransformer (see Fig. 1-10). By using the kilovolt peak (kVp) selector, the operator adjusts the autotransformer and converts the primary voltage from the input source into the desired secondary voltage. The selected secondary voltage is applied to the primary winding of the high-voltage transformer, which boosts the peak voltage of the incoming line current (110 V) up to 60,000 to 120,000 V (60 to 120 kV); this boosts the peak energy of the electrons passing through the tube to 60 to 120 keV and provides them sufficient energy to generate x rays. The kVp dial selects the peak operating voltage between the anode and cathode. Typically, intraoral, panoramic, and cephalometric machines (see Chapter 10) operate between 60 and 90 kVp, whereas cone-beam computed tomographic machines (see Chapter 11) operate at 90 to 120 kVp.

Because the polarity of the line current alternates (60 cycles per second), the polarity of the x-ray tube alternates at the same frequency (Fig. 1-11, *A*). Additionally, because the line voltage varies continuously, so does the voltage potential between the anode and cathode. When the polarity of the voltage applied across the tube causes the target anode to be positive and the filament to be negative, the electrons around the filament accelerate toward the positive target, and current flows through the tube (Fig. 1-11, *B*).

As the tube voltage is increased, the speed of the electrons moving toward the anode increases. When the electrons strike the focal spot of the target, some of their energy converts to x-ray photons. X rays are produced at the target with greatest efficiency when the voltage applied across the tube is high. Therefore the intensity of x-ray pulses tends to be sharply peaked at the center of each cycle (Fig. 1-11, *C*). During the following half (or negative half) of each cycle, the filament becomes positive, and the target becomes negative (see Fig. 1-11, *B*). At these times, the electrons do not flow across the gap between the two elements of the tube. This half of the cycle is called inverse voltage or reverse bias (see Fig. 1-11, *B*). No x rays are generated during this half of the voltage cycle (see Fig. 1-11, *C*). When an x-ray tube is powered with 60-cycle AC, 60 pulses of x rays are generated each second, each having a duration of $\frac{1}{120}$ second. This type of power supply circuitry, in which the alternating high voltage is applied directly across the x-ray tube, limits x-ray production to half the AC cycle and is called self-rectified or half-wave rectified. Almost all conventional dental x-ray machines are self-rectified.

Some dental x-ray manufacturers produce machines that replace the conventional 60-cycle AC, half-wave rectified power supply with a full-wave rectified, high-frequency power supply. This results in an essentially constant potential between the anode and cathode. The result is that the mean energy of the x-ray beam produced by these x-ray machines is higher than the mean energy from a conventional half-wave rectified machine operated at the same voltage. For a given voltage setting and radiographic density, the images resulting from these constant-potential machines have a longer contrast scale, and the patient receives a lower dose compared with conventional x-ray machines.

Figure 1-11, *C*, also shows that the tube current is dependent on the tube voltage; as the voltage increases between the anode and cathode, so does the current flow. The reason for this is subtle. When the hot filament releases electrons, it creates a cloud of electrons around the filament, a negative space charge. This negative space charge impedes the further release of electrons. The higher the voltage, the greater the removal of the electrons from the space charge, and the greater the tube current.

TIMER

A timer is built into the high-voltage circuit to control the duration of the x-ray exposure (see Fig. 1-10). The electronic timer controls the length of time that high voltage is applied to the tube and the time during which tube current flows and x rays are produced. However, before the high voltage is applied across the tube, the filament must be brought to operating temperature to ensure an adequate rate of electron emission. Subjecting the filament to continuous heating at normal operating current shortens its life. To minimize filament damage, the timing circuit first sends a current through the filament for about half a second to bring it to the proper operating temperature and then applies power to the high-voltage circuit. In some circuit designs, a continuous low-level current passing through the filament maintains it at a safe low temperature, further shortening the delay to preheat the filament. For these reasons, an x-ray machine may be left on continuously during working hours.

Some x-ray machine timers are calibrated in fractions of a second, whereas others are expressed as number of pulses in an

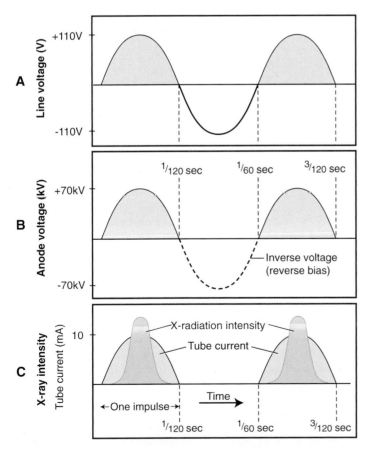

FIGURE 1-11 **A,** A 60-cycle AC line voltage at autotransformer. **B,** Voltage at the anode varies from zero up to the kVp setting (70 kVp in this case). **C,** The intensity of radiation produced at the anode (blue) is strongly dependent on the anode voltage and is highest when the tube voltage is at its peak. (*Modified from Johns HE, Cunningham JR: The physics of radiology, ed 3, Springfield, IL, 1974, Charles C Thomas.*)

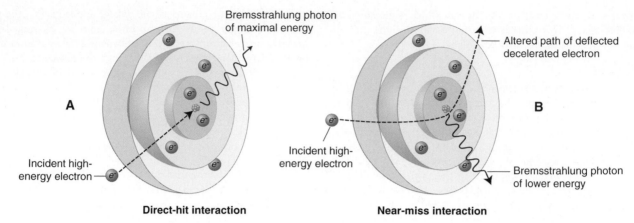

FIGURE 1-12 Bremsstrahlung radiation is produced by the direct hit of an electron on a nucleus in the target **(A)** or, much more frequently, by the passage of an electron near a nucleus, which results in electrons being deflected and decelerated **(B)**. For the sake of clarity, this diagram and other similar figures in this chapter show only the 1s, 2s, or 3s orbitals.

exposure (e.g., 3, 6, 9, 15). The number of pulses divided by 60 (the frequency of the power source) gives the exposure time in seconds. A setting of 30 pulses means that there will be 30 pulses of radiation, equivalent to a 0.5-second exposure.

TUBE RATING AND DUTY CYCLE

X-ray tubes produce heat at the target while in operation. The heat buildup at the anode is measured in heat units (HU), where HU = kVp × mA × seconds. The heat storage capacity for anodes of dental diagnostic tubes is approximately 20 kHU. Heat is removed from the target by conduction to the copper anode and then to the surrounding oil and tube housing and by convection to the atmosphere.

Each x-ray machine comes with a tube rating chart that describes the longest exposure time the tube can be energized for a range of voltages (kVp) and tube current (mA) values without risk of damage to the target from overheating. These tube ratings generally do not impose any restrictions on tube use for intraoral radiography. However, if a dental x-ray unit is used for extraoral exposures, it is wise to mount the tube-rating chart by the machine for easy reference. Duty cycle relates to the frequency with which successive exposures can be made without overheating the anode. The interval between successive exposures must be long enough for heat dissipation. This characteristic is a function of the size of the anode, the exposure kVp and mA, and the method used to cool the tube. A typical duty cycle is 1:60, meaning that one could make a 0.25-second exposure every 15 seconds.

PRODUCTION OF X RAYS

Most high-speed electrons traveling from the filament to the target interact with target electrons and release their energy as heat. Occasionally, these electrons convert their kinetic energy into x-ray photons by the formation of bremsstrahlung radiation and characteristic radiation.

BREMSSTRAHLUNG RADIATION

The sudden stopping or slowing of high-speed electrons by tungsten nuclei in the target produces bremsstrahlung photons, the primary source of radiation from an x-ray tube. (*Bremsstrahlung* means "braking radiation" in German.) Occasionally, electrons from the filament directly hit the nucleus of a target atom. When

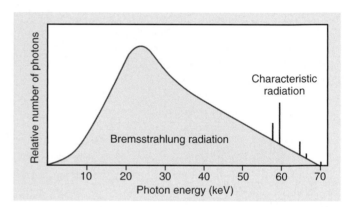

FIGURE 1-13 Spectrum of photons emitted from an x-ray machine operating at 70 kVp. The vast preponderance of radiation is bremsstrahlung (blue), with a minor addition of characteristic radiation.

this happens, all the kinetic energy of the electron is transformed into a single x-ray photon (Fig. 1-12, *A*). The energy of the resultant photon (in keV) is numerically equal to the energy of the electron—that is, the voltage applied across the x-ray tube at that instant.

More frequently, high-speed electrons pass by tungsten nuclei with near or wide misses (Fig. 1-12, *B*). In these interactions, the electron is attracted toward the positively charged nuclei, its path is altered toward the nucleus, and it loses some of its velocity. This deceleration causes the electron to lose kinetic energy that is given off in the form of many new photons. The closer the high-speed electron approaches the nuclei, the greater the electrostatic attraction between the nucleus and the electron, the braking effect, and the energy of the resulting bremsstrahlung photons. The efficiency of this process is proportional to the square of the atomic number of the target; high Z metals are more effective in deflecting the path of the incident electrons.

Bremsstrahlung interactions generate x-ray photons with a continuous spectrum of energy. The energy of an x-ray beam is usually described by identifying the peak operating voltage (in kVp). For example, a dental x-ray machine operating at a peak voltage of 70 kVp applies a fluctuating voltage of up to 70 kVp across the tube. This tube therefore produces a continuous spectrum of x-ray photons with energies ranging to a maximum of 70 keV (Fig. 1-13). The reasons for this continuous spectrum are as follows:

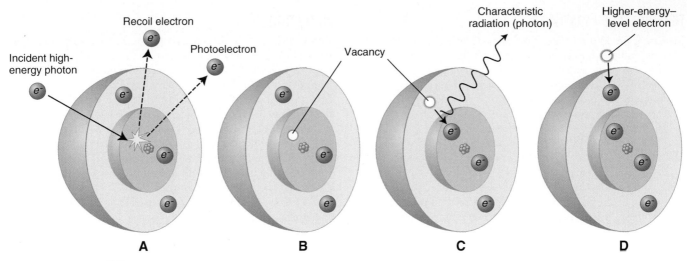

FIGURE 1-14 Production of characteristic radiation An incident electron **(A)** ejects an electron from an inner orbital creating a photoelectron, a recoil electron, and an electron vacancy **(B)**. **C,** An electron from an outer orbital fills this vacancy, and a photon is emitted with energy equal to the difference in energy levels between the two orbitals. **D,** Electrons from various orbitals may be involved, giving rise to other characteristic photons. The energies of the photons released are characteristic of the target atom.

- The continuously varying voltage difference between the target and filament causes the electrons striking the target to have varying levels of kinetic energy.
- The bombarding electrons pass at varying distances around tungsten nuclei and are thus deflected to varying extents. As a result, they give up varying amounts of energy in the form of bremsstrahlung photons.
- Most electrons participate in multiple bremsstrahlung interactions in the target before losing all their kinetic energy. As a consequence, an electron carries differing amounts of energy after successive interactions with tungsten nuclei.

CHARACTERISTIC RADIATION

Characteristic radiation contributes only a small fraction of the photons in an x-ray beam. It is made when an incident electron ejects an inner electron from the tungsten target. When this happens, an electron from an outer orbital is quickly attracted to the void in the deficient inner orbital (Fig. 1-14). When the outer orbital electron replaces the displaced electron, a photon is emitted with energy equivalent to the difference in the binding energies of the two orbitals. The energies of characteristic photons are discrete because they represent the difference of the energy levels of specific electron orbitals and are characteristic of the target atoms.

FACTORS CONTROLLING THE X-RAY BEAM

An x-ray beam may be modified by altering the beam exposure duration (timer), exposure rate (mA), energy (kVp and filtration), shape (collimation), or intensity (target-patient distance).

EXPOSURE TIME (s)

Changing the exposure time–typically measured in fractions of a second (s)–modifies the duration of the exposure and thus the number of photons generated (Fig. 1-15). When the exposure time is doubled, the number of photons generated at all energies in the x-ray emission spectrum is doubled. The range of photon energies is unchanged.

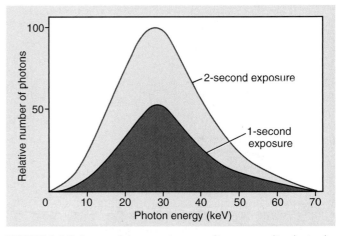

FIGURE 1-15 Spectrum of photon energies generated in an x-ray machine showing that as exposure time increases (kVp and tube voltage held constant), so does the total number of photons. The mean energy and maximal energies of the beams are unchanged.

TUBE CURRENT (mA)

The quantity of radiation produced by an x-ray tube (i.e., the number of photons that reach the patient and film) is directly proportional to the tube current (mA) and the time the tube is operated (Fig. 1-16). As the mA setting is increased, more power is applied to the filament, which heats up and releases more electrons that collide with the target to produce radiation. Thus the quantity of radiation produced is proportional to the product of time and tube current. The quantity of radiation remains constant regardless of variations in mA and time as long as their product remains constant. For instance, a machine operating at 10 mA for 1 second (10 mAs) produces the same quantity of radiation when operated at 20 mA for 0.5 second (10 mAs). In practice, some dental x-ray machines fall slightly short of this ideal constancy. The term beam quantity or beam intensity refers to the number of photons in an x-ray beam.

TUBE VOLTAGE PEAK (kVp)

Increasing the kVp increases the potential difference between the cathode and the anode, increasing the energy of each electron when it strikes the target. The greater the energy of an electron, the greater the probability it will be converted into x-ray photons. Increasing the kVp of an x-ray machine increases:

- The number of photons generated.
- The mean energy of the photons.
- The maximal energy of the photons (Fig. 1-17).

The term beam quality refers to the mean energy of an x-ray beam.

Exposure time, tube current (mA), and tube voltage are the three controls found on many x-ray machines. In some machines, the setting of the tube current, the setting of the tube voltage, or both is fixed. It is recommended that if the tube current is variable, the operator select the highest mA value available and always operate the machine at this setting; this allows the shortest exposure time and minimizes the chance of patient movement. Similarly, if tube voltage can be adjusted, it is recommended that the operator select a desired voltage, perhaps 70 kVp, and leave the machine at this setting. This protocol simplifies selecting the proper patient exposure settings by using just exposure time as the means to adjust for anatomic location within the mouth and patient size.

FILTRATION

Although an x-ray beam consists of a continuous spectrum of x-ray photon energies, only photons with sufficient energy to penetrate through anatomic structures and reach the image receptor (digital or film) are useful for diagnostic radiology. Low-energy photons that cannot reach the receptor contribute to patient risk but do not offer any benefit. Consequently, it is desirable to remove these low-energy photons from the beam. This removal can be accomplished in part by placing a metallic disk (filter) in the beam path. A filter preferentially removes low-energy photons from the beam, while allowing high-energy photons that are able to contribute to making an image to pass through (Fig. 1-18).

Inherent filtration consists of the materials that x-ray photons encounter as they travel from the focal spot on the target to form the usable beam outside the tube enclosure. These materials include the glass wall of the x-ray tube, the insulating oil that surrounds many dental tubes, and the barrier material that prevents the oil from escaping through the x-ray port. The inherent filtration of most x-ray machines ranges from the equivalent of 0.5 to 2 mm of aluminum. Added filtration may be supplied in the form of aluminum disks placed over the port in the head of the x-ray machine. Total filtration is the sum of the inherent and added

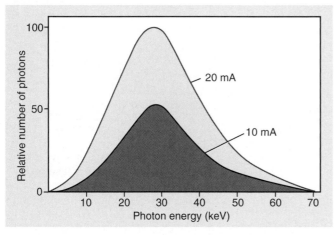

FIGURE 1-16 Spectrum of photon energies generated in an x-ray machine showing that as tube current (mA) increases (kVp and exposure time held constant), so does the total number of photons. The mean energy and maximal energies of the beams are unchanged.

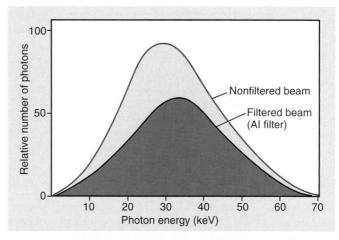

FIGURE 1-18 Spectrum of filtered x-ray beam generated in an x-ray machine showing that an aluminum filter preferentially removes low-energy photons, reducing the beam intensity, while increasing the mean energy of the residual beam. Compare with Figures 1-15, 1-16, and 1-17.

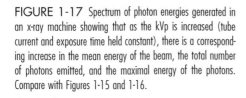

FIGURE 1-17 Spectrum of photon energies generated in an x-ray machine showing that as the kVp is increased (tube current and exposure time held constant), there is a corresponding increase in the mean energy of the beam, the total number of photons emitted, and the maximal energy of the photons. Compare with Figures 1-15 and 1-16.

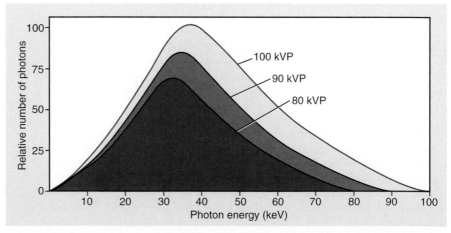

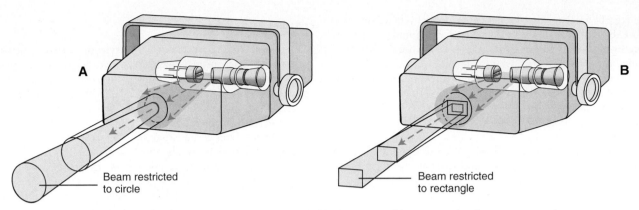

FIGURE 1-19 Collimation of an x-ray beam (blue) is achieved by restricting its useful size. **A,** Circular collimator. **B,** Rectangular collimator restricts area of exposure to just larger than the detector size and thereby reduces unnecessary patient exposure.

filtration. Governmental regulations require the total filtration in the path of a dental x-ray beam to be equal to the equivalent of 1.5 mm of aluminum for a machine operating at up to 70 kVp and 2.5 mm of aluminum for machines operating at higher voltages (see Chapter 3).

COLLIMATION

A collimator is a metallic barrier with an aperture in the middle used to restrict the size of the x-ray beam and the volume of tissue irradiated (Fig. 1-19). Round and rectangular collimators are most frequently used in dentistry. Dental x-ray beams are usually collimated to a circle 2¾ inches (7 cm) in diameter at the patient's face. A round collimator (see Fig. 1-19, *A*) is a thick plate of radiopaque material (usually lead) with a circular opening centered over the port in the x-ray head through which the x-ray beam emerges. Typically, round collimators are built into open-ended aiming cylinders. Rectangular collimators (see Fig. 1-19, *B*) further limit the size of the beam to just larger than the x-ray film, further reducing patient exposure. Some types of film-holding instruments also provide rectangular collimation of the x-ray beam (see Chapters 3 and 7).

Collimators also improve image quality. When an x-ray beam is directed at a patient, the hard and soft tissues absorb about 90% of the photons, and about 10% pass through the patient to reach the film. Many of the absorbed photons generate scattered radiation within the exposed tissues by a process called Compton scattering (see later in chapter). These scattered photons travel in all directions, and some reach the film and degrade image quality. Collimating the x-ray beam thus reduces the exposed volume and thereby the number of scattered photons reaching the film, resulting in reduced patient exposure and improved images.

INVERSE SQUARE LAW

The intensity of an x-ray beam (the number of photons per cross-sectional area per unit of exposure time) depends on the distance of the measuring device from the focal spot. For a given beam, the intensity is inversely proportional to the square of the distance from the source (Fig. 1-20). The reason for this decrease in intensity is that an x-ray beam spreads out as it moves from its source. The relationship is as follows:

$$\frac{I_1}{I_2} = \frac{(D_2)^2}{(D_1)^2}$$

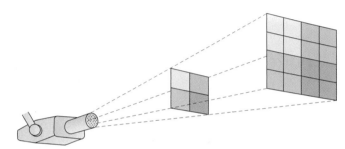

FIGURE 1-20 Intensity of an x-ray beam is inversely proportional to the square of the distance between the source and the point of measure. When the distance from the source to a target is doubled, the intensity of the beam decreases to one quarter.

where *I* is intensity and *D* is distance. If a dose of 1 Gy is measured at a distance of 2 m, a dose of 4 Gy would be found at 1 m, and a dose of 0.25 Gy would be found at 4 m.

Changing the distance between the x-ray tube and the patient, such as by switching from a machine with a short aiming tube to one with a long aiming tube, has a marked effect on skin exposure. Such a change requires a corresponding modification of the kVp or mA to keep constant the exposure to the film or digital sensor.

INTERACTIONS OF X RAYS WITH MATTER

In dental imaging, the x-ray beam enters the face of a patient, interacts with hard and soft tissues, and strikes a digital sensor or film. The incident beam contains photons of many energies but is spatially homogeneous. That is, the intensity of the beam is essentially uniform from the center of the beam outward. As the beam goes through the patient, it is reduced in intensity (attenuated). This attenuation results from absorption of individual photons in the beam by atoms in the absorbing tissues or by photons being scattered out of the beam. In absorption interactions, photons ionize absorber atoms, convert their energy into kinetic energy of the ejected electron, and cease to exist. In scattering interactions, photons also interact with absorber atoms but then move off in another direction. The frequency of these interactions depends on the type of tissue exposed (e.g., bone vs. soft tissue). Bone is more likely to absorb x-ray photons, whereas soft tissues are more likely to let them pass through. Although the incident beam striking the patient is spatially homogeneous, the remnant beam—the attenuated beam that exits the patient—is spatially heterogeneous because of differential absorption by the anatomic structures through which it has passed. This differential exposure of the film or digital sensor forms a radiographic image.

In a dental x-ray beam, there are three means of beam attenuation:
- Coherent scattering
- Photoelectric absorption
- Compton scattering

In addition, about 9% of the primary photons pass through the patient's tissues without interaction and strike the sensor to form an image (Fig. 1-21 and Table 1-4).

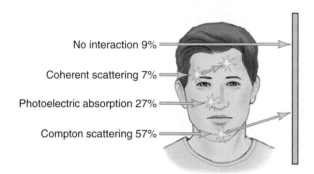

No interaction 9%
Coherent scattering 7%
Photoelectric absorption 27%
Compton scattering 57%

FIGURE 1-21 Photons in an x-ray beam interact with the object primarily by Compton scattering (57% of primary interactions), in which case the scattered photon may strike the film and degrade the radiographic image by causing fog. The next most frequent interaction is photoelectric absorption (27%), in which the photons cease to exist. A radiographic image is produced by photons passing through low atomic number structures (soft tissue) and preferentially undergoing photoelectric absorption by high atomic number structures (bone, teeth, and metallic restorations). Relatively few photons undergo coherent scattering (7%) within the object or pass through the object without interaction (9%) and expose the image receptor.

TABLE 1-4   Fate of 1 Million Incident Photons in Bitewing Projection

Interaction	Fate of Incident Photon	Primary Photons	Scattered Photons*	Total†
Coherent scattering	Scatters from atom	74,453	78,117	152,570
Photoelectric absorption	Ejects inner electron and ceases to exist; releases characteristic photon	268,104	261,041	529,145
Compton scattering	Ejects outer electron, both scatter	565,939	549,360	1,115,300
No interaction	Passes through patient	91,504	379,350	470,855
Total		1,000,000	1,267,868	2,267,869

From Gibbs SJ: Personal communication, 1986.

*The fate of scattered photons resulting from primary Compton, photoelectric, and coherent interactions.

†The sum of the total number of photoelectric interactions and photons that exit the patient equals the total number of incident photons.

COHERENT SCATTERING

Coherent scattering (also known as Rayleigh, classical, or elastic scattering) may occur when a low-energy incident photon (<10 keV) interacts with a whole atom. The incident photon causes it to become momentarily excited at the same frequency as the incoming photon (Fig. 1-22). The incident photon then ceases to exist. The excited atom quickly returns to the ground state and generates another x-ray photon with the same frequency (energy) as the incident photon. Usually the secondary photon is emitted in a different direction than the path of the incident photon. The net effect is that the direction of the incident x-ray photon is altered (scattered). Coherent scattering accounts for only about 7% of the total number of interactions in a dental exposure (see Table 1-4). Coherent scattering contributes little to film fog because the number of scattered photons is small, and their energy is too low for many of them to reach the film or sensor.

PHOTOELECTRIC ABSORPTION

Photoelectric absorption is critical in diagnostic imaging because it is the primary contributor to the image. This process occurs when an incident photon interacts with an electron in an inner orbital of an atom in the patient. The photon ejects the electron from its inner orbital, and it becomes a recoil electron (photoelectron) (Fig. 1-23). The incident photon gives up all of its energy and ceases to exist. The kinetic energy imparted to the recoil electron is equal to the energy of the incident photon minus the binding energy of the electron. In the case of atoms with low atomic numbers (e.g., atoms in most biologic molecules), the binding energy is small, and the recoil electron acquires most of the energy of the incident photon. Most photoelectric interactions occur in the 1s orbital because the density of the electron cloud is greatest in this region, and there is a higher probability of interaction. About 27% of interactions in a dental x-ray beam exposure involve photoelectric absorption.

An atom that has participated in a photoelectric interaction is ionized as a result of the loss of an electron. This electron deficiency (usually in the 1s orbital) is instantly filled, usually by a 2s or 2p electron, with the release of characteristic radiation (see Fig. 1-14). Whatever the orbital of the replacement electron, the characteristic photons generated are of such low energy that they are absorbed within the patient and do not fog the film. Recoil

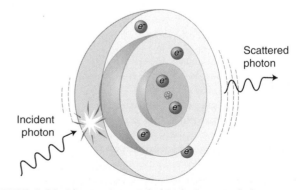

Scattered photon

Incident photon

FIGURE 1-22 Coherent scattering results from the interaction of a low-energy incident photon with a whole atom, causing it to be momentarily excited. After this interaction, the atom quickly returns to the ground state and emits a scattered photon of the same energy but at a different angle from the path of the incident photon.

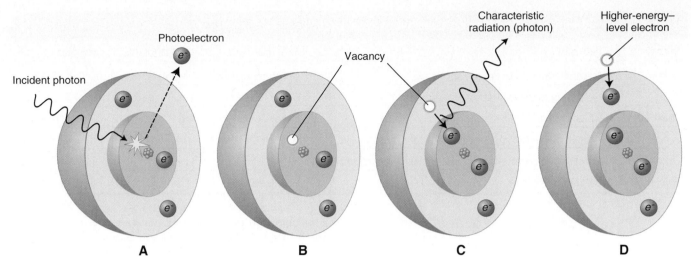

FIGURE 1-23   Photoelectric absorption. **A,** Photoelectric absorption occurs when an incident photon gives up all of its energy to an inner electron, which is ejected from the atom (a photoelectron). The incident electron ceases to exist at this point. **B,** The ionized atom now has an electron vacancy in the inner orbital. **C,** An electron from a higher energy level fills the vacancy and emits characteristic radiation. **D,** All orbitals are subsequently filled, completing the energy exchange.

electrons ejected during photoelectric absorption travel only short distances in the absorber before they give up their energy through secondary ionizations.

The clinical significance of photoelectric absorption—its usefulness in forming an image—depends on the fact that the frequency of photoelectric interaction varies directly with the third power of the atomic number of the absorber. Because the effective atomic number of compact bone ($Z = 13.8$) is greater than that of soft tissue ($Z = 7.4$), the probability that a photon will be absorbed by a photoelectric interaction in bone is approximately 6.5 times ($13.8^3/7.4^3 = 6.5$) greater than in an equal thickness of soft tissue. This great difference in the absorption of x-ray photons by the soft and hard tissues makes the production of a radiographic image possible. This differential photoelectric absorption is readily seen on dental radiographs as different optical densities of enamel, dentin, pulp, bone, and soft tissue.

COMPTON SCATTERING

Compton scattering occurs when a photon interacts with an outer orbital electron (Fig. 1-24). About 57% of interactions in a dental x-ray beam exposure involve Compton scattering. In this interaction, the incident photon collides with an outer electron, which receives kinetic energy and recoils from the point of impact. The path of the incident photon is deflected by this interaction and is scattered in a new direction from the site of the collision. The energy of the scattered photon equals the energy of the incident photon minus the sum of the kinetic energy gained by the recoil electron and its binding energy. As with photoelectric absorption, Compton scattering results in the loss of an electron and ionization of the absorbing atom. Scattered photons continue on their new paths, causing further ionizations and often exiting the patient. The recoil electrons also give up their energy by ionizing other atoms.

The probability of a Compton interaction is directly proportional to the electron density of the absorber. The density of electrons in bone ($5.55 \times 10^{23}/cm^3$) is greater than in soft tissue ($3.34 \times 10^{23}/cm^3$); therefore the probability of Compton scattering is correspondingly greater in bone than in tissue. As a result,

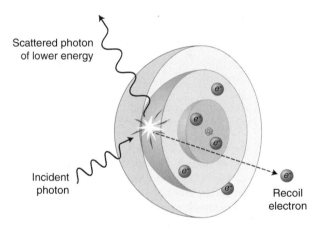

FIGURE 1-24   Compton scattering occurs when an incident photon interacts with an outer electron, producing a scattered photon of lower energy than the incident photon and a recoil electron ejected from the target atom. The new scattered photon travels in a different direction from the incident photon.

Compton interactions also contribute to the formation of an image.

The scattered photons travel in all directions. The scattered photons that exit the patient and strike the film or digital sensor carry no useful information and degrade the image by reducing contrast.

BEAM ATTENUATION

As an x-ray beam travels through matter, its intensity is reduced primarily through photoelectric absorption and Compton scattering. The extent of absorption of the beam depends primarily on the energy of the beam and the thickness and density of the absorber. High-energy x-ray photons have a greater probability of penetrating matter, whereas lower energy photons have a greater probability of being absorbed. The higher the kVp setting, the greater the penetrability of the resulting beam through matter. A useful way to characterize the penetrating quality of an x-ray beam

TABLE 1-5   Summary of Radiation Quantities and Units

Quantity	Description	SI Unit	Traditional Unit	Conversion
Exposure	Amount of ionization of air by x or γ rays	coulomb/kg (C/kg)	roentgen (R)	1 C/kg = 3876 R
Kerma	Kinetic energy transferred to charged particles	gray (Gy)	—	—
Absorbed dose	Total energy absorbed by a mass	gray (Gy)	rad	1 Gy = 100 rad
Equivalent dose	Absorbed dose weighted by biologic effectiveness of radiation type used	sievert (Sv)	rem	1 Sv = 100 rem
Effective dose	Sum of equivalent doses weighted by radiosensitivity of exposed tissue or organ	sievert (Sv)	—	—
Radioactivity	Rate of radioactive decay	becquerel (Bq)	curie (Ci)	1 Bq = 2.7×10^{-11} Ci

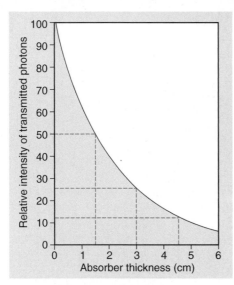

FIGURE 1-25 Intensity of an energetically homogeneous x-ray beam declines exponentially as it travels through an absorber. In this instance, the HVL of the beam is 1.5 cm of absorber—that is, every 1.5 cm of the absorber reduces the intensity of the beam by half. The curve for a heterogeneous x-ray beam (e.g., a dental x-ray beam) does not drop quite as precipitously because of the preferential removal of low-energy photons by the absorber and the increased mean energy of the resulting beam.

is by its half-value layer (HVL). The HVL is the thickness of an absorber, such as aluminum, required to reduce by one half the number of x-ray photons passing through it. As the mean energy of an x-ray beam increases, so does the amount of material required to reduce the beam intensity by half (its HVL).

The reduction of beam intensity also depends on physical characteristics of the absorber. Increasing the density of an absorber increases the attenuation of a beam because of greater photoelectric absorption and Compton scattering with increasing density. Also, increasing the thickness of an absorber increases the number of interactions. A monochromatic beam of photons, a beam in which all the photons have the same energy, provides a useful example. When only the primary (not scattered) photons are considered, a constant fraction of the beam is attenuated as the beam moves through each unit thickness of an absorber. For example, if 1.5 cm of water reduces a beam intensity by 50%, then the next 1.5 cm reduces the beam intensity by another 50% (to 25% of the original intensity), and so on. This is an exponential pattern of absorption (Fig. 1-25). The HVL described earlier is a measure of beam energy describing the amount of an absorber that reduces the beam intensity by half; in the preceding example, the HVL is 1.5 cm of water.

In contrast to the previous example, there is a wide range of photon energies in an x-ray beam. Low-energy photons are much more likely than high-energy photons to be absorbed. As a consequence, the superficial layers of an absorber tend to remove the low-energy photons and transmit the higher energy photons. As an x-ray beam passes through matter, the intensity of the beam decreases, but also the mean energy of the residual beam increases as a consequence of preferential removal of low-energy photons. In contrast to the absorption of a monochromatic beam, an x-ray beam is absorbed less and less by each succeeding unit of absorber thickness. For example, the first 1.5 cm of water might absorb 50% of the photons in an incident x-ray beam having a mean energy of 50 kVp. The mean energy of the residual beam might increase 20% as a result of the loss of lower energy photons. The next 1.5 cm of water removes only about 40% of the photons, and the average energy of the beam increases another 10%. This process results in beam hardening, an increase in the mean energy of the beam by preferential removal of lower energy photons.

As the energy of an x-ray beam increases, so does the transmission of the beam through an absorber. However, when the energy of the incident photon is increased to match the binding energy of the 1s orbital electrons of the absorber, the probability of photoelectric absorption increases sharply, and the number of transmitted photons is greatly decreased. This is called K-edge absorption. The probability that a photon will interact with an orbital electron is greatest when the energy of the photon equals the binding energy of the electron; it decreases as the photon energy increases. Photons with energy less than the binding energy of 1s orbital electrons interact photoelectrically only with electrons in the 2s or 2p orbitals and in orbitals even farther from the nucleus. Rare earth elements are sometimes used as filters because their 1s orbital binding energies, or K edges (e.g., 50.24 keV for gadolinium), greatly increase the absorption of high-energy photons. This is desirable because these high-energy photons degrade image contrast and are not as likely as midenergy photons to contribute to a radiographic image.

DOSIMETRY

Table 1-5 presents some frequently used units for measuring quantities of radiation. The traditional units have been in use since the earliest days of radiology. However, a move has occurred in recent years to use a modernized version of the metric system, called the SI system (*Système International d'Unités*), for measuring radiation.* This book uses SI units for radiation.

*The NIST Reference on Constants, Units, and Uncertainty: http://physics.nist.gov/cuu/Units/.

EXPOSURE

Exposure is a measure of the capacity of x rays or γ rays to ionize air. It is measured as the amount of charge per mass of air—coulombs/kg. Traditionally, this unit was called the roentgen (R), where 1 R = 2.58×10^{-4} C/kg. One R will produce 2.08×10^{8} ion pairs in 1 cm^3 of air. This unit measures the intensity of the radiation field as opposed to the amount of radiation absorbed, although there is a direct relationship. The roentgen has been largely replaced by the SI equivalent unit of air kerma.

AIR KERMA

When radiation interacts with matter, it produces kinetic energy of electrons through photoelectric absorption and Compton scattering. The kerma, an acronym for *kinetic energy released in matter*, measures the kinetic energy transferred from photons to electrons and is expressed in units of dose (gray [Gy]), where 1 Gy equals 1 J/kg. Kerma is the sum of the initial kinetic energies of all the charged particles liberated by uncharged ionizing radiation (e.g., x rays) in a sample of matter divided by the mass of the sample. Kerma values made in air are called air kerma. The kerma is rapidly replacing exposure measured in coulombs/kg or R. An exposure of 1 R results in an air kerma of about 8.73 mGy.

ABSORBED DOSE

Absorbed dose is a measure of the total energy absorbed by any type of ionizing radiation per unit of mass of any type of matter. It varies with the type and energy of radiation and the type of matter absorbing the energy. The SI unit is the gray, where 1 Gy equals 1 J/kg. The traditional unit of absorbed dose is the rad (radiation absorbed dose), where 1 rad is equivalent to 100 ergs per gram of absorber; 1 Gy equals 100 rad.

EQUIVALENT (RADIATION-WEIGHTED) DOSE

The equivalent dose (H_T) is used to compare the biologic effects of different types of radiation on a tissue or organ. Particulate types of radiation have a high LET and are more damaging to tissue than radiation with low LET, such as x rays. This relative biologic effectiveness of different types of radiation is called the radiation-weighting factor (W_R). For instance, deposition of 1 Gy of high-energy protons causes five times as much damage as 1 Gy of x-ray photons. The W_R of photons, the reference, is 1. The W_R of 5-keV neutrons and high-energy protons is 5, and the W_R of α particles is 20. To account for this difference, the H_T is computed as the product of the absorbed dose (D_T) averaged over a tissue or organ and the W_R:

$$H_T = W_R \times D_T$$

The unit of equivalent dose is the sievert (Sv). For diagnostic x-ray examinations, 1 Sv equals 1 Gy. The traditional unit of equivalent dose is the rem (roentgen equivalent man); 1 Sv equals 100 rem.

EFFECTIVE DOSE

The effective dose (E) is used to estimate the risk in humans. It is hard to compare the risk from a dental exposure with, for example, the risk from a radiographic chest examination because different tissues with different radiosensitivities are exposed. To allow such comparisons, the effective dose is a calculation that considers the relative biologic effectiveness of different types of radiation and the radiosensitivity of different tissues exposed in terms of the risk for cancer formation or heritable effect. The comparative radiosensitivities of different tissues are measured by the W_T. The tissue-weighting factors (ICRP 2007) include red bone marrow, breast, colon, lung, and stomach, all 0.12; gonads, 0.08; bladder, esophagus, liver, and thyroid, all 0.04; bone surface, brain, salivary glands, and skin, all 0.01; and other specified tissues, totaling 0.12. E is the sum of the products of the equivalent dose to each organ or tissue (H_T) and the tissue-weighting factor (W_T):

$$E = \Sigma W_T \times H_T$$

The unit of effective dose is the Sv.

RADIOACTIVITY

The measurement of radioactivity (*A*) describes the decay rate of a sample of radioactive material. The SI unit is the becquerel (Bq); 1 Bq equals 1 disintegration per second. The traditional unit is the curie (Ci), which corresponds to the activity of 1 g of radium (3.7×10^{10} disintegrations/s); 1 mCi equals 37 megaBq, and 1 Bq equals 2.7×10^{-11} Ci.

BIBLIOGRAPHY

Bushberg JT: *The essential physics of medical imaging*, ed 3, Philadelphia, 2012, Lippincott Williams & Wilkins.

Bushong SC: *Radiologic science for technologists: physics, biology, and protection*, ed 10, St Louis, 2012, Mosby.

Greene B: *The elegant universe*, ed 1, New York, 1999, Vintage.

Sacks O: *Uncle Tungsten: memories of a chemical boyhood*, New York, 2002, Vintage.

Wolbarst AB: *Physics of radiology*, ed 2, Madison, WI, 2005, Medical Physics.

The 2007 recommendations of the International Commission on Radiological Protection. IRCP Publication 103, *Ann ICRP* 37:1–332, 2007.

Radiobiology is the study of the effects of ionizing radiation on living systems. This discipline studies many levels of organization within biologic systems spanning broad ranges in size and time (Fig. 2-1). The initial interaction between ionizing radiation and matter occurs at the level of the electron within the first 10^{-13} seconds after exposure. These changes result in modification of biologic molecules within the following seconds to hours. The molecular changes may lead to alterations in cells and organisms that persist for hours, decades, and possibly generations. These changes may result in injury or death.

RADIATION CHEMISTRY

Radiation acts on living systems through direct and indirect effects. When the energy of a photon or secondary electron ionizes biologic macromolecules, the effect is termed *direct*. Alternatively, a photon may be absorbed by water in an organism, ionizing some of its water molecules. The resulting ions form free radicals that interact with and produce changes in biologic molecules. Because intermediate changes involving water molecules are required to alter the biologic molecules, this series of events is termed *indirect*.

DIRECT EFFECT

In direct effects, biologic molecules (RH, where R is the molecule and H is a hydrogen atom) absorb energy from ionizing radiation and form unstable free radicals (atoms or molecules having an unpaired electron in the valence orbital). Generation of free radicals occurs in less than 10^{-10} seconds after interaction with a photon. Free radicals are extremely reactive and have very short lives, quickly reforming into stable configurations by dissociation (breaking apart) or cross-linking (joining of two molecules). Free radicals play a dominant role in producing molecular changes in biologic molecules.

Free radical production:

$$\text{x-radiation} + RH \rightarrow R^{\bullet} + H^{+} + e^{-}$$

Free radical fates:
- Dissociation:

$$R^{\bullet} \rightarrow X + Y^{\bullet}$$

- Cross-linking:

$$R^{\bullet} + S^{\bullet} \rightarrow RS$$

Because the altered biologic molecules differ structurally and functionally from the original molecules, the consequence is a biologic change in the irradiated organism. *Approximately one third of the biologic effects of x-ray exposure result from direct effects.*

INDIRECT EFFECTS

Because water is the predominant molecule in biologic systems (about 70%), it frequently participates in the interactions between x-ray photons and biologic molecules. A complex series of chemical changes occurs in water after exposure to ionizing radiation. Collectively, these reactions result in the radiolysis of water:

$$\text{x-radiation} + H_2O \rightarrow H^{\bullet} + OH^{\bullet}$$

Although the radiolysis of water is complex, on balance, water is largely converted to hydrogen and hydroxyl free radicals.

Indirect effects are effects in which hydrogen and hydroxyl free radicals, produced by the action of radiation on water, interact with organic molecules. The interaction of hydrogen and hydroxyl free radicals with organic molecules results in the formation of organic free radicals. About two thirds of radiation-induced biologic damage results from indirect effects. Such reactions may involve the removal of hydrogen:

$$RH + OH^{\bullet} \rightarrow R^{\bullet} + H_2O$$

$$RH + H^{\bullet} \rightarrow R^{\bullet} + H_2$$

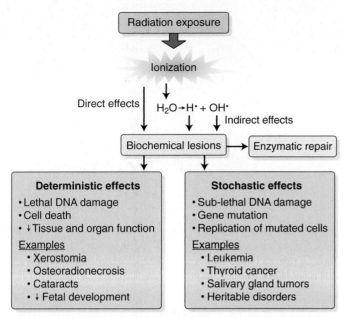

FIGURE 2-1 Overview of events after exposure of humans to ionizing radiation. The initial ionization, direct and indirect effects, and initial molecular changes in organic molecules occur in less than a second. The enzymatic repair or development of further biochemical lesions occurs in minutes to hours. The deterministic and stochastic effects occur over a time scale of months to decades to generations.

The OH⁻ free radical is more important than H⁻ in forming organic free radicals (R⁻). The resulting organic free radicals are unstable and transform into stable, altered molecules as described in the previous section on direct effects. These altered molecules have different chemical and biologic properties from the original molecules.

Radiation effects are thus caused primarily by direct effects and the diffusion of OH⁻. Both direct effects and indirect effects are completed within 10^{-5} seconds. The resulting damage may take hours to decades to become evident.

When dissolved oxygen is present, as is the case in normal tissues, hydroperoxyl free radicals may also be formed:

$$H^{\bullet} + O_2 \rightarrow HO_2^{\bullet}$$

Hydroperoxyl free radicals contribute to the formation of hydrogen peroxide in tissues:

$$HO_2^{\bullet} + H^{\bullet} \rightarrow H_2O_2$$

$$HO_2^{\bullet} + HO_2^{\bullet} \rightarrow O_2 + H_2O_2$$

Both peroxyl radicals and hydrogen peroxide are oxidizing agents and are the primary toxins produced in the tissues by ionizing radiation. The reactions of these oxidizing agents with organic molecules are another form of indirect effects.

DNA CHANGES

Damage to a cell's deoxyribonucleic acid (DNA) is the primary cause of radiation-induced cell death, heritable (genetic) mutations, and cancer formation (carcinogenesis). Radiation produces many different types of alterations in DNA, including the following:

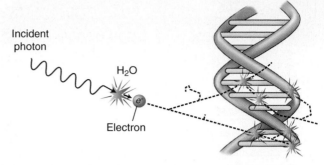

FIGURE 2-2 DNA damage cluster. A single photon may cause multiple ionizations in DNA, resulting in a cluster of double-strand breakage. In this instance, an incident photon causes ionization of a water molecule, and the recoil electron causes a cluster of damage to multiple sites in a DNA molecule. Such cluster damage is difficult to repair and is believed to be responsible for most radiation cell killing, carcinogenesis, and heritable effects.

- Breakage of one or both DNA strands
- Cross-linking of DNA strands within the helix to other DNA strands or to proteins
- Change or loss of a base
- Disruption of hydrogen bonds between DNA strands

The most important of these types of damage are single-strand and double-strand breakage. Most single-strand breakage is of little biologic consequence because the broken strand is readily repaired by using the intact second strand as a template. Radiation may also cause clusters of double-strand damage in DNA (Fig. 2-2). A cluster is defined as two or more double-strand breaks within two turns of DNA. Such double-strand breakage is believed to be responsible for most cell killing, carcinogenesis, and heritable effects. A single photon may cause these damage clusters. When damage clusters may result in cell killing, it is good for killing tumor cells. However, when there are not enough clusters to cause cell killing, there is the risk that they will induce mutations that may lead to cancer.

DETERMINISTIC AND STOCHASTIC EFFECTS

Radiation injury to organisms results from either the killing of large numbers of cells (deterministic effects) or sublethal damage to the genome of individual cells (stochastic effects) that results in cancer formation or heritable mutation. The differences between deterministic and stochastic effects are summarized in Table 2-1. Deterministic effects of radiation are effects seen when the radiation exposure to an organ or tissue exceeds a particular threshold level. The severity of this change is proportional to the dose; greater exposure leads to greater cell killing. At doses below the threshold, the effect does not occur. Stochastic effects are caused by sublethal radiation-induced damage to DNA. They have no minimum threshold for causation. Any dose of radiation has the potential to induce a stochastic effect. The probability of causing a stochastic effect increases as the radiation dose is increased.

DETERMINISTIC EFFECTS ON CELLS

INTRACELLULAR STRUCTURES

The effects of radiation on intracellular structures result from radiation-induced changes in their macromolecules. These changes are seen as structural and functional changes in cellular organelles. The changes may cause cell death.

TABLE 2-1	Comparison of Deterministic and Stochastic Effects of Radiation	
	Deterministic Effects	**Stochastic Effects**
Examples	Mucositis resulting from radiation therapy to oral cavity	Radiation-induced cancer
	Radiation-induced cataract formation	Heritable effects
Caused by	Killing of many cells	Sublethal damage to DNA
Threshold dose?	Yes: Sufficient cell killing required to cause a clinical response	No: Even one photon could cause a change in DNA that leads to a cancer or heritable effect
Severity of clinical effects and dose	Severity of clinical effects is proportional to dose; the greater the dose, the greater the effect	Severity of clinical effects is independent of dose; all-or-none response—an individual either has effect or does not
Probability of having effect and dose	Probability of effect independent of dose; all individuals show effect when dose is above threshold	Frequency of effect proportional to dose; the greater the dose, the greater the chance of having the effect

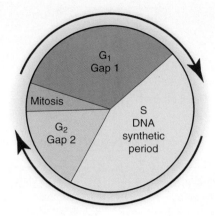

FIGURE 2-3 Cell cycle. A proliferating cell moves in the cycle from mitosis phase when chromosomes are condensed and visible to gap 1 (G_1) to the period of DNA synthesis (S) to gap 2 (G_2) to the next mitosis. Cells are most radiosensitive in the G_2 and mitosis phase, less sensitive in the G_1 phase, and least sensitive during the latter part of the S phase.

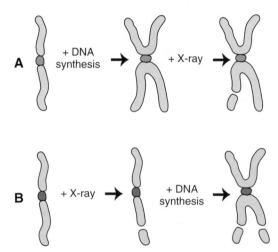

FIGURE 2-4 Chromosome aberrations. **A,** Irradiation of a cell after DNA synthesis results in a single-arm (chromatid) aberration. **B,** Irradiation before DNA synthesis results in a double-arm (chromosome) aberration because the damage is replicated in the next S phase and becomes visible in the next mitosis phase.

Nucleus

A wide variety of radiobiologic data indicate that the nucleus is far more radiosensitive (in terms of lethality) than the cytoplasm, especially in dividing cells. *The sensitive site in the nucleus is the DNA within chromosomes.*

Chromosome Aberrations

Chromosomes serve as useful markers for radiation injury. They may be easily visualized and quantified, and the extent of their damage is related to cell survival. Chromosome aberrations are observed in irradiated cells at the time of mitosis when the DNA condenses to form chromosomes. The type of damage that may be observed depends on the stage of the cell in the cell cycle at the time of irradiation.

Figure 2-3 shows the stages of the cell cycle. If radiation exposure occurs after DNA synthesis (i.e., in late S or G_2 phase), only one arm of the affected chromosome is broken (chromatid aberration) (Fig. 2-4, *A*). However, if the radiation-induced break occurs before the DNA has replicated (i.e., in G_1 or early S phase), the damage is seen as a break in both arms (chromosome aberration) at the next mitosis (Fig. 2-4, *B*). Most simple breaks are repaired by biologic processes and go unrecognized. Figure 2-5 illustrates several common forms of chromosome aberrations resulting from incorrect repair. Formation of rings (Fig. 2-5, *A*) and dicentrics (Fig. 2-5, *B*) is lethal because the cell cannot complete mitosis. Translocations (Fig. 2-5, *C*) result in unequal distribution of chromatin material to daughter cells, and they may prevent completion of a subsequent mitosis. Chromosome aberrations have been detected in peripheral blood lymphocytes of patients exposed to medical diagnostic procedures. Additionally, the

survivors of the atomic bombings of Hiroshima and Nagasaki have demonstrated chromosome aberrations in circulating lymphocytes more than 2 decades after the radiation exposure. The frequency of aberrations is generally proportional to the radiation dose received.

CELL REPLICATION

Radiation is especially damaging to rapidly dividing cell systems, such as skin and intestinal mucosa, and hematopoietic tissues (Table 2-2). Irradiation of such cell populations causes a reduction in size of the irradiated tissue as a result of mitotic delay (inhibition of progression of the cells through the cell cycle) and reproductive cell death (usually during mitosis). The three mechanisms of reproductive death are DNA damage, bystander effect, and apoptosis.

DNA Damage

Cell death is caused by damage to DNA, which causes chromosome aberrations that cause the cell to die during the first few

TABLE 2-2 Relative Radiosensitivity of Various Cells

	High	Intermediate	Low
Characteristics	Divide regularly Long mitotic futures Undergo no or little differentiation between mitoses	Divide occasionally in response to demand for more cells	Highly differentiated When mature are incapable of division
Examples	Spermatogenic and erythroblastic stem cells Basal cells of oral mucous membrane	Vascular endothelial cells Fibroblasts Acinar and ductal salivary gland cells Parenchymal cells of liver, kidney, and thyroid	Neurons Striated muscle cells Squamous epithelial cells Erythrocytes

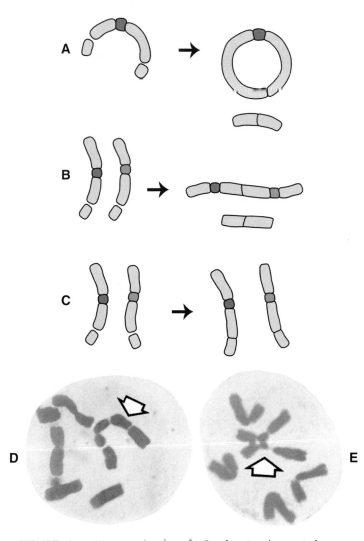

FIGURE 2-5 Chromosome aberrations. **A,** Ring formation plus acentric fragment. **B,** Dicentric formation. **C,** Translocation. **D** and **E,** Tetracentric exchange and chromatid exchange *(arrows)* taking place in *Trandescantia,* a New World perennial having a small number of large chromosomes. *(**D** and **E,** Courtesy Dr. M. Miller, Rochester, NY.)*

Bystander Effect

Cells that are damaged by radiation release into their immediate environment molecules that kill nearby cells. This bystander effect can cause chromosome aberrations, cell killing, gene mutations, and carcinogenesis.

Apoptosis

Apoptosis, also known as programmed cell death, occurs during normal embryogenesis. Cells round up, draw away from their neighbors, and condense nuclear chromatin. This characteristic pattern, which is different from necrosis, can be induced by radiation in both normal tissue and some tumors. Apoptosis is particularly common in hematopoietic and lymphoid tissues.

Recovery

Cell recovery from DNA damage and the bystander effect involves enzymatic repair of single-strand breaks of DNA. Because of this repair, a higher total dose is required to achieve a given degree of cell killing when multiple fractions are used (e.g., in radiation therapy) than when the same total dose is given in a single brief exposure. Damage to both strands of DNA at the same site is usually lethal to the cell.

DETERMINISTIC EFFECTS ON TISSUES AND ORGANS

The radiosensitivity of a tissue or organ is measured by its response to irradiation. Loss of moderate numbers of cells does not affect the function of most organs. However, with the loss of large numbers of cells, all affected organisms display an observable result. The severity of this change depends on the dose and thus the amount of cell loss. The following discussion pertains to the effect of irradiation of tissues and organs when the exposure is restricted to a small area, such as in radiation therapy. Comparable doses to the whole animal may result in death from damage to the most radiation-sensitive systems.

SHORT-TERM EFFECTS

The short-term effects of radiation on a tissue (effects seen in the first days or weeks after exposure) are determined primarily by the sensitivity of its parenchymal cells. When continuously proliferating tissues (e.g., bone marrow, oral mucous membranes) are irradiated with a moderate dose, cells are lost primarily by reproductive death, bystander effect, and apoptosis. The extent of cell loss depends on damage to the stem cell pools and the proliferative rate of the cell population. The effects of irradiation

mitoses after irradiation. The rate of cell replication in various tissues—and thus the rate of reproductive death—accounts for the varying radiosensitivity of tissues. When a population of slowly dividing cells is irradiated, larger doses and longer time intervals are required for induction of deterministic effects than when a rapidly dividing cell system is involved.

on such tissues become apparent quickly as a reduction in the number of mature cells in the series. Tissues composed of cells that rarely or never divide (e.g., neurons or muscle) demonstrate little or no radiation-induced hypoplasia over the short-term. The relative radiosensitivities of various tissues and organs are shown in Box 2-1.

LONG-TERM EFFECTS

The long-term deterministic effects of radiation on tissues and organs (seen months and years after exposure) are a loss of parenchymal cells and replacement with fibrous connective tissue. These changes are caused by reproductive death of replicating cells and by damage to the fine vasculature. Damage to capillaries leads to narrowing and eventual obliteration of vascular lumens. This impairs the transport of oxygen, nutrients, and waste products and results in death of all cell types dependent on this vascular supply. Thus both dividing (radiosensitive) and nondividing (radioresistant) parenchymal cells are replaced by fibrous connective tissue, a progressive fibroatrophy of the irradiated tissue.

MODIFYING FACTORS

The response of cells, tissues, and organs to irradiation depends on exposure conditions and the cell environment.

Dose

The severity of deterministic damage seen in irradiated tissues or organs depends on the amount of radiation received. Often a clinical threshold dose exists below which no adverse effects are seen. In all individuals receiving doses above the threshold level, the amount of damage is proportional to the dose.

Dose Rate

The term dose rate indicates the rate of exposure. For example, a total dose of 5 Gy may be given at a high dose rate (1 Gy/min) or a low dose rate (1 mGy/min). Exposure of biologic systems to a given dose at a high dose rate causes more damage than exposure to the same total dose given at a lower dose rate. When organisms are exposed at lower dose rates, a greater opportunity exists for repair of damage, resulting in less net damage. Although the dose from diagnostic exposures is low, they are given at a high dose rate compared with natural background exposure.

Oxygen

The radioresistance of many biologic systems increases by a factor of 2 or 3 when the exposure is made with reduced oxygen (hypoxia). The greater cell damage sustained in the presence of oxygen is related to the increased amounts of hydrogen peroxide and hydroperoxyl free radicals formed (described earlier). This is important clinically because hyperbaric oxygen therapy may be used during radiation therapy of tumors having hypoxic cells.

Linear Energy Transfer

In general, the dose required to produce a certain biologic effect is reduced as the linear energy transfer (LET) of the radiation is increased. Higher LET radiations (e.g., α particles) are more efficient in damaging biologic systems because their high ionization density is more likely than x rays to induce double-strand breakage in DNA. Low LET radiations such as x rays deposit their energy more sparsely, or uniformly, in the absorber and thus are more likely to cause single-strand breakage and less biologic damage.

RADIOTHERAPY IN THE ORAL CAVITY

RATIONALE

The oral cavity is exposed to large doses of radiation when radiation therapy is used to treat oral cancer, usually squamous cell carcinoma. Radiation therapy for malignant lesions in the oral cavity is usually indicated when the lesion is radiosensitive, advanced, or deeply invasive and cannot be approached surgically. Combined surgical and radiotherapeutic treatment often provides optimal treatment. Chemotherapy is increasingly being combined with radiation therapy and surgery.

The radiation treatment is administered as many daily small doses (fractions). Such fractionation of the total x-ray dose provides greater tumor destruction than is possible with a large single dose. Fractionation also allows increased cellular repair of surrounding normal tissues that are unavoidably exposed. Fractionation also increases the mean oxygen tension in an irradiated tumor, rendering the tumor cells more radiosensitive. This results from killing rapidly dividing tumor cells and shrinking the tumor mass after the first few fractions, reducing the distance that oxygen must diffuse from the fine vasculature through the tumor to reach the remaining viable tumor cells.

EFFECT ON ORAL TISSUES

The following sections describe the complications (deterministic effects) of a course of radiotherapy on the normal tissue of the oral cavity (Fig. 2-6). Typically, 2 Gy is delivered daily for a weekly exposure of 10 Gy. The radiotherapy course continues for 6 to 7 weeks until a total of 60 to 70 Gy is administered. In recent years, a new three-dimensional technique called intensity-modulated radiotherapy (IMRT) has been used to control the dose distribution with high accuracy, minimizing exposure to adjacent normal tissues. The effects described in the next section result only from therapeutic exposures, not from the far lower levels of radiation used for diagnostic imaging.

Oral Mucous Membrane

The oral mucous membrane contains a basal layer composed of rapidly dividing, radiosensitive stem cells. Near the end of the second week of therapy, as some of these cells die, the mucous membranes begin to show areas of redness and inflammation (mucositis). As the therapy continues, the irradiated mucous membrane begins to separate from the underlying connective tissue, with the formation of a white-to-yellow pseudomembrane (the desquamated epithelial layer) (Fig. 2-7). At the end of therapy, the mucositis is usually most severe, discomfort is at a maximum, and

BOX 2-1	Relative Radiosensitivity of Various Organs	
High	**Intermediate**	**Low**
Lymphoid organs	Fine vasculature	Neurons
Bone marrow	Growing cartilage	Muscle
Testes	Growing bone	
Intestines	Salivary glands	
Mucous membranes	Lungs	
	Kidney	
	Liver	

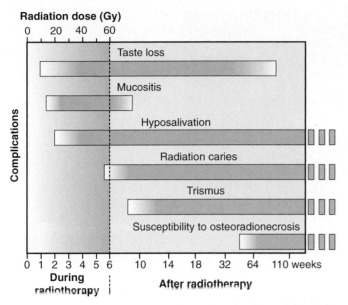

FIGURE 2-6 Oral complications. Typical time course of complications seen during and after a course of radiation therapy to the head and neck. Shaded area in first 6 weeks represents accumulated dose. Shading within bars indicates severity of complication. Note recovery of taste and healing of mucositis. Changes persisting after 2 years pose lifelong risks. *(Adapted from Kielbassa AM, Hinkelbein W, Hellwig E, et al: Radiation-related damage to dentition, Lancet Oncol 7:326–335, 2006.)*

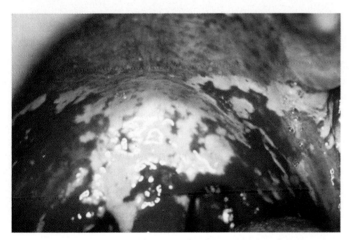

FIGURE 2-7 Mucositis of hard and soft palate. This patient is at the end of a course of radiotherapy and demonstrates an inflammatory response in the oral mucosa and areas of white pseudomembrane, areas where the oral epithelium separated from the underlying connective tissue.

food intake is difficult. Good oral hygiene minimizes infection. Topical anesthetics may be required at mealtimes. Secondary yeast infection by *Candida albicans* is a common complication and may require treatment.

After irradiation is completed, the mucosa begins to heal rapidly. Healing is usually complete by about 2 months. However, the mucous membrane later tends to become atrophic, thin, and relatively avascular. This long-term atrophy results from fibrosis of the underlying connective tissue. These atrophic changes complicate denture wearing because they may cause oral ulcerations of the compromised tissue. Ulcers may also result from radiation necrosis or tumor recurrence. A biopsy may be required to make the differentiation.

Taste Buds

Taste buds are sensitive to radiation. Doses in the therapeutic range cause extensive degeneration of the normal histologic architecture of taste buds. Patients often notice a loss of taste acuity during the second or third week of radiotherapy. Bitter and acid flavors are more severely affected when the posterior two thirds of the tongue is irradiated, and salt and sweet flavors are affected more when the anterior third of the tongue is irradiated. Taste acuity usually decreases by a factor of 1000 to 10,000 during the course of radiotherapy. Alterations in the saliva may partly account for this reduction, which may proceed to a state of virtual insensitivity. Taste loss is reversible, and recovery takes 60 to 120 days.

Salivary Glands

The major salivary glands are sometimes unavoidably exposed to 20 to 30 Gy during radiotherapy for cancer in the oral cavity or oropharynx. The parenchymal component of the salivary glands is radiosensitive (parotid glands more so than submandibular or sublingual glands). A marked and progressive loss of saliva is usually seen in the first few weeks after initiation of radiotherapy. The extent of reduced flow is dose dependent and may reach essentially zero at 60 Gy. The mouth becomes dry (xerostomia) and tender, and swallowing is difficult and painful. Histologically, an acute inflammatory response may occur soon after the initiation of therapy, particularly involving the serous acini. In the months after irradiation, the inflammatory response becomes more chronic, and the glands demonstrate marked loss of acini and ducts and a progressive fibrosis (Fig. 2-8). The loss of saliva-producing acini results in xerostomia. Patients with irradiation of both parotid glands are more likely to complain of dry mouth and difficulty with chewing and swallowing than patients with unilateral irradiation. Various saliva substitutes are available to help restore function. Use of intensity-modulated radiotherapy has helped to spare the contralateral salivary glands and thus minimize the loss of salivary function.

The reduced volume of saliva in patients receiving radiation therapy that includes the major salivary glands is altered from normal. Because serous cells are more radiosensitive than mucous cells, the residual saliva is more viscous than usual. The small volume of viscous saliva that is secreted usually has a pH value 1 unit below normal (i.e., an average of 5.5 in irradiated patients compared with 6.5 in unexposed individuals). This pH is low enough to initiate decalcification of normal enamel. In addition, the buffering capacity of saliva decreases up to 44% during radiation therapy. If some portions of the major salivary glands are spared, dryness of the mouth usually subsides in 6 to 12 months because of compensatory hypertrophy of residual salivary gland tissue. Reduced salivary flow that persists beyond 1 year is unlikely to show significant recovery. Patients with persistent xerostomia typically take frequent sips of water they carry with them.

Teeth

Children receiving radiation therapy to the jaws may show defects in the permanent dentition, such as retarded root development, dwarfed teeth, or failure to form one or more teeth (Fig. 2-9). If exposure precedes calcification, irradiation may destroy the tooth bud. Irradiation after calcification has begun may inhibit cellular differentiation, causing malformations and arresting general growth. Such exposure may retard or abort root formation, but the eruptive mechanism of teeth is relatively radiation

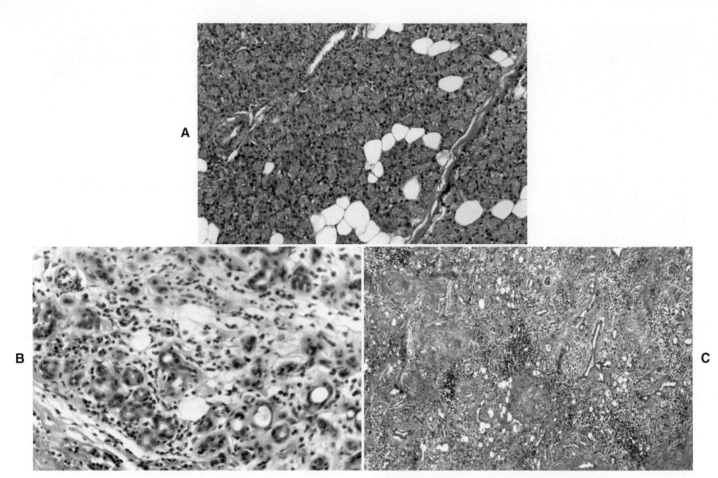

FIGURE 2-8 Radiation effects on human parotid salivary gland. **A,** Normal gland demonstrating mostly serous glandular cells (purple) with ducts and occasional adipocytes (clear). **B,** Gland 6 months after exposure to radiotherapy. Note the loss of acini and the presence of chronic inflammatory cells (dark). **C,** Gland 1 year after exposure to radiotherapy. Note the loss of acini, extensive fibrosis (pink), and persistent inflammatory cells (dark).

resistant. Irradiated teeth with altered root formation typically erupt, even if rootless. In general, the severity of the damage is dose dependent.

Radiation Caries

Radiation caries is a rampant form of dental decay that may occur in individuals who receive a course of radiotherapy that includes exposure of the salivary glands. Patients receiving radiation therapy to oral structures have increases in *Streptococcus mutans, Lactobacillus,* and *Candida.* Caries results from changes in the salivary glands and saliva, including reduced flow, decreased pH, reduced buffering capacity, increased viscosity, and altered flora. The residual saliva in individuals with xerostomia also has a low concentration of Ca^{2+} ion; this results in greater solubility of tooth structure and reduced remineralization. Because of the reduced or absent cleansing action of normal saliva, debris accumulates quickly. There is also growing evidence that radiation has direct effects on teeth that make them more prone to breakdown with flaking of enamel, particularly in areas of occlusal loading or stress, such as at the incisal, cuspal, and cervical regions of teeth. The destruction is seen with doses greater than 30 Gy and is pronounced when the teeth receive more than 60 Gy.

Clinically, three types of radiation caries exist. The most common is widespread superficial lesions attacking buccal, occlusal, incisal, and palatal surfaces (Fig. 2-10). Another type involves primarily the cementum and dentin in the cervical region. These lesions may progress around the teeth circumferentially and result in loss of the crown. The third type appears as a dark pigmentation of the entire crown. The incisal edges may be markedly worn. Combinations of all these lesions develop in some patients. The location, rapid course, and widespread attack distinguish radiation caries. There is also evidence that radiation caries is more likely to lead to periapical inflammatory lesions (see Chapter 20) if the periapical bone received a high dose of radiation.

The best method of reducing radiation caries is daily application of a viscous topical 1% neutral sodium fluoride gel in custom-made applicator trays. The best results are achieved from a combination of restorative dental procedures, excellent oral hygiene, a diet restricted in cariogenic foods, and topical applications of sodium fluoride. Patient cooperation in maintaining oral hygiene is extremely important because radiation caries is a lifelong threat. Teeth with gross caries or periodontal involvement are often extracted before irradiation.

Bone

Treatment of cancers in the oral region often includes irradiation of the mandible or maxilla. The primary damage to mature bone results from radiation-induced damage to the vasculature of the periosteum and cortical bone, which are normally already sparse. Radiation also acts by destroying osteoblasts and, to a lesser extent,

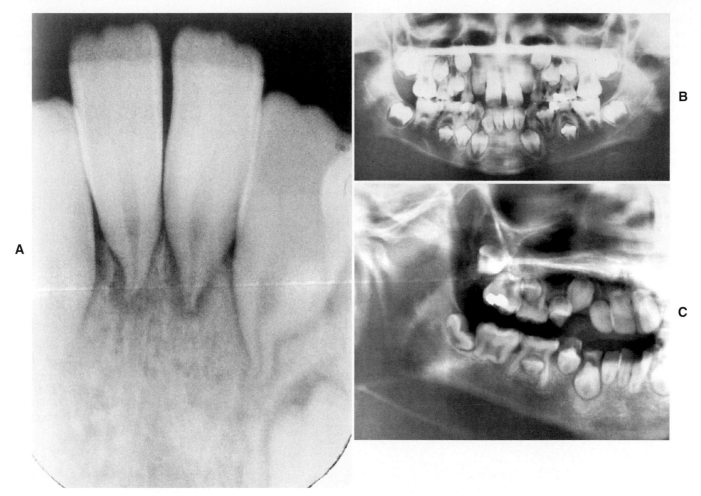

FIGURE 2-9 Dental abnormalities after radiotherapy in two patients. The first patient, a 9-year-old girl who received 35 Gy at age 4 years because of Hodgkin's disease, had severe stunting of the incisor roots with premature closure of the apices at 8 years (**A**) and retarded development of the mandibular second premolar crowns with stunting of the mandibular incisor, canine, and premolar roots at 9 years (**B**). The second patient (**C**), a 10-year-old boy who received 41 Gy to the jaws at age 4 years, had severely stunted root development of all permanent teeth with a normal primary molar. (**A** and **B**, Courtesy Mr. P. N. Hirschmann, Leeds, UK; **C**, Courtesy Dr. James Eischen, San Diego, CA.)

osteoclasts. In addition, the endosteum becomes atrophic, showing a lack of osteoblastic and osteoclastic activity. The degree of mineralization may be reduced, leading to brittleness. Typically, the oral mucosa breaks down with exposure of the underlying bone. This condition is termed osteoradionecrosis. It is the most serious clinical complication that occurs in bone after irradiation. The decreased vascularity of the mandible renders it easily infected by microorganisms from the oral cavity. This bone infection may result from radiation-induced breakdown of the oral mucous membrane, from mechanical damage to the weakened oral mucous membrane such as by a denture sore or tooth extraction, through a periodontal lesion, or from radiation caries. This infection may cause a nonhealing wound in irradiated bone that is treated with débridement with varying degrees of success (Fig. 2-11). It is more common in the mandible than in the maxilla, probably because of the richer vascular supply to the maxilla and the fact that the mandible is more frequently irradiated. The higher the radiation dose absorbed by the bone, especially more than 60 Gy, the

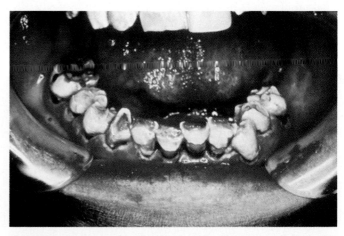

FIGURE 2-10 Radiation caries. Note the extensive loss of structure on the occlusal surface of the mandibular teeth resulting from radiation-induced xerostomia.

greater the risk for osteoradionecrosis. The risk is also greater in the presence of odontogenic or periodontal disease and in individuals with poor oral hygiene or ill-fitting dentures. Patients with osteoradionecrosis typically also have numerous other complications, including trismus, loss of taste, difficulty in swallowing, and xerostomia.

Patients should be referred for dental care before undergoing a course of radiation therapy to minimize radiation caries and osteoradionecrosis. Radiation caries can be minimized by restoring all carious lesions before radiation therapy and initiating preventive techniques of good oral hygiene and daily topical fluoride. The risk for osteoradionecrosis and infection can be minimized by removing teeth with extensive caries or with poor periodontal support (allowing 2 to 3 weeks for the extraction wounds to heal before beginning radiation therapy) and adjusting dentures to minimize the risk of denture sores. Removal of teeth after irradiation should be avoided when possible.

Patients who have had radiation therapy often require a radiographic examination to supplement clinical examinations. Radiographs are especially important to detect caries early. The amount of radiation from such diagnostic exposures is negligible compared with the amount received during therapy and should not serve as a reason to defer radiographs. However, whenever possible, it is desirable to avoid taking radiographs during the first 6 months after completion of radiotherapy to avoid injury to the mucous membrane by the sensor.

Musculature

Radiation may cause inflammation and fibrosis resulting in contracture and trismus in the muscles of mastication. The masseter or pterygoid muscles usually are involved. Restriction in mouth opening usually starts about 2 months after radiotherapy is completed and progresses thereafter. An exercise program may be helpful in increasing opening distance.

DETERMINISTIC EFFECTS OF WHOLE-BODY IRRADIATION

ACUTE RADIATION SYNDROME

The acute radiation syndrome is a collection of signs and symptoms experienced by individuals after a brief whole-body exposure to radiation (Table 2-3). Information about this syndrome comes from animal experiments and human exposures from medical radiotherapy, the atom bomb blasts in 1945, and radiation accidents such as at Chernobyl in 1986.

Prodromal Period

Within the first minutes to hours after exposure to whole-body irradiation of about 1.5 Gy, an individual may have anorexia, nausea, vomiting, diarrhea, weakness, and fatigue. These early symptoms constitute the prodromal period of the acute radiation syndrome. The higher the dose, the more rapid the onset, and the greater the severity of symptoms.

Latent Period

After the prodromal reaction comes a latent period, during which the exposed person shows no signs or symptoms of radiation sickness. The extent of the latent period is also dose related, lasting hours or days after supralethal exposures (approximately >5 Gy) to a few weeks after exposures of about 2 Gy.

Hematopoietic Syndrome

Whole-body exposures of 2 to 7 Gy cause injury to the mitotically active hematopoietic stem cells in the bone marrow and spleen.

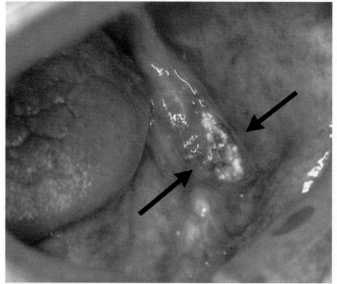

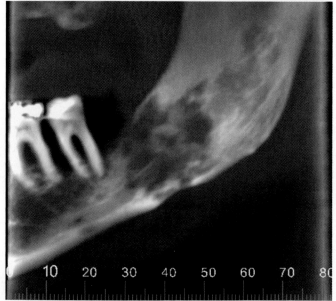

FIGURE 2-11 Osteoradionecrosis. **A,** Area of exposed mandible after radiotherapy. Note the loss of oral mucosa *(arrows)*. **B,** Destruction of irradiated bone resulting from infection.

TABLE 2-3	Acute Radiation Syndrome
Dose (Gy)	Manifestation
1–2	Prodromal symptoms
2–4	Mild hematopoietic symptoms
4–7	Severe hematopoietic symptoms
7–15	Gastrointestinal symptoms
50	Cardiovascular and central nervous system symptoms

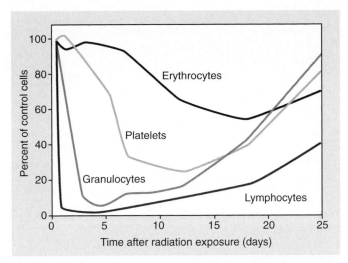

FIGURE 2-12 Radiation effects on blood cells. Whole-body exposure inhibits replication of blood stem cell precursors in bone marrow. This inhibits the replacement of circulating cells. As a result, the duration of the circulating cells' survival is largely determined by their life span in circulation. In this instance, the bone marrow damage is incomplete, and recovery is evident after 1 to 2 weeks.

Doses in this range cause a rapid decrease in the numbers of circulating granulocytes, platelets, and finally erythrocytes (Fig. 2-12). Although mature circulating granulocytes, platelets, and erythrocytes are radioresistant, nonreplicating cells, their paucity in the peripheral blood after irradiation reflects the radiosensitivity of their precursors. Granulocytes, with short lives in circulation, fall off in a few days, whereas red blood cells, with long lives in circulation, fall off slowly.

The clinical signs of the hematopoietic syndrome include infection (from lymphopenia and granulocytopenia), hemorrhage (from loss of platelets), and anemia (from erythrocyte depletion). The probability of death is low after exposures at the low end of this range but much higher at the high end. When death results from the hematopoietic syndrome, it usually occurs 10 to 30 days after irradiation.

Gastrointestinal Syndrome

Gastrointestinal syndrome is caused by whole-body exposures of 7 to 15 Gy. Exposures in this range cause extensive damage to the gastrointestinal system in addition to the hematopoietic damage described previously. Exposure in this dose range causes considerable injury to the rapidly proliferating basal epithelial cells of the intestinal villi and leads to rapid loss of the epithelial layer of the intestinal mucosa. Because of the denuded mucosal surface, there is loss of plasma and electrolytes, loss of efficient intestinal absorption, and ulceration of the mucosal lining with hemorrhaging into the intestines. These changes are responsible for diarrhea, dehydration, and weight loss. Endogenous intestinal bacteria readily invade the denuded surface, producing septicemia.

At about the time that developing damage to the gastrointestinal system reaches a maximum, the effect of bone marrow depression begins to manifest. The result is a marked lowering of the body's defense against bacterial infection and a decrease in effectiveness of the clotting mechanism. The combined effects of damage to these hematopoietic and gastrointestinal stem cell systems cause death within 2 weeks from fluid and electrolyte loss, infection, and possibly nutritional impairment. Of the plant staff and firefighters at the Chernobyl accident, 28 died within the first

few months of development of the hematopoietic or gastrointestinal syndrome.

Cardiovascular and Central Nervous System Syndrome

Exposures greater than 50 Gy usually cause death in 1 to 2 days. The few humans who have been exposed at this level showed collapse of the circulatory system with a precipitous fall in blood pressure in the hours preceding death. Autopsy revealed necrosis of cardiac muscle. Victims also may present with intermittent stupor, incoordination, disorientation, and convulsions suggestive of extensive damage to the nervous system. Although the precise mechanism is not fully understood, these latter symptoms most likely result from damage to the neurons and fine vasculature of the brain.

Management of Acute Radiation Syndrome

The presenting clinical problems govern the management of different forms of acute radiation syndrome. Antibiotics are indicated when the granulocyte count decreases. Fluid and electrolyte replacement is used as necessary. Whole-blood transfusions are used to treat anemia, and platelets may be administered to arrest bleeding.

RADIATION EFFECTS ON EMBRYOS AND FETUSES

The effects of radiation on human embryos and fetuses have been studied in animals, women exposed to diagnostic or therapeutic radiation during pregnancy, and women exposed to radiation from the atomic bombs dropped at Hiroshima and Nagasaki. Embryos and fetuses are considerably more radiosensitive than adults because most embryonic cells are relatively undifferentiated and rapidly mitotic.

Exposures of 1 to 3 Gy during the first few days after conception are thought to cause undetectable death of the embryo because many of these embryos fail to implant in the uterine wall. The period of organogenesis, when the major organ systems form, is 3 to 8 weeks after conception. The most common abnormalities among the Japanese children exposed early in gestation were reduced growth that persisted through life and reduced head circumference (microcephaly), often associated with mental retardation. Other abnormalities included small birth size, cataracts, genital and skeletal malformations, and microphthalmia. The period of maximal sensitivity of the brain is 8 to 15 weeks after conception. These effects are deterministic in nature and are believed to have a threshold of about 0.1 Gy. This threshold dose is 400 times higher than the fetal exposure from a dental examination (0.25 mGy from a full-mouth examination when a leaded apron is used). By comparison, the dose to an embryo and fetus from natural background radiation is approximately 2250 mGy during the 9 months of gestation.

Radiation has been shown to increase the probability of leukemia and other types of cancer (see later) during childhood of individuals exposed *in utero*. It is assumed that embryos and fetuses have approximately the same risk for carcinogenic effects as children (about three times that of the population as a whole). There is no known threshold for leukemia or other cancers. Because of these considerations, it is important to consider effects on the embryo and fetus when ordering dental radiographs for a pregnant patient. It is recommended to defer optional imaging until the end of pregnancy (e.g., bitewings only indicated by the length of time since the previous examination) but to make radiographs when there is a specific indication based on the patient's history or clinical findings.

LATE EFFECTS

Numerous late deterministic effects have been found in the survivors of the atomic bombing of Hiroshima and Nagasaki.

Growth and Development

Children exposed in the bombings showed impairment of growth and development, including reduced height, weight, and skeletal development. The younger the individual was at the time of exposure, the more pronounced the effects.

Cataracts

The threshold for induction of cataracts (opacities in the lens of the eye) is unclear, but it is now believed to be in the range of 0.5 Gy. Although these cataracts are clinically detectable, most affected individuals are unaware of their presence. Although exposures to the eye from dental radiography are quite small, they nonetheless should be avoided when possible during radiographic examinations.

Shortened Life Span

The survivors of the atomic bombings show a clear decrease in median life expectancy with increasing radiation dose (other than shortened life expectancy caused by cancer). The reduction in life span ranges from 2 months to 2.6 years by dose group, with an overall mean of 4 months. Survivors demonstrate increased frequency of heart disease, stroke, and noncancer diseases of the digestive, respiratory, and hematopoietic systems. It is believed that number of noncancer deaths resulting from radiation exposure is about half as many as deaths from cancer.

STOCHASTIC EFFECTS

Stochastic effects result from sublethal changes in the DNA of individual cells. The most important consequence of such damage is radiation-induced cancer. The severity of radiation-induced cancer does not vary with dose—either it is present or it is not. Many studies show increased cancer incidence in humans after exposure to radiation. Heritable effects, although much less likely, can also occur.

CARCINOGENESIS

Radiation causes cancer by modifying DNA. The most likely mechanism is a multistep process including accumulation of radiation-induced gene mutation. These mutations are usually base substitutions, insertions and deletions of bases, rearrangements caused by breakage and abnormal rejoining of DNA strands, or changes in the copy number of DNA segments. When the mutations involve growth-regulating genes—activation of oncogenes or inactivation of tumor suppressor genes—they can deregulate cell growth or differentiation or both and ultimately lead to neoplastic development. In principle, even one radiation photon may initiate cancer formation.

Estimation of the number of cancers induced by radiation is difficult. Radiation-induced cancers are not distinguishable from cancers produced by other causes. This means that the number of cancers can be estimated only as the number of excess cases found in exposed groups compared with the number in unexposed groups of people. The group of individuals most intensively studied for estimating the cancer risk from radiation is the Japanese atomic bomb survivors. These bombings occurred in 1945. Approximately 200,000 people died with the first 2 months as a

result of blast or burn injury or of the acute radiation syndrome (described earlier). Starting in 1950, systematic studies were initiated to follow the health of the survivors, children exposed *in utero*, and the offspring of exposed parents. In the survivor cohort, the histories of more than 120,000 individuals have been followed since 1950. The in utero study involved 3600 subjects, and the offspring study involved about 77,000 subjects. The incidences of deaths from leukemias and solid cancers in the survivor study are shown in Table 2-4 and Figure 2-13. The risk for most solid cancers increases linearly with dose and lasts for the lifetime of the exposed individual. The risk from exposure during childhood is two to three times as great as the risk during adulthood. The number of cancers induced by radiation is most likely a multiple of their spontaneous frequency. Box 2-2 shows the radiosensitivity of various tissues in

TABLE 2-4	Cancer Mortality Rate in 86,611 Atomic Bomb Survivors Having 50,620 Deaths from All Causes (1950–2003)	
	Leukemias	Solid Cancers
Deaths	296	10,929
Radiation induced	93	527

Data adapted from Preston DL, Pierce DA, Shimizu Y, et al: Effect of recent changes in atomic bomb survivor dosimetry on cancer mortality risk estimates, *Radiat Res* 162:377-389, 2004 (through 2000 for leukemias) and Ozasa K, Shimizu Y, Suyama A, Kasagi F, Soda M, Grant EJ, et al: Studies of the mortality of atomic bomb survivors, Report 14, 1950-2003: an overview of cancer and noncancer diseases. *Radiat Res* 177:229-243, 2012 (for solid cancers).

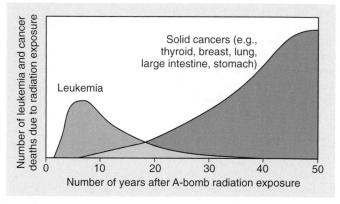

FIGURE 2-13 Schematic model of incidence of leukemia (orange plus pale green) and solid cancers (pale green plus dark green) shown by years after radiation exposure. Leukemias are initially seen in the first few years after exposure and cease after 3 decades. In contrast, solid tumors have a latent period of about a decade and remain in excess for the remainder of the exposed person's life. *(Adapted from Introduction to the Radiation Effects Research Foundation:* http://www.rerf.jp/shared/introd/introRERFe.pdf.*)*

BOX 2-2	Susceptibility of Different Organs to Radiation-Induced Cancer	
High	**Intermediate**	**Low**
Colon	Bladder	Bone surface
Stomach	Liver	Brain
Lung	Thyroid	Salivary glands
Bone marrow (leukemia)		Skin
Female breast		

terms of susceptibility to radiation-induced cancer. The following discussion pertains primarily to organs exposed in the course of dental radiography.

Leukemia

The incidence of leukemia (other than chronic lymphocytic leukemia) increases after exposure of the bone marrow to radiation. Atomic bomb survivors and patients irradiated for ankylosing spondylitis show a wave of leukemias beginning soon after exposure, peaking at around 7 years, and ceasing after about 30 years.

Thyroid Cancer

The incidence of thyroid carcinomas (arising from the follicular epithelium) increases in humans after exposure. Only about 10% or less of individuals with such cancers die of their disease. The best-studied groups are Israeli children irradiated to the scalp for ringworm, children irradiated to the thymus gland, survivors of the atomic bombs in Japan, and individuals exposed after the accident at Chernobyl. Susceptibility to radiation induced thyroid cancer is greater early in childhood than at any time later in life, and children are more susceptible than adults. Females are two to three times more susceptible than males to radiogenic and spontaneous thyroid cancers. The fallout from the accident at the Chernobyl nuclear power plant, primarily iodine-131, is thought to have caused about 7000 cases of thyroid cancer in children and 15 fatalities.

Esophageal Cancer

Excess numbers of esophageal cancers are found in the Japanese atomic bomb survivors and in patients treated with x radiation for ankylosing spondylitis.

Brain and Nervous System Cancers

Patients exposed to diagnostic x-ray examinations in utero and to therapeutic doses in childhood or as adults (average midbrain dose of about 1 Gy) show excess numbers of malignant and benign brain tumors. Additionally, case-control studies have shown an association between intracranial meningiomas and previous medical or dental radiography. If the association is real, it is most likely that the nature of the association is that more dental images were made in response to facial pain referred from the tumor rather than the radiation causing more meningiomas.

Salivary Gland Cancer

The incidence of salivary gland tumors is increased in patients treated with irradiation for diseases of the head and neck, in Japanese atomic bomb survivors, and in persons exposed to diagnostic x radiation. An association between tumors of the salivary glands and dental radiography has been shown. As with meningiomas, the association most likely is explained by dental radiographs made in response to the presence of the tumors.

Other Organs

Other organs, such as the skin, paranasal sinuses, and bone marrow, also show excess neoplasia after exposure. However, the mortality and morbidity rates expected after head and neck exposure are much lower than for the organs described previously.

HERITABLE EFFECTS

Heritable effects are changes seen in the offspring of irradiated individuals. They are the consequence of damage to the genetic material of reproductive cells. The basic findings of radiation-induced heritable effects are listed in Box 2-3. At low levels of

BOX 2-3 Basic Principles of Radiation Genetics

- Radiation causes increased frequency of spontaneous mutations rather than inducing new mutations.
- Frequency of mutations increases in direct proportion to dose, even at very low doses, with no evidence of a threshold.
- Most mutations are deleterious to the organism.
- Dose rate is important; at low dose rates, the frequency of induced mutations is greatly reduced.
- Males are much more radiosensitive than females.
- Rate of mutations is reduced as the time between exposure and conception increases.

exposure, such as encountered in dentistry, they are far less important than carcinogenesis.

Our knowledge of heritable effects of radiation on humans comes largely from the atomic bomb survivors. To date, no such radiation-related genetic damage has been demonstrated. No increase has occurred in adverse pregnancy outcome, leukemia or other cancers, or impairment of growth and development in the children of atomic bomb survivors. Similarly, studies of the children of patients who received radiotherapy show no detectable increase in the frequency of genetic diseases. These findings do not exclude the possibility that such damage occurs but do show that it must be at a very low frequency.

BIBLIOGRAPHY

Bushong SC: *Radiologic science for technologists: physics, biology, and protection*, ed 9, St Louis, 2008, Mosby.

Gusev I, Guskova A, Mettler F: *Medical management of radiation accidents*, ed 2, Boca Raton, FL, 2001, CRC.

Hall EJ, Giaccia AJ: *Radiobiology for the radiologist*, ed 7, Philadelphia, 2011, Lippincott Williams & Wilkins.

Joiner M, van der Kogel A: *Basic clinical radiobiology*, ed 4, London, 2002, Hodder Arnold.

SUGGESTED READINGS

Genetic Effects

United Nations Scientific Committee on the Effects of Atomic Radiation: Hereditary effects of radiation (2001): http://www.unscear.org/unscear/en/publications/2001.html.

Odontogenesis

Dahllof G: Craniofacial growth in children treated for malignant diseases, *Acta Odontol Scand* 56:378, 1998.

Kielbassa AM, Hinkelbein W, Hellwig E, et al: Radiation-related damage to dentition, *Lancet Oncol* 7:326–335, 2006.

Oral Sequelae of Head and Neck Radiotherapy

Chopra S, Kamdar D, Ugur OE, et al: Factors predictive of severity of osteoradionecrosis of the mandible, *Head Neck* 33:1600–1605, 2011.

Chung EM, Sung EC: Dental management of chemoradiation patients, *J Calif Dent Assoc* 34:735–742, 2006.

Hommez GM, De Meerleer GO, De Neve WJ, et al: Effect of radiation dose on the prevalence of apical periodontitis—a dosimetric analysis, *Clin Oral Invest* 16:1543–1547, 2012.

Jacobson AS, Buchbinder D, Hu K, et al: Paradigm shifts in the management of osteoradionecrosis of the mandible, *Oral Oncol* 46:795–801, 2010.

Sciubba JJ, Goldenberg D: Oral complications of radiotherapy, *Lancet Oncol* 7:175–183, 2006.

Teng MS, Futran ND: Osteoradionecrosis of the mandible, *Curr Opin Otolaryngol Head Neck Surg* 13:217–221, 2005.

Walker MP, Wichman B, Cheng A-L, et al: Impact of radiotherapy dose on dentition breakdown in head and neck cancer patients, *Pract Radiat Oncol* 1:142–148, 2011.

Somatic Effects

Committee to Assess Health Risks from Exposure to Low Levels of Ionizing Radiation: *Health risks from exposure to low levels of ionizing radiation: BEIR VII–phase 2*, Washington, DC, 2006, National Research Council, National Academies Press.

Neriishi K, Nakashima E, Akahoshi M, et al: Radiation dose and cataract surgery incidence in atomic bomb survivors, 1986–2005, *Radiology* 265:167–174, 2012.

Ozasa K, Shimizu Y, Suyama A, et al: Studies of the mortality of atomic bomb survivors, Report 14, 1950-2003: an overview of cancer and noncancer diseases, *Radiat Res* 177:229–243, 2012.

Preston DL, Shimizu Y, Pierce DA, et al: Studies of mortality of atomic bomb survivors. Report 13: solid cancer and noncancer disease mortality: 1950-1997, *Radiat Res* 160:381–407, 2003.

Sources and effects of ionizing radiation, UNSCEAR 2008 report: volumes I and II, New York, 2008, UNSCEAR (United Nations Publications vol I released in 2010 and vol II released in 2011). https://unp.un.org/details.aspx?pid=20417 and https://unp.un.org/Details.aspx?pid=21556.

The 2007 recommendations of the International Commission on Radiological Protection. IRCP Publication 103, *Ann ICRP* 37:1–332, 2007.

Safety and Protection

Dentists must be prepared to discuss intelligently with patients the benefits and possible hazards involved with the use of x rays and to describe the steps taken to reduce these hazards. This chapter considers sources of exposure, estimates of risks from dental radiography, and means to minimize exposure from dental examinations.

SOURCES OF RADIATION EXPOSURE

The general population is exposed to radiation primarily from natural background and medical sources (Table 3-1). Understanding these exposure sources provides a useful framework for considering dental exposure.

BACKGROUND RADIATION

All life on earth has evolved in a continuous exposure to natural background radiation (Fig. 3-1; see Table 3-1). Background radiation from space and various terrestrial sources yields an average annual effective dose of about 3.1 mSv in the United States.

Radon and Its Progeny

Radon is a gas (radon 222) released from the ground that enters homes and buildings. By itself, radon does little harm, but it decays, releasing α particles, to polonium 218 and lead 214. These isotopes decay further, emitting more α particles. Radon and its decay products may become attached to dust particles that can be inhaled and deposited on the bronchial epithelium in the respiratory tract. Radon is estimated to be responsible for approximately 73% of the background exposure of the world's population. Exposure to this quantity of radiation may cause 10,000 to 20,000 lung cancer deaths per year in the United States, mostly in smokers.

Space Radiation

Radiation from space comes from the sun or from cosmic rays. It is composed primarily of protons, helium nuclei, and nuclei of heavier elements as well as other particles generated by the interactions of primary space radiation with the earth's atmosphere. Exposure from space radiation is primarily a function of altitude, almost doubling with each 2000-m increase in elevation because less atmosphere is present to attenuate the radiation. At sea level, the exposure from space radiation is about 0.33 mSv/y; at an elevation of 1600 m (approximately 1 mile, the elevation of Denver, Colorado), it is about 0.50 mSv/y. Space radiation contributes about 11% of background exposure.

Internal Radionuclides

Another source of background radiation is radionuclides that are ingested. The greatest internal exposure comes from foods containing uranium and thorium and their decay products, primarily potassium 40 but also rubidium 87, carbon 14, tritium, and others. The total exposure from ingestion contributes about 9% of background exposure.

Terrestrial Radiation

The final source of background radiation comes from exposure from radioactive nuclides in the soil, primarily potassium 40 and the radioactive decay products of uranium 238 and thorium 232. Most of the γ radiation from these sources comes from the top 20 cm of soil. Indoor exposure from radionuclides is close to the exposure occurring outdoors because the shielding provided by structural materials balances the exposure from radioactive nuclides contained within these shielding materials. Terrestrial exposure contributes approximately 7% of background exposure.

MEDICAL EXPOSURE

Humans have contributed many additional sources of radiation to the environment (Fig. 3-2). The largest of these sources is medical imaging, with much smaller contributions from consumer products and other minor sources.

Approximately 400 million x-ray examinations are performed annually in the United States; about one quarter of these are dental. More recent estimates suggest that medical exposure in developed countries has grown rapidly in recent decades,

TABLE 3-1   Average Annual Effective Dose of Ionizing Radiation

Source	Dose (mSv)
Natural background	
Radon	2.3
Space	0.3
Internal radionuclides	0.3
Terrestrial	0.2
Subtotal background	*3.1*
Medical	
CT	1.5
Nuclear medicine	0.8
Interventional fluoroscopy	0.4
Conventional radiography and fluoroscopy	0.3
Dental	0.007
Subtotal medical	*3.0*
Consumer products and other	0.1
Grand total	6.2

Data from National Council on Radiation Protection and Measurements: *Ionizing radiation exposure of the population of the United States,* NCRP Report 160, Bethesda, MD, 2009, National Council on Radiation Protection and Measurements.

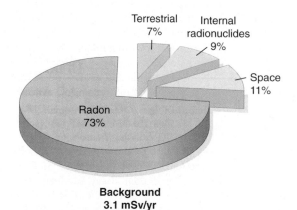

**Background
3.1 mSv/yr**

FIGURE 3-1 Natural background radiation contributes 3.1 mSv on average per year. Most exposure comes from radon, but there are significant contributions from space, ingested radionuclides, and terrestrial sources including external radionuclides in the soil and building materials. (*Data from National Council on Radiation Protection and Measurements:* Ionizing radiation exposure of the population of the United States, *NCRP Report 160, Bethesda, MD, 2009, National Council on Radiation Protection and Measurements.*)

particularly computed tomography (CT) of the chest and abdomen and increased use of cardiac nuclear medicine studies. The average doses from medical exposures are comparable to natural background exposure. CT (see Chapter 14) contributes more than half of medical exposure. In contrast to background radiation exposures, which affect everyone relatively uniformly, the distribution of medical exposures is highly skewed with older and sicker individuals receiving most medical exposures. Dental x-ray examinations, although made relatively frequently, are responsible for only 0.26% of the total exposure from medical imaging.

CONSUMER PRODUCTS

Consumer products contain some of the most interesting and unsuspected sources. This group includes, in order of importance,

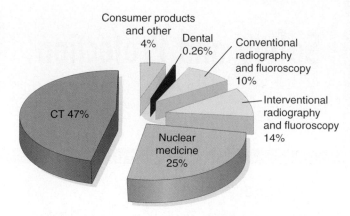

**Medical, consumer products and other
3.1 mSv/yr**

FIGURE 3-2 Sources of radiation in the United States from medical examinations and consumer products. The average person in the United States receives about as much radiation from medical and consumer products sources (3.0 mSv/y) as from natural background exposure. Most medical x-ray exposures come from CT, nuclear medicine (primarily cardiac imaging), fluoroscopy, and conventional radiography. Exposures from dental examinations and from occupational, fallout, and nuclear power sources are small. Although individuals with exposures from natural background are fairly evenly distributed in the population, most medically exposed individuals are relatively old and sick.

exposure from cigarette smoking, building materials, air travel, mining and agriculture, and combustion of fossil fuels. As more people travel frequently above the protection of the earth's atmosphere, cosmic radiation becomes a more significant contributor to exposure. An airline flight of 5 hours in the middle latitudes at an altitude of 12 km may result in an exposure of about 25 µSv. Other minor sources of exposure from consumer products include dental porcelain, television receivers, and smoke alarms. In total, consumer products contribute only about 1.6% of the total average annual exposure.

OTHER SOURCES

Other sources of exposure affect caregivers or others in contact with patients receiving nuclear medicine treatments; people who work in nuclear power generation; individuals involved in areas of industrial, medical, educational, or research activities; workers in medical and dental x-ray facilities; workers in airport inspection systems; and commercial pilots. All these sources of radiation combined contribute only about 0.1% of the total average annual exposure.

DOSE LIMITS, EXPOSURES, AND RISK

This section considers governmental dose limits for individuals who are occupationally exposed to radiation and for members of the general population. It also covers the amounts of radiation received by patients in dental and medical radiography and the estimated risks from these exposures.

DOSE LIMITS

Recognition of the harmful effects of radiation and the risks involved with its use led the International Commission on Radiological Protection (ICRP) to establish guidelines for limitations on the amount of radiation received by both occupationally exposed individuals and the public (Table 3-2). These limits pertain to planned exposure situations, not to background radiation and not

TABLE 3-2	International Commission on Radiological Protection Recommended Dose Limits for Human Exposure to Ionizing Radiation	
Type of Limit	**Occupational**	**Public**
Effective dose	20 mSv per year, averaged over defined periods of 5 years with a maximum of 50 mSv in any one year	1 mSv in a year
Annual equivalent dose to		
Lens of eye	20 mSv, averaged over defined periods of 5 years with a maximum of 50 mSv in any one year	15 mSv
Skin	500 mSv	50 mSv
Hands and feet	500 mSv	—

Data from the 2007 recommendations of the International Commission on Radiological Protection. IRCP Publication 103, *Ann ICRP* 37:1-332, 2007; and ICRP Statement on Tissue Reactions, ICRP ref 4825-3093-1464, 2011: http://www.icrp.org/docs/icrp%20statement%20on%20tissue%20reactions.pdf.

to emergency situations. Since their establishment in the 1930s, these dose limits have been revised downward several times reflecting increased knowledge concerning the harmful effects of radiation and the increased ability to use radiation more efficiently. Occupationally exposed individuals include dentists and their staffs. Individuals in the reception area or who are walking in a corridor outside a dental office are members of the public. Dose limits for members of the public—individuals not exposed occupationally—are generally set at 10% of occupationally exposed individuals. The current occupational exposure limits have been established to ensure that no individuals will have deterministic effects and that the probability for stochastic effects is as low as reasonably and economically feasible.

Dentists and their staff are occupationally exposed workers and are allowed to receive an average of 20 mSv of whole-body radiation exposure per year. Although this level of exposure is considered to present only a minimal risk, every effort should be made to keep the radiation dose to all individuals as low as practical. The dental profession does well in this area. The average dose for individuals occupationally exposed in the operation of dental x-ray equipment is 0.2 mSv—1% of the allowable exposure.

There are no limits on the exposure a patient can receive from diagnostic examinations, interventional procedures, or radiation therapy; this is because these exposures are made intentionally and for the direct benefit of the recipient. Individual circumstances make the setting of limits inappropriate. However, increasing concern for minimizing patient exposure has led multiple institutions, including the National Council on Radiation Protection and Measurement (NCRP) to issue diagnostic reference levels (DRL) for medical and dental diagnostic imaging. DRL exposure values represent the acceptable upper limits for patient exposure (75th percentile of general practice), whereas achievable doses represent the median dose (50th percentile) in general practice. The NCRP recommends a DRL of 1.6 mGy entrance skin dose for intraoral periapical and bitewing radiography. The NCRP further recommends an achievable dose of 1.2 mGy for intraoral

radiography. These standards require that most users of D-speed film convert to E/F-speed film or a digital system. Multiple means to minimize unnecessary patient and operator exposure are described next.

PATIENT EXPOSURE

Patient dose from dental radiography is usually reported as effective dose, a measure of the amount of radiation received by various radiosensitive organs during the radiographic examination. Table 3-3 shows typical effective doses from common dental intraoral, extraoral, and medical examinations. The equivalent exposure in terms of days of natural background radiation is shown. Dental exposures are a small fraction of the annual average background exposure.

ESTIMATING RISK

The primary risk from dental radiography is the unlikely chance of radiation-induced cancer. Cancer is a common disease, affecting about 40% of people at some time during their lives and accounting for about 20% of all deaths. There is an extensive body of literature linking relatively large exposures of radiation to cancer formation (both solid tumors and leukemias) in humans and research animals. Human epidemiologic studies include individuals exposed as survivors of the atomic bombings in Hiroshima and Nagasaki, in the course of diagnostic radiology, through multiple fluoroscopies or radiation therapy, occupationally or environmentally. However, there is great uncertainty regarding the risk from low-dose diagnostic procedures. Analysis of this literature has led to the development of the linear nonthreshold (LNT) hypothesis (Fig. 3-3). This hypothesis holds that there is a linear relationship between dose and the risk of inducing a new cancer, even at very low doses. In this hypothesis, there is no threshold or "safe dose" below which there is no added risk.

The LNT is a hypothesis that has been accepted widely for setting policy in radiation safety and protection. It is not a demonstrated scientific fact. There is a solid body of work demonstrating increased risk of tumors in individuals exposed to more than about 100 mGy. However, there are relatively few studies showing a risk in the diagnostic range. In this low-dose range, the LNT has been consistently neither verified nor falsified. A major difficulty in such studies is that at doses less than 100 mGy, epidemiologic studies require such large sample sizes as to be impractical. Thus the validity of the model is uncertain. This situation is not expected to change in the near future.

Despite its uncertainties in the low-dose range, there are several reasons for using the LNT. First, there needs to be a policy to set exposure limits for individuals exposed in the low-dose range, including from diagnostic radiology, in nuclear power plants, on long airline flights, and from other exposures. Second, several lines of evidence indicate that the LNT is scientifically plausible. The dose-response at doses greater than 100 mGy is linear. Complex damage to DNA, the basis of cancer formation, may occur with even one x-ray photon (see Fig. 2-2). Although sophisticated DNA repair mechanisms exist, some types of complex damage to DNA may be beyond the enzymatic repair. Finally, much epidemiologic data are consistent with, and do not exclude, a risk at very low doses. Most radiation protection organizations believe that it is prudent to assume that risk is proportional to dose, even for diagnostic exposures, and that there is no safe threshold. It is fairly common to see in the literature estimates of numbers of fatalities that may be caused by various radiographic examinations. Such estimates are based on the LNT and are highly speculative and at

TABLE 3-3　Effective Dose from Radiographic Examinations and Equivalent Background Exposure

Examination	Effective Dose (µSv)	Equivalent Background Exposure (days)
INTRAORAL[1]		
Rectangular collimation		
Posterior bitewings: PSP or F-speed film	5	0.6
Full-mouth: PSP or F-speed film	35	4
Full-mouth: CCD sensor (estimated)	17	2
Round collimation		
Full-mouth: D-speed film	388	46
Full-mouth: PSP or F-speed film	171	20
Full-mouth: CCD sensor (estimated)	85	10
EXTRAORAL		
Panoramic[1-3]	9–24	1–3
Cephalometric[1,2,4]	2–6	0.3–0.7
Cone-beam CT[5,6]		
Large field of view	68–1073	8–126
Medium field of view	45–860	5–101
Small field of view	19–652	2–77
Multislice CT		
Head: Conventional protocol[6-9]	860–1500	101–177
Head: Low-dose protocol[6,8]	180–534	21–63
Abdomen[7]	5300	624
Chest[7]	5800	682
Plain films[10]		
Skull	70	8
Chest	20	2
Barium enema	7200	847

CCD, Charge-coupled device; *PSP,* photostimulable phosphor.

1. Data from Ludlow JB, Davies-Ludlow LE, White SC: Patient risk related to common dental radiographic examinations: the impact of 2007 international commission on radiological protection recommendations regarding dose calculation, *J Am Dent Assoc* 139:1237-1243, 2008.
2. Data from Lecomber AR, Yoneyama Y, Lovelock DJ et al: Comparison of patient dose from imaging protocols for dental implant planning using conventional radiography and computed tomography, *Dentomaxillofac Radiol* 30:255-259, 2001.
3. Data from Ludlow JB, Davies-Ludlow LE, Brooks SL: Dosimetry of two extraoral direct digital imaging devices: NewTom cone beam CT and Orthophos Plus DS panoramic unit, *Dentomaxillofac Radiol* 32:229-234, 2003.
4. Data from Gijbels F, Sanderink G, Wyatt J et al: Radiation doses of indirect and direct digital cephalometric radiography, *Br Dent J* 197:149-152, 2004.
5. Data from Pauwels R, Beinsberger J, Collaert B et al: Effective dose range for dental cone beam computed tomography scanners, *Eur J Radiol* 81:267-271, 2012.
6. Data from Ludlow JB, Ivanovic M: Comparative dosimetry of dental CBCT devices and 64-slice CT for oral and maxillofacial radiology, *Oral Surg Oral Med Oral Pathol Oral Radiol Endod* 106:106-114, 2008.
7. Data from Shrimpton PC, Hillier MC, Lewis MA et al: National survey of doses from CT in the UK: 2003, *Br J Radiol* 79:968-980, 2006.
8. Data from Loubele M, Jacobs R, Maes F et al: Radiation dose vs. image quality for low-dose CT protocols of the head for maxillofacial surgery and oral implant planning, *Radiat Prot Dosimetry* 117:211-216, 2005.
9. Data from Loubele M, Bogaerts R, Van Dijck E et al: Comparison between effective radiation dose of CBCT and MSCT scanners for dentomaxillofacial applications, *Eur J Radiol* 71:461-468, 2009.
10. Data from European Commission: *Referral guidelines for imaging,* Radiation Protection 118, 2007.
http://www.sergas.es/Docs/Profesional/BoaPraticaClinica/RP118.pdf

best represent the probable upper limits. The actual numbers may be substantially lower or even zero. Although the LNT is the consensus opinion of most radiation safety groups around the world, there is controversy about whether there really is a risk. Some experts argue that there is no demonstrated risk at doses less than 100 mGy, and on balance patients may not reap the full diagnostic benefits by avoiding diagnostic imaging because of inappropriate fear. If the actual risk is significantly less than predicted by the LNT, there is a risk of harm to patients from making too few exposures. It is most reasonable to make radiographs only when there is a diagnostic need and to use all reasonable means to reduce patient exposure during the examination.

REDUCING DENTAL EXPOSURE

There are three guiding principles in radiation protection:
1. Justification
2. Optimization
3. Dose limitation

The principle of justification means the dentist should identify situations where the benefit to a patient from the diagnostic exposure likely exceeds the risk of harm. In practice, this principle influences what patients are selected for radiographic examinations and what examinations are chosen. These matters are considered in Chapter 16.

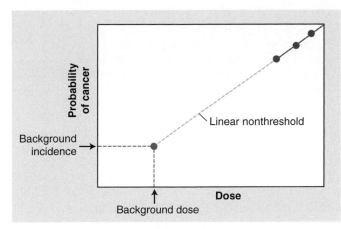

FIGURE 3-3 Linear nonthreshold hypothesis. There is a certain natural prevalence of cancer and a certain natural background radiation exposure *(gray-blue dot)*. Doses of radiation greater than about 100 mSv *(green dots)* result in a dose-dependent increase in the cancer rate. The linear nonthreshold hypothesis posits that at doses less than 100 mSv down to the background level, there is a linear relationship between dose and risk *(orange dashed line)* and that there is no threshold dose below which there is no additional risk.

BOX 3-1   Means for Reducing X-Ray Exposure

Use selection criteria to assist in determining type and frequency of radiographic examinations
Use E/F-speed film or digital sensors
Use holders to support film or digital sensors intraorally
Make exposures with 60 to 70 kVp
Replace short pointed aiming tubes with open-ended aiming cylinders
Use rectangular collimation for periapical and bitewing images
Use thyroid collars
Stand at least 6 feet (2 m) away from patient and away from the x-ray machine (preferably out of x-ray room) when making exposure
With film, use time-temperature film processing rather than "sight" processing, or use an automatic processor
Use rare-earth screens for panoramic and cephalometric film imaging or use digital systems
Reduce cone-beam CT beam field of view to region of interest

The principle of optimization holds that dentists should use every reasonable means to reduce unnecessary exposure to their patients, their staffs, and themselves. This philosophy of radiation protection is often referred to as the principle of ALARA (*A*s *L*ow *A*s *R*easonably *A*chievable). ALARA holds that exposures to ionizing radiation should be kept as low as reasonably achievable, economic and social factors being taken into account. The means to accomplish this end are considered by dentists every day in their practices and are discussed later in this chapter (Box 3-1).

The principle of dose limitation provides dose limits for occupational and public exposures to ensure that no individuals are exposed to unacceptably high doses. This principle applies to dentists and their staff who are exposed occupationally but not to patients because there are no dose limits for individuals exposed for diagnostic purposes. Many of the steps described in the following sections that optimize exposures of the patient also reduce exposure to dentists and their staff.

The dentist in each facility is responsible for the design and conduct of the radiation protection program. In this section, methods of exposure and dose reduction are described that can be used in dental radiography. Each subsection begins with a recommendation of the American Dental Association (ADA) Council on Scientific Affairs. This recommendation is followed by a discussion of ways in which the recommendation can be satisfied. All methods that reduce exposure to patients also reduce exposure to the dental staff and usually improve the quality of the radiographs made.

PATIENT SELECTION CRITERIA

Radiographic screening for the purpose of detecting disease before clinical examination should not be performed. A thorough clinical examination, consideration of the patient history, review of any prior radiographs, caries risk assessment and consideration of both the dental and the general health needs of the patient should precede radiographic examination (ADA 2012)

The most effective means to reduce unnecessary exposure is to reduce unnecessary radiographic examinations. Radiographs should be made only when there is a specific indication for a specific patient. The ADA has published radiographic selection criteria—clinical or historical findings that identify patients for whom a high probability exists that a radiographic examination would provide information affecting their treatment or prognosis. These criteria satisfy the principle of justification and are considered in Chapter 16.

When a decision is made to obtain a radiograph, the dentist should obtain the lowest dose image that would satisfy the task. Table 3-3 shows that there is a wide range of patient exposures from various common dental examinations.

CONDUCTING THE EXAMINATION

When a decision has been made that a radiographic examination is justified (using patient selection criteria), the way in which the examination is conducted, or the principle of optimization, greatly influences patient exposure to radiation. The conduct of the examination may be divided into choice of equipment, choice of technique, operation of equipment, and processing and interpreting the radiographic image.

Film and Digital Imaging

Good radiologic practice includes use of the fastest image receptor compatible with the diagnostic task (F-speed film or digital) (ADA 2012).

Intraoral dental x-ray film is available in two speed groups: D and E/F (see Chapter 5). Clinically, film of speed group E/F is approximately twice as fast (sensitive) as film of group D and thus requires only half the exposure (see Fig. 5-30). Fast films are desirable from the standpoint of exposure reduction. Multiple studies have found that E/F-speed film is preferred because it has the same useful density range, latitude, contrast, and image quality as D-speed films and can be used in routine intraoral radiographic examinations without sacrifice of diagnostic information. Current digital sensors (see Chapter 4) offer equal or greater dose savings than E/F-speed film and comparable diagnostic utility.

Intensifying Screens and Film

Rare-earth intensifying screens are recommended … combined with high-speed film of 400 or greater (ADA 2006).

Contemporary intensifying screens used in extraoral radiography use the rare earth elements gadolinium and lanthanum (see Chapter 5). These rare earth phosphors emit green light on interaction with x rays. Compared with the older calcium tungstate screens, rare earth screens decrease patient exposure by 55% in panoramic and cephalometric radiography.

In contrast to intraoral digital imaging, there is no significant dose reduction to be gained by replacing fast extraoral screen-film systems with digital imaging. Image resolution with digital systems is comparable to that obtained with rare earth screens matched with appropriate film.

Source-to-Skin Distance

Use of long source-to-skin distances of 40 cm, rather than short distances of 20 cm, decreases exposure by 10 to 25 percent. Distances between 20 cm and 40 cm are appropriate, but the longer distances are optimal (ADA 2006).

Two standard focal source-to-skin distances have evolved over the years for use in intraoral radiography, one 20 cm (8 inches) and the other 41 cm (16 inches). Use of the distance results in a reduction in exposed tissue volume because the x-ray beam is less divergent (Fig. 3-4). The use of a longer source-to-object distance also results in a smaller apparent focal spot size increasing the resolution of the radiograph (see Chapter 6).

Rectangular Collimation

Since a rectangular collimator decreases the radiation dose by up to fivefold as compared with a circular one, radiographic equipment should provide rectangular collimation for exposure of periapical and bitewing radiographs (ADA 2012).

Most state regulations require that the x-ray beam used in intraoral radiography be collimated so that the field of radiation at the patient's skin surface is no more than 7 cm (2.75 inches) in diameter. In view of the dimensions of No. 2 intraoral film (3.2 cm × 4.1 cm) or digital sensor, the area of such a field size is almost three times larger than necessary to expose the image. Consequently, limiting the size of the x-ray beam to the size of the image receptor significantly reduces unnecessary patient exposure. If the tissue volume exposed is decreased, the amount of scattered radiation is decreased, image fogging is decreased, and the resultant image has improved diagnostic quality.

There are several means to limit the size of the x-ray beam. First, a rectangular position-indicating device (PID) may be attached to the radiographic tube housing (Fig. 3-5). Use of a rectangular PID having an exit opening of 3.5 cm × 4.4 cm (1.38 inches × 1.34 inches) reduces the area of the patient's skin surface exposed by 60% over that of a round (7 cm) PID (see Fig. 3-4, C). However, this reduction in beam size may make aiming the beam difficult. To avoid the possibility of unsatisfactory radiographs (cone cutting), a film-holding instrument that centers the beam over the film or sensor is recommended (Fig. 3-6). Alternatively, film-positioning and sensor-positioning devices with rectangular collimators may be used with round aiming cylinders (Figs. 3-7 and 3-8). These holders reduce patient exposure to the same degree as rectangular PIDs.

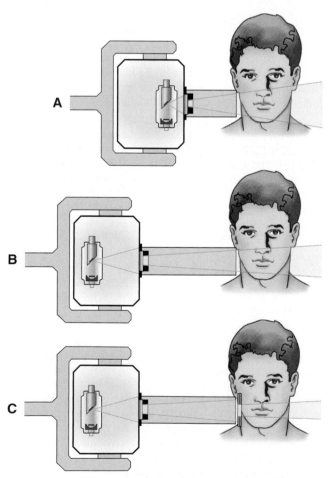

FIGURE 3-4 Effect of source-to-skin distance and collimation on the volume of tissue irradiated. A larger volume of irradiated tissue results with use of a short source-to-skin distance **(A)** compared with use of a longer source-to-skin distance **(B)**, which produces a less divergent beam. Using a rectangular collimator between the round PID and the patient **(C)** results in a smaller, less divergent beam and a smaller volume of tissue irradiated than in **A** or **B**.

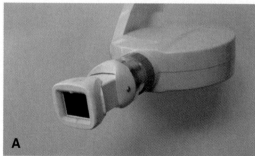

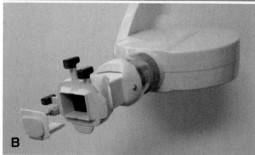

FIGURE 3-5 **A,** A rectangular PID mounted on an x-ray machine provides a means to limit the shape of the x-ray beam to just larger than the film or digital sensor, thus minimizing the volume of tissue exposed. It may rotate to accommodate to the patient. **B,** An external guide attaches to the end of the rectangular PID. The red, blue and yellow connectors on the guide allow the user to attach a bite block with a film or sensor to the external guide using a Rinn XCP-ORA arm to obtain positive alignment to the x-ray machine and thereby prevent cone cuts. (*Courtesy Margraf Dental Manufacturing, Inc., www.margrafdental.com.*)

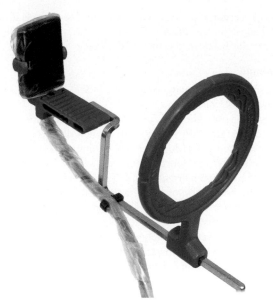

FIGURE 3-6 XCP film-holding instrument. The aiming ring aligns a circular aiming cylinder from an x-ray machine with the sensor to ensure that the image plane is perpendicular to the central ray and in the middle of the beam. Note notches to align rectangularly collimated aiming devices, such as shown in Figures 3-5 or 3-7. The digital sensor and cord is in a plastic bag to prevent contamination from saliva. *(Courtesy Dentsply Rinn: http://rinncorp.com.)*

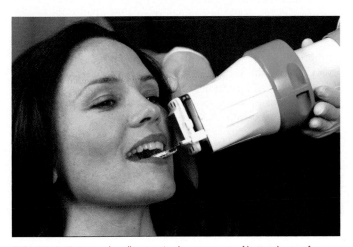

FIGURE 3-7 Rectangular collimation. An alternative means of limiting the size of an x-ray beam to a rectangle is to attach a device shown here into the end of a circular aiming cylinder that restricts the beam field to a rectangle and provides guidance in aligning the film holder. *(Courtesy Interactive Diagnostic Imaging: http://www.idixray.com.)*

Filtration

The x-ray beam emitted from the radiographic tube consists of a spectrum of x-ray photons. Low-energy photons, which have little penetrating power, are absorbed mainly by the patient and contribute nothing to the information on the image. The purpose of filtration is to remove these low-energy x-ray photons preferentially from the x-ray beam. Filtration results in decreased patient exposure with no loss of radiographic information.

When an x-ray beam is filtered with 3 mm of aluminum, the surface exposure is reduced to about 20% of the exposure with no filtration. In light of this and other information, the federal government has designated the specific amount of filtration, expressed as

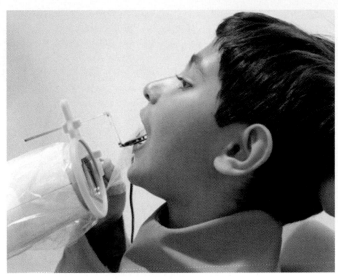

FIGURE 3-8 Rectangular collimation. Another means to collimate a round beam to a rectangle is to place a metallic shield in the path of the beam, limiting the size of the exposure field to an area just larger than the film or sensor. The JADRAD Dental X-Ray Shield is shown. *(Courtesy Dr. Jennifer Diederich, Farmington, CT.)*

minimum half-value layer, required for dental x-ray machines operating at various kilovoltages. Practically, these requirements can be met by having 1.5 mm of aluminum total filtration when operating from 50 to 70 kVp and 2.5 mm of aluminum total filtration when operating above 70 kVp.

Leaded Aprons and Thyroid Collars

The thyroid gland is more susceptible to radiation exposure during dental radiographic exams given its anatomic position, particularly in children. Protective thyroid collars and collimation substantially reduce radiation exposure to the thyroid during dental radiographic procedures. Because every precaution should be taken to minimize radiation exposure, protective thyroid collars should be used whenever possible (ADA 2012).

The function of leaded aprons and thyroid collars (Fig. 3-9) is to reduce radiation exposure of the gonads and thyroid gland. The NCRP 2003 recommendations referred to by the ADA are principally those already described—use of patient selection criteria, fast (E/F-speed film or digital sensors), and rectangular collimators. The NCRP and ADA concluded that leaded aprons are unnecessary because it is far more important in patient protection to place emphasis on reducing exposure of the primary beam to facial structures than to reduce the already very slight gonadal exposure. More recent research has shown that the risk of heritable effects from dental exposure is essentially insignificant (see Chapter 2). However, most states currently require the use of leaded aprons.

In recent years, lead-free aprons have been offered for sale. The virtues of these aprons are their lighter weight and avoiding the use of lead. These aprons include materials with high atomic numbers and low densities, such as antimony, tin, tungsten, or bismuth, to provide beam attenuation. These aprons typically attenuate about 98% as much as conventional aprons but weigh only about 60% as much.

There is reason to be concerned about radiation exposure to the thyroid gland. Multiple studies, including studies performed after the explosion of the Chernobyl reactor, have shown that the

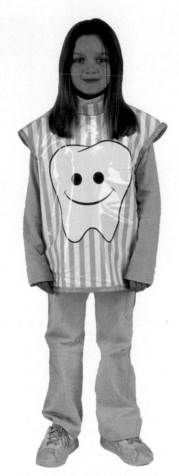

FIGURE 3-9 Leaded apron with a thyroid collar. Children are more sensitive to radiation than adults, and so the use of leaded aprons with thyroid collars is especially important for this population. *(Courtesy Dentsply Rinn: http://rinncorp.com/.)*

thyroid gland in children is especially sensitive to radiation. It is entirely appropriate to protect the thyroid glands of children during radiographic examinations. The best ways to accomplish this aim are to use fast receptors, rectangular collimation, and thyroid collars.

Film and Sensor Holders

Film holders that align the film precisely with the collimated beam are recommended for periapical and bitewing radiographs (ADA 2006).

Film or digital sensor holders should be used when intraoral radiographs are made because they improve the alignment of the film, or digital sensor, with teeth and x-ray machine. Their use results in a significant reduction in unacceptable images and thus avoidable retakes. The use of film and sensor holders allows the operator to control the position and alignment of the film or sensor with respect to the teeth and jaws. This is especially important when digital imaging (see Chapter 4) is used with the paralleling technique (see Chapter 6). In these cases, it is often desirable to position the receptor away from the teeth so as to get the best image and reduce patient discomfort. This requires the use of a film or sensor holder. Most such devices have an external guide that shows the operator where to align the aiming cylinder (PID). As a result, the x-ray beam is properly directed toward the receptors; this greatly reduces the chance of the beam partially missing

the image receptor (a "cone-cut") and reduces image distortion (see Chapter 6). As discussed earlier, many film holders also collimate the beam to the size of the image receptor.

Kilovoltage

The optimal operating potential of dental x-ray units is between 60 and 70 kVp (ADA 2012).

Although image diagnosis may be improved slightly with increased image contrast (low kVp) images, the patient dose is reduced with higher kVp exposures. Most intraoral machines use 60 to 70 kVp. The availability of constant-potential (fully rectified), high-frequency or direct current (DC) dental x-ray units has made possible the production of radiographs with lower kilovoltage and at reduced levels of radiation. The surface exposure required to produce a comparable radiographic density using a constant-potential unit is approximately 25% less than that of a conventional self-rectified unit operating at the same kilovoltage. At the present time, several manufacturers produce DC units.

Milliampere-Seconds

The operator should set the amperage and time settings for exposure of dental radiographs of optimal quality (ADA 2006).

Of the three settings on an x-ray machine (tube voltage, filtration, and exposure time), exposure time is the most crucial factor in influencing diagnostic quality. In terms of exposure, optimal image quality means that the radiograph is of diagnostic density, neither overexposed (too dark) nor underexposed (too light). Both overexposed and underexposed radiographs result in repeat exposures, leading to needless additional patient exposure. Image density is controlled by the quantity of x rays produced, which is best controlled by the combination of milliamperage and exposure time, termed milliampere-seconds (mAs) (see Chapter 1). Typically, a radiograph of correct density demonstrates very faint soft tissue outlines. Dentin has an optical density of about 1.0. If your x-ray machine has a variable milliampere control, it should be set at the highest choice. Proper exposure times should be determined empirically when using optimal film processing conditions (see Chapter 5) or manufacturer's recommendations for digital sensors. A chart showing optimal exposure times for each region of the arch in children and adults should be mounted by each x-ray machine. Because film-processing conditions are standardized and the mA and kVp settings are fixed, the only decision the dentist or the assistant needs to make is to select the proper exposure time for the age of the patient (less for young patients) and the region of the mouth being imaged (less in the anterior region).

Film Processing

All film should be processed following the film and processer manufacturer recommendations. Poor processing technique, including sight-developing, most often results in underdeveloped films, forcing the x-ray operator to increase the dose to compensate, resulting in patient and personnel being exposed to unnecessary radiation (ADA 2012).

A major cause of unnecessary patient exposure is the practice of overexposing films and compensating by underdevelopment. This procedure results in both needless exposure of the patient and in films that are of inferior diagnostic quality because of incomplete development. Time-temperature processing is the best way to ensure optimal film quality (see Chapter 5). To help ensure optimal image quality, the dental assistant should follow the film manufacturer's recommendation for processing solutions.

The use of automatic film processing machines has become widespread with more than 90% of dentists using such processors. They should be used in a darkroom. Although some units have daylight loaders, allowing film to be placed in the machine in room light, such loaders are difficult to keep clean and free of contamination. However, film processors can increase patient exposure if not correctly maintained. Approximately 30% of all films retaken because of incorrect film density are related to processor variability. Using a comprehensive maintenance program can reduce this retake rate significantly, resulting in a substantial savings in both patient exposure and operating costs.

Interpreting the Images

The dentist should view radiographs under appropriate conditions for analysis and diagnosis (ADA 2006).

Radiographs are best viewed in a semidarkened room with light transmitted through the films; all extraneous light should be eliminated. In addition, radiographs should be studied with the aid of a magnifying glass to detect even the smallest change in image density. Similarly, digital images are best interpreted on a computer screen in a darkened environment. It is often useful to magnify them electronically.

PROTECTING PERSONNEL

The methods of dose reduction discussed so far have emphasized the effect on patient exposure. However, any procedure or technique that reduces radiation exposure to the patient also reduces the possibility of operator or office personnel exposure from scattered radiation. In addition to those mentioned, several other steps can be taken to reduce the chance of occupational exposure.

Operators of radiographic equipment should use barrier protection when possible, and barriers should contain a leaded glass window to enable the operator to view the patient during exposure. When shielding is not possible, the operator should stand at least two meters from the tube head and out of the path of the primary beam (ADA 2006).

Dental operatories should be designed and constructed to meet the minimal shielding requirement of the state regulations; this requires consultation with a qualified expert. This recommendation states that walls must be of sufficient density or thickness that the exposure to nonoccupationally exposed individuals (e.g., someone occupying an adjacent office) is no greater than 100 μGy per week. In most instances, it is not necessary to line the walls with lead to meet this requirement. Walls constructed of gypsum wallboard (drywall or sheet rock) are adequate for the average dental office.

Every effort should be made so that the operator can leave the room or take a position behind a suitable barrier or wall during an exposure. A leaded glass window or a mirror would be required so that the operator can monitor the patient during the exposure. If leaving the room or making use of some other barrier is impossible, strict adherence to what has been termed the position-and-distance rule is required: the operator should stand at least 6 feet (2 m) from the patient, at an angle of 90 to 135 degrees to the central ray of the x-ray beam (Fig. 3-10). When applied, this rule not only takes advantage of the inverse square law to reduce x-ray exposure to the operator but also takes advantage of the fact that in this position the patient's head absorbs most scatter radiation. All practitioners should check their state's regulations for use of ionizing radiation regarding operator position during x-ray exposures.

Second, the operator should never hold films or sensors in place. Film or sensor-holding instruments should be used (see earlier section on rectangular collimation). If correct film placement and retention are still not possible, a parent or other individual responsible for the patient should be asked to hold the sensor in place and be afforded adequate protection with a leaded apron. Under no circumstances should this person be one of the office staff.

Third, neither the operator nor the patient should hold the radiographic tube housing during the exposure. Suspension arms should be adequately maintained to prevent housing movement and drift.

The best way to ensure that personnel are following office safety rules such as those described previously is with personnel-monitoring devices. These devices provide a means to measure if the operator is accumulating any occupational exposure. The ADA recommends that workers who may receive an annual dose greater than 1 mSv should wear personal dosimeters to monitor their exposure levels. Pregnant dental personnel operating x-ray equipment should use personal dosimeters, regardless of anticipated exposure levels (ADA 2012). Use of personal dosimeters is not only recommended but also required by law in certain states. Several

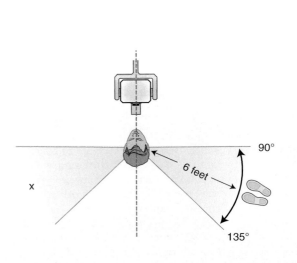

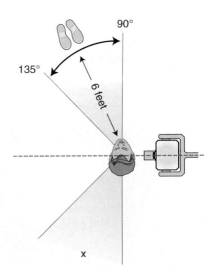

FIGURE 3-10 Position-and-distance rule. The operator may be exposed from leakage radiation from the x-ray tube head, scattered radiation from the patient, and primary photons passing through the patient. If no barrier is available, the operator should stand at least 6 feet from the patient, at an angle of 90 to 135 degrees to the central ray of the x-ray beam when the exposure is made because this region receives the least overall exposure.

companies in the United States offer dosimetry-monitoring services. These services provide badges that contain a radiosensitive crystal (Al_2O_3) that luminesces in proportion to the amount of radiation exposure (Fig. 3-11). These devices are sensitive to 10 μSv. A printed report of accumulated exposure may be obtained at regular intervals (Fig. 3-12). These reports indicate any undesirable change in work habits and help remove any apprehension office staff members may have about the possibility of exposure to x rays.

QUALITY ASSURANCE

Quality assurance protocols for the x-ray machine, imaging receptor, film processing, dark room, and patient shielding should be developed and implemented for each dental health care setting (ADA 2012).

Quality assurance may be defined as a program for periodic assessment of the performance of all parts of the radiologic procedure. It is intended to ensure that a dental office consistently produces high-quality images with minimum exposure to patients and personnel (see Chapter 15). Studies have indicated that dentists may be needlessly exposing their patients to compensate for improper exposure techniques, film processing practices, and darkroom procedures. One study reported that only 33% of panoramic radiographs that accompanied biopsy specimens were of acceptable diagnostic quality. However, when demands were placed on dentists to improve their techniques, the number of unsatisfactory radiographs was significantly reduced. Two studies by a dental insurance carrier demonstrated that after claims were rejected for unsatisfactory radiographs and the dentist was made aware of the errors and ways in which they could be corrected, the number of satisfactory radiographs submitted doubled. This study suggests that when the dentist is presented with guidelines for quality assurance, along with proper motivation, patient exposure can be dramatically reduced. Commercial mail-in devices are available to dentists and radiation protection agencies to measure dental image quality and dose of their radiographs.

Some states require dental offices to establish written guidelines for quality assurance and to maintain written records of quality assurance tests. Regardless of requirements, each dental office should establish maintenance and monitoring procedures as outlined in Chapter 15.

CONTINUING EDUCATION

Practitioners should remain informed about safety updates and the availability of new equipment, supplies and techniques that could farther improve the diagnostic quality of radiographs and decrease radiation exposure (ADA 2006).

Individuals who administer ionizing radiation must become familiar with the magnitude of exposure encountered in medicine, dentistry, and everyday life; the possible risks associated with such

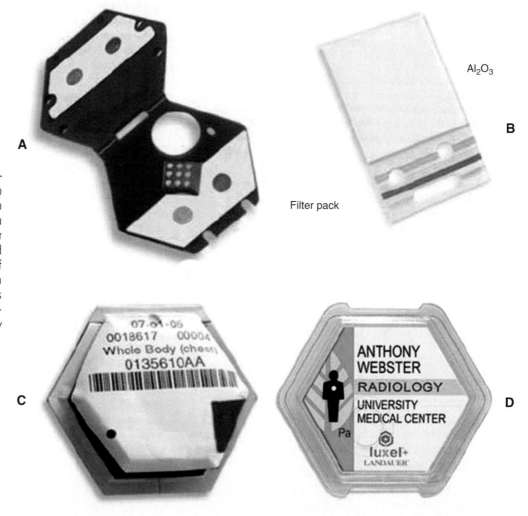

FIGURE 3-11 A personal optically stimulated luminescence dosimeter may contain a strip of Al_2O_3, which is sensitive to radiation. This strip is enclosed in a filter pack containing an open window and plastic, aluminum, and copper filters. These are packaged into a blister pack and worn by an operator. The amount and ratio of light output during the stimulation process from the regions of the Al_2O_3 under the filters allows determination of the energy and dose of radiation to which the badge was exposed. (Courtesy Landauer, Inc., Glenwood, IL.)

Al_2O_3

Filter pack

07-01-05
0018617   00004
Whole Body (chest)
0135610AA

ANTHONY WEBSTER
RADIOLOGY
UNIVERSITY MEDICAL CENTER
luxel+
LANDAUER

LANDAUER®

SAMPLE ORGANIZATION
RADIATION SAFETY OFFICER
2 SCIENCE ROAD
GLENWOOD, IL 60425

Landauer, Inc. 2 Science Road   Glenwood, Illinois 60425-1586
Telephone: (708) 755-7000   Facsimile: (708) 755-7016
www.landauerinc.com

RADIATION DOSIMETRY REPORT

luxel®

ACCOUNT NO.	SERIES CODE	ANALYTICAL WORK ORDER	REPORT DATE	DOSIMETER RECEIVED	REPORT TIME IN WORK DAYS	PAGE NO.
103702	RAD	992150087	06/13/03	06/09/03	4	1

PARTICIPANT NUMBER	NAME (ID NUMBER / BIRTH DATE / SEX)	DOSIMETER	USE	RADIATION QUALITY	DOSE EQUIVALENT (MREM) FOR PERIODS SHOWN BELOW			YEAR TO DATE DOSE EQUIVALENT (MREM)			LIFETIME DOSE EQUIVALENT (MREM)			RECORDS FOR YEAR	INCEPTION DATE (MMYY)
					DEEP DDE	EYE LDE	SHALLOW SDE	DEEP DDE	EYE LDE	SHALLOW SDE	DEEP DDE	EYE LDE	SHALLOW SDE		
FOR MONITORING PERIOD:					05/01/03 - 05/31/03			2003							
0000H	CONTROL	J	CNTRL		M	M	M							5	07/97
	CONTROL	P	CNTRL		M	M	M								07/97
	CONTROL	U	CNTRL				M								07/97
00189	ADAMS, HEATHER 336235619 08/31/1968 F	P	WHBODY		M	M	M	9	10	12	29	31	42	5	07/01
00191	ADDISON, JOHN 471563287 10/04/1968 M	J	WHBODY	PN	90	90	90	100	100	100	200	200	200	5	07/01
				P	60	60	60	70	70	70	170	170	170		
				NF	30	30	30	30	30	30	30	30	30		
00202	HARRIS, KATHY 587582144 06/09/1960 F	P	WHBODY		M	M	M	M	M	M	M	M	M	5	02/02
		U	RFINGR				M			30			30		02/92
00095	MEYER, STEVE 982778955 07/15/1964 M	P	COLLAR	PL	119	119	113							5	08/97
		P	WAIST	P	10	11	11								08/97
			ABDMN		19	119	113	33	185	174	1387	2308	2320		
			NOTE		ASSIGNED DOSE BASED ON EDE 1 CALCULATION										
		U	RFINGR				140			690			2180		08/97
00203	STEVENS, LEE 335478977 08/25/1951 M	P	WHBODY		ABSENT			M	M	M	M	M	M	4	07/02
		U	RFINGR		ABSENT					M			M		07/02
00204	WALKER, JANE 416995421 03/21/1947 F	P	WHBODY		3	3	3	12	11	11	22	21	21	5	11/02
00188	WEBSTER, ROBERT 355381469 05/15/1972 M	P	WHBODY		40	40	40	200	200	200	240	240	240	5	07/01
			NOTE		CALCULATED										

M: MINIMAL REPORTING SERVICE OF 1 MREM
ELECTRONIC MEDIA TO FOLLOW THIS REPORT

QUALITY CONTROL RELEASE: LMR

1 - PR   6774 - PT131 - N1   -21587

NVLAP®
NVLAP LAB CODE 100518-0**

FIGURE 3-12 Sample radiation dosimetry report showing exposure received by various individuals during the month reported as well as type of dosimeter, its location, and the dose distribution. The report also shows totals for the year to date and lifetime exposure. *(Courtesy Landauer, Inc., Glenwood, IL.)*

exposure; and the methods used to affect exposure and dose reduction. Although this chapter presents some of this information, acquiring knowledge and developing and maintaining skills is a lifelong process.

TALKING WITH YOUR PATIENT

Although most patients readily accept dental radiographs as part of their diagnosis, some have anxiety about radiation exposure for themselves or members of their families–usually their children. It is important to speak clearly and confidently with your patients if they bring up these concerns. The first step is to allow the patient to express his or her thoughts fully. Do not interrupt the patient's comments or belittle the patient's concerns. With all the discussion of radiation risks in the general media, it is completely reasonable that an individual may be concerned. After hearing your patient's remarks, you should first acknowledge them and show that you understand their apprehension. Next, you should tell the patient why you need radiographs as part of the patient's personal diagnosis–such as the detection of interproximal caries, the extent of bone loss from periodontal disease suggested by probing, periapical infections suggested by pain, or whatever radiologic investigation that is specific to the patient's condition. You should also describe the many measures you take to reduce patient exposure, such as using fast film or digital sensors, rectangular collimation, and thyroid collars. Finally, it may be helpful to point out that with these protective steps the exposure is small in terms of natural background radiation. With these assurances, including that you

will make only the exposures you specifically need for the patient's benefit, most patients will appreciate your attention to their concerns and accept radiographs.

In addition, assure new patients that you will contact their previous dentist to obtain previous radiographs that may assist you in their diagnosis. The approach described in the preceding paragraph is also appropriate for patients who are pregnant if you believe there may be a need for immediate treatment. Patients who have had radiation therapy for head and neck cancers should be told about the risk of caries and other problems that make it all the more important that they have regular follow-up examinations.

BIBLIOGRAPHY

American Dental Association Council on Scientific Affairs: The use of dental radiographs: update and recommendations, *J Am Dent Assoc* 137:1304–1312, 2006.

American Dental Association Council on Scientific Affairs: Dental radiographic examinations: recommendations for patient selection and limiting radiation exposure. Revised 2012: http://www.ada.org/sections/professionalResources/pdfs/Dental_Radiographic_Examinations_2012.pdf.

Code of Federal Regulations 21, Subchapter J: *Radiological health, part 1000*, Washington, DC, 1994, Office of the Federal Register, General Services Administration.

Committee to Assess Health Risks from Exposure to Low Levels of Ionizing Radiations: *Health risks from exposure to low levels of ionizing radiation: BEIR VII*, Washington, DC, 2006, National Academy Press.

Dental radiographs: Benefits and safety, *J Am Dent Assoc* 142:1101, 2011.

Environmental Protection Agency: Calculate your radiation dose: http://www.epa.gov/radiation/understand/calculate.html.

Hall EJ, Giaccia AJ: *Radiobiology for the radiologist*, ed 6, Baltimore, 2006, Lippincott Williams & Wilkins.

Horner K, Rushton VE, Walker A, et al: European guidelines on radiation protection in dental radiology: the safe use of radiographs in dental practice, *Radiat Protect* 136:1–115, 2004.

National Council on Radiation Protection and Measurements: *Control of radon in houses*, NCRP Report 103, Bethesda, MD, 1989, National Council on Radiation Protection and Measurements.

National Council on Radiation Protection and Measurements: *Quality assurance for diagnostic imaging*, NCRP Report 99, Bethesda, MD, 1990, National Council on Radiation Protection and Measurements.

National Council on Radiation Protection and Measurements: *Limitation of exposure to ionizing radiation*, NCRP Report 116, Bethesda, MD, 1993, National Council on Radiation Protection and Measurements.

National Council on Radiation Protection and Measurements: *Dental x-ray protection*, NCRP Report 145, Bethesda, MD, 2003, National Council on Radiation Protection and Measurements.

National Council on Radiation Protection and Measurements: *Ionizing radiation exposure of the population of the United States*, NCRP Report 160, Bethesda, MD, 2009, National Council on Radiation Protection and Measurements.

National Council on Radiation Protection and Measurements: *Reference levels and achievable doses in medical and dental imaging: recommendations for the United States*, NCRP Report 172, Bethesda, MD, 2012, National Council on Radiation Protection and Measurements.

Nationwide Evaluation of X-Ray Trends (NEXT): tabulation and graphical summary of the 1999 dental radiography survey, CRCPD Publication E-03-6, Bethesda, MD, 2003, Center for Devices and Radiological Health, U.S. Food and Drug Administration.

Preston RJ: Radiation biology: concepts for radiation protection, *Health Phys* 88:545–556, 2005.

SEDENTEXCT: Guidelines on CBCT for dental and maxillofacial radiology: http://www.sedentexct.eu/.

Sources and effects of ionizing radiation, UNSCEAR 2008 report: volumes I and II, New York, 2008, UNSCEAR (United Nations Publications vol I released in 2010 and vol II released in 2011). https://unp.un.org/details.aspx?pid=20417 and https://unp.un.org/Details.aspx?pid=21556.

The 2007 recommendations of the International Commission on Radiological Protection. IRCP Publication 103, *Ann ICRP* 37:1–332, 2007.

Wall BF, Kendall GM, Edwards AA, et al: What are the risks from medical x-rays and other low dose radiation? *Br J Radiol* 79:285–294, 2006.

CHAPTER

4

Digital Imaging

John B. Ludlow and André Mol

OUTLINE

The advent of digital imaging has revolutionized radiology. This revolution is the result of both technologic innovation in image acquisition processes and the development of networked computing systems for image retrieval and transmission. Dentistry is seeing a steady increase in the use of these technologies, improvement of software interfaces, and introduction of new products. Numerous forces are driving the shift from film to digital systems. The detrimental effects of inadequate film processing on diagnostic quality and the difficulty of maintaining high-quality chemical processing are well documented. Digital imaging eliminates chemical processing. Hazardous wastes in the form of processing chemicals and lead foil are eliminated with digital systems. Images can be electronically transferred to other health care providers without any alteration of the original image quality. In addition, digital intraoral receptors require less radiation than film, thus reducing patient exposure. Finally, digital imaging allows enhancements, measurements, and corrections not available with film.

Digital systems also have many disadvantages compared with film. The initial expense of setting up a digital imaging system is relatively high. Certain components, such as the electronic x-ray receptor used in some intraoral systems, are susceptible to rough handling and are costly to replace. Because digital systems use evolving technologies, there is a risk—perhaps even a likelihood—of systems becoming obsolete or manufacturers going out of business. The excellent image quality and comparatively low cost of a properly exposed and processed film keeps film-based radiography competitive with digital alternatives.

The trends are certain, however; computers play a role in most dental practices, and that role is expanding as various functions, including appointment scheduling, procedure billing, and patient charting, are integrated into seamless practice management software solutions. It is no longer a matter of *if* but rather *when* most dental practices will use digital imaging. Already during this time of transition, film-based practices are confronted with digital images from practices that have implemented digital radiography. This chapter describes the characteristics of digital images, image receptors, display options, and storage devices and discusses digital image processing.

ANALOG VERSUS DIGITAL

The term digital in digital imaging refers to the numeric format of the image content and its discreteness. Conventional film images can be considered an analog medium, in which differences in the size and distribution of black metallic silver result in a continuous density spectrum. Digital images are numeric and discrete in two ways: (1) in terms of the spatial distribution of the picture elements (pixels) and (2) in terms of the different shades of gray of each of the pixels. A digital image consists of a large collection of individual pixels organized in a matrix of rows and columns (Fig. 4-1). Each pixel has a row and column coordinate that uniquely identifies its location in the matrix. The formation of a digital image requires several steps, beginning with analog processes. At each pixel of an electronic detector, the absorption of x rays generates a small voltage. More x rays generate a higher voltage and vice versa. At each pixel, the voltage can fluctuate between a minimum and maximum value and is therefore an analog signal (Fig. 4-2, *A*).

Production of a digital image requires a process called analog-to-digital conversion (ADC). ADC consists of two steps: (1) sampling and (2) quantization. Sampling means that a small range of voltage values are grouped together as a single value (Fig. 4-2, *B*). Narrow sampling better mimics the original signal but leads to

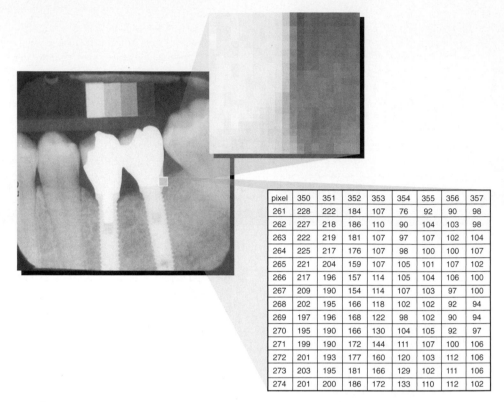

FIGURE 4-1 A digital image is made up of a large number of discrete picture elements (pixels). The size of the pixels is so small that the image appears smooth at normal magnification. The location of each pixel is uniquely identified by a row and column coordinate within the image matrix. The value assigned to a pixel represents the intensity (gray level) of the image at that location.

pixel	350	351	352	353	354	355	356	357
261	228	222	184	107	76	92	90	98
262	227	218	186	110	90	104	103	98
263	222	219	181	107	97	107	102	104
264	225	217	176	107	98	100	100	107
265	221	204	159	107	105	101	107	102
266	217	196	157	114	105	104	106	100
267	209	190	154	114	107	103	97	100
268	202	195	166	118	102	102	92	94
269	197	196	168	122	98	102	90	94
270	195	190	166	130	104	105	92	97
271	199	190	172	144	111	107	100	106
272	201	193	177	160	120	103	112	106
273	203	195	181	166	129	102	111	106
274	201	200	186	172	133	110	112	102

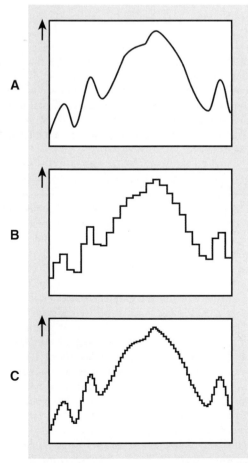

FIGURE 4-2 **A,** Illustration of an analog voltage signal generated by a detector. **B,** Sampling of the analog signal discards part of the signal. **C,** Sampling at a higher frequency preserves more of the original signal.

larger memory requirements for the resulting digital image (Fig. 4-2, *C*). Once sampled, the signal is quantized, which means that every sampled signal is assigned a value. These values are stored in the computer and represent the image. For the clinician to see the image, the computer organizes the pixels in their proper locations and displays a shade of gray that corresponds to the number that was assigned during the quantization step.

To understand the strengths and weaknesses of digital radiography, the clinician establishes which elements of the radiographic imaging chain stay the same and which ones change. The imaging chain can be conceptualized as a series of interconnecting links beginning with the generation of x rays. Exposure factors, patient factors, and the projection geometry determine how the x-ray beam is attenuated. A portion of the unattenuated x-ray beam is captured by the image receptor to form a latent image. This latent image is processed and converted into a real image, which is viewed and interpreted by the clinician. The use of digital detectors changes the way we acquire, store, retrieve, and display images. However, besides an adjustment of the exposure time, digital detectors do not fundamentally change the way in which x rays are selectively attenuated by the tissues of the patient. The physics of the interaction of x rays with matter and the effects of the projection geometry on the appearance of the radiographic image are unaltered and remain critically important for understanding image content and for optimizing image quality.

DIGITAL IMAGE RECEPTORS

Digital image receptors encompass numerous different technologies and come in many different sizes and shapes. Numerous different and sometimes confusing names are in use to identify these receptors in medicine and dentistry. The most useful distinction is that between two main technologies: (1) solid-state technology and (2) photostimulable phosphor (PSP) technology. Although solid-state detectors can be subdivided further, these detectors have in common certain physical properties and the ability to generate a digital image in the computer without any other external device. In medicine, the use of solid-state detectors is referred to as digital radiography. In dentistry, intraoral solid-state detectors are often called sensors. The other main technology, PSP, consists of a phosphor-coated plate in which a latent image is formed after x-ray exposure. The latent image is converted to a digital image by a scanning device through stimulation by laser light. This technology is sometimes referred to as storage phosphor on the basis of the notion that the image information is temporarily stored within the phosphor. Other times the term image plates is used to differentiate them from film and solid-state detectors. The use of PSP plates in medical radiology is referred to as computed radiography.

SOLID-STATE DETECTORS

Solid-state detectors collect the charge generated by x rays in a solid semiconducting material (Fig. 4-3). The key clinical feature of these detectors is the rapid availability of the image after

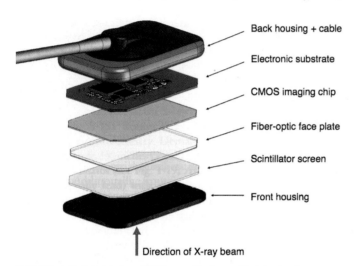

FIGURE 4-3 Exploded view of CMOS sensor. The front and back housings form a water-tight and light-tight barrier to protect the sensor components. The scintillator screen fluoresces when exposed to x-rays and forms a visible light radiographic image. The fiberoptic face plate couples the scintillator screen to the CMOS chip to reduce image noise. The CMOS imaging chip captures the light from the scintillator and creates a charge in each pixel proportional to the exposure. The sensor electronics read the charge in each pixel and transmits it to a computer. (Courtesy XDR Radiology.)

exposure. The matrix and its associated readout and amplifying electronics of intraoral detectors are enclosed within a plastic housing to protect them from the oral environment. These elements of the detector consume part of the real estate of the sensor so that the active area of the sensor is smaller than its total surface area. Sensor bulk, although reduced by continued miniaturization of the electronic components, is a potential drawback of intraoral solid-state detectors. In addition, most detectors incorporate an electronic cable to transfer data to the computer. The presence of a cable can make positioning of the sensor more challenging and requires some adaptation. It also results in increased vulnerability of the device. Manufacturers have addressed these issues in various ways. Some manufacturers have changed the location of the cable attachment to the corner of the sensor. Others offer sensors with magnetic connectors, induction connectors, or reinforced cables to reduce accidental damage to the device. Wireless radiofrequency transmission also has been introduced to eliminate the cable altogether. Wireless radiofrequency transmission frees the detector from a direct tether to the computer, but it necessitates some additional electronic components, thus increasing the overall bulk of the sensor.

Many manufacturers produce detectors with varying active sensor areas roughly corresponding to the different sizes of intraoral film. Detectors without flaws are relatively expensive to produce, and the expense of the detector increases with increasing matrix size (total number of pixels). Pixel size ranges from less than 20 to 70 micrometers (μm). Three types of solid-state sensors are in common use.

Charge-Coupled Device

The charge-coupled device (CCD), introduced to dentistry in 1987, was the first digital image receptor to be adapted for intraoral imaging. The CCD uses a thin wafer of silicon as the basis for image recording. The silicon crystals are formed in a pixel matrix (Fig. 4-4). When exposed to radiation, the covalent bonds between silicon atoms are broken, producing electron-hole pairs (Fig. 4-5). The number of electron-hole pairs that are formed is proportional to the amount of exposure that an area receives. The electrons are attracted toward the most positive potential in the device, where they create "charge packets." Each packet corresponds to one pixel. The charge pattern formed from the individual pixels in the matrix represents the latent image (Fig. 4-6). The image is read by transferring each row of pixel charges from one pixel to the next in a "bucket brigade" fashion. As a charge reaches the end of its row,

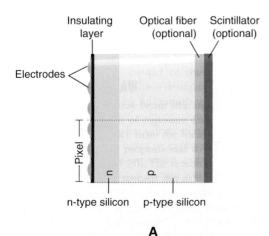

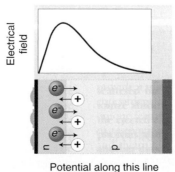

FIGURE 4-4 **A,** Basic structure of a CCD. The electrodes are insulated from an n-p silicon sandwich. The surface of the silicon typically incorporates a scintillating material to improve x-ray capture efficiency and fiberoptics to improve resolution. One pixel uses three electrodes. **B,** Excess electrons from the n-type layer diffuse into the p-type layer, whereas excess holes in the p-type layer diffuse into the n-type layer. The resulting charge imbalance creates an electric field in the silicon with a maximum just inside the n-type layer.

A

B

it is transferred to a readout amplifier and transmitted as a voltage to the analog-to-digital converter located within or connected to the computer. Voltages from each pixel are sampled and assigned a numeric value representing a gray level (ADC). Because CCD detectors are more sensitive to light than to x rays, most manufacturers use a layer of scintillating material coated directly on the CCD surface or coupled to the surface by fiberoptics. This scintillating material increases the x-ray absorption efficiency of the detector. Gadolinium oxybromide compounds similar to those used in rare earth radiographic screens or cesium iodide are examples of scintillators that have been used for this purpose.

CCDs have also been made in linear arrays of a few pixels wide and many pixels long for panoramic and cephalometric imaging. In the case of panoramic units, the CCD is fixed in position opposite to the x-ray source with the long axis of the array oriented parallel to the fan-shaped x-ray beam. Some manufacturers provide CCD sensors that may be retrofitted to older panoramic units. In contrast to film imaging, the mechanics for cephalometric imaging are different. Construction of a single CCD of a size that could simultaneously capture the area of a full skull would be prohibitively expensive. Combining a linear CCD array and a slit-shaped x-ray beam with a scanning motion permits scanning of the skull over several seconds. One disadvantage of this approach is the increased possibility of patient movement artifacts during the several seconds required to complete a scan.

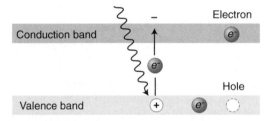

Photoelectric absorption in silicon

Electron

Conduction band

e⁻

Hole

Valence band

FIGURE 4-5 X-ray or light photons impart energy to electrons in the valence band, releasing them into the conduction band. This generates an "electron-hole" charge pair.

Complementary Metal Oxide Semiconductors

Complementary metal oxide semiconductor (CMOS) technology is the basis for typical consumer-grade digital cameras. These detectors are also silicon-based semiconductors but are fundamentally different from CCDs in the way that pixel charges are read. Each pixel is isolated from its neighboring pixels and is directly connected to a transistor. Similar to the CCD, electron-hole pairs are generated within the pixel in proportion to the amount of x-ray energy that is absorbed. This charge is transferred to the transistor as a small voltage. The voltage in each transistor can be addressed separately, read by a frame grabber, and stored and displayed as a digital gray value. CMOS technology is widely used in the construction of computer central processing unit chips and digital camera detectors, and the technology is less expensive than that used in the manufacturing of CCDs. Several manufacturers are using this technology for intraoral imaging applications (Fig. 4-7).

Flat Panel Detectors

Flat panel detectors are used for medical imaging but have also been used in several extraoral imaging devices. The detectors can provide relatively large matrix areas with pixel sizes less than 100 μm; this allows direct digital imaging of larger areas of the body, including the head. Two approaches have been taken in selecting x-ray–sensitive materials for flat panel detectors. Indirect detectors are sensitive to visible light, and an intensifying screen (gadolinium oxysulfide or cesium iodide) is used to convert x-ray energy into light. The performance of these devices is determined by the thickness of the intensifying screen. Thicker screens are more efficient but allow greater diffusion of light photons, leading to image unsharpness. Direct detectors use a photoconductor material (selenium) with properties similar to silicon and a higher atomic number, which permits more efficient absorption of x rays. Under the influence of an applied electrical field, the electrons that are freed during x-ray exposure of the selenium are conducted in a direct line to an underlying thin film transistor (TFT) detector element. Direct detectors using selenium ($Z = 34$) provide higher resolution but lower efficiency compared with indirect detectors

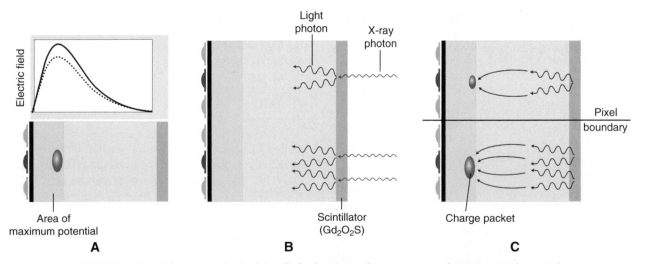

Light photon

X-ray photon

Electric field

Pixel boundary

Area of maximum potential

Scintillator (Gd₂O₂S)

Charge packet

A   **B**   **C**

FIGURE 4-6 **A,** Before exposure, the central electrode of each pixel is turned on, creating an area of maximum potential or potential well. **B,** X-ray photons are absorbed in the scintillating material and are converted to light photons. Light photons are absorbed in the silicon through photoelectric absorption. **C,** Electrons released from the valence band collect selectively near the n-p layer interface in the area of maximum potential to form a charge packet. During CCD readout, the electrical potential of the pixel electrodes is sequentially modulated to shift the charge packet from pixel to pixel.

using intensifying screens with gadolinium ($Z = 64$) or cesium ($Z = 55$). The electrical energy generated is proportional to the x-ray exposure and is stored at each pixel in a capacitor. The energy is released and read out by applying appropriate row and column voltages to a particular pixel's transistor. Flat panel detectors are expensive and likely to be limited to specialized imaging tasks, such as cone-beam computed tomography (CT).

PHOTOSTIMULABLE PHOSPHOR

PSP plates absorb and store energy from x rays and release this energy as light (phosphorescence) when stimulated by another light of an appropriate wavelength. To the extent that the stimulating light and phosphorescent light wavelengths differ, the two may be distinguished, and the phosphorescence can be quantified as a measure of the amount of x-ray energy that the material has absorbed.

The PSP material used for radiographic imaging is "europium-doped" barium fluorohalide. Barium in combination with iodine, chlorine, or bromine forms a crystal lattice. The addition of europium (Eu^{+2}) creates imperfections in this lattice. When exposed to a sufficiently energetic source of radiation, valence electrons in europium can absorb energy and move into the conduction band. These electrons migrate to nearby halogen vacancies (F-centers) in the fluorohalide lattice and may become trapped there in a metastable state. While in this state, the number of trapped electrons

is proportional to x-ray exposure and represents a latent image. When stimulated by red light of around 600 nm, the barium fluorohalide releases trapped electrons to the conduction band. When an electron returns to the Eu^{+3} ion, energy is released in the green spectrum between 300 and 500 nm (Fig. 4-8). Fiberoptics conduct light from the PSP plate to a photomultiplier tube. The photomultiplier tube converts light into electrical energy. A red filter at the photomultiplier tube selectively removes the stimulating laser light, and the remaining green light is detected and converted to a varying voltage. The variations in voltage output from the photomultiplier tube correspond to variations in stimulated light intensity from the latent image. The voltage signal is quantified by an analog-to-digital converter and stored and displayed as a digital image. In practice, the barium fluorohalide material is combined with a polymer and spread in a thin layer on a base material to create a PSP. For intraoral radiography, a polyester base similar to radiographic film is used.

When they are manufactured in standard intraoral sizes, these plates provide handling characteristics similar to intraoral film. PSP plates are also made in sizes commonly used for panoramic and cephalometric imaging. Some PSP processors accommodate a full range of intraoral and extraoral plate sizes. Other processors are limited to intraoral or extraoral formats.

Before exposure, PSP plates must be erased to eliminate residual images from prior exposures. This erasure is accomplished by

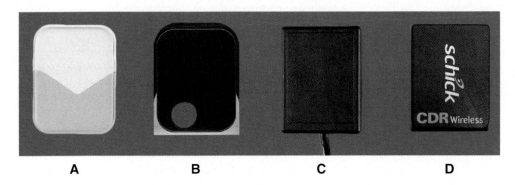

FIGURE 4-7 **A,** Kodak (Courtesy Carestream Health, Inc., exclusive manufacturer of Kodak dental systems.) No. 2 film. **B,** Soredex (Milwaukee, WI) OpTime No. 2 PSP plate (outlined in red) placed on a barrier envelope to demonstrate packaged size. **C,** Gendex (Hatfield, PA) No. 2 CCD sensor. **D,** Schick (Sirona Dental Inc., Charlotte, NC) No. 2 CMOS wireless sensor.

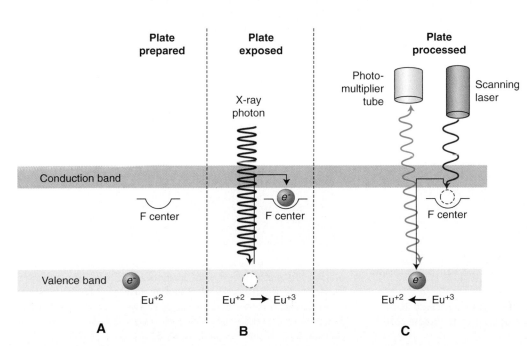

FIGURE 4-8 PSP image formation. **A,** Initially, the PSP plate is flooded with white light to return all electrons to the valence band. **B,** Exposure to x rays imparts energy to europium valence electrons, moving them into the conduction band. Some electrons become trapped at "F centers." **C,** A red scanning laser imparts energy to electrons at the F centers, promoting them to the conduction band from which many return to the valence band. With the electron's return to the valence band, energy is released in the form of light photons in the green spectrum. This light is detected by a photomultiplier tube or diode with a red filter to screen out the scanning laser light.

flooding the plate with a bright light; this is done by placing plates on a dental viewbox with the phosphor side of the plates facing the light for 1 or 2 minutes. More intense light sources can be used for shorter periods of time. Inadequate plate erasure results in double images and usually renders the image undiagnostic. Some PSP systems integrate automatic plate-erasing lights. Erased plates are placed in light-tight containers before exposure. In the case of intraoral plates, sealable polyvinyl envelopes that are impervious to oral fluids and light are used for packaging. For large-format plates, conventional cassettes without intensifying screens are used. After exposure, plates should be processed as soon as possible because trapped electrons spontaneously release over time. The rate of loss of electrons is greatest shortly after exposure. The rate varies depending on the composition of the storage phosphor and the environmental temperature. Some phosphors lose 23% of their trapped electrons after 30 minutes and 30% after 1 hour. Because loss of trapped electrons is uniform across the plate surface, early loss of charge does not typically result in clinically meaningful image deterioration. However, underexposed images may have noticeable image degradation. Adequately exposed images may be stored for 12 to 24 hours and retain acceptable image quality. A more important source of latent image fading is exposure to ambient light during plate preparation for processing. A semidark environment is recommended for plate handling. The more intense the background light and the longer the exposure of the plate to this light, the greater the loss of trapped electrons and the more degraded the resultant image. Red safelights found in most darkrooms are not safe for exposed PSP plates, which are most sensitive to the red light spectrum.

Stationary Plate Scans

Numerous approaches have been adopted for "reading" the latent images on PSP plates. Soredex (Milwaukee, WI) in its Digora and OpTime systems and Air Techniques (Melville, NY) in its ScanX system use a rapidly rotating multifaceted mirror that reflects a beam of red laser light. As the mirror revolves, the laser light sweeps across the plate. The plate is advanced, and the adjacent line of phosphor is scanned. The direction of the laser scanning the plate is termed the fast scan direction. The direction of plate advancement is termed the slow scan direction.

These scanners as well as the Carestream (Atlanta, GA) CS 7600 scanner also include automatic plate clearance after scanning. This plate clearance improves work flow and reduces potential plate damage from manual erasing. The mechanism used for plate intake in the Soredex OpTime scanner requires a metal disk on the back of the plate. This disk also serves as a marker to indicate when a plate was exposed backward.

Rotating Plate Scans

An alternative approach to plate reading used by Gendex (Hatfield, PA) in the DenOptix system and by Carestream in the CR 7400 system involves a rapidly rotating drum that can hold multiple plates. The rotation of the drum past a fixed laser provides a rapid scan. Incremental movement of the laser in the slow scan direction allows image data to be acquired line by line.

DIGITAL DETECTOR CHARACTERISTICS

CONTRAST RESOLUTION

Contrast resolution is the ability to distinguish different densities in the radiographic image; this is a function of the interaction of the following:

- Attenuation characteristics of the tissues imaged
- Capacity of the imaging system to distinguish differences in numbers of x-ray photons and translate them into gray values
- Ability of the computer display to portray differences between gray levels
- Ability of the observer to recognize those differences

Current digital detectors capture data at 8, 10, 12, or 16 bits. The bit depth is a power of 2 (Fig. 4-9). This means that the detector can theoretically capture 256 (2^8) to 65,536 (2^{16}) different attenuation levels. In practice, the actual number of meaningful attenuation levels that can be captured is limited by inaccuracies in image acquisition—that is, noise. Regardless of the number of attenuation differences that a detector can capture, conventional computer monitors are capable of displaying a gray scale of only 8 bits. Because operating systems such as Windows reserve many gray levels for the display of system information, the actual number of gray levels that can be displayed on a monitor is 242. A more important limiting factor is the human visual system, which is capable of distinguishing only about 60 gray levels at any time under ideal viewing conditions. Considering the typical viewing environment in the dental operatory, the actual number of gray levels that can be distinguished decreases to less than 30. Human visual limitations are also present for film viewing; however, the luminance (brightness) of a typical radiograph viewbox is much greater than that of a typical computer display. Therefore the ambient lighting of the room in which the image is viewed theoretically has a lower impact on film than on digital displays.

SPATIAL RESOLUTION

Spatial resolution is the capacity for distinguishing fine detail in an image. Resolution is often measured and reported in units of line pairs per millimeter. Test objects consisting of sets of very fine radiopaque lines separated from each other by spaces equal to the width of a line are constructed with a variety of line widths (Fig. 4-10). A line and its associated space are called a line pair (lp). At least two columns of pixels are required to resolve a line pair, one for the dark line and one for the light space. Typical observers are able to distinguish about 6 lp/mm without benefit of magnification. Intraoral film is capable of providing more than 20 lp/mm of resolution. Unless a film image is magnified, the observer is unable to appreciate the extent of the detail in the image.

With solid-state digital imaging systems, the theoretic resolution limit is determined by pixel size: the smaller the size of the

FIGURE 4-9 Contrast resolution. Examples of gray-scale ramps representing distinct gray levels from black to white. Bit depth controls the number of possible gray levels in the image. The actual number of distinct gray levels that are displayed depends on the output device and image processing. The perceived number of gray levels is influenced by viewing conditions and the visual acuity of the observer. **A,** 6 bits/pixel—64 gray levels. **B,** 5 bits/pixel—32 gray levels. **C,** 4 bits/pixel—16 gray levels. **D,** 3 bits/pixel—8 gray levels.

pixel, the higher the maximally attainable resolution. A sensor with 20-μm pixels can obtain a maximum theoretical resolution of 25 lp/mm: one line pair requires two pixels, in this case 2 × 20 μm, which equals 40 μm. Thus, the maximum resolution would be one line pair per 40 μm, which is equal to 25 lp/mm (Box 4-1). Alternatively, resolution can be expressed in dots per inch (DPI) or points per inch (PPI). At best, there is one dot or point per pixel. Thus, if the pixel size is 20 μm, there is one dot or point per 20 μm. This is equal to 1270 DPI or PPI because there are 25,400 μm in 1 inch (25,400/20 = 1270). However, in practice, actual detector resolution is lower than these theoretical limits for a variety of reasons, including: (1) electronic noise; (2) diffusion of photons in the scintillator coating; and (3) potentially imperfect optical coupling between the scintillator, the fiberoptic screen (when present), and the photodetector. At the present time, the highest resolution intraoral solid-state detector for dentistry has a measured resolution of approximately 20 lp/mm; however, this does not mean that this level of resolution is obtained clinically. Clinical spatial resolution not only depends on detector characteristics, but also is determined by the size of the focal spot, the source-to-object distance, and the object-to-image distance (see Chapter 6).

Resolution in PSP systems is influenced by the thickness of the phosphor material. Thicker phosphor layers cause more diffusion and yield a lower resolution. A thicker layer enhances x-ray absorption efficiency, resulting in a faster image receptor. Resolution is also inversely proportional to the diameter of the laser beam. Effective beam diameter is increased by vibration in the rotating mirror and drum scanner designs. Slow scan motion influences resolution by the increment of plate advancement. This increment may be adjusted to increase or reduce resolution in some systems. Current PSP systems are capable of providing more than 7 lp/mm of resolution.

Software displays of all digital images permit magnification of images. A periapical image filling the display of a computer monitor may be magnified by a factor of 10 times or more. At this level of magnification, the image takes on a building block pattern or pixelated appearance, and the limits of resolution of the imaging system are evident.

DETECTOR LATITUDE

The ability of an image receptor to capture a range of x-ray exposures is termed latitude. A desirable quality in intraoral image receptors is the ability to record a broad range of tissue attenuation differences—from gingiva to enamel. At the same time, subtle differences in attenuation within these tissues should be visually apparent. The useful range of densities in film radiography is two orders of magnitude, from 0.5 to 2.5. The dynamic range of film actually extends for more than four orders of magnitude, but densities of 3 and 4, which transmit only $\frac{1}{1000}$ to $\frac{1}{10,000}$ of the incident light, require intensified illumination or hot lighting to be distinguished from a density of 2.5. Such devices are not commonly used in general practice. The latitude of CCD and CMOS detectors is similar to the latitude of film and can be extended with digital enhancement of contrast and brightness. PSP receptors enjoy larger latitudes and have a linear response to five orders of magnitude of x-ray exposure (Fig. 4-11).

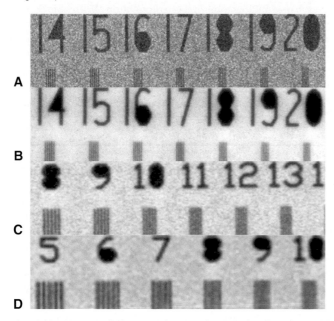

FIGURE 4-10 Images of a line-pair resolution test phantom made with various receptors. **A,** Kodak (Atlanta, GA) InSight film. **B,** Trophy RVGui (Kodak) high-resolution CCD. **C,** Gendex (Hatfield, PA) DenOptix PSP scanned at 600 DPI. **D,** Gendex DenOptix PSP scanned at 300 DPI.

BOX 4-1 Conversion between Pixel Size and Theoretical Limit of Resolution

Pixel Size (μm)	Theoretical Limit of Resolution	
	Line pairs per millimeter (lp/mm)	Dots or Points per inch (DPI or PPI)
20	25	1270
50	10	508
A	1000/(A × 2)	25,400/A
1000/(B × 2)	B	B × 2 × 25.4
25,400/C	C/(2 × 25.4)	C

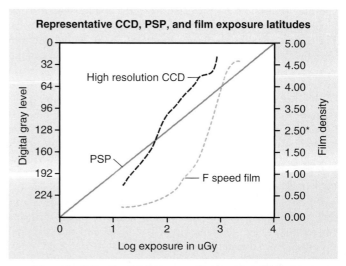

*An optical density of 2.5 is generally considered the upper limit of useful clinical density in the absence of special illumination or "hot lighting" of films.

FIGURE 4-11 Representative exposure latitudes of CCD, PSP, and intraoral film sensors. The clinically useful optical density of film has an upper limit of 2.5. Use of a more intense viewbox or "hot lighting" can extend the upper end of the usable density range and expand useful film latitude. PSP plates are unique in responding linearly to exposure.

DETECTOR SENSITIVITY

The sensitivity, or speed, of a detector is its ability to respond to small amounts of radiation. Intraoral film speed is classified according to speed group by criteria developed by the International Organization for Standardization. Extraoral screen-film combinations use a classification system developed by Eastman Kodak. At the present time, there are no classification standards for dental digital x-ray receptors. As a result, the reported sensitivity of systems by equipment manufacturers may exaggerate the performance that can be achieved in routine practice. The useful sensitivity of digital receptors is affected by numerous factors, including detector efficiency, pixel size, and system noise. Current PSP systems for intraoral imaging allow dose reductions of about 50% compared with F-speed film with similar diagnostic performance. Subjectively, most observers prefer intraoral PSP images with a higher level of x-ray exposure. Paradoxically, patient doses may increase if the level of x-ray exposure is determined by image criteria that are based on the subjective perception of "attractiveness." Additionally, patient exposure may increase with CCD systems because of the ease of making repeat exposures. In general, solid-state detectors require less exposure than PSP systems or film. CCD and PSP systems for extraoral imaging require exposures similar to exposures needed for 200-speed screen-film systems.

DIGITAL IMAGE VIEWING

ELECTRONIC DISPLAYS

Computer and television displays originally used a cathode ray tube (CRT) design. Issues of monitor bulk and image distortion associated with this technology have been reduced with the widespread adoption of TFT displays. TFT technology, which is used in flat panel detectors, is also used in laptop and flat panel computer displays. The process involves sending signals to the transistor associated with each pixel, which causes the associated liquid crystal display (LCD) to transmit light with an intensity proportional to the transistor voltage. Subpixels composed of red, green, and blue phosphors are subjected to varied voltages and in combination create a pixel output of a particular hue and intensity. The output of laptop displays is limited in intensity and does not have the dynamic range or contrast found in conventional desktop CRT or LCD displays. The viewing angle of laptop displays is also limited, and the observer needs to be positioned squarely in front of the display for optimum viewing quality. Current laptop displays are of sufficient quality to be used for typical dental diagnostic tasks. Desktop versions of TFT LCD displays have overcome brightness and viewing angle problems but consume more power and thus are not suited for laptop configurations. An increasing number of flat panel displays are brighter than conventional CRT displays and have viewing angles of 160 degrees. Some flat panel displays incorporate a digital video interface, which allows direct display of digital information without digital-to-analog conversion. These displays virtually eliminate signal loss and distortion from digital-to-analog conversion.

DISPLAY CONSIDERATIONS

The display of digital images on electronic devices is a straightforward engineering issue. Positioning an image in the context of other diagnostic and demographic information and in useful relationships with other images is a more complex challenge that may vary according to diagnostic task, practice pattern, and practitioner preference. These challenges are answered with varying degrees of success by image display software. The quality, capabilities, and ease of use of display software vary from vendor to vendor. Even with the same software, the display of images can vary dramatically, depending on how the software handles resizing of windows or the size and resolutions of different displays. For instance, on some displays, it may be impossible to view a full-mouth series of images on a single screen at normal magnification (100%). Software may permit reduction in image size or scrolling around the window to compensate for smaller display areas. These approaches are not as fast or flexible as shifting a film mount around on a viewbox. The visibility of electronic displays is degraded by many of the same elements that degrade viewing of film images. Bright background illumination from windows or other sources of ambient light reduces visual contrast sensitivity. Light reflecting off a monitor surface may reduce the visibility of image contrast further. Images are best viewed in an environment in which lighting is subdued and indirect.

HARD COPIES

Until all dental health care providers and third parties are able to send, receive, store, and display digital images from a variety of acquisition sources, there will be a need for a universal medium to exchange radiographic image information. With the development of digital photography as a mainstream technology, digital image printing has become an economical solution for making digital radiographs transferable. The question is whether the printed image provides adequate image quality to prevent loss of diagnostic information. Any time a digital image is modified, including the process of printing it in hard copy, there needs to be sufficient assurance that the image retains relevant diagnostic information. The requirements for quality vary with the diagnostic task at hand. For instance, assessment of the impaction status of a third molar puts a lower demand on the image quality than caries detection. There is limited scientific evidence to support the diagnostic efficacy of printed images. The large number of variables that influence the quality of the printed image (e.g., printing technology, printer quality, printer settings, and type of media) makes the printing process a much more complicated process than it initially appears to be. When images must be printed, it is imperative to use a printing system that is designed for its intended use and to follow the manufacturer's recommendations. It is always preferable to transfer images digitally when possible. The main types of printing technologies available for image printing include laser, inkjet, and dye sublimation with the use of either film or paper.

Film Printers

Radiologists have traditionally relied on film images for common interpretive tasks. Some radiologists still prefer film even for inherently digital technologies such as magnetic resonance imaging and CT. High-quality film printers that use laser or dye sublimation technologies are expensive, and low-cost alternatives have reduced diagnostic quality. Current film transparencies produced with inkjet technology appear to be suboptimal for tasks such as caries diagnosis.

Paper Printers

Although printing on film allows radiographs to be evaluated in a traditional manner with the transmitted light of a viewbox, paper-printed digital radiographs require reflective light from a normally lit room. Because most dental operatories are not well equipped to control the ambient light level for viewing film images on a viewbox, paper-printed digital radiographs offer a substantial advantage. Printing digital radiographs on paper allows the dentist to use technologies developed for the digital photography domain.

Photographic printers vary widely in price and quality. Although more costly models usually provide higher print resolution, printer resolution is only one of many factors determining the final quality of the printed image. Inkjet printers are the most dominant in the market and offer the most economical alternative. Dye sublimation printers provide excellent image quality but are generally more expensive.

For any printing technology, the printing resolution is usually defined as the number of DPI the printer can print. A printer with a higher DPI number is capable of laying the ink down more tightly than a printer with a lower DPI number. As a result, printers with a higher DPI number can print smaller objects and thus are said to have "higher resolution." The resolution of the digital radiograph can never be increased by a printer that prints at a higher resolution than that of the image itself. Printing digital radiographs at a lower resolution may reduce the final resolution of the image, unless the printed size of the image is increased. Spatial resolution is preserved as long as the image prints pixel for pixel.

The same cannot be said of contrast resolution, which is always reduced by the printing process. The reason for this reduction in contrast resolution is that the printer is not printing with shades of gray but instead is printing varying numbers of black dots. Typically, an 8 × 8 pixel page array is assigned to each image pixel (Fig. 4-12). The number of elements in the array that are filled with a black ink dot determines the relative gray level of the array. The 8 × 8 array provides for 0 to 64 ink dots or 65 gray values. With an 8 × 8 dot array, it may not be possible to print all pixels of an image on a single page. For instance, a PSP panoramic image with a physical size of 15 cm × 30 cm might be scanned at 150 DPI. For each pixel of this image to print within the same dimensions, a printer resolution of 1200 DPI (8 × 150) is required. If the maximum resolution of the printer is 1200 DPI, images with higher resolutions must be printed at a larger size to obtain full spatial resolution. Likewise, a bitewing image scanned at 300 DPI must be printed at twice its physical size of 30 mm × 40 mm to preserve the original resolution. Resizing of an image to fit on a printed page leads to interpolation of pixels and can result in a significant loss of resolution.

A final drawback of paper prints is the limited contrast ratio owing to the physics of the reflective process used for viewing images. The darkest inks absorb at most 96% on incident visible light. If the paper were able to reflect 100% of the incident light, the maximum reflective contrast ratio achievable is only 25 : 1.

IMAGE PROCESSING

Any operation that acts to improve, restore, analyze, or in some way change a digital image is a form of image processing. The use of digital imaging in dental radiography involves various image processing operations. Some of these operations are integrated in the image acquisition and image management software and are hidden from the user. Others are controlled by the user with the intention to improve the quality of the image or to analyze its contents. The fact that some of the image processing steps are hidden from the user may have consequences that have no analog in film. One such consequence is the difficulty in assessing underexposure or overexposure in digital radiographs. For film, this condition is readily apparent, but a suboptimally exposed digital image rarely appears too light or too dark because image processing usually includes automatic data leveling. Other metrics, such as the data histogram or noise measurements, should be employed.

IMAGE RESTORATION

When the raw image data enter the computer, they are usually not yet ready for storage or display. A number of preprocessing steps need to be performed to correct the image for known defects and to adjust the image intensities so that they are suitable for viewing. For example, some of the pixels in a CCD sensor are always defective. The image is restored by substituting the gray values of the defective pixels with some weighted average of the gray values from the surrounding pixels. Depending on the quality of the sensor and the choices made by the manufacturer, various other operations may be applied to the image before it becomes visible on the display. These operations are executed very rapidly and are unnoticed by the user. Most preprocessing operations are set by the manufacturer and cannot be changed.

IMAGE ENHANCEMENT

The term image enhancement implies that the adjusted image is an improved version of the original one. Most image enhancement operations are applied to make the image visually more appealing (subjective enhancement). This can be accomplished by increasing contrast, optimizing brightness, and reducing unsharpness and noise. Subjective image enhancement does not improve the accuracy of image interpretation. Image enhancement operations are often task specific: what benefits one diagnostic task may reduce the image quality for another task. For example, increasing contrast between enamel and dentin for caries detection may make it more difficult to identify the contour of the alveolar crest. Image enhancement operations are also dependent on viewer preference.

Brightness and Contrast

Digital radiographs do not always use the full range of available gray values effectively. They can be relatively dark or light, and they can show too much contrast in certain areas or not enough. Although the brightness and contrast can be judged visually, the image histogram is a convenient tool to examine which of the available gray values the image is using (Fig. 4-13). The minimum and maximum values and the shape of the histogram indicate the potential benefit of brightness and contrast enhancement operations.

Digital imaging software commonly includes a histogram tool and tools for the adjustment of brightness and contrast. Some tools

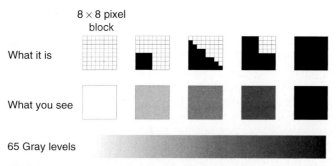

FIGURE 4-12 Gray scale printing. Each image pixel is assigned to an 8 × 8 pixel array on the printed page. From 0 to 64 black ink dots can be used to fill each array, resulting in 65 potential gray levels. This means that an 8-bit (256 gray levels) image is reduced to 6 bits with a concomitant loss of contrast resolution during the printing process.

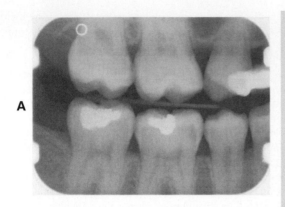
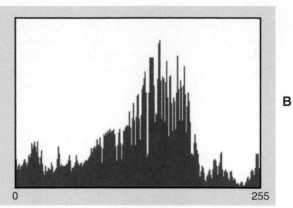

FIGURE 4-13 Digital image **(A)** with image histogram **(B)**. Horizontal axis represents image gray levels (8 bits—256 levels); vertical axis represents number of pixels. Each bar indicates the number of pixels in the image with that particular gray level.

also allow adjustment of the gamma value. Changing the gamma value of an image selectively enhances image contrast in either the brighter or the darker areas of the image. Adjustment of brightness, contrast, and gamma value changes the original intensity values of the image (input) to new values (output). The operator can choose to make these changes permanent or to restore the image to its original settings. Figure 4-14 is a graphic representation of the relationship between input values (horizontal axis) and output values (vertical axis) with the corresponding images and their histograms. Digital imaging software usually also includes tools for histogram equalization and contrast inversion. Histogram equalization is an enhancement operation that increases contrast between the image intensities abundantly present within the image, while reducing contrast between image intensities that are used only sparsely. The actual effect of histogram equalization depends on the image content and may sometimes lead to unexpected degradation of image quality. Contrast inversion changes a radiographic positive image into a radiographic negative image. Although this may affect the subjective perception of the image content, the altered appearance is foreign to interpretive practice and is little used.

The effect of contrast enhancement on the diagnostic value of digital radiographs is controversial. Some studies show substantial benefits of contrast enhancement operations, whereas others have found only limited value or no improvement at all. The effect of contrast enhancement cannot be predicted easily. The key to successful image enhancement is to enhance relevant radiographic signs selectively without simultaneously enhancing distracting features.

SHARPENING AND SMOOTHING

The purpose of sharpening and smoothing filters is to improve image quality by removing blur or noise. Noise represents random intensity variation and is often categorized as high-frequency noise (small-scale intensity variations) or low-frequency noise (gradual or large-scale intensity variations). Speckling is a special type of high-frequency noise that is characterized by isolated small regions surrounded by lighter or darker regions. Filters that smooth an image are sometimes called noise or despeckling filters because they are designed to remove high-frequency noise. Filters that sharpen an image either remove low-frequency noise or enhance boundaries between regions with different intensities (edge enhancement). For the purposeful application of filters, it is

important to know what type of noise the filters reduce and how that affects radiographic features of interest. Without this knowledge, important radiographic features may degrade or disappear as noise is removed. Similarly, edge enhancement of radiographic features of interest may enhance noise or enhance local contrast to the extent that it simulates disease. Sharpening and smoothing filters may make the dental radiographic images subjectively more appealing; however, there is no scientific evidence suggesting an increase in diagnostic value. The indiscriminate use of filters made available in most imaging software packages should be avoided if there is no scientific support for their clinical usefulness.

Color

Most digital systems on the market provide opportunities for color conversion of gray-scale images, also called pseudocolor. Humans can distinguish many more colors than shades of gray. Transforming the gray values of a digital image into various colors theoretically could enhance the detection of objects within the image; however, this works only if all the gray values representing an object are unique for that object. Because this is rarely the case, boundaries between objects may change, and new boundaries may be created. In most cases, these changes distract the observer from seeing the real content of the image and result in degraded image interpretation. Therefore color conversion of radiographs is neither diagnostically nor educationally useful. Some useful applications of color do exist. When objects can be uniquely identified on the basis of a set of image features, color can be used to label or highlight these objects. The development of such criteria is a complex task, and only a few successful studies have been reported in the literature.

Digital Subtraction Radiography

When two images of the same object are registered, and the image intensities of corresponding pixels are subtracted, a uniform difference image is produced. If there is a change in the radiographic attenuation between the baseline and follow-up examinations, this change shows up as a brighter area when the change represents gain and as a darker area when the change represents loss, such as loss of enamel and dentin owing to caries or loss of alveolar bone height with periodontitis. The strength of digital subtraction radiography (DSR) is that it cancels out the complex anatomic background against which this change occurs and reveals subtle changes. However, for DSR to be diagnostically useful the baseline

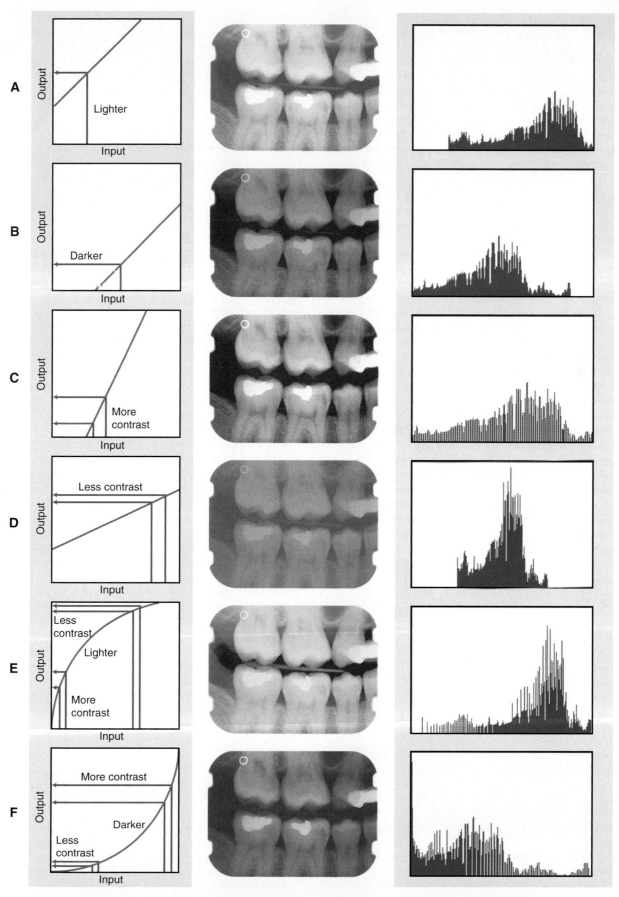

FIGURE 4-14 Effect of brightness, contrast, and gamma adjustment as illustrated by image transformation graphs *(left column)*, digital images *(middle column)*, and image histograms *(right column)*. The image adjustments are relative to those of Figure 4-13. **A,** Increase in brightness. **B,** Decrease in brightness. **C,** Increase in contrast. **D,** Decrease in contrast. **E,** Increase in gamma. **F,** Decrease in gamma.

projection geometry and image intensities must be closely reproduced—a requirement that is difficult to achieve clinically.

IMAGE ANALYSIS

Image analysis operations are designed to extract diagnostically relevant information from the image. This information can range from simple linear measurements to fully automated diagnosis. The use of image analysis tools brings with it the responsibility to understand their limitations. The accuracy and precision of a measurement are limited by the extent to which the image is a truthful and reproducible representation of the patient and by the operator's ability to make an exact measurement.

Measurement

Digital imaging software provides numerous tools for image analysis. Digital rulers, densitometers, and various other tools are readily available. These tools are usually digital equivalents of existing tools used in endodontics, orthodontics, periodontology, implantology, and other areas of dentistry (Fig. 4-15). Digital imaging has also added new tools that were not available with film-based radiography. The size and image intensity of any area within a digital radiograph can be measured. Tools are also being developed for measuring the complexity of the trabecular bone pattern. Such measurements can be useful as screening tools for osteoporosis assessment and for detecting other diseases.

Diagnosis

One of the most challenging areas of research is the development of tools and procedures that automate the detection, classification, and quantification of radiographic signs of disease. The rationale for the use of such methods is early and accurate disease detection through use of reproducible and objective criteria. The development of automated image analysis operations is very complex and requires a thorough understanding of anatomy, pathology, and radiographic image formation. The three basic steps of image analysis are segmentation, feature extraction, and object classification. Of these, segmentation is the most critical step. The goal of

segmentation is to simplify the image and reduce it to its basic components. This involves subdividing the image, thus separating objects from the background. Objects of interest are defined by the diagnostic task (e.g., a tooth, a carious lesion, a bone level, or an implant). When image segmentation results in the detection of an object, a variety of features can be measured that assist in determining what the object represents. Such features may include measures of size and shape, relative location, average density, homogeneity, and texture. A unique set of values for a certain combination of features can lead to classification of the object. Automated cephalometric landmark identification is an example of this technology. Other dental examples include caries detection, classification of periodontal disease, and detection and quantification of periapical bone lesions. The success of many of these applications is highly dependent on specific imaging parameters; very few provide reliable results when used clinically. This situation underscores the complexity of the radiographic image interpretation process.

IMAGE STORAGE

The use of digital imaging in dentistry requires an image archiving and management system that is very different from that used for conventional radiography. Storage of diagnostic images on magnetic or optical media raises new issues that must be considered. The file size of dental digital radiographs varies considerably, ranging from approximately 200 kilobytes for intraoral images to 6 megabytes for extraoral images. Storage and retrieval of these images in an average-sized dental practice is not a trivial issue. The development of new storage media and the continuing decrease in the price of a unit of storage has alleviated the capacity issue in dental radiography. The hard drive capacities of modern computers already exceed the storage needs of most dental practices.

The simplicity with which digital images can be modified through image processing poses a potential risk with respect to ensuring the integrity of the diagnostic information. Once in a digital format, critical image data can be deleted or modified. It is important that the software prevents the user from permanently deleting or modifying original image data, whether intentionally or unintentionally. Not all software programs provide such a safeguard. As the use of digital imaging in dentistry continues to expand, the implementation of standards for preserving original image data becomes urgent. It is also imperative that images and other important patient-related information are regularly stored on secondary external media. The use of computers for storing critical patient information mandates the design and use of a backup protocol. Box 4-2 shows some issues that need to be considered when a backup protocol is designed. Backup media suitable for external storage of digital radiographs include external hard drives,

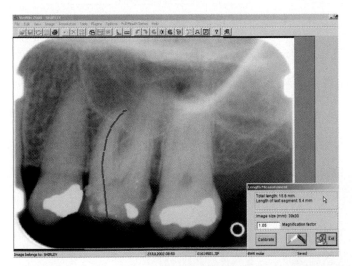

FIGURE 4-15 Example of a measurement tool to determine the length of the crown and mesiobuccal root of the first molar. The measurement has been calibrated for a magnification factor of 1.05. The digital measurement tool is more versatile than the analog ruler; however, for both types of measurement tools, the apparent length remains dependent on the projection geometry.

BOX 4-2 Digital Image Backup Considerations

- Type of backup media
- Time and method of backup
- Backup interval
- Storage location of backup media
- Recovery time
- Recovery reliability
- Future compatibility of backup technology

digital tapes, CDs, and DVDs. Downloading of data by telephone or dedicated data lines to off-site commercial storage sites is available through many vendors and provides essentially unlimited storage and backup. All these technologies are low in cost and have demonstrated reasonable reliability.

The purpose of image compression is to reduce the size of digital image files for archiving or transmission. In particular, storing extraoral images in a busy clinic may pose a challenge to storage capacity and speed of image access. The purpose of file compression is to reduce the file size significantly, while preserving critical image information.

Compression methods are generally classified as lossless or lossy. Lossless methods do not discard any image data, and an exact copy of the image is reproduced after decompression. Most compression techniques take advantage of redundancies in the image, which can be expressed in simpler terms. The maximum compression rate for lossless compression is usually less than 3:1. Lossy compression methods achieve higher levels of compression by discarding image data; empiric evidence suggests that this does not affect the diagnostic quality of an image. Compression rates of 12:1 and 14:1 were shown to have no appreciable effect on caries diagnosis. For determining endodontic file length, a rate of 25:1 was diagnostically equivalent to the uncompressed image. A compression rate of 28:1 was acceptable for the subjective evaluation of image quality and the detection of artificial lesions in panoramic radiographs.

Version 3.0 of the Digital Imaging and Communications in Medicine (DICOM) standard adopted JPEG (Joint Photographic Experts Group) as the compression method, which provides a range of compression levels. Other types of image compression methods, such as wavelet compression, are being investigated for their use in medical imaging. Although low and medium levels of lossy compression appear to have little effect on the diagnostic value of dental images, lossy compression should be used with caution and only after its effect for specific diagnostic tasks has been evaluated. With the continuing increase in the capacity of storage media and the widespread use of high-speed data communication lines, lossy compression of dental radiographs is rapidly becoming obsolete. At the same time, new digital image receptors are generating images with more and more pixels and more bits per pixel, thus increasing storage needs. Image compression negates to some extent the gain from such high-end detectors. Diagnostic criteria should dictate the need for high-resolution detectors and use of image compression. Current evidence suggests that detector quality and moderate image compression have a limited impact on diagnostic outcomes.

SYSTEMS COMPATIBILITY

The development of digital imaging systems for dental radiography has largely been driven by industry. Manufacturers have adopted and developed technologies according to individual needs and philosophies. As a result, image formats among systems from different vendors are not standardized, and image archival, retrieval, and display systems are often incompatible. Despite the proprietary nature of imaging software, it is possible to transfer images from one vendor's system to the other. Most systems provide image export and import tools using a variety of generic image formats, such as JPEG and TIFF (tagged image file format). However, the process of transferring images through export-import procedures is cumbersome. It requires many steps, and the operator needs to ensure that the right images are imported into the proper patient folder. Also, it cannot be assumed that the display and calibration of imported and native images will be the same.

Exporting and importing is not the method of choice when digital imaging is going to be used on a large scale. It has long been recognized that the adoption of a standard for transferring images and associated information between digital imaging devices in medicine and dentistry is necessary. The American College of Radiology and the National Electrical Manufacturers Association formed a joint committee to develop a standard for digital imaging systems. Numerous professional organizations have contributed to this complex development process, which has resulted in the current DICOM standard. Various dental organizations, including the American Dental Association, are playing an active role in defining aspects of the DICOM standard related to dentistry. The DICOM standard is not a static set of rules dictating to manufacturers how to build imaging devices. Rather, it is an evolving document addressing the interoperability of medical and dental imaging and information systems. Manufacturers of digital imaging systems for dental radiography are responding to the call to adopt the DICOM standard. At the present time, not all systems conform to the DICOM standard, and systems that do may not conform to every aspect of the standard. The successful adoption of digital imaging in dentistry requires interoperability of all devices. It is likely that manufacturers do not want to be left behind and that the market will weed out the systems that are noncompliant. Dentists using different vendors with DICOM-compliant imaging devices are able to exchange images seamlessly.

CLINICAL CONSIDERATIONS

Some fundamental differences from film in the clinical handling of digital receptors should be noted (Tables 4-1 and 4-2). Because digital receptors are intended to be reusable, they must be handled with greater care than their film counterparts. In certain situations film may be intentionally damaged through bending to accommodate patient anatomy. This situation never occurs with digital receptors as bending sensors would damage them. Instead, allowances must be made for sensor rigidity, such as placement of the sensor toward the midline to allow for greater clearance or to modify beam angulation to account for the smaller imaging area of digital sensors. Examples of common image artifacts found on images made with solid-state or PSP systems are presented in Box 4-3. PSP plates are susceptible to bending and scratching during handling that induce permanent artifacts in the receptor. These artifacts obscure information of potential diagnostic importance and may necessitate disposal of the receptor and repeat imaging of the patient. Because of the inability of digital detectors to be bent to accommodate patient anatomy, new imaging strategies must be used for some patients. It may not be possible to capture consistently the distal surface of the canine on premolar views. An additional projection may be required to visualize this surface adequately.

A significant potential problem with most PSP systems is the inability to distinguish images from plates that have been exposed backward. In contrast to film packets, which incorporate a lead foil with a characteristic embossed pattern that results in an underexposed image of the anatomy with the pattern artifact when exposed backward, PSP images have little x-ray attenuation from the polyester base. It is much too easy for inattentive radiographers to mount these digital images on the contralateral position from their true side. One can imagine the liability that could occur from diagnosing and treating disease on the opposite side of the actual

TABLE 4-1   Clinical Comparison of Intraoral Imaging Alternatives

Imaging Step	Film	CCD/CMOS	PSP
Receptor preparation	None	(1) Place protective plastic sleeve over receptor envelope (2) Receptor must be connected to computer and patient identifying information entered for acquisition/archiving software	(1) "Erase" plates (2) Package plates in protective plastic
Receptor placement	(1) Numerous generic film holding devices are available (2) Film may be bent to accommodate anatomy	(1) Specialized receptor holder specific for manufacturer's receptor may limit options (2) Receptor inflexibility and bulk limit placement options (3) Receptor cable must be carefully routed out of patient mouth (4) Patient discomfort more likely than with film or PSP	(1) Many receptor holders used for film may be adapted for PSP plates (2) Bending of receptor may irreversibly damage it
Exposure	Simple exposure	Computer must be activated before exposure	Simple exposure
Processing	(1) Dark, light-safe environment in form of darkroom or daylight loader required (2) Processor chemistry must be prepared or replenished (3) Chemical temperature must be warmed, or processing time must be adjusted to accommodate temperature (4) Films must be removed from wrapper; lead foil must be separated for recycling	(1) Image acquisition and display almost immediate	(1) Dimly light environment desirable to prevent loss of image information (2) Processor must be programmed with patient and detector information so that images are identified, preprocessed, and stored properly (3) Protective wrapper must be removed from plates (4) Plates must be loaded on drum systems
Display preparation	(1) Films may be placed in a variety of film mounts (2) Mounts must be labeled with patient-identifying information	(1) Software may be configured to place image in appropriate position in digital mount when exposures are made in a predetermined sequence; otherwise, images must be individually placed in mount	(1) Images must be individually placed in mount (2) Images may need to be digitally rotated to achieve proper orientation
Display	(1) A room with subdued lighting and a masked viewbox are optimal (2) Any light source (including the operatory window or ceiling light) permits quick evaluation of the image	Same considerations apply to all digital receptor types: (1) A room with subdued lighting is optimal for interpretation activities (2) Computer and display with appropriate software are necessary; viewing is restricted to the location of the computer (3) Laptop computers increase flexibility of computer placement but may reduce display quality (4) Size of display restricts the numbers of images that may be viewed simultaneously; more time is required to open/close or expand/contract images when interpreting a series of images	
Image duplication	(1) Quality of duplication is always inferior to original and is sometimes nondiagnostic	(1) Electronic copies may be stored on various media without loss of image quality (2) Output on film or paper is inferior and is often nondiagnostic unless appropriate combinations of expensive printers and papers or film are used	

lesion. To date, only the Soredex OpTime system has addressed this issue by incorporating a round metal disk on the back of intraoral plates (see Fig. 4-7). This marker becomes visible on the image if the imaging plate is exposed backward. The appearance of the marker on the image does not fully obscure the anatomic information, and these images can be "mirrored" with imaging software tools without the need for repeated exposure.

Infection control is also an issue with digital receptors. Digital receptors cannot be sterilized by conventional means. They may be disinfected by wiping with mild agents such as isopropyl alcohol but should not be immersed in disinfecting solutions. The adage that "you can autoclave a digital receptor … once" stems from the fact that heat ruins electronic components in CCD and CMOS sensors and distorts the polyester base of PSP plates. Another potential drawback to drum-based PSP systems is the 2- to 5-minute cycle time required by some devices for plate scanning. During this time, no additional plates may be processed. With film and non–drum-based PSP scanners, there is less delay between the times when additional films or plates may be "fed" into the

Text continued on p. 61

TABLE 4-2   Comparison of Physical Properties of Film, Charge-Coupled Device, Complementary Metallic Oxide Semiconductor, and Photostimulable Phosphor Receptors

Feature	Technical Comment	Clinical Comment
Spatial resolution	Intraoral systems: Film > CCD = CMOS > PSP Panoramic systems: Film = CCD = PSP Cephalometric systems: Film > CCD = PSP	Limits of resolution for digital systems are readily appreciated when magnifying these images. With magnification, a "blocky" or "pixelated" appearance is evident. Resolution of panoramic systems is limited by mechanical motion to about 5 lp/mm
Exposure latitude	PSP $\gg$ CCD $\geq$ CMOS > film	Because of the wide latitude of PSP and the automatic brightness and contrast "optimization" by image acquisition software, use of more x-ray exposure than is necessary is possible
Receptor dimensions	For equivalent imaged area, Film = PSP < CCD = CMOS	"Active area" of CCD and CMOS receptors is smaller than surface area because of other electronic components within the plastic housing
Time for image acquisition	CCD = CMOS $\ll$ PSP = film	Rapid image acquisition may be important for endodontic procedures or during implant placement
Image quality	Subjective quality is best with film when carefully exposed and well processed	Digital and film imaging are not significantly different when used for common diagnostic tasks
Image adjustment/processing	Improves appearance of digital images	Takes time; may not improve diagnostic performance
Cost	Initial costs of digital systems are greater than film. Subsequent costs vary greatly depending on receptor wear and tear or abuse	Manufacturers' estimates of life expectancy of reusable receptors may be overly optimistic
Reliability	Mechanical problems affect digital PSP and film systems. Software reliability varies greatly among manufacturers. Changes in unrelated computer components and software can cause digital systems to malfunction	Digital systems fail when problems occur with receptors during image acquisition or with computers during image processing, archiving, and display
Image storage and retrieval	Data backup is critical for digital systems	Films can be misfiled and lost or be damaged by poor storage conditions. Digital data can be lost as a result of failures in power supplies or storage media and operator error
Transmitting images to others	Rapidly done with digital images	Facilitates communication between colleagues or with insurance companies

---

BOX 4-3   Common Problems in Digital Image Receptor Exposure, Processing, and Handling

Enrique Platin

NOISY IMAGES

Although the brightness of these images has been adjusted to display similar average gray values, notice the noisy appearance of the underexposed periapical radiograph (Fig. 4-16, *A*, 0.032 second) compared with the properly exposed radiograph (Fig. 4-16, *B*, 0.32 second).

PSP image degradation as a result of excessive exposure to ambient light between image acquisition and plate scanning (Fig. 4-17). This type of noise resembles that of x-ray underexposure.

NONUNIFORM IMAGE DENSITY

Partial exposure of PSP plates to excessive ambient light before scanning results in nonuniform image density (Fig. 4-18, *A*). This happens when plates are overlapped while exposed to ambient light (Fig. 4-18, *B*).

DISTORTED IMAGES

Bending of PSP plates during intraoral placement: moderate bending (Fig. 4-19, *A*), retake of image *A* (Fig. 4-19, *B*), severe bending (Fig. 4-19, *C*), and retake of image *C* (Fig. 4-19, *D*).

DOUBLE IMAGES

PSP double image on incisor periapical radiograph resulting from incomplete erasure of previous image of posterior periapical region (Fig. 4-20, *A*) and retake of image (Fig. 4-20, *B*).

More examples of double images resulting from incomplete erasure of PSP receptors: posterior periapical radiograph with double image (Fig. 4-21, *A*), retake of image *A* (Fig. 4-21, *B*), anterior periapical radiograph with double image (Fig. 4-21, *C*), and retake of image *C* (Fig. 4-21, *D*).

DAMAGED IMAGE RECEPTORS

Scratched phosphor surface mimicking root canal filling (Fig. 4-22, *A*) and retake of image (Fig. 4-22, *B*).

Image artifacts resulting from excessive bending of the PSP plate (Fig. 4-23, *A*). Excessive bending has resulted in permanent damage to the phosphor plate (Fig. 4-23, *B*).

PSP circular artifact as a result of plate damage (Fig. 4-24, *A*) and localized swelling of the protective coating from disinfectant solution on work surface (Fig. 4-24, *B*).

PSP image artifact resulting from plate surface contamination (Fig. 4-25, *A*). This artifact was caused by a glove powder smudge that prevented proper scanning of the

Continued

BOX 4-3   Common Problems in Digital Image Receptor Exposure, Processing, and Handling—cont'd

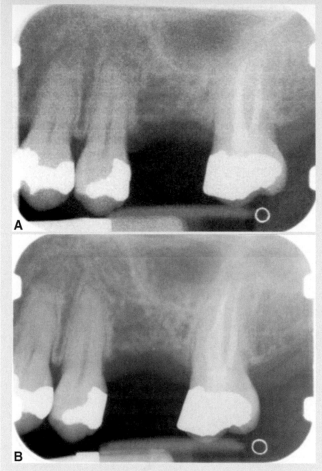

FIGURE 4-16

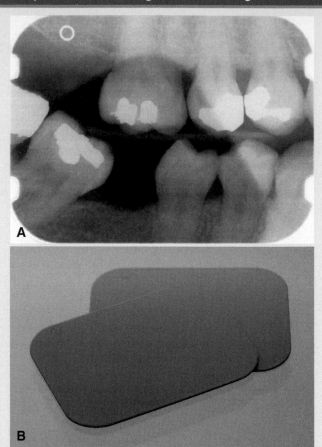

FIGURE 4-18

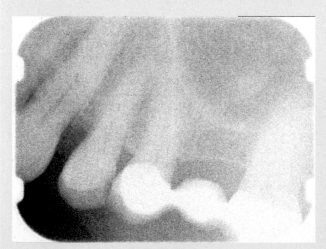

FIGURE 4-17

affected area of the PSP plate (Fig. 4-25, *B*). Contaminants combined with skin oils may permanently damage the phosphor plate surface.

Malfunctioning CCD sensor resulting from rough handling (dropped sensor). The sensor produces geometric image artifacts (Fig. 4-26, *A* and *B*).

IMPROPER USE OF IMAGE PROCESSING

Improper use of image processing tools, such as filters, may result in false-positive findings. An edge enhancement filter was applied to the panoramic image, which produced radiolucencies at restoration edges simulating recurrent caries (Fig. 4-27, *A*). These radiolucencies are not present in a follow-up intraoral image (Fig. 4-27, *B*).

EFFECT OF IMAGE SCANNING RESOLUTION

PSP scanning resolution settings may have a significant impact on image quality. Scanning at 150 DPI (Fig. 4-28, *A*) produces an image that lacks detail and appears pixelated when magnified. Scanning at 300 DPI provides increased detail through higher resolution (Fig. 4-28, *B*). Box 4-1 shows how to convert from DPI (scanner) to lp/mm (image resolution).

BOX 4-3 Common Problems in Digital Image Receptor Exposure, Processing, and Handling—cont'd

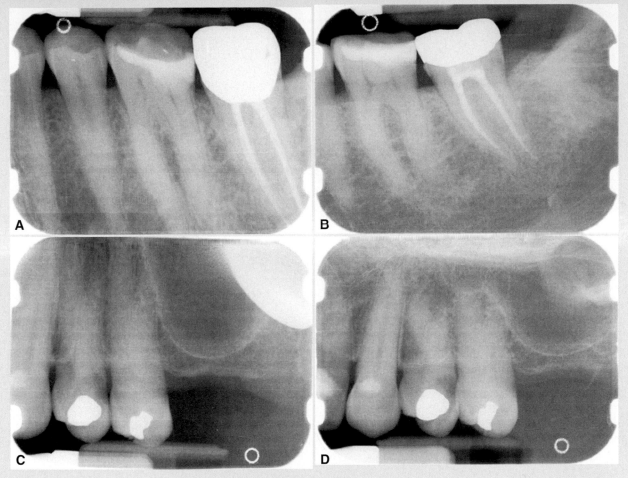

FIGURE 4-19

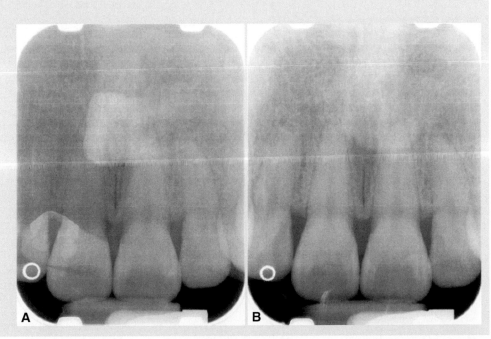

FIGURE 4-20

Continued

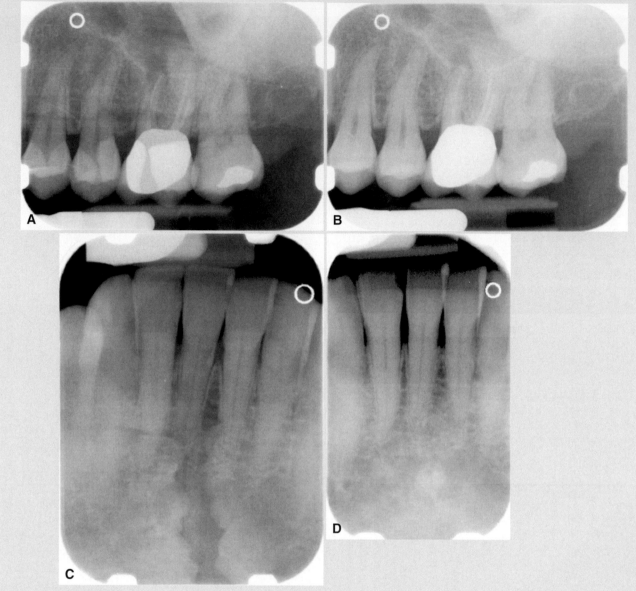

FIGURE 4-21

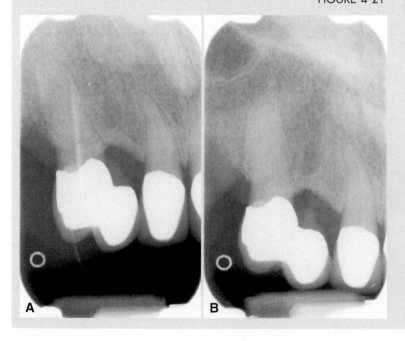

FIGURE 4-22

BOX 4-3 Common Problems in Digital Image Receptor Exposure, Processing, and Handling—cont'd

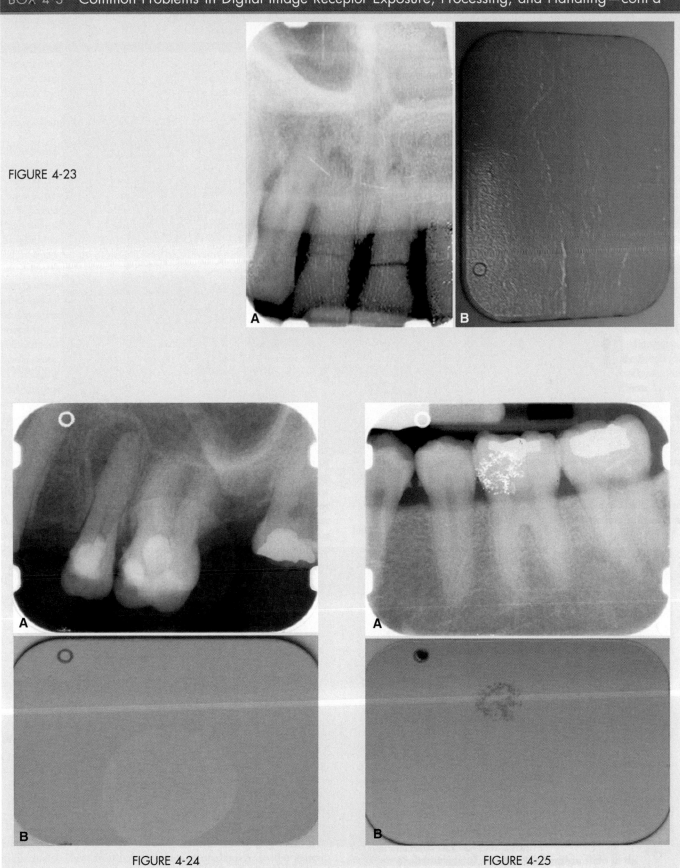

FIGURE 4-23

FIGURE 4-24

FIGURE 4-25

Continued

BOX 4-3   Common Problems in Digital Image Receptor Exposure, Processing, and Handling—cont'd

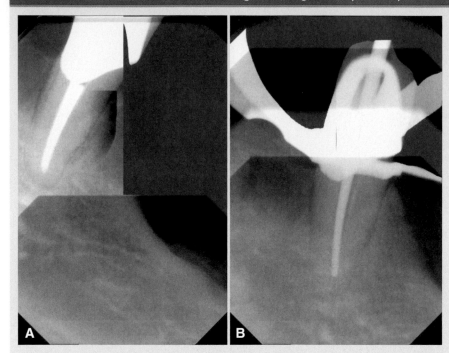

FIGURE 4-26

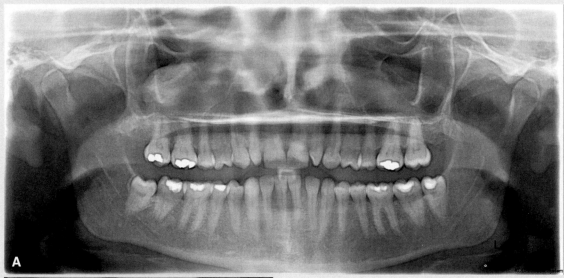

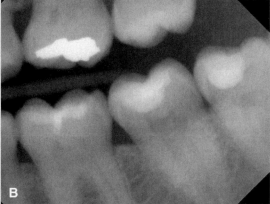

FIGURE 4-27

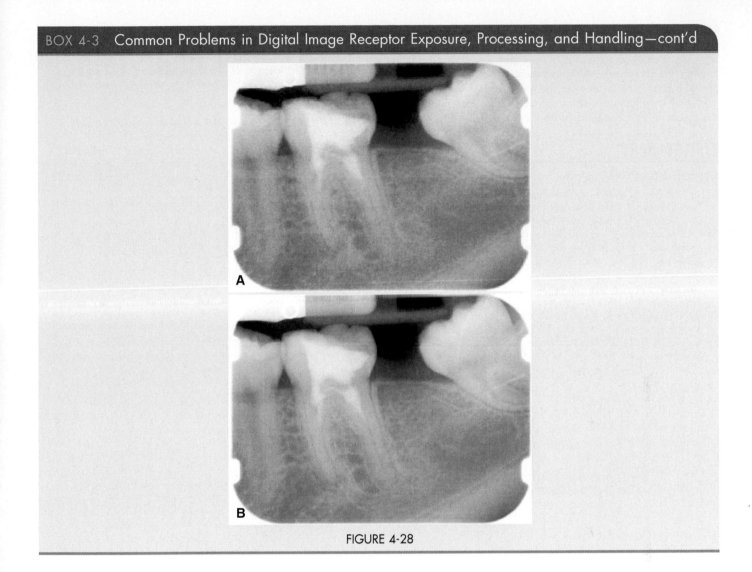

FIGURE 4-28

processor. Although each of the preceding concerns is of potential importance, the advantage of eliminating chemical processing in digital systems should not be overlooked. The time required to monitor and maintain a film processor properly is significant. Too often, insufficient attention is paid to this critical aspect of film radiography. Digital systems may not save the time gained by eliminating film processing, but they do eliminate the loss in diagnostic quality that occurs when insufficient time and effort are spent on film processing quality assurance.

CONCLUSION

Dental practitioners commonly ask, "Which is better, film or digital imaging?" There is no simple answer to this question (see Tables 4-1 and 4-2). Reported technical properties of resolution, contrast, and latitude are confounded by a lack of standardization in the assessment of these characteristics. From a diagnostic standpoint, most studies suggest that digital performance is not clinically different from film for typical diagnostic tasks, such as caries diagnosis. The "look and feel" of digital displays is distinctly different from film viewing, and some practitioners may find this

difference disconcerting. A basic understanding of computers and a mastery of common computing skills are essential for viewing digital images. Beyond this, learning the peculiarities and vagaries of a particular acquisition and display software takes time and may not be intuitive. Multiple mouse clicks through multiple menus may be required to view a full-mouth series of images. This activity may modestly increase the time required to complete the interpretative process.

In selecting an imaging system, other issues should be considered. Digital images avoid environmental pollutants encountered with film processing, but what about the environmental impact associated with the disposal of broken or obsolete electronic equipment? The initial financial outlay for digital imaging hardware makes these systems more expensive than film. Manufacturers point out that the costs of film or digital systems should be amortized over the life of the equipment and consumables; however, the life expectancy of newer digital systems is highly speculative. Mishandling of digital system components can catastrophically shorten any projected life expectancy. Additionally, what price should we place on the ability to transmit images instantly and to integrate them into a fully electronic record? There are no universal answers to these questions. They must be asked and answered according to the needs and objectives of individual dental practices. As practice patterns and technology change with time, the answers will also change. Although the details of the image in our crystal ball have yet to resolve, the trends of increasing adoption of digital imaging and continuing technologic innovation make the future of digital imaging in dentistry certain.

BIBLIOGRAPHY

Digital Detectors and Displays

Abreu M Jr, Mol A, Ludlow JB: Performance of RVGui sensor and Kodak Ektaspeed Plus film for proximal caries detection, *Oral Surg Oral Med Oral Pathol Oral Radiol Endod* 91:381–385, 2001.

Butt A, Mahoney M, Savage NW: The impact of computer display performance on the quality of digital radiographs: a review, *Aust Dent J* 57(Suppl 1):16–23, 2012.

Couture RA, Hildebolt C: Quantitative dental radiography with a new photostimulable phosphor system, *Oral Surg Oral Med Oral Pathol Oral Radiol Endod* 89:498–508, 2000.

Hildebolt CF, Couture RA, Whiting BR: Dental photostimulable phosphor radiography, *Dent Clin North Am* 44:273–297, 2000.

Sanderink GC, Miles DA: Intraoral detectors: CCD, CMOS, TFT, and other devices, *Dent Clin North Am* 44:249–255, 2000.

Vandenberghe B, Jacobs R, Bosmans H: Modern dental imaging: a review of the current technology and clinical applications in dental practice, *Eur Radiol* 20:2637–2655, 2010.

Van der Stelt PF: Principles of digital imaging, *Dent Clin North Am* 44:237–248, 2000.

Image Processing

Analoui M: Radiographic image enhancement, I: spatial domain techniques, *Dentomaxillofac Radiol* 30:1–9, 2001.

Analoui M: Radiographic digital image enhancement, II: transform domain techniques, *Dentomaxillofac Radiol* 30:65–77, 2001.

Gonzalez R, Wood R: *Digital image processing*, ed 3, Upper Saddle River, NJ, 2007, Prentice Hall.

Mol A: Image processing tools for dental applications, *Dent Clin North Am* 44:299–318, 2000.

Russ JC: *The image process handbook*, ed 5, Boca Raton, FL, 2006, CRC Press.

Clinical Considerations

Wenzel A: A review of dentists' use of digital radiography and caries diagnosis with digital systems, *Dentomaxillofac Radiol* 35:307–314, 2006.

Wenzel A, Møystad A: Work flow with digital intraoral radiography: a systematic review, *Acta Odontol Scand* 68:106–114, 2010.

Film Imaging

A beam of x-ray photons that passes through the dental arches is reduced in intensity (attenuated) by absorption and scattering of photons out of the primary beam. The pattern of the photons that exits the patient, the remnant beam, conveys information about the patient's anatomy. For this information to be useful diagnostically, the remnant beam must be recorded on an image receptor. The image receptor most often used in dental radiography is x-ray film. This chapter describes x-ray film and film processing and the use of intensifying screens. Digital radiographic systems, which also may be used to make radiographs, are described in Chapter 4.

X-RAY FILM

COMPOSITION

X-ray film has two principal components: (1) emulsion and (2) base. The emulsion, which is sensitive to x rays and visible light, records the radiographic image. The base is a plastic supporting material onto which the emulsion is coated (Fig. 5-1).

Emulsion

The two principal components of emulsion are silver halide grains, which are sensitive to x radiation and visible light, and a vehicle matrix in which the crystals are suspended. The silver halide grains are composed primarily of crystals of silver bromide. The composition of a dental film emulsion is shown in Table 5-1. The silver halide grains in INSIGHT film and Ultra-speed film (Carestream Dental, a division of Carestream Health, Inc.) are flat, tabular crystals with a mean diameter of about 1.8 µm (Fig. 5-2). The

tabular grains are oriented parallel with the film surface to offer a large cross-sectional area to the x-ray beam (Fig. 5-3). INSIGHT film has about twice the number of silver grains so that it requires only half the exposure of Ultra-speed film.

The silver halide grains are suspended in a surrounding vehicle that is applied to both sides of the supporting base. During film processing (described later in this chapter) the vehicle absorbs processing solutions, allowing the chemicals to reach and react with the silver halide grains. An additional layer of vehicle is added to the film emulsion as an overcoat. This barrier helps protect the film from damage by scratching, contamination, or pressure from rollers when an automatic processor is used.

Film emulsions are sensitive to both x-ray photons and visible light. Film intended to be exposed by x rays is called direct exposure film. All intraoral dental film is direct exposure film. Screen film is used with intensifying screens (described later in this chapter) that emit visible light. Screen film and intensifying screens are used for extraoral projections, such as panoramic and cephalometric radiographs.

Base

The function of the film base is to support the emulsion. The base for dental x-ray film is made of polyester polyethylene terephthalate, which provides the proper degree of flexibility to allow easy handling of the film. The film base must also withstand exposure to processing solutions without becoming distorted. The base is uniformly translucent and casts no pattern on the resultant radiograph.

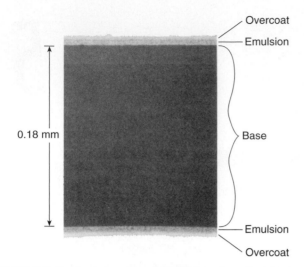

FIGURE 5-1 Scanning electron micrograph of INSIGHT dental x-ray film (original magnification 300×). Note the overcoat, emulsion, and base on this double-emulsion film. (Courtesy Carestream Dental, a division of Carestream Health, Inc.)

TABLE 5-1	Typical Coating Weights per Film Side (mg/cm^2)				
Film Type	Silver	Bromide	Emulsion Vehicle	Overcoat Vehicle	
InSight (E/F speed)	0.8–1.1	0.6–0.75	0.6–0.8	0.1–0.2	
Ultra-Speed (D speed)	0.4–0.55	0.6–0.75	0.4–0.7	0.1–0.2	

Data from Carestream Health, Inc., exclusive manufacturer of Kodak dental systems.

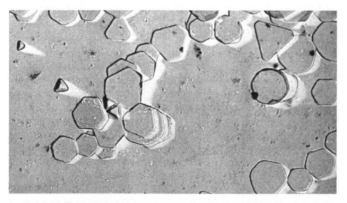

FIGURE 5-2 Scanning electron micrograph of emulsion of INSIGHT film showing flat tabular silver bromide crystals, which capture incident photons. (Courtesy Carestream Dental, a division of Carestream Health, Inc.)

INTRAORAL X-RAY FILM

Intraoral dental x-ray film is made as a double-emulsion film—that is, both sides of the base are coated with an emulsion. With a double layer of emulsion, less radiation is required to produce an image. Direct exposure film is used for intraoral examinations because it provides higher resolution images than screen-film combinations. Some diagnostic tasks, such as detection of incipient caries or early periapical disease, require this higher resolution.

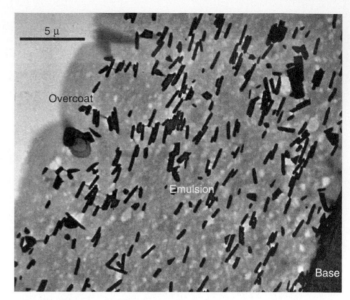

FIGURE 5-3 Cross-sectional electron microscope image of emulsion of INSIGHT film. The orientation of the tabular crystals in the emulsion is essentially parallel to the film surface to increase the exposure surface of the crystals to the incident x-ray beam. (Courtesy Carestream Dental, a division of Carestream Health, Inc.)

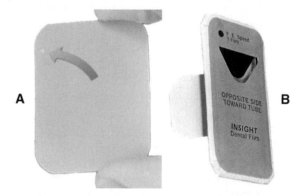

FIGURE 5-4 A, The raised film dot (arrow) indicates the tube side of the film and identifies the patient's right and left sides. B, The location of this dot is clearly marked with a black circle on the outside of every film packet. (Courtesy of Carestream Dental, a division of Carestream Health, Inc.)

One corner of each dental film has a small, raised dot that is used for film orientation (Fig. 5-4). The manufacturer orients the film in the packet so that the convex side of the dot is toward the front of the packet and faces the x-ray tube. The side of the film with the depression is thus oriented toward the patient's tongue. After the film has been exposed and processed, the dot is used to orient the patient's right and left side images properly. When mounting radiographs, each film is oriented with the convex side of the dot toward the viewer, and on the basis of the features of the teeth and anatomic landmarks in the adjacent bone, the films are arranged in their normal sequential relationship in the mount.

Intraoral x-ray film packets contain either one or two sheets of film (Fig. 5-5). When double-film packs are used, the second film serves as a duplicate record that can be sent to insurance companies or to a colleague. The film is encased in a protective black paper wrapper and then in an outer white paper or plastic wrapping, which is resistant to moisture. The outer wrapping clearly

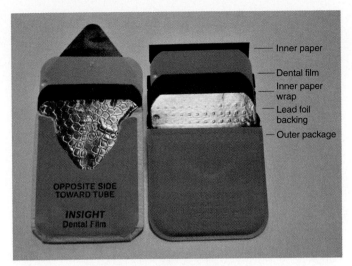

FIGURE 5-5 Moisture-proof and lightproof packets, paper on the left and vinyl on right, contain an opening tab on the side opposite the tube. Inside is an interleaf paper wrapper that is folded around the film as well as a sheet of lead foil. Film is packaged with one or two sheets of film. The foil is positioned between the back side of the packet and the paper wrapper. In this position, it absorbs radiation that has passed through the film and prevents scatter radiation from blurring the image. If the film packet is inadvertently placed backward in the patient's mouth, the mottled image of the foil shows on the resultant image. *(Courtesy of Carestream Dental, a division of Carestream Health, Inc.)*

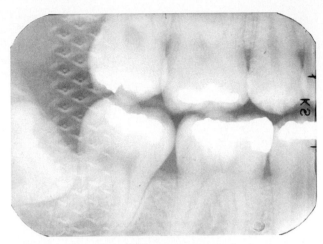

FIGURE 5-6 Placing a film backward in the patient's mouth when the exposure was made results in a radiograph that is too light and shows the characteristic markings caused by exposure through the lead foil in the film packaging. In such an image, the left and right sides of the patient are reversed when using the dot as the orientation guide.

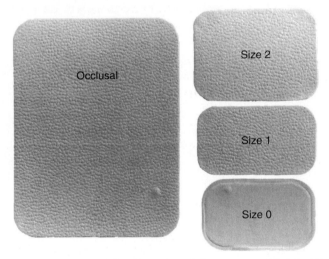

FIGURE 5-7 Dental x-ray film is commonly supplied in various sizes. *Left,* Occlusal film. *Top right,* Size 2 for adult posterior film. *Middle right,* Size 1 for adult anterior film. *Bottom right,* Size 0 for child-size film (in vinyl wrapping).

indicates the location of the raised dot and identifies which side of the film should be directed toward the x-ray tube.

A thin lead foil backing with an embossed pattern is between the wrappers in the film packet. The foil is positioned in the film packet behind the film, away from the tube. This lead foil serves several purposes. It shields the film from backscatter (secondary) radiation, which fogs the film and reduces subject contrast (image quality). It also reduces patient exposure by absorbing some of the residual x-ray beam. Most importantly, if the film packet is placed backward in the patient's mouth so that the tube side of the film is facing away from the x-ray machine, the lead foil will be positioned between the subject and the film. In this circumstance, most of the radiation is absorbed by the lead foil, and the resulting radiograph is light and shows the embossed pattern in the lead foil (Fig. 5-6). This combination of a light film with the characteristic pattern indicates that the film packet was exposed backward in the patient's mouth and that the patient's right side–left side designation indicated by the film dot is reversed.

Periapical View

Periapical views are used to record the crowns, roots, and surrounding bone. Film packs come in three sizes: (1) size 0 for small children (22 mm × 35 mm); (2) size 1, which is relatively narrow and used for views of the anterior teeth (24 mm × 40 mm); and (3) size 2, the standard film size used for adults (30.5 mm × 40.5 mm) (Fig. 5-7).

Bitewing View

Bitewing (interproximal) views are used to record the coronal portions of the maxillary and mandibular teeth in one image. They are useful for detecting interproximal caries and evaluating the height of alveolar bone. Size 2 film is normally used in adults; the smaller size 1 is preferred in children. In small children, size 0 may be used. A relatively long size 3 is also available.

Bitewing films often have a paper tab projecting from the middle of the film on which the patient bites to support the film (Fig. 5-8). This tab is rarely visualized and does not interfere with the diagnostic quality of the image. Film-holding instruments for bitewing projections also are available.

Occlusal View

Occlusal film, size 4, is more than three times larger than size 2 film (see Fig. 5-7). It is used to show larger areas of the maxilla or mandible than may be seen on a periapical film. These films also are used to obtain right-angle views to the usual periapical view. The name derives from the fact that the film is held in position by having the patient bite lightly on it to support it between the occlusal surfaces of the teeth (see Chapter 7).

SCREEN FILM

The extraoral projections used most frequently in dentistry are panoramic and cephalometric views. For these projections, screen

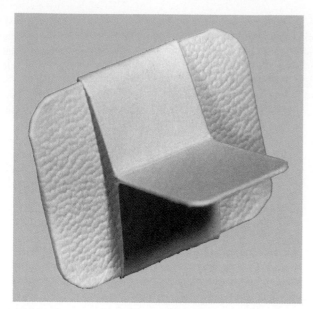

FIGURE 5-8 Paper loop placed around a size 2 adult film to support the film when the patient bites on the tab for a bitewing projection. This projection reveals the tooth crowns and alveolar crests.

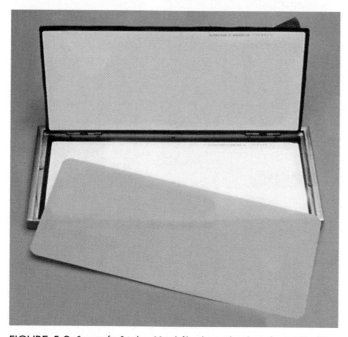

FIGURE 5-9 Cassette for 8 inch × 10 inch film along with a sheet of screen film. When the cassette is closed, the film is supported in close contact between the two white intensifying screens seen on the inside of the cassette. These intensifying screens absorb most of the incident x-ray beam and then fluoresce and expose the film.

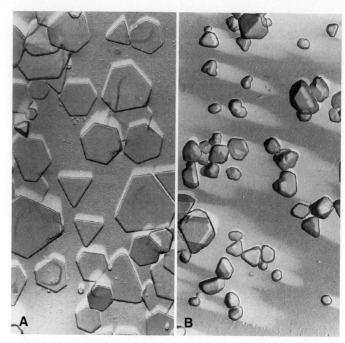

FIGURE 5-10 Tablet grains of silver halide in an emulsion of T-MAT film **(A)** are larger and flatter than the smaller, thicker crystals in an emulsion of older conventional film **(B)**. The flat surfaces of the tablet grains are oriented parallel with the film surface, facing the radiation source. *(Courtesy of Carestream Dental, a division of Carestream Health, Inc.)*

film is used with intensifying screens (described later in this chapter) to reduce patient exposure (Fig. 5-9). Screen film is different from dental intraoral film. It is designed to be sensitive to visible light because it is placed between two intensifying screens when an exposure is made. The intensifying screens absorb x rays and emit visible light, which exposes the film. Silver halide crystals are inherently sensitive to ultraviolet (UV) and blue light (300 to 500 nm) and thus are sensitive to screens that emit UV and blue light. When film is used with screens that emit green light, the

silver halide crystals are coated with sensitizing dyes to increase absorption. It is important to use the appropriate screen-film combination recommended by the screen and film manufacturer so that the emission characteristics of the screen match the absorption characteristics of the film.

Contemporary screen films use tabular-shaped (flat) grains of silver halide (Fig. 5-10) to capture the image. The tabular grains are oriented with their relatively large, flat surfaces facing the radiation source, providing a larger cross section (target) and resulting in increased speed without loss of sharpness. To increase the sharpness of images, some manufacturers add an absorbing dye in the film emulsion. This dye reduces light from one screen crossing through the film to reach the emulsion on the opposite side. EVG film from Carestream Dental is an example of this type of film.

INTENSIFYING SCREENS

Early in the history of radiography, scientists discovered that various inorganic salts or phosphors fluoresce (emit visible light) when exposed to an x-ray beam. The intensity of this fluorescence is proportional to the x-ray energy absorbed. These phosphors are incorporated into intensifying screens for use with screen film. The sum of the effects of the x rays and the visible light emitted by the screen phosphors exposes the film in an intensifying cassette (see Fig. 5-9).

FUNCTION

The presence of intensifying screens creates an image receptor system that is 10 to 60 times more sensitive to x rays than the film alone. Consequently, use of intensifying screens substantially reduces the dose of x radiation to the patient. Intensifying screens are used with films for virtually all extraoral radiography, including panoramic, cephalometric, and skull projections. Generally, the resolving power of screens is related to their speed: the slower the speed of a screen, the greater its resolving power, and vice versa. Intensifying screens are not used intraorally with periapical or occlusal films because their use would reduce the resolution of the resulting image below that necessary for diagnosis of much dental disease.

COMPOSITION

Intensifying screens are made of a base supporting material, a phosphor layer, and a protective polymeric coat (Fig. 5-11). In all dental applications, intensifying screens are used in pairs, one on each side of the film, and they are positioned inside a cassette (see Fig. 5-9). The purpose of a cassette is to hold each intensifying screen in contact with the x-ray film to maximize the sharpness of the image.

Base

The base material of most intensifying screens is some form of polyester plastic that is about 0.25 mm thick. The base provides mechanical support for the other layers. In some intensifying screens, the base also is reflective; thus it reflects light emitted from the phosphor layer back toward the x-ray film. This reflective base increases the light emission of the intensifying screen but also results in some image "unsharpness" because of the divergence of light rays reflected back to the film.

Phosphor Layer

The phosphor layer is composed of phosphorescent crystals suspended in a polymeric binder. When the crystals absorb x-ray photons, they fluoresce (see Fig. 5-11). The phosphor crystals often contain rare earth elements, most commonly lanthanum and gadolinium. Their fluorescence can be increased by the addition of small amounts of elements, such as thulium, niobium, or terbium. Common phosphor combinations used in intensifying screens are shown in Table 5-2. Rare earth screens convert each absorbed x-ray photon into about 4000 lower energy, visible light (green or blue) photons. These visible photons expose the film.

Different phosphors fluoresce in different portions of the spectrum. For example, light emission from Lanex rare earth intensifying screens ranges from 375 to 600 nm and peaks sharply at 545 nm (green). Figure 5-12 shows the spectral emission of a rare earth screen and the spectral sensitivity of an appropriate film. Other intensifying screens have a major peak at 350 nm (UV) and at 450 nm (blue). It is important to match green-emitting screens with green-sensitive films and blue-emitting screens with blue-sensitive films.

Fast screens have large phosphor crystals and efficiently convert x-ray photons to visible light but produce images with lower resolution. As the size of the crystals or the thickness of the screen decreases, the speed of the screen also declines, but image sharpness increases. Fast screens also have a thicker phosphor layer and a reflective layer, but these properties also decrease sharpness. In deciding on the combination to use, the practitioner must consider the resolution requirements of the task for which the image will be used. Screen-film combinations are rated for speed, a measure of the amount of radiation required for a proper exposure. For dental extraoral diagnostic tasks, it is recommended to use screen-film combinations that have a speed of 400 or faster.

Protective Coat

A protective polymer coat (≤15 μm thick) is placed over the phosphor layer to protect the phosphor and to provide a surface that can be cleaned. The intensifying screens should be routinely cleaned because any debris, spots, or scratches may cause light spots on the resultant radiograph.

TABLE 5-2	Rare Earth Elements Used in Intensifying Screens
Emission	**Phosphor**
Green	Gadolinium oxysulfide, terbium activated
Blue and UV	Yttrium tantalite, niobium activated

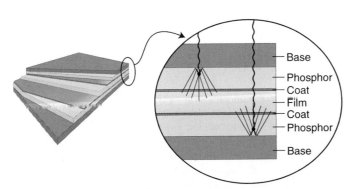

FIGURE 5-11 Image on the *left* shows a schematic of two intensifying screens enclosing a film (yellow). An intensifying screen is composed of a supporting base (purple), a layer containing the phosphors (light blue), and a protective coat (orange). The detailed view on the *right* shows x-ray photons entering at the top, traveling through the base, and striking phosphors in the base. The phosphors emit visible light, exposing the film. Some visible light photons may reflect off the reflecting layer of the base.

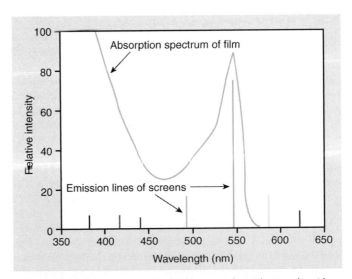

FIGURE 5-12 Relative sensitivity of T-MAT film (*orange line*) and emission lines (shown in their visual colors) of Carestream Dental LANEX and EV screens (gadolinium oxysulfide, terbium activated). Intensifying screens emit light as a series of relatively narrow line emissions. The maximal emission of the screen at 545 nm (*green*) corresponds well to a high-sensitivity region of the film. (*Data from Carestream Dental, a division of Carestream Health, Inc.*)

FORMATION OF THE LATENT IMAGE

When a beam of photons exits an object and exposes an x-ray film (either direct-exposure film or screen film exposed by light photons), it chemically changes the photosensitive silver halide crystals in the film emulsion. These chemically altered silver bromide crystals constitute the latent (invisible) image on the film. Before exposure, film emulsion consists of photosensitive crystals containing primarily silver bromide (Fig. 5-13, *A*). These silver halide crystals also contain a few free silver ions (interstitial silver ions) and trace amounts of sulfur compounds bound to the surface of the crystals. Along with physical irregularities in the crystal produced by iodide ions, sulfur compounds create sensitivity sites, sites in the crystals that are sensitive to radiation. Each crystal has many sensitivity sites. When the silver halide crystals are irradiated, x-ray photons release electrons from the bromide ions (Fig. 5-13, *B*). The free electrons move through the crystal until they reach a sensitivity site, where they become trapped and impart a negative charge to the site. The negatively charged sensitivity site attracts positively charged free interstitial silver ions (Fig. 5-13, *C*). When a silver ion reaches the negatively charged sensitivity site, it is reduced and forms a neutral atom of metallic silver (Fig. 5-13, *D*). The sites containing these neutral silver atoms are now called latent image sites. This process occurs numerous times within a crystal. The overall distribution of crystals with latent image sites

in a film after exposure constitutes the latent image. Processing the exposed film in developer and fixer converts the latent image into the visible radiographic image.

PROCESSING SOLUTIONS

Film processing involves the following procedures:
1. Immerse exposed film in developer.
2. Rinse developer off film in water bath.
3. Immerse film in fixer.
4. Wash film in water bath to remove fixer.
5. Dry film and mount for viewing.

Following exposure, each grain of silver halide in film emulsion (Fig. 5-14, *A*) contains neutral silver atoms at their latent image sites (Fig. 5-14, *B*). These latent image sites render the crystals sensitive to development and image formation. Developer converts silver bromide crystals with neutral silver atoms deposited at the latent image sites into black, solid silver metallic grains (Fig. 5-14, *C*). These solid silver grains block light from a viewbox. Fixer removes unexposed, undeveloped silver bromide crystals (crystals without latent image sites), leaving the film clear in unexposed areas (Fig. 5-14, *D*). Thus the radiographic image is composed of light (radiopaque) areas, where few photons reached the film, and dark (radiolucent) areas of the film that were struck by many photons.

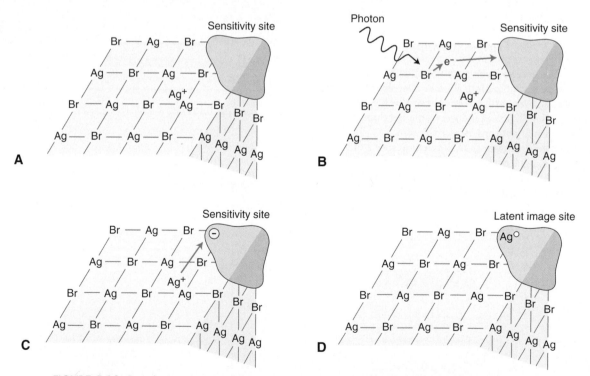

FIGURE 5-13 **A,** A silver bromide crystal in the emulsion of an x-ray film contains mostly silver and bromide ions in a crystal lattice. There are also free interstitial silver ions and areas of trace chemicals that form sensitivity sites. **B,** Exposure of the crystal to photons in an x-ray beam results in the release of electrons, usually by interaction of the photon with a bromide ion. The recoil electrons have sufficient kinetic energy to move about in the crystal. When electrons reach a sensitivity site, they impart a negative charge to this region. **C,** Free interstitial silver ions (with a positive charge) are attracted to the negatively charged sensitivity site. **D,** When the silver ions reach the sensitivity site, they acquire an electron and become neutral silver atoms. These silver atoms now constitute a latent image site. The collection of latent image sites over the entire film constitutes the latent image. Developer causes the neutral silver atoms at the latent image sites to initiate the conversion of all the silver ions in the crystal into one large grain of metallic silver. The bromine dissolves in the developer.

DEVELOPING SOLUTION

The developer reduces all silver ions in the exposed crystals of silver halide (crystals with a latent image) to metallic silver grains (see Fig. 5-14). To produce a diagnostic image, this reduction process must be restricted to crystals containing latent image sites; to accomplish this, the reducing agents used as developers are catalyzed by the neutral silver atoms at the latent image sites (see Fig. 5-14, *B*). Individual crystals are developed completely or not at all during the recommended developing times (see Fig. 5-14, *C*). Variations in density on the processed radiographs are the result of different ratios of developed (exposed) and undeveloped (unexposed) crystals. Areas with many exposed crystals are darker because of their higher concentration of black metallic silver grains after development.

When an exposed film is developed, the developer initially has no visible effect (Fig. 5-15). After this initial phase, the density increases, rapidly at first and then more slowly. Eventually, all the exposed crystals develop (are converted to black metallic silver), and the developing agent starts to reduce the unexposed crystals.

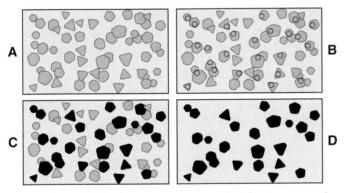

FIGURE 5-14 Emulsion changes during film processing. **A,** Before exposure, many silver bromide crystals (gray) are present in the emulsion. **B,** After exposure, the exposed crystals containing neutral silver atoms at latent image sites (orange dots within some crystals) constitute the latent image. **C,** The developer converts the exposed crystals containing neutral silver atoms at the latent image sites into solid grains of metallic silver (black). **D,** The fixer dissolves the unexposed, undeveloped silver bromide crystals, leaving only the solid silver grains that form the radiographic image.

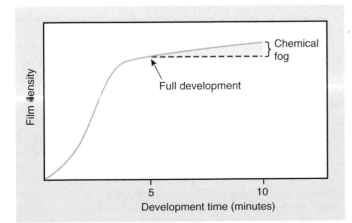

FIGURE 5-15 Relationship between film density and development time. The density of film increases quickly initially in the developer. After full development, the density continues to increase slowly because of chemical fogging.

The development of unexposed crystals results in chemical fog on the film. The interval between maximal density and fogging explains why a properly exposed film does not become overdeveloped, although it may be in contact with the developer longer than the recommended interval.

The developing solution contains four components, all dissolved in water: (1) developer, (2) activator, (3) preservative, and (4) restrainer.

Developer

Developer converts exposed silver halide crystals into metallic silver grains. Two developing agents, usually phenidone and hydroquinone, are used in dental radiology. Phenidone serves as the first electron donor that converts silver ions to metallic silver at the latent image site. This electron transfer generates the oxidized form of phenidone. Hydroquinone provides an electron to reduce the oxidized phenidone back to its original active state so that it can continue to reduce silver halide grains to metallic silver. Unexposed crystals—crystals without latent images are unaffected during the time required for reduction of the exposed crystals.

Activator

The developers are active only at pH values around 10. This pH is achieved with the addition of alkali compounds (activators) such as sodium or potassium hydroxide. Buffers are used to maintain this condition. The activators also cause the gelatin to swell so that the developing agents can diffuse more rapidly into the emulsion to reach silver bromide crystals.

Preservative

The developing solution contains an antioxidant or preservative, usually sodium sulfite, which extends the useful life of the solution. The preservative also combines with oxidized developer to produce a compound that subsequently stains images brown if not washed out.

Bromide-containing compounds are added to the developing solution to restrain development of unexposed silver halide crystals. Restrainers act as antifog agents and increase contrast.

DEVELOPER REPLENISHER

The developing solution of both manual and automatic developers should be replenished with fresh solution each morning to prolong the life of the used developer. The recommended amount to be added daily is 8 ounces of fresh developer (replenisher) per gallon of developing solution. This assumes the development of an average of 30 periapical or 5 panoramic films per day. Some of the used solution may need to be removed to make room for the replenisher.

RINSING

After development, the film emulsion swells and becomes saturated with developer. At this point, the films are rinsed in water for 30 seconds with continuous, gentle agitation before they are placed in the fixer. Rinsing dilutes the developer, slowing the development process. It also removes the alkali activator, preventing neutralization of the acid fixer. This rinsing process is typical for manual processing but is not used with most automatic processors.

FIXING SOLUTION

Fixing solution removes undeveloped silver halide crystals from the emulsion (see Fig. 5-14, *D*). If these crystals are not removed, the image on the resultant radiograph is dark and nondiagnostic (Fig. 5-16). Figure 5-17 is a photomicrograph of film emulsion showing the solid silver grains after fixer has removed the unexposed silver bromide crystals. (Compare it with Fig. 5-2, which shows the unprocessed emulsion.) Fixer also hardens and shrinks the film emulsion. As with developer, fixer should be replenished daily at the rate of 8 ounces per gallon.

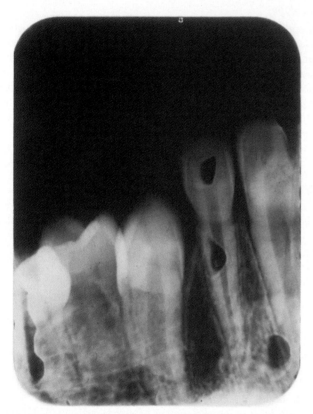

FIGURE 5-16 Incomplete fixation results in images that are dark and discolored, making them diagnostic. This film was also poorly positioned in the patient's mouth, cutting off most apices of the teeth. Staining may also be caused by using depleted developer or fixer or using contaminated solutions.

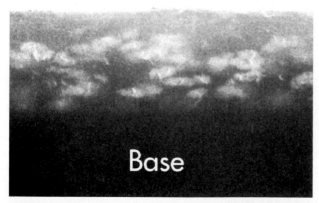

FIGURE 5-17 Scanning electron micrograph of a processed emulsion of Ultra-speed dental x-ray film (500×). Note the white-appearing solid silver grains above the base. (Courtesy of Carestream Dental, a division of Carestream Health, Inc.)

Fixing solution also contains four components, all dissolved in water: (1) clearing agent, (2) acidifier, (3) preservative, and (4) hardener.

Clearing Agent

An aqueous solution of ammonium thiosulfate ("hypo") dissolves the unexposed silver halide grains. It forms stable, water-soluble complexes with silver ions, which diffuse from the emulsion. Excessive fixation (hours) results in a gradual loss of film density because the grains of silver slowly dissolve in the acetic acid of the fixing solution.

Acidifier

The fixing solution contains an acetic acid buffer system (pH 4 to 4.5) to keep the fixer pH constant. The acidic pH is required to promote good diffusion of thiosulfate into the emulsion and of silver thiosulfate complex out of the emulsion. The acid-fixing solution also inactivates any residual developing agents in the film emulsion, blocking continued development of any unexposed crystals while the film is in the fixing tank.

Preservative

Ammonium sulfite is the preservative in the fixing solution, as it is in the developer. It prevents oxidation of the thiosulfate clearing agent, which is unstable in the acid environment of the fixing solution.

Hardener

A hardening agent, usually aluminum sulfate, complexes with the gelatin during fixing and prevents damage to the gelatin during subsequent handling. The hardeners also reduce swelling of the emulsion during the final wash. This reduction of swelling lessens mechanical damage to the emulsion and shortens drying time.

WASHING

After fixing, the processed film is washed in water to remove all thiosulfate ions and silver thiosulfate complexes. Washing efficiency declines rapidly when the water temperature decreases to less than 60° F. Any silver compound or thiosulfate that remains because of improper washing discolors and causes stains, which are most apparent in the radiopaque (light) areas.

DARKROOM AND EQUIPMENT

A conventional darkroom with manual wet processing tanks should be convenient to the x-ray machines and dental operatories and should be at least 4 feet × 5 feet (1.2 m × 1.5 m) (Fig. 5-18).

DARKROOM

One of the most important requirements is that the darkroom be lightproof. If it is not, stray light can cause film fogging and loss of contrast. To make the darkroom lightproof, a light-tight door or doorless maze (if space permits) is used. The door should have a lock to prevent accidental opening, which might allow an unexpected flood of light that can ruin opened films. The darkroom must also be well ventilated for the comfort of people working in the area and to exhaust moisture from drying films. Also, a comfortable room temperature helps maintain optimal conditions for developing, fixing, and washing solutions.

SAFELIGHTING

The processing room should have both white illumination and safelighting. Safelighting is low-intensity illumination of relatively long wavelength (red) that does not rapidly affect open film but permits one to see well enough to work in the area (Fig. 5-19). To minimize the fogging effect of prolonged exposure, the safelight should have a frosted 15-watt bulb or a clear 7.5-watt bulb and should be mounted at least 4 feet above the surface where opened films are handled.

X-ray films are very sensitive to the blue-green region of the spectrum and are less sensitive to red wavelengths. The red GBX-2 filter is recommended as a safelight in darkrooms where either intraoral or extraoral films are handled because this filter transmits light only at the red end of the spectrum (Fig. 5-20). Film handling under a safelight should be limited to about 5 minutes because film emulsion shows some sensitivity to light from a safelight with prolonged exposure. The older ML-2 filters (yellow light) are not appropriate for fast intraoral dental film or extraoral panoramic or cephalometric film.

MANUAL PROCESSING TANKS

It is wise for dental offices to have the capability to develop film by tank processing, if only as a backup for an automatic processor or digital imaging system. The tank must have hot and cold running water and a means of maintaining the temperature between 60° F and 75° F. A practical size for a dental office is a master tank about 20 cm × 25 cm (8 inches × 10

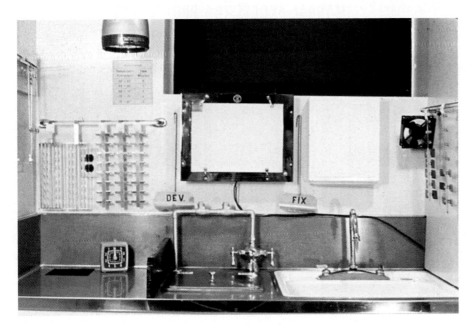

FIGURE 5-18 Darkroom work area. *Left,* Film mounting area, timer, film racks, and safelight above. *Middle,* Developing and fixing tanks below the viewbox and stirring paddles. *Right,* Sink and drying racks with fan. *(Courtesy C. L. Crabtree, DDS, Bureau of Radiological Health, Rockville, MD.)*

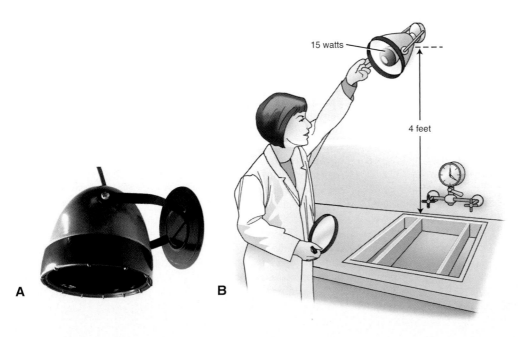

15 watts

4 feet

FIGURE 5-19 **A,** A safelight may be mounted on the wall or ceiling in the darkroom and should be at least 4 feet from the work surface. **B,** The safelight uses a GBX-2 filter and 15-watt bulb.

A   B

inches) that can serve as a water jacket for two removable inserts that fit inside (Fig. 5-21). The insert tanks usually hold 3.8 L (1 gallon) of developer or fixer and are placed within the outer, larger master tank. The outer tank holds the water for maintaining the temperature of the developer and fixer in the insert tanks and for washing films. The developer customarily is placed in the insert tank on the left side of the master tank, and the fixer is placed in the insert tank on the right. All three tanks should be made of stainless steel, which does not react with the processing solutions and is easy to clean. The master tank should have a cover to reduce oxidation of the processing solutions, protect the developing film from accidental exposure to light, and minimize evaporation of the processing solutions.

THERMOMETER

The temperature of the developing, fixing, and washing solutions should be closely controlled. A thermometer can be left in the water circulating through the master tank to monitor the temperature and ensure that the water temperature regulator is working properly. The most desirable thermometers clip onto the side of the tank. Thermometers may contain alcohol or metal, but they should not contain mercury because they could break and contaminate the processor or solutions.

TIMER

The x-ray film must be exposed to the processing chemicals for specific intervals. An interval timer is indispensable for controlling development and fixation times.

DRYING RACKS

Two or three drying racks can be mounted on a convenient wall for film hangers. Drip trays are placed underneath the racks to catch water that may run off the wet films. An electric fan can be used to circulate the air and speed the drying of films, but it should not be pointed directly at the films.

MANUAL PROCESSING PROCEDURES

Manual processing of film requires the following eight steps:
1. *Replenish solutions.* The first step in manual tank processing is to replenish the developer and fixer. Check the solution levels to

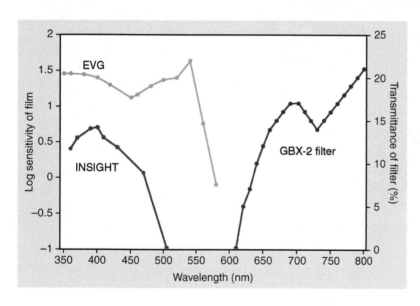

FIGURE 5-20 Spectral sensitivities of EVG film *(green line)* and INSIGHT film *(blue line)* shown with the transmission characteristics of a GBX-2 filter *(red line)*. The films are more sensitive in the blue-green portion of the spectrum (shorter than 600 nm), whereas the GBX-2 filter transmits primarily at the red end of the spectrum (longer than 600 nm).

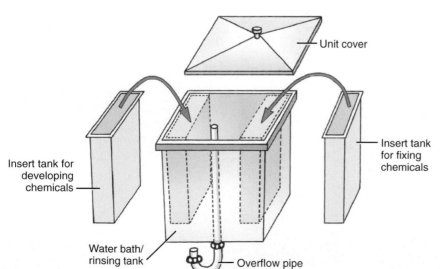

FIGURE 5-21 Processing tank. The developing and fixing tanks are inserted into a bath of running water with an overflow drain. The water bath may be maintained at a stable and optimal temperature for film processing.

ensure that the developer and fixer cover the films on the top clips of the film hangers.

2. *Stir solutions.* Stir the developer and fixing solution to mix the chemicals and equalize the temperature throughout the tanks. To prevent cross-contamination, use a separate paddle for each solution. It is best to label one paddle for the developer and the other for the fixer.

3. *Mount films on hangers.* Using only safelight illumination in the darkroom, remove the exposed film from its lightproof packet or cassette. Hold the films by their edges only to avoid damage to the film surface. Clip the bare film onto a film hanger, one film to a clip (Fig. 5-22). Label the film racks with the patient's name and the exposure date.

4. *Set timer.* Check the temperature of the developer, and set the interval timer to the time indicated by the manufacturer for the solution temperature, typically:

Temperature (°F)	Development Time (minutes)
68	5
70	4½
72	4
76	3
80	2½

Processing films at either higher or lower temperatures and for longer or shorter times than recommended by the manufacturer reduces the contrast of the processed film.

5. *Develop.* Start the timer mechanism, and immerse the hanger and films immediately in the developer. Agitate the hanger mildly for 5 seconds to remove air bubbles from the film. Do not agitate the film during development.

6. *Rinse.* After development, remove the film hanger from the developer, draining excess into the water bath, and place in the running water bath for 30 seconds. Agitate the films continuously in the rinse water to remove excess developer, thus slowing development and minimizing contamination of the fixer.

7. *Fix.* Place the hanger and film in the fixer solution for 2 to 4 minutes and agitate for 5 of every 30 seconds. Agitation eliminates bubbles and brings fresh fixer into contact with the emulsion. When the films are removed, drain the excess fixer into the wash bath.

8. *Wash.* After fixation of the films is complete, place the hanger in running water for at least 10 minutes to remove residual processing solutions. After the films have been washed, remove surface moisture by gently shaking excess water from the films and hanger.

9. *Dry.* Dry the films in circulating, moderately warm air. After drying, the films are ready to mount.

RAPID-PROCESSING CHEMICALS

Rapid-processing solutions typically develop films in 15 seconds and fix them in 15 seconds at room temperature. They have the same general formulation as conventional processing solutions but often contain a higher concentration of hydroquinone. They also have a more alkaline pH than conventional solutions, which causes the emulsion to swell more, thus providing greater access to developer. These solutions are especially advantageous in endodontics and in emergency situations, when short processing time is essential. Although the resultant images may be satisfactory, they often do not achieve the same degree of contrast as films processed conventionally, and they may discolor over time if not fully washed. After viewing, rapidly processed films are placed in conventional fixing solution for 4 minutes and washed for 10 minutes; this improves the contrast and helps keep them stable in storage. Conventional solutions are preferred for most routine use.

CHANGING SOLUTIONS

All processing solutions deteriorate as a result of continued use and exposure to air. Although regular replenishment of the developer and fixer prolongs their useful life, the buildup of reaction products eventually causes these solutions to cease functioning properly. Exhaustion of the developer results from oxidation of the developing agents, depletion of the hydroquinone, and buildup of bromide. With regular replenishment, solutions may last 3 or 4 weeks before they must be changed.

A simple procedure can help determine when solutions should be changed. A double film packet is exposed on one projection for the first patient radiographed after new solutions have been prepared. One film is placed in the patient's chart, and the other is mounted on a corner of a viewbox in the darkroom. As successive films are processed, they are compared with this reference film. Loss of image contrast and density become evident as the solutions deteriorate, indicating when it is time to change them. The fixer is changed when the developer is changed.

AUTOMATIC FILM PROCESSING

Equipment that automates all processing steps is available (Fig. 5-23). Although automatic processing has numerous advantages, the most important is the time saved. Depending on the equipment and the temperature of operation, an automatic processor requires only 4 to 6 minutes to develop, fix, wash, and dry a film. Many dental automatic processors have a light-shielded (daylight loading) compartment in which the operator can unwrap films and feed them into the machine without working in a darkroom.

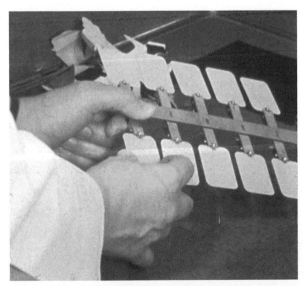

FIGURE 5-22 Films are mounted securely on film clips. Film is always held by its edges to avoid fingerprints on the image. *(Courtesy C. L. Crabtree, DDS, Bureau of Radiological Health, Rockville, MD.)*

However, special care must be taken to maintain infection control when using these daylight-loading compartments (see Chapter 15).

When extraoral films are processed, the light-shielded compartment is removed to provide room for feeding the larger film into the processor. Another attractive feature of the automatic system is that the density and contrast of the radiographs tend to be consistent. However, because of the higher temperature of the developer and the artifacts caused by rollers, the quality of films processed automatically often is not as high as the quality of films carefully developed manually. With automatically processed films, if more grain is evident in the final image, the correct choice of processing solutions may be able to help minimize the issue.

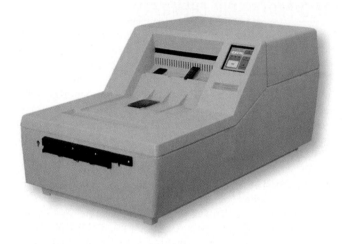

FIGURE 5-23   Dent-X 810 AR film automatic film processor. The operator opens the film packet in a darkroom and inserts the film into the opening on the left end of the machine. The exposed film is carried on a roller apparatus through processing solutions, and the processed and dried film is returned through the upper right opening in 4.5 minutes. (Courtesy Image-Works, Elmsford, NY.)

Whether automatic processing equipment is appropriate for a specific practice depends on the dentist and the nature and volume of the practice. The equipment is expensive and must be cleaned frequently, as described by the processor manufacturer. Also, automated equipment may break down, and conventional darkroom equipment may still be needed as a backup system.

MECHANISM

Automatic processors have an in-line arrangement consisting of a transport mechanism that picks up exposed, unwrapped film and passes it through the developing, fixing, washing, and drying sections (Fig. 5-24). The transport system most often used is a series of rollers driven by a motor that operates through gears, belts, or chains. The rollers often consist of independent assemblies of multiple rollers in a rack, with one rack for each step in the operation. Although these assemblies are designed and positioned so that the film crosses over from one roller to the next, the operator may remove them independently for cleaning and repairing.

The primary function of the rollers is to move the film through the developing solutions, but they also serve at least three other purposes. First, their motion helps keep the solutions agitated, which contributes to the uniformity of processing. Second, in the developer, fixer, and water tanks, the rollers press on the film emulsion, forcing some solution out of the emulsion. The emulsions rapidly fill again with solution, thus promoting solution exchange. Finally, the top rollers at the crossover point between the developer and fixer tanks remove developing solution, minimizing carryover of developer into the fixer tank. This feature helps maintain the uniformity of processing chemicals.

The chemical compositions of the developer and fixer are modified to operate at higher temperatures than the temperatures used for manual processing and to meet the more rapid development, fixing, washing, and drying requirements of automatic processing. The quality of the fixer is very important. High quality fixers

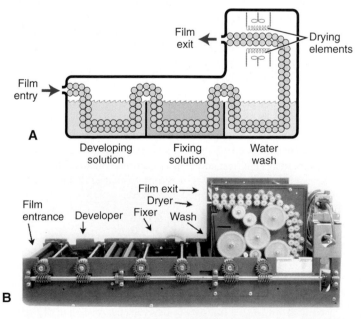

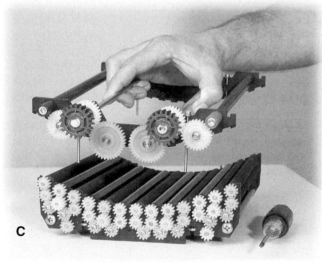

FIGURE 5-24   **A,** Automatic film processors typically consist of a roller assembly that transports the film through developing, fixing, washing, and drying stations. **B,** Assembly of film transport mechanism. **C,** One roller assembly. (**B** and **C,** Courtesy ImageWorks, Elmsford, NY.)

contain an additional hardener that helps the emulsion withstand the rigors of the transport system and improves transport. Poor quality fixers containing no hardener produce more film artifacts, and film may slip and jam during transport.

OPERATION

Successful operation of an automatic processor requires standardized procedures and regular maintenance. The processor and surrounding area should always be kept clean so that no chemicals contaminate hands or films. The solution level and temperature should be checked each morning before films are processed. Hands should be dry when handling film, and films should be touched on their edges only. The better processors have automatic replenishment systems. A daily, weekly, and quarterly maintenance routine (see Chapter 15) should be followed, including cleaning the rollers and other working parts. It is vital to run a large roller transport clean-up film daily through the processor to clean the top and bottom rollers.

ESTABLISHING CORRECT EXPOSURE TIMES

When radiographs are first made with a new x-ray machine, it is important to examine the exposure guidelines that come with the machine. Typically, such guidelines provide a table listing the various anatomic regions (incisors, premolars, or molars), patient size (adult or child), and the length of the aiming cylinder. For each of these combinations, there is a suggested exposure time. It is also important to start out using fresh processing chemicals and optimal processing conditions as previously described. After the first images are made on patients, it may be necessary to adjust exposure time. If optimal film processing techniques are being followed and the images are consistently dark, exposure times should be decreased until optimal images are obtained. If images are consistently light, exposure times should be increased. When the optimal times have been determined, these values should be posted by the control panel.

MANAGEMENT OF RADIOGRAPHIC WASTES

To prevent environmental damage, many communities and states have passed laws governing the disposal of wastes. Such laws often derive from the federal Resource Conservation and Recovery Act of 1976. Although dental radiographic waste constitutes only a small potential hazard, it should be discarded properly. The primary ingredient of concern in processing solutions is the dissolved silver found in used fixer. Another material of concern is the lead foil found in film packets. Dental offices also should consider using companies licensed to pick up waste materials.

IMAGE CHARACTERISTICS

Processing an exposed x-ray film causes it to become dark in the exposed area. The degree and pattern of film darkening depend on numerous factors, including the energy and intensity of the x-ray beam, composition of the subject imaged, film emulsion used, and characteristics of film processing. This section describes the major imaging characteristics of x-ray film.

RADIOGRAPHIC DENSITY

When a film is exposed by an x-ray beam (or by light, in the case of screen-film combinations) and then processed, the silver halide

crystals in the emulsion that were struck by the photons are converted to grains of metallic silver. These silver grains block the transmission of light from a viewbox and give the film its dark appearance. The degree of darkening or opacity of an exposed film is referred to as optical density. The optical density of an area of an x-ray film can be measured as follows:

$$\text{Optical density} = \text{Log}_{10}\frac{I_o}{I_t}$$

where I_o is the intensity of incident light (e.g., from a viewbox), and I_t is the intensity of the light transmitted through the film. With an optical density of 0, 100% of the light is transmitted; with a density of 1, 10% of the light is transmitted; with a density of 2, 1% of the light is transmitted; and so on.

A plot of the relationship between film optical density and exposure is called a characteristic curve (Fig. 5-25). It usually is shown as the relationship between the optical density of the film and the logarithm of the corresponding exposure. As exposure of the film increases, its optical density increases. A film is of greatest diagnostic value when the structures of interest are imaged on the relatively straight portion of the graph, between 0.6 and 3.0 optical density units. The characteristic curves of films reveal much information about film contrast, speed, and latitude.

An unexposed film, when processed, shows some density. This appearance is caused by the inherent density of the base and added tint and the development of a few unexposed silver halide crystals. This minimal density is called base plus fog and typically is 0.2 to 0.3. Radiographic density is influenced by exposure and the thickness and density of the subject.

Exposure

The overall film density depends on the number of photons absorbed by the film emulsion. Increasing the milliamperage (mA), peak kilovoltage (kVp), or exposure time increases the number of photons reaching the film and thus increases the density of the radiograph. Reducing the distance between the focal spot and film also increases film density.

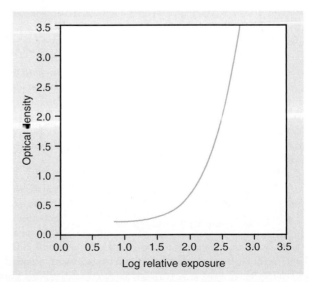

FIGURE 5-25 Characteristic curve of direct exposure film. The contrast (slope of the curve) is greater in the high-density region than in the low-density region.

Subject Thickness

The thicker the subject, the more the beam is attenuated, and the lighter the resultant image (Fig. 5-26). If exposure factors intended for adults are used on children or edentulous patients, the resultant films are dark because a smaller amount of absorbing tissue is in the path of the x-ray beam. The dentist should vary exposure time according to the patient's size to produce radiographs of optimal density.

Subject Density

Variations in the density of the subject exert a profound influence on the image. The greater the density of a structure within the subject, the greater the attenuation of the x-ray beam directed through that subject or area. In the oral cavity, the relative densities of various natural structures, in order of decreasing density, are enamel, dentin and cementum, bone, muscle, fat, and air. Metallic objects (e.g., restorations) are far denser than enamel and hence better absorbers. Because an x-ray beam is differentially attenuated by these absorbers, the resultant beam carries information that is recorded on the radiographic film as light and dark areas. Dense objects (which are strong absorbers) cause the radiographic image to be light and are said to be radiopaque. Objects with low

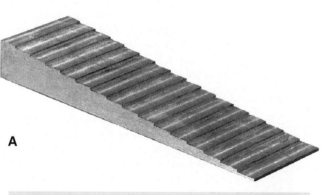

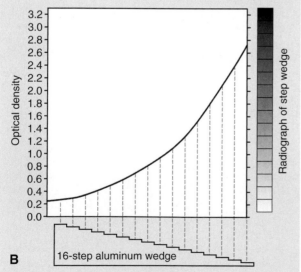

FIGURE 5-26 **A,** Aluminum step wedge. **B,** Graph of the optical density of a radiograph made by exposing the step wedge. As the thickness of the aluminum decreases, more photons are passed through the wedge and are available to expose the film, and the image becomes progressively darker.

densities are weak absorbers. They allow most photons to pass through, and they cast a dark area on the film that corresponds to the radiolucent object.

RADIOGRAPHIC CONTRAST

Radiographic contrast is a general term that describes the range of densities on a radiograph. It is defined as the difference in densities between light and dark regions on a radiograph. An image that shows both light areas and dark areas has high contrast; this also is referred to as a short gray scale of contrast because few shades of gray are present between the black-and-white images on the film. Alternatively, a radiographic image composed only of light gray and dark gray zones has low contrast, also referred to as having a long gray scale of contrast (Fig. 5-27). The radiographic contrast of an image is the result of the interplay of subject contrast, film contrast, scattered radiation, and beam energy.

Subject Contrast

Subject contrast is the range of characteristics of the subject that influences radiographic contrast. It is influenced largely by the subject's thickness, density, and atomic number. The subject contrast of a patient's head and neck exposed in a lateral cephalometric view is high. The dense regions of the bone and teeth absorb most of the incident radiation, whereas the soft tissue facial profile transmits most of the radiation.

Subject contrast also is influenced by beam energy and intensity. The energy of the x-ray beam, selected by the kVp, influences image contrast. Figure 5-28 shows an aluminum step wedge exposed to x-ray beams of differing energies. Because increasing the kVp increases the overall density of the image, the exposure time has been adjusted so that the density of the middle step in each case is comparable. As the kVp of the x-ray beam increases, subject contrast decreases. Similarly, when relatively low kVp energies are used, subject contrast increases. Most clinicians select a kVp in the range of 60 to 80. At higher values, the exposure time is reduced, but the loss of contrast may be objectionable because subtle changes may be obscured. Changing the time or mA of the exposure (and holding the kVp constant) also influences subject contrast. If the film is excessively light or dark, contrast of anatomic structures is diminished.

Film Contrast

Film contrast describes the inherent capacity of radiographic films to display differences in subject contrast—that is, variations in the intensity of the remnant beam. A high-contrast film reveals areas of small difference in subject contrast more clearly than a low-contrast film. Film contrast usually is measured as the average slope of the diagnostically useful portion of the characteristic curve (Fig. 5-29): the greater the slope of the curve in this region, the greater the film contrast. In Figure 5-29, film *A* has a higher contrast than film *B*. When the slope of the curve in the useful range is greater than 1, the film exaggerates subject contrast. This desirable feature, which is found in most diagnostic film, allows visualization of structures that differ only slightly in density. For example, the remnant beam in the region of a tooth pulp chamber is more intense (greater exposure) than the beam from the surrounding enamel crown. A high-contrast film shows a greater contrast (difference in optical density) between these structures than a low-contrast film. As can be seen in Figure 5-25, film contrast also depends on the density range being examined. With dental direct-exposure film, the slope of the curve continually increases with increasing exposure. As a result, properly exposed films have more

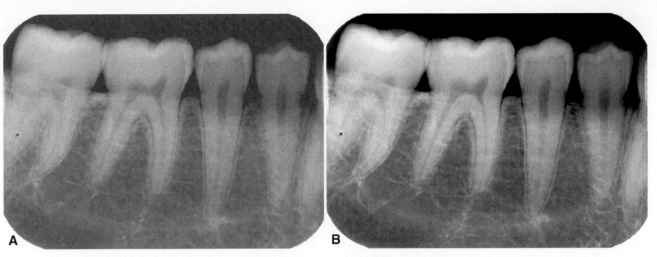

FIGURE 5-27 Radiograph of a dried mandible revealing low contrast **(A)** and high contrast **(B)**.

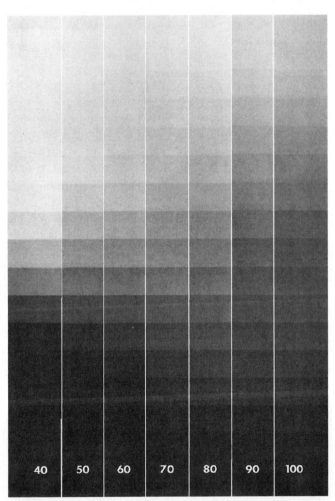

FIGURE 5-28 Seven radiographs of a step wedge made at 40 to 100 kVp shown side by side. As the kVp increased, the mA was reduced to maintain a roughly uniform middle-step density. Note the long gray scale (low contrast) image with high kVp and the short scale (high contrast) image when using low kVp. *(Courtesy of Carestream Dental, a division of Carestream Health, Inc.)*

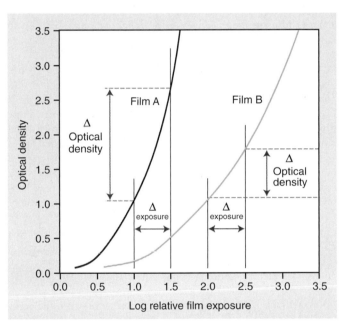

FIGURE 5-29 Characteristic curves of two films demonstrating the greater inherent contrast of film *A* compared with film *B*. The slope of film *A* is greater than the slope of film *B*; film *A* shows a greater change in optical density than film *B* for a constant change in exposure. The fact that film *A* is faster than film *B* in this figure is unrelated to film contrast.

contrast than underexposed (light) films. Films used with intensifying screens typically have a slope in the range of 2 to 3.

Film processing is another factor that influences film contrast. Film contrast is maximized by optimal film processing conditions. Mishandling of the film through incomplete or excessive development diminishes contrast of anatomic structures. Also, storage at too high a temperature, exposure to excessively bright safelights, and light leaks in the darkroom degrade film contrast.

Fog on an x-ray film results in increased film density arising from causes other than exposure to the remnant beam. Film contrast is reduced by the addition of this undesirable density. Common causes of film fog are improper safelighting, storage of film at too high a temperature, expired film, poor chemistry quality, and development of film at an excessive temperature or for a prolonged period. Film fog can be reduced by proper film processing and storage.

Scattered Radiation

Scattered radiation results from photons that have interacted with the subject by Compton or coherent interactions. These interactions cause the emission of photons that travel in directions other than that of the primary beam. This scattered radiation causes fogging of a radiograph—an overall darkening of the image—and results in loss of radiographic contrast. In most dental applications, the best means of reducing scattered radiation are to use a relatively low kVp and to collimate the beam to the size of the film to prevent scatter from an area outside the region of the image.

RADIOGRAPHIC SPEED

Radiographic speed refers to the amount of radiation required to produce an image of a standard density. Film speed frequently is expressed as the reciprocal of the exposure (in roentgens) required to produce an optical density of 1 above base plus fog. A fast film requires a relatively low exposure to produce a density of 1, whereas a slower film requires a longer exposure for the processed film to have the same density. Film speed is controlled largely by the size of the silver halide grains and their silver content.

The speed of dental intraoral x-ray film is indicated by a letter designating a particular group (Table 5-3). The fastest dental film available at the present time has a speed rating of E/F; that is, it is right on the border between the E- and F-speed categories. Only films with a D or faster speed rating are appropriate for intraoral radiography. The types of film used most often in the United States are Ultra-speed (group D) and INSIGHT (high end of the E speed range with manual processing and F with automatic processing conditions). INSIGHT film is preferred because it requires approximately half the exposure time and thus half the radiation dose of Ultra-speed film. INSIGHT film also provides a wider range of processing conditions and should exhibit more detail and a wider range of contrast. INSIGHT F-speed film is faster than Ultra-speed D-speed film because it has double the amount of tabular crystal grains. The characteristic curves in Figure 5-30 show that INSIGHT film (curve on the left) is faster than Ultra-speed film (curve on the right) because less exposure is required to produce the same level of density, although the two films have similar contrast.

FILM LATITUDE

Film latitude is a measure of the range of exposures that can be recorded as distinguishable densities on a film. A film optimized to display wide latitude can record a subject with a wide range of subject contrast. A film with a characteristic curve that has a long straight-line portion and a shallow slope has wide latitude (Fig. 5-31). As a consequence, wide variations in the amount of radiation exiting the subject can be recorded. Films with wide latitude

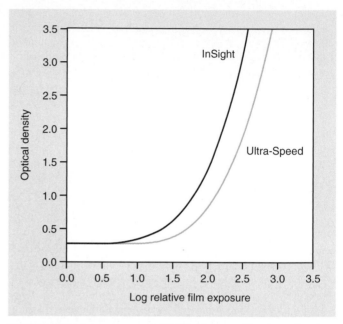

FIGURE 5-30 Characteristic curves for INSIGHT and Ultra-speed film. INSIGHT film is faster and has essentially the same contrast (slope) as Ultra-speed film. INSIGHT film requires only half as much patient exposure and is the preferred film. *(Courtesy of Carestream Dental, a division of Carestream Health, Inc.)*

TABLE 5-3	Intraoral Film Speed Classification per ISO 3665 and ISO 5799
Film Speed Group	**Speed Range (Reciprocal Roentgens*)**
C	No longer listed as no longer offered
D	14–27.9
E	28–55.9
F	56–111.9

Data from National Council on Radiation Protection and Measurements, Report No. 145, Appendix E, 2004.

*Reciprocal roentgens are the reciprocal of the exposure in roentgens required to obtain a film with an optical density of 1.0 above base plus fog after processing. ISO 3665, Third edition, 2011-09-01.

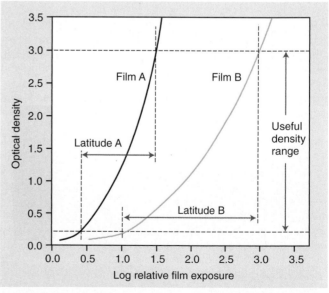

FIGURE 5-31 Characteristic curves for two films demonstrating greater inherent latitude of film *B* compared with film *A*. The slope of film *B* is less steep than the slope of film *A*; film *B* records a greater range of exposures within the useful density range than film *A*.

have lower contrast than films with a narrow latitude. Wide-latitude films are useful when both the osseous structures of the skull and the soft tissues of the facial region must be recorded.

RADIOGRAPHIC NOISE

Radiographic noise is the appearance of uneven density of a uniformly exposed radiographic film. It is seen on a small area of film as localized variations in density. The primary causes of noise are radiographic mottle and radiographic artifact. Radiographic mottle is uneven density resulting from the physical structure of the film or intensifying screens. Radiographic artifacts are defects caused by errors in film handling, such as fingerprints or bends in the film, or errors in film processing, such as splashing developer or fixer on a film or marks or scratches from rough handling.

On intraoral dental film, mottle may be seen as film graininess, which is caused by the visibility of silver grains in the film emulsion, especially when magnification is used to examine an image. Film graininess is most evident when high-temperature processing is used.

Radiographic mottle is also evident when the film is used with fast intensifying screens. Two important causes of the phenomenon are quantum mottle and screen structure mottle. Quantum mottle is caused by a fluctuation in the number of photons per unit of the beam cross-sectional area absorbed by the intensifying screen. Screen structure mottle is graininess caused by screen phosphors. Quantum mottle and screen structure mottle are each most evident when fast film-screen combinations are used.

RADIOGRAPHIC SHARPNESS AND RESOLUTION

Sharpness is the ability of a radiograph to define an edge precisely (e.g., the dentin-enamel junction, or a thin trabecular plate). Resolution, or resolving power, is the ability of a radiograph to record separate structures that are close together. It usually is measured by radiographing an object made up of a series of thin lead strips with alternating radiolucent spaces of the same thickness. The groups of lines and spaces are arranged in the test target in order of increasing numbers of lines and spaces per millimeter (Fig. 5-32). The resolving power is measured as the highest number of line pairs (a line pair being the image of an absorber and the adjacent lucent space) per millimeter that can be distinguished on the resultant radiograph when examined with low-power magnification. Typically, panoramic film-screen combinations can resolve about five lp/mm; periapical film, which has better resolving power, can delineate clearly more than 20 lp/mm.

Radiographic blur is the loss of sharpness. It can be caused by image receptor (film and screen) blurring, motion blurring, or geometric blurring.

Image Receptor Blurring

With intraoral dental x-ray film, the size and number of the silver grains in the film emulsion determines image sharpness: the finer the grain size, the finer the sharpness. In general, slow-speed films have fine grains, and faster films have larger grains.

Use of intensifying screens in extraoral radiography has an adverse effect on image sharpness. Some degree of sharpness is lost because visible light and UV radiation emitted by the screen spread out beyond the point of origin and expose a film area larger than the phosphor crystal (see Fig. 5-11). The spreading light causes a blurring of fine detail on the radiograph. Intensifying screens with large crystals are relatively fast, but image sharpness is diminished. Fast intensifying screens have a relatively thick phosphor layer, which contributes to dispersion of light and loss of image sharpness. Diffusion of light from a screen can be minimized and image sharpness maximized by ensuring as close a contact as possible between the intensifying screen and the film.

The presence of an image on each side of a double-emulsion film also causes a loss of image sharpness through parallax (Fig. 5-33). Parallax results from the apparent change in position or size of a subject when it is viewed from different perspectives. Because dental film has a double coating of emulsion and the x-ray beam is divergent, the images recorded on each emulsion vary slightly in size. When intensifying screens are used, parallax distortion contributes to image unsharpness because light from one screen may cross the film base and reach the emulsion on the opposite side. This problem can be solved by incorporating dyes into the base that absorb the light emitted by the screens.

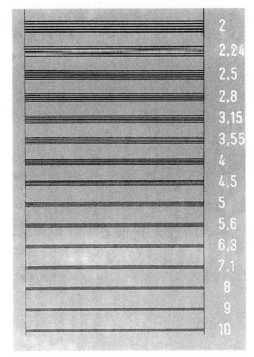

FIGURE 5-32 Radiograph of a resolving power target consisting of groups of radiopaque lines and radiolucent spaces. Numbers at each group indicate the number of line pairs per millimeter represented by the group.

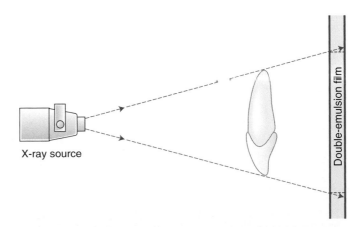

FIGURE 5-33 Parallax unsharpness results when double-emulsion film is used because of the slightly greater magnification of the object on the side of the film away from the x-ray source. Parallax unsharpness is a minor problem in clinical practice.

Motion Blurring

Image sharpness also can be lost through movement of the film, subject, or x-ray source during exposure. Movement of the x-ray source in effect enlarges the focal spot and diminishes image sharpness. Patient movement can be minimized by stabilizing the patient's head with the chair headrest during exposure. Use of a higher mA and correspondingly shorter exposure times also helps resolve this problem.

Geometric Blurring

Several geometric factors influence image sharpness. Loss of image sharpness results in part because photons are not emitted from a point source (focal spot) on the target in the x-ray tube. The larger the focal spot, the greater the loss of image sharpness. Also, image sharpness is improved by increasing the distance between the focal spot and the object and reducing the distance between the object and the image receptor. Various means of optimizing projection geometry are discussed in Chapter 6.

IMAGE QUALITY

Image quality describes the subjective judgment by the clinician of the overall appearance of a radiograph. It combines the features of density, contrast, latitude, sharpness, resolution, and perhaps other parameters. Various mathematic approaches have been used to evaluate these parameters further, but a thorough discussion of them is beyond the scope of this text. The detective quantum efficiency (DQE) is a basic measure of the efficiency of an imaging system. It encompasses image contrast, blur, speed, and noise. Often a system can be optimized for one of these parameters, but this usually is achieved at the expense of others. For instance, a fast system typically has a high level of noise. However, even with these and other sophisticated approaches, more information is needed for complete understanding of all the factors responsible for the subjective impression of image quality.

COMMON CAUSES OF FAULTY RADIOGRAPHS

Although film processing can produce radiographs of excellent quality, inattention to detail may lead to many problems and images that are diagnostically suboptimal. Poor radiographs contribute to a loss of diagnostic information and loss of professional and patient time. Box 5-1 presents a list of common causes of faulty radiographs. The steps necessary for correction are self-evident.

BOX 5-1 Common Problems in Film Exposure and Development

LIGHT RADIOGRAPHS (Fig. 5-34)

Processing Errors
Underdevelopment (temperature too low; time too short; thermometer inaccurate)
Depleted developer solution
Diluted or contaminated developer
Excessive fixation

Underexposure
Insufficient mA
Insufficient kVp
Insufficient time
Film-source distance too great
Film packet reversed in mouth (see Fig. 5-6)

DARK RADIOGRAPHS (Fig. 5-35)

Processing Errors
Overdevelopment (temperature too high; time too long)
Developer concentration too high
Inadequate time in fixer
Accidental exposure to light
Improper safelighting
Storage of films without shielding, at too high a temperature, or past expiration date

Overexposure
Excessive mA
Excessive kVp
Excessive time
Film-source distance too short

INSUFFICIENT CONTRAST (Fig. 5-36)
Underdevelopment
Underexposure
Excessive kVp
Excessive film fog

FILM FOG (Fig. 5-37)
Improper safelighting (improper filter; excessive bulb wattage; inadequate distance between safelight and work surface; prolonged exposure to safelight)
Light leaks (cracked safelight filter; light from doors, vents, or other sources)
Overdevelopment
Contaminated solutions
Deteriorated film (stored at high temperature; stored at high humidity; exposed to radiation; outdated)

DARK SPOTS OR LINES (Fig. 5-38)
Fingerprint contamination
Protective wrapping paper sticking to film surface
Film in contact with tank or another film during fixation
Film contaminated with developer before processing
Excessive bending of film
Static discharge to film before processing
Excessive roller pressure during automatic processing
Dirty rollers in automatic processing

LIGHT SPOTS (Fig. 5-39)
Film contaminated with fixer before processing
Film in contact with tank or another film during development
Excessive bending of film

YELLOW OR BROWN STAINS (see Fig. 5-16)
Depleted developer
Depleted fixer
Insufficient washing
Contaminated solutions

BLURRING (Fig. 5-40)
Movement of patient
Movement of x-ray tube head
Double exposure

BOX 5-1   Common Problems in Film Exposure and Development—cont'd

PARTIAL IMAGES (Fig. 5-41)
Top of film not immersed in developing solution
Misalignment of x-ray tube head ("cone cut")

EMULSION PEEL
Abrasion of image during processing
Excessive time in wash water

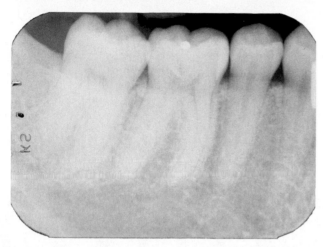

FIGURE 5-34 Radiograph that is too light because of inadequate processing or insufficient exposure.

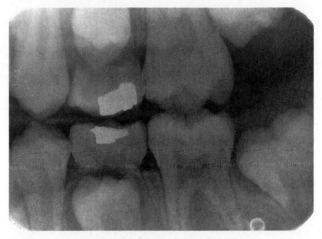

FIGURE 5-36 Radiograph with insufficient contrast, showing gray enamel and gray pulp chambers.

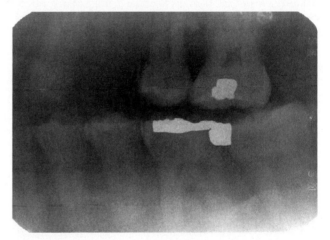

FIGURE 5-37 Fogged radiograph marked by darkening and lack of image detail.

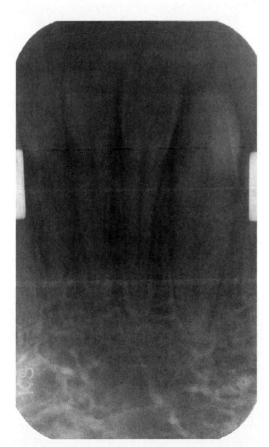

FIGURE 5-35 Radiograph that is too dark because of overdevelopment or overexposure.

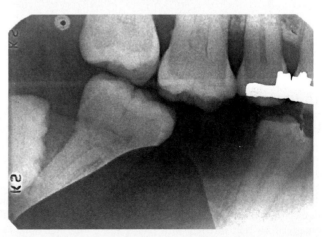

FIGURE 5-38 Dark spot on an x-ray film caused by film contact with the tank wall during fixation. This contact prevented the fixer from dissolving the unexposed silver bromide crystals on the emulsion in contact with the tank wall.

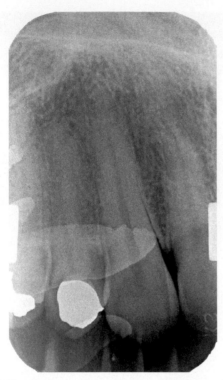

FIGURE 5-39 Light spots on an x-ray film caused by film contact with drops of fixer before processing. The fixer removed the unexposed silver bromide grains on one emulsion but did not affect the opposite side, so there is still an image.

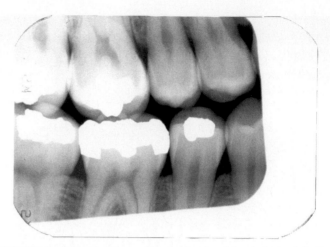

FIGURE 5-41 Partial image caused by poor alignment of the tube head with the film rectangular collimator.

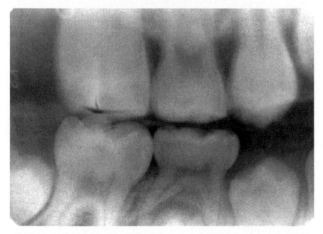

FIGURE 5-40 Blurred radiograph caused by movement of the patient during exposure.

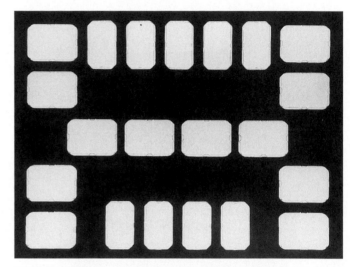

FIGURE 5-42 Film mount for holding nine narrow anterior periapical views, eight posterior periapical views, and four bitewing views. An opaque film mount blocks extraneous light from a viewbox when examining the radiographs.

MOUNTING RADIOGRAPHS

Radiographs must be preserved and maintained in the most satisfactory and useful condition. Periapical, interproximal, and occlusal films are best handled and stored in a film mount (Fig. 5-42). The operator can handle them with greater ease, and there is less chance of damaging the emulsion. Mounts are made of plastic or cardboard and may have a clear plastic window that covers and protects the film. However, the window may have scratches or imperfections that interfere with radiographic interpretation. The operator can arrange several films from the same individual in a film mount in the proper anatomic relationship. This facilitates correlation of the clinical and radiographic examinations. Opaque

mounts are best because they prevent stray light from the viewbox from reaching the viewer's eyes.

The preferred method of positioning periapical and occlusal films in the film mount is to arrange them so that the images of the teeth are in the anatomic position and have the same relationship to the viewer as when the viewer faces the patient. The radiographs of the teeth in the right quadrants should be placed in the left side of the mount, and the radiographs of the teeth of the left quadrants should be placed in the right side. This system, advocated by the American Dental Association, allows the examiner's gaze to shift from radiograph to tooth without crossing the midline. The alternative arrangement, with the images of the right quadrants on the right side of the mount and the images of the left quadrant on the left side, is not recommended.

DUPLICATING RADIOGRAPHS

Occasionally, radiographs must be duplicated; this is best accomplished with duplicating film. The film to be duplicated is placed against the emulsion side of the duplicating film, and the two films are held in position by a glass-topped cassette or photographic printing frame. The films are exposed to light, which passes through the clear areas of the original radiograph and exposes the duplicating film. The duplicating film is processed in conventional x-ray processing solutions. In contrast to conventional x-ray film, duplicating film gives a positive image. Thus areas exposed to light come out clear, as on the original radiograph. Duplication typically results in images with less resolution and more contrast than the original radiograph. The best images are obtained when a circular, UV light source is used. In contrast to the usual negative film, images on duplicating film that are too dark or too light are underexposed or overexposed, respectively.

BIBLIOGRAPHY

Bushberg JT: *The essential physics of medical imaging*, ed 3, Baltimore, 2012, Lippincott Williams & Wilkins.

Bushong SC: *Radiologic science for technologists: physics, biology, and protection*, ed 9, St Louis, 2009, Mosby.

Castro VM, Katz JO, Hardman PK, et al: In vitro comparison of conventional film and direct digital imaging in the detection of approximal caries, *Dentomaxillofac Radiol* 36:138–142, 2007.

Fitterman AS, Brayer FC, Cumbo PE: *Processing chemistry for medical imaging*, Technical and Scientific Monograph No. 5, N-327, Rochester, NY, 1995, Eastman Kodak.

Ludlow JB, Platin E, Mol A: Characteristics of Kodak InSight, an F-speed intraoral film, *Oral Surg Oral Med Oral Pathol Oral Radiol Endod* 91:120–129, 2001.

Mees DEK, James TH: *The theory of the photographic process*, New York, 1977, Macmillan.

Nair MK, Nair UP: An in-vitro evaluation of Kodak InSight and Ektaspeed Plus film with a CMOS detector for natural proximal caries: ROC analysis, *Caries Res* 35:354–359, 2001.

Pontual AA, de Melo DP, de Almeida SM, et al: Comparison of digital systems and conventional dental film for the detection of approximal enamel caries, *Dentomaxillofac Radiol* 39:431–436, 2010.

Revised American Dental Association Specification No. 22 for intraoral dental radiographic film adapted. Council on Dental Materials and Devices, *J Am Dent Assoc* 80:1066–1068, 1970.

Syriopoulos K, Velders XL, Sanderink GC, et al: Sensitometric evaluation of four dental x-ray films using five processing solutions, *Dentomaxillofac Radiol* 28:73–79, 1999.

Thunthy KH, Ireland EJ: A comparison of the visibility of caries on Kodak F-speed (InSight) and D-speed (Ultra-Speed) films, *LDA J* 60:31–32, 2001.

6 Projection Geometry

A conventional radiograph is made with a stationary x-ray source and displays a two-dimensional image of a part of the body. Such images are often called plain or projection views (in contrast to ultrasound, computed tomography [CT], magnetic resonance imaging, or nuclear medicine). In plain views, the entire volume of tissue between the x-ray source and the image receptor (digital sensor or film) is projected onto a two-dimensional image. To obtain the maximal value from a radiograph, a clinician must have a clear understanding of normal anatomy and mentally reconstruct a three-dimensional image of the anatomic structures of interest from one or more of these two-dimensional views. Using high-quality radiographs greatly facilitates this task. The principles of projection geometry describe the effect of focal spot size and relative position of the object and image receptor (digital sensor or film) on image clarity, magnification, and distortion. Clinicians use these principles to maximize image clarity, minimize distortion, and localize objects in the image field.

IMAGE SHARPNESS AND RESOLUTION

Several geometric considerations contribute to image sharpness and spatial resolution. Sharpness measures how well a boundary between two areas of differing radiodensity is revealed. Image spatial resolution measures how well a radiograph is able to reveal small objects that are close together. Although sharpness and resolution are two distinct features, they are interdependent, being influenced by the same geometric variables. For clinical diagnosis, it is desirable to optimize conditions that result in images with high sharpness and resolution.

When x rays are produced at the target in an x-ray tube, they originate from all points within the area of the focal spot. Because these rays originate from different points and travel in straight lines, their projections of a feature of an object do not occur at exactly the same location on an image receptor. As a result, the image of the edge of an object is slightly blurred rather than sharp and distinct. Figure 6-1 shows the path of photons that originate at the margins of the focal spot and provide an image of the edges of an object. The resulting blurred zone of unsharpness on an image causes a loss in image sharpness. The larger the focal spot area, the greater the unsharpness.

There are three means to maximize image sharpness:

1. *Use as small an effective focal spot as practical.* Dental x-ray machines preferably should have a effective focal spot size of 0.4 mm because this greatly adds to image clarity. As described

in Chapter 1, the size of the effective focal spot is a function of the angle of the target with respect to the long axis of the electron beam. A large angle distributes the electron beam over a larger surface and decreases the heat generated per unit of target area, thus prolonging tube life; however, this results in a larger effective focal spot and loss of image clarity (Fig. 6-2). A small angle has a greater wearing effect on the target but results in a smaller effective focal spot and increased image sharpness.

2. *Increase the distance between the focal spot and the object by using a long, open-ended cylinder.* Figure 6-3 shows how increasing the focal spot-to-object distance reduces image blurring by reducing the divergence of the x-ray beam. A longer focal spot-to-object distance minimizes blurring by using photons whose paths are almost parallel. The benefits of using a long focal spot-to-object distance support the use of long, open-ended cylinders as aiming devices on dental x-ray machines.

3. *Minimize the distance between the object and the image receptor.* Figure 6-4 shows that, as the object-to-image receptor distance is reduced, the zone of unsharpness decreases, resulting in enhanced image clarity. This is the result of minimizing the divergence of the x-ray photons.

IMAGE SIZE DISTORTION

Image size distortion (magnification) is the increase in size of the image on the radiograph compared with the actual size of the object. The divergent paths of photons in an x-ray beam cause enlargement of the image on a radiograph. Image size distortion results from the relative distances of the focal spot-to-image receptor and object-to-image receptor (see Figs. 6-3 and 6-4). Increasing the focal spot-to-image receptor distance and decreasing the object-to-image receptor distance minimizes image magnification. The use of a long, open-ended cylinder as an aiming device on an x-ray machine thus reduces the magnification of images on a periapical view. As previously mentioned, this technique also improves image sharpness by increasing the distance between the focal spot and the object.

IMAGE SHAPE DISTORTION

Image shape distortion is the result of unequal magnification of different parts of the same object. This situation arises when not all the parts of an object are at the same focal spot-to-object

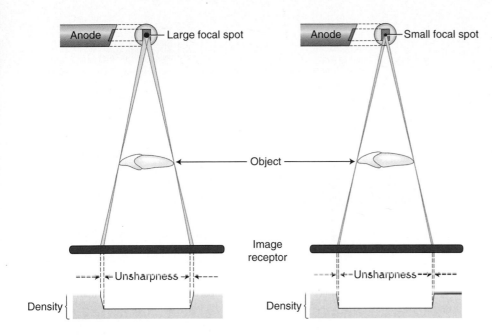

FIGURE 6-1 Photons originating at different places on the focal spot (red) result in a zone of unsharpness on the radiograph. The density of the image changes from a high background value to a low value in the area of an edge of enamel, dentin, or bone. On the left, a large focal spot size results in a wide zone of unsharpness compared with a small focal spot size on the right, which results in a sharper image (narrow zone of unsharpness).

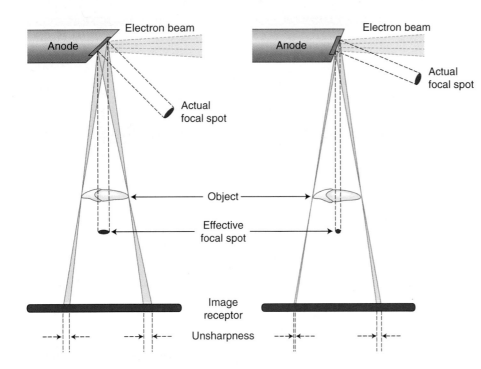

FIGURE 6-2 As the angle of the target becomes closer to perpendicular to the long axis of the electron beam (as shown on the right) the actual focal spot becomes smaller, which decreases heat dissipation and tube life. The more perpendicular angle also decreases the effective focal spot size, increasing the sharpness of the resulting image.

distance. The physical shape of the object may often prevent its optimal orientation, resulting in some shape distortion. Such a phenomenon is seen by the differences in appearance of the image on a radiograph compared with the true shape. To minimize shape distortion, the practitioner should make an effort to align the tube, object, and image receptor carefully according to the following guidelines:

1. *Position the image receptor parallel to the long axis of the object.* Image shape distortion is minimized when the long axes of the image receptor and tooth are parallel. Figure 6-5 shows that the central ray of the x-ray beam is perpendicular to the image receptor, but the object is not parallel to the image receptor. The resultant image is distorted because of the unequal distances of the various parts of the object from the image receptor. This type of shape distortion is called foreshortening because it causes the radiographic image to be shorter than the object. Figure 6-6 shows the situation when the x-ray beam is oriented at right angles to the object but not to the image receptor; this results in elongation, with the object appearing longer on the image receptor than its actual length.

2. *Orient the central ray perpendicular to the object and image receptor.* Image shape distortion occurs if the object and image receptor are parallel, but the central ray is not directed at right angles to each. This distortion is most evident on maxillary molar views (Fig. 6-7). If the central ray is oriented with an excessive vertical angulation, the palatal roots appear disproportionately longer than the buccal roots.

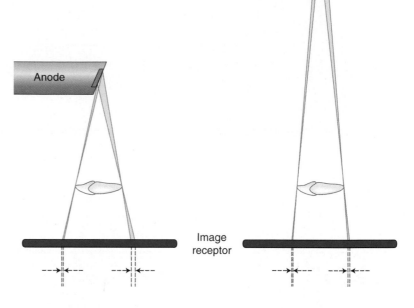

FIGURE 6-3 Increasing the distance between the focal spot and the object results in an image with increased sharpness and less magnification of the object as seen on the right.

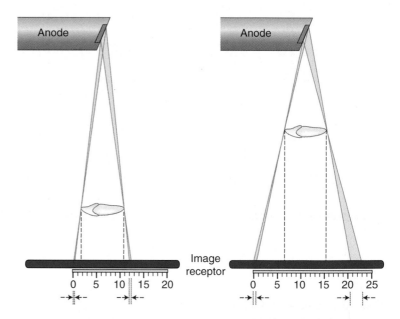

FIGURE 6-4 Decreasing the distance between the object and the image receptor increases the sharpness and results in less magnification of the object as seen on the left.

The practitioner can prevent shape distortion errors by aligning the object and image receptor parallel with each other and the central ray perpendicular to both.

PARALLELING AND BISECTING-ANGLE TECHNIQUES

From the earliest days of dental radiography, a clinical objective has been to produce accurate images of dental structures that are normally visually obscured. An early method for aligning the x-ray beam and image receptor with the teeth and jaws was the bisecting-angle technique (Fig. 6-8). In this method, the image receptor is placed as close to the teeth as possible without deforming it. However, when the image receptor is in this position, it is not parallel to the long axes of the teeth. This arrangement inherently causes distortion. Nevertheless, by directing the central ray perpendicular to an imaginary plane that bisects the angle between the teeth and the image receptor, the practitioner can make the length of the tooth's image on the image receptor correspond to the actual length of the tooth. This angle between a tooth and the image receptor is especially apparent when teeth are radiographed in the maxilla or anterior mandible. Although the projected length of a tooth is correct, these images display a distorted image of the

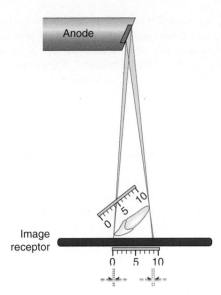

FIGURE 6-5 Foreshortening of a radiographic image results when the central ray is perpendicular to the image receptor but the object is not parallel with the image receptor.

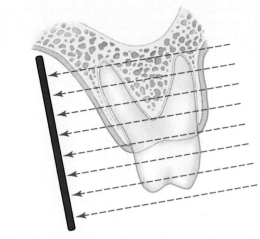

FIGURE 6-7 The central ray should be perpendicular to the long axes of both the tooth and the image receptor. If the direction of the x-ray beam is not at right angles to the long axis of the tooth, the appearance of the tooth is distorted, typically by apparent elongation of the length of the palatal roots of upper molars and distortion of the relationship of the height of the alveolar crest relative to the cementoenamel junction.

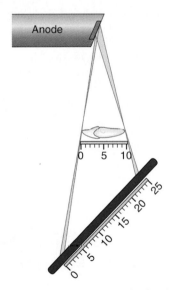

FIGURE 6-6 Elongation of a radiographic image results when the central ray is perpendicular to the object but not to the image receptor.

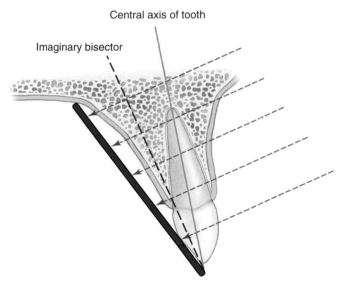

FIGURE 6-8 In the bisecting-angle technique, the central ray is directed at a right angle to the imaginary plane that bisects the angle formed by the image receptor and the central axis of the object. This method produces an image that is the same length as the object but results in some image distortion.

position of alveolar crest with respect to the cementoenamel junction of a tooth. In recent years, the bisecting-angle technique has been used less frequently for general periapical radiography as use of the paralleling technique has increased.

The **paralleling technique** is the preferred method for making intraoral radiographs. It derives its name as the result of placing the image receptor parallel to the long axis of the tooth (Fig. 6-9). This procedure minimizes image distortion and best incorporates the imaging principles described in the first three sections of this chapter.

To achieve this parallel orientation, the practitioner often must position the image receptor toward the middle of the oral cavity, away from the teeth. Although this allows the teeth and image receptor to be parallel, it results in some image magnification and

loss of sharpness. To overcome these limitations, the paralleling technique also uses a relatively long open-ended aiming cylinder ("cone") to increase the focal spot-to-object distance. This "cone" directs only the most central and parallel rays of the beam to the image receptor and teeth and reduces image magnification, while increasing image sharpness. Because it is desirable to position image receptors near the middle of the oral cavity with the paralleling technique, image receptor holders should be used to support the image receptor in the patient's mouth (see Chapter 7).

OBJECT LOCALIZATION

In clinical practice, the dentist often must derive from a radiograph three-dimensional information concerning patients. For example, the dentist may wish to use radiographs to determine the location of a foreign object or an impacted tooth within the jaw. Three methods are frequently used to obtain such three-dimensional information. The first is to examine two images projected at right angles to each other. The second method is to use the tube-shift technique employing conventional periapical views. Third, in recent years, the advent of cone-beam imaging has provided a new tool for obtaining three-dimensional information. In this chapter, we discuss the first two of these methods. These techniques are valuable because cone-beam CT may not be available or even necessary if the dentist already has multiple periapical views of the region of interest. Cone-beam CT is discussed in Chapters 11-13.

Figure 6-10 shows the first method, in which *two views made at right angles to one another* localize an object in or about the maxilla in three dimensions. In clinical practice, the position of an object on each radiograph is noted relative to the anatomic landmarks; this allows the observer to determine the position of the object or area of interest. For example, if a radiopacity is found near the apex of the mandibular first molar on a periapical radiograph, the dentist may take a mandibular occlusal view to identify its mediolateral position. The occlusal film may reveal a calcification in the soft tissues located laterally or medially to the body of the mandible. This information is important in determining the treatment required. The right-angle (or cross section) technique is best for the mandible (see Figs. 22-8, *A*, 22-15, and 22-23, *B*). On a maxillary occlusal view, the superimposition of features in the anterior part of the skull frequently obscures the area of interest.

The second method used to identify the spatial position of an object is the tube-shift technique. Other names for this procedure are the buccal-object rule and Clark's rule (Clark described this method in 1910). The rationale for this procedure derives from the manner in which the relative positions of radiographic images of two separate objects change when the projection angle at which the images were made is changed.

Figure 6-11 shows two radiographs of an object exposed at different angles. Compare the position of the object in question on each radiograph with the reference structures. If the tube is shifted and directed at the reference object (e.g., the apex of a tooth) from a more mesial angulation and the object in question also moves mesially with respect to the reference object, the object lies lingual to the reference object.

Alternatively, if the tube is shifted mesially and the object in question appears to move distally, it lies on the buccal aspect of the reference object (Fig. 6-12). These relationships can be easily remembered by the acronym *SLOB: s*ame *l*ingual, *o*pposite *b*uccal. Thus if the object in question appears to move in the *same* direction with respect to the reference structures as does the x-ray tube, it is on the *lingual* aspect of the reference object; if it appears to move in the *opposite* direction as the x-ray tube, it is on the *buccal* aspect. If it does not move with respect to the reference object, it lies at the same depth (in the same vertical plane) as the reference object.

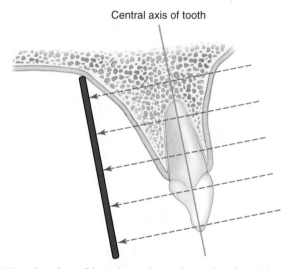

Central axis of tooth

FIGURE 6-9 In the paralleling technique, the central ray is directed at a right angle to the central axes of the object and the image receptor. This technique requires a device to support the film in position.

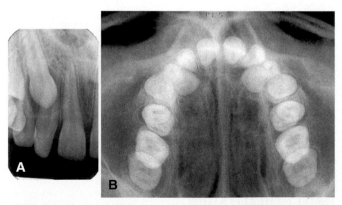

FIGURE 6-10 **A,** Periapical radiograph shows impacted canine lying apical to roots of lateral incisor and first premolar. **B,** Vertex occlusal view shows that the canine lies palatal to the roots of the lateral incisor and first premolar.

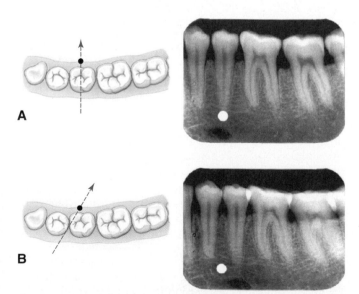

A

B

FIGURE 6-11 The position of an object may be determined with respect to reference structures with use of the tube shift technique. **A,** A radiopaque object on the lingual surface of the mandible (black dot) may appear apical to the second premolar. **B,** When another radiograph is made of this region angulated from the mesial, the object appears to have moved mesially with respect to the second premolar apex ("same lingual" in the acronym *SLOB*).

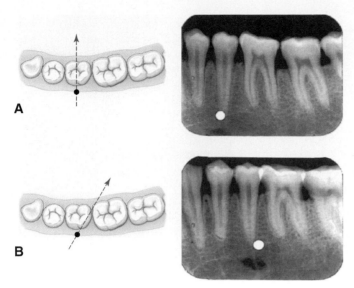

FIGURE 6-12 The position of an object can be determined with respect to reference structures with use of the tube shift technique. **A,** An object on the buccal surface of the mandible may appear apical to the second premolar. **B,** When another radiograph is made of this region angulated from the mesial, the object appears to have moved distally with respect to the second premolar apex ("opposite buccal" in the acronym *SLOB*).

Examination of a conventional set of full-mouth images with this rule in mind demonstrates that the incisive foramen is located lingual (palatal) to the roots of the central incisors and that the mental foramen lies buccal to the roots of the premolars. This technique assists in determining the position of impacted teeth, the presence of foreign objects, and other abnormal conditions. It works just as well when the x-ray machine is moved vertically as horizontally.

The dentist may have two radiographs of a region of the dentition that were made at different angles, but no record exists of the orientation of the x-ray machine. Comparison of the anatomy displayed on the images helps distinguish changes in horizontal or vertical angulation. The relative positions of osseous landmarks with respect to the teeth help identify changes in horizontal or vertical angulation. Figure 6-13 shows the inferior border of the zygomatic process of the maxilla over the molars. This structure lies buccal to the teeth and appears to move mesially as the x-ray beam is oriented more from the distal. Similarly, as the angulation of the beam is increased vertically, the zygomatic process is projected occlusally over the teeth.

EGGSHELL EFFECT

Plain images—images that project a three-dimensional volume onto a two-dimensional receptor—may produce an eggshell effect of corticated structures. Figure 6-14, *A*, shows a schematic view of an egg being exposed to an x-ray beam. The top photon has a tangential path through the apex of the egg and a much longer path through the shell of the egg than does the lower photon, which strikes the egg at right angles to the surface and travels through two thicknesses of the shell. As a result, photons traveling through the periphery of a curved surface are more attenuated

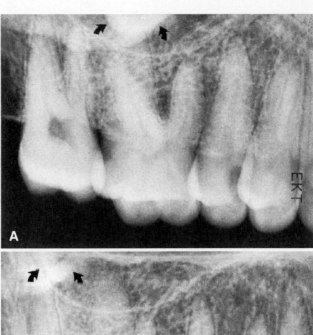

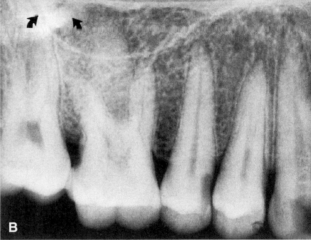

FIGURE 6-13 The position of the maxillary zygomatic process in relation to the roots of the molars can help in identifying the orientation of views. **A,** The inferior border of the zygomatic process lies over the palatal root of the first molar. **B,** The inferior border of the zygomatic process lies posterior to the palatal root of the first molar. This difference in position of the zygomatic process in relation to the palatal root indicates that when the image in **A** was made, the beam was oriented more from the posterior than when the image in **B** was made. The same conclusion can be reached independently by examining the roots of the first molar. The palatal root lies behind the distobuccal root in the image in **A**, but it lies between the two buccal roots in the image in **B**.

than photons traveling at right angles to the surface. Figure 6-14, *B*, shows an expansile lesion on the buccal surface of the mandible on an occlusal view. The periphery of the expanded cortex is more opaque than the region inside the expanded border. The cortical bone is not thicker on the cortex than over the rest of the lesion, but rather the x-ray beam is more attenuated in this region because of the longer path length of photons through the bony cortex on the periphery. This eggshell effect accounts for why normal structures such as the lamina dura, the border of the maxillary sinuses and nasal fossa, and abnormal structures, including the corticated walls of cysts and benign tumors, are well demonstrated on plain images. Soft tissue masses, such as the nose and tongue, do not show an eggshell effect because they are uniform rather than being composed of a dense layer surrounding a more lucent interior.

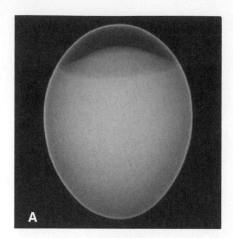
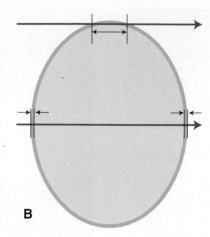
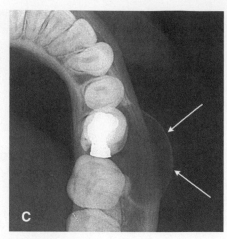

FIGURE 6-14 Eggshell effect. **A,** Radiograph of a hard-boiled egg. Note how the rim of the eggshell is opaque even though it is uniform in thickness. **B,** Schematic view of the egg being exposed to an x-ray beam. The top photon has a tangential path through the apex of the egg and a longer path through the shell of the egg than the lower photon. As a result, photons traveling through the periphery of a curved surface are more attenuated than the photons traveling at right angles to the surface. **C,** An expansile lesion on the buccal surface of the mandible on an occlusal view. The expanded cortex is more opaque than the region inside the border as a result of the eggshell effect.

BIBLIOGRAPHY

Buccal-Object Rule

Clark CA: A method of ascertaining the relative position of unerupted teeth by means of film radiographs, *Proc R Soc Med Odontol Sect* 3:87–90, 1910.

Gutmann JL, Endo C: Clark's rule vis a vis the buccal object rule: its evolution and application in endodontics, *J Hist Dent* 59(1):12–15, 2011.

Jacobs SG: Radiographic localization of unerupted maxillary anterior teeth using the vertical tube shift technique: the history and application of the method with some case reports, *Am J Orthod Dentofac Orthop* 116:415–423, 1999.

Jacobs SG: Radiographic localization of unerupted teeth: further findings about the vertical tube shift method and other localization techniques, *Am J Orthod Dentofac Orthop* 118:439–447, 2000.

Jaju PP: Localization of mandibular canal by buccal object rule, *Oral Surg Oral Med Oral Pathol Oral Radiol Endod* 109:799; author reply 800, 2010.

Katz JO, Langlais RP, Underhill TE, et al: Localization of paraoral soft tissue calcifications: the known object rule, *Oral Surg Oral Med Oral Pathol* 67:459–463, 1989.

Khabbaz MG, Serefoglou MH: The application of the buccal object rule for the determination of calcified root canals, *Int Endod J* 29:284–287, 1996.

Ludlow JB: The buccal object rule, *Dentomaxillofac Radiol* 28:258, 1999.

Richards AG: The buccal object rule, *Dent Radiogr Photogr* 53:37–56, 1980.

Richards AG: The buccal object rule: http://www.unc.edu/~jbl/BuccalObjectRule.html.

Paralleling Technique

Forsberg J: A comparison of the paralleling and bisecting-angle radiographic techniques in endodontics, *Int Endod J* 20:177–182, 1987.

Forsberg J: Radiographic reproduction of endodontic "working length" comparing the paralleling and the bisecting-angle techniques, *Oral Surg Oral Med Oral Pathol* 64:353–360, 1987.

Forsberg J, Halse A: Radiographic simulation of a periapical lesion comparing the paralleling and the bisecting-angle techniques, *Int Endod J* 27:133–138, 1994.

Rushton VE, Horner K: A comparative study of radiographic quality with five periapical techniques in general dental practice, *Dentomaxillofac Radiol* 23:37–45, 1994.

Rushton VE, Horner K: The acceptability of five periapical radiographic techniques to dentists and patients, *Br Dent J* 177:325–331, 1994.

Schulze RK, d'Hoedt B: A method to calculate angular disparities between object and receptor in "paralleling technique," *Dentomaxillofac Radiol* 31:32–38, 2002.

Intraoral Projections

Intraoral radiographic (imaging) examinations are the backbone of imaging for the general dentist. Intraoral images can be divided into three categories: (1) periapical projections, (2) bitewing projections, and (3) occlusal projections. Periapical radiographs should show all of a tooth, including the surrounding bone. Bitewing images show only the crowns of teeth and the adjacent alveolar crests. Occlusal images show an area of teeth and bone larger than periapical images.

A full-mouth set of radiographs consists of periapical and bitewing projections (Fig. 7-1). These projections, when well exposed and properly processed, can provide considerable diagnostic information to complement the clinical examination. As with any clinical procedure, the operator must clearly understand the goals of dental radiography and the criteria for evaluating the quality of performance.

Images should be made only when a clear diagnostic need exists for the information the radiograph may provide. The frequency of such examinations varies with the individual circumstances of each patient (see Chapter 16).

CRITERIA OF QUALITY

Every radiographic examination should produce images of optimal diagnostic quality, incorporating the following features:
- Radiographs should record the complete areas of interest on the image. In the case of intraoral periapical images, the full length of the roots and at least 2 mm of periapical bone must be visible. If evidence of a pathologic condition is present, the area of the entire lesion plus some surrounding normal bone should show on one radiograph. If this is not possible to achieve on a periapical radiograph, an occlusal projection may be required as well as an extraoral projection. Bitewing examinations should demonstrate each posterior proximal surface at least once.
- Radiographs should have the least possible amount of distortion. Most distortion is caused by improper angulation of the x-ray beam rather than by the curvature of the structures being

examined or inappropriate positioning of the receptor. Close attention to proper positioning of the receptor and x-ray tube results in diagnostically useful images.
- Images should have optimal density and contrast to facilitate interpretation. Although milliamperage (mA), peak kilovoltage (kVp), and exposure time are crucial parameters influencing density and contrast, faulty processing can adversely affect the quality of a properly exposed radiograph.

When evaluating images and considering whether to retake a view, the practitioner should consider the initial reason for making the image. When a full-mouth set is indicated, it is not necessary to retake a view that fails to open a contact or show a periapical region if the missing information is available on another view. If a single view or only a few views are needed, they should be repeated only if they fail to reveal the desired information.

PERIAPICAL IMAGING

Two intraoral projection techniques are commonly used for periapical imaging: (1) the paralleling technique and (2) the bisecting-angle technique. Most clinicians prefer the paralleling technique because it provides a less distorted view of the dentition. The paralleling technique is the most appropriate technique for digital imaging. The following discussion describes the principles and uses of the paralleling technique to obtain a full-mouth set of radiographs. When anatomic configuration (e.g., palate and floor of the mouth) precludes strict adherence to the paralleling concept, slight modifications may have to be made. If the anatomic constraints are extreme, some of the principles of the bisecting-angle technique may be used to accomplish the required receptor placement and determine the vertical angulation of the tube. The bisecting-angle technique is described later.

The term image receptor refers to any medium that can capture an image, including film, charge-coupled device (CCD) or complementary metal oxide semiconductor (CMOS) sensors, or storage phosphor plates. The principles for making images are the same

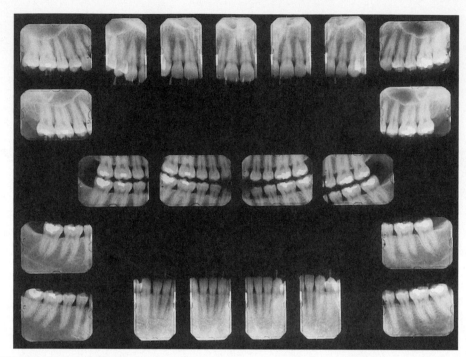

FIGURE 7-1 Mounted full-mouth set of film radiographs consisting of 17 periapical views and 4 bitewing views. Digital images may be positioned in various arrangements depending on the software and preferences of the user.

for each of these receptor types; thus this chapter uses the general term receptor to refer any of the image receptors.

GENERAL STEPS FOR MAKING AN EXPOSURE

- *Prepare unit for exposure.* Place barriers for universal infection control (see Chapter 15) and have receptors and receptor-holding instruments ready at chairside.
- *Greet and seat the patient.* Position the patient upright in the chair with the back and head well supported, and briefly describe the procedures that are to be performed. Position the dental chair low for maxillary projections and elevated for mandibular projections. Ask the patient to remove eyeglasses and all removable appliances. Drape the patient with a lead apron regardless of whether a single image or a full series is to be made. Do not comment on any discomfort the patient may feel during the procedure. If it seems necessary to apologize for any discomfort, do it after the examination.
- *Adjust the x-ray unit setting.* Set the x-ray machine for the proper kVp, mA, and exposure time. Generally, only the exposure time is adjusted for the various anatomic locations.
- *Wash hands thoroughly.* Wash your hands with soap and water, preferably in front of the patient or at least in an area where the patient can observe or be aware of the washing. Put on disposable gloves.
- *Examine the oral cavity.* Before placing any receptors in the mouth, examine the teeth to estimate their axial inclination, which influences the placement of the receptor. Also note tori or other obstructions that modify receptor placement.
- *Position the tube head.* Bring the tube head to the side to be examined so that it is readily available for final positioning after the receptor has been placed in the mouth.

- *Position the receptor.* Insert the receptor into the holding device, and position the receptor and holding device in the region of the patient's mouth to be examined. Angle the receptor holder such that the film or sensor is parallel to the occlusal plane. Leading with the apical end of the receptor, rotate it into the oral cavity. This technique avoids asking the patient to open wide. For maxillary views, place the receptor in the mouth as far from the teeth as possible, near the midline of the palate. This places the receptor in the midline where there is the maximal space available. The added space allows the receptor to be oriented parallel to the long axis of the teeth. With the receptor now in the mouth, place it gently on the palate or floor of the mouth. For all bitewing and mandibular periapical images, it is useful to shift the mandible to the side being imaged; this provides more patient comfort because there is now more room for the sensor on the lingual side of the mandible. After the sensor is positioned, rotate the receptor-holding instrument until the bite-block rests on the teeth to be radiographed, and place a cotton roll between the bite-block and the opposing teeth. The cotton roll helps stabilize the receptor-holding instrument and in many cases contributes to the patient's comfort. Ask the patient to close the mouth gently, holding the instrument and receptor in place. When placing a CCD or CMOS sensor, remember to account for the 2- to 4-mm nonimaging area found at the end of the sensor where the cord attaches.
- *Position the x-ray tube.* Adjust the vertical and horizontal angulation of the tube head to correspond to the receptor-holding instrument. The end of the aiming cylinder of the x-ray machine must be flush or parallel to the guide ring instrument. Alignment is satisfactory when the aiming cylinder covers the port

and is within the limits of the face shield. Caution the patient not to move.

- *Make the exposure.* Make the exposure with the preset exposure time. If the receptor is a film or storage phosphor plate, remove the receptor from the patient's mouth after exposure, dry it with a paper towel, and place it in an appropriate receptacle outside the exposure area. If the receptor is a CCD or CMOS sensor, you may be able to keep it in the patient's mouth and reposition it for the next view. Encourage the patient along the way.

A typical full-mouth set of radiographs consists of 21 images (Box 7-1; see also Fig. 7-1). Establish a regular sequence when making exposures to avoid overlooking individual projections. Make the anterior views before the posterior views because the former views cause less discomfort for the patient. The following description of procedures pertains to the paralleling technique.

BOX 7-1   Projections

ANTERIOR PERIAPICAL (USE NO. 1 RECEPTOR)

- Maxillary central incisors: one projection
- Maxillary lateral incisors: two projections
- Maxillary canines: two projections
- Mandibular centrolateral incisors: two projections
- Mandibular canines: two projections

POSTERIOR PERIAPICAL (USE NO. 2 RECEPTOR)

- Maxillary premolars: two projections
- Maxillary molars: two projections
- Maxillary distomolar (as needed): two projections
- Mandibular premolars: two projections
- Mandibular molars: two projections
- Mandibular distomolar (as needed): two projections

BITEWING (USE NO. 2 RECEPTOR)

- Premolars: two projections
- Molars: two projections

PARALLELING TECHNIQUE

The central concept of the paralleling technique (also called the right-angle technique or long-cone technique) is that the x-ray receptor is supported parallel to the long axis of the teeth, and the central ray of the x-ray beam is directed at right angles to the teeth and receptor (Fig. 7-2). This orientation of the receptor, teeth, and central ray minimizes geometric distortion and presents the teeth and supporting bone in their true anatomic relationships. To reduce geometric distortion, the x-ray source should be located relatively distant from the teeth. The use of a long source-to-object distance reduces the apparent size of the focal spot, thus increasing image sharpness, and provides images with minimal magnification. The paralleling method works equally well for film, CCD or CMOS sensors, or storage phosphor plates.

Receptor-Holding Instruments

Use instruments to allow precise positions of the receptor in the patient's mouth. Many of these receptor holders are specific for various brands of digital sensors, storage phosphor plates, or film. It is also important to use a receptor-holding instrument that has an external guiding ring. This guiding ring is used to align the x-ray aiming cylinder and ensures that the receptor is centered in the beam behind the teeth of interest and that the receptor and teeth are perpendicular to the x-ray beam (Fig. 7-3). These should be used with rectangular collimators to reduce patient exposure (see Chapter 3).

Receptor Placement

For the best images, the receptor should be positioned parallel to the teeth and deep in the patient's mouth; this is particularly important when rigid sensors are used because they may be larger than film. For maxillary projections, the superior border of the receptor generally rests at the height of the palatal vault in the midline. Similarly, for mandibular projections, the receptor should be used to displace the tongue posteriorly or toward the midline to allow the inferior border of the receptor to rest on the floor of the mouth away from the mucosa on the lingual surface of the mandible. Especially for digital sensors, patient acceptance and comfort are best when the receptor is placed in the center of the mouth.

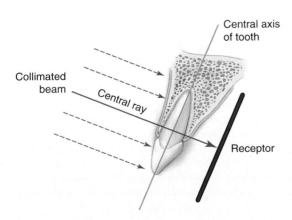

FIGURE 7-2 Paralleling technique illustrates the parallelism between the long axis of the tooth and the receptor. The central ray is directed perpendicular to each. This technique minimizes image distortion but requires a receptor holder.

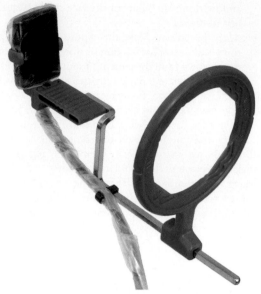

FIGURE 7-3 Receptor-holding instruments. XCP instrument for anterior views shown with sensor and cord wrapped in disposable sensor cover for infection control and to protect the sensor from saliva. *(Courtesy Dentsply Rinn, Elgin, IL.)*

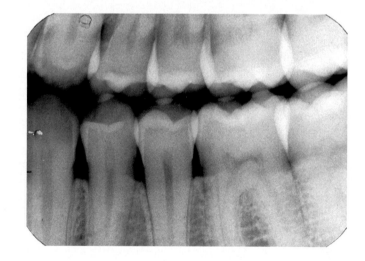

FIGURE 7-4 Horizontal overlapping of crowns results from misdirection of the central ray in the horizontal plane.

Angulation of the Tube Head

Orient the aiming cylinder of the x-ray machine in the vertical and horizontal planes to align with the aiming ring. The horizontal direction of the beam primarily influences the degree of overlapping of the images of the crowns at the interproximal spaces (Fig. 7-4).

BISECTING-ANGLE TECHNIQUE

The bisecting-angle technique was used often in the first half of the twentieth century but has been largely replaced by the paralleling technique. This method may be useful when the operator is unable to apply the paralleling technique because of large rigid sensors or the anatomy of the patient. The bisecting-angle technique is based on a simple geometric theorem, Cieszynski's rule of isometry, which states that two triangles are equal when they share one complete side and have two equal angles. Dental radiography applies the theorem as follows. The receptor is positioned as close as possible to the lingual surface of the teeth, resting in the palate or in the floor of the mouth (Fig. 7-5). The plane of the receptor and the long axis of the teeth form an angle with its apex at the point where the receptor is in contact with the teeth along an imaginary line that bisects this angle and directs the central ray of the beam at right angles to this bisector. This forms two triangles with two equal angles and a common side (the imaginary bisector). Consequently, when these conditions are satisfied, the images cast on the receptor theoretically are the same

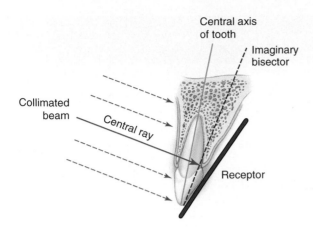

FIGURE 7-5 Bisecting-angle technique shows the central ray directed at a right angle to the plane that bisects the angle between the long axis of the tooth and the receptor. This technique results in an image with the correct length of the tooth but with distortions of the tooth and heights of the alveolar crests.

length as the projected object. To reproduce the length of each root of a multirooted tooth accurately, the central beam must be angled differently for each root. Another limitation of this technique is that the alveolar ridge often projects more coronally than its true position, thus distorting the apparent height of the alveolar bone around the teeth.

Receptor-Holding Instruments

Several methods can be used to support receptors intraorally for bisecting-angle projections. The preferred method is to use a receptor-holding, bisecting-angle instrument that provides an external device for localizing the x-ray beam. The bisecting-angle instrument uses a fixed average bisecting angle. It is undesirable to have the patient support the receptor from the lingual surface with his or her forefinger. Patients often use excessive force and bend the receptor, causing distortion of the image. Also, the receptor might slip without the operator's expertise, resulting in an improper image field. Finally, without an external guide to the position of the receptor, the x-ray beam may miss part of the receptor, resulting in a partial image (**cone cut**).

Positioning of the Patient

For images of the maxillary arch, the patient's head should be positioned upright with the sagittal plane vertical and the occlusal plane horizontal. When the mandibular teeth are to be radiographed, the head is tilted back slightly to compensate for the changed occlusal plane when the mouth is opened.

Receptor Placement

The projections described for the paralleling technique may also be used for the bisecting-angle technique. The receptor is positioned behind the area of interest, with the apical end against the mucosa on the lingual or palatal surface. The occlusal or incisal edge is oriented against the teeth with an edge of the receptor extending just beyond the teeth. If necessary for the patient's comfort, the anterior corner of a film can be softened by bending it before it is placed against the mucosa. Care must be taken not to bend the film excessively because this may result in considerable image distortion and pressure defects in the emulsion that are apparent on the processed film. Such bending is impossible with CCD or CMOS sensors or storage phosphor plates.

TABLE 7-1	Angulation Guidelines for Bisecting-Angle Projections*	
Projection	Maxilla	Mandible
Incisors	+40 degrees	−15 degrees
Canines	+45 degrees	−20 degrees
Premolars	+30 degrees	−10 degrees
Molars	+20 degrees	−5 degrees

Note: With a positive (+) angulation, the aiming tube is pointed downward, and with a negative (−) angulation, it is pointed upward.
*When the occlusal plane is oriented parallel with the floor.

Angulation of the Tube Head

Horizontal Angulation. When a receptor-holding device with a beam-localizing ring is used, the instrument is positioned horizontally so that when the tube is aligned with the ring, the central ray is directed through the contacts in the region being examined. If the receptor-holding device does not have a beam-localizing feature, the tube is pointed so as to direct the central ray through the contacts. In this situation, the radiation beam is also centered on the receptor. This angulation usually is at right angles (in the horizontal projection) to the buccal or facial surfaces of the teeth in each region.

Vertical Angulation. In practice, the clinician's goal is to aim the central ray of the x-ray beam at right angles to a plane bisecting the angle between the receptor and the long axis of the tooth. This principle works well with flat, two-dimensional structures, but teeth that have depth or are multirooted show evidence of distortion. Excessive vertical angulation results in foreshortening of the image, whereas insufficient vertical angulation results in image elongation. The angle that directs the central ray perpendicular to the bisecting plane varies with the individual's anatomy. Several measurements can be used as a general guide when the occlusal plane is oriented parallel with the floor (Table 7-1).

Text continued on p. 114

PARALLELING TECHNIQUE • **MAXILLARY CENTRAL INCISOR PROJECTION***

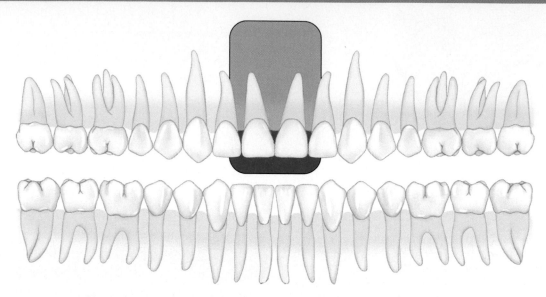

Image Field. The field of view on these radiographs *(shaded area)* should include both central incisors and their periapical areas.

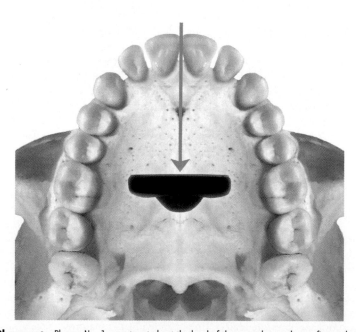

Receptor Placement. Place a No. 1 receptor at about the level of the second premolars or first molars to take advantage of the maximal palatal height so that the entire length of the teeth can be projected on it. Have the receptor resting on the palate with its midline centered with the midline of the arch. Position the packet's long axis parallel to the long axis of the maxillary central incisors.

PARALLELING TECHNIQUE • MAXILLARY CENTRAL INCISOR PROJECTION*—cont'd

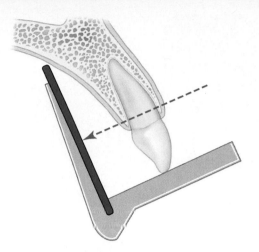

Projection of Central Ray.† Direct the central ray through the contact point of the central incisors and perpendicular to the plane of the receptors and roots of the teeth. Because the axial inclination of the maxillary incisors is about 15 to 20 degrees, the vertical angulation of the tube should be at the same positive angle. The tube should have 0 horizontal angulation.

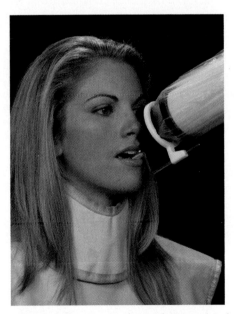

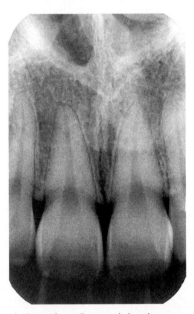

Point of Entry. Direct the point of entry of the central ray high on the lip, in the midline, just below the septum of the nostril. If the palatal vault is unusually low or a palatal torus is present, it may be necessary to tilt the receptor holder positively and compromise a completely parallel relationship between the receptor and the teeth to ensure that the periapical region is included on the image.

*Patient photos for the paralleling technique on pages 97, 99, 101, 103, 105, 107, 109, 111, and 113 are from Iannucci J, Jansen Howerton L: *Dental radiography: principles and techniques,* ed 4, St Louis, 2012, Saunders.
†Projection of the central ray and point of entry are described in the discussion of the paralleling technique for instances when a receptor-holding device without a tube alignment ring or face shield is used. When using a receptor-holding device with a tube-alignment ring or face shield, position the device in the mouth to give the appropriate horizontal and vertical angulation.

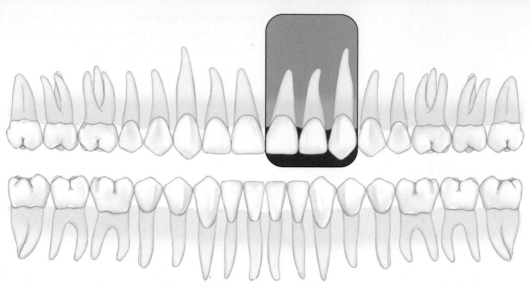

Image Field. This projection should show the lateral incisor and its periapical field centered on the radiograph. Include the mesial interproximal area with the distal aspect of the central incisor on the radiograph so that no overlap is evident.

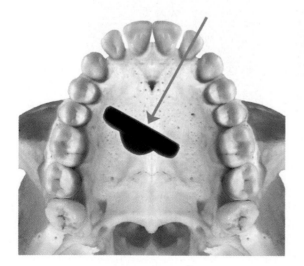

Receptor Placement. Place a No. 1 receptor deep in the oral cavity parallel with the long axis and the mesiodistal plane of the maxillary lateral incisor.

PARALLELING TECHNIQUE • **MAXILLARY LATERAL PROJECTION—cont'd**

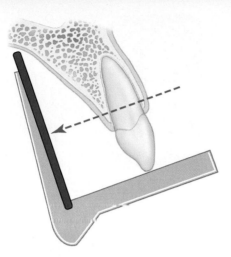

Projection of Central Ray. Direct the central ray through the middle of the lateral incisor, with no overlapping of the margins of the crowns at the interproximal space on its mesial aspect. Do not attempt to visualize the distal contact with the canine.

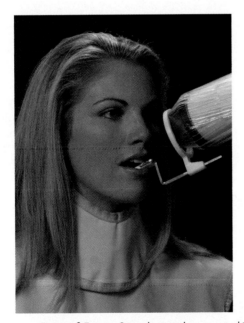

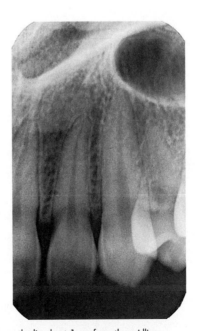

Point of Entry. Orient the central ray to enter high on the lip about 1 cm from the midline.

PARALLELING TECHNIQUE • MAXILLARY CANINE PROJECTION

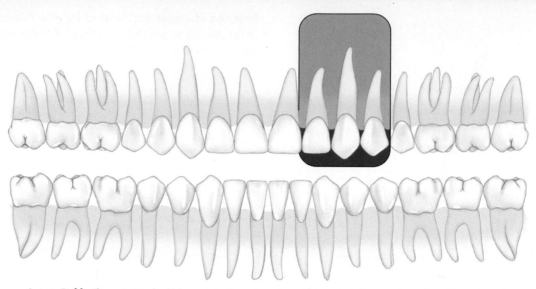

Image Field. This projection should demonstrate the entire canine, with its periapical area, in the midline of the radiograph. Open the mesial contact area. Ignore the distal contact because it will be visualized on other projections.

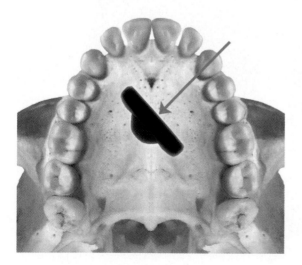

Receptor Placement. Place a No. 1 receptor against the palate, well away from the palatal surface of the teeth. Orient the receptor packet with its anterior edge at about the middle of the lateral incisor and its long axis parallel with the long axis of the canine.

PARALLELING TECHNIQUE • **MAXILLARY CANINE PROJECTION—cont'd**

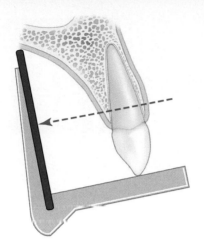

Projection of Central Ray. Position the holding instrument so that it directs the beam through the mesial contact of the canine. Do not attempt to open the distal contact.

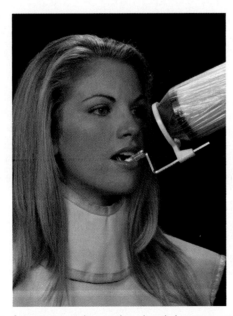
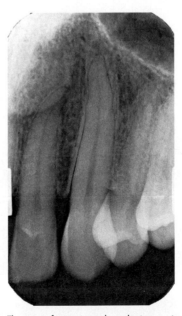

Point of Entry. Direct the central ray through the canine eminence. The point of entry is at about the intersection of the distal and inferior borders of the ala of the nose.

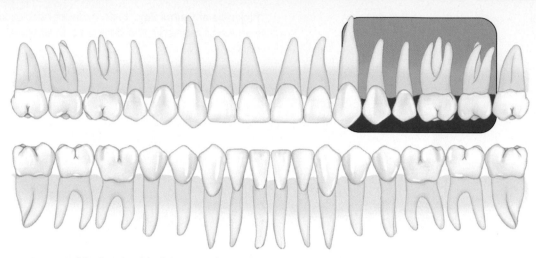

Image Field. The radiograph of this region should include the images of the distal half of the canine and the premolars, with room for at least the first molar.

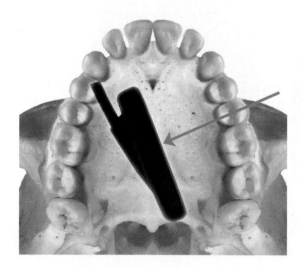

Receptor Placement. Place a No. 2 receptor in the mouth with the long dimension parallel with the occlusal plane and in the midline and near the palatal midline. The packet should extend far enough forward to cover the distal half of the canine. It should also include the premolars and the first molar and maybe the mesial portion of the second molar. The plane of the receptor should be nearly vertical to correspond with the long axis of the premolar teeth. Position the receptor-holding device so that the long axis of the receptor is parallel with the mean buccal plane of the premolars. This establishes the proper horizontal angulation.

PARALLELING TECHNIQUE • **MAXILLARY PREMOLAR PROJECTION—cont'd**

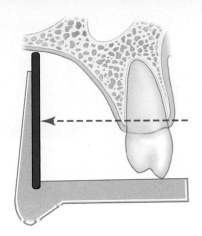

Projection of Central Ray. Direct the central ray perpendicular to the receptor. The horizontal angulation of the holding instrument should be adjusted to permit the beam to pass through the interproximal area between the first and second premolars.

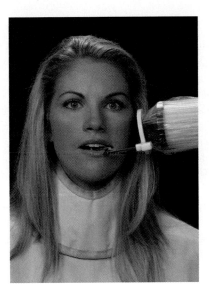

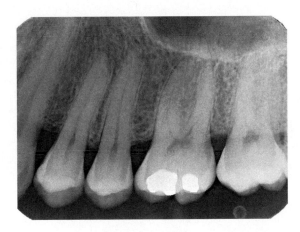

Point of Entry. Place the holding instrument so that the central ray passes through the center of the second premolar root. This point usually is below the pupil of the eye.

PARALLELING TECHNIQUE • **MAXILLARY MOLAR PROJECTION**

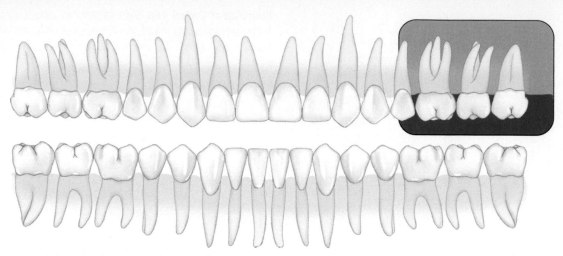

Image Field. The radiograph of this region should show the images of the distal half of the second premolar, the three maxillary permanent molars, and some of the tuberosity. Include the same area on the receptor even if some or all molars are missing. If the third molar is impacted in an area other than the region of the tuberosity, a distal oblique or extraoral projection (e.g., panoramic or oblique lateral jaw view) may be required.

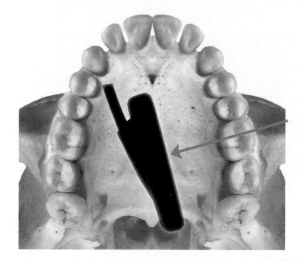

Receptor Placement. When placing the No. 2 receptor for this projection, position the wide dimension of the receptor nearly horizontal to minimize brushing the palate and dorsum of the tongue. When the receptor is in the region to be examined, rotate it into position with a firm and definite motion. This maneuver is important in avoiding the gag reflex, and resolute action by the operator enhances the patient's confidence. Place the receptor far enough posterior to cover the first, second, and third molar areas and some of the tuberosity. The anterior border should just cover the distal aspect of the second premolar. To cover the molars from crown to apices, place the receptor at the midline of the palate. In this position, room should be available to orient the receptor parallel with the molar teeth. The mesial or distal rotation of the receptor-holding device should ensure that the long axis of the receptor is parallel with the mean buccal plane of the molars (to establish the proper horizontal angulation). A shallow palate may require slight tipping of the holding instrument to avoid bending the receptor.

Note: In some cases, the size of the mouth (length of the arch) does not allow positioning of the receptor (holding device) as far posterior as recommended for the molar projection. However, by placing the receptor-holding device so that half the tube alignment ring or face shield is behind the outer canthus of the eye, the molars and part of the tuberosity usually can be included in the image of the molar projection.

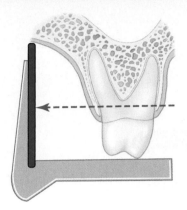

Projection of Central Ray. Direct the central ray perpendicular to the receptor. Adjust the horizontal angulation of the receptor-holding instrument to direct the beam at right angles to the buccal surfaces of the molar teeth.

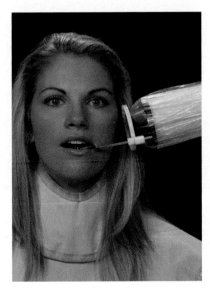

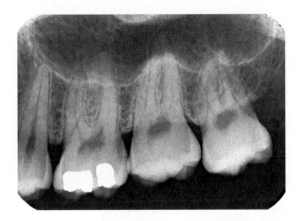

Point of Entry. The point of entry of the central ray should be on the cheek below the outer canthus of the eye and the zygoma at the position of the maxillary second molar.

PARALLELING TECHNIQUE • **MANDIBULAR CENTROLATERAL PROJECTION**

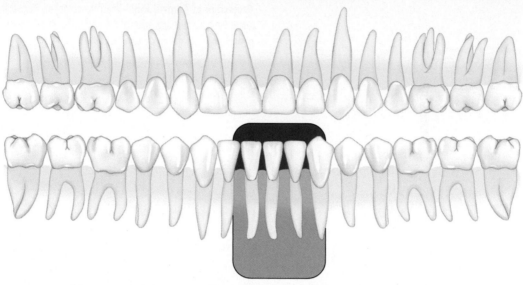

Image Field. Center the image of the mandibular central and lateral incisors and their periapical areas on the receptor. Because the space in this area frequently is restricted, use two of the narrower anterior periapical receptors for the incisors to provide good coverage with minimal discomfort. In addition, the incisor contact areas are better visualized on two narrower anterior receptors because the angulation of the central ray can be adjusted for the contact area on each side.

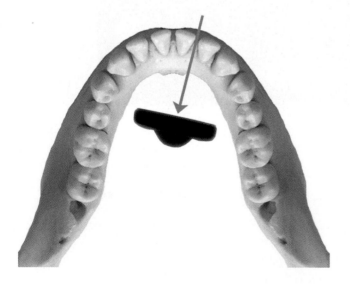

Receptor Placement. Place the long dimension of the No. 1 receptor vertically behind the central and lateral incisors with the contact area centered and the lower border below the tongue. Position the receptor posteriorly as far as possible, usually between the premolars. With the receptor resting gently on the floor of the mouth as the fulcrum, tip the instrument downward until the receptor-holder bite-block is resting on the incisors. Instruct the patient to close the mouth slowly. As the patient is closing slowly and the floor of the mouth is relaxing, rotate the instrument with the teeth as the fulcrum to align the receptor to be more parallel with the teeth.

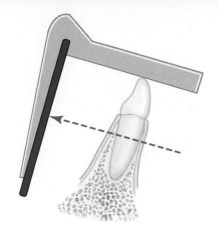

Projection of Central Ray.   Orient the central ray through the interproximal space between the central and lateral incisors.

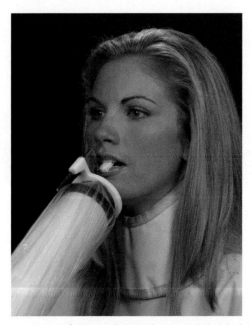
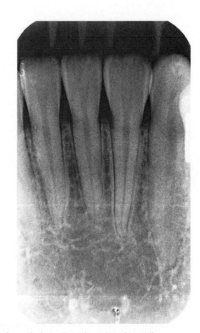

Point of Entry.   The central ray enters below the lower lip and about 1 cm lateral to the midline.

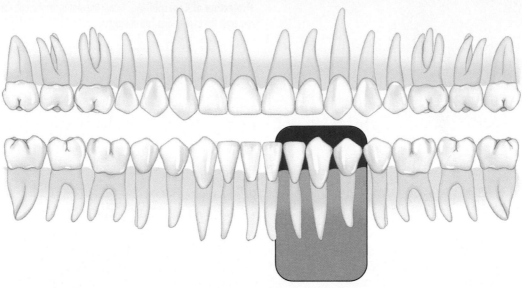

Image Field. This image should show the entire mandibular canine and its periapical area. Open its mesial contact area. The distal contact is included on other projections.

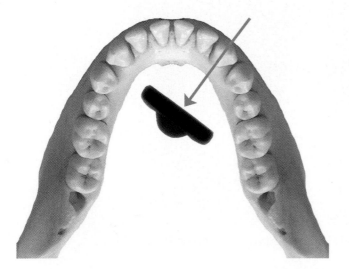

Receptor Placement. Place a No. 1 receptor packet in the mouth with its long dimension vertical and the canine in the midline of the receptor. Position it as far lingual as the tongue and contralateral alveolar process permit, with its long axis parallel and in line with the canine. The instrument must be tipped with the bite-block on the canine before the patient is asked to close.

PARALLELING TECHNIQUE • **MANDIBULAR CANINE PROJECTION—cont'd**

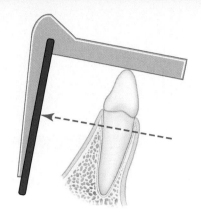

Projection of Central Ray. Direct the central ray through the mesial contact of the canine without regard to the distal contact.

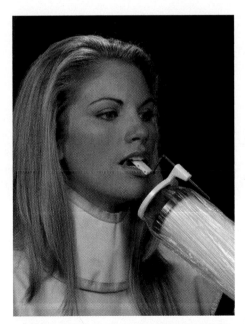

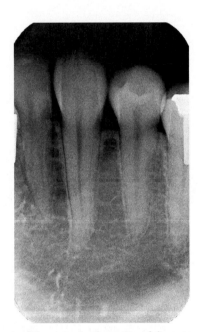

Point of Entry. The point of entry is nearly perpendicular to the ala of the nose, over the position of the canine, and about 3 cm above the inferior border of the mandible.

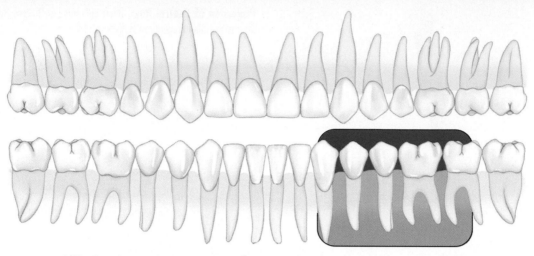

Image Field. The radiograph of this area should show the distal half of the canine, the two premolars, and the first molar.

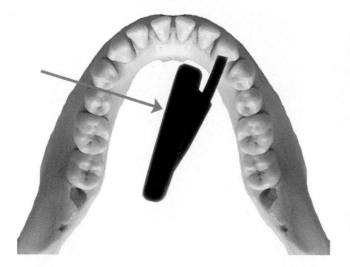

Receptor Placement. Bring the No. 2 receptor into the mouth with its plane nearly horizontal. Rotate the lead edge to the floor of the mouth between the tongue and the teeth with the anterior border near the midline of the canine. Place the receptor away from the teeth to position it in the deeper portion of the mouth. Placing the receptor toward the midline also provides more room for the anterior border of the receptor in the curvature of the jaw as it sweeps anteriorly. Prevent the anterior border from contacting the very sensitive attached gingiva on the lingual surface of the mandible.

PARALLELING TECHNIQUE • MANDIBULAR PREMOLAR PROJECTION—cont'd

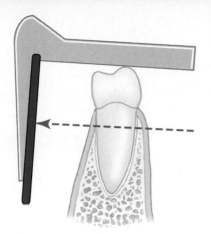

Projection of Central Ray. Position the receptor-holding instrument to project the central ray through the second premolar-molar area. The vertical angulation should be small, nearly parallel with the occlusal plane, to keep the receptor as nearly parallel with the long axis of the teeth as possible. Adjust the horizontal angulation and the placement of the receptor-holding device to direct the beam through the premolar contact points.

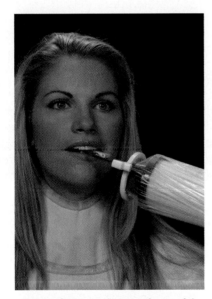

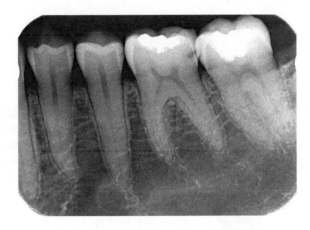

Point of Entry. The point of entry of the central ray is below the pupil of the eye and about 3 cm above the inferior border of the mandible.

PARALLELING TECHNIQUE • **MANDIBULAR MOLAR PROJECTION**

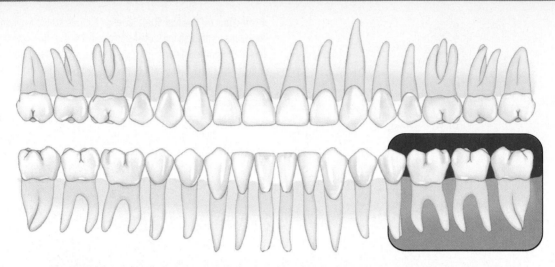

Image Field. The radiograph of this region should include the distal half of the second premolar and the three mandibular permanent molars. In the case of an impacted third molar or a pathologic condition distal to the third molar, a distal oblique molar projection or even additional extraoral projections (panoramic or lateral ramus) may be required to demonstrate the area adequately. If the molar area is edentulous, place the receptor far enough posterior to include the retromolar area in the examination.

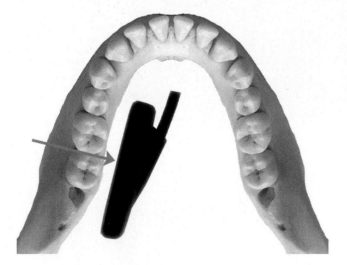

Receptor Placement. Place the No. 2 receptor in the mouth with its plane nearly horizontal. Rotate the inferior edge downward beneath the lateral border of the tongue, displacing it medially. The anterior edge of the receptor should be at about the middle of the second premolar. In most cases, the tongue forces the receptor near the alveolar process and molars, aligning it parallel with the long axis of the teeth and the line of occlusion.

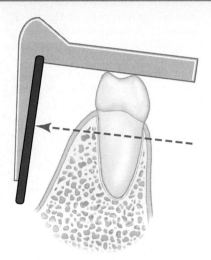

Projection of Central Ray. Proper placement of the holding instrument directs the central ray through the second molar. Adjust the horizontal angulation to project the beam through the contact areas. Because of the slight lingual inclination of the molars, the central ray may have some slight positive angulation (approximately 8 degrees).

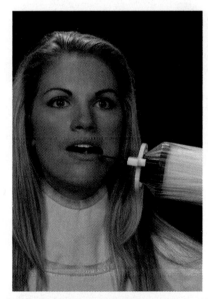

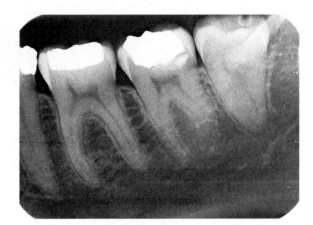

Point of Entry. Direct the point of entry of the central ray below the outer canthus of the eye about 3 cm above the inferior border of the mandible.

BITEWING EXAMINATIONS

Bitewing (also called interproximal) images include the crowns of the maxillary and mandibular teeth and the alveolar crest on the same receptor. Bitewing receptors are particularly valuable for detecting interproximal caries in the early stages of development before it becomes clinically apparent. Because of the horizontal angle of the x-ray beam, these radiographs also may reveal secondary caries below restorations that may escape recognition in the periapical views. Bitewing projections are also useful for evaluating the periodontal condition. They provide a good perspective of the alveolar bone crest, and changes in bone height can be assessed accurately through comparison with the adjacent teeth. In addition, because of the angle of projection directly through the interproximal spaces, the bitewing receptor is especially effective and useful for detecting calculus deposits in interproximal areas. (Because of its relatively low radiodensity, calculus is better visualized on images made with reduced exposure.) The long axis of bitewing receptors usually is oriented horizontally but may be oriented vertically.

Horizontal Bitewing Receptors

To obtain the desirable characteristics of the bitewing examination described, the beam is carefully aligned between the teeth and parallel with the occlusal plane. As the receptor or receptor-holding instrument is placed in the mouth, the portion of the mandibular quadrant that is being radiographed is in view. The position of the teeth in this segment of the mandibular quadrant is evaluated, and the beam is directed through the contacts. Some difference may exist in the curvature of the mandibular and maxillary arches. However, when the x-ray beam is accurately directed through the mandibular premolar contacts, overlapping is minimal or absent in the maxillary premolar segment. A few degrees of tolerance are available in the horizontal angulation before overlapping becomes critical. The contact between the maxillary first and second molars often is angled a few degrees more anteriorly than between the mandibular first and second molars. The aiming cylinder is positioned about +10 degrees to project the beam parallel with the occlusal plane (occlusal dentinoenamel junction). This orientation minimizes overlapping of the opposing cusps onto the occlusal surface and thus improves the probability of detecting early occlusal lesions at the dentinoenamel junction.

The XCP (Dentsply Rinn, Elgin, IL) bitewing instrument has an external guide ring for positioning the tube head. This guide ring reduces the possibility of cone cutting the receptor (Fig. 7-6). To position the XCP instrument properly, the guide bar is placed parallel with the direction of the beam that opens the contacts of the dentition being examined.

A receptor fitted with a bitewing tab or loop may be used instead of a holding device (Fig. 7-7). The receptor is placed in a

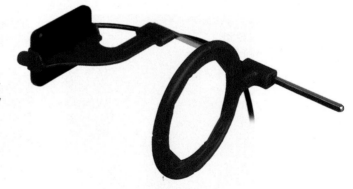

FIGURE 7-6 Receptor-holding device for bitewing images. Note the external localizing ring, which is used to position the aiming tube of the x-ray machine to ensure that the entire receptor is in the x-ray beam. Disposable barrier has been removed to show detector and wire. *(Courtesy Dentsply Rinn, Elgin, IL.)*

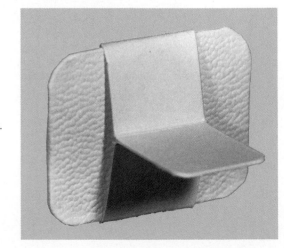

FIGURE 7-7 Bitewing loop, showing the tab that the patient bites on to support the receptor during exposure.

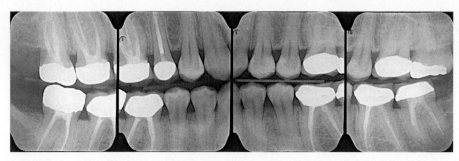

FIGURE 7-8 Set of vertical bitewing views. Orienting the length of the receptor vertically increases the likelihood that the residual alveolar crests in the maxilla and the mandible will be recorded on the radiograph even in patients with extensive alveolar bone loss.

comfortable position lingual to the teeth to be examined. The aiming cylinder is oriented in the predetermined direction that passes the x-ray beam through the interproximal spaces. To help prevent cone cutting, the central ray is directed toward the center of the bitewing tab, which protrudes to the buccal side. The beam is angulated +7 to +10 degrees vertically to preclude overlap of the cusps onto the occlusal surface.

Two posterior bitewing views, a premolar and a molar, are recommended for each quadrant. However, for children 12 years or younger, one bitewing receptor (No. 2 receptor) usually suffices. The premolar projection should include the distal half of the canines and the crowns of the premolars. Because the mandibular canines usually are more mesial than the maxillary canines, the mandibular canine is used as the guide for placement of the premolar bitewing receptor. The molar bitewing receptor is placed 1 or 2 mm beyond the most distally erupted molar (maxillary or mandibular).

Vertical Bitewing Receptors

Vertical bitewing receptors usually are used when the patient has moderate to extensive alveolar bone loss. Orienting the length of the receptor vertically increases the likelihood that the residual alveolar crests in the maxilla and the mandible will be recorded on the radiograph (Fig. 7-8). The principles for positioning the receptor and orienting the x-ray beam are otherwise the same as for horizontal bitewing projections.

Text continued on p. 126

PREMOLAR BITEWING PROJECTION*

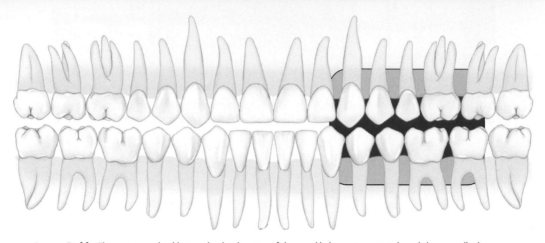

Image Field. This projection should cover the distal portion of the mandibular canine anteriorly and show equally the crowns of the maxillary and mandibular premolar teeth.

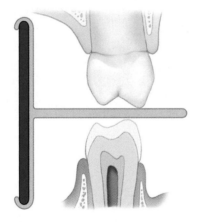

Receptor Placement. Place the receptor between the tongue and the teeth, far enough from the lingual surface of the teeth to prevent interference by the palate on closing and parallel to the long axes of the teeth. The anterior border of the receptor should extend beyond the contact area between the mandibular canine and the first premolar. Hold the receptor in place until the patient's mouth is completely closed. Holding the receptor while closing prevents it from being displaced distally.

PREMOLAR BITEWING PROJECTION—cont'd

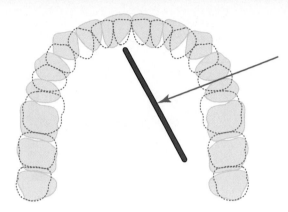

Projection of Central Ray. Adjust the horizontal angulation of the cone to project the central ray to the center of the receptor through the premolar contact areas. To compensate for the slight inclination of the receptor against the palatal mucosa, the vertical angulation should be about +5 degrees. (In the drawing, the mandibular teeth are shown in *dashed lines*.)

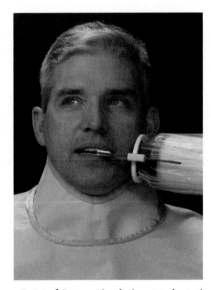

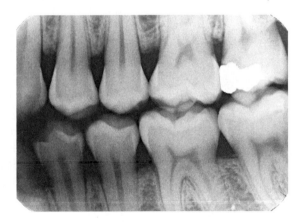

Point of Entry. Identify the point of entry by retracting the cheek and determining that the central ray will enter the line of occlusion at the point of contact between the second premolar and the first molar.

*Patient photos for the bitewing projections on pages 117 and 119 are from Iannucci J, Jansen Howerton L: *Dental radiography: principles and techniques,* ed 4, St Louis, 2012, Saunders.

MOLAR BITEWING PROJECTION

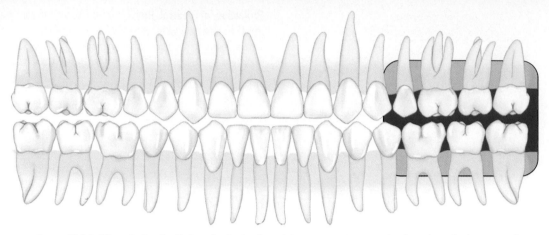

Image Field. This projection should show the distal surface of the most posterior erupted molar and equally the crowns of the maxillary and mandibular molars. Because the maxillary and mandibular molar contact areas may not be open from the same horizontal angulation, they may not be visible on one receptor. In this case, it may be desirable to open the maxillary molar contacts because the mandibular molar contacts usually are open on the periapical receptors.

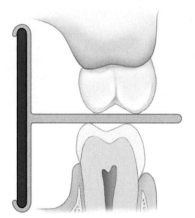

Receptor Placement. Place the receptor between the tongue and teeth as far lingual as practical to avoid contacting the sensitive attached gingiva. The distal margin of the receptor should extend 1 to 2 mm beyond the most posterior erupted molar. When using the XCP, adjust the horizontal angulation by placing the guide bar parallel with the direction of the central ray to open the contact area between the first and second molars.

MOLAR BITEWING PROJECTION—cont'd

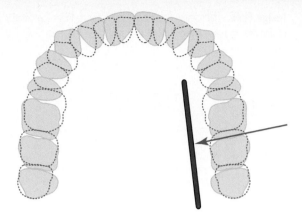

Projection of Central Ray. Project the central ray to the center of the receptor and through the contact of the first and second maxillary molars. Angle the central ray slightly from the anterior because the molar contacts usually are not oriented at right angles to the buccal surfaces of these teeth. A vertical angulation of +10 degrees is recommended. (In the drawing, the mandibular teeth are shown in *dashed lines*.)

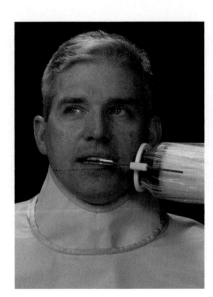

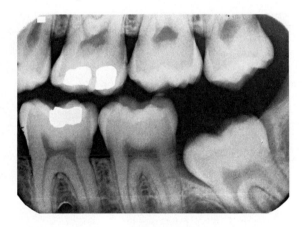

Point of Entry. The central ray should enter the cheek below the lateral canthus of the eye at the level of the occlusal plane.

ANTERIOR MAXILLARY OCCLUSAL PROJECTION

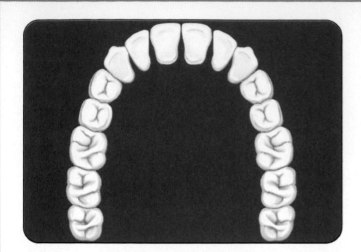

Image Field. The primary field of this projection includes the anterior maxilla and its dentition and the anterior floor of the nasal fossa and teeth from canine to canine.

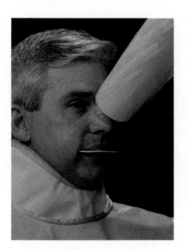

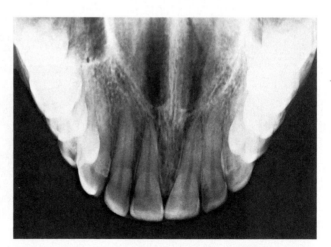

Receptor Placement. Adjust the patient's head so that the sagittal plane is perpendicular and the occlusal plane is horizontal to the floor. Place the receptor in the mouth with the exposure side toward the maxilla, the posterior border touching the rami, and the long dimension of the receptor perpendicular to the sagittal plane. The patient stabilizes the receptor by gently closing the mouth or using gentle bilateral thumb pressure.

Projection of Central Ray. Orient the central ray through the tip of the nose toward the middle of the receptor with approximately +45 degrees vertical angulation and 0 degrees horizontal angulation.

Point of Entry. The central ray enters the patient's face approximately through the tip of the nose.

*Patient photos for the occlusal projections on pages 120, 121, 122, 123, and 124 are from Iannucci J, Jansen Howerton L: *Dental radiography: principles and techniques*, ed 4, St Louis, 2012, Saunders.

TOPOGRAPHICAL MAXILLARY OCCLUSAL PROJECTION*

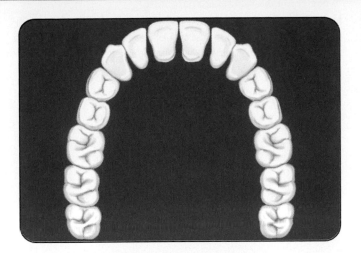

Image Field. This projection shows the palate, zygomatic processes of the maxilla, anteroinferior aspects of each antrum, nasolacrimal canals, teeth from second molar to second molar, and nasal septum.

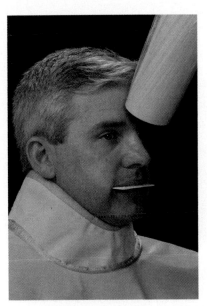

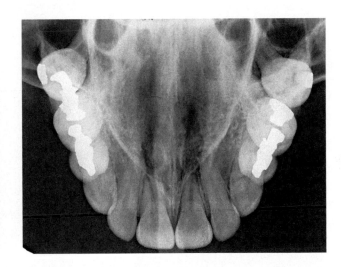

Receptor Placement. Seat the patient upright with the sagittal plane perpendicular to the floor and the occlusal plane horizontal. Place the receptor, with its long dimension perpendicular to the sagittal plane, crosswise in the mouth. Gently push the receptor in backward until it contacts the anterior border of the mandibular rami. The patient stabilizes the receptor by gently closing the mouth.

Projection of Central Ray. Direct the central ray at a vertical angulation of +65 degrees and a horizontal angulation of 0 degrees to the bridge of the nose just below the nasion, toward the middle of the receptor.

Point of Entry. Generally, the central ray enters the patient's face through the bridge of the nose.

LATERAL MAXILLARY OCCLUSAL PROJECTION*

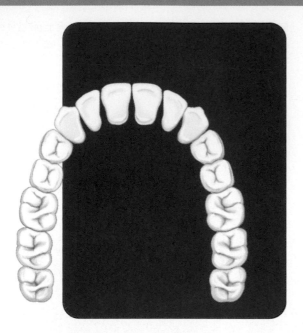

Image Field. This projection shows a quadrant of the alveolar ridge of the maxilla, inferolateral aspect of the antrum, tuberosity, and teeth from the lateral incisor to the contralateral third molar. In addition, the zygomatic process of the maxilla superimposes over the roots of the molar teeth.

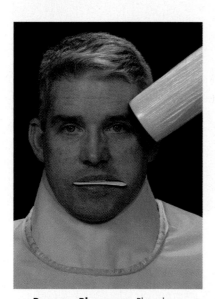

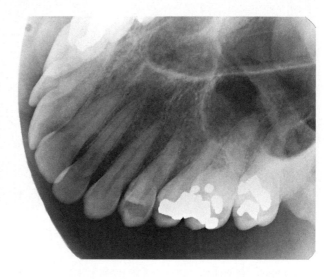

Receptor Placement. Place the receptor with its long axis parallel to the sagittal plane and on the side of interest, with the tube side toward the side of the maxilla in question. Push the receptor posteriorly until it touches the ramus. Position the lateral border parallel with the buccal surfaces of the posterior teeth, extending laterally approximately 1 cm past the buccal cusps. Ask the patient to close gently to hold the receptor in position.

Projection of Central Ray. Orient the central ray with a vertical angulation of +60 degrees, to a point 2 cm below the lateral canthus of the eye, directed toward the center of the receptor.

Point of Entry. The central ray enters at a point approximately 2 cm below the lateral canthus of the eye.

ANTERIOR MANDIBULAR OCCLUSAL PROJECTION*

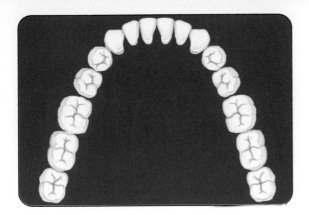

Image Field. This projection includes the anterior portion of the mandible, the dentition from canine to canine, and the inferior cortical border of the mandible.

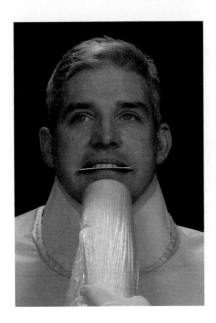

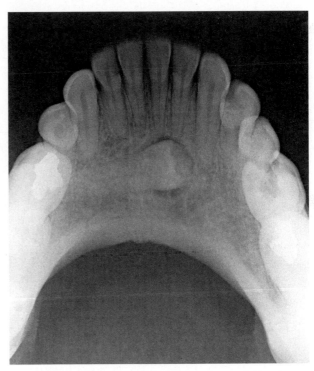

Receptor Placement. Seat the patient tilted back so that the occlusal plane is 45 degrees above horizontal. Place the receptor in the mouth with the long axis perpendicular to the sagittal plane and push it posteriorly until it touches the rami. Center the receptor with the pebbled side (tube side) down, and ask the patient to bite lightly to hold the receptor in position.

Projection of Central Ray. Orient the central ray with −10 degrees angulation through the point of the chin toward the middle of the receptor; this gives the ray −55 degrees of angulation to the plane of the receptor.

Point of Entry. The point of entry of the central ray is in the midline and through the tip of the chin.

TOPOGRAPHICAL MANDIBULAR OCCLUSAL PROJECTION*

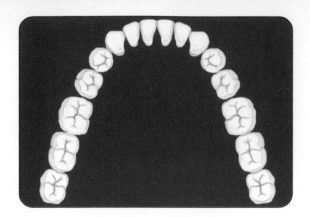

Image Field. This projection includes the soft tissue of the floor of the mouth and reveals the lingual and buccal plates of the mandible from second molar to second molar. When this view is made to examine the floor of the mouth (e.g., for sialoliths), the exposure time should be reduced to half the time used to create an image of the mandible.

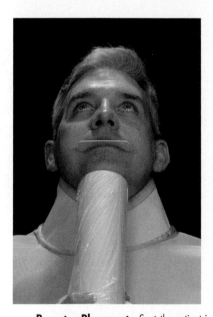
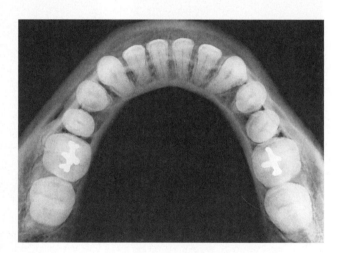

Receptor Placement. Seat the patient in a semireclining position with the head tilted back so that the ala-tragus line is almost perpendicular to the floor. Place the receptor in the mouth with its long axis perpendicular to the sagittal plane and with the tube side toward the mandible. The anterior border of the receptor should be approximately 1 cm beyond the mandibular central incisors. Ask the patient to bite gently on the receptor to hold it in position.

Projection of Central Ray. Direct the central ray at the midline through the floor of the mouth approximately 3 cm below the chin, at right angles to the center of the receptor.

Point of Entry. The point of entry of the central ray is in the midline through the floor of the mouth approximately 3 cm below the chin.

LATERAL MANDIBULAR OCCLUSAL PROJECTION

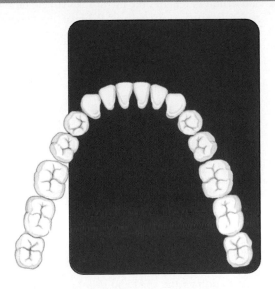

Image Field. This projection covers the soft tissue of half the floor of the mouth, the buccal and lingual cortical plates of half of the mandible, and the teeth from the lateral incisor to the contralateral third molar. When this view is used to provide an image of the floor of the mouth, the exposure time should be reduced to half that used to provide an image of the mandible.

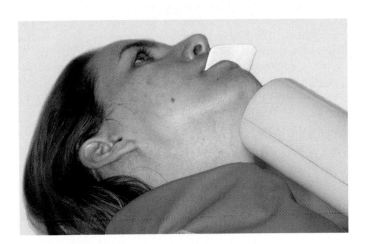

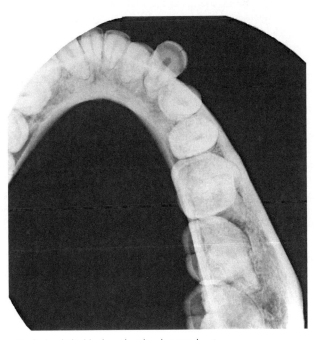

Receptor Placement. Seat the patient in a semireclining position with the head tilted back so that the ala-tragus line is almost perpendicular to the floor. Place the receptor in the mouth with its long axis initially parallel with the sagittal plane and with the pebbled side down toward the mandible. Place the receptor as far posterior as possible, then shift the long axis buccally (right or left) so that the lateral border of the receptor is parallel with the buccal surfaces of the posterior teeth and extends laterally approximately 1 cm.

Projection of Central Ray. Direct the central ray perpendicular to the center of the receptor through a point beneath the chin, approximately 3 cm posterior to the point of the chin and 3 cm lateral to the midline.

Point of Entry. The point of entry of the central ray is beneath the chin, approximately 3 cm posterior to the chin and approximately 3 cm lateral to the midline.

OCCLUSAL IMAGING

An occlusal radiograph displays a relatively large segment of a dental arch. It may include the palate or floor of the mouth and a reasonable extent of the contiguous lateral structures. Occlusal radiographs also are useful when patients are unable to open wide enough for periapical images or for other reasons cannot accept periapical receptors. Because occlusal radiographs are exposed at a steep angulation, they may be used with conventional periapical images to determine the location of objects in all three dimensions. Typically, the occlusal radiograph is especially useful in the following cases:

- To locate precisely roots and supernumerary, unerupted, and impacted teeth (this technique is especially useful for impacted canines and third molars)
- To localize foreign bodies in the jaws and stones in the ducts of sublingual and submandibular glands
- To demonstrate and evaluate the integrity of the anterior, medial, and lateral outlines of the maxillary sinus
- To aid in the examination of patients with trismus, who can open their mouths only a few millimeters; this condition precludes intraoral radiography, which may be impossible or at least extremely painful for the patient
- To obtain information about the location, nature, extent, and displacement of fractures of the mandible and maxilla
- To determine the medial and lateral extent of disease (e.g., cysts, osteomyelitis, malignancies) and to detect disease in the palate or floor of the mouth

To make an occlusal radiograph, a large receptor (7.7 cm × 5.8 cm [3 inches × 2.3 inches]) is inserted between the occlusal surfaces of the teeth. Occlusal receptors are made only of film or storage phosphor plates. Neither CCD nor CMOS sensors exist this large. As its name implies, the receptor lies in the plane of occlusion. The "tube" side of this receptor is positioned toward the jaw to be examined, and the x-ray beam is directed through the jaw to the receptor. Because of its size, the receptor allows examination of relatively large portions of the jaw. Standardized projections are used, which stipulate a desired relationship between the central ray, receptor, and region being examined. However, the clinician should feel free to modify these relationships to meet a specific clinical requirement.

IMAGING OF CHILDREN

Radiation protection is most important for children because of their greater sensitivity to irradiation. The best way to reduce unnecessary exposure is for the dentist to make the minimal number of receptors required for the individual patient. These judgments are based on a careful clinical examination and consideration of the patient's age, medical history, growth considerations, and general oral health as well as whether caries is present and the time elapsed since previous examinations. Prudence suggests making bitewing examinations for caries assessment at periodic intervals after the patient's contacts have closed. The frequency should be determined partly by the patient's caries rate. A periapical survey is often recommended for children early in the mixed dentition stage. Special attention should be paid to procedures that reduce exposure (see Chapter 3), including use of fast receptor, proper processing, beam-limiting devices, and leaded aprons and thyroid shields.

Radiography in a child can be an interesting and challenging experience. Although the principles of periapical radiography for children are the same as for adults, in practice children present special considerations because of their small anatomic structures and possible behavioral problems. The smaller size of the arches and dentition requires the use of smaller periapical receptors. The relatively shallow palate and floor of the mouth may require further modification of receptor placement. Special radiographic examinations using an occlusal receptor for extraoral projections have been suggested.

PATIENT MANAGEMENT

Children are often apprehensive about the radiographic examination, much as they are about many other types of dental procedures. The radiographic examination usually is the first manipulative procedure performed on a young patient. If this examination is nonthreatening and comfortable, subsequent dental experiences usually are accepted with little or no apprehension. This apprehension is best allayed by familiarizing children with the procedure, which is done by explaining it in a manner they can comprehend. It often is wise to describe the x-ray machine as a camera used to take pictures of teeth. The child can become more comfortable with the receptor and x-ray machine by touching them before the examination. The operator should carry on a conversation with the child to distract the child and gain his or her confidence. It may be advantageous for the child to watch an older brother or sister being radiographed or to have the parent or dental assistant serve as a model. For children who feel a gagging sensation, the clinician can have them breathe through the nose, curl their toes, or make a fist to distract their attention from the radiographic procedure. However, if the procedure is postponed until the next appointment, the gag reflex may not be encountered or often is much easier for the patient to control. It is especially important to explain to the patient that the procedure will be much easier the next time—plant the positive thought.

EXAMINATION COVERAGE

When a complete radiographic survey is necessary, it should show the periapical region of all teeth, the proximal surfaces of all posterior teeth, and the crypts of the developing permanent teeth. The number of projections required depends on the child's size. Also, an exposure appropriate to the child's size should be used. For example, a 50% reduction in the mA used for an average young adult gives the proper density for patients younger than 10 years. Exposure is reduced about 25% for children 10 to 15 years old.

Primary Dentition (3 to 6 Years)

A combination of projections can be used to provide adequate coverage for the pediatric dental patient. This examination may consist of two anterior occlusal receptors, two posterior bitewing receptors, and up to four posterior periapical receptors as indicated (Fig. 7-9). For the maxillary and interproximal projections, the child is seated upright with the sagittal plane perpendicular to and the occlusal plane parallel with the floor (horizontal plane). For mandibular projections, except the occlusal, the child is seated upright with the sagittal plane perpendicular. The tragus corner of the mouth line is oriented parallel to the floor. Some dentists find that a panoramic view, rather than the four periapicals, is more informative and results in less exposure to the child (see Chapter 3).

Maxillary Anterior Occlusal Projection.   A No. 2 receptor should be placed in the mouth with its long axis perpendicular to the sagittal plane and the pebbled surface toward the maxillary teeth. The receptor is centered on the midline with the anterior border

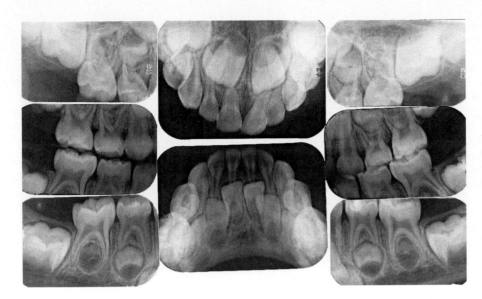

FIGURE 7-9 Radiographic examination of primary dentition consists of two anterior occlusal views, four posterior periapical views, and two bitewing views. Often it is preferable to make a bitewing and panoramic examination followed by selected periapical views as indicated.

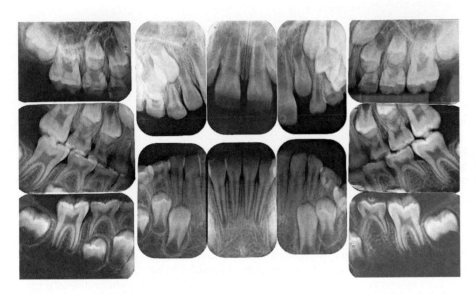

FIGURE 7-10 Radiographic examination of mixed dentition consists of two incisor views, four canine views, four posterior views, and two bitewing views. Often it is preferable to make a bitewing and panoramic examination followed by selected periapical views as indicated.

extending just beyond the incisal edges of the anterior teeth. The central ray is directed at a vertical angulation of +60 degrees through the tip of the nose toward the center of the receptor.

Mandibular Anterior Occlusal Projection.   The child should be seated with the head tipped back so that the occlusal plane is about 25 degrees above the plane of the floor. A No. 2 receptor is placed with the long axis perpendicular to the sagittal plane and the pebbled surface toward the mandibular teeth. The central ray is oriented at −30 degrees vertical angulation and through the tip of the chin toward the receptor.

Bitewing Projection.   A No. 0 receptor is used with a paper loop receptor holder. The receptor is placed in the child's mouth as in the adult premolar bitewing projection. The image field should include the distal half of the canine and the deciduous molars. A positive vertical angulation of +5 to +10 degrees should be used. The horizontal angle is oriented to direct the beam through the interproximal spaces.

Deciduous Maxillary Molar Periapical Projection.   A No. 0 receptor in a modified XCP or BAI (Dentsply Rinn, Elgin, IL) bite-block,

either with or without the aiming ring and indicator bar, is used. The receptor is positioned in the midline of the palate with the anterior border extending to the maxillary primary canine. The image field of this projection should include the distal half of the primary canine and both primary molars.

Deciduous Mandibular Molar Projection.   A No. 0 receptor is positioned in a modified XCP or BAI bite-block, with or without the aiming ring and indicator bar, between the posterior teeth and tongue. The exposed radiograph should show the distal half of the mandibular primary canine and the primary molar teeth.

Mixed Dentition (7 to 12 Years)

A complete examination of the mixed dentition, if indicated, consists of two incisor periapical views, four canine periapical views, four posterior periapical views, and two or four posterior bitewing views (Fig. 7-10). For the maxillary and interproximal projections, the child should be seated upright with the sagittal plane perpendicular and the occlusal plane parallel to the floor. For the mandibular projections, the child should be seated upright with the sagittal plane perpendicular and the ala-tragus line parallel to the floor. XCP instruments are used for larger children.

Bisecting-angle bite-blocks may be more comfortable for smaller individuals.

Maxillary Anterior Periapical Projection.   A No. 1 receptor should be centered on the embrasure between the central incisors in the mouth behind the maxillary central and lateral incisors. The receptor should be centered on the midline.

Mandibular Anterior Periapical Projection.   A No. 1 receptor should be positioned behind the mandibular central and lateral incisors.

Canine Periapical Projection.   A No. 1 receptor should be positioned behind each of the canines.

Deciduous and Permanent Molar Periapical Projection.   A No. 1 or No. 2 receptor (if the child is large enough) should be positioned with the anterior edge behind the canine.

Posterior Bitewing Projection.   Bitewing projections should be exposed in the premolar region with a No. 1 or No. 2 receptor as previously described, using either bitewing tabs or the Rinn bitewing instrument. Four bitewing projections should be exposed when the second permanent molars have erupted.

MOBILE IMAGING

Occasionally it is difficult to have a patient come to a conventional wall-mounted dental x-ray machine. For instance, in remote sites such as nursing homes, hospitals, or at disaster scenes, it could be highly advantageous to have a portable machine that could be taken directly to the patient. Combining such a portable x-ray generator with digital imaging provides rapid, self-contained imaging capability. Such a portable battery-powered x-ray generator has been approved more recently by the U.S. Food and Drug Administration (Fig. 7-11). Clinical trials have shown that this unit can be held stable and produces clinically acceptable images. This machine uses a high-frequency, constant potential x-ray generator (60 kilowatt constant potential) and has a short focal spot-to-skin distance (20 cm). Both of these factors allow for short exposure times compared with conventional units. It has a small focus spot (0.4 mm). The operator dose is mitigated by the use of internal

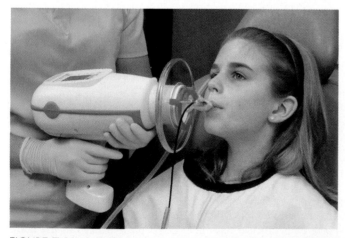

FIGURE 7-11 *Handheld x-ray machine useful for patients in remote situations. Operator dose is minimized by internal shielding and shield on aiming cylinder to reduce backscatter. (Courtesy Aribex, Inc., Orem, UT.)*

shielding materials in the unit to reduce leakage exposure and a shield on the aiming cylinder to minimize backscatter from the patient. These units are approved for use in many, but not all, states in the United States.

SPECIAL CONSIDERATIONS

The radiographic procedures that have been described in this chapter are for "well" patients. These procedures may need to be modified for patients who have unusual difficulties. Specific modifications depend on the patient's physical and emotional characteristics. However, as with any dental procedure, the dental assistant begins the examination by showing appreciation of the patient's condition and sympathy for any problems that might occur for either of them. If the assistant is kind but firm, the patient's confidence increases, which helps the patient relax and cooperate. Following are a few conditions and circumstances that may be encountered, with recommendations and suggestions that may help the clinician achieve an adequate radiographic examination.

INFECTION

Infection in the orofacial structures may result in edema and lead to trismus of some of the muscles of mastication. As a result, intraoral radiography may be painful to the patient and difficult for both the patient and the radiologist. Under such circumstances, extraoral or occlusal techniques may offer the only possibility of an examination. The choice of a specific extraoral projection depends on the condition and the areas to be examined. Although the resulting radiograph may not be ideal in many respects, it usually provides more useful information than the diagnostician would have without it. In the case of edema in an area to be examined, exposure time should be increased to compensate for the tissue swelling.

TRAUMA

A patient who has undergone trauma may have a dental or facial fracture. Dental fractures are best appreciated by using periapical or occlusal radiographs. Special care must be taken when making these views because of the condition of the patient. Skeletal fractures are usually best seen with panoramic or other extraoral views or a computed tomography examination. In some cases, patients with fractures of the facial skeleton may be bedridden because of other injuries. Consequently, an extraoral radiographic examination with the patient in the supine position is necessary. However, the circumstances need not compromise the techniques, and satisfactory intraoral images can be produced if the proper relative positions of the tube, patient, and receptor are observed.

PATIENTS WITH MENTAL DISABILITIES

Patients with mental disabilities may cause some difficulty for the radiologist who is attempting an examination. The difficulty usually is the result of the patient's lack of coordination or inability to comprehend what is expected. When the radiographic examination is performed speedily, unpredictable moves by the patient can be minimized. In some cases, sedation may be required.

PATIENTS WITH PHYSICAL DISABILITIES

Patients with physical disabilities (e.g., loss of vision, loss of hearing, loss of the use of any or all extremities, congenital defects such as cleft palate) may require special handling during a radiographic examination. These patients usually are cooperative and eager to assist. They may be accustomed to so much discomfort and inconvenience that their tolerance level is high, and they are not challenged by the relatively slight irritation represented by the x-ray procedures. Generally, intraoral and extraoral radiographic examinations may be performed for these patients if a good rapport between the patient and radiology technician is established and maintained. Members of the patient's family often are very helpful in assisting the patient into and out of the examination chair and in receptor positioning and holding, inasmuch as they usually are familiar with the patient's condition and accustomed to coping with it.

GAG REFLEX

Occasionally, patients who need a radiographic examination manifest a gag reflex at the slightest provocation. These patients usually are very apprehensive and frightened by unknown procedures; others simply seem to have very sensitive tissue that precipitates a gag reflex when stimulated. This sensitivity is manifested when the receptor is placed in the oral cavity. To overcome this disability, the radiologist should make an effort to relax and reassure the patient. The radiologist can describe and explain the procedures. Often gagging can be controlled if the operator bolsters the patient's confidence by demonstrating technical competence and showing authority tempered with compassion. The gag reflex often is worse when a patient is tired; therefore it is advisable to perform the examination in the morning, when the individual is well rested, especially in the case of children.

Stimulating the posterior dorsum of the tongue or the soft palate usually initiates the gag reflex. Consequently, during the placement of the receptor, the tongue should be very relaxed and positioned well to the floor of the mouth; this can be accomplished by asking the patient to swallow deeply just before opening the mouth for placement of the receptor. (The dentist should never mention the tongue or ask patients to relax the tongue; this usually makes them more conscious of it and precipitates involuntary movements.) The receptor is carried into the mouth parallel to the occlusal plane. When the desired area is reached, the receptor is rotated with a decisive motion, bringing it into contact with the palate or the floor of the mouth. Sliding it along the palate or tongue is likely to stimulate the gag reflex. Also, the dentist must keep in mind that the longer the receptor stays in the mouth, the greater the possibility that the patient will start to gag. The patient should be advised to breathe rapidly through the nose because mouth breathing usually aggravates this condition.

Any little exercise that can be devised that does not interfere with the x-ray examination but shifts the patient's attention from the receptor and the mouth is likely to relieve the gag reaction. Asking patients to hold their breath or to keep a foot or arm suspended during receptor placement and exposure often can create such a distraction. In extreme cases, topical anesthetic agents in mouthwashes or spray can be administered to produce temporary numbness of the tongue and palate to reduce gagging. However, in our experience, this procedure gives limited results. The most effective approach is to reduce apprehension, minimize tissue irritation, and encourage rapid breathing through the nose. If all measures fail, an extraoral examination may be the only means, short of administering general anesthesia, to examine the patient radiographically.

IMAGING FOR ENDODONTICS

Radiographs are essential to the practice of endodontics. Not only are they indispensable for determining the diagnosis and prognosis

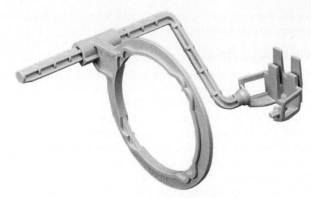

FIGURE 7-12 EndoRay receptor holder used for endodontic images. This device provides room for files to be in place when making the image. (Courtesy Dentsply Rinn, Elgin, IL.)

of pulp treatment, but also they are the most reliable method of managing endodontic treatment. The presence of a rubber dam, rubber dam clamp, and root canal instruments may complicate an intraoral periapical examination by impairing proper receptor positioning and aiming cylinder angulation. Despite these obstacles, certain requirements must be observed, as follows:

1. The tooth being treated must be centered in the image.
2. The receptor must be positioned as far from the tooth and apex as the region permits to ensure that the apex of the tooth and some periapical bone are apparent on the radiograph.

For maxillary projections, the patient is seated so that the sagittal plane is perpendicular and the occlusal plane is parallel to the floor. For mandibular projections, the patient is seated upright with the sagittal plane perpendicular and the tragus-to-corner of the mouth line parallel to the floor. Specially designed receptor holders for endodontic images are available (Fig. 7-12). These instruments fit over files, clamps, and the rubber dam without touching the subject tooth. The aiming cylinder is aligned so as to direct the central ray perpendicular to the center of the receptor.

Often a single radiograph of a multirooted tooth made at the normal vertical and horizontal projection does not display all the roots. In these cases, when it is necessary to separate the roots on multirooted teeth, a second projection may be made. The horizontal angulation is altered 20 degrees mesially for maxillary premolars, 20 degrees mesially or distally for maxillary molars, or 20 degrees distally for an oblique projection of mandibular molar roots.

If a sinus tract is encountered, its course is tracked by threading a No. 40 gutta-percha cone through the tract before the radiograph is made. It also is possible to localize and determine the depth of periodontal defects with this gutta-percha tracking technique.

A final radiograph of the treated tooth is made to demonstrate the quality of the root canal filling and the condition of the periapical tissues after removal of the clamp and rubber dam.

PREGNANCY

Although a fetus is sensitive to ionizing radiation, the amount of exposure received by an embryo or fetus during dental radiography is extremely low. There have been no reports of damage to a fetus from dental radiography. Regardless, prudence suggests that such radiographic examinations be kept to a minimum consistent with the mother's dental needs. As with any patient, radiographic examination is limited during pregnancy to cases with a specific diagnostic indication. With the low patient dose afforded by use of optimal radiation safety techniques (see Chapter 3), an intraoral or extraoral examination can be performed whenever a reasonable diagnostic requirement exists.

EDENTULOUS PATIENTS

Radiographic examination of edentulous patients is important, whether the area of interest is one tooth or an entire arch. These areas may contain roots, residual infection, impacted teeth, cysts, or other pathologic entities that may adversely affect the usefulness of prosthetic appliances or the patient's health. After a determination has been made that these entities are not present, repeated examinations to detect them are not warranted in the absence of signs or symptoms.

If available, a panoramic examination of the edentulous jaws is most convenient. If abnormalities of the alveolar ridges are identified, the higher resolution of periapical receptor is used to make intraoral projections to supplement the panoramic examination.

In a completely or partly edentulous patient, a receptor-holding device is used for intraoral radiography of the alveolar ridges. Placement of the receptor-holding instrument may be complicated by its tipping into the voids normally occupied by the crowns of the missing teeth. To manage this difficulty, cotton rolls are placed between the ridge and the receptor holder, supporting the holder in a horizontal position. An orthodontic elastic band to hold cotton rolls to the bite-block on the receptor holder often is useful when several such projections must be exposed. With elastics, it is simple to maneuver the cotton rolls into the areas that require support. The patient may steady the receptor-holding instrument with a hand or an opposing denture.

If panoramic equipment is unavailable, an examination consisting of 14 intraoral views provides an excellent survey. The exposure required for an edentulous ridge is approximately 25% less than that for a dentulous ridge. This examination consists of seven projections in each jaw (adult No. 2 receptor) as follows:

Central incisors (midline): one projection
Lateral canine: two projections
Premolar: two projections
Molar: two projections

BIBLIOGRAPHY

Adriaens PA, De Boever J, Vande Velde F: Comparison of intra-oral long-cone paralleling radiographic surveys and orthopantomographs with special reference to the bone height, *J Oral Rehabil* 9:355–365, 1982.

Biggerstaff RH, Phillips JR: A quantitative comparison of paralleling long-cone and bisection-of-angle periapical radiography, *Oral Surg Oral Med Oral Pathol* 62:673–677, 1976.

Dubrez B, Jacot-Descombes S, Cimasoni G: Reliability of a paralleling instrument for dental radiographs, *Oral Surg Oral Med Oral Pathol Oral Radiol Endod* 80:358–364, 1995.

Forsberg J, Halse A: Radiographic simulation of a periapical lesion comparing the paralleling and the bisecting-angle techniques, *Int Endod J* 27:133–138, 1994.

Iannucci J, Jansen Howerton L: *Dental radiography: principles and techniques*, ed 3, St Louis, 2006, Saunders.

Scandrett FR, Tebo HG, Miller JT, et al: Radiographic examination of the edentulous patient, 1: review of the literature and preliminary report comparing three methods, *Oral Surg Oral Med Oral Pathol* 35:266–274, 1973.

Schulze RK, d'Hoedt B: A method to calculate angular disparities between object and receptor in "paralleling technique," *Dentomaxillofac Radiol* 31:32–38, 2002.

Weclew TV: Comparing the paralleling extension cone technique and the bisecting angle technique, *J Acad Gen Dent* 22:18–20, 1974.

Intraoral Anatomy

The radiographic recognition of disease requires a sound knowledge of the radiographic appearance of normal structures. Intelligent diagnosis mandates an appreciation of the wide range of variation in the appearance of normal anatomic structures. Similarly, most patients demonstrate many of the normal radiographic landmarks, but it is a rare patient who shows them all. The absence of one or even several such landmarks in any individual should not necessarily be considered abnormal.

TEETH

Teeth are composed primarily of dentin, with an enamel cap over the coronal portion and a thin layer of cementum over the root surface (Fig. 8-1). The enamel cap characteristically appears more radiopaque than the other tissues because it is the most dense, naturally occurring substance in the body. Because it is 90% mineral, it causes the greatest attenuation of x-ray photons. Its radiographic appearance is uniformly opaque and without evidence of the fine structure. Only the occlusal surface reflects the complex gross anatomy. The dentin is about 75% mineralized, and because of its lower mineral content, its radiographic appearance is roughly comparable to bone. Dentin is smooth and homogeneous on radiographs because of its uniform morphologic features. The junction between enamel and dentin appears as a distinct interface that separates these two structures. The thin layer of cementum on the root surface has a mineral content (50%) comparable to dentin. Cementum is not usually apparent radiographically because the contrast between it and dentin is so low and the cementum layer is so thin.

Diffuse radiolucent areas with ill-defined borders may be apparent radiographically on the mesial or distal aspects of teeth in the cervical regions between the edge of the enamel cap and the crest

of the alveolar ridge (Fig. 8-2). This phenomenon, called **cervical burnout**, is caused by the normal configuration of the affected teeth, which results in decreased x-ray absorption in the areas in question. Close inspection reveals intact edges of the proximal surfaces. The perception of these radiolucent areas results from the contrast with the adjacent, relatively opaque enamel and alveolar bone. Such radiolucencies should be anticipated in almost all teeth and should not be confused with root surface caries, which frequently have a similar appearance.

The pulp of normal teeth is composed of soft tissue and consequently appears radiolucent. The chambers and root canals containing the pulp extend from the interior of the crown to the apices of the roots. Although the shape of most pulp chambers is fairly uniform within tooth groups, great variations exist among individuals in the size of the pulp chambers and the extent of pulp horns. The practitioner must anticipate such variations in the proportions and distribution of the pulp and verify them radiographically when planning restorative procedures.

In normal, fully formed teeth, the root canal may be apparent, extending from the pulp chamber to the apex of the root. An apical foramen is usually recognizable (Fig. 8-3). In other normal teeth, the canal may appear constricted in the region of the apex and not discernible in the last 1 mm or so of its length (Fig. 8-4). In this case, the canal may occasionally exit on the side of the tooth, just short of the radiographic apex. Lateral canals may occur as branches of an otherwise normal root canal. They may extend to the apex and end in a normal, discernible foramen or may exit the side of the root. In either case, two or more terminal foramina might cause endodontic treatment to fail if they are not identified.

At the end of a developing tooth root, the pulp canal diverges, and the walls of the root rapidly taper to a knife edge (Fig. 8-5). In the recess formed by the root walls and extending a

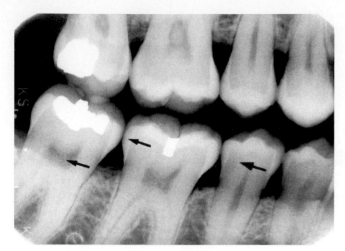

FIGURE 8-1 Teeth are composed of pulp (*arrow* on the second molar), enamel (*arrow* on the first molar), dentin (*arrow* on the second premolar), and cementum (usually not visible radiographically).

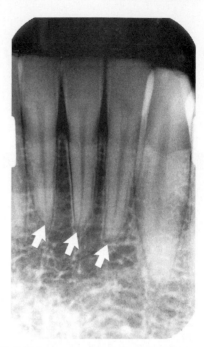

FIGURE 8-3 Root canals open at the apices of adult incisors (*arrows*).

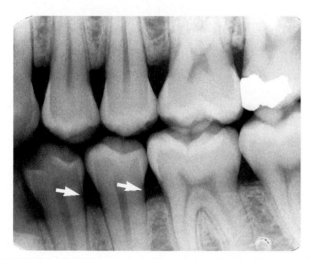

FIGURE 8-2 Cervical burnout is caused by overexposure of the lateral portion of roots between the enamel and the alveolar crest and results in an ill-defined radiolucent zone (*arrows*).

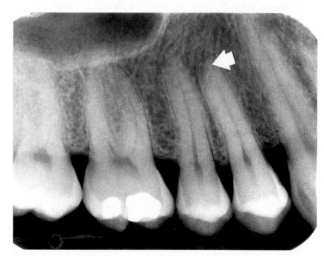

FIGURE 8-4 Although the root canal is typically not radiographically visible in the apical 2 mm of a tooth, anatomically it is present and contains vascular and neural supply to the pulp (*arrow*).

short distance beyond is a small, rounded, radiolucent area in the trabecular bone, surrounded by a thin layer of hyperostotic bone. This is the dental papilla bounded by its bony crypt. The papilla forms the dentin and the primordium of the pulp. When the tooth reaches maturity, the pulpal walls in the apical region begin to constrict and finally come into close apposition. Awareness of this sequence and its radiographic pattern is often useful in evaluating the stage of maturation of the developing tooth; it also helps avoid misidentifying the apical radiolucency as a periapical lesion.

In a mature tooth, the shape of the pulp chamber and canal may change. A gradual deposition of secondary dentin occurs with aging. This process begins apically, proceeds coronally, and may lead to pulp obliteration. Trauma to the tooth (e.g., from caries, a blow, restorations, attrition, or erosion) also may stimulate dentin production, leading to a reduction in size of the pulp chamber and canals. Such cases usually include evidence of the source of the pathologic stimulus. However, in the case of a blow to the teeth, only the patient's recollection may suggest the true reason for the reduced pulp chamber size.

SUPPORTING STRUCTURES

LAMINA DURA

A radiograph of sound teeth in a normal dental arch demonstrates that the tooth sockets are bounded by a thin radiopaque layer of dense bone (Fig. 8-6). Its name, lamina dura ("hard layer"), is derived from its radiographic appearance. This layer is continuous with the shadow of the cortical bone at the alveolar crest. It is only slightly thicker and no more highly mineralized than the trabeculae of cancellous bone in the area. Its radiographic appearance is caused by the fact that the x-ray beam passes tangentially through many times the thickness of the thin bony wall, which results in its observed attenuation (the eggshell effect). Developmentally, the lamina dura is an extension of the lining of the bony crypt that surrounds each tooth during development.

The appearance of the lamina dura on radiographs may vary. When the x-ray beam is directed through a relatively long expanse of the structure, the lamina dura appears radiopaque and well defined. When the beam is directed more obliquely, the lamina dura appears more diffuse and may not be discernible. In fact, even if the supporting bone in a healthy arch is intact, identification of a lamina dura completely surrounding every root on each film is frequently difficult, although it usually is evident to some extent about the roots on each film (Fig. 8-7). In addition, small variations and disruptions in the continuity of the lamina dura may result from superimpositions of cancellous bone and small nutrient canals passing from the marrow spaces to the periodontal ligament (PDL).

The thickness and density of the lamina dura on the radiograph vary with the amount of occlusal stress to which the tooth is subjected. The lamina dura is wider and more dense around the roots of teeth in heavy occlusion and thinner and less dense around teeth not subjected to occlusal function.

The appearance of the lamina dura is a valuable diagnostic feature. The presence of an intact lamina dura around the apex of a tooth strongly suggests a vital pulp. However, because of the variable appearance of the lamina dura, the absence of its image around an apex on a radiograph may be normal. Rarely, the lamina dura may be absent from a molar root extending into the maxillary sinus in the absence of disease. Therefore, the clinician is advised to consider other signs and symptoms as well as the integrity of the lamina dura when establishing a diagnosis and treatment.

ALVEOLAR CREST

The gingival margin of the alveolar process that extends between the teeth is apparent on radiographs as a radiopaque line—the alveolar crest (Fig. 8-8). The level of this bony crest is considered normal when it is not more than 1.5 mm from the cementoenamel junction of the adjacent teeth. The alveolar crest may recede

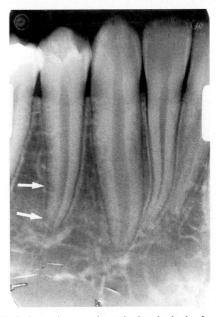

FIGURE 8-7 The lamina dura is poorly visualized on the distal surface of this premolar *(arrows)* but is clearly seen on the mesial surface. A broad, flat lamina dura oriented parallel to the x-ray beam produces a prominent lamina dura, whereas a curved, narrow lamina dura is less visible.

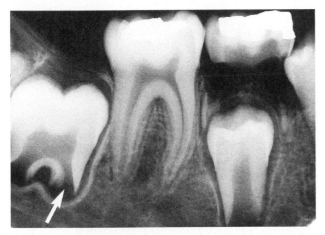

FIGURE 8-5 A developing root shown by a divergent apex around the dental papilla *(arrow)*, which is enclosed by an opaque bony crypt. The apices of the first molar are still open but nearing closure.

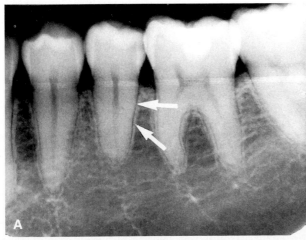
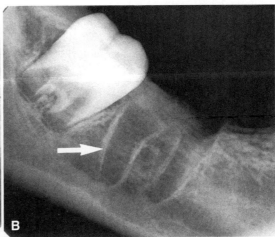

FIGURE 8-6 The lamina dura *(arrows)* appears as a thin opaque layer of bone around teeth **(A)** and around a recent extraction socket **(B)**.

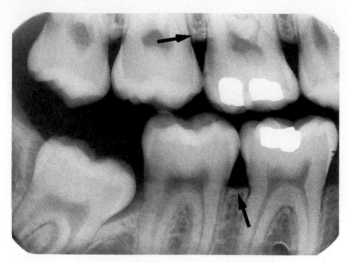

FIGURE 8-8 The alveolar crests *(arrows)* are seen as cortical borders of the alveolar bone. The alveolar crest is continuous with the lamina dura.

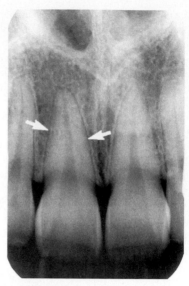

FIGURE 8-9 The periodontal ligament space *(arrows)* is seen as a narrow radiolucency between the tooth root and the lamina dura.

apically with age and show marked resorption with periodontal disease. Radiographs can demonstrate only the position of the crest; determining the significance of its level is primarily a clinical problem (see Chapter 19).

The length of the normal alveolar crest in a particular region depends on the distance between the teeth in question. In the anterior region, the crest is reduced to only a point of bone between the close-set incisors. Posteriorly, it is flat, aligned parallel with and slightly below a line connecting the cementoenamel junctions of the adjacent teeth. The crest of the bone is continuous with the lamina dura and forms a sharp angle with it. Rounding of these sharp junctions is indicative of periodontal disease.

The image of the crest varies from a dense layer of cortical bone to a smooth surface without cortical bone. In the latter case, the trabeculae at the surface are of normal size and density. In the posterior regions, this range of radiodensity of the crest is presumed to be normal if the bone is at a proper level in relation to the teeth. However, the absence of an image of cortex between the incisors is considered by many to be an indication of incipient disease, even if the level of the bone is not abnormal.

PERIODONTAL LIGAMENT SPACE

Because the PDL is composed primarily of collagen, it appears as a radiolucent space between the tooth root and the lamina dura. This space begins at the alveolar crest, extends around the portions of the tooth roots within the alveolus, and returns to the alveolar crest on the opposite side of the tooth (Fig. 8-9).

The PDL varies in width from patient to patient, from tooth to tooth in the individual, and even from location to location around one tooth (Fig. 8-10). It is usually thinner in the middle of the root and slightly wider near the alveolar crest and root apex, suggesting that the fulcrum of physiologic movement is in the region where the PDL is thinnest. The thickness of the ligament relates to the degree of function because the PDL is thinnest around the roots of embedded teeth and teeth that have lost their antagonists. The reverse is not true, however, because an appreciably wider space is not regularly observed in persons with especially heavy occlusion or bruxism.

The shape of the tooth creates the appearance of a double PDL space. When the x-ray beam is directed so that two convexities of a root surface appear on a film, a double PDL space is seen

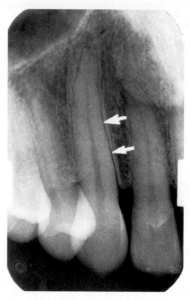

FIGURE 8-10 The periodontal ligament space appears wide on the mesial surface of this canine *(arrows)* and thin on the distal surface.

(Fig. 8-11). A common example of this double PDL space is seen on the buccal and lingual eminences on the mesial surface of mandibular first and second molar roots.

CANCELLOUS BONE

The cancellous bone (also called trabecular bone or spongiosa) lies between the cortical plates in both jaws. It is composed of thin radiopaque plates and rods (trabeculae) surrounding many small radiolucent pockets of marrow. The radiographic pattern of the trabeculae comes from two anatomic sources. The first is the cancellous bone itself. The second is the endosteal surface of the outer cortical bone where the cancellous bone fuses with the cortical bone. At this surface, trabecular plates are relatively thick and make a significant contribution to the radiographic image. The trabecular pattern shows considerable intrapatient and interpatient variability,

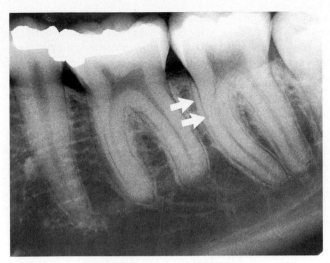

FIGURE 8-11 A double periodontal ligament space and lamina dura *(arrows)* may be seen when there is a convexity of the proximal surface of the root resulting in two heights of contour. Double PDL spaces may also be seen on the mesial surfaces of both roots of the first molar.

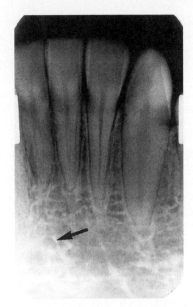

FIGURE 8-13 The trabecular pattern in the anterior mandible is characterized by coarser trabecular plates *(arrow)* and larger marrow spaces than in the anterior maxilla.

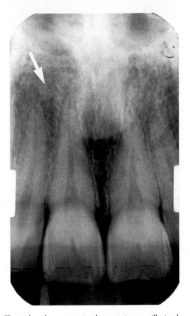

FIGURE 8-12 The trabecular pattern in the anterior maxilla is characterized by fine trabecular plates and multiple small trabecular spaces *(arrow)*.

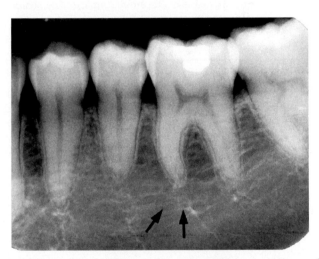

FIGURE 8-14 The trabecular pattern in the posterior mandible is quite variable, generally showing large marrow spaces and sparse trabeculation, especially inferiorly *(arrows)*.

which is normal and not a manifestation of disease. To evaluate the trabecular pattern in a specific area, the practitioner should examine the trabecular distribution, size, and density and compare them throughout both jaws and especially with the corresponding region on the opposite side. This comparison frequently demonstrates that a particularly suspect region is characteristic for the individual.

The trabeculae in the anterior maxilla are typically thin and numerous, forming a fine, granular, dense pattern (Fig. 8-12), and the marrow spaces are consequently small and relatively numerous. In the posterior maxilla, the trabecular pattern is usually quite similar to the pattern in the anterior maxilla, although the marrow spaces may be slightly larger.

In the anterior mandible, the trabeculae are thicker than in the maxilla, resulting in a coarser pattern (Fig. 8-13) with trabecular

plates that are oriented more horizontally. The trabecular plates are also fewer than in the maxilla, and the marrow spaces are correspondingly larger. In the posterior mandible, the periradicular trabeculae and marrow spaces may be comparable to those in the anterior mandible but are usually larger (Fig. 8-14). The trabecular plates also are oriented mainly horizontally in this region. Below the apices of the mandibular molars, the number of trabeculae dwindles still more. In some cases, the area from just below the molar roots to the inferior border of the mandible may appear to be almost devoid of trabeculae. The distribution and size of the trabeculae throughout both jaws show a relationship to the thickness (and strength) of the adjacent cortical plates. It may be speculated that where the cortical plates are thick (e.g., in the posterior region of the mandibular body), internal bracing by the trabeculae is not required, so there are relatively few except where required to support the alveoli. By contrast, in the maxilla and anterior region of the mandible, where the cortical plates are relatively thin and less rigid, trabeculae are more numerous and lend internal bolstering to the jaw. Occasionally, the trabecular spaces in this region are very irregular, with some so large that they mimic pathologic lesions.

If trabeculae are apparently absent, suggesting the presence of disease, it is often revealing to examine previous radiographs of the region in question. This helps determine whether the current appearance represents a change from a prior condition. An abnormality is more likely when the comparison indicates a change in the trabecular pattern. If prior films are unavailable, it is frequently useful to repeat the radiographic examination at a reduced exposure because this often demonstrates the presence of an expected but sparse trabecular pattern that was overexposed and burned out in the initial projection. Finally, if prior films are unavailable and reduced exposure does not allay the examiner's apprehension, it may be appropriate to expose another radiograph at a later time to monitor for ominous changes. Considerable variation may exist in trabecular patterns among patients, so examining all regions of the jaws is important in evaluating a trabecular pattern for any individual. This examination enables the dentist to determine the general nature of the particular pattern and whether any areas deviate appreciably from that norm.

The buccal and lingual cortical plates of the mandible and maxilla do not cast a discernible image on periapical radiographs.

MAXILLA

INTERMAXILLARY SUTURE

The intermaxillary suture (also called the median suture) appears on intraoral periapical radiographs as a thin radiolucent line in the midline between the two portions of the premaxilla (Fig. 8-15). It extends from the alveolar crest between the central incisors superiorly through the anterior nasal spine and continues posteriorly between the maxillary palatine processes to the posterior aspect of the hard palate. It is not unusual for this narrow radiolucent suture to terminate at the alveolar crest in a small rounded or V-shaped enlargement (Fig. 8-16). The suture is limited by two parallel

radiopaque borders of thin cortical bone on each side of the maxilla. The radiolucent region is usually of uniform width. The adjacent cortical margins may be either smooth or slightly irregular. The appearance of the intermaxillary suture depends on both anatomic variability and the angulation of the x-ray beam through the suture.

ANTERIOR NASAL SPINE

The anterior nasal spine is most frequently demonstrated on periapical radiographs of the maxillary central incisors (Fig. 8-17). Located in the midline, it lies approximately 1.5 to 2 cm above the alveolar crest, usually at or just below the junction of the inferior end of the nasal septum and the inferior outline of the nasal aperture. It is radiopaque because of its bony composition, and it is usually V-shaped.

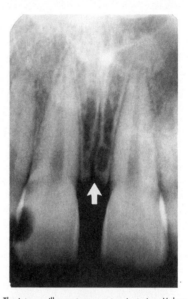

FIGURE 8-16 The intermaxillary suture may terminate in a V-shaped widening *(arrow)* at the alveolar crest. This is a normal variation and should not be confused with alveolar bone loss associated with periodontal disease.

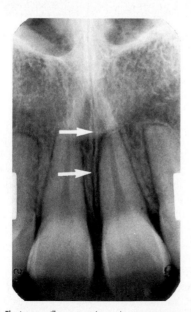

FIGURE 8-15 The intermaxillary suture *(arrows)* appears as a curved radiolucency in the midline of the maxilla.

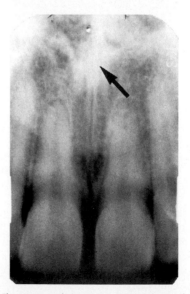

FIGURE 8-17 The anterior nasal spine is seen as an opaque, irregular or V-shaped projection from the floor of the nasal aperture in the midline *(arrow)*.

NASAL APERTURE

Because the air-filled nasal aperture (and cavity) lies just above the oral cavity, its radiolucent image may be apparent on intraoral radiographs of the maxillary teeth, especially in central incisor projections. On periapical radiographs of the incisors, the inferior border of the fossa aperture appears as a radiopaque line extending bilaterally away from the base of the anterior nasal spine (Fig. 8-18). Above this line is the radiolucent space of the inferior portion of the cavity. If the radiograph was made with the x-ray beam directed in the sagittal plane, the relatively radiopaque nasal septum is seen arising in the midline from the anterior nasal spine (Fig. 8-19). The shadow of the septum may appear wider than anticipated and not sharply defined because the image is a superimposition of septal cartilage and vomer bone. Also, the septum frequently deviates

slightly from the midline, and its plate of bone (the vomer) is curved.

The nasal cavity contains the opaque shadows of the inferior conchae extending from the right and left lateral walls for varying distances toward the septum. These conchae fill varying amounts of the lateral portions of the cavity (Fig. 8-20). The floor of the nasal aperture and a small segment of the nasal cavity are occasionally projected high onto a maxillary canine radiograph (Fig. 8-21).

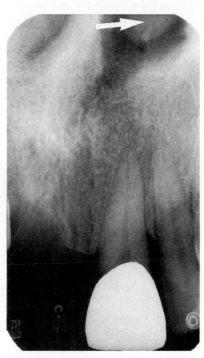

FIGURE 8-20 The mucosal covering of the inferior concha *(arrow)* is occasionally visualized in the nasal cavity.

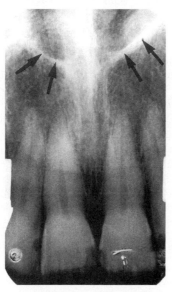

FIGURE 8-18 The anterior floor of the nasal aperture *(arrows)* appears as opaque lines extending laterally from the anterior nasal spine.

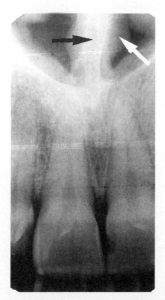

FIGURE 8-19 The nasal septum *(black arrow)* arises directly above the anterior nasal spine and is covered on each side by mucosa *(white arrow).*

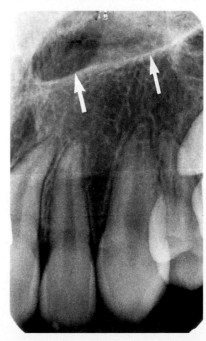

FIGURE 8-21 The floor of the nasal aperture *(arrows)* often may be seen extending posteriorly from the anterior nasal spine above the maxillary lateral incisor and canine.

Also, in the posterior maxillary region, the floor of the nasal cavity may be seen in the region of the maxillary sinus. (It is impossible to determine from a single radiograph which of two superimposed structures is in front of or behind the other, unless the conclusion is based on an awareness of the anatomic features and relationships.) It may falsely convey the impression of a septum in the sinus or a limiting superior sinus wall (Fig. 8-22).

INCISIVE FORAMEN

The incisive foramen (also called the nasopalatine foramen or anterior palatine foramen) in the maxilla is the oral terminus of the nasopalatine canal. This canal originates in the anterior floor of the nasal fossa. The incisive foramen transmits the nasopalatine vessels and nerves (which may participate in the innervation of the maxillary central incisors) and lies in the midline of the palate behind the central incisors at approximately the junction of the

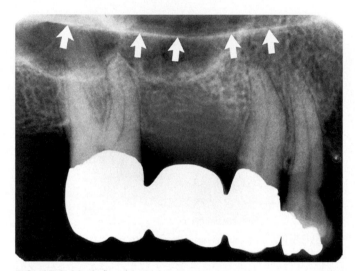

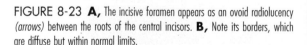
FIGURE 8-22 The floor of the nasal aperture *(arrows)* extends posteriorly, superimposed over the maxillary sinus.

median palatine and incisive sutures. The radiographic image is usually projected between the roots and in the region of the middle and apical thirds of the central incisors (Fig. 8-23). The foramen varies markedly in its radiographic shape, size, and sharpness. It may appear smoothly symmetric, with numerous forms, or very irregular, with a well-demarcated or ill-defined border. The position of the foramen is also variable and may be recognized at the apices of the central incisor roots, near the alveolar crest, anywhere in between, or extending over the entire distance. The great variability of its radiographic image is primarily the result of (1) the differing angles at which the x-ray beam is directed for the maxillary central incisors and (2) some variability in its anatomic size.

Familiarity with the incisive foramen is important because it is a potential site of cyst formation. An incisive canal cyst is radiographically discernible because it frequently causes a readily perceived enlargement of the foramen and canal. The presence of a cyst is presumed if the width of the foramen exceeds 1 cm or if enlargement can be demonstrated on successive radiographs. Also, if the radiolucency of the normal foramen is projected over the apex of one central incisor, it may suggest a pathologic periapical condition. The absence of disease is indicated by a lack of clinical symptoms and an intact lamina dura around the central incisor in question.

The lateral walls of the nasopalatine canal are not usually seen on periapical views but occasionally can be visualized on a projection of the central incisors as a pair of radiopaque lines running vertically from the superior foramina of the nasopalatine canal to the incisive foramen (Fig. 8-24, *A*). However, cone-beam images of this region regularly demonstrate the borders of the nasopalatine canal (Figs. 8-24, *B* and *C*). Visualization of these structures is important when placing an implant in this region is being considered.

SUPERIOR FORAMINA OF THE NASOPALATINE CANAL

The nasopalatine canal originates at two foramina in the floor of the nasal cavity. The openings are on each side of the nasal septum, close to the anteroinferior border of the nasal cavity, and each canal passes downward anteriorly and medially to unite with the

FIGURE 8-23 A, The incisive foramen appears as an ovoid radiolucency *(arrows)* between the roots of the central incisors. **B,** Note its borders, which are diffuse but within normal limits.

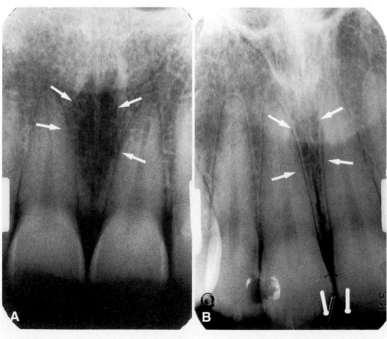

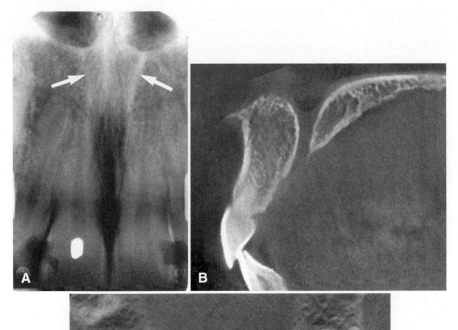

FIGURE 8-24 Nasopalatine canal. **A,** The lateral walls of the nasopalatine canal *(arrows)* extend from the incisive foramen to the floor of the nasal fossa. **B,** Cone-beam image in the sagittal plane shows superior foramina in the floor of the nasal fossa, the anterior and posterior borders of the canal, and the incisive foramen opening onto the hard palate. **C,** Cone-beam image in the axial plane at the level of the incisive foramen shows anterior and lateral borders of the incisive canal lying palatal to the incisor roots seen in cross section.

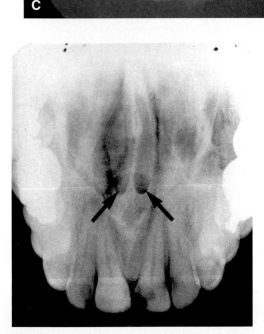

FIGURE 8-25 The superior foramina of the nasopalatine canal *(arrows)* appear just lateral to the nasal septum and posterior to the anterior nasal spine.

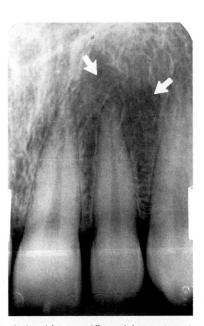

FIGURE 8-26 The lateral fossa is a diffuse radiolucency *(arrows)* in the region of the apex of the lateral incisor. It is formed by a depression in the maxilla at this location.

LATERAL FOSSA

The lateral fossa (also called incisive fossa) is a gentle depression in the maxilla near the apex of the lateral incisor (Fig. 8-26). It may appear diffusely radiolucent on periapical projections of this region. The image will not be misinterpreted as a pathologic

canal from the other side in a common opening, the incisive (nasopalatine) foramen. The superior foramina of the canal occasionally appear in projections of the maxillary incisors, especially when an exaggerated vertical angle is used (Fig. 8-25). They are usually round or oval, although they may make various outlines, depending on the angle of projection.

condition, however, if the radiograph is examined for an intact lamina dura around the root of the lateral incisor. This finding, coupled with absence of clinical symptoms, suggests normalcy of the bone.

NOSE

The soft tissue of the tip of the nose is frequently seen in projections of the maxillary central and lateral incisors, superimposed over the roots of these teeth. The image of the nose has a uniform, slightly opaque appearance with a sharp border (Fig. 8-27). Occasionally, the radiolucent nares can be identified, especially when a steep vertical angle is used.

NASOLACRIMAL CANAL

The nasal and maxillary bones form the nasolacrimal canal. It runs from the medial aspect of the anteroinferior border of the orbit inferiorly to drain under the inferior concha into the nasal cavity. Occasionally, it can be visualized on periapical radiographs in the region above the apex of the canine, especially when steep vertical angulation is used (Fig. 8-28). The nasolacrimal canals are routinely seen on maxillary occlusal projections (see Chapter 7) in the region of the molars (Fig. 8-29).

MAXILLARY SINUS

The maxillary sinus, similar to the other paranasal sinuses, is an air-containing cavity lined with mucous membrane. It develops by the invagination of mucous membrane from the nasal cavity. The largest of the paranasal sinuses, it normally occupies virtually the entire body of the maxilla. Its function is unknown.

The sinus may be considered as a three-sided pyramid, with its base the medial wall adjacent to the nasal cavity and its apex extending laterally into the zygomatic process of the maxilla. Its three sides are (1) the superior wall forming the floor of the orbit, (2) the anterior wall extending above the premolars, and (3) the posterior wall bulging above the molar teeth and maxillary tuberosity. The sinus communicates with the nasal cavity by the ostium, approximately 3 to 6 mm in diameter and positioned under the posterior aspect of the middle concha of the ethmoid bone.

The borders of the maxillary sinus appear on periapical radiographs as a thin, delicate, tenuous radiopaque line (actually a thin layer of cortical bone) (Fig. 8-30). In the absence of disease, it appears continuous, but on close examination it can be seen to have small interruptions in its smoothness or density. These discontinuities are probably illusions caused by superimposition of small marrow spaces. In adults, the sinuses are usually seen to extend from the distal aspect of the canine to the posterior wall of the maxilla above the tuberosity.

The maxillary sinuses show considerable variation in size. They enlarge during childhood, achieving mature size by age 15 to 18 years. They may change during adult life in response to environmental factors. The right and left sinuses usually appear similar in shape and size, although marked asymmetry is occasionally present. The floors of the maxillary sinus and nasal cavity are seen on dental

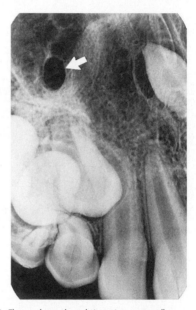

FIGURE 8-28 The nasolacrimal canal *(arrow)* is occasionally seen near the apex of the canine when steep vertical angulation is used. Note the mesiodens (supernumerary tooth) in the midline superior to the central incisor.

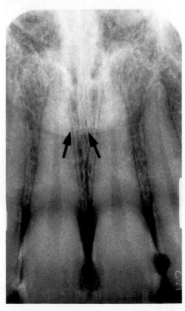

FIGURE 8-27 The soft tissue outline of the nose *(arrows)* is superimposed on the anterior maxilla.

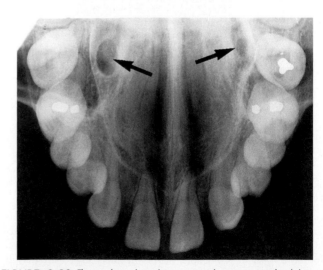

FIGURE 8-29 The nasolacrimal canals are commonly seen as ovoid radiolucencies *(arrows)* on maxillary occlusal projections. They should not be confused with the greater palatine foramina, which are not apparent on maxillary occlusal projections.

radiographs at approximately the same level around the age of puberty. In older individuals, the sinus may extend farther into the alveolar process; in the posterior region of the maxilla, its floor may appear considerably below the level of the floor of the nasal cavity. Anteriorly, each sinus is restricted by the canine fossa and is usually seen to sweep superiorly, crossing the level of the floor of the nasal cavity in the premolar or canine region. Consequently, on periapical radiographs of the canine, the floors of the sinus and nasal cavity are often superimposed and may be seen crossing one another, forming an inverted "Y" in the area (Fig. 8-31).

The outline of the nasal fossa is usually heavier and more diffuse than the outline of the thin, delicate cortical bone denoting the sinus. The degree of extension of the maxillary sinus into the alveolar process is extremely variable. In some projections, the floor of the sinus is well above the apices of the posterior teeth; in others, it may extend well beyond the apices toward the alveolar ridge. In response to a loss of function (associated with the loss of posterior teeth), the sinus may expand farther into the alveolar bone, occasionally extending to the alveolar ridge (Fig. 8-32).

The roots of the molars usually lie in close apposition to the maxillary sinus. Root apices may project anatomically into the floor of the sinus, causing small elevations or prominences. The thin layer of bone covering the root is seen as a fusion of the lamina dura and the floor of the sinus. Rarely, defects may be present in the bony covering of the root apices in the sinus floor, and a periapical radiograph fails to show lamina dura covering the apex.

When the rounded sinus floor dips between the buccal and palatal molar roots and is medial to the premolar roots, the projection of the apices is superior to the floor. This appearance conveys the impression that the roots project into the sinus cavity, which is an illusion. As the positive vertical angle of the projection is increased, the roots medial to the sinus appear to project farther into the sinus cavity. In contrast, the roots that are lateral to the sinus appear to move either out of the sinus or farther away from it as the angle is increased.

The intimate relationship between sinus and teeth leads to the possibility that clinical symptoms originating in the sinus may be perceived in the teeth and vice versa. This proximity of sinus and teeth is in part a consequence of the gradual developmental expansion of the maxillary sinus, which thins the sinus walls and opens

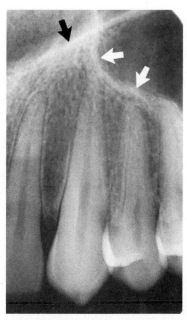

FIGURE 8-31 The anterior border of the maxillary sinus *(white arrows)* crosses the floor of the nasal fossa *(black arrow).*

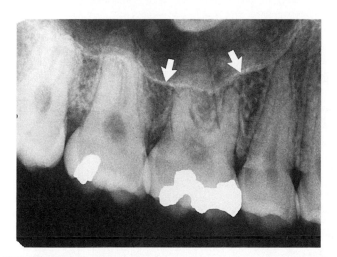

FIGURE 8-30 The inferior border of the maxillary sinus *(arrows)* appears as a thin radiopaque line near the apices of the maxillary premolars and molars.

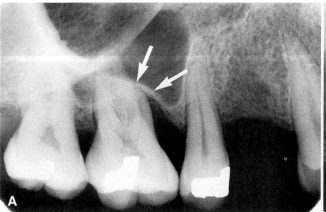

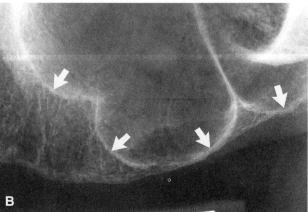

FIGURE 8-32 **A** and **B,** The floor of the maxillary sinus *(arrows)* often extends toward the crest of the alveolar ridge in response to missing teeth.

the canals that traverse the anterolateral and posterolateral walls and carry the superior alveolar nerves. The nerves are in intimate contact with the membrane lining the sinus. As a result, an acute inflammation of the sinus is frequently accompanied by pain in the maxillary teeth innervated by the portion of the nerve proximal to the insult. Subjective symptoms in the area of the maxillary posterior teeth may require careful analysis to differentiate tooth pain from sinus pain.

Frequently, thin radiolucent lines of uniform width are found within the image of the maxillary sinus (Fig. 8-33). These are the shadows of neurovascular canals or grooves in the lateral sinus walls that accommodate the posterior superior alveolar vessels, their branches, and the accompanying superior alveolar nerves. Although they may be found coursing in any direction (including vertically), they are usually seen running a curved posteroanterior course that is convex toward the alveolar process. Occasionally, they may be found to branch and rarely also to extend outside the image of the sinus and continue as an interradicular channel. Because such vascular markings are not seen in the walls of cysts, they may serve to distinguish a healthy sinus from a cyst.

Often one or several radiopaque lines traverse the image of the maxillary sinus (Fig. 8-34). These opaque lines are called septa. They are thin folds of cortical bone that project a few millimeters away from the floor and wall of the antrum, or they may extend across the sinus. They are usually oriented vertically and vary in number, thickness, and length. They appear on many periapical intraoral radiographs and frequently on cone-beam images. Although septa appear to separate the sinuses into distinct compartments, this is seldom the case. Rather, the septa typically extend only a few millimeters into the central volume of the sinus.

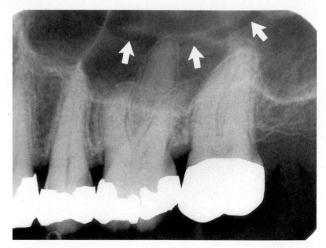

FIGURE 8-33 Neurovascular canals *(arrows)* in the lateral wall of the maxillary sinus. Such vascular canals, although typically less prominent, are commonly seen in the walls of the normal maxillary sinus.

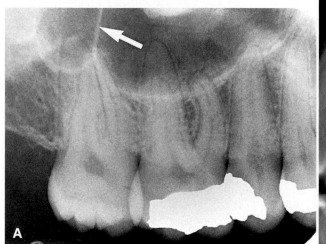

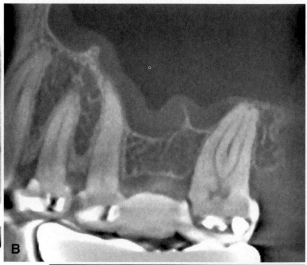

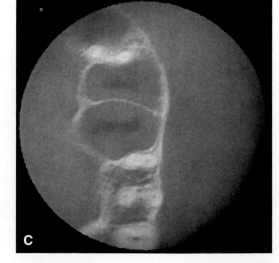

FIGURE 8-34 Maxillary sinus septa. **A,** Septum *(arrow)* in the maxillary sinus formed by a low ridge of bone on the sinus wall. (See also Fig. 8-32, *B.*) **B,** Sagittal section shows septa in the region of the missing first molar (different patient than **A**). Note also thickening of the sinus mucous membrane. **C,** Axial section of **B** at the level of the septum shows extension of septa from the buccal to palatal wall of the sinus.

Septa warrant attention because they sometimes mimic periapical disease, and the chambers they create in the alveolar recess may complicate the search for a root fragment displaced into the sinus.

The floor of the maxillary sinus occasionally shows small radiopaque projections, which are nodules of bone (Fig. 8-35). These must be differentiated from root tips, which they resemble in shape. In contrast to a root fragment, which is quite homogeneous in appearance, the bony nodules often show trabeculation; although they may be quite well defined, at certain points on their surface they blend with the trabecular pattern of adjacent bone. A root fragment may also be recognized by the presence of a root canal. It is common to see the floor of the nasal fossa in periapical views of the posterior teeth superimposed on the maxillary sinus (see Fig. 8-22). The floor of the nasal fossa is usually oriented more or less horizontally, depending on film placement, and is superimposed high on maxillary views. The image, a solid opaque line, frequently appears thicker than the adjacent sinus walls and septa.

ZYGOMATIC PROCESS AND ZYGOMA

The zygomatic process of the maxilla is an extension of the lateral maxillary surface that arises in the region of the apices of the first

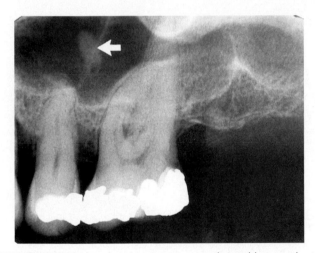

FIGURE 8-35 This bony mass (arrow) may represent a bony nodule, a normal variant of the floor of the maxillary sinus, but is most likely a retained root fragment from a prior extraction.

and second molars and articulates with the maxillary process of the zygoma. On periapical radiographs, the zygomatic process appears as a U-shaped radiopaque line with its open end directed superiorly. The enclosed rounded end is projected in the apical region of the first and second molars (Fig. 8-36). The size, width, and definition of the zygomatic process are quite variable, and its image may be large, depending on the angle at which the beam was projected. The maxillary antrum may expand laterally into the zygomatic process of the maxilla (and into the zygomatic bone after the maxillozygomatic suture has fused), resulting in a relatively increased radiolucent region within the U-shaped image of the process.

When the sinus is recessed deep within the process as in Fig. 8-36, B (and perhaps into the zygoma), the image of the air space within the process is dark. Typically the walls of the process are thin and well defined (in contrast to the very dark radiolucent air space). When the sinus exhibits relatively little penetration of the maxillary process as in Fig. 8-36, A (usually in younger individuals or individuals who have maintained their posterior teeth and vigorous masticatory function), the image of the walls of the zygomatic process of the maxilla tends to be thicker, and the appearance of the sinus in this region is smaller and more opaque.

The inferior border of the zygoma extends posteriorly from the inferior border of the zygomatic process of the maxilla to the zygomatic process of the temporal bone. It can be identified as a uniform radiopacity over the apices of the molars (Fig. 8-37). The zygomatic process of the temporal bone and the body of the zygoma compose the zygomatic arch. The prominence of the molar apices superimposed on the shadow of the zygoma and the amount of periapical detail supplied by the radiograph depend primarily on the extent of aeration (pneumatization) of the zygoma by the maxillary sinus and on the orientation of the x-ray beam.

NASOLABIAL FOLD

An oblique line demarcating a region that appears to be covered by a veil of slight radiopacity frequently traverses periapical radiographs of the premolar region (Fig. 8-38). The line of contrast is sharp, and the area of increased radiopacity is posterior to the line. The line is the nasolabial fold, and the opaque veil is the thick cheek tissue superimposed on the teeth and the alveolar process. The image of the fold becomes more evident with age as the repeated creasing of the skin along the line (where the elevator of

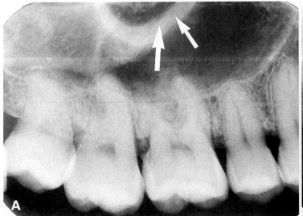
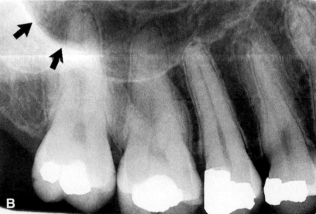

FIGURE 8-36 The zygomatic process of the maxilla (arrows) protrudes laterally from the maxillary wall. Its size may be quite variable: small with thick borders (A) or large with thin borders (B).

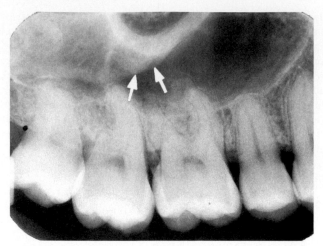

FIGURE 8-37 The inferior border of the zygoma *(arrows)* extends posteriorly from the inferior portion of the zygomatic process of the maxilla.

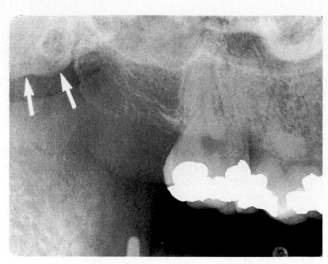

FIGURE 8-39 Pterygoid plates *(arrows)* located posterior to the maxillary tuberosity.

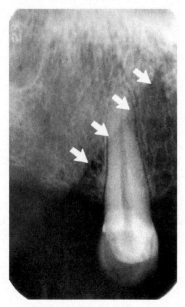

FIGURE 8-38 The nasolabial soft tissue fold *(arrows)* extends across the canine-premolar region.

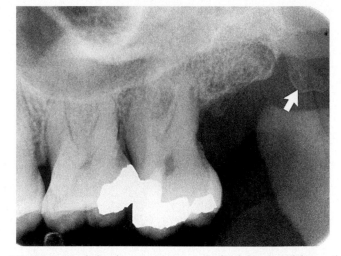

FIGURE 8-40 The hamular process *(arrow)* extends inferiorly from the medial pterygoid plate.

the lip, zygomatic head, and orbicularis all insert into the skin) and the degeneration of the elastic fibers finally lead to the formation and deepening of permanent folds. This radiographic feature frequently proves useful in identifying the side of the maxilla represented by a film of the area if it is edentulous and few other anatomic features are demonstrated.

PTERYGOID PLATES

The medial and lateral pterygoid plates lie immediately posterior to the tuberosity of the maxilla. The image of these two plates is extremely variable, and they do not appear at all on many intraoral radiographs of the third molar area. When they are apparent, they almost always cast a single radiopaque homogeneous shadow without any evidence of trabeculation (Fig. 8-39). Extending inferiorly from the medial pterygoid plate is the hamular process (Fig. 8-40), which on close inspection can show trabeculae.

MANDIBLE

SYMPHYSIS

Radiographs of the region of the mandibular symphysis in infants demonstrate a radiolucent line through the midline of the jaw between the images of the forming deciduous central incisors (Fig. 8-41). This suture usually fuses by the end of the first year of life, after which it is no longer radiographically apparent. It is not frequently encountered on dental radiographs because few young patients have cause to be examined radiographically. If this radiolucency is found in older individuals, it is abnormal and may suggest a fracture or a cleft.

GENIAL TUBERCLES

The genial tubercles (also called the mental spine) are located on the lingual surface of the mandible slightly above the inferior border and in the midline. They are bony protuberances, more or less spine-shaped, that often are divided into a right and left prominence and a superior and inferior prominence. They attach the

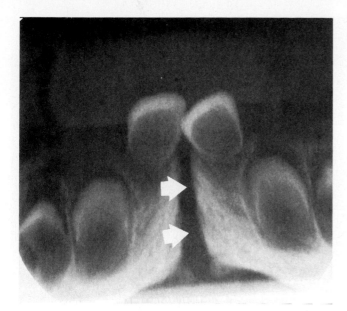

FIGURE 8-41 Mandibular symphysis *(arrows)* in a newborn infant. This suture closed within the first year. Note the erupted bilateral supernumerary primary incisors.

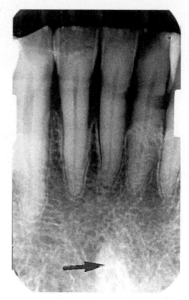

FIGURE 8-43 The genial tubercles *(arrow)* appear as a radiopaque mass, in this case without evidence of the lingual foramen.

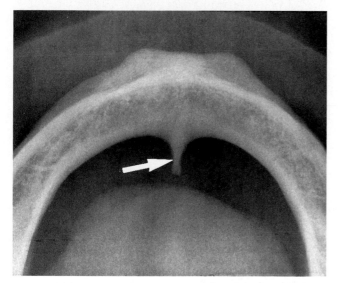

FIGURE 8-42 Genial tubercle *(arrow)* on the lingual surface of the mandible in this cross-sectional mandibular occlusal view. This tubercle is unusually prominent.

genioglossus muscles (at the superior tubercles) and the geniohyoid muscles (at the inferior tubercles) to the mandible. They are well visualized on mandibular occlusal radiographs as one or more small projections (Fig. 8-42). Their appearance on periapical radiographs of the mandibular incisor region is variable; often they appear as a radiopaque mass (3 to 4 mm in diameter) in the midline below the incisor roots (Fig. 8-43). They also may not be apparent at all.

LINGUAL FORAMEN

There is usually a foramen on the lingual surface of the midline of the mandible in the region of the genial tubercles—the lingual foramen. There are often two or even more such foramina. The superior foramen contains a neurovascular bundle from the lingual arteries and nerve, whereas the inferior foramen is supplied from

the sublingual or submental arteries and from the mylohyoid nerve. The lingual foramen (Fig. 8-44) is typically visualized as a single round radiolucent canal with a well-defined opaque border lying in the midline below the level of the apices of the incisors.

MENTAL RIDGE

On periapical radiographs of the mandibular central incisors, the mental ridge (protuberance) may occasionally be seen as two radiopaque lines sweeping bilaterally forward and upward toward the midline (Fig. 8-45). They are of variable width and density and may be found to extend from low in the premolar area on each side up to the midline, where they lie just inferior to or are superimposed on the mandibular incisor tooth roots. The image of the mental ridge is most prominent when the beam is directed parallel with the surface of the mental tubercle (as when using the bisecting-angle technique).

MENTAL FOSSA

The mental fossa is a depression on the labial aspect of the mandible extending laterally from the midline and above the mental ridge. Because of the resulting thinness of jawbone in this area, the image of this depression may be similar to that of the submandibular fossa (see later in chapter) and likewise may be mistaken for periapical disease involving the incisors (Fig. 8-46).

MENTAL FORAMEN

The mental foramen is usually the anterior limit of the inferior dental canal that is apparent on periapical radiographs (Fig. 8-47). Its image is quite variable, and it may be identified only about half of the time because the opening of the mental canal is directed superiorly and posteriorly (Fig. 8-48). As a result, the usual view of the premolars is not projected through the long axis of the canal opening. This circumstance is responsible for the variable appearance of the mental foramen. Although the wall of the foramen is of cortical bone, the density of the image of the foramen varies, as does the shape and definition of its border. It may be round, oblong, slitlike, or very irregular and partially or completely

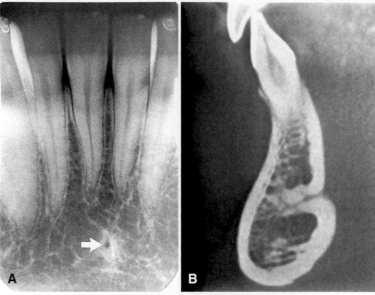

FIGURE 8-44 Lingual foramen. **A,** Lingual foramen on a periapical view *(arrow)*, with a sclerotic border, in the symphyseal region of the mandible. **B,** Cone-beam sagittal section through mandibular midline shows superior lingual foramen extending deep into the mandible from the lingual surface.

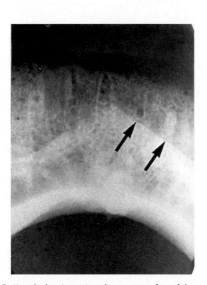

FIGURE 8-45 Mental ridge *(arrows)* on the anterior surface of the mandible, seen as a radiopaque ridge. The mental ridge is most prominent when the beam is angled from well below the occlusal plane.

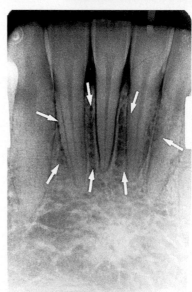

FIGURE 8-46 The mental fossa is a depression on the anterior surface of the mandible and is seen as a radiolucent area with ill-defined borders *(arrows)* in the region of the incisor roots.

corticated. The foramen is seen about halfway between the lower border of the mandible and the crest of the alveolar process, usually in the region of the apex of the second premolar. Also, because it lies on the surface of the mandible, the position of its image in relation to the tooth roots is influenced by projection angulation. It may be projected anywhere from just mesial of the permanent first molar roots to as far anterior as mesial of the first premolar root. The image of two mental foramina, one above the other, has also been observed.

When the mental foramen is projected over one of the premolar apices, it may mimic periapical disease (Fig. 8-49). In such cases, evidence of the inferior dental canal extending to the suspect radiolucency or a detectable lamina dura in the area would suggest the true nature of the dark shadow. However, the relative thinness of the lamina dura superimposed with the radiolucent foramen may result in considerable "burnout" of the lamina dura image, which complicates its recognition. Nevertheless, a

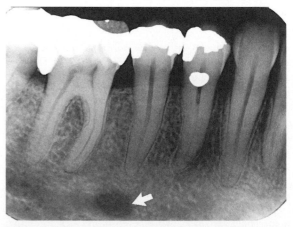

FIGURE 8-47 The mental foramen *(arrow)* appears as an oval radiolucency typically near the apex of the second premolar.

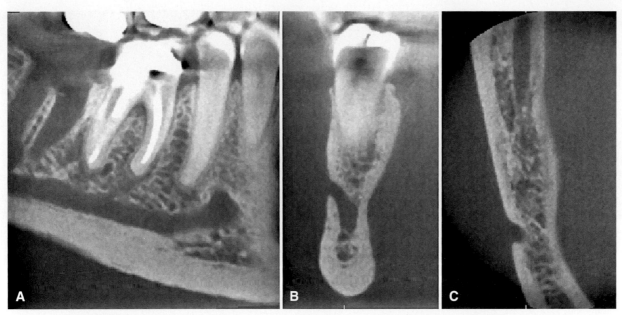

FIGURE 8-48 Cone-beam images through the mental foramen. **A,** Sagittal section through the body of the mandible shows the mandibular canal rising toward the mental foramen, which lies anterior to the apex of the second premolar. **B,** Coronal section through the mental foramen shows how the mandibular canal ascends to exit through the buccal cortex at the mental foramen. A clear understanding of this anatomy is important when implants are placed in this region. **C,** Axial section through the mental foramen demonstrates posterior inclination of the opening of the mental foramen on the mandibular buccal surface. Note also the section of the mandibular canal lying more posteriorly, inferior to the molars, and adjacent to the lingual cortex *(top of image)*.

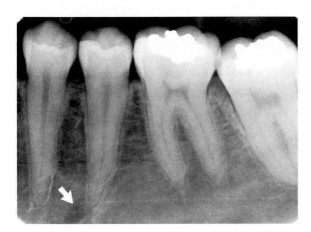

FIGURE 8-49 The mental foramen *(arrow)* (over the apex of the second premolar) may simulate periapical disease. However, continuity of the lamina dura around the apex indicates the absence of periapical abnormality.

second radiograph from another angle is likely to show the lamina dura clearly as well as some shift in position of the radiolucent foramen relative to the apex.

MANDIBULAR CANAL

The radiographic image of the mandibular canal is a dark linear shadow with thin radiopaque superior and inferior borders cast by the lamella of bone that bounds the canal (Fig. 8-50). Sometimes the borders are seen only partially or not at all. The width of the canal shows some interpatient variability but is usually constant anterior to the third molar region. The canal's course may be apparent between the mandibular foramen and the mental

foramen. Only rarely is the image of its anterior continuation toward the midline discernible on the radiograph.

The relationship of the mandibular dental canal to the roots of the lower teeth may vary, from one in which there is close contact with all molars and the second premolar to one in which the canal has no intimate relationship to any of the posterior teeth. In the usual picture, however, the canal is in contact with the apex of the third molar, and the distance between it and the other roots increases as it progresses anteriorly. When the apices of the molars are projected over the canal, the lamina dura may be overexposed, conveying the impression of a missing lamina or a thickened PDL space that is more radiolucent than apparently normal for the patient (Fig. 8-51). To ensure the soundness of such a tooth, other clinical testing procedures must be used (e.g., vitality testing). Because the canal is usually located just inferior to the apices of the posterior teeth, altering the vertical angle for a second film of the area is not likely to separate the images of the apices and canal.

Histologic studies have shown that the inferior alveolar nerve typically courses through the mandible as one major trunk with branches extending to the apices of the teeth. However, there are multiple smaller branches of the inferior alveolar nerve running roughly parallel to the major trunk. Occasionally, these branches are large enough that they have a secondary mandibular canal. Such bifid canals are seen most commonly on panoramic and cone-beam images (Fig. 8-52). Patients with bifid canals are at greater risk of inadequate anesthesia or difficulties with jaw surgery, including implants, or trauma.

NUTRIENT CANALS

Nutrient canals carry a neurovascular bundle and appear as radiolucent lines of fairly uniform width. They are most often seen on mandibular periapical radiographs running vertically from the

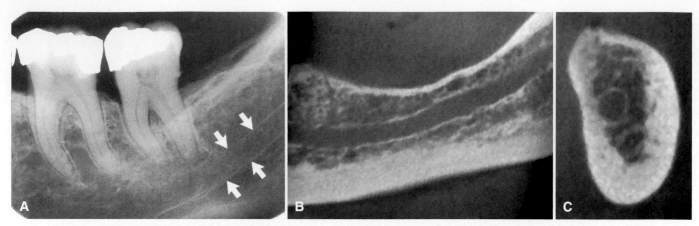

FIGURE 8-50 Mandibular canal. **A,** On periapical view, *arrows* denote radiopaque superior and inferior cortical borders. **B,** Cone-beam section through the body of the mandible (different patient) shows corticated borders of the mandibular canal. **C,** Cone-beam cross-sectional view shows the circular mandibular canal with corticated borders lying adjacent to the lingual plate.

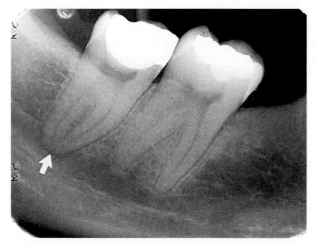

FIGURE 8-51 Superimposition of the mandibular canal over the apex of a molar causes the image of the periodontal ligament space to appear wider *(arrow)*. However, the presence of an intact lamina dura indicates that there is no periapical disease.

inferior dental canal directly to the apex of a tooth (Fig. 8-53) or into the interdental space between the mandibular incisors (Fig. 8-54). They are visible in about 5% to 40% of all patients and are more frequent in black patients; male patients; older patients; and patients with high blood pressure, diabetes mellitus, or advanced periodontal disease. They also indicate a thin ridge, useful in implant assessment. Because they are anatomic spaces with walls of cortical bone, their images occasionally have hyperostotic borders. Sometimes a nutrient canal is oriented perpendicular to the cortex and appears as a small round radiolucency simulating a pathologic radiolucency.

MYLOHYOID RIDGE

The mylohyoid ridge (also called the internal oblique ridge) is a slightly irregular crest of bone on the lingual surface of the mandibular body. Its anterior margin lies about 10 mm inferior to the alveolar ridge lingual to the second premolar and extends posteriorly to the area of the third molar about 5 mm below the alveolar crest. This ridge serves as an attachment for the mylohyoid muscle. Its radiographic image runs diagonally downward and forward

from the area of the third molars to the premolar region, at approximately the level of the apices of the posterior teeth (Fig. 8-55). This image is sometimes superimposed on the images of the molar roots. The margins of the image are not usually well defined but appear quite diffuse and of variable width. Occasionally, the ridge is relatively dense with sharply demarcated borders (Fig. 8-56). It is more evident on periapical radiographs when the beam is positioned with excessive negative angulation. Generally, as the ridge becomes less defined, its anterior and posterior limits blend gradually with the surrounding bone.

SUBMANDIBULAR GLAND FOSSA

On the lingual surface of the mandibular body, immediately below the mylohyoid ridge in the molar area, there is frequently a depression in the bone. This concavity accommodates the submandibular gland and often appears as a radiolucent area with the sparse trabecular pattern characteristic of the region (Fig. 8-57). This trabecular pattern is even less defined on radiographs of the area because it is superimposed on the relatively reduced mass of the concavity. The radiographic image of the fossa is sharply limited superiorly by the mylohyoid ridge and inferiorly by the lower border of the mandible but is poorly defined anteriorly (in the premolar region) and posteriorly (at about the ascending ramus). Although the image may appear strikingly radiolucent, accentuated as it is by the dense mylohyoid ridge and inferior border of the mandible, awareness of its possible presence should preclude its being confused with a bony lesion by inexperienced clinicians.

EXTERNAL OBLIQUE RIDGE

The external oblique ridge is a continuation of the anterior border of the mandibular ramus. It follows an anteroinferior course lateral to the alveolar process; it is relatively prominent in its upper part and juts considerably on the outer surface of the mandible in the region of the third molar (Fig. 8-58). This bony elevation gradually flattens and usually disappears at about where the alveolar process and mandible join below the first molar. The ridge is a line of attachment of the buccinator muscle. Characteristically, it is projected onto posterior periapical radiographs superior to the mylohyoid ridge, with which it runs an almost parallel course. It appears as a radiopaque line of varying width, density, and length, blending at its anterior end with the shadow of the alveolar bone.

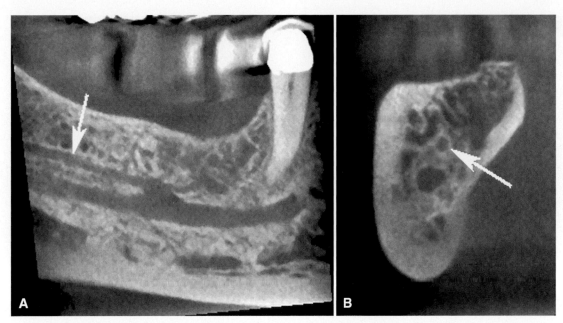

FIGURE 8-52 Bifid mandibular canals. **A,** Cone-beam sagittal section through the body of the mandible shows a bifid mandibular canal. The superior branch has a smaller diameter than the primary canal *(arrow).* **B,** Cross-sectional image shows primary canal and superior secondary canal *(arrow).*

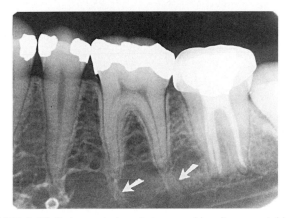

FIGURE 8-53 Nutrient canals *(arrows),* demonstrated by radiopaque cortical borders, descend from the mandibular first molar. Nutrient canals at this location are a common finding.

INFERIOR BORDER OF THE MANDIBLE

Occasionally, the inferior mandibular border is seen on periapical projections (Fig. 8-59) as a characteristically dense, broad radiopaque band of bone.

CORONOID PROCESS

The image of the coronoid process of the mandible is frequently apparent on periapical radiographs of the maxillary molar region as a triangular radiopacity, with its apex directed superiorly and anteriorly, superimposed on the region of the third molar (Fig. 8-60). In some cases, it may appear as far forward as the second molar and be projected above, over, or below these molars, depending on the position of the jaw and the projection of the x-ray beam. Usually the shadow of the coronoid process is homogeneous, although internal trabeculation can be seen in some cases. Its appearance on maxillary molar radiographs results from the

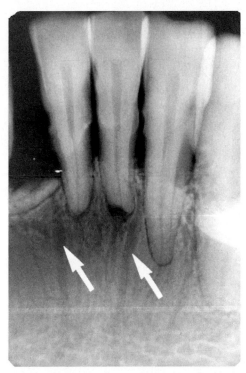

FIGURE 8-54 Nutrient canals seen as vertical radiolucent structures *(arrows)* in the anterior mandible are often associated with periodontal disease as in this patient.

downward and forward movement of the mandible when the mouth is open. Consequently, if the opacity reduces the diagnostic value of a film and the film must be remade, the second view should be acquired with the mouth minimally open. (This contingency must be considered whenever this area is radiographically

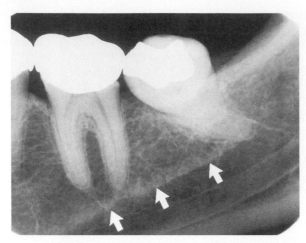

FIGURE 8-55 Mylohyoid ridge *(arrows)* running at the level of the molar apices and above the mandibular canal.

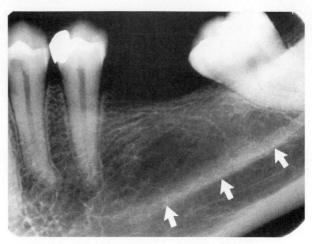

FIGURE 8-56 The mylohyoid ridge *(arrows)* may be dense, especially when a radiograph is exposed with excessive negative angulation.

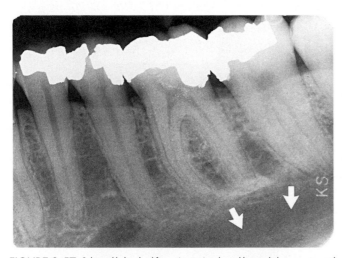

FIGURE 8-57 Submandibular gland fossa *(arrows)*, indicated by a radiolucent region with ill-defined borders and sparse trabecular bone lying inferiorly to the mandibular molars.

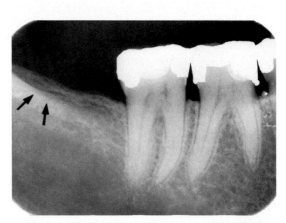

FIGURE 8-58 External oblique ridge *(arrows)* on the buccal surface of the mandible, seen as a radiopaque line near the alveolar crest in the mandibular third molar region.

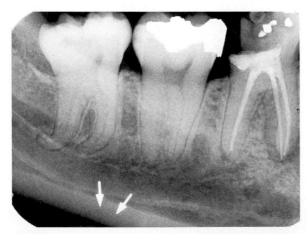

FIGURE 8-59 The inferior border of the mandible *(arrows)* is seen as a dense, broad radiopaque band.

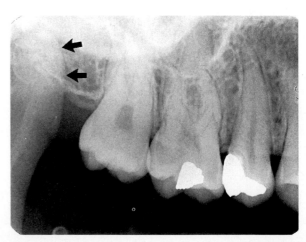

FIGURE 8-60 Coronoid process of the mandible *(arrows)* superimposed on the maxillary tuberosity.

examined.) Occasionally, especially when its shadow is dense and homogeneous, the coronoid process is mistaken for a root fragment by a neophyte clinician. The true nature of the shadow can be easily demonstrated by obtaining two radiographs with the mouth in different positions and noting the change in position of the suspect shadow.

RESTORATIVE MATERIALS

Restorative materials vary in their radiographic appearance, depending primarily on their thickness, density, and atomic number. Of these, the atomic number is most influential.

A variety of restorative materials may be recognized on intraoral radiographs. The most common, silver amalgam, is completely radiopaque (Fig. 8-61). Gold is equally opaque to x rays, whether cast as a crown (Fig. 8-62) or an inlay or condensed as gold foil. Stainless steel pins also appear radiopaque (Fig. 8-63). Often a calcium hydroxide base is placed in a deep cavity to protect the pulp. Although such base material may be radiolucent, most is radiopaque (Fig. 8-64). Another material of comparable radiopacity is gutta-percha, a rubber-like substance used to fill tooth canals during endodontic therapy (Fig. 8-65). Silver points were previously used to obliterate canals during endodontic therapy (Fig. 8-66). Composite restorations are typically partially radiopaque, as are porcelain restorations, which are usually fused to a metallic coping (Fig. 8-67). In addition, stainless steel crowns (Fig. 8-68) and orthodontic appliances around teeth (Fig. 8-69) are relatively radiopaque.

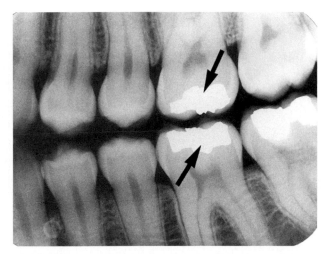

FIGURE 8-61 Amalgam restorations appear completely radiopaque *(arrows).*

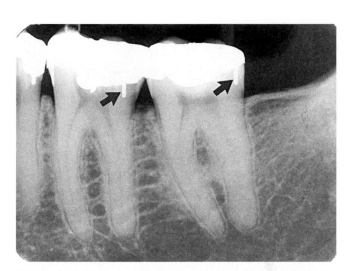

FIGURE 8-63 Stainless steel pins *(arrows)* provide retention for amalgam restorations.

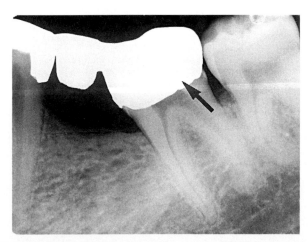

FIGURE 8-62 A cast gold crown, appearing completely radiopaque *(arrow),* serves as the terminal abutment of a bridge.

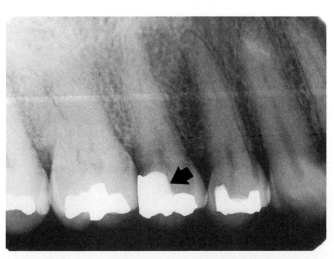

FIGURE 8-64 Base material *(arrow)* is usually radiopaque but less opaque than the amalgam restoration.

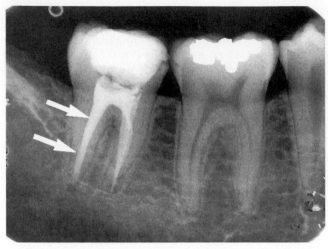

FIGURE 8-65 Gutta-percha *(arrows)* is a radiopaque rubber-like material used in endodontic therapy.

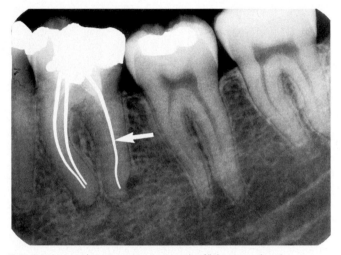

FIGURE 8-66 Silver points *(arrow)* were used to fill the root canals in this patient.

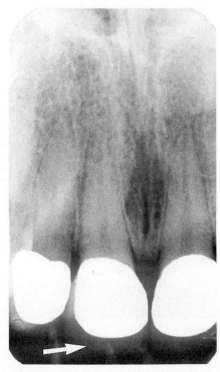

FIGURE 8-67 Porcelain appears radiolucent *(arrow)* over a metal coping.

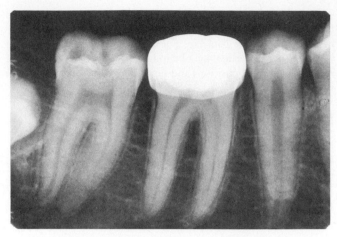

FIGURE 8-68 Stainless steel crowns appear mostly radiopaque.

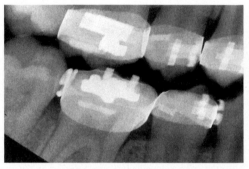

FIGURE 8-69 Orthodontic appliances have a characteristic radiopaque appearance.

BIBLIOGRAPHY

Berkovitz BKB, Holland GR, Moxham BL: *Oral anatomy, histology and embryology,* ed 4, London, 2009, Mosby.

Claeys V, Waskens G: Bifid mandibular canal: literature review and case report, *Dentomaxillofac Radiol* 34:55–58, 2005.

Jacobs R, Mraiwa N, van Steenberghe D, et al: Appearance, location, course, and morphology of the mandibular incisive canal: an assessment on spiral CT scan. *Dentomaxillofac Radiol* 31:322–327, 2002.

Kasle MJ: *An atlas of dental radiographic anatomy,* ed 4, Philadelphia, 1994, Saunders.

Liang X, Jacobs R, Lambrichts I, et al: Lingual foramina on the mandibular midline revisited: a macroanatomical study, *Clin Anat* 20:246–251, 2007.

Lusting JP, London D, Dor BL, et al: Ultrasound identification and quantitative measurement of blood supply to the anterior part of the mandible, *Oral Surg Oral Med Oral Pathol Oral Radiol Endod* 96: 625–629, 2003.

Mraiwa N, Jacobs R, van Steenberghe D, et al: Clinical assessment and surgical implications of anatomic challenges in the anterior mandible, *Clin Implant Dent Relat Res* 5:219–225, 2003.

Extraoral Projections and Anatomy

Sotirios Tetradis and Mel L. Kantor

OUTLINE

In extraoral radiographic examinations, both the x-ray source and the image receptor (film or electronic sensor) are placed outside the patient's mouth. This chapter describes the most common extraoral radiographic examinations in which the source and sensor remain static. These include the lateral cephalometric projection of the sagittal or median plane; the submentovertex (SMV) projection of the transverse or horizontal plane; and the Waters, posteroanterior (PA) cephalometric, and reverse-Towne projections of the coronal or frontal plane. Panoramic radiography is described in Chapter 10, and other more complex imaging modalities are described in Chapters 11 through 14.

SELECTION CRITERIA

Extraoral radiographs are used to examine areas not fully covered by intraoral films or to evaluate the cranium, face (including the maxilla and mandible), or cervical spine for diseases, trauma, or abnormalities. Standardized extraoral (cephalometric) radiographs also assist in evaluating the relationship between various orofacial and dental structures, growth and development of the face, or treatment progression.

Before obtaining an extraoral radiograph, it is essential to evaluate the patient's complaints and clinical signs in detail. The clinician first must decide which anatomic structures need to be evaluated and then select the appropriate projection or projections. Selecting the appropriate extraoral radiographic examination for the diagnostic task at hand is the *first* step in obtaining and interpreting a radiograph. For spatially localizing pathology, usually at least two radiographs taken at right angles to each another are obtained.

TECHNIQUE

Extraoral radiographs are produced with conventional dental x-ray machines, certain models of panoramic machines, or higher capacity medical x-ray units. Cephalometric and skull views require at least a 20 cm × 25 cm (8 inch × 10 inch) image receptor. It is critical to label the right and left sides of the image correctly and clearly. This usually is done by placing a metal marker (an *R* or an *L*) on the outside of the cassette in a corner in which the marker does not obstruct diagnostic information.

The proper exposure parameters depend on the patient's size, anatomy, and head orientation; image receptor speed; x-ray source-to-receptor distance; and whether or not grids are used. In cases of known or suspected disease, medium-speed or high-speed rare-earth screen-film combinations provide optimal balance between diagnostic information and patient exposure. For orthodontic purposes, high-speed combinations reduce patient exposure without compromising the identification of anatomic landmarks necessary for cephalometric analysis. Although radiographic grids reduce scattered radiation and improve contrast and resolution, they result in higher patient exposure. Cephalometry does not require the use of grids. However, grids could improve the radiographic appearance of fine structures, such as trabecular architecture, and aid in the diagnosis of disease.

Proper positioning of the x-ray source, patient, and image receptor requires patience, attention to detail, and experience. The main anatomic landmark used in patient positioning during extraoral radiography is the canthomeatal line, which joins the central point of the external auditory canal to the outer canthus of the eye. The canthomeatal line forms approximately a 10-degree angle with the Frankfort plane, the line that connects the superior border of the external auditory canal with the infraorbital rim. The image receptor and patient placement, central beam direction, and resultant image for the lateral, submentovertex, Waters, posteroanterior, and reverse-Towne projections are summarized in Table 9-1 and are described in detail in the text. Table 9-1 is organized to show the progressive head rotation in relation to the x-ray beam in the frontal views and thus clarify the resultant projected anatomy.

EVALUATION OF THE IMAGE

Extraoral images should first be evaluated for overall quality. Proper exposure and processing result in an image with good contrast and density. Proper patient positioning prevents unwanted

TABLE 9-1   Technical Aspects of Extraoral Radiographic Projections and Resultant Images

	LATERAL CEPH	SMV	WATERS	PA CEPH	REVERSE TOWNE
Patient placement	Film parallel to midsagittal plane	Canthomeatal line parallel to film	Canthomeatal line at 37° with film	Canthomeatal line at 10° with film	Canthomeatal line at −30° with film
Central beam	Beam perpendicular to film	Beam perpendicular to film	Beam perpendicular to film	Beam perpendicular to film	Beam perpendicular to film
Diagram of patient placement					
Illustration of patient placement					
Skull view					
Resultant image					

superimpositions and distortions and facilitates identification of anatomic landmarks. Interpreting poor-quality images can lead to diagnostic errors and subsequent treatment errors.

The first step in the interpretation of radiographic images is the identification of anatomy. A thorough knowledge of normal radiographic anatomy and the appearance of normal variants is critical for the identification of pathology. Abnormalities cause disruptions of normal anatomy. Detecting the altered anatomy precedes classifying the type of change and developing a differential diagnosis. What is not detected cannot be interpreted.

Interpretation of extraoral radiographs should be thorough, careful, and meticulous. Images should be interpreted in a room with reduced ambient light, and peripheral light from the viewbox or monitor should be masked. A systematic, methodical approach should be used for the visual exploration or interrogation of the diagnostic image. A method for the visual interrogation of extraoral radiograph of the head and neck is illustrated for the lateral and PA projections but can be applied to the remaining projections

as well. These methods are not the only approach to examining radiographic images. Any technique that reliably ensures that the entire image will be examined is equally appropriate.

LATERAL SKULL PROJECTION (LATERAL CEPHALOMETRIC PROJECTION)

Of the extraoral radiographs described in this chapter, the lateral cephalometric projection is the most commonly used in dentistry. All cephalometric radiographs, including the lateral view, are taken with a cephalostat that helps maintain a constant relationship among the skull, the film, and the x-ray beam. Skeletal, dental, and soft tissue anatomic landmarks delineate lines, planes, angles, and distances that are used to generate measurements and to classify patients' craniofacial morphology. At the beginning of treatment, these measurements are often compared with an established standard; during treatment, the measurements are usually compared with measurements from previous cephalometric radiographs of

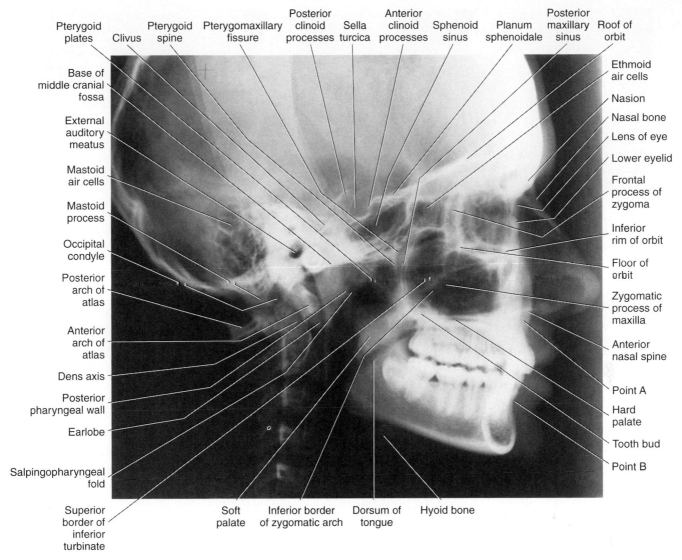

Pterygoid plates
Clivus
Pterygoid spine
Pterygomaxillary fissure
Posterior clinoid processes
Sella turcica
Anterior clinoid processes
Sphenoid sinus
Planum sphenoidale
Posterior maxillary sinus
Roof of orbit

Base of middle cranial fossa
External auditory meatus
Mastoid air cells
Mastoid process
Occipital condyle
Posterior arch of atlas
Anterior arch of atlas
Dens axis
Posterior pharyngeal wall
Earlobe
Salpingopharyngeal fold
Superior border of inferior turbinate

Ethmoid air cells
Nasion
Nasal bone
Lens of eye
Lower eyelid
Frontal process of zygoma
Inferior rim of orbit
Floor of orbit
Zygomatic process of maxilla
Anterior nasal spine
Point A
Hard palate
Tooth bud
Point B

Soft palate
Inferior border of zygomatic arch
Dorsum of tongue
Hyoid bone

FIGURE 9-1 Anatomic landmarks identified in the lateral cephalometric projection.

the same patient to monitor growth and development as well as treatment.

Image Receptor and Patient Placement

The image receptor is positioned parallel to the patient's midsagittal plane. The site of interest is placed toward the image receptor to minimize distortion. In cephalometric radiography, the patient is placed with the left side toward the image receptor (U.S. standards), and a wedge filter at the tube head is positioned over the anterior aspect of the beam to absorb some of the radiation and allow visualization of soft tissues of the face. Additional information about lateral cephalometry is provided at the end of this section.

Position of Central X-Ray Beam

The central beam is perpendicular to the midsagittal plane of the patient and the plane of the image receptor and is centered over the external auditory meatus.

Resultant Image (Fig. 9-1)

Exact superimposition of right and left sides is impossible because the structures on the side near to the image receptor are magnified

less than the same structures on the side far from the image receptor. Bilateral structures close to the midsagittal plane demonstrate less discrepancy in size compared with bilateral structures farther away from the midsagittal plane. Structures close to the midsagittal plane (e.g., the clinoid processes and inferior turbinates) should be nearly superimposed.

Interpretation

Although the lateral cephalometric radiograph is obtained to evaluate the relationship of the oral and facial structures, this radiograph is still a lateral *skull* film providing significant diagnostic information for the head and neck anatomy. As such, lateral cephalometric radiographs should first be evaluated for possible pathology and for anatomic variants that might simulate disease, before cephalometric analysis. It is not sufficient to limit the interpretation to the cephalometric analysis. To ensure that all anatomic structures are assessed, a systematic visual interrogation of lateral cephalometric radiographs should be followed. Such an approach is presented next (Fig. 9-2):

Step 1. Evaluate the base of the skull and calvaria. Identify the mastoid air cells, clivus, clinoid processes, sella turcica, sphenoid sinuses, and roof of the orbit. In the calvaria, assess vessel

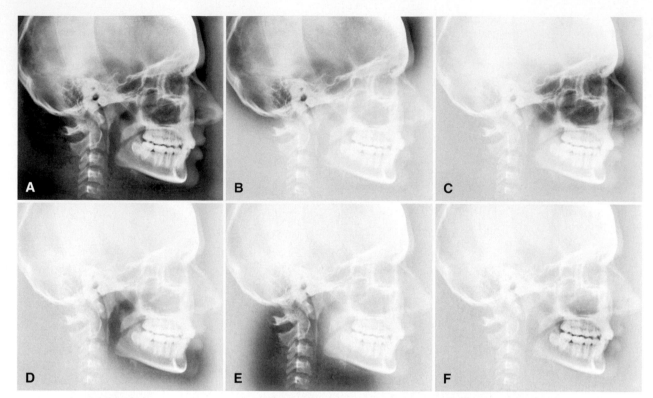

FIGURE 9-2 Interrogating the lateral cephalometric projection. The radiograph in the upper left demonstrates the whole image. Subsequent radiographs correspond to the steps of interrogation.

grooves, sutures, and diploic space. Look for intracranial calcifications.

Step 2. Evaluate the upper and middle face. Identify the orbits, sinuses (frontal, ethmoid, and maxillary), pterygomaxillary fissures, pterygoid plates, zygomatic processes of the maxilla, anterior nasal spine, and hard palate (floor of the nose). Evaluate the soft tissues of the upper and middle face, nasal cavity (turbinates), soft palate, and dorsum of tongue.

Step 3. Evaluate the lower face. Follow the outline of the mandible: from the condylar and coronoid processes; to the rami, angles, and bodies; and finally to the anterior mandible. Evaluate the soft tissue of the lower face.

Step 4. Evaluate the cervical spine, airway, and area of the neck. Identify each individual vertebra, confirm that the skull-C1 and C1-C2 articulations are normal, and assess the general alignment of the vertebrae. Assess soft tissues of the neck, hyoid bone, and airway.

Step 5. Evaluate the alveolar bone and teeth.

Figure 9-3 presents incidental findings identified on lateral cephalometric radiographs of asymptomatic orthodontic patients. Calcification of the intraclinoid ligament and formation of a bridged sella is a common normal variant that does not warrant any further evaluation (Fig. 9-3, *A*). Alternatively, expansion, irregular outlines, and destruction of the sella floor (Fig. 9-3, *B*) raise suspicion of an invasive lesion, such as a pituitary tumor, and require further investigation with advanced imaging and referral to a medical specialist. Multiple opacities throughout patient's calvaria are the result of superimposed hair braids (Fig. 9-3, *C*). Well-defined opacities at the superior aspect of the calvaria represent calcifications of arachnoid granulations and are a normal variant (Fig. 9-3, *D*). Enlargement of the pharyngeal adenoids and palatal tonsils (Fig. 9-3, *E*) is a common

finding in young patients but can cause narrowing of the airway and breathing difficulties. Finally, partial agenesis of the ring of atlas (Fig. 9-3, *F*) is a developmental anomaly that can cause instability of the atlanto-occipital and atlanto-odontoid articulation and requires further evaluation. The fusion of the body and transverse process of the dens with the third cervical vertebrae (see Fig. 9-3, *F*), which is a rare normal variant, should also be noted.

After evaluation of the whole lateral skull radiograph for possible pathology, cephalometric evaluation of the patient follows. There are many cephalometric analyses based on a variety of anatomic landmarks. Steiner and Ricketts analyses are two commonly used analyses that employ the skeletal, dental, and soft tissue landmarks listed in Box 9-1. Precise identification of the various landmarks on the lateral cephalometric radiograph is necessary to generate accurate cephalometric measurements. The landmarks in Box 9-1 are shown in Figure 9-4, *A*, on a side view of a skull and in Figure 9-4, *B*, on a 5-mm-wide midline section of an orthodontic patient imaged by cone-beam computed tomographic imaging. Finally, Figure 9-4, *C*, depicts the projected landmark position on the lateral cephalogram of an orthodontic patient.

POSTEROANTERIOR SKULL PROJECTION (POSTEROANTERIOR CEPHALOMETRIC PROJECTION)

The second most common skull radiograph used in dentistry is the PA cephalometric projection. The PA cephalogram is mainly used for evaluation of facial asymmetries and for assessment of orthognathic surgery outcomes involving the patient's midline or mandibular-maxillary relationship.

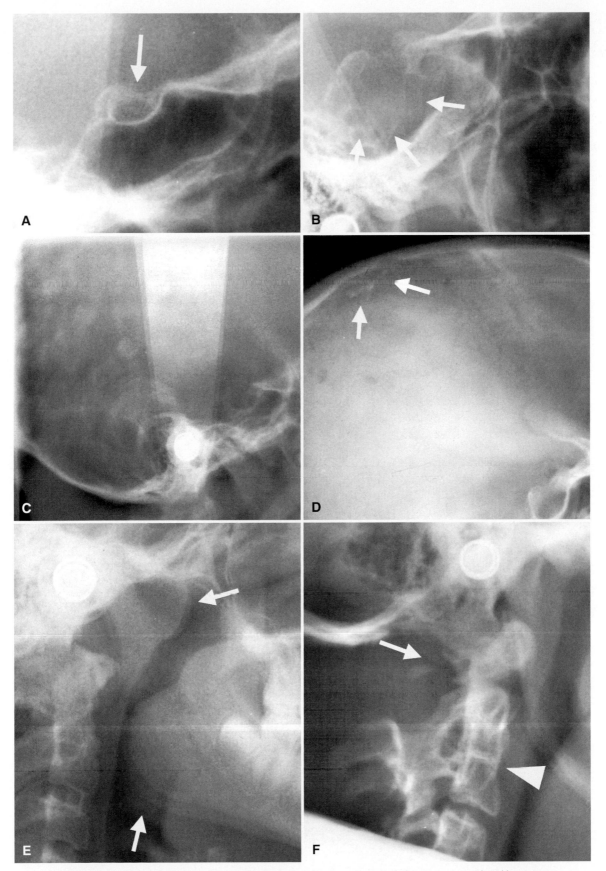

FIGURE 9-3 Incidental findings on lateral cephalometric radiographs of asymptomatic orthodontic patients are indicated by *arrows*.
A, Intraclinoid ligament calcification appearing as a bridged sella. **B,** Irregular and erosive expansion of the floor and anterior and posterior walls of sella turcica. **C,** Hair braid shadows are superimposed over the patient's calvaria. **D,** Calcification of arachnoid granulations is a normal variant. **E,** Enlarged pharyngeal adenoids and palatal tonsils can be a normal finding depending on the patient's age but can compromise nasal breathing. **F,** Cervical spine anomalies, such as agenesis of the posterior ring of atlas (C1) *(arrow)*, can cause spine instability, whereas vertebrae fusion of dens (C2) and C3 *(arrowhead)* is a normal variant.

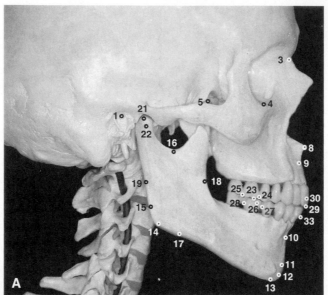

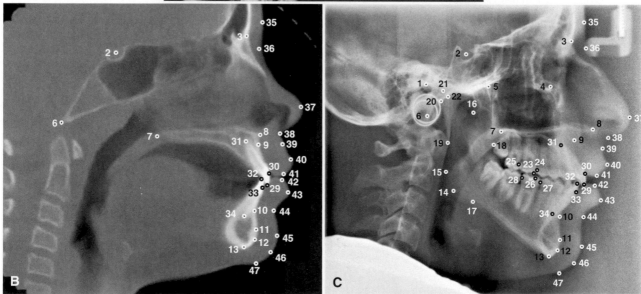

FIGURE 9-4 **A,** Anatomic cephalometric landmarks shown on a side view of the skull. **B,** Midline anatomic cephalometric landmarks depicted on a 5-mm-wide cone-beam computed tomographic section of an orthodontic patient. **C,** Cephalometric landmarks used in Steiner and Ricketts cephalometric analyses *(see Box 9-1).*

BOX 9-1   Definition of Cephalometric Landmarks

SKELETAL LANDMARKS

1. Porion (P): Most superior point of the external auditory canal
2. Sella (S): Center of the hypophyseal fossa
3. Nasion (N): Frontonasal suture
4. Orbitale (O): Most inferior point of the infraorbital rim
5. PT point: Most posterior point of the pterygomaxillary fissure
6. Basion (Ba): Most anterior point of the foramen magnum
7. PNS: Tip of the posterior nasal spine
8. ANS: Tip of the anterior nasal spine
9. A point (A): Deepest point of the anterior border of the maxillary alveolar ridge concavity
10. B point (B): Deepest point in the concavity of the anterior border of the mandible
11. Pogonion (Po): Most anterior point of the symphysis
12. Gnathion: Midpoint of the symphysis outline between pogonion and menton
13. Menton (M): Most inferior point of the symphysis
14. Gonion: Most convex point along the interior border of the mandibular ramus
15. Ramus point: Most posterior point of the posteroinferior border of the mandibular ramus
16. R1: Most inferior point of the sigmoid notch
17. R2: Arbitrary point on the lower border of the mandible below R1
18. R3: Most concave point of the anterior border of the mandibular ramus
19. R4: Most convex point of the posterior border of the mandibular ramus
20. Articulare (Ar): Point of intersection between the basisphenoid and the posterior border of the condylar head
21. Condyle top: Most superior point of the condyle
22. DC point: Center of the condylar head

DENTAL LANDMARKS

23. U6 mesial cusp: Tip of the maxillary first molar mesial buccal cusp
24. U6 mesial: Contact point on the mesial surface of the maxillary first molar
25. U6 distal: Contact point on the distal surface of the maxillary first molar
26. L6 mesial cusp: Tip of the mandibular first molar mesial buccal cusp
27. L6 mesial: Contact point on the mesial surface of the mandibular first molar
28. L6 distal: Contact point on the distal surface of the mandibular first molar
29. UI incisal: Incisal edge of maxillary central incisor
30. UI facial: Most convex point of the buccal surface of the maxillary central incisor
31. UI root: Root tip of the maxillary central incisor
32. LI incisal: Incisal edge of mandibular central incisor
33. LI facial: Most convex point of the buccal surface of the mandibular central incisor
34. LI root: Root tip of the mandibular central incisor

SOFT TISSUE LANDMARKS

35. Soft tissue glabella: Most anterior point of the soft tissue covering the frontal bone
36. Soft tissue nasion: Most concave point of soft tissue outline at the bridge of the nose
37. Tip of nose: Most anterior point of the nose
38. Subnasale: Soft tissue point where the curvature of the upper lip connects to the floor of the nose
39. Soft tissue A point: Most concave point of the upper lip between the subnasale and the upper lip point
40. Upper lip: Most anterior point of the upper lip
41. Stomion superius: Most inferior point of the upper lip
42. Stomion inferius: Most superior point of the lower lip
43. Lower lip: Most anterior point of the lower lip
44. Soft tissue B point: Most concave point of the lower lip between the chin and lower lip point
45. Soft tissue pogonion: Most anterior point of the soft tissue of the chin
46. Soft tissue gnathion: Midpoint of the chin soft tissue outline between the soft tissue pogonion and soft tissue menton
47. Soft tissue menton: Most inferior point of the soft tissue of the chin

See Figure 9-4.

Image Receptor and Patient Placement

The image receptor is placed in front of the patient, perpendicular to the midsagittal plane and parallel to the coronal plane. For the PA cephalometric radiograph, the patient is placed so that the canthomeatal line forms a 9-degree angle with the horizontal plane and the Frankfurt plane is perpendicular to the image receptor. For the standard PA skull projection, the canthomeatal line is perpendicular to the image receptor.

Position of Central X-Ray Beam

The central beam is perpendicular to the image receptor, directed from the posterior to the anterior (hence the name posteroanterior), parallel to the patient's midsagittal plane, and is centered at the level of the bridge of the nose.

Resultant Image (Fig. 9-5)

The midsagittal plane (represented by an imaginary line extending from the interproximal space of the central incisors through the nasal septum and the middle of the bridge of the nose) should divide the skull image into two symmetric halves. The superior border of the petrous ridge should lie in the lower third of the orbit.

Interpretation

Similar to the lateral cephalometric projection, the PA cephalogram should be viewed as a skull film first, before any cephalometric analysis. A systematic review of the radiograph, ensuring evaluation of all structures, should be followed. Such an approach is presented next (Fig. 9-6):

Step 1. Evaluate the calvaria, sutures, and diploic space starting in the area of the left external auditory meatus, over the top of the calvaria, to the right external auditory meatus. Look for intracranial calcifications. Identify the mastoid air cells and petrous ridge of the right and left temporal bones. In this and all subsequent steps, compare the right and left sides and look for symmetry.

Step 2. Evaluate the upper and middle face. Identify the orbits, sinuses (frontal, ethmoid, and maxillary), and zygomatic processes of the maxilla. Assess the nasal cavity, middle and inferior turbinates, nasal septum, and hard palate.

Step 3. Evaluate the lower face. Follow the outline of the mandible starting from the right condylar and coronoid processes, ramus, angle, and body through the anterior mandible to the left body, angle, ramus, coronoid process, and condyle.

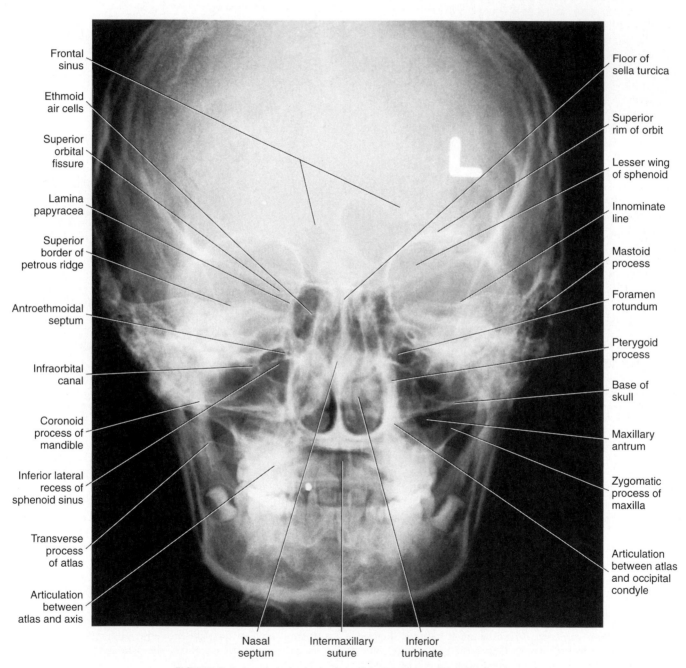

Frontal sinus

Ethmoid air cells

Superior orbital fissure

Lamina papyracea

Superior border of petrous ridge

Antroethmoidal septum

Infraorbital canal

Coronoid process of mandible

Inferior lateral recess of sphenoid sinus

Transverse process of atlas

Articulation between atlas and axis

Floor of sella turcica

Superior rim of orbit

Lesser wing of sphenoid

Innominate line

Mastoid process

Foramen rotundum

Pterygoid process

Base of skull

Maxillary antrum

Zygomatic process of maxilla

Articulation between atlas and occipital condyle

Nasal septum

Intermaxillary suture

Inferior turbinate

FIGURE 9-5 Anatomic landmarks identified in the posteroanterior cephalometric projection.

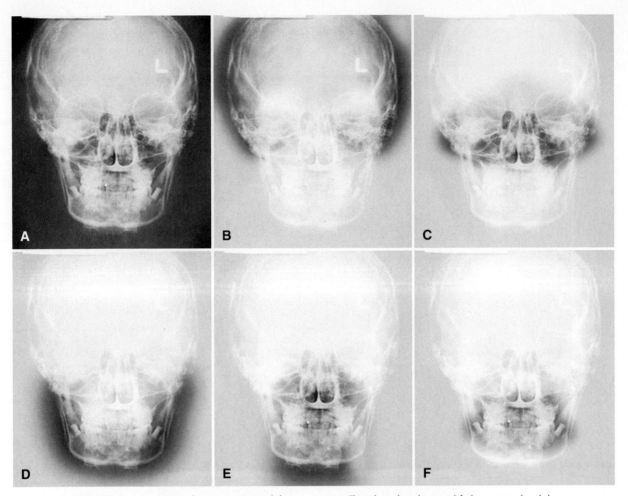

FIGURE 9-6 Interrogating the posteroanterior cephalometric projection. The radiograph in the upper left demonstrates the whole image. Subsequent radiographs correspond to the steps of interrogation.

Step 4. Evaluate the cervical spine. Identify the dens, the superior border of C2, and the inferior border of C1.

Step 5. Evaluate the alveolar bone and teeth.

SUBMENTOVERTEX (BASE) PROJECTION

Image Receptor and Patient Placement

The image receptor is positioned parallel to the patient's transverse plane and perpendicular to the midsagittal and coronal planes. To achieve this position, the patient's neck is extended as far backward as possible, with the canthomeatal line forming a 10-degree angle with the image receptor.

Position of Central X-Ray Beam

The central beam is perpendicular to the image receptor, directed from below the mandible toward the vertex of the skull (hence the name submentovertex), and centered about 2 cm anterior to a line connecting the right and left condyles.

Resultant Image (Fig. 9-7)

The midsagittal plane (represented by an imaginary line extending from the interproximal space of the maxillary central incisors through the nasal septum, to the middle of the anterior arch of the atlas, and to the dens) should divide the skull image into two symmetric halves. The buccal and lingual cortical plates of the mandible should be projected as uniform opaque lines. An underexposed view is required for the evaluation of the zygomatic arches because they will be overexposed or "burned out" on radiographs obtained with normal exposure factors.

Interpretation

As described earlier for the lateral and PA cephalometric projections, a systematic approach that ensures interrogation of the complete image and evaluation of all anatomic structures is paramount in the interpretation of the SMV projection.

WATERS PROJECTION

Image Receptor and Patient Placement

The image receptor is placed in front of the patient and perpendicular to the midsagittal plane. The patient's head is tilted upward so that the canthomeatal line forms a 37-degree angle with the image receptor. If the patient's mouth is open, the sphenoid sinus is seen superimposed over the palate.

Position of Central X-Ray Beam

The central beam is perpendicular to the image receptor and centered in the area of the maxillary sinuses.

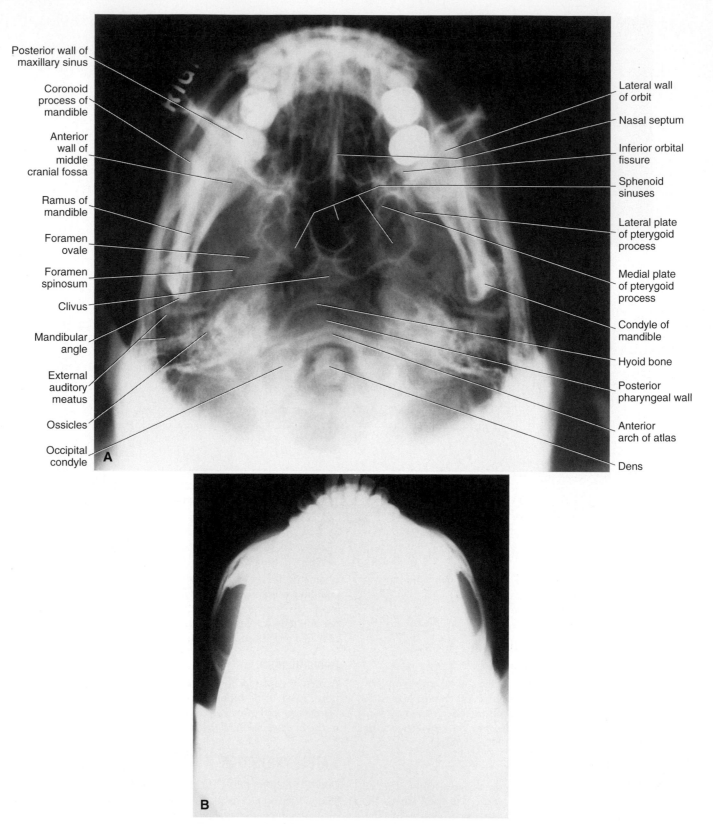

Posterior wall of maxillary sinus

Coronoid process of mandible

Anterior wall of middle cranial fossa

Ramus of mandible

Foramen ovale

Foramen spinosum

Clivus

Mandibular angle

External auditory meatus

Ossicles

Occipital condyle

Lateral wall of orbit

Nasal septum

Inferior orbital fissure

Sphenoid sinuses

Lateral plate of pterygoid process

Medial plate of pterygoid process

Condyle of mandible

Hyoid bone

Posterior pharyngeal wall

Anterior arch of atlas

Dens

FIGURE 9-7 A, Anatomic landmarks identified in the submentovertex (SMV) projection. **B,** Underexposed SMV view reveals the zygomatic arches.

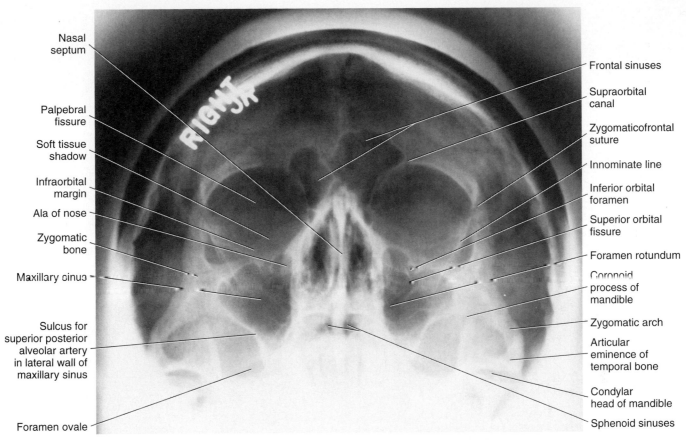

Nasal septum

Palpebral fissure

Soft tissue shadow

Infraorbital margin

Ala of nose

Zygomatic bone

Maxillary sinus

Sulcus for superior posterior alveolar artery in lateral wall of maxillary sinus

Foramen ovale

Frontal sinuses

Supraorbital canal

Zygomaticofrontal suture

Innominate line

Inferior orbital foramen

Superior orbital fissure

Foramen rotundum

Coronoid process of mandible

Zygomatic arch

Articular eminence of temporal bone

Condylar head of mandible

Sphenoid sinuses

FIGURE 9-8 Anatomic landmarks identified in the Waters projection.

Resultant Image (Fig. 9-8)

The midsagittal plane (represented by an imaginary line extending from the interproximal space of the maxillary central incisors through the nasal septum and the middle of the bridge of the nose) should divide the skull image into two symmetric halves. The petrous ridge of the temporal bone should be projected below the floor of the maxillary sinus.

Interpretation

As described earlier for the lateral and PA cephalometric projections, a systematic approach that ensures interrogation of the complete image and evaluation of all anatomic structures is paramount in the interpretation of the Waters projection.

REVERSE-TOWNE PROJECTION (OPEN-MOUTH)

Image Receptor and Patient Placement

The image receptor is placed in front of the patient, perpendicular to the midsagittal plane and parallel to the coronal plane. The patient's head is tilted downward so that the canthomeatal line forms a 25-degree to 30-degree angle with the image receptor. To improve the visualization of the condyles, the patient's mouth is opened so that the condylar heads are located inferior to the articular eminence. When requesting this image to evaluate the condyles, it is necessary to specify "open-mouth, reverse-Towne"; otherwise, a standard Towne view of the occiput may result.

Position of Central X-Ray Beam

The central beam is perpendicular to the image receptor and parallel to the patient's midsagittal plane and is centered at the level of the condyles.

Resultant Image (Fig. 9-9)

The midsagittal plane (represented by an imaginary line extending from the middle of the foramen magnum and the posterior arch of the atlas through the middle of the bridge of the nose and the nasal septum) should divide the skull image in two symmetric halves. The petrous ridge of the temporal bone should be superimposed at the inferior part of the occipital bone, and the condylar heads should be projected inferior to the articular eminence.

Interpretation

As described earlier for the lateral and PA cephalometric projections, a systematic approach that ensures interrogation of the complete image and evaluation of all anatomic structures is paramount in the interpretation of the reverse-Towne projection.

CONCLUSIONS

Extraoral radiography can provide valuable information for the evaluation of the dental and craniofacial complex. After assessing the patient's signs and symptoms, the clinician should choose the proper projection that provides the appropriate diagnostic information for the evaluation of the anatomic structures in question.

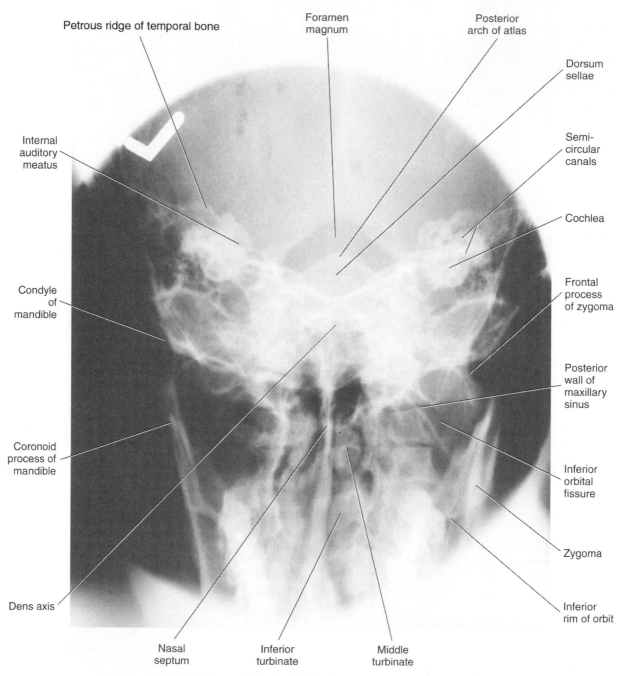

Petrous ridge of temporal bone

Foramen magnum

Posterior arch of atlas

Dorsum sellae

Semi-circular canals

Cochlea

Frontal process of zygoma

Posterior wall of maxillary sinus

Inferior orbital fissure

Zygoma

Inferior rim of orbit

Internal auditory meatus

Condyle of mandible

Coronoid process of mandible

Dens axis

Nasal septum

Inferior turbinate

Middle turbinate

FIGURE 9-9 Anatomic landmarks identified in the open-mouth reverse-Towne projection.

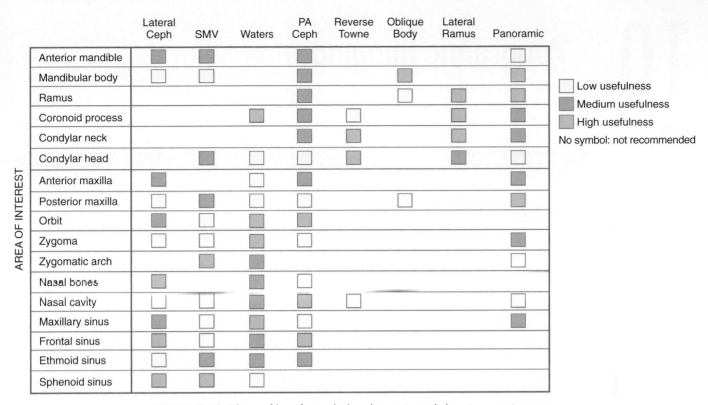

FIGURE 9-10 Relative usefulness of extraoral radiographic projections to display various anatomic structures.

Figure 9-10 summarizes the use of extraoral radiographs for the evaluation of various anatomic structures. Although panoramic radiography is the subject of Chapter 10, it is included in Figure 9-10 for comparison.

Although most extraoral radiographs in dentistry are cephalometric projections obtained for orthodontic and orthognathic assessment of asymptomatic patients, anatomic variants that can simulate disease or affect treatment or even occult pathology can be identified. As such, cephalometric radiographs should be viewed as skull radiographs first, and interpreted following a systematic, thorough, and knowledgeable approach.

BIBLIOGRAPHY

Kantor ML, Norton LA: Normal radiographic anatomy and common anomalies seen in cephalometric films, *Am J Orthod Dentofac Orthop* 91:414–426, 1987.

Keats TE, Anderson MW: *Atlas of normal roentgen variants that may simulate disease*, ed 9, St Louis, 2012, Mosby.

Long BW, Ballinger PW, Smith BJ, et al: *Merrill's atlas of radiographic positions and radiologic procedures*, vol 2, ed 11, St Louis, 2007, Mosby.

Miyashita K: *Contemporary cephalometric radiography*, Tokyo, 1996, Quintessence Publishing Co.

Shapiro R: *Radiology of the normal skull*, Chicago, 1981, Year Book Medical Publishers.

Swischuk LE: *Imaging of the cervical spine in children*, New York, 2001, Springer-Verlag.

10 Panoramic Imaging

Sanjay M. Mallya and Alan G. Lurie

OUTLINE

Panoramic imaging (also called pantomography) is a technique for producing a single image of the facial structures that includes both the maxillary and the mandibular dental arches and their supporting structures (Fig. 10-1). This technique produces a tomographic image in that it selectively images a specific body layer. In panoramic radiography, an x-ray source and an image receptor rotate around the patient's head (Fig. 10-2) and create a curved focal trough, a zone in which the included objects are displayed clearly. Objects in front of or behind this focal trough are blurred and largely not seen. The panoramic machine thus creates a focal trough through the dentition and adjacent structures.

Panoramic images are most useful clinically for diagnostic problems requiring broad coverage of the jaws (Box 10-1). Common examples include evaluation of trauma including jaw fractures, location of third molars, extensive dental or osseous disease, known or suspected large lesions, tooth development and eruption (especially in the mixed dentition), retained teeth or root tips (in edentulous patients), temporomandibular joint (TMJ) pain, and developmental anomalies. Panoramic imaging is often used as the initial evaluation image that can provide the required insight or assist in determining the need for other projections. Panoramic images are also useful for patients who do not tolerate intraoral procedures well.

The main disadvantage of panoramic radiology is that the image does not display the fine anatomic detail available on intraoral periapical radiographs. Thus, it is not as useful as periapical radiography for detecting small carious lesions, fine structure of the marginal periodontium, or periapical disease. The proximal surfaces of premolars also typically overlap. The availability of a panoramic radiograph for an adult patient often does not preclude the need for intraoral films for the diagnoses of most commonly encountered dental diseases. When a full-mouth series of radiographs is available for a patient requiring only general dental care, typically little or no additional useful information is gained from a simultaneous panoramic examination. Other problems associated with panoramic radiography include unequal magnification and geometric distortion across the image. Occasionally, the presence of overlapping structures, such as the cervical spine, can hide odontogenic lesions, particularly in the incisor regions. Clinically important objects may be situated outside the focal trough and may appear distorted or not be seen at all.

PRINCIPLES OF PANORAMIC IMAGE FORMATION

Paatero and, independently, Numata were the first to describe the principles of panoramic radiography. Figure 10-2 shows a schematic view of the relationships between the x-ray source, the patient, the secondary collimator, and the image receptor during panoramic image formation. The following illustrations explain the formation of the focal trough in a panoramic machine. Imagine an assembly containing a disk with upright physical objects (represented by letters) and an image receptor (Fig. 10-3). The receptor travels upward through the beam at the same speed as objects A through C rotate through the beam. A lead collimator in the shape of a slit located at the x-ray source limits the x-rays to a narrow vertical beam. Another collimator between the objects and the image receptor reduces scattered radiation from the objects to the image receptor. Consider first radiopaque objects A through C. As the disk rotates, their radiographic images are recorded sharply on the receptor that also moves through the beam at the same direction and speed. The spatial relationship of the shadows of these objects correctly represents the relationship of the actual objects. Because the source-receptor distance is constant and the object-receptor distance is the same for each object, all objects are magnified equally. Now consider objects D through F. They are located on the opposite side of the disk, between the x-ray source and the center of rotation of the disk. These objects move in the opposite direction of the receptor, so their shadows are reversed on the receptor. Because these objects are much closer to the x-ray source, their images are greatly magnified.

Figure 10-4 shows that the same relationship between the rotating receptor and objects can be achieved if the disk is held stationary but the x-ray source and the receptor are rotated around the center of rotation in the disk. The x-ray beam still passes through the center of the disk and sequentially through objects A through C. Similarly, the receptor is still moved through the beam and at the same rate as the beam passes through A through C. In this

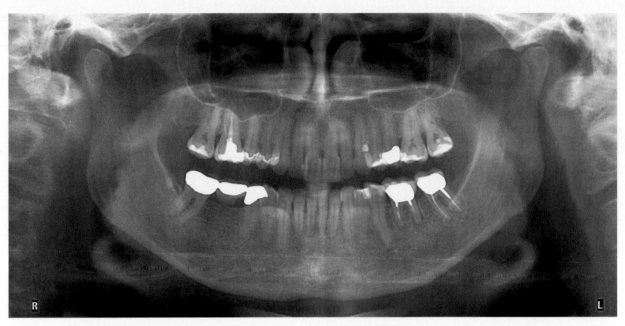

FIGURE 10-1 Panoramic image demonstrating broad coverage of hard and soft tissues of adult orofacial region including maxilla, mandible, dentition, and adjacent structures. Panoramic images are made with a much lower dose than a full-mouth set and have broader coverage, but they have lower resolution.

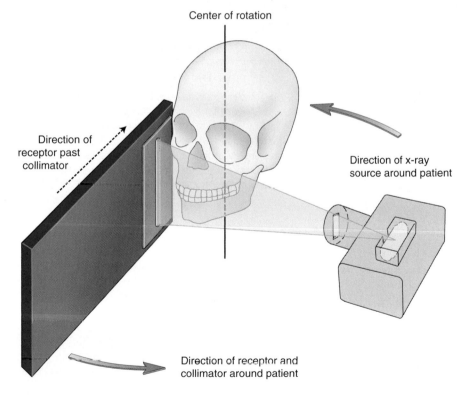

Center of rotation

Direction of receptor past collimator

Direction of x-ray source around patient

Direction of receptor and collimator around patient

FIGURE 10-2 Schematic view of relationships between the x-ray source, the patient, the secondary collimator, and film or storage phosphor image receptor. As the x-ray tube head moves around one side of the patient, the receptor assembly moves on the opposite side. The image receptor slides past the collimator sequentially producing a latent image. With a charge-coupled device (CCD) image receptor, there is a vertical CCD linear array behind the collimator that continuously reads out the exposure to produce an image.

situation, as before, objects *A* through *C* move through the x-ray beam in the same direction and at the same rate as the receptor. Objects *D* through *F* continue to be blurred, just as before.

Figure 10-5 shows that a patient may replace the disk and objects *A* through *F* represent teeth and surrounding bone. The illustration demonstrates the positions of the x-ray source and the receptor early in an exposure cycle. The center of rotation is located off to the side of the arch, away from the objects being imaged. The rate of movement of the receptor is regulated to be the same as that of the x-ray beam sweeping through the dentoal-veolar structures on the side of the patient nearest the receptor. Structures on the opposite side of the patient (near the x-ray tube) are distorted and appear out of focus because the x-ray beam sweeps through them in the direction opposite that in which the image receptor is moving. In addition, structures near the x-ray source are so magnified (and their borders so blurred) that they are not seen as discrete images on the resultant image. These structures appear only as diffuse phantom or ghost images. Because of both of these circumstances, only structures near the receptor are usefully captured on the resultant image.

Contemporary panoramic machines use a continuously moving center of rotation rather than multiple fixed locations (Fig. 10-6).

BOX 10-1   Panoramic Imaging

INDICATIONS

- Overall evaluation of dentition
- Examine for intraosseous pathology, such as cysts, tumors, or infections
- Gross evaluation of temporomandibular joints
- Evaluation of position of impacted teeth
- Evaluation of eruption of permanent dentition
- Dentomaxillofacial trauma
- Developmental disturbances of maxillofacial skeleton

ADVANTAGES COMPARED WITH A FULL-MOUTH EXAMINATION

- Broad coverage of facial bones and teeth
- Low radiation dose
- Ease of panoramic radiographic technique
- Can be used in patients with trismus or in patients who cannot tolerate intraoral radiography
- Quick and convenient radiographic technique
- Useful visual aid in patient education and case presentation

DISADVANTAGES

- Lower resolution images that do not provide the fine details provided by intraoral radiographs
- Magnification across image is unequal, making linear measurements unreliable
- Image is superimposition of real, double, and ghost images and requires careful visualization to decipher anatomic and pathologic details
- Requires accurate patient positioning to avoid positioning errors and artifacts.
- Difficult to image both jaws when patient has severe maxillomandibular discrepancy

---

This feature optimizes the shape of the focal trough to reveal best the teeth and supporting bone. This center of rotation is initially near the lingual surface of the right body of the mandible when the left TMJ region is being imaged. The rotation center moves anteriorly along an arc that ends just lingual to the symphysis of the mandible when the midline is imaged. The arc is reversed as the opposite side of the jaws is imaged.

This basic principle of image formation remains the same, regardless of the type of detector used to record the image. In the case where the receptor is a charge-coupled device (CCD) array, the film is replaced by a two-dimensional CCD array. Each column of the array is read out to construct the image. The key is to read out the columns at the same rate as an imaginary moving film would move past the array. The CCD array is read out continuously as the x-ray source and receptor travel around the patient. The resulting geometric projection characteristics are the same as if film or a photostimulable phosphor plate (PSP) had been used; this holds true for geometric distortions such as magnification and elongation, the presence of ghost images, superimposition of the

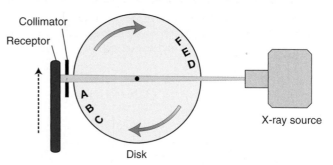

FIGURE 10-3 Producing a panoramic image. In this conceptual view, the x-ray source and collimator are held stationary. The receptor moves through the beam, and the rotating disk also carries objects A-F through the beam. Objects A-C move through the beam at the same rate and direction as the image receptor and are imaged well. Objects D-F move through the beam at the same rate as the receptor but in the opposite direction, and so their images are blurred. In the case of CCD panoramic radiography, the principles of image formation are the same as with film or storage phosphor receptors.

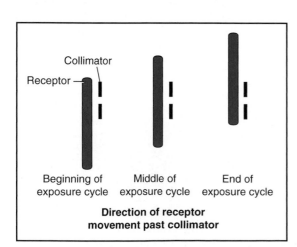

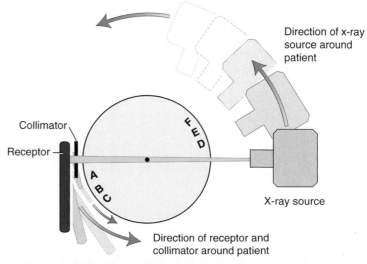

FIGURE 10-4 Producing a panoramic image. The disk is held stationary while the x-ray source, receptor, and collimator rotate around the center of the disk. Nonetheless, the x-ray beam still passes through the objects to the image receptor in the same direction as in Figure 10-3, and the same imaging results are obtained. The *inset* emphasizes how the receptor moves past the collimator during their motion around the disk.

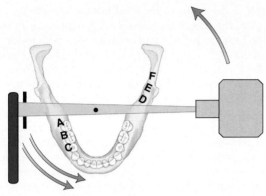

FIGURE 10-5 Producing a panoramic image. The imaging geometry is the same as Figures 10-3 and 10-4, but the disk and objects are replaced with a patient. The rate the receptor moves through the beam is the same as the rate the beam passes through objects *A-C*; thus, only the dentition in the mandible near the receptor (objects *A-C*) are imaged well. Structures on the opposite side of the mandible (objects *D-F*) are blurred beyond recognition.

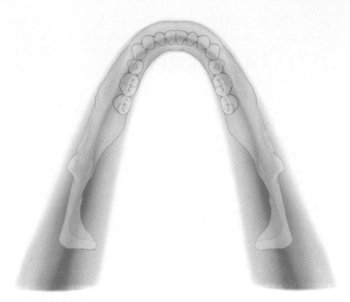

FIGURE 10-7 Focal trough. The moving source and receptor generate a zone of sharpness, known as the focal trough. The closer an anatomic structure is positioned to the center of the trough, the more clearly it is imaged on the resulting radiograph. Panoramic machines typically provide laser lights to allow the operator to position the patient's dentition optimally in the focal trough.

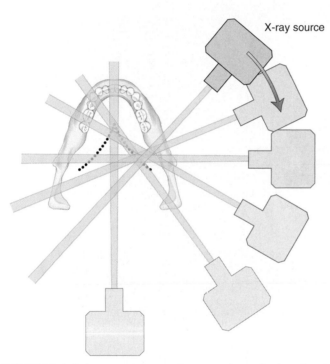

X-ray source

FIGURE 10-6 Producing a panoramic image. In contrast to the preceding three schematic drawings shown in Figures 10-3 through 10-5, the center of rotation of the x-ray source moves continuously as the tube and receptor rotate around the patient. Initially, the x-ray beam rotates on the end of the dotted arc on the tube side of the patient. As the x-ray source moves behind the patient, the center of rotation moves forward along the arc *(dotted line)*. The drawing shows the directions of the x-ray beam at various intervals for the first half of the exposure cycle. The x-ray source then continues to move around the patient to image the opposite side.

cervical spine over midline structures, overlap of teeth, and left-right size variations from lack of proper positioning of the patient's sagittal plane in the instrument.

FOCAL TROUGH

The focal trough is a three-dimensional curved zone, or "image layer," where the structures lying within this zone are reasonably well defined on the final panoramic image (Fig. 10-7). The

structures seen on a panoramic image are primarily those located within the focal trough. Images are most clear in the middle and become less clear further from the central line. Objects outside the focal trough are blurred, magnified, or reduced in size and are sometimes distorted to the extent of not being recognizable. The shape of the focal trough varies with the brand of equipment used as well as with the imaging protocol selected within each unit. The shape and width of the focal trough is determined by the path and velocity of the receptor and x-ray tube head, alignment of the x-ray beam, and collimator width. The location of the focal trough can change with extensive machine use, so recalibration may be necessary if consistently suboptimal images are being produced.

In some panoramic machines, the shape of the focal trough can be adjusted to conform better to the shape of the patients' maxillomandibular anatomy or to show specific anatomic areas better, such as the TMJ or the maxillary sinuses. This adjustment is accomplished through varying the shape of the moving center of rotation and allows better imaging of children, unusually shaped patients, or specific anatomic sites of interest. For example, in some units, the rotational arc of the x-ray source-receptor movement is decreased to modify the focal trough size to pediatric jaws. The decreased rotational arc also results in reduced patient radiation exposure. In some panoramic units, the projection angle of the x-ray beam is modified to yield images with decreased overlap of adjacent teeth and with minimal superimposition of structures from the opposite side of the jaw.

IMAGE DISTORTION

The panoramic image necessarily produces distortion of the size and shape of the object. These distortions make the panoramic image highly unreliable for linear or angular measurements. The image distortion is influenced by several factors, including x-ray beam angulation, x-ray source-to-object distance, path of rotational center, and position of the object within the focal trough. These parameters vary among panoramic units and among different regions of the jaws for the same unit. They are also strongly dependent on patient anatomy and positioning of the patient in the unit. These variables make it impossible to apply preset magnification factors that can be used to make reliable measurements on panoramic radiographs.

Horizontal magnification is determined by the position of the object within the focal trough. The magnitude of the horizontal distortion depends on the distance of the object from the center of the focal trough and thus is strongly influenced by patient positioning. Figure 10-8 illustrates the influence of patient positioning on image size and shape. Figure 10-8, *A* and *B*, shows a mandible supporting a brass ring properly aligned in the middle of the focal trough. Note the even magnification of the ring and the images of the anterior teeth in proper proportion. Figure 10-8, *C* and *D*, shows the same mandible positioned 5 mm posterior to

the middle of the center of the focal trough. This position causes distortion of the ring in the horizontal dimension, with the ring appearing broader and a commensurate increased width of the images of the teeth. Figure 10-8, *E* and *F*, shows the same mandible positioned 5 mm anterior to the middle of the focal trough. The horizontal distortion results in the ring appearing narrow and a commensurate decreased width of the projected teeth. On these images, the vertical dimension, in contrast to the horizontal dimension, is little altered. These distortions result from the horizontal movements of the receptor and x-ray source. Thus, as a general rule, when the structure of interest, in this case the mandible, is displaced to the lingual side of its optimal position in the focal trough, toward the x-ray source, the beam passes more slowly through it than the speed at which the receptor moves. Consequently, the images of the structures in this region are elongated

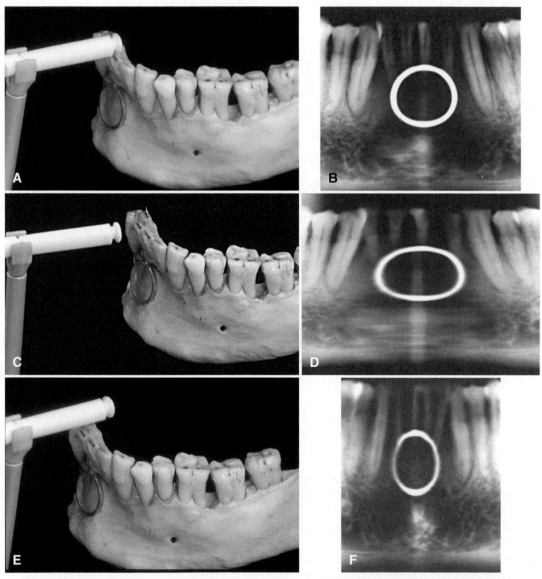

FIGURE 10-8 Influence of an object's position on its radiographic size. **A,** A mandible is supporting a metal ring positioned at the center of the focal trough. The mandible is positioned at the center of the focal trough by placing the incisal edges of the central incisors in a notch at the end of a bite rod-positioning device. **B,** Resultant panoramic radiograph shows minimal distortion of the metal ring. **C,** The mandible and ring are positioned 5 mm away from the focal trough. **D,** Resultant panoramic radiograph demonstrates horizontal magnification of both the ring and the mandibular teeth. **E,** The mandible and ring are positioned 5 mm in front of the notch in bite-block. **F,** Resultant panoramic radiograph demonstrates the horizontal minification of both the ring and the mandibular teeth.

horizontally on the image, and they appear wider. Alternatively, when the mandible is displaced toward the buccal aspect of the focal trough, the beam passes at a rate faster than normal through the structures. In the example shown, because the receptor is moving at the proper rate, the representations of the anterior teeth are compressed horizontally on the image, and they appear thinner.

The same principle applies to the patient's sagittal plane being rotated in the focal trough. The posterior structures on the side to which the patient's head is rotated are magnified in the horizontal dimension because the posterior structures are moved away from the image receptor, whereas posterior structures on the opposite side are moved closer to the image receptor and are reduced in horizontal dimension. The resulting image has horizontally large molar teeth and mandibular ramus and severe premolar overlap on one side and horizontally smaller molar teeth and mandibular ramus on the other side. This imaging appearance must not be confused with a congenital or developmental facial asymmetry (this positioning artifact is demonstrated in Fig. 10-9).

The magnitude of horizontal distortion varies between the anterior and posterior regions of the jaws. In the anterior region, horizontal magnification increases markedly as the object moves away from the center of the focal trough. The degree of this magnification in the posterior regions is less than that in the anterior region. Two identical objects located in the anterior and posterior regions may have different horizontal magnifications. Thus, overall horizontal measurements made on panoramic radiographs are unreliable. Special attention must be paid to these considerations in following the progress of a bony lesion, especially in the anterior region. As a result of improper patient positioning, the lesion may appear greater (enlarging) (see Fig. 10-8, *D*) or reduced (healing) (see Fig. 10-8, *F*) on successive images. The importance of careful alignment and positioning of the patient's dental arches within the area of the focal trough is apparent.

Vertical magnification is determined by distance between the x-ray source and the object, similar to conventional radiography. In some panoramic radiographs, this distance is maintained constant through the exposure cycle, and the vertical magnification is relatively constant through the different areas of the image in these units. However, despite this, assessment of vertical relationships in a panoramic radiograph is unreliable.

The orientation of the panoramic x-ray beam has a slight caudocranial inclination. As a result of this beam angulation, structures that are positioned closer to the source are projected higher up on the image, relative to structures that are positioned further away from the source of radiation. Thus, the spatial relationships between the objects in the vertical dimension may not accurately represent true anatomic relationships. Figure 10-10 shows a mandibular molar and the mandibular canal. Three different positions of the mandibular canal are indicated, from lingual to buccal. All three positions are in the same horizontal plane (see Fig. 10-10, *A*). However, owing to the angulation of the x-ray beam, the image of the lingually positioned canal (orange) is projected closer to the apex of the molar, whereas the image of the buccally positioned canal (green) is projected further away from the root apex. Thus, the distance between the root apex and the mandibular canal can be misrepresented on a panoramic radiograph.

REAL, DOUBLE, AND GHOST IMAGES

Because of the rotational nature of the x-ray source and receptor, the x-ray beam intercepts some anatomic structures twice during each exposure cycle. Depending on their location, objects may cast three different types of images, as follows:

- *Real images:* Objects that lie between the center of rotation and the receptor form a real image. Within this zone, objects that lie within the focal trough cast relatively sharp images, whereas images of objects located away from the focal trough are

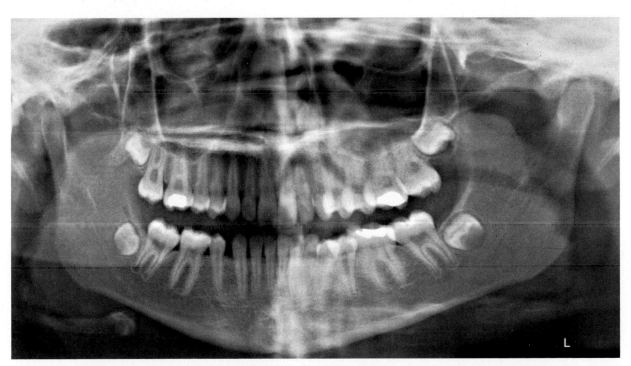

FIGURE 10-9 Panoramic image shows positioning error—rotation of the sagittal plane. The patient's head was rotated to the right, placing the right jaws buccal to the focal trough and the left jaws lingual to the focal trough. As a consequence, the images of the right jaws are minimized, whereas the images of the left jaws are magnified. Note also the severe overlaps of the left posterior teeth. It is important to recognize this common distortion and not to mistake it for skeletal asymmetry.

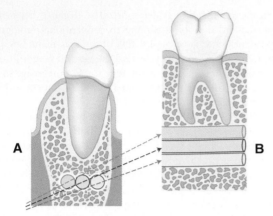

FIGURE 10-10 Influence of projection geometry on spatial relationships in the vertical dimension. **A,** Diagrammatic representation of a coronal cross section through the mandible. Three potential locations of the mandibular canal are shown. The locations lie in the same horizontal plane but differ in their buccolingual position. The x-ray beam *(dotted lines)* is angulated relative to the horizontal plane. **B,** Apparent locations of the mandibular canals in the resultant image. When lingually positioned (orange), the canal is projected more superiorly than when the canal is located buccally (green).

blurred. Figure 10-11, *A* and *C*, shows the positions of the x-ray source during imaging of the left and right sides of the mandibular ramus, respectively. In Figure 10-11, *A*, the left ramus lies between the center of rotation and the receptor and casts a real image. Because it is within the focal trough, its image is sharp. Also demonstrated in Figure 10-11, *A*, is the formation of the real images of the hyoid bone and cervical spine. However, because these structures are away from the focal trough and closer to the x-ray source, their images are blurred and magnified. Figure 10-11, *D*, shows in blue the anatomic region that makes real images.

- *Double images:* Objects that lie posterior to the center of rotation and that are intercepted twice by the x-ray beam form double images (green region in Fig. 10-11, *E*). This region includes the hyoid bone, epiglottis, and cervical spine, all of which cast images on both sides and form double images.

- *Ghost images*: Some objects are located between the x-ray source and the center of rotation. These objects cast ghost images. On the panoramic image, ghost images appear on the image on the opposite side of its true anatomic location and at a higher level because of the upward inclination of the x-ray beam. Because

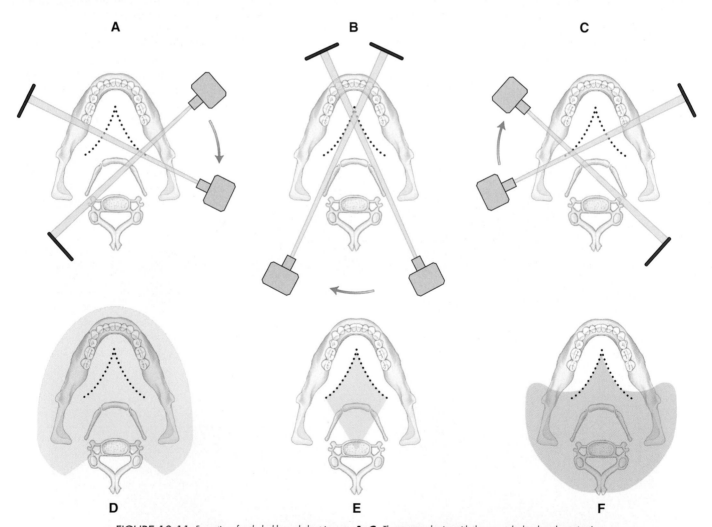

FIGURE 10-11 Formation of real, double, and ghost images. **A-C,** The exposure begins with the x-ray tube head on the patient's right side and continues with the tube head moving behind the patient and ending up on the left side. The *dotted line* represents the path of the moving center of rotation during the exposure cycle. **D,** Structures between the moving center of rotation and the receptor form real images (blue zone). **E,** Structures lying between the moving centers of rotation and the receptor that are imaged twice (green zone) cast double images. **F,** Structures located between the x-ray source and moving center of rotation (orange zone) cast ghost images.

the object is located outside of the focal plane and close to the x-ray source, the ghost image is blurred and significantly magnified. Several anatomic structures cast ghost images (orange region in Fig. 10-11, *F*). For example, in Figure 10-11, *A*, the right mandibular ramus lies between the x-ray source and the center of rotation, and its ghost image is superimposed over the left side of the image. Similarly, the ghost image of the left ramus is superimposed over the right side of the image (see Fig. 10-11, *C*). The hyoid bone and cervical spine also form ghost images when the anterior regions of the jaws are imaged (see Fig. 10-11, *B*). Additionally, metallic accessories, such as earrings, necklaces, and hairpins, form ghost images, which appear as blurred radiopaque images that can obscure anatomic details, mask pathologic changes, or mimic pathologic changes. Figure 10-12 shows a panoramic image of half a cadaver head and all the associated ghost images.

Some anatomic zones form both real double and ghost images.

PANORAMIC MACHINES

Many companies manufacture high-quality film-based and digital panoramic machines. The Veraviewepocs (Fig. 10-13, *A*) (J. Morita Mfg Co, Kyoto, Japan), GXDP-700 (Fig. 10-13, *B*) (Gendex Dental Systems, Hatfield, PA), and ProOne (Fig. 10-13, *C*) (Planmeca Inc, Wood Dale, IL) are all highly versatile. In addition to producing standard panoramic images of the jaws, they have the capability of adjusting to patients of various sizes and making frontal and lateral images of TMJs. Some of these machines also are capable of producing tomographic views through the sinuses and cross-sectional views of the maxilla and mandible. These views are acquired by having special tube head and film movements programmed into the machine. Each machine also has the capability for adding on a cephalometric attachment to allow exposure of standardized skull views. Some machines have the capability of automated exposure control; this is accomplished by measuring the amount of radiation passing through the patient's mandible during the initial part of the exposure and adjusting the imaging factors (peak kilovoltage [kVp], milliamperage [mA], and speed of imaging movements) to obtain a correctly exposed image. Finally, all of these machines are available in CCD-digital configurations, and some have cone-beam imaging capability (see Chapters 11-13).

PATIENT POSITIONING AND HEAD ALIGNMENT

To obtain diagnostically useful panoramic radiographs, it is necessary to prepare patients properly and to position their heads carefully in the focal trough. Dental appliances, earrings, necklaces, hairpins, and any other metallic objects in the head and neck region should be removed. It may also be wise to demonstrate the machine to the patient by cycling it while explaining the need to remain still during the procedure. This is particularly important for children, who may be anxious. Children should be instructed to look forward and not to follow the tube head with their eyes.

The anteroposterior position radiograph of the patient is achieved typically by having patients place the incisal edges of their maxillary and mandibular incisors into a notched positioning device (bite-block). Patients should not shift the mandible to either side when making this protrusive movement. The midsagittal plane must be centered within the focal trough of the particular x-ray unit. Most panoramic units have laser beams to facilitate alignment of the patient's midsagittal plane, Frankfort plane, and anteroposterior position within the focal trough.

Placement of the patient either too far anterior or too far posterior results in significant dimensional aberrations in the images. Too far posterior results in magnified mesiodistal dimensions through the anterior sextants and resulting "fat" teeth (see Fig. 10-8, *D*). Too far anterior results in reduced mesiodistal dimensions through the anterior sextants and resulting "thin" teeth (see Fig. 10-8, *F*). Failure to position the midsagittal plane in the rotational midline of the machine results in a radiograph showing right and left sides that are unequally magnified in the horizontal dimension (see Fig. 10-9).

Poor midline positioning is a common error, causing horizontal distortion in the posterior regions; excessive tooth overlap in the premolar regions; and occasionally, nondiagnostic, clinically unacceptable images. A simple method for evaluating the degree of horizontal distortion of the image is to compare the apparent width of the mandibular first molars bilaterally. The smaller side is too close to the receptor, and the larger side is too close to the x-ray source.

The patient's chin and occlusal plane must be properly positioned to avoid distortion. The occlusal plane is aligned so that it is lower anteriorly, angled 20 to 30 degrees below the horizontal. A general guide for chin positioning is to place the patient so that a line from the tragus of the ear to the outer canthus of the eye is parallel with the floor. If the chin is tipped too high, the occlusal plane on the radiograph appears flat or inverted, and the image of the mandible is distorted (Fig. 10-14, *A*). In addition, a radiopaque shadow of the hard palate is superimposed on the roots of the maxillary teeth. If the chin is tipped too low, the teeth become severely overlapped, the symphyseal region of the mandible may be cut off the film, and both mandibular condyles may be projected off the superior edge of the film (Fig. 10-14, *B*). Patients are positioned with their backs and spines as erect as possible and their necks extended. Having patients place their feet on a foot support and using a cushion for back support may facilitate proper back positioning in seated units. These devices help straighten the spine, minimizing the artifact produced by a shadow of the spine.

Proper neck extension is best accomplished by using a gentle upward force on the mastoid eminences when positioning the head in a manner similar to applying cervical traction. Allowing patients to slump their heads and necks forward causes a large opaque artifact in the midline created by the superimposition of an increased mass of cervical spine. This shadow obscures the entire symphyseal region of the mandible and may require that the radiograph be retaken (Fig. 10-15). Finally, after patients are positioned in the machine, they should be instructed to swallow and hold the tongue on the roof of the mouth. This raises the dorsum of the tongue to the hard palate, eliminating the air space and providing optimal visualization of the apices of the maxillary teeth.

IMAGE RECEPTORS

Digital receptors are being used increasingly for making panoramic images. One option is to use a film-sized PSP plate (see Chapter 4). After exposing the plate, the image is processed by reading the latent image off of the PSP plate yielding a digital image. Alternatively, most manufacturers have developed direct digital acquisition panoramic machines. The receptor on such a machine is an array of solid-state detector (CCD or complementary metal oxide semiconductor sensors). The sensor array transmits an electronic signal to the controlling computer, which displays the image on the viewscreen as it is being acquired. Both of these digital modalities allow the user to modify the image

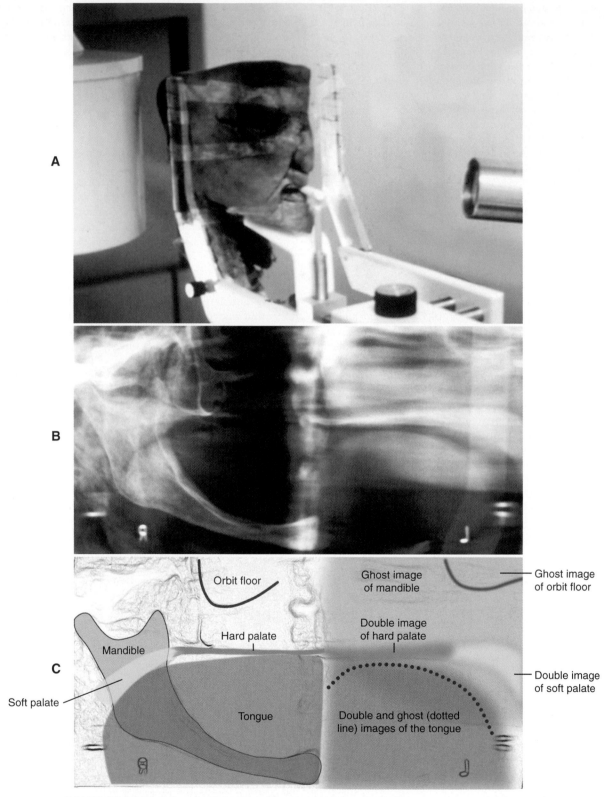

FIGURE 10-12 **A,** Half a cadaver head supported in a panoramic machine. **B,** Resulting panoramic image with real images of right-side structures and double or ghost images shown on the opposite side. **C,** Schematic representation of the real, double, and ghost images of key anatomic structures. (**A** and **B,** Courtesy Dr. Barton Gratt, Redmond, WA.)

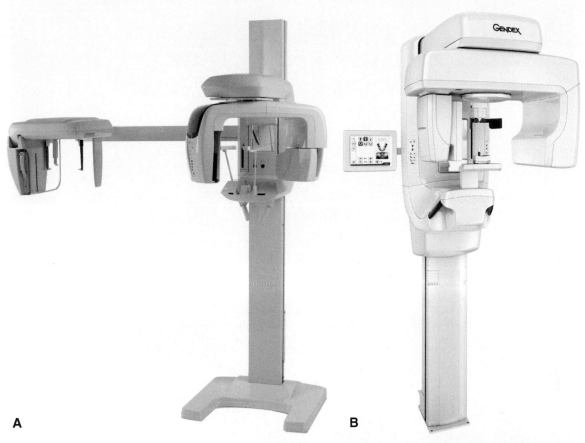

A

B

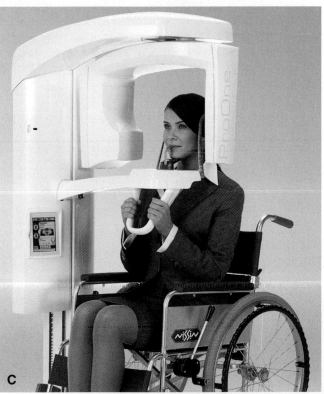

C

FIGURE 10-13 **A,** Veraviewepocs two-dimensional panoramic unit with cephalometric arm attachment. **B,** GXDP-700 panoramic unit. **C,** ProOne panoramic machine. In a clinical situation a leaded apron would be used to protect the patient. (**A,** *Courtesy J. Morita Mfg Corp, Kyota, Japan;* **B,** *Courtesy Gendex Dental Systems, Hatfield, PA;* **C,** *Courtesy Planmeca Inc, Wood Dale, IL.*)

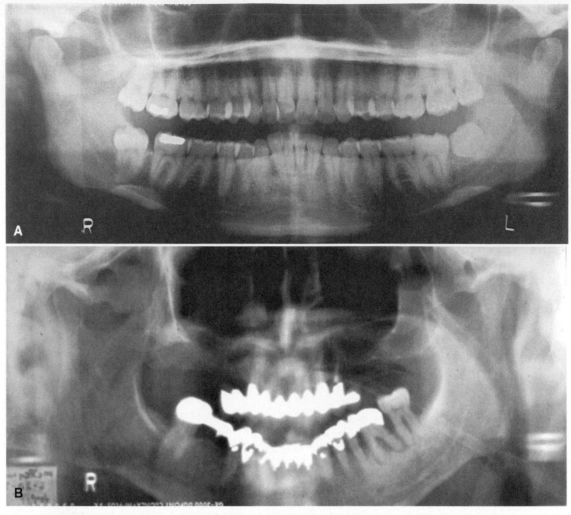

FIGURE 10-14 Panoramic radiographs demonstrating poor patient head alignment. **A,** The chin and occlusal plane are rotated upward, resulting in overlapping images of the teeth and an opaque shadow (the hard palate) obscuring the roots of the maxillary teeth. **B,** The chin and occlusal plane are rotated downward, cutting off the symphyseal region on the radiograph and distorting the anterior teeth.

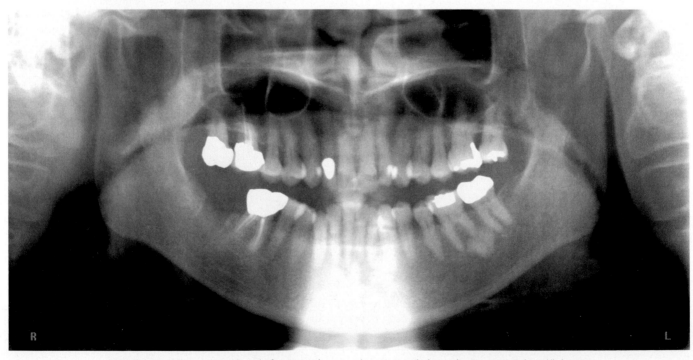

FIGURE 10-15 Panoramic radiograph of an improperly positioned patient. Note the large radiopaque region in the middle because the patient has the neck angled forward. This ghost image of the cervical spine could have been eliminated by having the patient sit straight and align or stretch the neck.

characteristics, including contrast and density adjustments, black/white reversal, area of interest magnification, edge enhancement, and color rendering. Most units are capable of exporting the digital image in DICOM (Digital Imaging and Communications in Medicine) format or in a variety of standard image formats, such as Tagged Image File Format (tiff) or Joint Photography Experts Group (jpeg), allowing easy exchange of radiographic images. DICOM is a standard that specifies handling, storage, printing, and transmission of medical images. The American Dental Association endorses the use of DICOM as the standard for exchange of all dental digital images and recommends that all new digital x-ray units be DICOM compliant.

Intensifying screens (see Chapter 5) are used in film-based panoramic radiography because they significantly reduce the amount of radiation required for properly exposing a radiograph. Fast films combined with high-speed (rare earth) screens are indicated for most examinations. In most cases, the manufacturer provides panoramic machines with intensifying screens. The type of screen (manufacturer and model) is printed in black letters on each screen and clearly projected onto the radiograph. With rare earth screens and fast films, the patient's skin exposure from panoramic radiography is approximately equivalent to four bitewing views made with F-speed film.

All panoramic images should have some mechanism for automatically marking the patient's left or right sides on the image. Also, the patient's name and age and the date the image was acquired should be indicated, with markers, photographic imprinting, or glued labels. The dentist's name must be on the image. No significant anatomic structures should be obscured by any of these labels or markings. Also, no parts of the image should be trimmed to make the film fit the patient's chart.

PANORAMIC FILM DARKROOM TECHNIQUES

Special darkroom procedures are needed when panoramic film is being processed. These films are far more light sensitive than intraoral films, especially after they have been exposed. A reduction in darkroom lighting from that used for conventional intraoral film is necessary. A Kodak GBX-2 (Carestream Dental LLC, Atlanta, GA) filter can be installed with a 15-watt bulb at least 4 feet from the working surface. An ML-2 (Carestream Dental LLC, Atlanta, GA) filter should not be used because it fogs panoramic film. Panoramic film should be developed either manually or in automatic film processors according to the manufacturer's recommendations. Obtaining optimal results relies on the same care to develop, rinse, fix, and wash panoramic films as is taken with intraoral films.

INTERPRETING PANORAMIC IMAGES

As with all image viewing, one should mask out extraneous light from around the image, dim the room lights, and, when possible, work seated in a quiet room. These recommendations apply equally to viewing digital images on a computer display and traditional film radiographs on a viewbox. When interpreting the image, the starting points are systematic analysis of the image and a thorough understanding of the appearances of the normal anatomic structures and their variants on the image. Panoramic images are quite different from intraoral images and demand a disciplined and focused approach to their interpretation. Recognizing normal anatomic structures on panoramic radiographs is challenging because of the complex anatomy of the midface, the superimposition of various anatomic structures, and the changing projection orientation with real, double, and ghost images. The many potential artifacts associated with machine and patient movement, patient positioning, and unusual patient anatomy must be identified and understood. *The absence of a normal anatomic structure may be the most important finding on the image.* Thus, it is essential to identify the presence and integrity of all the major anatomic structures.

Most images in dentistry are two-dimensional representations of three-dimensional structures. On a posteroanterior skull film, orbital rims, nasal conchae, teeth, cervical vertebrae, and petrous ridges are all in sharp focus on the image, although they may be 8 inches apart from each other. As panoramic views are curved image "slices" of the mandibulofacial tissues, there is less superimposition of structures and thus less of an interpretation problem. There is still a thickness to the tomogram that must be considered, however, and the clinician must relate the structures on the image to their relative positions in the midfacial skeleton. An example of this three-dimensionality is the relative positioning of the external oblique and mylohyoid ridges in the mandible: on the panoramic image, they generally both appear sharp, whereas physically the external oblique ridge is on the mandibular buccal surface and the mylohyoid ridge is on the mandibular lingual surface, separated by several millimeters. When panoramic images are viewed, it is important for the clinician to remember this principle and to attempt to visualize the structures three-dimensionally in his or her mind.

It is helpful to view the image as if looking at the patient, with the structures on the patient's right side positioned on the viewer's left (Fig. 10-16). Thus, the image is presented in the same orientation as that of periapical and bitewing images, making the interpretation more comfortable. It is extremely important to recognize the planes of the patient that are represented in different parts of the panoramic image. The panoramic image represents the curved jaw that is unfolded onto a flat plane. In the posterior regions, the panoramic image depicts a sagittal (lateral) view of the jaws, whereas in the anterior sextant, it represents a coronal (anteroposterior) view.

DENTITION

A strength of the panoramic image is the demonstration of the complete dentition. Although there is a rare situation where positioning of the patient or an ectopic tooth places the tooth out of the focal trough, all the teeth are generally seen on the image. Thus, the interpretation must always include identification of all erupted and developing teeth (Fig. 10-17). The teeth should be examined for abnormalities of number, position, and anatomy. Existing dentistry, including endodontic obturations, crowns, and other fixed restorations, should be noted. Excessively wide or narrow anterior teeth suggest malposition of the patient in the focal trough. Similarly, teeth that are wider on one side than the other suggest that the patient's sagittal plane was rotated. Gross caries and periapical and periodontal disease may be evident. However, the resolution of a panoramic radiograph is lower than that of intraoral radiographs, and additional intraoral radiographs may be needed to detect subtle disease. The proximal surfaces of the premolar teeth often overlap, which interferes with caries interpretation.

It is particularly important to examine impacted third molars closely. The orientation of the molars; the numbers and configurations of the roots; the relationships of the tooth components to critical anatomic structures, such as the mandibular canal, floor

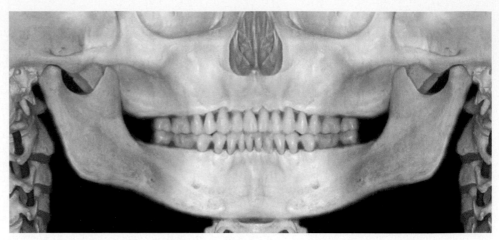

FIGURE 10-16 The bones of the mandible, midface, cervical spine, and skull base as they appear on a panoramic image. The image is composed of left and right lateral views of the facial bones posterior to the canines and a view anterior to the premolars.

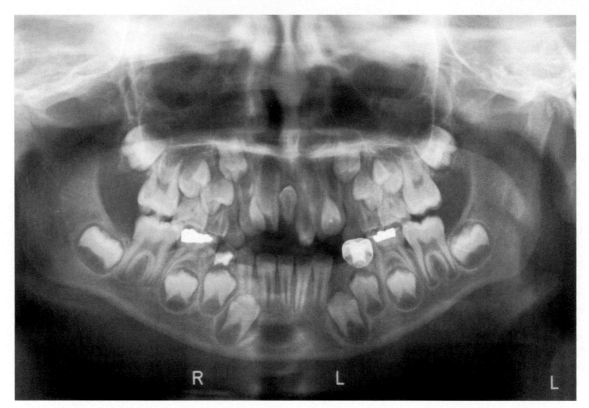

FIGURE 10-17 Panoramic image showing late mixed dentition of an 8-year-old patient. The panoramic image can be useful in identifying the presence or absence of the permanent dentition as well as assessing its developmental status. Note impacted and inverted mesiodens in the maxillary midline and malalignment of incisors.

and posterior wall of the maxillary sinus, maxillary tuberosity, and adjacent teeth; and the presence of abnormalities in the pericoronal or periradicular bone must be carefully studied. However, given the two-dimensional nature of the panoramic image, such findings may need additional imaging with cone-beam computed tomographic (CT) imaging to define precisely the spatial relationships of the roots of the impacted molars to the vital structures.

MIDFACIAL REGION

The midface is a complex mixture of bones, air cavities, and soft tissues, all of which appear on panoramic images (Fig. 10-18). Individual bones that may appear on the panoramic image of the midface include temporal, zygoma, mandible, frontal, maxilla, sphenoid, ethmoid, vomer, nasal, nasal conchae, and palate; thus, it is a misnomer to refer to the midfacial region on the panoramic image as "the maxilla." Maintaining the discipline and focus of a systemic examination of all aspects of the midfacial images is difficult and critical in the overall examination of the panoramic image.

The maxilla can be compartmentalized into major sites for examination (see Fig. 10-18), as follows:
- Cortical boundary of the maxilla, including the posterior border and the alveolar ridge
- Pterygomaxillary fissure

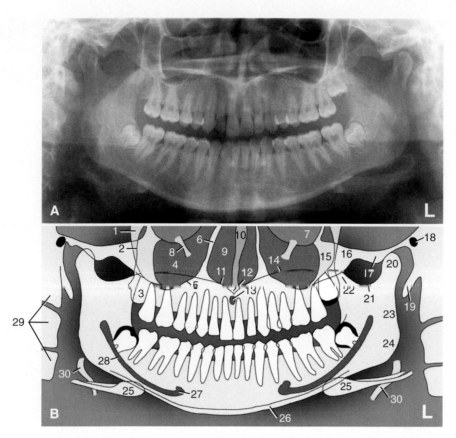

1. Pterygomaxillary fissure
2. Posterior border of maxilla
3. Maxillary tuberosity
4. Maxillary sinus
5. Floor of the maxillary sinus
6. Medial border of maxillary sinus/ lateral border of the nasal cavity
7. Floor of the orbit
8. Infraorbital canal
9. Nasal cavity
10. Nasal septum
11. Floor of the nasal cavity
12. Anterior nasal spine
13. Incisive foramen
14. Hard palate/floor of the nasal cavity
15. Zygomatic process of the maxilla
16. Zygomatic arch
17. Articular eminence
18. External auditory meatus
19. Styloid process
20. Mandibular condyle
21. Sigmoid notch
22. Coronoid process
23. Posterior border of ramus
24. Angle of mandible
25. Hyoid bone
26. Inferior border of mandible
27. Mental foramen
28. Mandibular canal
29. Cervical vertebrae
30. Epiglottis

FIGURE 10-18 **A,** Properly acquired and displayed panoramic image of an adult patient. The patient's left side is indicated on the image, and the image is oriented as if the clinician were facing the patient. This is the same orientation used with a full-mouth series, making it easier for the clinician to orient himself or herself and to interpret the image. **B,** Drawing of the same panoramic radiograph identifying midfacial and mandibular anatomic structures.

- Maxillary sinuses
- Zygomatic complex, including inferior and lateral orbital rims, zygomatic process of maxilla, and anterior portion of zygomatic arch
- Nasal cavity and conchae
- TMJ (also viewed in the mandible, but visualizing important structures multiple times is always a good idea in image interpretation)
- Maxillary dentition and supporting alveolus

Examining the cortical outline of the maxilla is a good way to center the examination of the midface. The posterior border of the maxilla extends from the superior portion of the pterygomaxillary fissure down to the tuberosity region and around to the other side. The posterior border of the pterygomaxillary fissure is the pterygoid spine of the sphenoid bone (the anterior border of the pterygoid plates). Occasionally, the sphenoid sinus may extend into this structure. The pterygomaxillary fissure itself has an inverted

teardrop appearance; it is very important to identify this area on both sides of the image because maxillary sinus mucoceles and carcinomas characteristically destroy the posterior maxillary border, which is manifested as loss of the anterior border of the pterygomaxillary fissure. Also, Le Fort fractures of the maxilla by definition involve the pterygoid plates, and a Le Fort fracture often is initially diagnosed by disturbances of the integrity of the pterygomaxillary fissure on the panoramic image. These disturbances may be the only evidence for such a fracture on the panoramic image. To clarify the three-dimensional anatomy of the pterygomaxillary fissure, Figure 10-19 shows this structure in a dried skull, in an axial CT image, and in the panoramic image.

The maxillary sinuses are usually well visualized on panoramic images. The clinician should identify each of the borders (posterior, anterior, floor, roof) and note whether they are entirely outlined with cortical bone, roughly symmetric, and comparable in radiographic density. The borders should be present and intact.

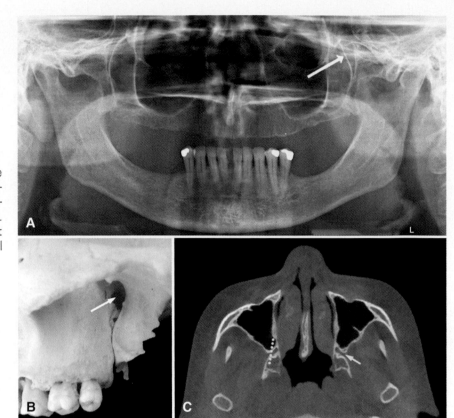

FIGURE 10-19 Pterygomaxillary fissure, a space between the posterior surface of the maxilla and the anterior border of the pterygoid plates. **A,** Inverted teardrop shape of the fissure on a panoramic image *(arrow).* **B,** The fissure on a dried skull *(arrow).* **C,** The approximate image section *(dotted line)* of the panoramic focal trough through the pterygomaxillary fissure *(arrow)* on an axial computed tomographic (CT) section.

The medial border of the maxillary sinus is the lateral border of the nasal cavity; however, this interface is not demonstrated on the panoramic image. The superior border, or roof, of the maxillary sinus is the floor of the orbit; this interface is demonstrated on the panoramic image in its most anterior aspect. Although it is useful to compare right and left maxillary sinuses when looking for abnormalities, it is important to remember that the sinuses are frequently nonpathologically asymmetric relative to size, shape, and presence and numbers of septa. The posterior aspect of the sinus is more opaque because of superimposition of the zygoma. Each sinus should be examined for evidence of a mucous retention cyst, mucoperiosteal thickening, and other sinus abnormalities.

The zygomatic complex, or "buttress" of the midface, is a very complex anatomic area, with contributions from the frontal, zygomatic, and maxillary bones. It includes the lateral and inferior orbital rims, the zygomatic process of the maxilla, and the zygomatic arch. The zygomatic process of the maxilla arises over the maxillary first and second molars. The maxillary sinus can pneumatize the zygomatic process of the maxilla up to the zygomaticomaxillary suture. This can result in the appearance of an elliptical, corticated radiolucency in the maxillary sinus, possibly superimposed over the roots of a molar tooth, on a panoramic image. The inferior border of the zygomatic arch extends posteriorly from the inferior portion of the zygomatic process of the maxilla and continues posteriorly to the articular tubercle and glenoid fossa of the temporal bone. The superior border of the zygomatic arch, which curves anterosuperiorly to form the lateral aspect of the lateral orbital rim, should also be noted. The zygomaticotemporal suture lies in the middle of the zygomatic arch and may simulate a fracture if visualized on the image. Additionally, the mastoid air cells occasionally pneumatize the temporal bone all the way to the zygomaticotemporal suture, giving the glenoid fossa of the TMJ

the appearance of having a multilocular, or "soap-bubbly," radiolucency, which is a variant of normal.

The nasal fossa may show the nasal septum and inferior concha, including both the bone and its mucosal covering. In the anterior region, the lateral border and anterior rim of the nasal cavity are seen as a radiopaque line. The anterior nasal spine and the incisive foramen also may be seen. The floor of the nasal cavity or hard palate is seen as a horizontal radiopacity, superimposed over the maxillary sinus in the posterior regions; this is often seen as two radiopaque lines (Fig. 10-20). The lower line is sharp and represents the junction between the lateral wall of the nasal cavity and hard palate on the tube side. The upper line is more diffuse and represents the junction on the opposite side. The conchae, composed of an internal bone, the turbinate, and covering cartilage and mucosa, are seen in a coronal manner in the anterior portion of the image and in a sagittal manner in the posterior portions of the panoramic image. They can appear as very large, homogeneous, soft tissue densities superimposed over the maxillary sinuses and occasionally the anterior nasopharynx.

MANDIBLE

Studying the mandible (see Fig. 10-18) can be compartmentalized into the major anatomic areas of this curved bone, as follows:

- Condylar process and TMJ
- Coronoid process
- Ramus
- Body and angle
- Anterior sextant
- Mandibular dentition and supporting alveolus

The clinician should be able to follow a cortical border around the entire bone, with the exception of the dentate areas. This border should be smooth, without interruptions ("step

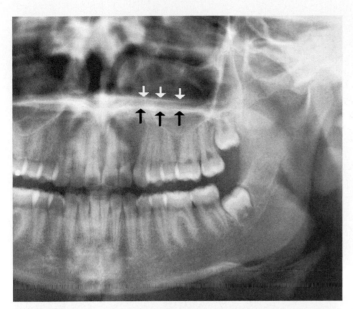

FIGURE 10-20 Panoramic radiograph cropped to show the left posterior midfacial region. The hard palate appears as two radiopaque lines. The lower line *(black arrows)* represents the junction between the hard palate and lateral nasal wall on the receptor side of the patient. The upper line *(white arrows)* represents the junction between the nasal wall and hard palate on the tube side.

deformities") and should have symmetric thicknesses in comparable anatomic areas (e.g., angles, inferior borders of bodies, posterior borders of rami). The trabeculation of the mandible tends to be more plentiful in the anterior regions, whereas the marrow compartment increases toward the angle and into the ramus; however, these trabecular patterns and densities should be relatively symmetric. This is especially true in children, who have very sparse trabeculation throughout the deciduous and mixed dentition stages.

The mandibular condyle is generally positioned slightly anteroinferior to its normal closed position because the patient has to open and protrude the mandible slightly to engage the positioning device in most panoramic machines. The TMJ can be assessed for gross anatomic changes of the condylar head and glenoid fossa; the soft tissues, such as the articular disc and posterior ligamentous attachment, cannot be evaluated. The glenoid fossa is part of the temporal bone, and it can be pneumatized by the mastoid air cells. This can result in the appearance of a multilocular radiolucency in the articular eminence and the roof of the glenoid fossa, which is a variant of normal. More definitive osseous assessment of the TMJ is accomplished by using cone-beam CT imaging and CT scan. Magnetic resonance imaging is the examination of choice for evaluation of the disc and pericondylar soft tissues.

Shadows of other structures that can be superimposed over the mandibular ramal area include the following:
- Pharyngeal airway shadow, especially when the patient is unable to expel the air and place the tongue in the palate during the exposure
- Posterior wall of the nasopharynx
- Cervical vertebrae, especially in patients with pronounced anterior lordosis, typically seen in severely osteoporotic individuals
- Earlobe and ear decorations
- Nasal cartilage and nasal decorations
- Soft palate and uvula

- Dorsum of the tongue and tongue decorations
- Ghost shadows of the opposite side of the mandible and metallic jewelry or piercings

From the angle of the mandible, viewing should be continued anteriorly toward the symphyseal region. A fracture often manifests as a discontinuity (step deformity) in the inferior border; a sharp change in the level of the occlusal plane indicates that the fracture passes through the tooth-bearing area, whereas a cant in the entire occlusal table without a step deformity in the occlusal plane indicates that the fracture is posterior to the tooth-bearing area. The width of the cortical bone at the inferior border of the mandible should be at least 3 mm in adults and of uniform density. The bone may be thinned locally by an expansile lesion such as a cyst or thinned generally by systemic diseases such as hyperparathyroidism and osteoporosis. The outlines of both sides of the mandible should be compared for symmetry, noting any changes. Asymmetry of size may result from improper patient positioning or conditions such as hemifacial hyperplasia or hypoplasia. The hyoid bone may be projected below or onto the inferior border of the mandible.

Trabeculation is most evident within the alveolar process. The mandibular canals and mental foramina are usually clearly visualized in the ramus and body regions of the body of the mandible. Typically, the canals exhibit uniform width or gentle tapering from the mandibular foramina to the mental foramina. They may be less well seen in the first molar and premolar regions. When only one border of the canal is seen, it is typically the inferior border. The canals usually rise to meet the mental foramina, often looping several millimeters anterior of the mental foramina; this is termed the "anterior loop" of the mandibular canal, and its position and extent are considerations when planning dental implants in the mandibular canine regions. A bulging of the canal suggests a neural tumor; however, slight widening at the point that the canal bends to enter the body of the mandible from the ramus is a variation of normal. The mandible should be examined for radiolucencies or opacities. The midline is more opaque because of the mental protuberance, increased trabecular numbers, and attenuation of the beam as it passes through the cervical spine. Many modern panoramic machines automatically increase the exposure factors as they pass across the cervical spine region in an attempt to minimize this opacity; nevertheless, some opacity is generally seen in the anterior regions of the image. There are often depressions on the lingual surfaces of the mandible, which are occupied by the submandibular and sublingual glands. These depressions are termed the lingual salivary gland depressions, or fossae, and are often more radiolucent. This anatomic feature is shown on a panoramic image, periapical image, coronal CT section, and dry skull in Figure 10-21.

SOFT TISSUES

Numerous opaque soft tissue structures may be identified on panoramic radiographs, including the tongue arching across the image under the hard palate (roughly from the region of the right angle of the mandible to the left angle), lip markings (in the middle of the film), the soft palate extending posteriorly from the hard palate over each ramus, the posterior wall of the oral and nasal pharynx, the nasal septum, the earlobes, the nose, and the nasolabial folds (Fig. 10-22). Radiolucent airway shadows superimpose on normal anatomic structures and may be demonstrated by the borders of adjacent soft tissues. They include the nasal fossa, nasopharynx, oral cavity, and oropharynx. The epiglottis and thyroid cartilage are often seen in panoramic images (Fig. 10-23). Occasionally, the

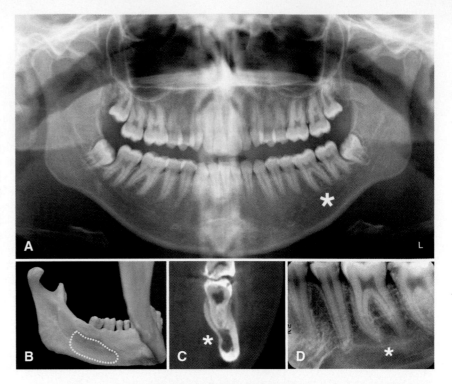

FIGURE 10-21 The submandibular fossa (lingual salivary gland depression) is a concavity often found on the posterior lingual surface of the mandible. This triangularly shaped area is bounded by the mylohyoid ridge superiorly and the inferior border of the mandibular body and lies in the region of the roots of the molars and premolars. *Asterisk* indicates the area of the submandibular fossa on the various images. **A,** Panoramic image. **B,** Photograph of the lingual side of a dried mandible. **C,** Coronal computed tomographic (CT) scan through the molar region of the mandible. **D,** Mandibular molar periapical image.

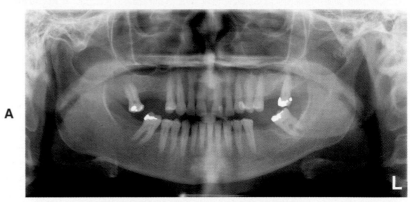

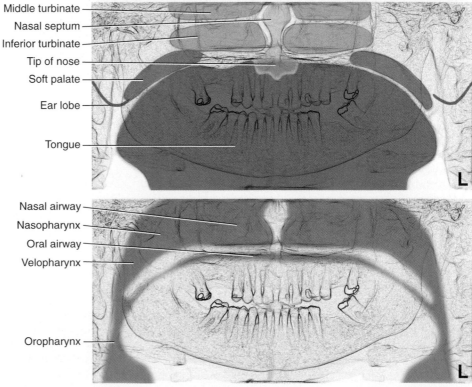

FIGURE 10-22 Soft tissue images on a panoramic radiograph. **A,** Properly acquired panoramic radiograph. **B,** The same panoramic image (processed with an edge filter) with an overlay showing the position of the radiographically evident orofacial soft tissues. **C,** The same panoramic image with an overlay indicating the components of the airway. The nasal airway surrounds the turbinates. The nasopharynx is posterior to the turbinates and above the level of the hard palate. The velopharynx is posterior to the soft palate. The oropharynx is below the uvula.

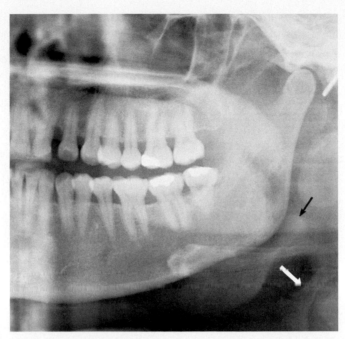

FIGURE 10-23 Normal structures occasionally seen in the neck region on panoramic images. The superior aspect of the thyroid cartilage *(white arrow)* can be mistaken for a vascular calcification. The epiglottis *(black arrow)* lies posterior to the dorsum of the tongue. Also note the ear decoration posterior to the mandibular condylar head.

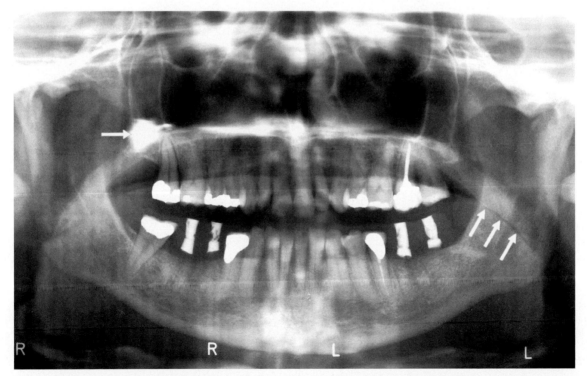

FIGURE 10-24 Airway shadow superimposed over the mandibular ramus may be mistaken for a fracture *(three white arrows)*. Also, the ghost image of a metallic earring on the patient's left side is superimposed over the right maxillary tuberosity region *(single white arrow)*.

air space between the dorsum of the tongue and the soft palate simulates a fracture through the ramus or angle of the mandible (Fig. 10-24).

BIBLIOGRAPHY

Brooks SL, Brand JW, Gibbs SJ, et al: Imaging of the temporomandibular joint: a position paper of the American Academy of Oral and Maxillofacial Radiology, *Oral Surg Oral Med Oral Pathol Oral Radiol Endod* 83:609–618, 1997.

Chomenko AG: *Atlas for maxillofacial pantomographic interpretation*, Chicago, 1985, Quintessence.

Farman AG, editor: *Panoramic radiology: seminars on maxillofacial imaging and interpretation*, Berlin, 2007, Springer.

Langland OE, Langlais RP, McDavid WD, et al: *Panoramic radiology*, ed 2, Philadelphia, 1989, Lea & Febiger.

McDavid WD, Dove SB, Welander U, et al: Dimensional reproduction in direct digital rotational panoramic radiography, *Oral Surg Oral Med Oral Pathol* 75:523–527, 1993.

McDavid WD, Langlais RP, Welander U, et al: Real, double and ghost images in rotational panoramic radiography, *Dentomaxillofac Radiol* 12:122–128, 1983.

Numata H: Consideration of the parabolic radiography of the dental arch, *J Shimazu Stud* 10:13, 1933.

Paatero YV: The use of a mobile source of light in radiography, *Acta Radiol* 29:221, 1948.

Paatero YV: A new tomographic method for radiographing curved outer surfaces, *Acta Radiol* 32:177, 1949.

Rushton VE, Rout J: *Panoramic radiology*, London, 2006, Quintessence Publishing Co.

Cone-Beam Computed Tomography: Volume Acquisition

William C. Scarfe and Allan G. Farman

OUTLINE

Cone-beam computed tomographic (CBCT) imaging is the most significant technologic advance in maxillofacial imaging since the introduction of panoramic radiography. CBCT imaging was initially developed commercially for angiography in the early 1980s. It uses a divergent cone-shaped or pyramid-shaped source of ionizing radiation and a two-dimensional area detector fixed on a rotating gantry to provide multiple sequential transmission images that are integrated directly, forming volumetric information (Fig. 11-1). In the early 1990s, four technologic developments converged to facilitate construction of affordable CBCT units small enough to be used in the dental office for maxillofacial imaging:

- Introduction of x-ray detectors capable of rapid acquisition of multiple basis images
- Development of suitably high-output x-ray generators
- Evolution of suitable image acquisition and integration algorithms
- Availability of inexpensive computers powerful enough to process the enormous amount of acquired image data

The introduction of CBCT imaging has heralded a shift from a two-dimensional to a volumetric approach in maxillofacial imaging. There are three main components to CBCT imaging: (1) image production, (2) visualization, and (3) interpretation. This chapter addresses the technical issues of image production including image data set acquisition and "for presentation" reconstruction.

PRINCIPLES OF CONE-BEAM COMPUTED TOMOGRAPHIC IMAGING

All computed tomographic (CT) scanners consist of an x-ray source and detector mounted on a rotating gantry (see Chapter 14). During rotation of the gantry, the x-ray source produces radiation, while the receptor records the residual x rays after attenuation by the patient's tissues. These recordings constitute the "raw data" that is reconstructed by a computer algorithm to generate cross-sectional images. The basic component of these grayscale images is the picture element (pixel) values. The grayscale value or intensity of each pixel is related to the intensity of the photons incident on the detector. Although providing similar images, CBCT imaging represents a separate evolutionary arm to CT imaging employing multidetector computed tomographic (MDCT) imaging equipment.

The geometric configuration and acquisition mechanics for the CBCT technique are theoretically simple (Fig. 11-2). CBCT imaging is performed using a rotating platform or gantry carrying an x-ray source and detector. A divergent cone-shaped or pyramidal source of radiation is directed through the region of interest (ROI), and the residual attenuated radiation beam is projected onto an area x-ray detector on the opposite side. The x-ray source and detector rotate around a rotation center, fixed within the center of the ROI. This rotational center becomes the center of the final acquired image volume. During the rotation, multiple sequential planar projection images are obtained while the x-ray source and detector move through an arc of 180 to 360 degrees. These single-projection images constitute the raw primary data and are individually referred to as basis, frame, or raw images. Basis images appear similar to cephalometric radiographic images except that each is slightly offset from the next. There are usually several hundred two-dimensional basis images from which the image volume is calculated and constructed. The complete series of images is referred to as the projection data. Because CBCT exposure incorporates the entire ROI, only one rotational scan of the gantry of 180 to 360 degrees is necessary to acquire enough data for volumetric image construction. Software programs incorporating sophisticated algorithms including filtered back projection are applied to these projection data to generate a volumetric data set that can be used to provide primary reconstruction images in three orthogonal planes (axial, sagittal, and coronal). Cone-beam geometry captures volumetric data quickly, and this configuration affords significant cost savings compared with MDCT imaging because multiple patients can be imaged with CBCT imaging in the time taken for one patient to be imaged with MDCT imaging.

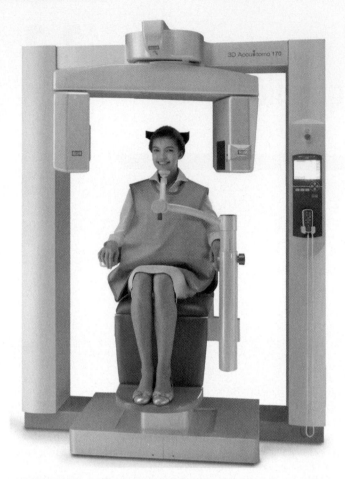

FIGURE 11-1 Example of CBCT unit. Imaging may be performed with the patient seated, supine, or standing. The patient's head is positioned and stabilized between the x-ray generator and detector by a head-holding apparatus. The detector may be a flat panel (this example) or image intensifier. During exposure, the generator and detector rotate fully or partially around the patient's head. Scan time may be as fast as 5 seconds. A separate exposure parameter control panel may be displayed either on the computer screen or on the equipment itself (as shown). Most CBCT units have a small "footprint" enabling in-office placement. *(Image of 3D Accuitomo 170 shown courtesy of J. Morita Mfg Corp, Kyoto, Japan.)*

COMPONENTS OF IMAGE PRODUCTION

There are three major components to CBCT image production:
- X-ray generation
- X-ray detection
- Image reconstruction

The x-ray generation and detection specifications of currently available CBCT systems (Tables 11-1 and 11-2) reflect proprietary variations in these parameters.

X-RAY GENERATION

Although CBCT imaging is technically simple in that only a single scan of the patient is made to acquire a projection data set, numerous clinically important parameters in x-ray generation affect both image quality and patient radiation dose.

Patient Stabilization

Depending on the unit, CBCT examinations are made with the patient sitting, standing, or supine. Supine units are physically larger, have a greater physical footprint, and may not be accessible for patients with some physical disabilities. Standing units may not be able to be adjusted to a height low enough to accommodate wheelchair-bound patients. Although seated units are the most comfortable, they may not allow scanning of physically disabled or wheelchair-bound patients. With all systems, immobilization of the patient's head is more important than patient positioning because any head movement degrades the final image. Immobilization of the head is accomplished by using some combination of a chin cup, bite fork, or other head-restraint mechanism.

X-Ray Generator

During the scan rotation, each projection image set is made by sequential single-image capture of the remnant x-ray beam by the detector. X-ray generation may be continuous or pulsed to coincide with the detector activation. It is preferable to pulse the x-ray beam to coincide with the detector sampling; this means that actual exposure time is up to 50% less than scanning time. This technique reduces patient radiation dose considerably.

FIGURE 11-2 Cone-beam imaging geometry. A three-dimensional cone (this example) or pyramidal (if collimation is rectangular) divergent x-ray beam is directed through the patient onto a detector (either solid-state flat panel detector or II/charge-coupled device). After a single two-dimensional projection is acquired by the detector, the x-ray source and detector rotate a small distance around a trajectory arc. At this second angular position, another basis projection image or frame is captured. This sequence continues around the object for the entire 360 degrees (full trajectory) capturing hundreds of individual images or along a reduced or partial trajectory.

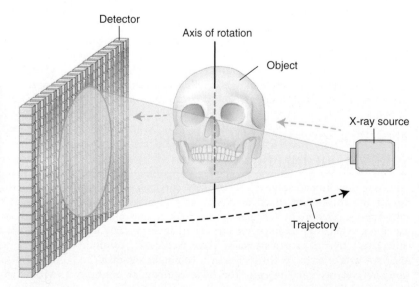

TABLE 11-1	Summary of Specifications for Cone-Beam Computed Tomographic Systems	
Specification	**Variable**	**Parameter**
Unit type	Patient position during image acquisition	Supine; standing; seated
	Functionality	CBCT only; multimodal (CBCT/pan or CBCT/pan/ceph)
	Geometry	Full; partial arc trajectory (degrees)
	Number of basis projections	Fixed; variable (number)
		Scan time (s)
X-ray generator	mA/kVp	Fixed; variable (settings available)
	X-ray source	Constant; pulsed
	AEC	Present/absent
	Focal spot size	Millimeters
Scan volume	Shape	Spherical; cylindrical; convex triangular; other
	Dimensions	Diameter; height × diameter (cm)
Detector	Type	II/CCD; CsI/a-Si; PST; CsI/CMOS
	Voxel size	Fixed; variable (range)
	Grayscale (bit depth)	Acquired; displayed; archived (2^n)
Software	Primary reconstruction time	<1 min, 1-3 min, >3 min

AEC, Automatic exposure control; *CBCT*, cone-beam computed tomographic; *ceph*, cephalometric radiography; *CMOS*, complementary metal oxide semiconductor; *CsI/a-Si*, cesium iodide/amorphous silicon flat panel; *II/CCD*, area image intensifier/charge-coupled device; *kVp*, kilovolt peak; *mA*, milliamperes; *n*, bit-depth; *pan*, panoramic radiography; *PST*, proprietary Siemens Technology.

TABLE 11-2	Representative Cone-Beam Computed Tomographic Imaging Systems	
Products; Models		**Distributor**
3D Accuitomo 80/170; Veraviewpocs 3D R100; Veraviewepocs 3De; Accuitomo FPD60/80		J. Morita Mfg Corp, Kyoto, Japan
Art 3D/Digi-X 3D		Oy Ajat, Espoo, Finland
Auge/Auge Solio/Alioth/Alphard series		Asahi Roentgen, Kyoto, Japan/Belmont, Somerset, NJ
CB MercuRay; CB Throne		Hitachi Medical Systems, Kyoto, Japan
Galileos; Galileos Comfort/Compact		Sirona Dental Systems GmbH, Bensheim Germany
GXCB-500 HD/GXDP-700 S; KaVo 3D eXam		Gendex Dental Systems, Hatfield, PA,/ KaVo Dental Systems, GmbH, Bensheim Germany
i-CAT Classic/Next Generation/Precise		Imaging Sciences, Hatfield, PA
CS 9000 3D/9000 C 3D/9300/9300 Select/9500		Carestream Dental, Atlanta, GA
NewTom 9000/3G/VGi/VGi-Flex/ Giano/5G		QR srl,/Cefla Dental Group, Verona, Italy
OP300		Instrumentarium Dental, Tuusula, Finland
Orion		Ritter Imaging, Ulm, Germany
Master 3Ds/PaX-Flex 3D/PaX-Duo 3D/PaX-Zenith 3D		VATECH Co Ltd, Gyeonggi-Do, Republic of Korea
PreXion 3D Elite		PreXion Inc, San Mateo, CA
Promax 3Ds/3D/3DMid/Max		Planmeca Oy, Helsinki, Finland
Scanora 3D/Cranex 3D		Soredex, Tuusulu, Finland
DaVinci D3D; Hyperion 9		My-Ray Dental Imaging, Cefla Dental Group, Imola, Italy
Suni 3D HD		Suni Medical Imaging, Inc, San Jose, CA

The ALARA (*As Low As Reasonably Achievable*) principle of dose optimization necessitates that CBCT exposure factors should be adjusted on the basis of patient size. This adjustment can be achieved by appropriate selection of tube current (milliamperes [mA]), tube voltage (kilovolt peak [kVp]), or both. In some cases, time also can be adjusted with faster scans producing images with fewer basis images (see later section on scan factors). Although both kVp and mA may be fixed on some units, they are automatically modulated in near real time on other units by a feedback mechanism detecting the intensity of the transmitted beam, a process known as automatic exposure control. On other units, exposure settings are automatically determined by the initial scout exposure. This feature is highly desirable because it is operator independent. The variation in exposure parameters together with the presence of pulsed x-ray beam and size of the image field are the primary determinants of patient exposure.

Scan Volume

The dimensions of the field of view (FOV) or scan volume able to be covered primarily depend on the detector size and shape, the beam projection geometry, and the ability to collimate the beam. The shape of the scan volume can be either cylindrical or spherical. Collimating the primary x-ray beam limits x radiation exposure to the ROI. It is desirable to limit the field size to the smallest volume that images the ROI. This field size must be

selected for each patient based on individual needs. This procedure reduces unnecessary exposure to the patient and produces the best images by minimizing scattered radiation, which degrades image quality. CBCT units are classified according to the maximum FOV incorporated from the scan or scans (Fig. 11-3).

Two approaches have been introduced to enable scanning of an ROI greater than the FOV of the detector. One method involves obtaining data from two or more separate scans and superimposing the overlapping regions of the CBCT data volumes using corresponding fiducial reference landmarks (referred to as either "bioimage registration" or "mosaicing"). Software is used to fuse adjacent image volumes ("stitching" or "blending") to create a larger volumetric data set either in the horizontal or in the vertical dimension (Fig. 11-4). The disadvantage of stitching overlapped regions is that such overlapped regions are imaged twice, resulting in double the

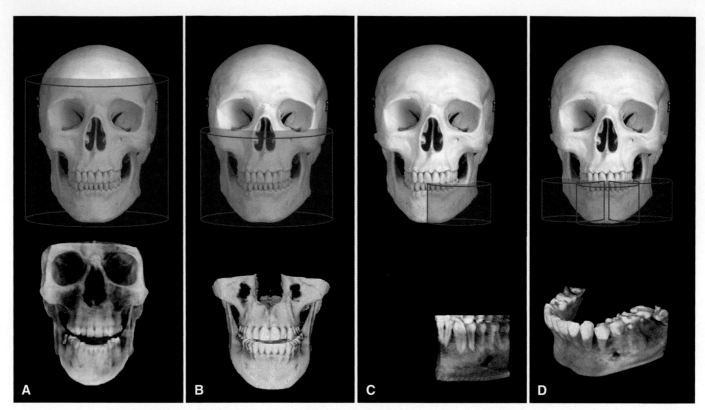

FIGURE 11-3 Classification of CBCT units according to the FOV. **A,** Large FOV scans provide images of the entire craniofacial skeleton, enabling cephalometric analysis. **B,** Medium FOV scans image the maxilla or mandible or both. **C,** Focused or restricted FOV scans provide high-resolution images of limited regions. **D,** Stitched scans from multiple focused FOV scans provide larger regions of interest to be imaged from superimposition of multiple scans. *(Skull image courtesy and copyright of Primal Pictures, Ltd, London, UK: http://www.primalpictures.com.)*

radiation dose to such regions. A second method to increase the height or width of the FOV using a small area detector is to offset the position of the detector, collimate the beam asymmetrically, and scan only half the patient's ROI in each of the two offset scans (Fig. 11-5).

Scan Factors

The number of images constituting the projection data throughout the scan is determined by the detector frame rate (number of images acquired per second), the completeness of the trajectory arc (180 to 360 degrees), and the rotation speed of the source and detector. The number of basis images making up a single scan set may be fixed or variable. Higher frame rates have both desirable and undesirable effects. Higher frame rates increase the signal-to-noise ratio, producing images with less noise and reducing metallic artifacts. However, a higher frame rate is associated with a longer scan time and higher patient dose. In addition, more data are obtained, and primary reconstruction time is increased.

CBCT imaging systems often use a complete circular trajectory or a scan arc to acquire adequate projection data for volumetric software reconstruction. However, increasingly, CBCT units are based on panoramic platforms, which have scan arcs less than 360 degrees. Most CBCT units have fixed scan arcs; however, some provide a choice of manual controls to reduce the scan arc further. A limited scan arc potentially reduces the scan time and patient

radiation dose and is mechanically easier to perform. However, images produced by this method may have greater noise and reconstruction interpolation artifacts.

It is desirable to reduce CBCT scan times to as short as possible to reduce motion artifact resulting from patient movement. Patient movement can be substantial and may be a limiting factor in image resolution. Decreased scanning times may be achieved by increasing the detector frame rate, reducing the number of projections, or reducing the scan arc. The first method provides images of the highest quality, whereas the latter methods increase image noise.

IMAGE DETECTORS

Current CBCT units can be divided into two groups based on detector type: (1) image intensifier tube/charge-coupled device (II/CCD) combination or (2) flat panel detectors (FPDs). II/CCD units are usually larger and bulkier and result in circular basis image areas (spherical volumes) rather than rectangular ones (cylindrical volumes) produced by FPDs. Most, but not all, contemporary CBCT units use FPDs. FPDs employ an "indirect" detector based on a large-area solid-state sensor panel coupled to an x-ray scintillator layer (see Chapter 4). The most common flat panel configuration consists of a cesium iodide scintillator applied to a thin film transistor made of amorphous silicon. More recently, large complementary metal oxide semiconductor technology arrays have also been used.

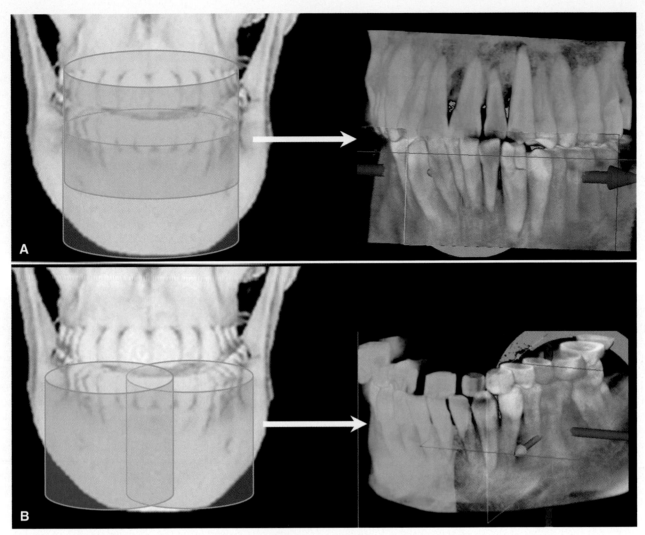

FIGURE 11-4 Increasing FOV by "stitching" volumetric data sets. Larger ROI can be acquired by small FOV CBCT units by "stitching" adjacent limited area volumetric data sets. This process requires acquisition of separate scans *(left)*, registration of each volume by super-imposition of fiducial landmarks, and fusion to provide a larger FOV *(right)*. Units may use this technique to increase either the vertical **(A)** or the horizontal **(B)** FOV. Shown here are adjacent (orange and blue) volumetric data sets (KODAK CS 9000 Carestream Dental, Atlanta, GA) stitched manually using proprietary software (InVivoDental software; Anatomage, San Jose, CA).

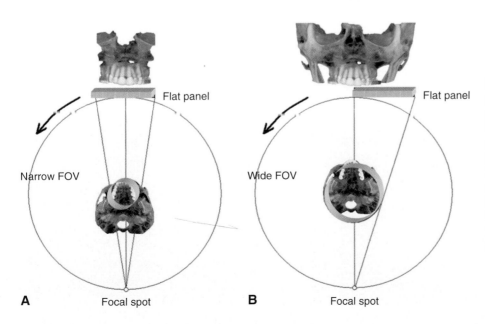

FIGURE 11-5 Schematic of asymmetric CBCT geometric configuration to increase FOV using a FPD. **A,** Conventional geometric arrangement whereby the central ray of the x-ray beam from the focal source is directed through the middle of the object to the center of the FPD. The resultant image is limited to the region of the detector (dentition in this case). **B,** Alternative method increasing image size involves shifting the location of the flat panel imager and collimating the x-ray beam laterally to extend the FOV object. In this instance, the FPD is shifted to the opposite side of the midline halfway through the exposure. The resulting image doubles the horizontal ROI. *(Adapted courtesy of SOREDEX, Tuusula, Finland.)*

Voxel Size

The spatial resolution—and therefore detail of a CBCT image—is determined by the individual volume elements (voxels) produced in formatting the volumetric data set. CBCT units in general provide voxel resolutions that are isotropic—equal in all three dimensions. The principal determinants of nominal voxel size in a CBCT image are the matrix and pixel size of the detector. Detectors with smaller pixels capture fewer x-ray photons per voxel and result in more image noise. Consequently, CBCT imaging using higher resolutions may be designed to use higher dosages to achieve a reasonable signal-to-noise ratio for improved diagnostic image quality.

Both the focal spot size and the geometric configuration of the x-ray source are important to determine the degree of geometric unsharpness, a limiting factor in spatial resolution. The cost of x-ray tubes—and therefore of the CBCT unit—increases substantially with small focal spot size tubes. Reducing the object-to-detector distance and increasing source-to-object distance also minimizes geometric unsharpness. In maxillofacial CBCT imaging, the detector position is limited because it must be located far enough from the patient's head so that it freely rotates and clears the patient's shoulders. Limitations also exist in extending the source-to-object distance because this increases the size of the CBCT unit. However, reducing source-to-object distance produces a magnified projected image on the detector, increasing potential spatial resolution. Additional factors influencing image resolution include motion of the patient's head during the exposure, the type of scintillator used in the detector, and the image reconstruction algorithms applied.

Grayscale

The ability of CBCT imaging to display differences in attenuation is related to the ability of the detector to reveal subtle contrast differences. This parameter is called the bit depth of the system and determines the number of shades of gray available to display the attenuation. All currently available CBCT units use detectors capable of recording grayscale differences of 12 bits or greater. A 12-bit detector provides 2^{12} or 4096 shades to display contrast. A 16-bit detector provides 2^{16} or 65,536 shades of gray. Although higher bit-depth images in CBCT imaging are possible, this added information comes at the expense of increased computational time and substantially larger file sizes.

RECONSTRUCTION

After the basis projection frames are acquired, it is necessary to process these data to create a volumetric data set. This process is called primary reconstruction. Although a single cone-beam rotation may take less than 20 seconds, it produces 100 to more than 600 individual projection frames, each with more than 1 million pixels with 12 to 16 bits of data assigned to each pixel. These data are processed to create a volumetric data set composed of cuboidal volume elements (voxels) by a sequence of software algorithms in a process called reconstruction. Subsequently, visual orthogonal (i.e., perpendicular) images sectioning the volumetric data set are secondarily reconstructed. The reconstruction of these data is computationally complex. To facilitate data handling, data are usually acquired by one computer (acquisition computer) and transferred by an Ethernet connection to a processing computer (workstation). In contrast to conventional CT imaging, cone-beam data reconstruction is performed by personal computer–based, rather than workstation platforms.

The reconstruction process consists of two stages, each comprising numerous steps (Fig. 11-6):

1. Preprocessing stage (Fig. 11-7). The preprocessing stage is performed at the acquisition computer. After the multiple planar projection images are acquired, these images must be corrected for inherent pixel imperfections, variations in sensitivity across the detector, and uneven exposure. Image calibration should be performed routinely to remove these defects.

2. Reconstruction stage. The remaining data-processing steps are performed on the reconstruction computer. The corrected images are converted into a special representation called a sinogram, a composite image developed from multiple projection images (Fig. 11-8). The horizontal axis of a sinogram represents individual rays at the detector, whereas the vertical axis represents projection angles. If there are 300 projections, the sinogram will have 300 rows. This process of generating a sinogram is referred to as the Radon transformation. The resulting image comprises multiple sine waves of different amplitude, as individual objects are projected onto the detector at continuously varying angles. The final image is reconstructed

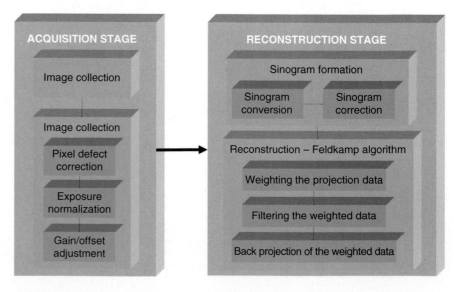

FIGURE 11-6 Image acquisition and reconstruction. The acquisition stage involves acquisition of individual basis projections and subsequent modification of these images to correct for inconsistencies. Image correction is sequential and consists of the removal of signal voids from individual or linear pixel defects, image normalization by histogram equalization so that a full range of voxel intensity values are used, and removal of inherent electronic detector artifacts. After correction, images undergo reconstruction, which includes converting the corrected basis projection images into sinograms and application of the Feldkamp reconstruction to the corrected filters to the image and use of back-projection techniques to reconstitute the image.

ACQUISITION STAGE

Image collection

Image collection
Pixel defect correction
Exposure normalization
Gain/offset adjustment

RECONSTRUCTION STAGE

Sinogram formation
Sinogram conversion   Sinogram correction
Reconstruction – Feldkamp algorithm
Weighting the projection data
Filtering the weighted data
Back projection of the weighted data

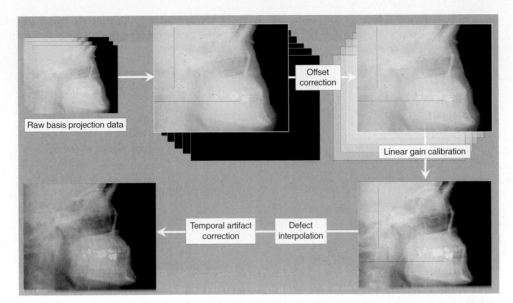

FIGURE 11-7 CBCT detector preprocessing. The first step of CBCT detector preprocessing is offset correction. This is accomplished by pixel-wise subtraction of an individual offset value computed by averaging over a series of up to 30 dark images. The second step is the linear gain calibration, consisting of dividing each pixel by its individual gain factor. The gain factors are obtained by averaging a sequence with up to 30 images of homogeneous exposures without any object between x-ray source and detector. The gain sequence is first offset corrected with its own sequence of dark images. The next procedure is the defect interpolation. Each pixel that shows unusual behavior, either in the gain image or in the average dark sequence, is marked in a defect map. The gray values of pixels classified as defective in this way are computed by linear interpolation along the least gradient descent. For FPDs, there is usually an additional procedure to correct for temporal artifacts. These arise in such detectors because both the scintillator and the photodiodes exhibit residual signals.

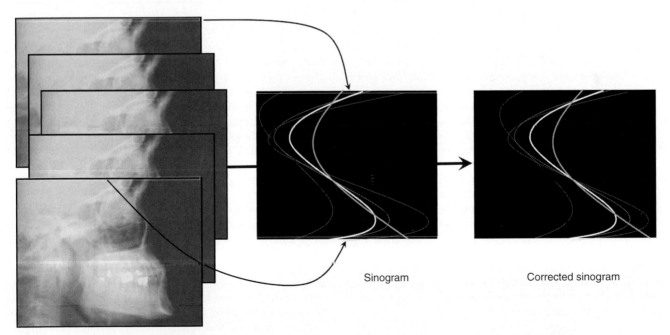

FIGURE 11-8 Radon transformation—construction and correction of sinograms. Specific projections of an object, at a few sample projection angles, are shown on the left. A sinogram is a special image that captures the projection information of an object in a different spatial format. The horizontal axis of a sinogram represents the attenuation of each ray of the x-ray beam. The center of the horizontal axis corresponds to the center of the beam and the center of the detector. The vertical axis of a sinogram represents each projection angle. The resulting sinusoidal waves within the sinogram represent projections of off-center features in the object over the range of continuously varying projection angles. Before reconstruction, sinograms must be corrected for blurring that ordinarily occurs as a result of the back-projection reconstruction process. A specific filter is applied to the sinogram data to reduce this blurring effect. When corrected, the sinogram is ready to be processed by the appropriate reconstruction algorithm.

from the sinogram with a filtered back-projection algorithm for volumetric data acquired by CBCT imaging; the most widely used algorithm is the Feldkamp algorithm. This process is referred to as inverse Radon transformation. When all slices have been reconstructed, they are combined into a single volume for visualization.

Reconstruction times vary depending on the acquisition parameters (voxel size, size of the image field, and number of projections), hardware (processing speed, data throughput from acquisition to reconstruction computer), and software (reconstruction algorithms) used. Reconstruction should be accomplished in an acceptable time (<5 minutes) to complement patient flow.

CLINICAL CONSIDERATIONS

Operation of CBCT equipment is technically straightforward and similar, in many respects, to the performance of panoramic radiography. However, in contrast to panoramic imaging, numerous image acquisition settings may be adjusted, depending on the CBCT unit used (see Table 11-1). Practitioners and operators using CBCT must have a thorough understanding of the operational parameters and the effects of these parameters on image quality and radiation safety.

PATIENT SELECTION CRITERIA

Cone-beam exposure provides a radiation dose to the patient higher than radiation doses of other dental radiographic procedures. The principal tenet of the ALARA principle must be applied: there should be justification of the exposure to the patient so that the total potential diagnostic benefits are greater than the individual detriment radiation exposure might cause. Generally, a CBCT image should be used only when a lower dose examination, such as a periapical or panoramic view, cannot provide the necessary information for patient diagnosis and treatment. Numerous consensus-derived statements providing guidelines on the clinical use of CBCT have been published. General use guidelines from the American Academy of Oral and Maxillofacial Radiology (AAOMR) and more recently the American Dental Association (ADA) provide general statements on performing and interpreting diagnostic CBCT imaging. These documents provide guidance on the appropriate use and prescription of CBCT imaging, detail the responsibilities of practitioners and licensed operators in performing the examination, outline the appropriate documentation and radiation safety considerations, and provide recommendations for quality control and patient education. In addition, specific use guidelines are available for endodontics and implant dentistry from the AAOMR. Essentially, CBCT imaging should be used as an adjunctive diagnostic tool to existing dental imaging techniques for specific clinical applications, not as a screening procedure. It is advisable that the indication for the CBCT examination be documented by entry in the patient's chart or on the written request or prescriptive order for the CBCT examination.

PATIENT PREPARATION

Patients should be escorted into the scanner unit and provided with appropriate personal radiation barrier protection before head stabilization. Although the mandatory use of these devices is regulated by regional (state) or federal legislation, it is recommended that at least a leaded torso apron be applied correctly (above the collar) to the patient. Use of a leaded apron is particularly advisable for pregnant patients and for children. It is highly recommended that a lead thyroid collar also be used, provided that it would not interfere with the scan, to reduce thyroid exposure.

Immediately before the scan, the patient should be asked to remove all metallic objects from the head and neck areas, including eyeglasses, jewelry (including earrings and piercings), and metallic partial dentures. It is not necessary to remove completely removable plastic prostheses.

Each CBCT unit has a unique method of head stabilization, varying from chin cups to posterior or lateral head supports to head restraints. Patient motion can be minimized by application of one or more methods simultaneously. Image quality is severely degraded by head movement, so it is important to obtain patient compliance.

Alignment of the area of interest with the x-ray beam is critical to image the appropriate field. Often facial topographic reference planes (e.g., the midsagittal plane, Frankfort horizontal) or internal references (e.g., occlusal plane, palatal plane) are adjusted to align with external laser lights to position the patient correctly.

Unless specifically indicated otherwise (e.g., closed temporomandibular joint views or orthodontic views), it is desirable that the dentition be separated but held together firmly during the scan; this can be done with a tongue depressor or cotton rolls. Separation of the teeth is particularly useful in single arch scans where scatter from metallic restorations in the opposing arch can be reduced.

The patient should be directed to remain as still as possible before exposure, to breathe slowly through the nose, and to close the eyes. The last suggestion reduces the possibility of the patient moving as a result of following the detector as it passes in front of the face.

IMAGING PROTOCOL

An imaging protocol is a set of technical exposure parameters for CBCT imaging that depend on the specified purpose of the examination. An imaging protocol is developed to produce images of optimal quality with the least amount of radiation exposure to the patient. For specific cone-beam units, manufacturer-provided imaging protocols are usually available. Most commonly, they involve modifications in imaging field, number of basis projections, and voxel resolution. Operators should be aware of the effects of all parameters on image quality and patient dose when choosing imaging protocols.

Exposure Settings

The quality and quantity of the x-ray beam depend on tube voltage (kVp) and tube current (mA). CBCT unit manufacturers approach setting exposure factors in one of two ways. They either provide a selection of "fixed" exposure settings or allow operator "manual" adjustment of kVp or mA or both. Operators who use CBCT units with operator-adjustable exposure settings must understand that these parameters affect both image quality (Fig. 11-9) and patient radiation dose and that careful selection is required to fulfill the ALARA principle. Although mA may be increased on some units and is suggested to compensate for increases in patient size, the effective dose increases proportionately. Adjustment of kVp has an even greater effect on dose than mA, with each increase in 5 kVp approximately doubling the dose if all other parameters remain the same. Exposure parameters should be appropriate for both the given patient size and the diagnostic task that motivated image selection.

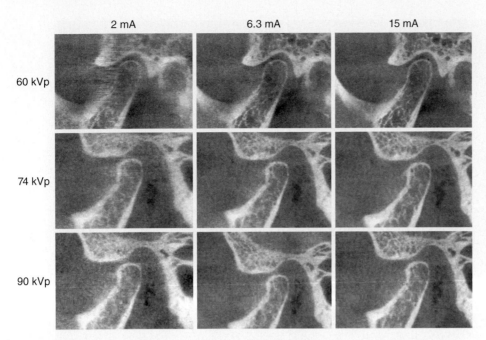

2 mA   6.3 mA   15 mA

60 kVp

74 kVp

90 kVp

FIGURE 11-9 Effect of exposure parameters on image quality. Representative 0.076-mm parasagittal slices of the left temporomandibular joint of a cadaver demonstrate the effect of changing mA (columns) and kVp (rows) on image quality for high-density (cortical bone) and low-density (cancellous bone) structures. Although all images are adequate for visualization of gross morphologic changes at all values, there is increased graininess (noise) of the images made at low kVp and mA, making discernment of the fine trabecular pattern or surface irregularities of cortical plates more difficult. Little improvement in subjective image quality is achieved at settings greater than 74 kVp and 6.3 mA despite appreciable associated increases in dose. *(Images acquired with a CS 9000 S; courtesy of Carestream Dental, a division of Carestream Health, Inc.)*

Spatial Resolution

Spatial resolution refers to the ability of an image to reveal fine detail. It is determined primarily by detector nominal pixel size, beam projection geometry, patient scatter, detector motion blur, fill factor (the fraction of a pixel's area capable of collecting light), focal spot size, number of basis images, and reconstruction algorithm. The voxel size with which projection images are acquired varies from manufacturer to manufacturer. In addition, CBCT units may offer a selection of voxel sizes. For these choices, the image detector collects information over a series of pixels in the horizontal and vertical directions and averages the data. This collation or pixel binning results in a substantial reduction in data processing, reducing secondary reconstruction times. Therefore, voxel size should be specified as either acquisition or reconstruction. Although increased image resolution in some CBCT units does not affect changes in exposure parameters, some manufacturers incorporate reduced-dose exposure protocols for low-resolution settings.

Scan Time and Number of Projections

Adjusting the detector frame rate to increase the number of basis image projections results in reconstructed images with fewer artifacts and better image quality (Fig. 11-10). However, increasing the number of projections requires longer primary reconstruction times and increases patient radiation exposure proportionately.

Scanning Trajectory

Reconstructed images from incomplete, limited, or truncated scanning trajectories of less than 360 degrees may have limited-angle artifacts because of missing information. These include greater peripheral unidirectional streaking artifacts and more pronounced midplane cupping and photon starvation artifacts. Missing data can be compensated for with many approaches, including use of statistical knowledge of the patient's anatomy and use of numerous algorithm projection completion techniques.

Field of View

Collimation of the CBCT primary x-ray beam by adjustment of the FOV enables limitation of the x radiation to the ROI.

Reduction in the FOV usually can be accomplished mechanically or, in some instances, electronically. Mechanical reduction in the dimensions of the x-ray beam can be achieved by either preirradiation (reducing primary radiation dimensions) or postirradiation (reducing the dimensions of the transmitted radiation, before it is detected) collimation. Electronic collimation involves elimination of data recorded on the detector that are peripheral to the area of interest. Electronic collimation is undesirable because it results in greater exposure of the patient to radiation than is necessary for the imaging task.

Reduction of the FOV to the ROI improves image quality because of reduced scattered radiation (see Fig. 11-10). More importantly, a reduction in FOV is usually associated with patient dose reductions ranging from 25% to 66% depending on machine, type of collimation (vertical or horizontal), amount of mechanical collimation, and location (maxilla vs. mandible; anterior vs. posterior).

ARCHIVING, EXPORT, AND DISTRIBUTION

The process of CBCT imaging produces two data products: (1) the volumetric image data from the scan and (2) the image report generated by the operator. Both sets of data must be archived and distributed. Scan data backup is usually performed in its native or proprietary image format. However, export of image data is usually in the Digital Imaging and Communications in Medicine standard version 3 (DICOM v3) file format. This is the International Standards Organization–referenced standard for all diagnostic imaging, including medical, dental, and veterinary imaging, and includes all modalities, such as x ray, visible light, and ultrasound. It is the dental image standard in the United States, adopted by the ADA. CBCT DICOM data can be imported into third-party application-specific software programs that provide virtual simulations that can be used to plan treatment and predict dental implant and prosthetic, surgical orthognathic, orthodontic, or prosthetic outcomes (see Chapter 12).

IMAGE ARTIFACTS

The fundamental factor that impairs CBCT image quality is image artifact. An artifact is any distortion or error in the image that is

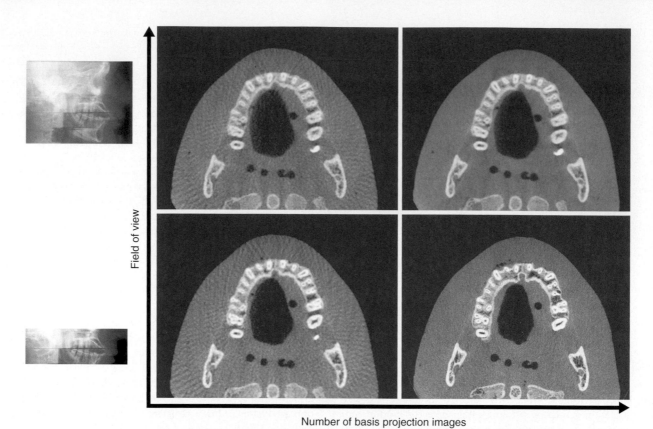

Field of view

Number of basis projection images

FIGURE 11-10 Pictorial plot of the effect of number of basis projection images and size of FOV on image quality. Increasing number of projections in one 360-degree scan (x-axis) provides more data and reduces image noise; however, it increases patient dose proportionately. Reducing the number of projections creates undersampling and produces streaks. Minimizing the FOV (y-axis) reduces patient exposure and resultant scatter radiation and results in images with increased contrast and decreased noise.

unrelated to the subject being studied. CBCT images inherently have more artifacts than MDCT images because the lower energy spectra used; cone-beam geometry; and the introduction of additional considerations such as aliasing artifacts caused by the cone-beam divergence, scatter, and a generally higher noise level. Artifacts can be classified according to their etiology.

INHERENT ARTIFACTS

Artifacts can arise from limitations in the physical processes involved in the acquisition of CBCT data. The beam projection geometry of CBCT, reduced trajectory rotational arcs, and image reconstruction methods produce the following three types of cone-beam–related artifacts:

- Scatter
- Partial volume averaging
- Cone-beam effect

Scatter results from x-ray photons that are diffracted from their original path after interaction with matter. Because CBCT uses area detectors, they capture scattered photons that contribute to overall image degradation or "quantum noise" compared with MDCT imaging (Fig. 11-11). Scatter causes streak artifacts similar to artifacts of beam hardening.

Partial volume averaging is a feature of both MDCT and CBCT imaging. It occurs when the selected voxel size of the scan is larger than the size of the object being imaged. For instance, a voxel 1 mm on one side may contain both bone and adjacent soft

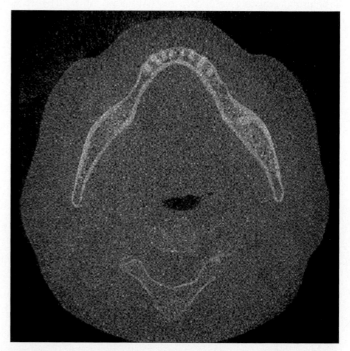

FIGURE 11-11 Quantum noise CBCT artifacts. Axial high-resolution CBCT image at default resolution (0.125 mm nominal voxel size) shows marked graininess or quantum noise caused by contamination of detector signal by scatter radiation.

tissue. In this case, the displayed pixel is not representative of either bone or soft tissue but rather becomes an average of the brightness values of the different tissues. Boundaries in the resultant image may have a "step" appearance or homogeneity of pixel intensity levels. Partial volume averaging artifacts occur in regions where surfaces are rapidly changing in the Z direction, for example, in the temporal bone. Selection of the smallest acquisition voxel can reduce the presence of these effects.

The cone-beam effect is a potential source of artifacts, especially in the peripheral portions of the scan volume. Because of the divergence of the x-ray beam as it rotates around the patient in a horizontal plane, structures at the top or bottom of the image field are exposed only when the x-ray source is on the opposite side of the patient (Fig. 11-12). The result is image distortion, streaking artifacts, and greater peripheral noise. This effect is minimized by incorporation by manufacturers of various forms of cone-beam reconstruction. Clinically, the effect can be reduced by positioning the ROI in the horizontal plane of the x-ray beam.

PROCEDURE-RELATED ARTIFACTS

Undersampling of the object can occur when too few basis projections are provided for image reconstruction or when rotational trajectory arcs are incomplete. A reduced data sample leads to misregistration, sharp edges, and noisier images as a result of aliasing, which appear as fine striations in the image (Fig. 11-13). Because increasing the number of basis projections or a complete

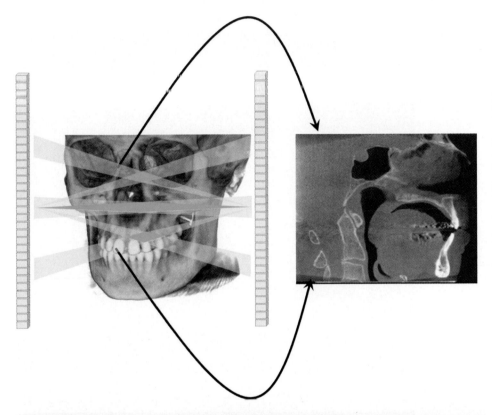

FIGURE 11-12 Schematic of cone-beam artifact. Exaggerated projection of three representative x-ray beams (one perpendicular, one angled inferiorly, and one angled superiorly) from the focal spot point of origin is shown at two positions of the x-ray tube rotation, 180 degrees apart. The optimal amount of data collected by the detector for reconstruction corresponds to the solid blue volume between the overlapping projections. Centrally, the amount of data acquired is maximal, whereas peripherally (transparent blue), the amount of data collected is appreciably less. The midsagittal section image demonstrates the visual effects of data interpolation by the reconstruction algorithm owing to inadequate data obtained at the peripheral superior and inferior extensions of the volumetric data set producing a peripheral "V" artifact of increased noise, distortion, and reduced contrast.

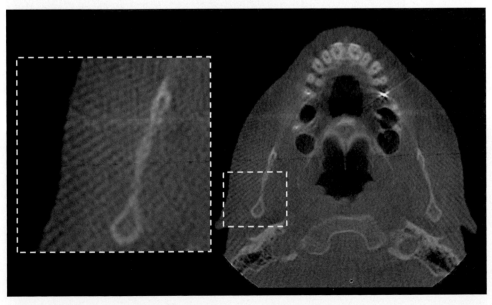

FIGURE 11-13 Moire artifact. Too great an interval between basis projections (undersampling) or an incomplete scanning trajectory can result in misregistration of data by the reconstruction software, known as aliasing. On the CBCT image, particularly on the periphery (inset), fine alternating hyperdense and hypodense stripes appear to be radiating from the edge of the volumetric data, resulting in a characteristic "Moire" pattern, a type of aliasing artifact.

trajectory arch rotation is proportional to patient exposure, the importance of this artifact should be considered in relation to the diagnostic information.

Typically, scanner-related artifacts appear as circular or ring streaks resulting from imperfections in scanner detection or poor calibration (Fig. 11-14). Either of these problems results in a consistently repetitive reading at each angular position of the detector, resulting in a circular artifact.

Misalignment of the x-ray source to the detector creates a double contour artifact, similar to that created by patient motion. Repeated use of CBCT equipment over time may result in slight configuration changes, and components may need to be periodically realigned.

INTRODUCED ARTIFACTS

As an x-ray beam passes through an object, lower energy photons are absorbed in preference to higher energy photons. This phenomenon, called beam hardening, results in two types of artifact: (1) distortion of metallic structures as a result of differential absorption, known as a cupping artifact, and (2) streaks and dark bands, which, when present between two dense objects, create extinction or missing value artifacts (Fig. 11-15). In clinical practice, it is advised to reduce the field size, modify patient position, or separate the dental arches to avoid scanning regions susceptible to beam hardening (e.g., metallic restorations, dental implants). It is also important to remove metallic objects such as jewelry before

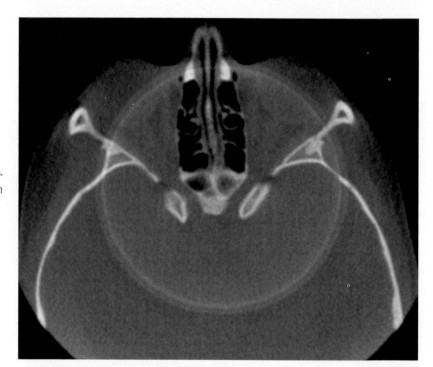

FIGURE 11-14 Circular or ring artifacts. Visual appearance of scanner-related artifacts as circular rings on an axial image suggests imperfections in scanner detection as a result of poor calibration.

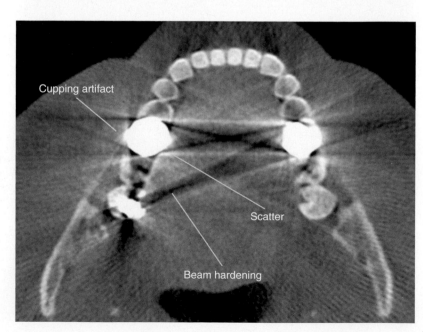

FIGURE 11-15 Introduced artifacts. Axial view demonstrating beam hardening (dark bands), scatter (white streaks), and cupping (image distortion) artifacts.

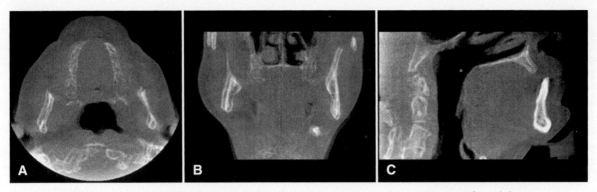

FIGURE 11-16 Motion artifacts. Patient motion during the scanning exposure can result in misregistration artifacts, which appear as double contours in the reconstructed image as demonstrated in the axial (**A**), coronal (**B**), and sagittal (**C**) planes.

scanning to reduce peripheral beam hardening effects superimposed on the ROI.

PATIENT MOTION ARTIFACTS

Patient motion can cause misregistration of data, which appear as double contours in the reconstructed image (Fig. 11-16). The smaller the voxel size (i.e., the higher the spatial resolution), the smaller the movement necessary to cause misalignment of structures. This problem can be minimized by restraining the head and using as short a scan time as possible.

STRENGTHS AND LIMITATIONS

Cone-beam imaging has numerous features that make it suitable for many dental applications, but it also has a number of limitations.

STRENGTHS

Size and Cost
CBCT equipment has a greatly reduced size and physical footprint compared with conventional CT equipment, and it is approximately one fourth to one fifth the cost. Both of these features make it available for the dental office.

Fast Acquisition
With more recent advances in solid-state detector achievable frame rates, computer processing speed, and units incorporating reduced trajectory arcs, most CBCT scanning is performed in less than 30 seconds.

Submillimeter Resolution
All CBCT units currently use megapixel solid-state devices for x-ray detection, which provide submillimeter voxel resolution in all orthogonal planes. Some CBCT units are capable of high-resolution imaging (nominal 0.076- to 0.125-mm voxel resolution) and may be required for tasks requiring discernment of fine detail structures and disease processes, such as the periodontal space, root canal morphology, and root resorption or fracture.

Relatively Low Patient Radiation Dose
Published reports indicate that the effective dose (ICRP 2007) for various CBCT devices ranges from 25 to 1025 μSv depending on the type and model of CBCT equipment and imaging protocol used. These values are approximately equivalent to 1 to 42 digital panoramic radiographs (approximately 24 μSv) or 3 to 123 days' equivalent per capita natural background radiation (approximately 3000 μSv in the United States). Patient radiation dose can be reduced by collimating the beam, elevating the chin, and using protective eyewear and thyroid and cervical spine shielding. CBCT imaging provides a range of potentially substantial dose reductions compared with conventional head MDCT imaging (range, 430 to 1160 μSv).

Interactive Analysis
CBCT data reconstruction and viewing is performed natively by use of a personal computer. In addition, some manufacturers provide software with extended functionality for specific applications, such as implant placement or orthodontic analysis (see Chapter 12). Finally, the availability of cursor-driven measurement algorithms provides the practitioner with an interactive capability for real-time dimensional assessment, annotation, and measurements.

LIMITATIONS

CBCT images have limitations compared with conventional CT images.

Image Noise
The cone-beam projection acquisition geometry results in a large volume being irradiated with every basis image projection. A large portion of the photons undergo Compton scattering interactions and produce scattered radiation. Most scattered radiation is produced omnidirectionally and recorded by pixels on the cone-beam area detector. The number of photons detected at each pixel does not reflect the actual attenuation of an object along a specific path of the x-ray beam. This additional recorded x-ray detection is called noise and contributes to image degradation. The amount of scattered radiation is generally proportional to the total mass of tissue contained within the primary x-ray beam; this increases with increasing object thickness and field size. The contribution of this scattered radiation to production of the CBCT image may be greater than the primary beam. In clinical applications, the scatter-to-primary ratios are about 0.01 for single-ray CT imaging and 0.05 to 0.15 for fan-beam and spiral CT imaging and may be 0.4 to 2 in CBCT imaging. For these reasons, it is always desirable to use the smallest FOV possible when making a CBCT image.

Additional sources of image noise in CBCT are statistical variations in the homogeneity of the incident x-ray beam (quantum mottle) and added noise of the detector system (electronic). The inhomogeneity of x-ray photons depends on the number of the primary and scattered x rays absorbed, the primary and scattered x-ray spectra incident on the detector, and the number of basis projections. Electronic noise is due to the inherent degradations of the detector system related to the x-ray absorption efficiency of energy at the detector.

In addition, because of the increased divergence of the x-ray beam over the area detector, there is a pronounced heel effect. This effect produces a large variation or nonuniformity of the incident x-ray beam on the patient and resultant nonuniformity in absorption with greater signal-to-noise ratio (noise) on the cathode side of the image relative to the anode side.

Poor Soft Tissue Contrast

Contrast resolution is the ability of an image to reveal subtle differences in image density. Variations in image intensity are a result of differential attenuation of x rays by tissues that differ in density, atomic number, or thickness. Two principal factors limit the contrast resolution of CBCT. First, although scattered radiation contributes to increased noise of the image, it is also a significant factor in reducing the contrast of the cone-beam system. Scattered x-ray photons reduce subject contrast by adding background signals that are not representative of the anatomy, reducing image quality. CBCT units have noticeably less soft tissue contrast than MDCT units.

Second, there are numerous inherent FPD-based artifacts that affect linearity or response to x radiation. Saturation (nonlinear pixel effects above a certain exposure), dark current (charge that accumulates over time with or without exposure), and bad pixels (pixels that do not react to exposure) contribute to nonlinearity. In addition, the sensitivity of different regions of the panel to radiation (pixel-to-pixel gain variation) may not be uniform over the entire region.

CONCLUSIONS

CBCT imaging is an effective volumetric diagnostic imaging technology that produces accurate, submillimeter resolution images of diagnostic quality in formats enabling volumetric visualization of the osseous structures of the maxillofacial region at lower doses and costs compared with MDCT imaging. Although technically easy to perform, CBCT imaging should be considered an adjunctive diagnostic modality to the history and clinical examination. Imaging should be "task specific" with exposure and scan factor protocols adjusted and image formatting options tailored to optimize image display and minimize patient radiation dose.

BIBLIOGRAPHY

Principles of Cone-Beam Computed Tomographic Imaging

Angelopoulos C, Scarfe WC, Farman AG: A comparison of maxillofacial CBCT and medical CT, *Atlas Oral Maxillofac Surg Clin North Am* 20:1–17, 2012.

Scarfe WC, Farman AG: What is cone-beam CT and how does it work? *Dent Clin North Am* 52:707–730, 2008.

Scarfe WC, Li Z, Aboelmaaty W, et al: Maxillofacial cone beam computed tomography: essence, elements and steps to interpretation, *Aust Dent J* 57(Suppl 1):46–60, 2012.

Radiation Dose

Carrafiello G, Dizonno M, Colli V, et al: Comparative study of jaws with multislice computed tomography and cone-beam computed tomography, *Radiol Med* 115:600–611, 2010.

Loubele M, Bogaerts R, Van Dijck E, et al: Comparison between effective radiation dose of CBCT and MSCT scanners for dentomaxillofacial applications, *Eur J Radiol* 71:461–468, 2009.

Ludlow JB, Ivanovic M: Comparative dosimetry of dental CBCT devices and 64-slice CT for oral and maxillofacial radiology, *Oral Surg Oral Med Oral Pathol Oral Radiol Endod* 106:106–111, 2008.

Okano T, Harata Y, Sugihara Y, et al: Absorbed and effective doses from cone beam volumetric imaging for implant planning, *Dentomaxillofac Radiol* 38:79–85, 2009.

Pauwels R, Beinsberger J, Collaert B, et al; SEDENTEXCT Project Consortium: effective dose range for dental cone beam computed tomography scanners, *Eur J Radiol* 81:267–271, 2012.

Theodorakou C, Walker A, Horner K, et al; SEDENTEXCT Project Consortium: estimation of paediatric organ and effective doses from dental cone beam CT using anthropomorphic phantoms, *Br J Radiol* 85:153–160, 2012.

The 2007 recommendations of the International Commission on Radiological Protection. IRCP Publication 103, *Ann ICRP* 37:1–332, 2007.

Image Reconstruction

Endo M, Tsunoo T, Nakamori N, et al: Effect of scattered radiation on image noise in cone beam CT, *Med Phys* 28:469–474, 2001.

Feldkamp LA, Davis LC, Kress JW: Practical cone-beam algorithm, *J Opt Soc Am* 1:612–619, 1984.

Siewerdsen JH, Jaffray DA: Cone-beam computed tomography with a flat-panel imager: magnitude and effects of x-ray scatter, *Med Phys* 28:220–231, 2001.

Patient Selection Criteria

American Association of Endodontists; American Academy of Oral and Maxillofacial Radiology: Use of cone-beam-computed tomography in endodontics. Joint Position Statement of the American Association of Endodontists; American Academy of Oral and Maxillofacial Radiography, *Oral Surg Oral Med Oral Pathol Oral Radiol* 111:234–237, 2011.

Carter L, Farman AG, Geist J, et al; American Academy of Oral and Maxillofacial Radiology: American Academy of Oral and Maxillofacial Radiology executive opinion statement on performing and interpreting diagnostic cone beam computed tomography, *Oral Surg Oral Med Oral Pathol Oral Radiol Endod* 106:561–562, 2008.

The American Dental Association Council on Scientific Affairs: The use of cone-beam computed tomography in dentistry: an advisory statement from the American Dental Association Council on Scientific Affairs, *J Am Dent Assoc* 143:899–902, 2012.

Tyndall DA, Price JB, Tetradis S, et al: Position statement of the American Academy of Oral and Maxillofacial Radiology on selection criteria for the use of radiology in dental implantology with emphasis on cone beam computed tomography, *Oral Surg Oral Med Oral Pathol Oral Radiol* 113:817–826, 2012.

Image Artifacts

Benic GI, Sancho-Puchades M, Jung RE, et al: In vitro assessment of artifacts induced by titanium dental implants in cone beam computed tomography, *Clin Oral Implants Res* 24:378–383, 2013.

Esmaeili F, Johari M, Haddadi P, et al: Beam hardening artifacts: comparison between two cone-beam computed tomography scanners, *J Dent Res Dent Clin Dent Prospects* 6:49–53, 2012.

Schulze R, Heil U, Gross D, et al: Artefacts in CBCT: a review, *Dentomaxillofac Radiol* 40:265–273, 2011.

Cone-Beam Computed Tomography: Volume Preparation

William C. Scarfe and Allan G. Farman

OUTLINE

As cone-beam computed tomographic (CBCT) imaging is inherently a digital volumetric image-capture technology, image visualization should also be by digital display. This demands that clinicians move from static hard copy (printed) images to software-assisted volumetric review. Image display should be dynamic and formatted according to task-specific display protocols. Expanding the use of volumetric data for treatment planning and image guidance of operative and surgical procedures is facilitated by the use of appropriate application of software.

Chapter 11 detailed technical aspects of CBCT image production—creating and caring for volumetric CBCT data. This chapter focuses on the interaction and use of the subsequent volumetric data, including image display, image interpretation, and task-specific applications.

STAGES IN VOLUMETRIC DATA DISPLAY

The default presentation of the CBCT volumetric data set by most software programs is usually as secondary two-dimensional contiguous reconstructed images in three orthogonal planes (axial, sagittal, and coronal) at a defaulted thickness (Fig. 12-1). Each panel of the display software presents one of a series of contiguous images in that plane. Each image is interrelational such that the location of each image in the sequence can be identified in the other two planes. CBCT data should be considered as a volume to be explored from which selected images are extracted. Technically, four stages provide an efficient and consistent systematic methodologic approach to optimize CBCT image display before image interpretation:

1. Reorient the data
2. Optimize the data
3. View the data
4. Format the data

REORIENT DATA

One of the advantages of CBCT acquisition is that the resultant volumetric data set can be reoriented in all three planes using PC-based software. Initial adjustment of the volumetric data set should include reorientation such that the patient's anatomic features are realigned symmetrically or according to a reference plane (Fig. 12-2). This stage is particularly important for aligning subsequent cross-sectional, transaxial images perpendicular to the structure of interest, such as to visualize single tooth pathology, to measure the maximal height and width of the residual alveolar ridge in an edentulous segment for implant site assessment (Fig. 12-3), to compare temporomandibular joint (TMJ) condylar morphology, or to perform a craniofacial analysis.

OPTIMIZE DATA

Great variability can exist in the overall density and contrast of orthogonal images between CBCT units and within the same unit depending on patient images and scan parameters selected. Therefore, to optimize image presentation and facilitate diagnosis, it is often necessary to adjust contrast (window) and brightness (level) parameters to favor bony structures. Although CBCT proprietary software may provide for window and level presets, it is advisable that these parameters be optimized for each scan. After these parameters are set, further enhancements can be performed by the application of sharpening, filtering, and edge algorithms. The use of these functions must be weighed against the visual effects of increased noise in the image (Fig. 12-4). After these adjustments, secondary algorithms (e.g., annotation, measurement, magnification) can be applied with confidence.

VIEW DATA

Because there are numerous component orthogonal images in each plane, it is impractical to display all slices on one display format. Therefore, it is necessary to review each series dynamically by scrolling through the consecutive orthogonal image "stack." This is referred to as a "cine" or "paging" mode. It is recommended that scrolling be performed craniocaudally (i.e., from head to toe) and then in reverse, slowing down in areas of greater complexity (e.g., TMJ articulations and skull base). This scrolling process should be performed at least in the coronal and axial planes. Viewing orthogonal projections at this stage is recommended as an overall survey for disease and to establish the presence of any asymmetry.

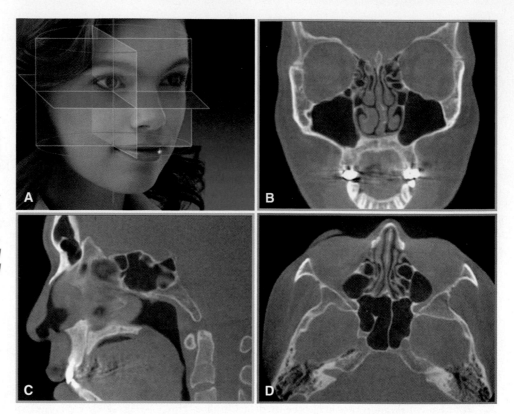

FIGURE 12-1 Standard display modes of CBCT volumetric data. **A,** Cylindrical three-dimensional volumetric data set superimposed on the head showing the three orthogonal planes in relation to the reconstructed volumetric data set: coronal (teal), sagittal (green), and axial (pink). **B-D,** Corresponding representative coronal (teal) **(B),** sagittal (green) **(C),** and axial (pink) **(D)** images. Each orthogonal plane has multiple contiguous thin slice sections, which are interrelational. *(Image of head and superimposed volumetric data set and orthogonal orientation courtesy of J. Morita Mfg Corp, Kyoto, Japan.)*

FORMAT DATA

CBCT software provides many formatting options, each directed toward visualizing specific components of the volumetric data set. Protocols incorporating field of view (FOV) scan exposure parameters and display modes should be applied selectively to highlight anatomic features or functional characteristics within a specific diagnostic task. Overall, selection should be based on applying thin sections to show detail and thicker sections to demonstrate relationships. There are three basic format options (Fig. 12-5):
- Multiplanar reformation
- Ray sum
- Volumetric rendering

Multiplanar Reformation

Because of the isotropic nature of acquisition, the volumetric data set can be sectioned nonorthogonally to provide nonaxial two-dimensional planar images referred to as multiplanar reformation (MPR). MPR modes include linear oblique, curved planar, and serial transaxial reformations. Several anatomic structures are not particularly well visualized and represented as displayed in orthogonal planes, and oblique reformatting can be useful in these instances (Fig. 12-6). Oblique images are most often used to transect the mandibular condyle. Curved planar images are generated by manually drawing a planning line or spline by selecting multiple nodes along the centerline corresponding to the jaw arch on an appropriate axial image; this creates a "simulated" or reconstructed dental panoramic image. Because clinicians are familiar with them and they are distortion-free, panoramic MPR reconstructions are useful for jaw evaluation. Such reconstructions must be thick enough to include the entire mandible to avoid missing disease. Serial transaxial images provide sequential images perpendicular to an arbitrary linear oblique or curved planar MPR. They are most commonly called cross-sectional images. The slice width (slice thickness) of the image and the distance between adjacent cross-sectional images (interslice interval) can often be defined. Cross-sectional images are optimal for examining teeth and alveolar bone.

Ray Sum

The slice thickness of orthogonal or MPR images can be "thickened" by increasing the number of adjacent voxels included in the display (Fig. 12-7). This creates an image slab that represents a specific volume of the patient, referred to as a ray sum. The thickness of the slab is usually variable and determined by the thickness of the structure to be imaged. Full-thickness perpendicular ray sum images can be used to generate simulated projections, such as lateral cephalometric images (Fig. 12-8). In contrast to conventional radiographs, these ray sum images are without magnification and parallax distortion. However, this technique uses the entire volumetric data set, and interpretation is negatively affected by "anatomic noise"–the superimposition of multiple structures–also inherent in conventional projection radiography.

Volume Rendering

Volume rendering allows visualization of volumetric data by selective display of voxels within a data set. Two specific techniques are commonly used: indirect volume rendering and direct volume rendering.

Indirect volume rendering is a complex process requiring selection of the intensity or density of the grayscale level of the voxels to be displayed within an entire data set (called "segmentation"). This process is technically demanding and computationally difficult, requiring specific software; however, it provides a volumetric surface reconstruction with depth (Fig. 12-9). Two types of views are possible: views that are solid (surface rendering) and views that are transparent (volumetric rendering). This volumetric

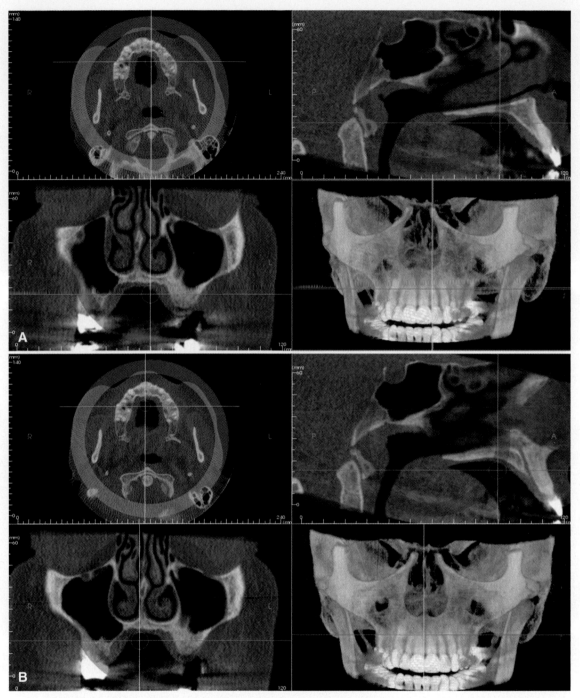

FIGURE 12-2 CBCT volumetric data reorientation. Axial, sagittal, and coronal orthogonal sectional images and three-dimensional volumetric rendering before **(A)** and after **(B)** reorientation of the CBCT data set. The circular rotational tool superimposed on the respective images is selected with the cursor and adjusted to align images according to specific reference lines. In this case, axial and sagittal orthogonal images were realigned such that the maxillary jaw was symmetrically aligned, and the palatal plane was parallel to the floor. (Screen view of case made with InVivoDental software, Anatomage, San Jose, CA.)

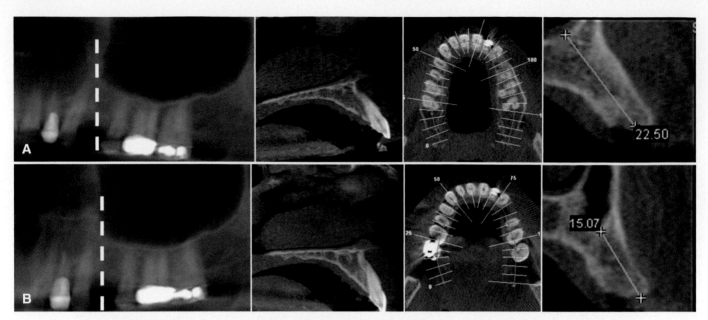

FIGURE 12-3 Reorientation of sagittal plane to internal reference (occlusal plane). *(From left to right)* Reformatted panoramic, midsagittal, axial, and cross-sectional images of the same data set at original orientation **(A)** and after down tilt of the volumetric data set in the sagittal plane such that the residual alveolar ridge is parallel to the occlusal plane **(B)**. The lower set of images reveals the appropriate relationship of the maxillary sinus to the alveolar ridge and a substantial difference in measured height of the alveolar bone.

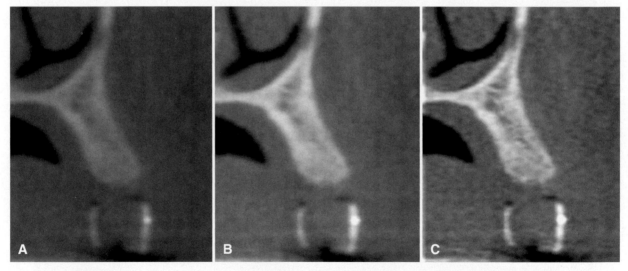

FIGURE 12-4 Effect of image enhancement on CBCT images. The visual effect of three sequential adjustments on corrected MPR cross-sectional images. **A,** Default image after interpolation algorithm — smoothens edges of cortical bone but adds blur to high-contrast structures. **B,** Adjustment of window level and width to bone preset (W/L: 3000/500). **C,** Addition of mild sharpen algorithm. *(Images created with i-CAT, ISI, Hatfield, PA, created with XoranCat software, Xoran Technologies, Inc, Ann Arbor, MI.)*

procedure is optimal for visualization and analysis of craniofacial conditions and determination of relationships of various anatomic features, such as the inferior alveolar canal to the mandibular third molar.

Direct volume rendering is a much simpler process that involves selecting an arbitrary threshold of voxel intensities, below or above which all gray values are eliminated. Numerous techniques are available; however, the most commonly used is maximum intensity projection (MIP). MIP visualizations are achieved by evaluating each voxel value along an imaginary projection ray from the observer's eyes within a particular volume of interest and representing only the highest value as the display value. Voxel intensities that are below an arbitrary threshold are eliminated (Fig. 12-10). MIP images have great utility for demonstration of the location of impacted teeth, for TMJ evaluation, for identification of fractures, for craniofacial analysis, for surgical follow-up, for assessment of cervical spine anomalies, and for demonstration of soft tissue dystrophic calcifications.

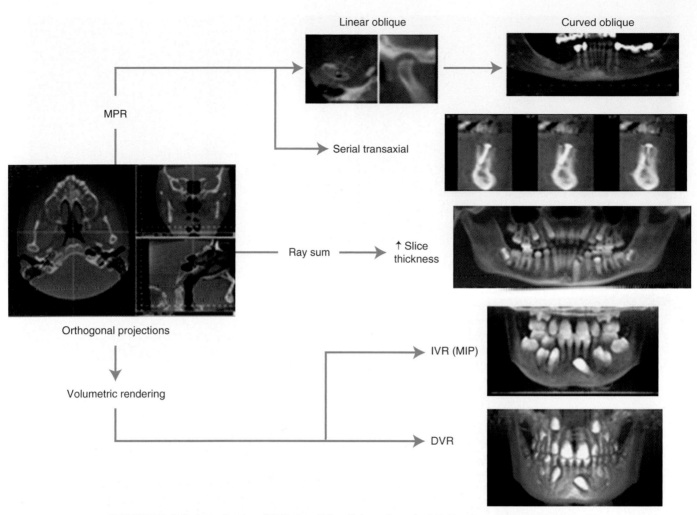

FIGURE 12-5 Display mode options of CBCT volumetric data. Display modes can be divided into three categories: MPR consisting of linear, curved oblique and serial transaxial images; ray sum comprising images of increased section thickness; and volumetric images consisting of indirect volume rendering *(IVR)*, the most common of which being MIP and direct volume rendering *(DVR)*.

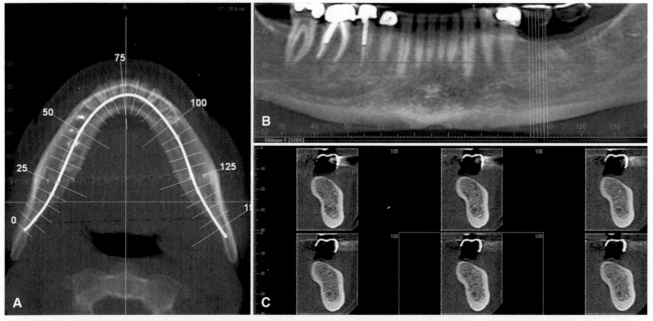

FIGURE 12-6 MPR. A thick axial image **(A)** simulating an occlusal image with an MPR oblique curved line *(white solid line)* and resultant "panoramic" image **(B)** and serial cross-sectional, 1-mm-thick images **(C)** of a potential implant site in the lower left mandible. The axial and panoramic images are used as reference images to show the location of the cross-sectional images. The cross-sectional images demonstrate the amount of lingual undercut and location of the inferior alveolar canal.

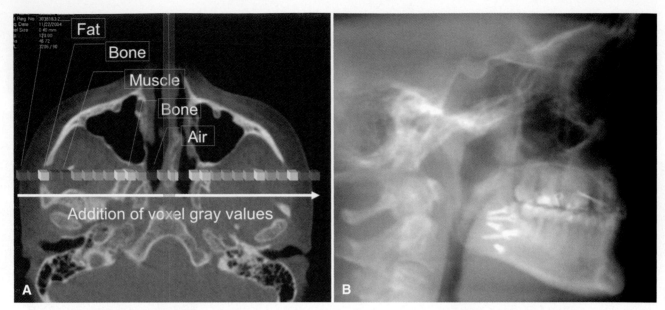

FIGURE 12-7 Ray sum images. **A,** An axial projection is used as the reference image. A section slice is identified that in this case corresponds to the midsagittal plane, and the thickness of this slice is increased to include both left and right sides of the volumetric data set. As the thickness of the "slab" increases, adjacent voxels representing elements such as air, bone, and soft tissues are added. **B,** The resultant image generated from a full-thickness ray sum provides a simulated lateral cephalometric image.

FIGURE 12-8 Two-dimensional projections generated with cone-beam data set. This patient had an asymmetry of one side of the face. Ray sum reformation of the CBCT data was performed to provide multiple conventional images, such as the lateral cephalometric **(A)**, frontal cephalometric or postero-anterior **(B)**, and panoramic **(C)** projections. *(Images generated with Dolphin 3D Imaging Software, Chatsworth, CA.)*

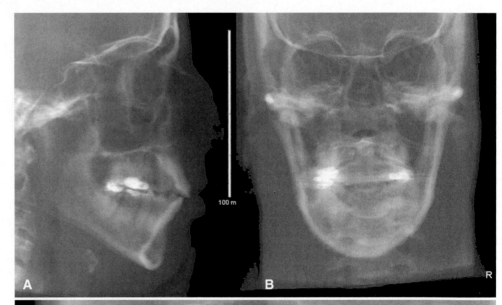

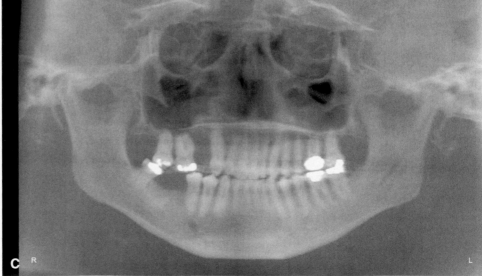

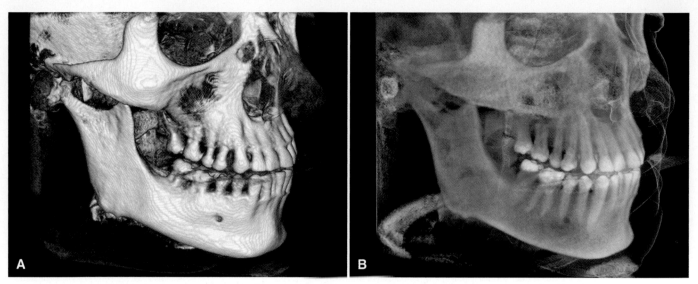

FIGURE 12-9 Three-dimensional volumetric surface rendering. Manual segmentation is often accomplished by an adjustable scale determining the upper and lower limit and range of intensity values to include in the segmentation. The visual result of changes in this scale is displayed in "real time" so that the effects of incremental changes can be visualized. The segmentation may be optimized to reveal the objects of interest, including bone as a solid surface or shaded surface display **(A)** and bone and the dentition under the bone as a transparency **(B)** using volumetric imaging. *(Segmentation performed with InVivoDental software, Anatomage, San Jose, CA.)*

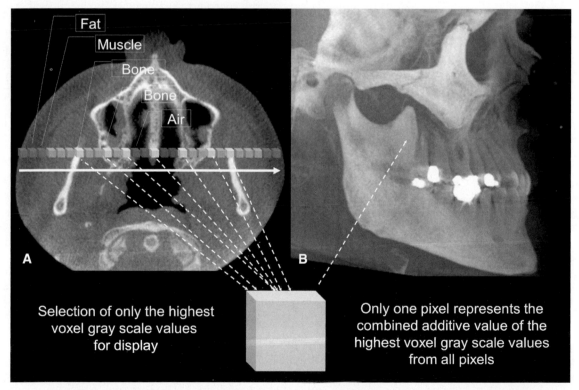

FIGURE 12-10 MIP. This method produces a "pseudo"–three-dimensional image by evaluating each voxel value along an imaginary projection ray from the observer's eyes within the data set and then representing only the highest value as the display value. In this example, an axial projection **(A)** is used as the reference image. A projection ray is identified throughout the entire volumetric data set along which individual voxels are identified, each with varying grayscale intensity corresponding to various tissue densities, such as fat, muscle, air, and bone. The MIP algorithm selects only the values along the projection ray that have the highest values (usually corresponding to bone or metal) and represents this as only one pixel on the resultant image **(B)**.

TABLE 12-1 Essential Elements of a Cone-Beam Computed Tomographic Radiologic Report

Outline	Details
Patient information	Patient name, unique identifier code, date of birth, referring practitioner's name, rationale for procedure
Scan information	Succession number, date of procedure, date report was generated, location of facility, equipment used, scan parameters, and images provided Problems encountered during procedure (e.g., patient motion)
Radiologic findings	General findings should include reference to gnathic (dental status including specific missing teeth, restorative status, root canal, filled teeth, periapical lesions, general marginal alveolar bone status, and status of edentulous regions) and extragnathic (TMJ, paranasal sinuses, nasopharyngeal airway, soft tissue of the neck, intracranial calcifications) structures Specific findings should provide observations addressing rationale for procedure Significant incidental findings should be identified
Radiologic impression	Definitive or differential diagnosis, related to rationale for imaging examination or clinically significant incidental findings Correlation to patient presentation addressing pertinent clinical issues Comparison with previous imaging studies, if available Recommendations for follow-up or additional diagnostic or clinical studies, as appropriate, to clarify, confirm, or exclude diagnosis

INTERPRETIVE REPORT

Cone-beam imaging comprises the technical component of patient exposure. It is the professional duty of a practitioner who operates a CBCT unit or who requests a CBCT study to provide a written interpretive report describing the imaging findings based on examination of the entire image data set. Documentation of the CBCT procedure by the inclusion of an interpretive report is an essential element of CBCT imaging and should form part of a patient's record. Patient diagnosis may often be complex, and management may involve numerous practitioners. An interpretation report serves as the optimal method of communication of interpretation findings for CBCT. Often this report includes selected images that best document significant findings.

It is imperative that all image data be systematically reviewed for disease. Competency in interpretation of both anatomic and pathologic findings on CBCT images varies depending principally on practitioner experience and the FOV of the scan. Qualified specialist oral and maxillofacial radiologists may be able to assist diagnostically when practitioners are unwilling to accept the responsibility to review the whole exposed tissue volume. The essential elements of a CBCT radiologic report are outlined in Table 12-1.

TASK-SPECIFIC APPLICATIONS

CBCT technology has been applied to diagnosis in all areas of dentistry. CBCT imaging is not a replacement for panoramic or conventional projection radiographic applications but rather is best used as a complementary modality for specific applications.

DIAGNOSIS AND PREOPERATIVE ASSESSMENT

Implant Site Assessment

Perhaps the greatest impact of CBCT has been on the planning of dental implant placements. CBCT provides cross-sectional images of the alveolar bone height, width, and angulation and accurately depicts vital structures, such as the inferior alveolar dental nerve canal in the mandible or the sinus in the maxilla. The most useful series of images for implant site assessment include the axial, reformatted panoramic, and cross-sectional images at the specific location (Fig. 12-11). In many instances, a diagnostic stent is made with radiographic markers and inserted at the time of the scan (Fig. 12-12). This stent provides a precise reference of the location of the proposed implants or teeth.

Endodontics

The use of CBCT imaging in endodontics should be limited to the assessment and treatment of complex endodontic conditions (Fig. 12-13), such as the following:

- Identification of potential accessory canals in teeth with suspected complex morphology
- Identification of root canal system anomalies and determination of root curvature
- Diagnosis of dental periapical pathosis in patients who present with contradictory or nonspecific clinical signs and symptoms or conventional radiographic findings
- Diagnosis of pathosis of nonendodontic origin
- Intraoperative or postoperative assessment of endodontic treatment complications
- Diagnosis and management of dentoalveolar trauma
- Localization and differentiation of external from internal root resorption or invasive cervical resorption
- Presurgical case planning to determine the exact location of root apex or apices and to evaluate the proximity of adjacent anatomic structures

Orthodontics and Three-Dimensional Cephalometry

CBCT imaging is being used in the diagnosis, assessment, and analysis of maxillofacial orthodontic and orthopedic anomalies. The diagnostic advantages of CBCT imaging have been most commonly reported in the identification of dental structural anomalies, such as root resorption and display of the position of impacted and supernumerary teeth and their relationships to adjacent roots or other anatomic structures. CBCT imaging facilitates surgical exposure and planning of subsequent movement. Other applications include the assessment of palatal morphologic features and dimensions, tooth inclination and torque, characterization of alveolar bone for orthodontic mini-implant placement, and determining available alveolar bone width for buccolingual movement of teeth. CBCT imaging also provides adequate visualization of the TMJ, pharyngeal airway space, and soft tissue relationships.

CBCT imaging provides two unique contributions to orthodontic practice. The first is that numerous linear images currently used in orthodontic diagnosis, cephalometric analysis, and treatment planning can be created from a single CBCT scan (see Table 9-1). This capability provides for greater clinical efficacy. The second and more important contribution is that CBCT data can be reconstructed to provide unique, previously unavailable images. Specific software provides three-dimensional visualization and

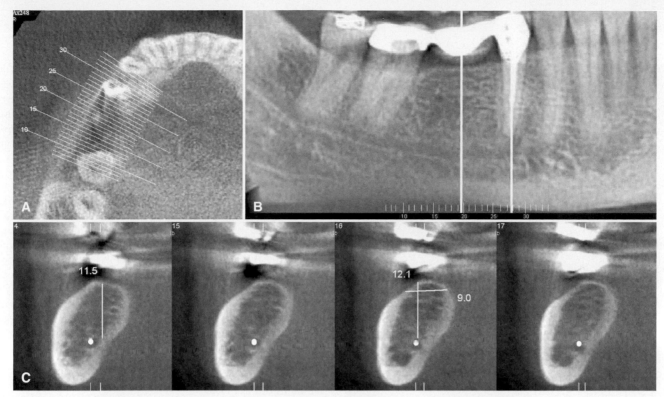

FIGURE 12-11 CBCT imaging for implant site assessment. A curved planar MPR is accomplished by aligning the long axis of the imaging plane with the dental arch **(A)**, providing a regional panorama-like thin slice image **(B)**. In addition, serial thin-slice transplanar images are often generated **(C)**, which are useful in the assessment of specific morphologic features, such as the location of the inferior alveolar canal (shown with a *white dot*) for implant site assessment and for allowing measurement of the available alveolar bone height and width *(solid line)*. *(Images created with Newtom 3G, AFP Imaging Corp, Elmsford, NY.)*

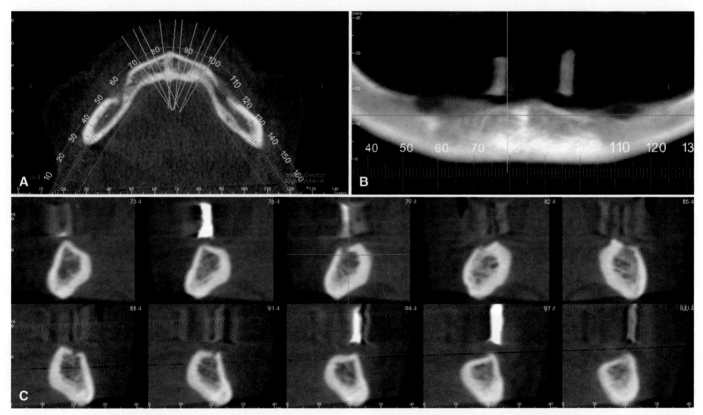

FIGURE 12-12 Use of a diagnostic stent. Stents provide fiducial radiographic landmarks that can be used to correlate proposed clinical location and angulation of implants with the available alveolar bone. The axial **(A)** and panoramic **(B)** projections provide an overview of location, whereas serial cross-sectional images **(C)** indicate alveolar bone height. In this example of an edentulous mandible with a stent with two radiographic markers at proposed sites, the 10 1-mm-thick transplanar images at 3-mm intervals of the mandibular anterior region indicate that although the right trajectory is optimal (upper left cross-sectional image), the proposed placement trajectory of the right implant (lower left) is too far buccal to engage the available bone. *(Images generated on InVivoDental software, Anatomage, San Jose, CA.)*

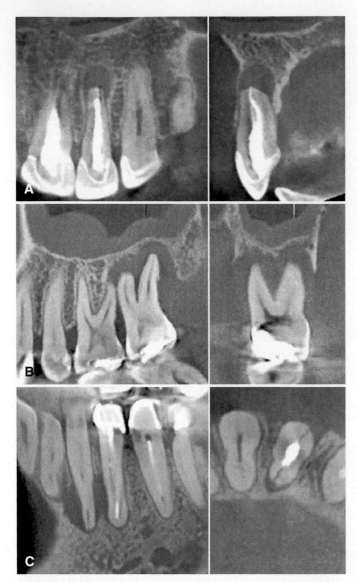

FIGURE 12-13 CBCT imaging for endodontics. Numerous endodontically related conditions can be demonstrated in high resolution with restricted FOV CBCT imaging, including periapical conditions **(A);** periodontal, periapical, and sinus disease **(B);** and root fracture and associated alveolar bone loss **(C)**. Images taken created with a 3DX Accuitomo, J. Morita Mfg Corp, Kyoto, Japan.)

analysis of the maxillofacial skeleton and soft tissue boundaries, such as the airway and facial outline. The numerous potential benefits to three-dimensional cephalometry include demonstrating and characterizing asymmetry and anteroposterior, vertical, and transverse dentoskeletal discrepancies, incorporating the soft tissue integument, and the potential for assessment of growth and development.

Mandibular Third Molar Position

The relationship of the inferior alveolar canal (IAC) to the roots of mandibular third molar teeth is important when considering extractions and attempting to minimize the likelihood of nerve damage that may lead to permanent loss of sensation to one side to the lower lip. Accurate assessment of the position of the IAC in relation to the impacted third molar may reduce injuries to this nerve. Traditional panoramic imaging may be adequate when the third molar is clear of the canal, but in the case of radiographic superimposition it is advisable to use a three-dimensional imaging approach. Volumetric rendering with IAC annotation or "tracing" in combination with cross-sectional imaging provides useful visualization of the relationships of anatomic structures in these circumstances (Fig. 12-14).

Temporomandibular Joint

CBCT imaging provides multiplanar and potentially three-dimensional images of the condyle and surrounding structures to facilitate analysis and diagnosis of bone morphologic features and joint space and function, which are critical keys to providing appropriate treatment outcomes in patients with TMJ signs and symptoms. Imaging can depict the features of degenerative joint disease (Fig. 12-15) and developmental anomalies of the condyle, ankylosis, and rheumatoid arthritis. Appropriate imaging protocols should include reformatted panoramic and axial reference images; corrected parasagittal and paracoronal cross-sectional slices; and for cases in which asymmetry is suspected or surgery is contemplated, volumetric reconstructions.

Maxillofacial Pathoses

CBCT imaging can assist in the assessment of many conditions of the jaws, most notably dental conditions such as impacted canines and supernumerary teeth, fractured or split teeth, periapical lesions, and periodontal disease. Benign calcifications (e.g., tonsilloliths, lymph nodes, salivary gland stones) can also be identified by location and differentiated from potentially significant calcifications, such as may occur in carotid artery atheroma. Although CBCT imaging does not provide suitable soft tissue contrast to distinguish the contents of paranasal soft tissue attenuations, the morphologic characteristics and extent of these lesions are particularly well seen (e.g., mucous extravasation cyst). CBCT imaging has been found to be particularly useful for assessment of trauma (Fig. 12-16) and for visualizing the extent and degree of involvement of benign odontogenic (Fig. 12-17) or nonodontogenic conditions as well as osteomyelitis.

TREATMENT PLANNING AND VIRTUAL SIMULATIONS

The key feature of CBCT image output that makes systems interoperable is the use of image files that are conformant with the Digital Imaging and Communications in Medicine (DICOM) standard file format.

Treatment planning for a potential implant site involves an interplay of considerations of both surgical and prosthetic requirements. Implant planning software allows greater sophistication in analysis and planning, providing interactive methods of translating prosthetic planning to the surgical site (Fig. 12-18). In implant planning, software can be used to select and direct the placement of implant fixtures either directly by the use of image-guided navigation or indirectly via the construction of restrictive surgical guides.

Image fusion is the process of integration of two imaging data sets. Most commonly, CBCT volumes are fused with extraoral facial (photographic) (Fig. 12-19) or intraoral (impression) optical data. After registration, numerous options allow interaction with the data sets either independently or in toto. Composite data sets provide holistic assessment of the interaction of hard tissue base with the soft tissue integument; monitoring and evaluation of changes over time; and, in combination with simulation software, predictive modeling.

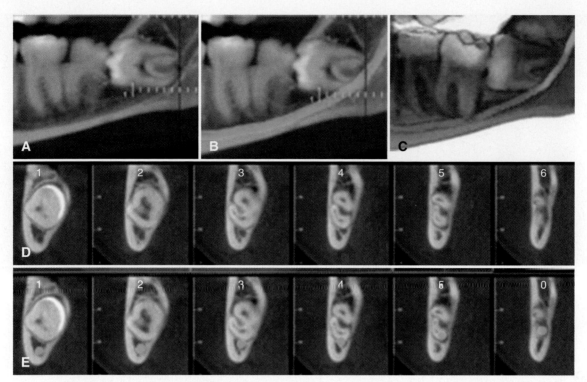

FIGURE 12-14 Cone-beam imaging for third molar assessment. Third-party software used to demonstrate the location of the IAC (green). Nonannotated **(A)** annotated **(B)** panoramic MPR reformatted, volumetric transparency reconstruction **(C)** images with corresponding nonannotated **(D)** and annotated **(E)** cross-sectional images at 1-mm intervals. Cross-sectional slices with the IAC traced (green). **All** images demonstrate the close proximity and course of the IAC in relation to the root of the left mandibular, horizontally bony impacted and unerupted third molar. *(Images created with Dolphin 3D Imaging Software, Chatsworth, CA.)*

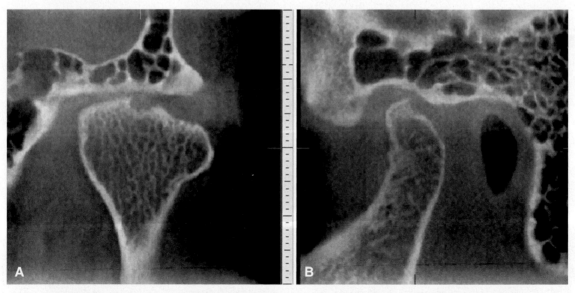

FIGURE 12-15 CBCT imaging of the TMJ. Corrected coronal **(A)** and sagittal **(B)** images of a right TMJ with erosive defects on the superior surface of the condyle associated with mild degenerative joint disease. *(Images created with 3DX Accuitomo, J. Morita Mfg Corp, Kyoto, Japan.)*

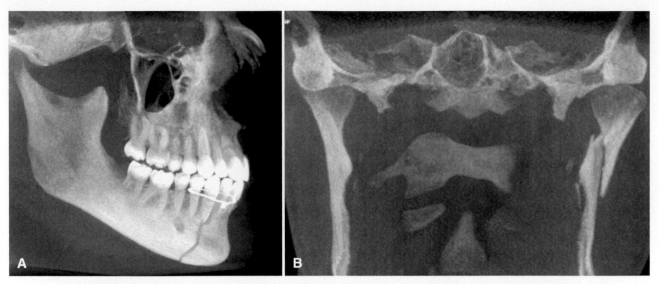

FIGURE 12-16 CBCT imaging of mandibular fractures. Use of MIP in the assessment of complex mandibular fractures. **A,** Oblique thin slab MPR image with MIP application demonstrates a simple, slightly displaced fracture of the right parasymphyseal region. **B,** Coronal thin slab MIP image demonstrates a comminuted displaced left subcondylar neck fracture. *(Images created with i-CAT, ISI, Hatfield, PA, created using XoranCat software, Xoran Technologies, Inc, Ann Arbor, MI.)*

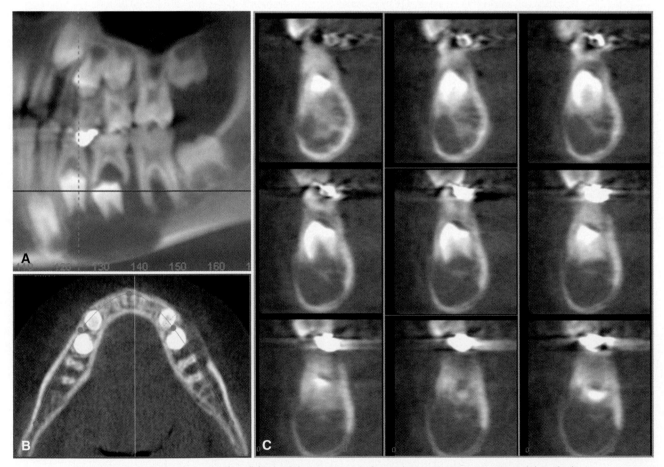

FIGURE 12-17 CBCT imaging of maxillofacial pathology. **A,** Cropped reformatted ray sum panoramic view. **B,** Axial slice at level of red horizontal line on panoramic view and outline for midportion of cross-sectional images. **C,** Nine serial 1-mm-thick cross-sectional slices (of unilocular well-defined hypodensity) in the left premolar mandibular body of a patient in the mixed dentition phase.

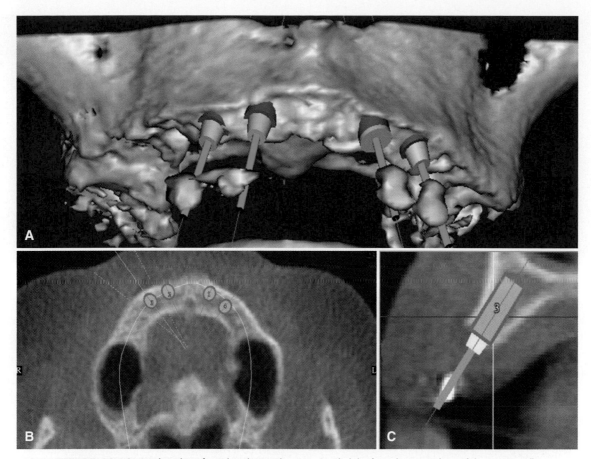

FIGURE 12-18 Virtual simulation for implant planning placement. **A,** Shaded-surface volumetric rendering of the anterior totally edentulous maxilla shows the alignment of the four virtual implant fixtures in relation to the radiographic markers providing the planned incisal edges of the lateral incisor and canine teeth bilaterally. **B,** Anterior-posterior spread of the position of the implants can be determined on the axial image. **C,** Cross-sectional image of the right maxillary canine shows the buccopalatal emergence profile (green line) and position (implant in light pink). Software also allows the use of overlay prosthetic tools, such as (1) surgical confidence marker (dark pink outline around each implant used to identify 0.5-mm surgical tolerance limits); (2) tapering drill confidence limit, shown on the apical portion of the implant (tapering dark pink outline); (3) 2-mm soft tissue collar (yellow); and (4) desirable prosthetic space, given by the length of the emergence profile line. *(Images created with Virtual Implant Placement (VIP), Biohorizons IPH, Inc, Birmingham, AL.)*

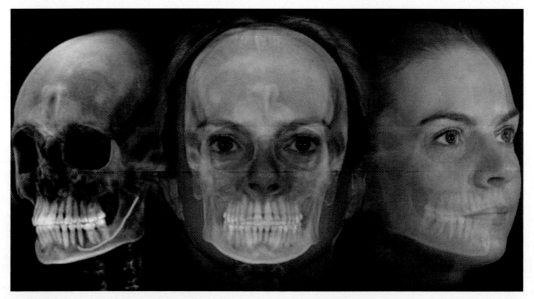

FIGURE 12-19 Fusion image. Three-dimensional anatomic views demonstrate imaging possibilities with fusion of CBCT data and photographic image sets. *(Images created with 3DMD, Atlanta, GA; courtesy Dr. Chester Wang.)*

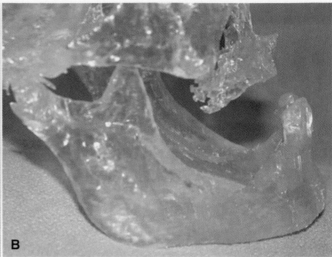

FIGURE 12-20 Rapid prototype. **A,** Three-dimensional volumetric reconstruction from CBCT data. **B,** Rapid prototype constructed model of patient with right-sided bisphosphonate-related osteonecrosis of the jaws. Modeling was performed to provide a physical model on which surgical plates were premolded before surgical resection and reconstruction.

IMAGE-GUIDED SURGERY AND RAPID PROTOTYPING

Imaged-guided surgery refers to techniques that translate software-derived virtual surgical plans developed from virtual simulations to the surgical environment. Two concepts for image-guided surgery have been developed. The first concept involves the fabrication of a plastic drilling and surgical template based on a virtual treatment plan. Numerous systems are available; some systems are for oral and maxillofacial surgery; however, most are for dental implant placement (Fig. 12-20). The surgical templates can be a modification of a laboratory imaging stent or created directly from image data using rapid prototyping techniques. The second concept incorporates expensive navigation systems that implement the techniques of frameless stereotaxy. This real-time, in operatory, display-driven virtual guidance of surgical tools is based on the registration of the surgical instrument with the virtual patient as demonstrated by CBCT data.

Rapid prototyping is a broad term used to describe a group of related processes and techniques that are used to fabricate physical scale models directly from three-dimensional computer-assisted design data. The purpose of rapid prototyping in maxillofacial imaging is to create a life-size, dimensionally accurate model of an anatomic structure. These models are also referred to as biomodels. DICOM data imported to proprietary software can be used to compute three-dimensional images generated by thresholding the intensity of the voxel values to be displayed and segmenting these from the background. The resulting models are used for presurgical planning of numerous complex maxillofacial surgical cases, including craniofacial reconstruction for correction of deformity caused by trauma, tumor resection, distraction osteogenesis, and, more widely, dental implants. The models provide the practitioner with a higher level of confidence before performing a surgical procedure and may reduce surgical and anesthetic time.

CONCLUSIONS

Further applications and increasing availability of CBCT imaging are expected to extend maxillofacial CBCT imaging from diagnosis to image guidance of operative and surgical procedures. CBCT will undoubtedly affect the expected standards of care, and this has implications for increased practitioner responsibility in the performance, optimal visualization, and interpretation of volumetric data sets.

BIBLIOGRAPHY

Radiologic Reports

American College of Radiology: ACR practice guideline for communication of diagnostic imaging findings. In: *Practice guidelines and technical standards (2005)*, 2005, American College of Radiology. http://www.acr.org. Accessed December 22, 2012.

Carter L, Farman AG, Geist J, et al: American Academy of Oral and Maxillofacial Radiology executive opinion statement on performing and interpreting diagnostic cone beam computed tomography, *Oral Surg Oral Med Oral Pathol Oral Radiol Endod* 106:561–562, 2008.

European Society of Radiology (ESR): Good practice for radiological reporting. Guidelines from the European Society of Radiology, *Insights Imaging* 2:93-96, 2011.

Clinical Applications

Abou-Elfetouh A, Barakat A, Abdel-Ghany K: Computed-guided rapid-prototyped templates for segmental mandibular osteotomies: a preliminary report, *Int J Med Robot* 7:187–192, 2011.

American Association of Endodontists; American Academy of Oral and Maxillofacial Radiology: use of cone-beam-computed tomography in endodontics. Joint Position Statement of the American Association of Endodontists; American Academy of Oral and Maxillofacial Radiography, *Oral Surg Oral Med Oral Pathol Oral Radiol* 111:234–237, 2011.

Cevidanes LH, Alhadidi A, Paniagua B, et al: Three-dimensional quantification of mandibular asymmetry through cone-beam computerized tomography, *Oral Surg Oral Med Oral Pathol Oral Radiol Endod* 111:757–770, 2011.

D'Urso PS, Barker TM, Earwaker WJ, et al: Stereolithography biomodelling in cranio-maxillofacial surgery: a prospective trial, *J Craniomaxillofac Surg* 27:30–37, 1999.

Kapila S, Conley RS, Harrell WE Jr: The current status of cone beam computed tomography imaging in orthodontics, *Dentomaxillofac Radiol* 40:24–34, 2011.

Scarfe WC, Farman AG, Sukovic P: Clinical applications of cone-beam computed tomography in dental practice, *J Can Dent Assoc* 72:75–80, 2006.

Scarfe WC, Levin MD, Gane D, et al: Use of cone beam computed tomography in endodontics, *Int J Dent* 2009:634567, 2009.

Swennen GR, Schutyser F: Three-dimensional cephalometry: spiral multislice vs cone-beam computed tomography, *Am J Orthod Dentofacial Orthop* 130:410–416, 2006.

The American Dental Association Council on Scientific Affairs: The use of cone-beam computed tomography in dentistry: an advisory statement from the American Dental Association Council on Scientific Affairs, *J Am Dent Assoc* 143:899–902, 2012.

Tyndall DA, Price JB, Tetradis S, et al: Position statement of the American Academy of Oral and Maxillofacial Radiology on selection criteria for the use of radiology in dental implantology with emphasis on cone beam computed tomography, *Oral Surg Oral Med Oral Pathol Oral Radiol* 113:817–826, 2012.

13 Cone-Beam Computed Tomography: Anatomy

Sanjay M. Mallya and Sotirios Tetradis

OUTLINE

Cone-beam computed tomographic (CBCT) imaging is an advanced imaging modality that provides excellent visualization of the dental hard tissues and osseous structures in three dimensions. CBCT imaging has become widely used over the last decade because it has multiple applications in dentomaxillofacial diagnosis. The anatomic coverage of CBCT imaging may be limited to the dentoalveolar arch or may extend to encompass a large part of the craniofacial skeleton. Clinicians who use CBCT imaging must be competent in recognizing radiographic manifestations of disease throughout the volume imaged. Similar to two-dimensional images, radiographic identification of abnormalities requires a thorough knowledge of the radiographic appearance of anatomic structures.

GENERAL PRINCIPLES OF EVALUATION

Although the region of immediate diagnostic interest may be limited to a specific site, it is important to evaluate all structures imaged. Many instances have been reported of benign and malignant tumors being detected serendipitously—that is, in part of the volume unrelated to the reason for which the image was made. Accordingly, it is critical to evaluate the imaged volume systematically in the axial, coronal, and sagittal planes. The anatomic structures must be identified and, where applicable, the symmetry and continuity of the bony outlines assessed.

CBCT images are displayed as multiplanar reconstructions of the imaged structures in three orthogonal planes (Fig. 13-1). For ease of visualization, the imaged volume may have to be reoriented, for example, to align the midsagittal plane to correct for any slight positioning errors during image acquisition; this is particularly important when examining for symmetry of structures. Many software programs used for CBCT image visualization allow for reorientation of all three planes. It is useful to reorient the axial plane to facilitate viewing of specific structures—for example, parallel to the Frankfort plane when examining the skull base or parallel to the occlusal plane when examining the dentoalveolar arches. To decipher the complete morphology of the imaged region, it is critical to view the entire image volume in all three orthogonal planes. Depending on the diagnostic task, it may be necessary to make additional custom reconstructions in specific planes, such as cross sections to evaluate the teeth and dentoalveolar ridges. In

any single section, the plane of section may be oblique and incomplete through an anatomic site and may cause the structure to appear abnormal.

TEETH AND SUPPORTING STRUCTURES

The detailed anatomy of the teeth and the supporting periodontium is best depicted on limited field-of-view (FOV) scans. Similar to intraoral radiographs, the teeth demonstrate a radiopaque enamel cap, a homogeneously radiopaque dentin, and radiolucent pulp chambers and pulp canals (see Fig. 13-1). As in periapical radiographs, cementum is typically not radiographically apparent because of the lack of radiographic contrast between cementum and dentin. Because CBCT scans provide three-dimensional information, they portray the morphology of the roots, pulp chambers, and pulp canals more accurately than intraoral radiographs. Thus a pulpal canal that is not evident in periapical radiographs owing to superimposition often can be clearly depicted on CBCT scans. CBCT imaging is particularly useful to evaluate multirooted teeth and roots with multiple pulp canals. The number and morphology of pulp canals and their course through the roots in all three planes can be examined. For multirooted teeth, reconstruction of the image volume along the long axis of each root may also be required. The individual canals are best identified on axial sections, whereas the course of the canal through the length of the root and its exit through the apex are typically assessed on coronal and sagittal sections (Fig. 13-2). Frequently, morphologic variations, such as root dilacerations in the buccolingual dimension, are not apparent on periapical and panoramic radiographs but are well demonstrated on CBCT examinations (Fig. 13-3). Detection of normal variations of the radicular and pulpal morphology is vital to endodontic treatment planning and presurgical assessment of the relationship of the roots to adjacent neurovascular structures. CBCT scans also reveal the proximity of the root surface to the cortical plates of the alveolar bone and detect anatomic variations, such as fenestrations or dehiscence defects (Fig. 13-4).

When viewing dentoalveolar structures, it is often useful to make cross-sectional reconstruction—slices in the buccolingual direction that are parallel to the long axis of the tooth. Additional curved planar reformatting can be used to generate a "panoramic"

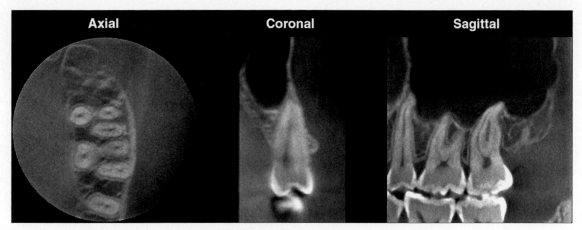

FIGURE 13-1 Multiplanar reconstructions with a limited FOV CBCT scan showing high-resolution axial, coronal, and sagittal sections through the dentoalveolar region of the posterior maxilla.

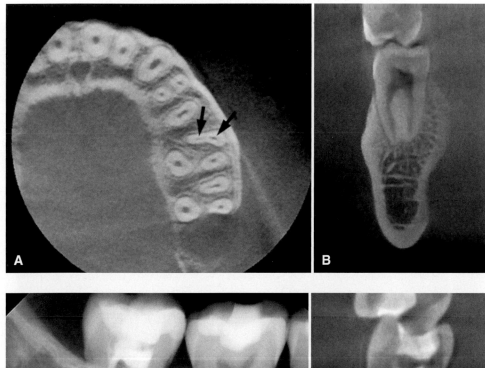

FIGURE 13-2 Limited CBCT scans demonstrating pulpal morphology. **A,** Axial section through the roots of the maxillary teeth. Two pulp canals *(arrows)* are visible in the mesiobuccal root of the first molar. **B,** Cross-sectional slice through the long axis of the mesial root of the mandibular first molar demonstrating the course of two pulp canals.

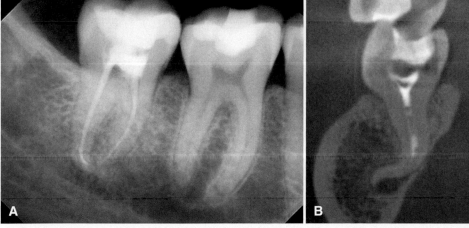

FIGURE 13-3 A, Periapical radiograph of the mandibular right posterior region showing close proximity of the root apices to the mandibular canal. **B,** Cross section through the distal root demonstrating severe dilaceration that was not apparent on the periapical radiograph. Also, the lingual location of the mandibular canal relative to the root apex is evident.

reconstruction, which also depicts the locations of the individual cross-sectional slices.

MAXILLA AND MIDFACIAL BONES

The maxilla and palatine bones form the upper jaw. The maxilla comprises a pyramidal-shaped body and four processes—alveolar, palatine, zygomatic, and frontal. The alveolar and palatine processes articulate in the midline to form the intermaxillary suture between the central incisors, best evaluated on coronal and axial sections. Examine the alveolar process, which forms the bone around the maxillary teeth, along with the maxillary teeth and supporting periodontal structures. In particular, owing to their three-dimensional nature, CBCT scans demonstrate the relationship of

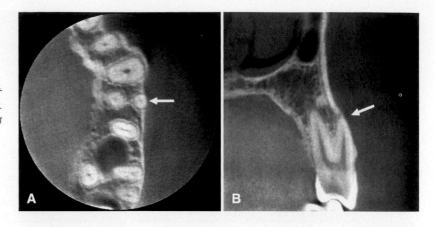

FIGURE 13-4 Axial **(A)** and coronal **(B)** CBCT sections demonstrating the proximity of the roots of the first premolar to the buccal cortical plate. Note the fenestration defect adjacent to the buccal root of the first premolar *(arrows)*.

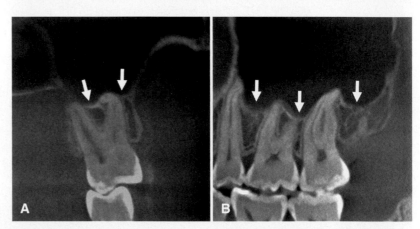

FIGURE 13-5 Coronal **(A)** and sagittal **(B)** CBCT sections through the maxillary posterior region demonstrating the relationship between the teeth and the maxillary sinus floor *(arrows)*. The corticated border of the sinus dips in between the tooth roots. Dilaceration of the mesiobuccal root of the maxillary molar is depicted on the coronal image.

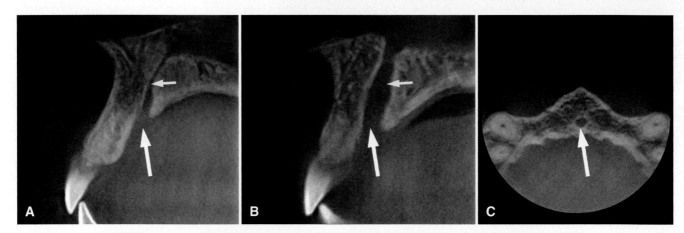

FIGURE 13-6 **A** and **B,** Sagittal CBCT sections through the midsagittal plane showing the course of the nasopalatine canal *(yellow arrow)* and the opening of the incisive foramen *(white arrow)*. Note the range of normal variation in the size of these structures. **C,** Axial section through the level of the incisive foramen *(arrow)*.

the molar and premolar teeth to the floor of the maxillary sinus better than periapical and panoramic radiographs. A common anatomic finding is pneumatization of the alveolar process by the maxillary sinus, which may invaginate between tooth roots (Fig. 13-5).

The palatine processes are thick horizontal bony projections that form the anterior three-fourths of the hard palate and the floor of the nasal cavity. The integrity and symmetry of the cortical bony contour are best visualized on coronal sections (see Plates 13-4 and 13-5). Disruption of the hard palate suggests developmental disturbances, such as a cleft palate. Areas of bony protuberances or tori

are frequently noted, especially in the midline. Numerous nutrient canals also may be observed perforating the cortical outline of the hard palate on high-resolution scans.

The incisive foramen is located in the midline on the anterior aspect of the palatine process, immediately palatal to the maxillary central incisors (Fig. 13-6; see Plate 13-7). Within this foramen are two lateral canals—the incisive canals or foramina of Stensen—that transmit the terminal branch of the descending palatine artery and the nasopalatine nerve. Occasionally, there may be two additional midline canals—the foramina of Scarpa, which transmit the naso-palatine nerves. The shape and size of the incisive foramen is appreciated on axial sections (see Plates 13-2 and 13-3). There is considerable variation in the size of the nasopalatine canal and incisive foramen. It is important to differentiate between a large incisive foramen and an incisive canal cyst because the latter can cause localized dilation of the canal or widening of the incisive foramen and may cause displacement of teeth (see Chapter 21).

The maxillary sinus occupies a major portion of the maxillary body. When evaluating the maxilla, the continuity of the sinus walls should be examined (see Plates 13-2, 13-4, 13-5, and 13-7). This examination includes the anterior wall, lateral wall (or infratemporal wall), medial wall (lateral wall of nasal fossa), and superior wall (orbital floor). Additionally, the symmetry of the right and left sinuses is evaluated. The zygomatic processes of the maxilla, which emanates from the junction of the anterior and lateral walls of the maxillary body, articulate posteriorly with the maxillary process of the zygoma. These two processes form the anterior segment of the zygomatic arch. The zygomaticomaxillary suture is visualized as a thin radiolucent, jagged line in this portion of the arch. Disruptions of the integrity or symmetry of the arch may be associated with craniofacial developmental abnormalities or facial trauma.

The medial and lateral pterygoid plates lie immediately posterior to the maxilla. These structures are best visualized on coronal and axial sections (see Plates 13-2 and 13-5) and must be carefully evaluated when assessing a patient with facial trauma. Involvement of the pterygoid plates is an essential feature of Le Fort fractures (see Chapter 30).

NASAL CAVITY AND PARANASAL SINUSES

The nasal cavity and paranasal sinuses aerate the maxillary, sphenoid, ethmoid, and frontal bones. The paranasal sinuses communicate directly with, and drain into, the nasal cavity via ostia. The nasal cavity is divided by the nasal septum in the midline (see Plates 13-2, 13-4, and 13-5). The cribriform plate of the ethmoid bone and the ethmoidal air cells form the roof of the nasal cavity. The hard palate forms the floor. The lateral walls contain thin bony projections called conchae. The conchae plus their mucosal covering are called turbinates (see Plates 13-2, 13-4, and 13-5). There are three nasal turbinates: superior, middle, and inferior, which define spaces termed superior, middle, and inferior meati (see Plate 13-4). Pneumatization of the concha is termed concha bullosa and is a common variant with a reported frequency of 14% to 53% (Fig. 13-7).

The paranasal sinuses consist of four pairs of air-filled cavities—maxillary, frontal, and sphenoid sinuses and the ethmoid air cells. The maxillary sinus is bordered by a roof, floor, and three walls—medial, anterior, and lateral. The roof separates the maxillary sinus from the orbit, and the medial wall forms the lateral wall of the nasal cavity. The floor of the maxillary sinus often undulates around the roots of the premolar and molar teeth. Occasionally, the maxillary sinuses also cause pneumatization of the hard palate and the zygomatic process of the maxilla.

The ethmoidal sinuses are divided into the anterior, middle, and posterior ethmoidal air cells, and the number of air cells per side ranges from 3 to 18. Frequently, extramural air cells—air cells outside of the ethmoid bone—can be visualized. These include agger nasi air cells, causing pneumatization of the lacrimal bone, and Haller's cells, which cause pneumatization of the orbital floor.

The sphenoid sinuses are midline structures in the body of the sphenoid bone and start to develop at approximately 4 months in utero. The sinuses vary considerably in size, and the right and left

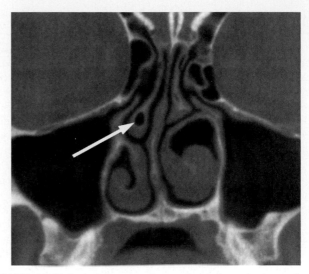

FIGURE 13-7 Concha bullosa. Coronal section through the nasal turbinates showing pneumatization of the middle concha (arrow), or concha bullosa.

sphenoid sinuses are often asymmetric and separated by a bony septum. Often multiple septa are present, giving the sinus a "locular" appearance. The sphenoid sinuses may extend inferiorly, resulting in pneumatization of the pterygoid bones.

The frontal sinuses are the last paranasal sinuses to develop, usually starting at approximately 6 to 7 years of age. They are typically symmetric. Hypoplasia of the frontal sinus is a common normal variant, and aplasia of the frontal sinuses is noted in approximately 4% of the population.

In a normal paranasal sinus, the epithelial lining is relatively thin and barely visualized. Thus the sinuses appear radiolucent, with a well-corticated bony outline. Inflammatory and neoplastic changes in the sinus lining appear as a soft tissue density, contrasted against the air-filled cavity. Thus the sinuses are evaluated for the presence of soft tissue thickening, the integrity of the borders, and the patency of the drainage paths of the paranasal sinuses. Evaluation of the paranasal sinuses should include a critical examination of the following anatomic structures:

- *Osteomeatal complex:* The maxillary sinus drains via the ostium into the infundibulum—a channel between the uncinate process of the ethmoid bone and the inferomedial wall of the orbit (see Plates 13-1, 13-2, 13-4, and 13-5). The infundibulum channels drainage to the hiatus semilunaris (see Plate 13-4) and then into the middle meatus. The complex of the maxillary ostium, infundibulum, uncinate process, hiatus semilunaris, ethmoidal bulla, and middle meatus is referred to as the osteomeatal complex. This region is the common drainage path for the frontal and maxillary sinuses and anterior ethmoidal air cells and thus must be carefully inspected for patency. This complex is best visualized on the coronal and axial sections.
- *Frontal recess:* This is the path for the drainage of the frontal sinus into the middle meatus. This recess is best visualized on sagittal and coronal sections (see Plate 13-4).
- *Sphenoethmoidal recess:* This is the drainage path for the sphenoid sinus and posterior ethmoidal air cells, in the superior meatus at the posterior region of the nasal cavity. This recess is located between the posterior ethmoidal cells and the sphenoid sinus (see Plate 13-1). It is best appreciated in axial and sagittal sections.

MANDIBLE

As with the maxillary arch, the dentoalveolar region of the mandibular body is best evaluated along with the mandibular teeth on cross-sectional and panoramic reconstructions. In addition to the periradicular bone, the mandible is evaluated in all three planes to assess for continuity and intact contours of the cortical outlines as well as for symmetry. A radiologic assessment includes evaluating the neurovascular canals and foramina; the integrity, radiodensity, and shapes of the cortical outline; and the density and architecture of the trabecular bone. The borders of the mandible appear as radiodense thick lines, predominantly along the inferior and posterior borders.

Sagittal and axial sections demonstrate the bony protuberances of the genial tubercles (see Plates 13-3, *D*, and 13-8, *A*), the site of attachment of the geniohyoid and genioglossus muscles. These tubercles may be seen as four discrete protuberances—one superior and one inferior tubercle on each side—or may be fused into a single tubercle. Midline lingual foramina are present in 96% to 100% of individuals, located in the region of the genial tubercles (see Plate 13-8, *B*). Typically, there are two individual foramina, but the number may vary from one to four. The number, location, and course of the neurovascular canals should be noted. This anatomic information is essential in presurgical treatment planning because damage to the neurovascular bundle in the course of implant bed preparation, for example, may lead to excessive bleeding.

The course of the mandibular canal is traced through the mandibular ramus and body, starting from the lingula on the lingual aspect of the ramus to the mental foramen on the buccal aspect of the mandibular body (see Plate 13-8, *C-F*). In cross-sectional and coronal slices, the mandibular canal is typically seen as an oval or round radiolucency with corticated borders. Sometimes, the cortication may be thin or imperceptible. The relationship of the canal to the tooth roots should be assessed. This relationship varies greatly among patients, especially in the molar region, with the mandibular canal occupying a position from close to the root apices to adjacent to the inferior border of the mandible. Other variations include bifid mandibular canals, with a reported frequency of about 15%. The mandibular canal exits to the buccal surface of the mandible, via the mental foramen, usually at the premolar region. There is significant variation in the size, shape, and location of the mental foramen. An important anatomic variation to detect when placing implants in the premolar region is the anterior loop, where the mandibular canal extends anterior to the mental foramen before it loops posteriorly to exit through the mental foramen. The incidence of an accessory mental foramen is about 7%. Sometimes the mandibular incisive canal is visible, extending anteriorly beyond the mental foramen.

In the posterior body and ramus of the mandible, the lingual surface of the mandible is concave below the mylohyoid ridge. The extent and depth of this concavity, or undercut, varies greatly (see Plate 13-8, *D*). The identification of this anatomic feature is crucial when examining mandibular anatomy for implant treatment planning.

Mandibular symmetry is best assessed on axial (see Plates 13-3 to 13-5) and coronal images. When comparing the ramal heights and shapes, custom reconstructions through the rami can be made to assess ramal dimensions qualitatively and quantitatively. Additionally, the gonial angle and the presence of any antegonial notching bilaterally are noted because these are frequently altered by abnormal mandibular growth.

TEMPOROMANDIBULAR JOINT

The temporomandibular joint (TMJ) is the articulation between the glenoid fossa of the temporal bone and the condyle of the mandible. The glenoid fossa is a concave depression located in the squamous portion of the temporal bone (see Plates 13-6 and 13-7). It is bordered anteriorly by the articular eminence and posteriorly by the squamotympanic and petrotympanic fissures. The articular eminence is usually described as a posterior slope, adjacent to the fossa, and the crest, which is the inferior-most tip of the eminence. The condyle is typically ellipsoid and is longer in the mediolateral dimension than in the anteroposterior dimension. The condyle is angulated with the medial pole being positioned posterior to the lateral pole, typically forming an angle of 15 to 30 degrees with the sagittal plane. When viewing sections through the TMJ, it is useful to make custom reconstructions through the axial long axis of the condylar head. The resulting oblique sections are referred to as "corrected" sagittal and frontal sections (Fig. 13-8).

- In the sagittal view, the fossa and eminence form an inverted "S" shape, characteristically seen as a smooth radiopaque line (see Fig. 13-8). The angle of the posterior slope of the eminence can vary considerably and is typically 30 to 60 degrees to the Frankfort plane. Anatomic variations such as a steep eminence (angle >60 degrees) have been suggested to predispose to TMJ internal derangements.

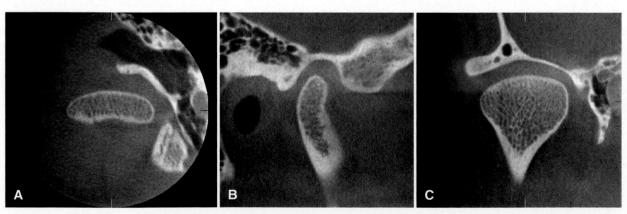

FIGURE 13-8 Limited FOV CBCT image of the TMJ. Axial **(A)**, corrected sagittal **(B)**, and frontal **(C)** sections. Note intact cortical borders on all articular surfaces.

- The superior surface of the condylar head is usually rounded or convex, but anatomic variations, such as slight flattening or marked convexity, are frequently observed. The size and shape of the right and left condylar heads should be compared. When an asymmetry is observed, the symmetry of the entire mandible should be assessed, including the intercuspation of the teeth and any deviation of the mandible on opening.
- In adults, the articular surfaces of the condyle, glenoid fossa, and articular eminence have a corticated border. Pathologic conditions, such as osteoarthritis, often cause a thinning or loss of this normal cortication. However, this corticated border is not visualized during periods of condylar growth and thus is not seen until approximately age 18 years.
- With the teeth in maximal intercuspation, the condyle is normally seated concentrically within the glenoid fossa. Although considerable deviation from this position is observed in radiographs of asymptomatic individuals, the condyle is frequently retruded in individuals with TMJ dysfunction.

BASE OF THE SKULL

The skull base is best evaluated on axial and coronal sections. To facilitate viewing of the anatomic structures, it is useful to orient the CBCT volume to the Frankfort plane—with the axial slices parallel to this plane and coronal slices perpendicular to this plane. Five bones form the skull base: ethmoid, sphenoid, occipital, frontal (paired), and temporal (paired).

The entire cranial base is evaluated for symmetry, integrity, and continuity. For example, infections or neoplasms may extend from the ethmoid air cells into the cranial fossa through the cribriform plate, disrupting this anatomic structure. Furthermore, it is important to be familiar with the various foramina and canals in the skull base.

The anterior cranial base is formed by the frontal bones (laterally), the cribriform plate and crista galli of the ethmoid bone (medially), and the lesser wing of the sphenoid bone (posteriorly). These bones also contribute to the roof of the nasal cavity, ethmoid air cells, and orbits. The anterior cranial base is best visualized on coronal and sagittal sections (see Plates 13-4, 13-5, and 13-7).

The middle cranial base is formed by the body and greater wings of the sphenoid bone and the petrous and squamous portions of the temporal bones and overlies the sphenoid sinuses and the mastoid air cells, middle and inner ears, and infratemporal fossae (see Plates 13-5 to 13-7). The sella turcica is a depression in the body of the sphenoid and contains the pituitary gland. This depression, together with the anterior and posterior clinoid processes, forms a U-shaped corticated line on sagittal sections and is saddle-shaped on coronal sections. There is a broad range in the dimensions of the sella turcica, with the anteroposterior dimension ranging from 6 to 11 mm and the depth ranging from 3 to 11 mm. On either side of the sella turcica is the carotid groove, seen extending posteriorly to the carotid canal that passes vertically through the petrous portion of the temporal bone. The clivus is a triangular bone formed by the union of the basisphenoid and basiocciput bones and extends posteriorly and caudally from the sella turcica. The union between these bones—the spheno-occipital synchondrosis—is completed by 16 to 20 years. Thus, an open synchondrosis, seen as a gap in the clivus, is a normal appearance for children younger than 16 years old (Fig. 13-9).

There are several key communications between the middle cranial fossa and the extracranial space, as follows:

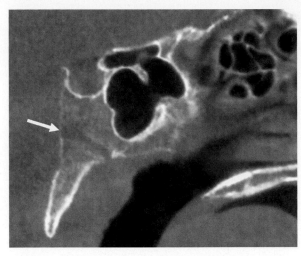

FIGURE 13-9 Clivus showing incomplete spheno-occipital synchondrosis. This is a normal appearance until the synchondrosis is completed, typically by 16 to 20 years.

- *Superior orbital fissure* (see Plate 13-1): Located lateral to the sphenoid body and immediately below the anterior clinoid processes and transmits cranial nerves III, IV, V, and VI and the superior ophthalmic vein.
- *Foramen rotundum:* Canal that traverses through the greater wing of the sphenoid bone and transmits the maxillary division of the trigeminal nerve to the pterygopalatine fossa. The course of this canal is best visualized on coronal sections (see Plate 13-5).
- *Foramen ovale:* Located in the sphenoid body and transmits the mandibular division of the trigeminal nerve to the infratemporal fossa. It is adequately visualized on axial and coronal sections (see Plates 13-2 and 13-5). There is considerable variation in the size of this foramen.
- *Foramen spinosum:* Located posterior and lateral to the foramen ovale and is best visualized on axial sections (see Plate 13-2).

An important anatomic region to examine is the pterygopalatine fossa. This is a funnel shaped fossa located below the skull base and has communications with the middle cranial fossa, the nasal cavity, the orbit, the infratemporal fossa, and the oral cavity. This fossa is bordered anteriorly by the posterior wall of the maxilla and posteriorly by the pterygoid process of the sphenoid bone. The opening to the pterygopalatine fossa from the lateral aspect is the pterygomaxillary fissure. On sagittal sections, the fossa is seen as an inverted pear-shaped radiolucency (see Plate 13-7); on axial and coronal sections, it appears as a rectangular-shaped area (see Plates 13-1 and 13-5).

The styloid process is noted as a bony projection from the inferior surface of the petrous temporal bone, adjacent to the stylomastoid foramen. The length of this process ranges from 5 to 50 mm. The stylohyoid ligament is often calcified, with reported frequencies of up to 30%. The mastoid process is another protuberance from the inferior surface of the temporal bone. Pneumatization of this bony process by the mastoid air cells occurs starting at age 3 to 5 years. As a result of the presence of air, the mastoid air cells appear as radiolucent air spaces, and opacification of these air cells often indicates disease. Sometimes pneumatization may extend anteriorly into the articular eminence and even into the zygoma or the occipital bone adjacent to the mastoid process.

AIRWAY

Medium to full FOV CBCT scans often encompass the airway space from the nasal cavity to the pharynx. The pharynx is typically considered in four zones: the nasopharynx, velopharynx, oropharynx, and hypopharynx (see Plate 13-7). The nasopharynx lies behind the nasal cavity and extends to the level of the hard palate. The velopharynx extends from the level of the hard palate to the caudal tip of the uvula. The oropharynx spans the region between the tongue and the pharyngeal wall, extending from the uvula to the base of the epiglottis. The hypopharynx is the most caudal part of the pharynx, below the epiglottis. The airway should be evaluated for symmetry and patency. Anatomic variations in the size of the soft palate or tongue or pathologic enlargements of the palatine tonsils can cause narrowing of the airway dimensions.

BIBLIOGRAPHY

Harnesberger HR, Osborn AG, Ross J, et al, editors: *Diagnostic and surgical imaging anatomy: brain, head and neck, spine*, Salt Lake City, 2006, Amirsys.

Naitoh M, Hiraiwa Y, Aimiya H, et al: Accessory mental foramen assessment using cone-beam computed tomography, *Oral Surg Oral Med Oral Pathol Oral Radiol Endod* 107:289–294, 2009.

Von Arx T, Matter D, Buser D, et al: Evaluation of the location and dimensions of lingual foramina using limited cone-beam computed tomography, *J Oral Maxillofac Surg* 69:2777–2785, 2011.

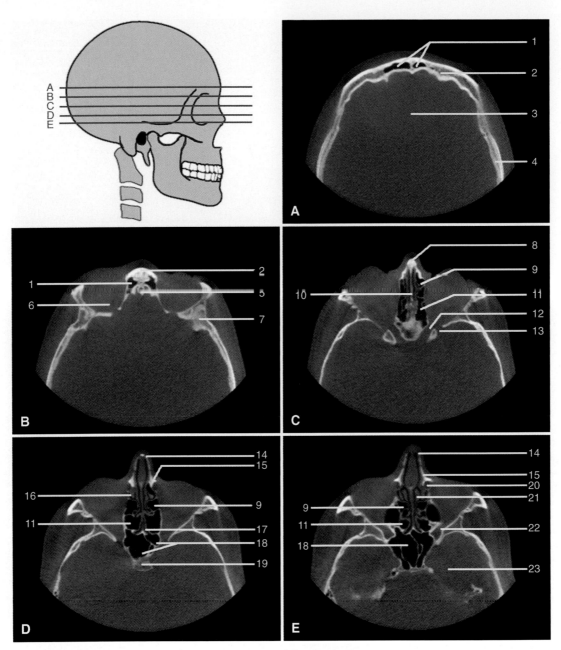

1. Frontal sinus
2. Frontal bone
3. Anterior cranial fossa
4. Squamous portion of temporal bone
5. Crista galli
6. Orbit
7. Greater wing of sphenoid bone
8. Nasal bone
9. Anterior ethmoid air cells
10. Perpendicular plate of ethmoid bone
11. Posterior ethmoid air cells

12. Optic canal
13. Superior orbital fissure
14. Nasal bone
15. Nasal process of maxillary bone
16. Uncinate process
17. Sphenoethmoid recess
18. Sphenoid sinus
19. Floor of sella turcica
20. Nasolacrimal duct
21. Superior turbinate
22. Inferior orbital fissure
23. Middle cranial fossa

PLATE 13-1

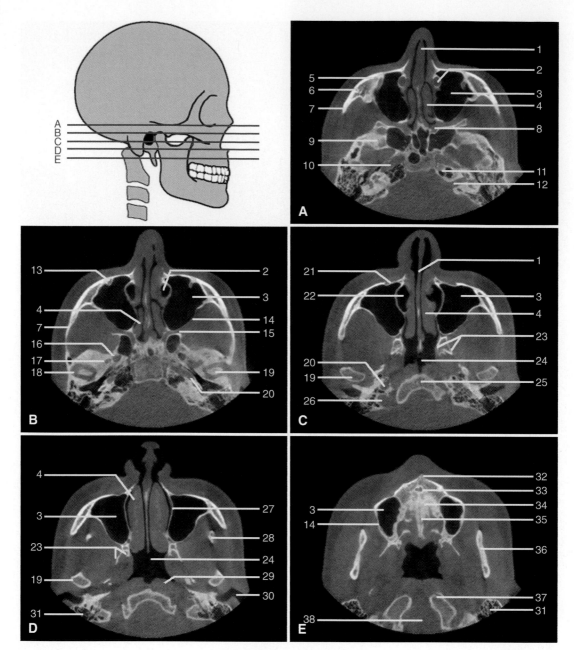

1. Nasal septum
2. Nasolacrimal duct
3. Maxillary sinus
4. Nasal turbinate
5. Zygomatic process of maxilla
6. Zygomatico-maxillary suture
7. Zygomatic arch
8. Pterygopalatine fossa
9. Greater wing of sphenoid bone
10. Carotid canal
11. Petrous portion of temporal bone
12. Internal auditory canal
13. Infraorbital canal

14. Lateral wall of maxillary sinus
15. Pterygomaxillary fissure
16. Foramen ovale
17. Foramen spinosum
18. Glenoid fossa
19. Mandibular condylar head
20. Carotid canal
21. Infraorbital foramen
22. Nasal cavity
23. Pterygoid plates
24. Nasopharyngeal airway
25. Occipital bone
26. Jugular bulb

27. Medial wall of maxillary sinus
28. Coronoid process
29. Pharyngeal wall
30. External auditory meatus
31. Mastoid process
32. Anterior nasal spine
33. Nasopalatine canal
34. Hard palate
35. Intermaxillary suture
36. Ramus of mandible
37. Anterior arch of atlas (C1)
38. Foramen magnum

PLATE 13-2

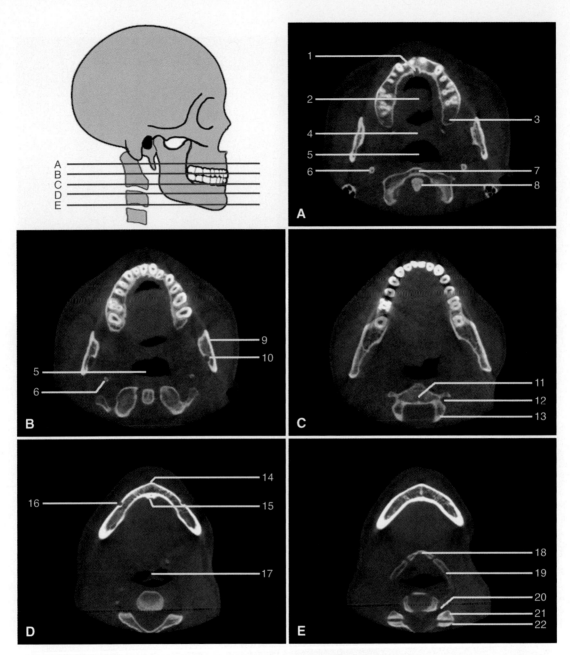

1. Incisive foramen
2. Tongue
3. Maxillary tuberosity
4. Soft palate
5. Oropharyngeal airway space
6. Styloid process
7. Anterior arch of atlas (C1)
8. Odontoid process of C2
9. Ramus of mandible
10. Lingula
11. Inferior body of C2
12. Transverse foramen
13. Lamina of C2
14. Mandibular symphysis
15. Genial tubercles
16. Mental foramen
17. Epiglottis
18. Body of hyoid bone
19. Greater cornu of hyoid bone
20. C2-C3 neural foramen
21. Superior articular process of C3
22. Inferior articular process of C2

PLATE 13-3

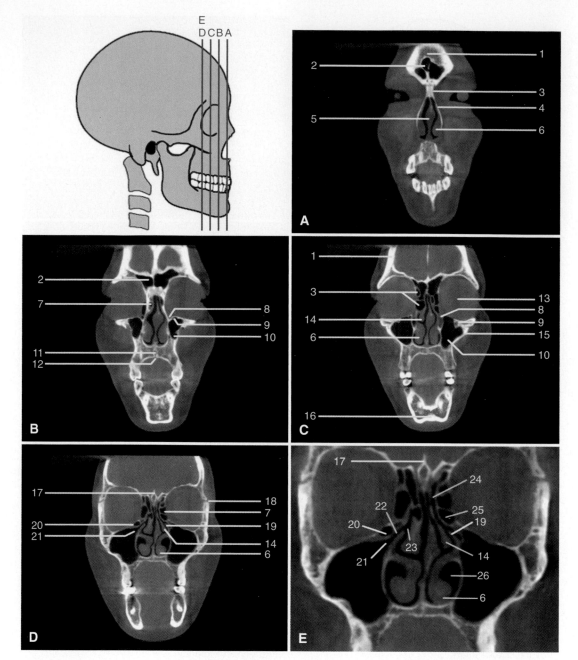

1. Frontal bone
2. Frontal sinus
3. Nasal bone
4. Maxillary bone
5. Nasal septum
6. Inferior nasal turbinate
7. Ethmoid air cells
8. Nasolacrimal duct
9. Infraorbital canal

10. Maxillary sinus
11. Nasopalatine canal
12. Incisive foramen
13. Orbit
14. Middle nasal turbinate
15. Zygomatic process of the maxilla
16. Mandible
17. Crista galli of ethmoid bone
18. Fronto-zygomatic suture

19. Uncinate process
20. Infraorbital ethmoid air cells
    (Haller's cells)
21. Ostium of maxillary sinus
22. Infundibulum
23. Hiatus semilunaris
24. Frontal recess
25. Ethmoid bulla
26. Inferior meatus

PLATE 13-4

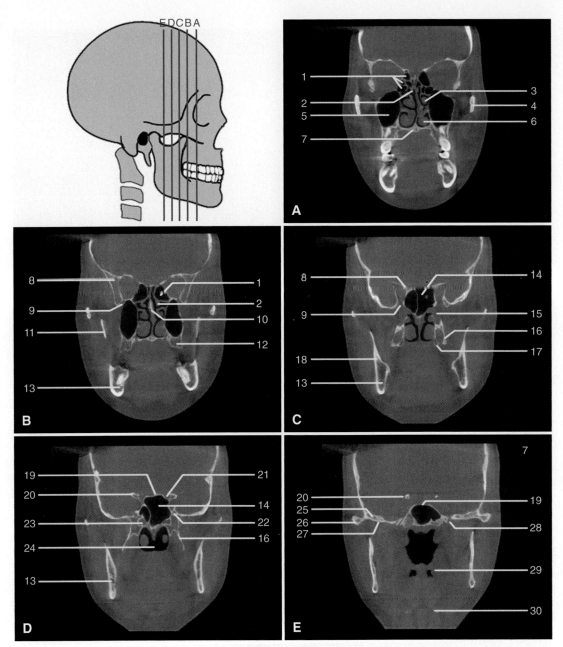

1. Ethmoid air cells
2. Superior nasal turbinate
3. Middle nasal turbinate
4. Zygomatic arch
5. Maxillary sinus
6. Inferior nasal turbinate
7. Hard palate (floor of nasal cavity)
8. Sphenoid bone
9. Inferior orbital fissure
10. Perpendicular plate of ethmoid bone
11. Coronoid process of mandible
12. Maxillary tuberosity
13. Mandibular canal
14. Sphenoid sinus
15. Pterygopalatine fossa
16. Lateral pterygoid plate
17. Medial pterygoid plate
18. Mandibular ramus
19. Floor of sella turcica
20. Anterior clinoid process
21. Optic canal
22. Foramen rotundum
23. Pterygoid (vidian) canal
24. Nasopharyngeal airway
25. Squamous temporal bone
26. Zygomatic process of
    temporal bone
27. Sphenosquamosal suture
28. Foramen ovale
29. Palatine tonsils
30. Hyoid bone

PLATE 13-5

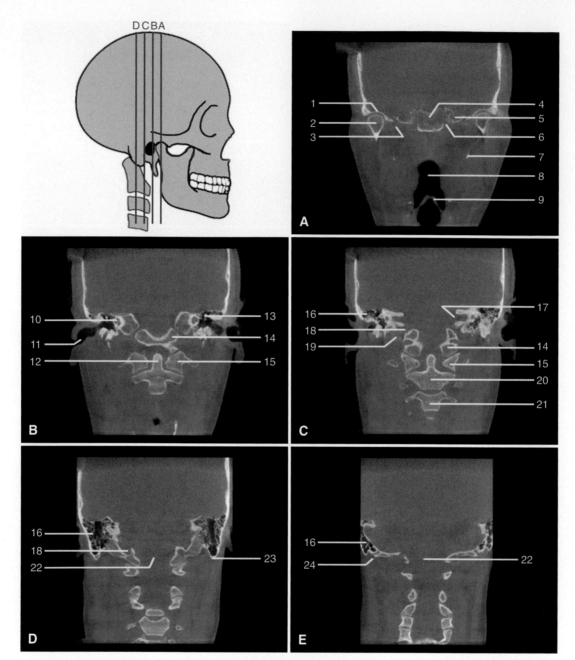

1. Glenoid fossa
2. Mandibular condyle
3. Foramen spinosum
4. Basiocciput
5. Carotid canal
6. Petrooccipital suture
7. Styloid process
8. Oropharyngeal airway space
9. Epiglottis
10. Semicircular canal
11. External auditory meatus
12. Odontoid process of C2
13. Ossicles of ear
14. Occipital condyles
15. Lateral mass of C1
16. Mastoid air cells
17. Internal auditory meatus
18. Jugular foramen
19. Jugular bulb
20. Body of C2
21. Body of C3
22. Foramen magnum
23. Mastoid process
24. Occipito-mastoid suture

PLATE 13-6

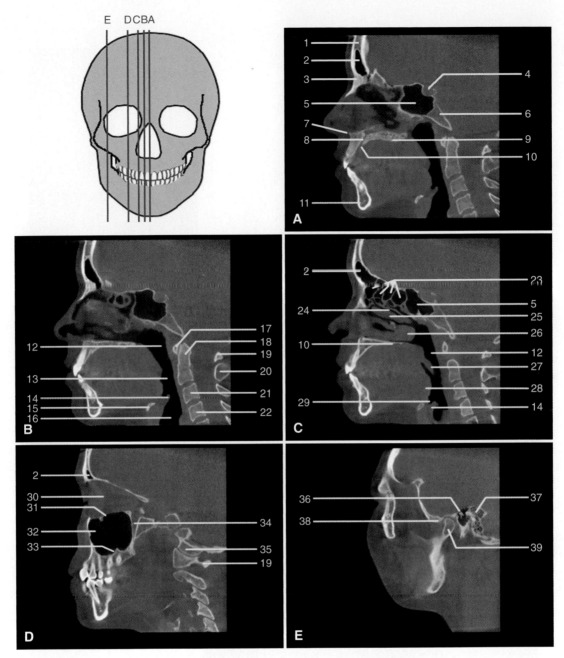

1. Frontal bone
2. Frontal sinus
3. Nasal bone
4. Sella turcica
5. Sphenoid sinus
6. Clivus
7. Anterior nasal spine
8. Nasopalatine canal
9. Incisive foramen
10. Hard palate
11. Mandibular symphysis
12. Velopharynx
13. Oropharynx

14. Epiglottis
15. Hyoid bone
16. Hypopharynx
17. Anterior arch of C1
18. Odontoid process of C2
19. Posterior arch of C1
20. Spinous process of C2
21. Body of C3
22. Body of C4
23. Ethmoid air cells
24. Hiatus semilunaris
25. Middle turbinate
26. Inferior turbinate

27. Soft palate
28. Base of tongue
29. Vallecula
30. Orbit
31. Floor of orbit/roof of maxillary sinus
32. Maxillary sinus
33. Floor of maxillary sinus
34. Pterygopalatine fossa
35. Occipital condyle
36. Ossicle of middle ear
37. Mastoid process
38. Articular eminence
39. Mandibular condyle

PLATE 13-7

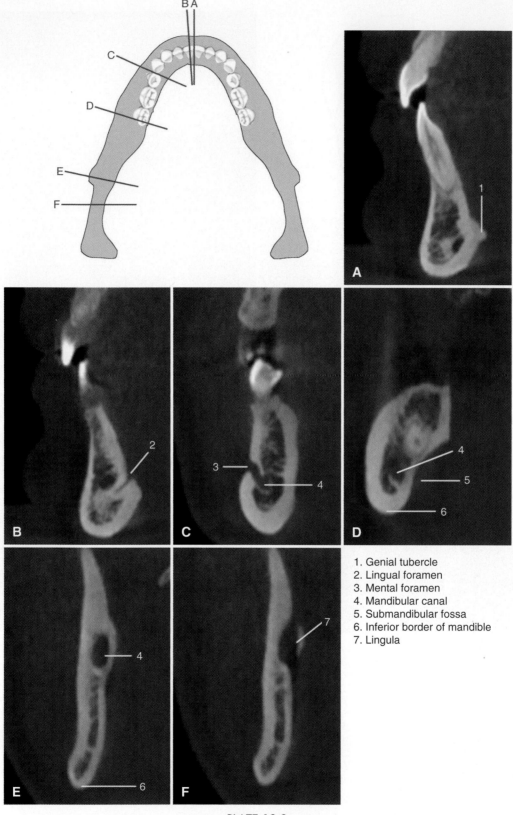

1. Genial tubercle
2. Lingual foramen
3. Mental foramen
4. Mandibular canal
5. Submandibular fossa
6. Inferior border of mandible
7. Lingula

PLATE 13-8

Other Imaging Modalities

The imaging modalities described in this chapter employ equipment and techniques that are beyond the routine needs of most general dental practitioners. Each of these techniques makes a tomographic image–that is, a slice through tissue–rather than a simple projection image. The most versatile of these modalities are computed tomographic (CT) scanning and magnetic resonance (MR) imaging. Nuclear medicine, ultrasonography, and positron emission tomographic (PET) imaging are used for more specialized applications. Film tomography, a mainstay imaging technique during the twentieth century, has been largely replaced by CT scanning, MR imaging, and cone-beam imaging (see Chapters 11–13). Each of these imaging modalities is used to aid in the diagnosis of conditions in the oral cavity. Thus, dentists should have a basic understanding of their operating principles and clinical applications.

COMPUTED TOMOGRAPHIC SCANNING

In 1972, Hounsfield, an engineer, announced the invention of a revolutionary imaging technique that used image reconstruction mathematics developed by Cormack in the 1950s and 1960s to produce cross-sectional images of the head. This form of imaging is called computed tomographic (CT) scanning. Hounsfield and Cormack shared the Nobel Prize in Physiology or Medicine in 1979 for their pioneering work.

COMPUTED TOMOGRAPHIC SCANNERS

In its simplest form, a CT scanner consists of an x-ray tube that emits a finely collimated, fan-shaped x-ray beam directed through a patient to a series of scintillation detectors or ionization chambers (Fig. 14-1, *A*). These detectors measure the number of photons that exit the patient. This information can be used to construct a cross-sectional image of the patient. In early versions of CT scanners, both the x-ray tube and the detectors rotated synchronously around the patient. In more recent designs, the detectors form a continuous ring around the patient, and the x-ray tube moves in a circle within the fixed detector ring (Fig. 14-1, *B*). Originally, patients would lie on a stationary table while the x-ray source rotated one cycle around them. Then the table would move 1 to 5 mm for the next scan. CT scanners that used this type of "step and shoot" movement for image acquisition are called **incremental scanners**. The final image set consists of a series of contiguous or overlapping axial images, made at right angles to the long axis of the patient's body. These two-dimensional slices are cross sections, typically 1 mm thick.

In 1989, CT scanners were introduced that acquire image data in a helical fashion (Fig. 14-2). With helical scanners, the gantry, containing the attached x-ray tube and detectors, continuously revolves around the patient, while the table on which the patient is lying continuously advances through the gantry. A continuous helix of data is acquired as the x-ray beam moves down the patient. Helical CT imaging is now the standard. In helical CT scanners, **pitch** refers to the amount of patient movement compared with the width of the image acquired. More precisely, the equation is as follows:

$$\text{Pitch} = \frac{\text{Table travel per x-ray tube rotation}}{\text{Image thickness}}$$

A pitch of 1 means that the image width is equal to the amount of patient movement per slice. A pitch of 2 means that the patient moves twice as far as the detector is wide, and only half the tissue

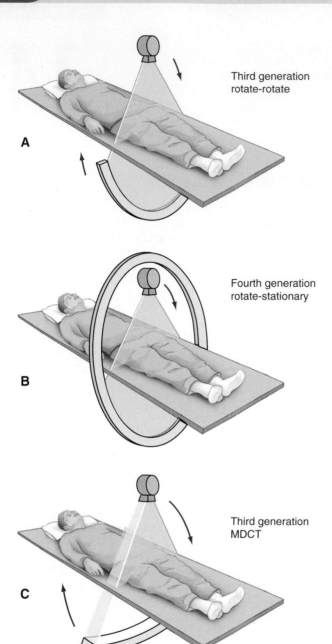

FIGURE 14-1 Geometry of CT scanners. **A,** In CT scanners, the x-ray source emits a fan beam. In third-generation CT scanners, both the x-ray source and the detector array rotate around the patient in a circular path. The patient is moved incrementally between each rotation of the source. **B,** In fourth-generation CT scanners, the x-ray tube rotates around the patient, and the remnant beam is detected by a fixed circular array. **C,** Most contemporary CT scanners use a third-generation design with a relatively wide multidetector helical computed tomographic (MDCT) array having 64 to 128 rows. In these scanners, all parts of the detector array arc are equidistant from the x-ray source.

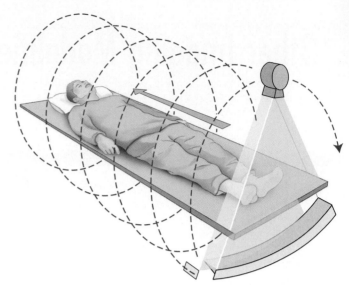

FIGURE 14-2 Helical CT imaging. In helical scanners, the patient is moved continuously through the gantry, and the x-ray source moves continuously around the patient in a circle. The net effect is to describe a helical beam—and image—path through the patient. True axial sections are reconstructed in the software.

imaging and multirow CT imaging. MDCT imaging has become widely used and has had a pronounced clinical impact. With this method, usually 64 or 128 adjacent detector arrays are used in conjunction with a helical CT scanner (see Fig. 14-1, *C*). Additionally, the time for the x-ray tube to make a full cycle around the patient has been reduced to 0.25 second (four rotations per second). These developments allow images from multiple slices to be captured quickly and simultaneously, thus greatly reducing both exposure time and motion artifact from breathing, peristalsis, or heart contractions; this is important for patients who cannot hold their breath for long periods and for pediatric and trauma patients. The quality of axial, reformatted, and three-dimensional images is also greatly improved with MDCT scanners compared with single-slice scanners. The meaning of pitch with MDCT scanners varies with the individual manufacturer but often means table travel per x-ray tube rotation divided by total active detector width. In general, the patient dose is higher with MDCT scanners than with single-slice scanners.

X-RAY TUBES

CT scanners use x-ray tubes with rotating anodes (see Fig. 1-9). These tubes have a high heat capacity, up to 8 million heat units (compare with dental tubes of 20,000 heat units). They operate at typically 120 kVp (range, 80 to 140 kVp) and 200 to 800 mA. Focal spot sizes range from 0.5 to 2.0 mm. The high x-ray output minimizes exposure time and improves image quality by increasing the signal-to-noise ratio. The high kVp also provides a wide dynamic range by reducing bone absorption compared with soft tissue and extends tube life by reducing tube loading. The tubes operate continuously by using three-phase or high-frequency generators. To minimize patient exposure the beam is collimated to a thin fan beam before it enters the patient. Some of the x-ray photons interact with the patient and are scattered. To improve image quality the residual beam is again collimated to remove the scattered photons. Postpatient collimation controls slice thickness. Slice thickness is typically 1 to 3 mm. Thinner slices result in

is exposed. A pitch of 0.5 means that half the image is overlapped in each slice. Overlapping reconstructions result in the highest spatial resolution but also the highest patient dose. Compared with incremental CT scanners, helical scanners provide improved multiplanar image reconstructions, reduced examination time, and a reduced radiation dose.

The most recent major advance was the introduction of multidetector helical computed tomographic (MDCT) scanners in 1998. Alternative terms for the same technology are multislice CT

higher spatial resolution and contrast, less partial volume effect (see later), and higher patient dose.

DETECTORS

The x-ray beam exiting the patient is captured by an array of solid-state detectors. These detectors are usually made of rare earth materials, such as Gd_2S_2O. The spaces between the ceramic scintillators or crystals are heated into a ceramic, sawn into small elements, and coupled to a photodiode. The ceramic is scored with a saw or laser, and the spaces are filled with an opaque material to create individual pixels 0.625 mm across. These detectors are about 80% efficient. The signal from the detector is amplified, digitized, and sent to a computer for analysis.

IMAGE RECONSTRUCTION

The photons recorded by the detectors represent a composite of the absorption characteristics of all elements of the patient in the path of the x ray beam. Computer algorithms use these photon counts to construct one or, more often, many digital cross-sectional images. The CT image is recorded and displayed as a matrix of individual blocks called voxels (volume elements) (Fig. 14-3). Each square of the image matrix is a pixel. Images are typically 512 × 512 pixels or 1024 × 1024 pixels. Although the size of the pixel

(about 0.6 mm) is determined partly by the computer program used to construct the image, the length of the voxel (about 1 to 20 mm) is determined by the width of the x-ray beam, which is controlled by the prepatient and postpatient collimators. An interpolator algorithm is used to correct for the helical motion of the scanner and to construct planar cross sections from the helical information.

The methods used to reconstruct images are complex. Initially, an object with four compartments, as shown in Figure 14-4, should be pictured. The linear attenuation coefficients (densities) of each of the four cells can be computed by using four simultaneous equations to solve for four unknowns. This method becomes computationally impracticable when there are 512^2 or 1024^2 cells. Instead, methods called filtered back-projection algorithms involving Fourier transformations are used for rapid image reconstruction. A modification of these methods, called the Feldkamp reconstruction, is used for MDCT and cone-beam reconstructions to account for the diverging x-ray beam. This same principle is used in cone-beam imaging (see Chapter 11). After reconstruction, various image processing filters are applied. Typically, these are smoothing filters to minimize noise in low-contrast objects such as soft tissue and edge-sharpening filters to improve visualization of fine bony detail. In recent years, an image processing technique

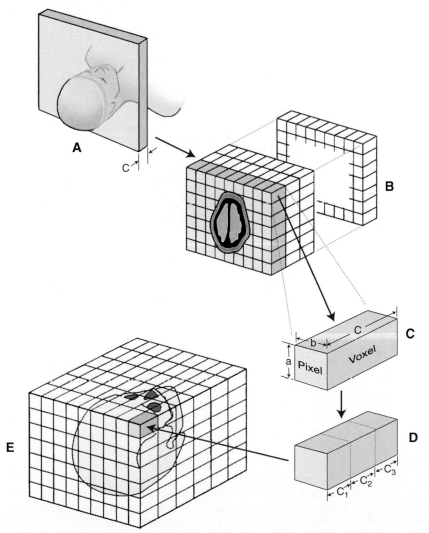

FIGURE 14-3 CT image formation. **A,** Data for a single-plane image are acquired from multiple projections made during the course of a 360-degree rotation around the patient. Slice thickness (c) is controlled by the width of the postpatient collimator. **B,** A single-plane image is constructed from absorption characteristics of the subject and displayed as differences in optical density, ranging from −1000 to +1000 HU. Several planes may be imaged from multiple contiguous scans. **C,** The image consists of a matrix of individual pixels representing the face of a volume called a voxel. Although dimensions *a* and *b* are determined partly by the computer program used to construct the image, dimension *c* is controlled by the collimator as in **A. D,** Cuboid voxels can be created from the original rectangular voxel by computer interpolation. This allows the formation of multiplanar and three-dimensional images **(E)**.

FIGURE 14-4 Image reconstruction. **A,** Assume four volumes with differing linear attenuation coefficients (μ). A beam entering the object with N_0 photons is reduced in intensity by object. The intensity of the remnant beam is measured by the detector array. The value of each cell in the object can be determined by solving four (or more) independent simultaneous equations. Such a brute-force approach is computationally intensive, and in practice much faster algorithms are used to reconstruct images. **B,** This task is conceptually similar to sudoku problems in that the exposure to the detector is known, and the filtered back-projection algorithms estimate the exposure intensity at each voxel.

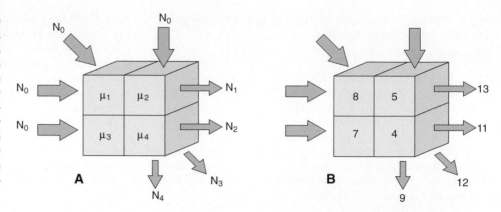

called iterative reconstruction has been used instead of filtered back-projection to reduce noise from images. This technique allows the use of low-dose protocols yet still produces images with comparable or better image quality. More recent research in CT imaging includes using dual-energy CT imaging and spectral CT imaging to remove bone from soft tissue images and to facilitate tissue characterization.

COMPUTED TOMOGRAPHIC IMAGE

For image display, each pixel is assigned a CT number representing tissue density. This number is proportional to the degree to which the material within the voxel has attenuated the x-ray beam. CT numbers, also known as Hounsfield units (HU), in honor of the inventor Hounsfield, range from −1000 to +1000, each corresponding to a different level of beam attenuation (Table 14-1). Some newer CT machines have a range of up to 4000 HU. Because the human eye can detect only about 40 shades of gray, it is useful to adjust the range and mean of CT numbers displayed on a monitor (Fig. 14-5). An image optimized for viewing bone, a "bone window," may have a range (window width [WW]) of 700 units and mean (window level [WL]) of 500 units. Alternatively, an image optimized to view soft tissues may have a WW of 400 units and a WL of 40 units. In these images, bone is white or light grey, soft tissue is medium gray, and air is dark grey to black. By convention, these images are displayed as if the clinician is standing at the feet of the patient who is lying on his or her back. Thus, the patient's anterior structures appear at the top (Fig. 14-6, *A*), and the patient's right side appears on the left (Fig. 14-6, *B* and *C*).

CT imaging has several advantages over conventional film radiography and tomography. First, CT imaging eliminates the superimposition of images of structures outside the area of interest. Second, because of the inherent high-contrast resolution of CT imaging, differences between tissues that differ in physical density by less than 1% can be distinguished; conventional radiography requires a 10% difference in physical density to distinguish between tissues. Third, data from a single CT imaging procedure, consisting of either multiple contiguous or one helical scan, can be viewed as images in the axial, coronal, or sagittal planes or in any arbitrary plane depending on the diagnostic task; this is referred to as multiplanar reformatted imaging. Having the capability of viewing normal anatomy or pathologic processes simultaneously in three orthogonal planes often facilitates radiographic interpretation (see Fig. 14-6).

Multiplanar images are two-dimensional and require a certain degree of mental integration by the viewer for interpretation. This

TABLE 14-1	Typical Hounsfield Units for Air and Tissues
Tissue	Hounsfield Units (CT Numbers)
Bone	+400 to +1000
Soft tissue	+40 to +80
Water	0
Fat	−60 to −100
Lung	−400 to −600
Air	−1000

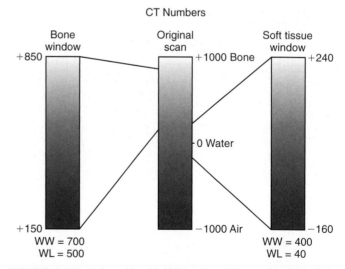

FIGURE 14-5 Window width and level. CT numbers (HU) are scaled on cortical bone (+1000), water (0), and air (−1000). Viewing bone or soft tissue is optimized by improving the contrast of the appropriate region of the original image. Window width *(WW)* is the range of CT numbers used, and window level *(WL)* is the midportion of the range. Bone and soft tissue window views are used to enhance visualization of those tissues. In this example, a bone window may have a range of 700 units and a mean of 500 units, whereas a soft tissue window may have a range of 400 units and a mean of 40 units.

limitation has led to the development of computer programs that reformat data acquired from axial CT scans into three-dimensional images. The use of three-dimensional images has been boosted by the use of MDCT imaging as a means of reviewing large amounts of information collected at each examination.

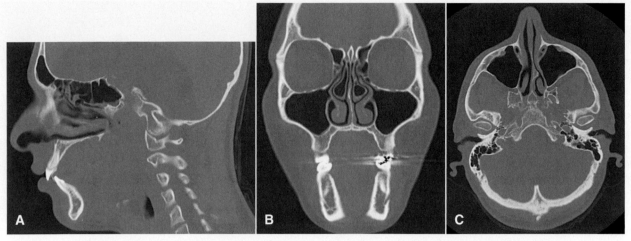

FIGURE 14-6 Multiplanar reconstruction views facilitate interpretation of complex anatomy. **A,** CT images demonstrating the sagittal plane through lateral incisors and foramen lacerum. Note the frontal, ethmoid, and sphenoid sinuses. **B,** Coronal view through the ethmoid and maxillary sinuses and mental foramen in the left mandible. **C,** Axial view through the level of maxillary sinuses and mandibular condyles. The patient's right side appears on the left side of the coronal and sagittal images as if the patient is lying on the back with the toes pointed toward the observer.

Three-dimensional reformatting requires that each original voxel, shaped as a rectangular solid, be dimensionally altered into multiple cuboidal voxels. This process, called interpolation, creates sets of evenly spaced cuboidal voxels (cuberilles) that occupy the same volume as the original voxel (see Fig. 14-4, *D*). The CT numbers of the cuberilles represent the average of the original voxel CT numbers surrounding each of the new voxels. Isotropic voxels 0.24 mm in size can be achieved. Creation of these new cuboidal voxels allows the image to be reconstructed in any plane without loss of resolution by locating the position of each voxel in space relative to one another. In constructing the three-dimensional CT image, only cuberilles representing the surface of the object scanned are displayed on the monitor. The surface formed by these cuberilles, either solid or partially transparent, is made to appear as if illuminated by a light source located behind the viewer (Fig. 14-7). In this manner, the visible surface of each pixel is assigned a gray-level value, depending on its distance from and orientation to the light source. Thus, pixels that face the light source or are closer to it appear brighter than pixels that are turned away from the source or are farther away. After construction, three-dimensional CT images may be manipulated further by rotation around any axis to display the structure imaged from any angle. Also, external surfaces of the image can be removed electronically to reveal concealed deeper anatomy.

ARTIFACTS

Different types of artifacts may degrade CT images. Partial volume artifact occurs because a voxel has finite dimensions. When a voxel contains tissues of differing densities (e.g., bone and soft tissue), the resulting CT number for that voxel is an intermediate value that does not represent either tissue. The resulting image may be a blurring of the junction of the tissues or a loss of part of a thin cortical layer of bone. Beam-hardening artifact results by the preferential absorption of lower energy photons in the heterogeneous x-ray beam. Because the distance through the center of the head is longer than along a path closer to the surface, there is beam hardening seen as darkening in the middle of an axial slice. Software algorithms may minimize this artifact. Metal streaking

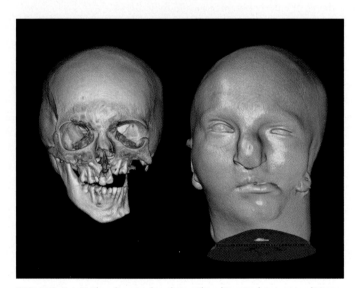

FIGURE 14-7 Three-dimensional rendering. Three-dimensional images can be reconstructed from the cuberilles, thresholded for bone *(left)* or soft tissue *(right)*, oriented in any arbitrary direction, and made to appear to have depth by highlighting structures near the front and shadowing structures near the back. This patient has hemifacial microsomia and demonstrates incomplete development of the left frontal, sphenoid, temporal maxillary, zygomatic, and mandibular bones. Note also the reduced size of the left orbit, depression of the tip of the nose, missing and incompletely erupted left maxillary teeth, deviation of the right mandible to the left, sunken left midface, and malformation of the left ear. *(Images courtesy Dr. P.-L. Westesson, University of Rochester, NY).*

artifacts occur because of the near-complete absorption of x-ray photons by metallic restorations. They appear as opaque streaks in the occlusal plane (see Figs. 14-6, *B*, and 14-7).

CONTRAST AGENTS

Contrast agents are substances used to improve visualization of structures. CT imaging frequently uses iodine, administered intravenously, to enhance soft tissue and vascular image detail. The iodine in the contrast medium has a large atomic number and

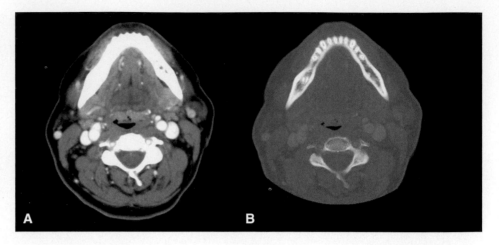

FIGURE 14-8 Contrast agents. Iodine may be administered intravenously to enhance blood vessels and structures with a rich vascular supply, including the periphery of some tumors. **A,** CT image through the mandible in the soft tissue window and after administration of iodine. Note prominent great vessels lying just anterior and lateral to the cervical vertebrae and muscles of the floor of the mouth and neck. **B,** The same axial slice displayed in the bone window. Note the presence of fine detail in the mandible and cervical spine, such as cortical and cancellous bone and teeth, including their pulp chambers, but loss of soft tissue contrast.

effectively absorbs x rays (Fig. 14-8). Malignant facial tumors often are more vascularized than surrounding normal tissues; thus, the presence of the iodine perfusing these tissues increases their radiographic density and makes their margins more detectable. Contrast medium also helps to visualize enlarged lymph nodes containing metastatic carcinoma. However, contrast dye can be toxic to the kidneys in elderly patients with kidney disease.

APPLICATIONS

CT imaging is useful for diagnosing and determining the extent of a wide variety of infections, osteomyelitis, cysts, benign and malignant tumors, and trauma in the maxillofacial region. The ability of CT imaging to display fine bone detail makes it an ideal modality for lesions involving bone. Three-dimensional CT imaging has been applied to trauma cases and craniofacial reconstructive surgery and has been used for treatment of both congenital and acquired deformities. The availability of data in a three-dimensional format also has allowed the construction of life-sized models that can be used for trial surgeries and the construction of surgical stents for guiding dental implant placement and for the creation of accurate implanted prostheses.

MAGNETIC RESONANCE IMAGING

Lauterbur described the first MR image in 1973, and Mansfield further developed use of the magnetic field and the mathematical analysis of the signals for image reconstruction. MR imaging was developed for clinical use around 1980, and Lauterbur and Mansfield were awarded the Nobel Prize in Physiology or Medicine in 2003.

To make an MR image, the patient is first placed inside a large magnet. This magnetic field causes the nuclei of many atoms in the body, particularly hydrogen, to align with the magnetic field. The scanner directs a radiofrequency (RF) pulse into the patient, causing some hydrogen nuclei to absorb energy (resonate). When the RF pulse is turned off, the stored energy is released from the body and detected as a signal in a coil in the scanner. This signal is used to construct the MR image—in essence, a map of the distribution of hydrogen.

MR imaging has the particular advantages of being noninvasive, using nonionizing radiation, and making high-quality images of soft tissue resolution in any imaging plane. Disadvantages of MR imaging include high cost, long scan times, and the fact that various metals in the imaging field either distort the image or may move into the strong magnetic field, injuring the patient.

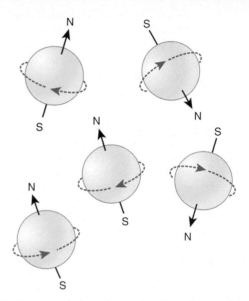

FIGURE 14-9 Magnetic dipoles. Hydrogen nuclei within a patient normally have randomly oriented dipoles and thus no net magnetic vector.

PROTONS

Individual protons and neutrons (nucleons) in the nuclei of all atoms possess a spin, or angular momentum. In nuclei having equal numbers of protons and neutrons, the spin of each nucleon cancels that of another, producing a net spin of zero. However, nuclei containing an unpaired proton or neutron have a net spin. Because spin is associated with an electrical charge, a magnetic field is generated in nuclei with unpaired nucleons, causing these nuclei to act as magnets with north and south poles (magnetic dipoles) and having a magnetic moment. The most common of these atoms, the MR active nuclei, are hydrogen, carbon 13, nitrogen 15, oxygen 17, fluorine 19, sodium 23, and phosphorus 31. Hydrogen is the most abundant of these atoms in the body.

A hydrogen nucleus consists of a single unpaired proton and therefore acts as a magnetic dipole. Normally, these magnetic dipoles are randomly oriented in space (Fig. 14-9). When an external magnetic field is applied, the hydrogen nuclear axes align in the direction of the magnetic field (Fig. 14-10). Two states are possible: **spin-up**, which parallels the external magnetic field, and **spin-down**, which is antiparallel with the field. Because more energy is required to align antiparallel with the magnetic field, antiparallel hydrogen nuclei are considered to be at a higher energy state than hydrogen nuclei aligned parallel with the field. Nuclei prefer to be in a lower energy state, and usually more are aligned parallel with the magnetic field. This situation results in a net magnetization vector in the direction of the magnetic field. Increasing the magnetic field strength increases the magnitude of the net magnetization vector.

PRECESSION

The magnetic moments of hydrogen nuclei in a magnetic field do not align exactly with the direction of the magnetic field. Instead, the orientations of the axes of spinning protons actually oscillate with a slight tilt from a position absolutely parallel with the flux of the external magnet (Fig. 14-11). This tilting of the spin axis,

called precession, is similar to a spinning toy top, which rotates around an upright position as it slows down. Similarly, the presence of the magnetic field causes the axis of the spinning proton to wobble (or precess) around the lines of the applied magnetic field (Fig. 14-12). The rate or frequency of precession is called the precessional frequency, resonance frequency, or Larmor frequency. The precessional frequency depends on the species of nucleus (i.e., hydrogen nucleus or other) and is proportional to the strength of the external magnetic field. The magnetic field in an MR scanner is provided by an external permanent magnet. MR field strengths range from 0.1 to 4 Tesla (T) with 1.5 T being the most common (1.5 T is about 30,000 times the strength of the earth's magnetic field). The Larmor precession frequency of hydrogen is 63.86 MHz in a magnetic field of 1.5 T. Other MR active nuclei precess at different frequencies in the same magnetic field.

RESONANCE

Nuclei can be made to undergo transition from one energy state to another by absorbing or releasing energy. Energy required for transition from the lower to the higher energy level can be supplied

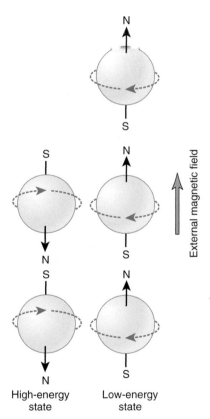

FIGURE 14-10 Hydrogen nuclei in an external magnetic field. In the presence of an applied strong external magnetic field, most nuclei are in the lower energy state and are aligned parallel with the magnetic field, whereas others align in the higher energy state antiparallel to the magnetic field.

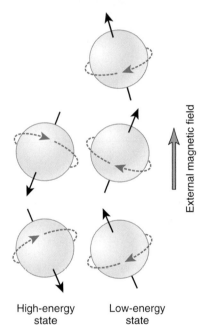

FIGURE 14-11 Hydrogen nuclei in an external magnetic field. The magnetic dipoles are not aligned exactly with the external magnetic field. Instead, the axes of spinning protons actually oscillate or wobble with a slight tilt from being absolutely parallel with the flux of the external magnet.

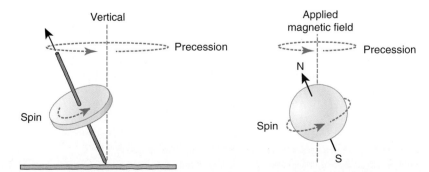

FIGURE 14-12 Precession. Much as a top rotates around a vertical axis when spinning, the spin axis of a spinning hydrogen nucleus rotates around the direction of the external magnetic field. This movement is called precession, and the rate or frequency of precession is called the precessional, resonance, or Larmor frequency. The Larmor frequency depends on the strength of the external magnetic field and is specific for the nuclear species.

by electromagnetic energy in the RF portion of the electromagnetic spectrum. In an MR imaging scanner, the RF broadcast from an antenna coil is directed to tissue with protons (hydrogen nuclei) aligned in the Z axis (long axis of a patient) by the external static magnetic field (Fig. 14-13). When the frequency of the RF pulse matches the Larmor frequency of the protons in the tissue, the protons resonate and absorb the RF energy. This absorbance causes some of the low-energy nuclei (parallel) to gain energy to convert to the high-energy (antiparallel) state. As a consequence, the longitudinal magnetic vector is reduced. The longer the RF pulse is applied, the less the longitudinal magnetic vector. The RF pulse also causes the protons to precess in phase with each other, resulting in a net tissue magnetization vector in the transverse plane (XY plane) perpendicular to longitudinal alignment (Z axis) (Fig. 14-14).

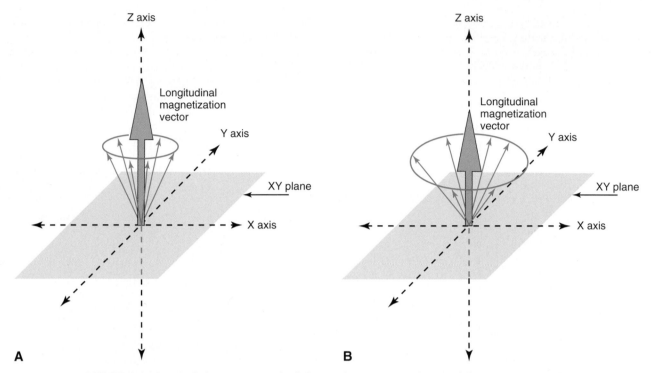

FIGURE 14-13 Longitudinal magnetic vector. When hydrogen nuclei are in an external magnetic field, two energy states result: spin-up, which is parallel to the direction of the field, and spin-down, which is antiparallel to the direction of the field. **A,** The combined effect of these two energy states is a weak net magnetic moment, or magnetization vector parallel with the applied magnetic field. **B,** When the frequency of the RF pulse matches the Larmor frequency, the protons absorb the RF energy causing some low-energy nuclei to convert to the high-energy state, reducing the net longitudinal magnetic vector (vertical black arrow in Z axis).

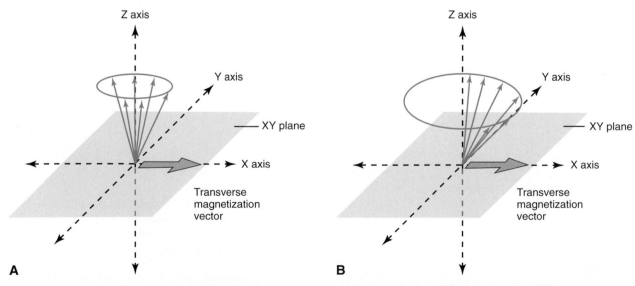

FIGURE 14-14 Transverse magnetic vector. **A,** RF pulse also causes the protons to precess in phase with each other, resulting in a net tissue magnetization vector in the transverse plane (XY plane). **B,** Increasing the intensity and duration RF of the pulse increases the transverse magnetization vector because the nuclei are more nearly in phase (horizontal black arrow in X axis).

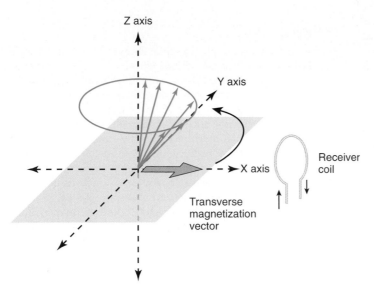

Z axis

Y axis

X axis

Receiver coil

Transverse magnetization vector

FIGURE 14-15 Receiver coil. The precession of the net transverse magnetic vector in the XY plane induces a current flow in a receiver coil, the MR signal. The frequency of this induced alternating current signal matches the frequency of the RF pulse and the Larmor precessional frequency of hydrogen nuclei.

If the RF pulse is of sufficient intensity and duration, the longitudinal magnetic vector is reduced to zero. An RF pulse that accomplished this is called a 90-degree RF pulse or having a flip angle of 90 degrees. At this time, the net magnetic vector in the transverse plane is maximized because the magnetic moments of all nuclei are in phase.

MAGNETIC RESONANCE SIGNAL

The precession of the net magnetic vector—that is, the precession of the magnetic moments of the hydrogen nuclei in phase in the transverse plane—induces a current flow in a receiver coil (Fig. 14-15), the MR signal. The frequency of this alternating current signal matches the frequency of the RF pulse and the Larmor precessional frequency of hydrogen nuclei. The magnitude of this signal is proportional to the overall concentration of hydrogen nuclei (proton density) in the tissue. This strength of the signal also depends on the degree to which hydrogen is bound within a molecule. Tightly bound hydrogen atoms, such as hydrogen atoms present in bone, do not align themselves with the external magnetic field and produce only a weak signal. Loosely bound or mobile hydrogen atoms, such as those in soft tissues and liquids, react to the RF pulse and produce a detectable signal at the end of the RF pulse. The concentration of loosely bound hydrogen nuclei available to create the signal is referred to as the proton density or spin density of the tissue in question. The higher the concentration of these nuclei of loosely bound hydrogen atoms, the stronger the net transverse magnetization, the more intense the recovered signal, and the brighter the corresponding part of the MR image.

When the RF pulse is turned off, the nuclei begin to return to their original lower energy spin state, a condition called relaxation. As they give up the energy absorbed by the RF pulse, some of the high-energy nuclei return to the low-energy state, and the net longitudinal magnetic vector returns to its original state. Additionally, and independently, the individual magnetic moments of the protons begin to interact with each other and dephase. This dephasing results in reduction of the magnetization in the transverse plane, a condition called decay. As a result of the loss of transverse magnetization and the dephasing of the hydrogen nuclei, there is a loss of intensity of the MR signal. The reduced voltage induced in the receiving coil is called the free induction

Tissue Type	T1 Time (ms)	T2 Time (ms)
Fat	240–250	60–80
Bone marrow	550	50
White matter of cerebrum	780	90
Gray matter of cerebrum	920	100
Muscle	860–900	50
CSF (similar to water)	2200–2400	500–1400

TABLE 14-2   T1 and T2 Relaxation Times in a Main Field of 1.5 Tesla

CSF, Cerebrospinal fluid.

decay signal. The free induction decay of the MR signal results from the loss of the transverse net magnetization vector; this results from return of the net magnetization vector to the longitudinal plane and dephasing of the hydrogen nuclei.

T1 AND T2 RELAXATION

Relaxation at the end of the RF pulse results in recovery of the longitudinal magnetization; this is accomplished by a transfer of energy from individual hydrogen nuclei (spin) to the surrounding molecules (lattice). This is an exponential process, and the time required for 63% of the net magnetization to return to equilibrium (the time constant) by this transfer of energy is called the T1 relaxation time or spin-lattice relaxation time. The T1 relaxation time varies with different tissues and reflects the ability of their nuclei to transfer their excess energy to surrounding molecules (Table 14-2). Tissues with a high fluid content, such as cerebrospinal fluid (CSF), tend to have long T1 times because the high inherent energy of water inhibits the transfer of energy from excited hydrogen nuclei. However, tissues with a high fat content, such as bone marrow, tend to have short T1 times reflecting the low inherent energy of fat and the relative ease by which energy is transferred from excited hydrogen nuclei.

Additionally, at the end of the RF pulse, the magnetic moments of adjacent hydrogen nuclei begin to interfere with one another, causing the nuclei to dephase with a resultant loss of transverse magnetization. The time constant that describes the exponential rate of loss of transverse magnetization is called the T2 relaxation time or the spin-spin relaxation time. As the transverse magnetization rapidly decays to zero, so does the amplitude and duration of the detected radio signal. T2 relaxation occurs more rapidly than T1 relaxation. Similar to T1 times, T2 times are also a feature of the tissues being examined. Fatty tissues have short T2 relaxation times, whereas tissues containing more fluid have long T2 relaxation times. The closely packed molecular structure of fat results in more potent dephasing interactions between adjacent hydrogen nuclei compared with the spaced molecular arrangement of water.

RADIOFREQUENCY PULSE SEQUENCES (AND IMAGE CONTRAST)

The components of the RF pulse sequence are set by the operator and determine the appearance of the resultant image. The most basic features of a pulse sequence are the repetition time (TR) and echo time (TE). The TR is the duration between repeat RF pulses (Fig. 14-16). The time between pulse repetitions determines the amount of T1 relaxation that has occurred at the time the signal is collected. The TE is the time after application of the RF pulse when the MR signal is read. It controls the amount of T2 relaxation that has occurred when the signal is collected. There are many sequences that can be used to emphasize various features of the tissues being examined.

TISSUE CONTRAST

Image contrast between tissues is governed both by intrinsic features of the tissues, including the proton density and T1 and T2 times of the issues being imaged, and by extrinsic parameters of a given pulse sequence, such as the TR and TE, which can be adjusted to emphasize those features. For instance, a tissue that has a high proton density and strong transverse magnetization vector (protons precessing in phase) at TE produces a strong MR signal that appears bright on an MR image. Conversely, a tissue with a low proton density or low transverse magnetization vector at TE produces a weak signal and appears dark on an MR image.

T1-Weighted Image

A T1-weighted image emphasizes differences in T1 values of tissues (Fig. 14-17, A); this is accomplished by use of short TR (typically 300 to 700 ms) and short TE (20 ms). In such images, tissues with short T1 times, such as fat, appear bright, whereas tissues with long T1 times, such as CSF (water), appear dark. T1-weighted images are more commonly used to demonstrate anatomy.

T2-Weighted Image

A T2-weighted image emphasizes differences in T2 values of tissues (Fig. 14-17, B); this is accomplished by use of long TR (2000 ms) and long TE (typically ≥60 ms). In such images, tissues with long T2 times, such as CSF or temporomandibular joint (TMJ) fluid, appear bright, whereas tissues with short T2 times, such as fat, appear dark. Images with T2 weighting are most commonly used for identifying pathology because pathologic tissue usually contains more water than surrounding tissues, owing to inflammation.

There are many pulse sequences varying the strength and timing of the RF pulses that emphasize or suppress various tissues in the resultant images. Techniques such as turbo spin echo and gradient echo allow images to be captured rapidly. Other techniques allow the signal from fat or water to be enhanced or suppressed. A technique called fat saturation, seen commonly in short tau inversion recovery (STIR) sequences, minimizes the signal from fat allowing improved visualization of adjacent structures. Similarly, fluid attenuated inversion recovery (FLAIR) sequences minimize the signal from fluid, allowing for better visualization of pathology adjacent to the CSF.

Contrast Agents

Contrast agents, most commonly gadolinium, may be administered intravenously to improve tissue contrast (Fig. 14-17, C). Gadolinium is not imaged itself, but rather it shortens the T1 relaxation times of enhancing tissues, making them appear brighter. Tissues that enhance include normal tissues, such as vessels with slow-flowing blood, sinus mucosa, and muscle. Pathologic tissues often enhance allowing them to be better differentiated from surrounding normal tissue. Pathologic tissues include tumors, infections, inflammations, and posttraumatic lesions. For imaging the head and neck, it is common practice to obtain T1 images, T1 images after gadolinium administration and with fat saturation, and T2 images with fat saturation. There is more recent evidence that gadolinium-based contrast media could be a cause of a debilitating disease called nephrogenic systemic fibrosis in some patients with renal dysfunction. The implications of this finding are under active study.

SCANNER GRADIENTS

To generate an image, an MR signal must be collected from a discrete slice of tissue in the patient. Image production is accomplished by using three gradient coils within the bore of the imaging magnet oriented in the X (left to right), Y (anterior to posterior), and Z (head to toe) planes. The intensity of the magnetic field

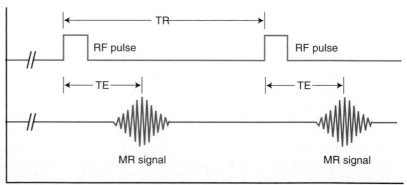

FIGURE 14-16 RF pulse sequences. The most basic features of a pulse sequence are the TR, the replication time, the duration between repeat RF pulses, and the TE, the echo time, the time after application of the RF pulse when the MR signal is read. TR determines the amount of T1 relaxation that has occurred at the time the signal is collected, whereas TE controls the amount of T2 relaxation that has occurred when the signal is collected.

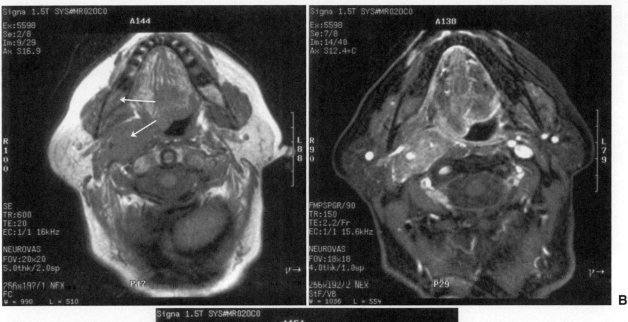

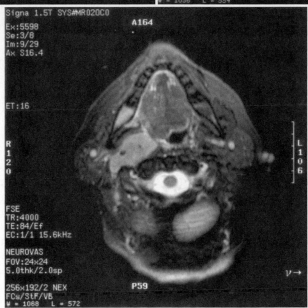

FIGURE 14-17 MR images. MR imaging examination performed to evaluate a neck mass in a patient with a known diagnosis of multiple myeloma. **A,** Axial T1 precontrast (no fat saturation) image through the mandible. Note abnormally dark marrow in the posterior right mandible (*upper arrow,* compare with left side) and mass in the right carotid space (*lower arrow*). **B,** Axial T1 postcontrast image with fat saturation. Note abnormal enhancement of the mass in the right carotid space. **C,** Axial T2 with fat saturation demonstrating an abnormally bright signal in both the marrow in the right mandible and the mass in the right carotid space. *(Courtesy Dr. Thomas Underhill, Radiology Associates, Richmond, VA.)*

surrounding a patient may be modified with these gradient coils. When one of the coils is turned on, it creates a gradient in the intensity of the magnetic field. Thus, in a 1.5 T scanner, when the Z-axis gradient is turned on, the strength of the magnetic field at the head might be 1.4 T and at the toe might be 1.6 T. When this gradient field is applied, the precessional frequency of hydrogen nuclei varies linearly along the magnetic gradient. When an RF pulse is applied, only nuclei precessing at the same frequency as the applied signal resonate; this allows selecting the desired slice of tissue along the patient's long axis (Z gradient). The slope of the gradient applied and the bandwidth of the RF pulse determine the thickness of this slice. The location of the signal within the X and

Y (transverse) planes of the selected longitudinal plane is derived by switching off the Z-gradient coil followed by rapidly turning on the X-gradient and then the Y-gradient coils (phase encoding and frequency encoding, respectively). This sequence alters the phase and precessional frequencies of the nuclei in the selected slice. The resulting MR signal from the patient is read out while the frequency-encoding gradient is applied. The signal from the patient contains many frequencies that are decomposed by the fast Fourier transform into amplitude and frequency. This information, which reflects the number of hydrogen nuclei and their T1 and T2 properties at each X and Y location in the selected longitudinal plane, is reconstructed into MR images.

MAGNETIC RESONANCE IMAGES

MR imaging has several advantages over other diagnostic imaging procedures. First, it offers the best contrast resolution of soft tissues. Although x-ray attenuation coefficients of soft tissues may vary by no more than 1%, T1 and T2 relaxation times may vary by up to 40%. Second, no ionizing radiation is involved with MR imaging. Third, because the region of the body imaged in MR imaging is controlled with the gradient coils, direct multiplanar imaging is possible without reorienting the patient.

Disadvantages of MR imaging include relatively long imaging times and the potential hazard imposed by the presence of ferromagnetic metals in the vicinity of the imaging magnet. This latter disadvantage excludes from MR imaging any patient with implanted metallic foreign objects or medical devices that consist of or contain ferromagnetic metals (e.g., cardiac pacemakers, some cerebral aneurysm clips, or ferrous foreign bodies in the eye). The strong magnetic fields may harm patients if they move these objects, cause excessive heating, or induce strong electrical currents. Gold and stainless steel are considered to be ferromagnetic, whereas nickel, titanium, amalgam restorations, and silver-palladium are not. Metals used in dental restorations or orthodontics do not move but may significantly distort the image in their vicinity. Accordingly, archwires and any removable appliances should be removed before scanning. Stainless steel brackets and bands should be checked to ensure that they are well cemented and, if so, may be left in place unless they interfere with the region of the image being examined. Titanium implants cause only minor local image degradation. Finally, some patients have claustrophobia when positioned in an MR imaging machine.

APPLICATIONS

Because of its excellent soft tissue contrast resolution, MR imaging is useful in evaluating soft tissue conditions, such as the position and integrity of the disk in the TMJ (Fig. 14-18); evaluating soft tissue disease, especially neoplasia involving the soft tissues, such as tongue, cheek, salivary glands, and neck; determining malignant involvement of lymph nodes; and determining perineural invasion by malignant neoplasia. In cases of osteomyelitis, it may be used to visualize edematous changes in the fatty marrow as well as the surrounding soft tissue. It also may be useful in identifying the location of the mandibular nerve in cases where it is not clearly seen on panoramic or CBCT images. A technique known as sweep imaging with Fourier transform (SWIFT) has proved useful in revealing the extent of penetration of carcinoma into the cortex of the mandible. Similar to CT imaging, a contrast agent such as gadolinium can be added to enhance the image resolution of neoplasia (Fig. 14-19). Also, it is customary to remove the high signal of surrounding fat tissue (fat suppression) to enhance the appearance of the neoplasm. A typical protocol would include T1 images, T1 images after gadolinium (with fat suppression), and T2 images (with fat suppression). More recently, high-resolution SWIFT MR images of the dentition have been made with a 4 T system (Fig. 14-20). Although currently in the research phase, this method holds promise for future clinical use for dental imaging without ionizing radiation.

MR angiography is used to visualize the blood flowing through vessels. Although there are multiple pulse sequences that produce bright images of the vessels, most techniques currently use gadolinium as an intravenous contrast agent. MR angiography is mostly used to image arteries, including in the head and neck, to examine for occlusion, aneurysms, or arteriovenous malformation (Fig. 14-21).

NUCLEAR MEDICINE

Film radiography, CT imaging, MR imaging, and diagnostic ultrasonography are morphologic imaging techniques in that each requires a macroscopic anatomic change for information to be recorded by an image receptor. However, in some human diseases, abnormal biochemical processes occur without anatomic change. Radionuclide imaging (a form of functional imaging) provides a means of assessing such physiologic change. Nuclear medicine examinations are commonly used to assign function of the brain, thyroids, heart, lungs, and gastrointestinal system as well as for diagnosis and follow-up of metastatic disease, bone tumors, and infection (Fig. 14-22).

Radionuclide imaging uses radioactive atoms or molecules that emit γ (gamma) rays. These atoms behave in an organism in a manner comparable to their stable counterparts because they are chemically indistinguishable. Radionuclides allow measurement of tissue function in vivo and provide an early marker of disease through measurement of biochemical change. After the radionuclides are administered, they distribute in the body according to their chemical properties. The gamma camera detects γ rays and forms planar images showing the locations of the radionuclides in the body. Single photon emission computed tomographic (SPECT) imaging and PET imaging are advanced nuclear medicine techniques that form tomographic views. More recently, molecular imaging of individual gene expression is being performed in the laboratory. As with CT imaging, iterative reconstruction techniques improve the diagnostic quality of the images.

RADIONUCLIDES

The ideal radionuclide has a short half-life, emits γ rays but no charged particles, and is capable of binding to various pharmaceuticals. Although many gamma-emitting isotopes are used in radionuclide imaging, including iodine (^{131}I), gallium (^{67}Ga), and selenium (^{74}Se), the most commonly used is technetium 99m (^{99m}Tc). ^{99m}Tc has a half-life of 6 hours and emits primarily 140 keV photons. As technetium pertechnetate, ^{99m}Tc mimics iodine distribution when injected intravenously and is concentrated by the salivary and thyroid glands and gastric mucosa. When it is attached to various carrier molecules, it can be used to examine virtually every organ of the body.

To image bone, ^{99m}Tc is typically bound to methylene diphosphonate (MDP), and a dose of 20 to 30 mCi (740 to 1110 megabecquerels [MBq]) is injected intravenously. Immediately after injection, the tracer distributes intravascularly. Images made during this flow phase, the first 60 to 90 seconds, are called radionuclide angiography. In the second, or blood pool, phase, the tracer quickly moves into the extracellular space. The third, or bone scintigraphy, phase, is made 2 to 3 hours after injection. The MDP deposition in the skeleton depends both on osteoblastic activity and on blood flow (see Fig. 14-22). Images made 2 to 3 hours after injection show most of the tracer activity in the skeleton, kidneys, and bladder. Most metastatic tumors in bone induce formation of new bone and may be detected on such an examination.

Radionuclide-labeled tracers are used in quantities well below amounts that are lethal to cells. However, although radionuclide imaging is considered noninvasive, the radiation dose the patient receives as a result of intravenous injection of radionuclide-labeled tracers should be considered. Injection of 740 MBq of ^{99m}Tc pertechnetate delivers a whole-body radiation dose of 2 mGy. This quantity is less than the average annual effective dose resulting from natural radiation (see Chapter 3).

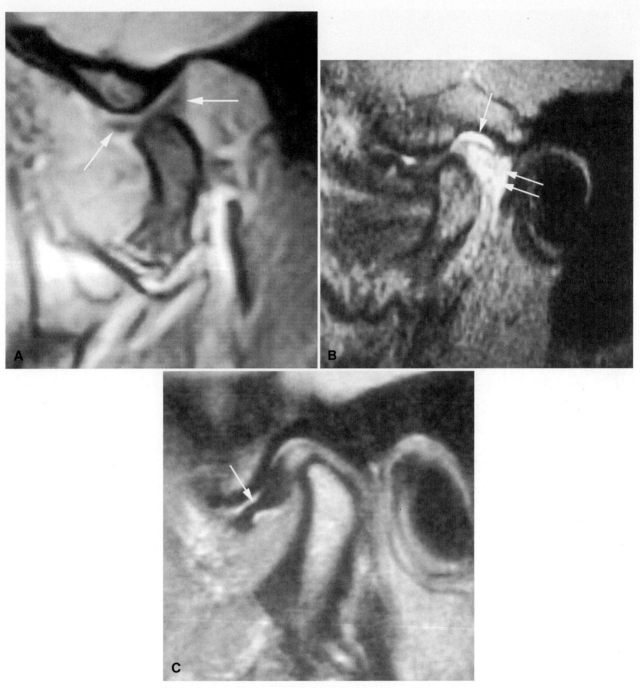

FIGURE 14-18 MR imaging of TMJ. **A,** T1-weighted MR image of the TMJ. In this image, the jaw is partly open, as indicated by the location of the condyle relative to the articular eminence. The articular disk, which has a "bow tie" appearance *(arrows)*, is in a normal position relative to the translating condyle. **B,** T2-weighted MR image of the TMJ illustrates both inflammatory effusion into the superior joint space *(arrow)* and hyperemia caused by increased vasculature in the retrodiskal tissues *(double arrows)*. **C,** In this proton or spin density MR image of the TMJ, the disk is anteriorly displaced *(arrow)*, with the posterior band in the 9 o'clock position relative to the condylar head. (**B** and **C,** *Courtesy Richard Harper, DDS, Dallas, TX.*)

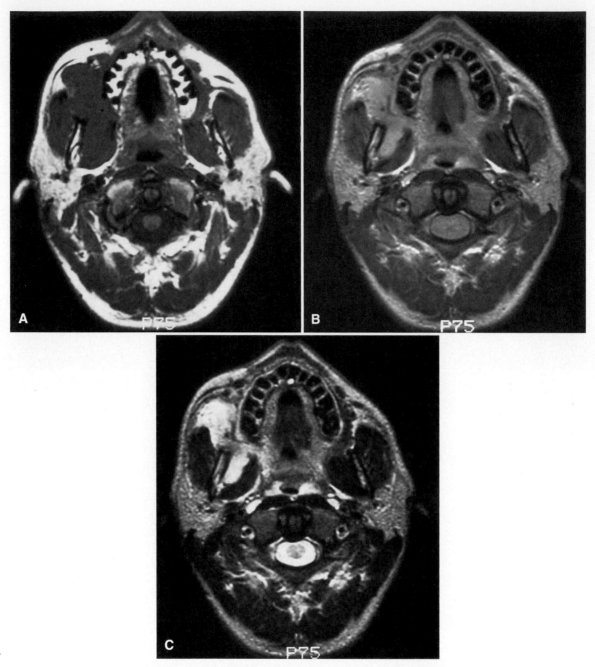

FIGURE 14-19 Gadolinium enhancement of MR image. **A,** Axial T1 MR image of a rhabdomyosarcoma involving the soft tissues of the right face. The tumor cannot be distinguished from the adjacent masseter and pterygoid muscles because both have the same tissue signal. **B,** Axial T1 postgadolinium MR image. The tumor now has a brighter signal (lighter) than the adjacent muscles because of its greater vascularity, enhanced by gadolinium. **C,** Axial T2 MR image. The tumor has a brighter signal than adjacent muscles because of greater fluid content of the tumor.

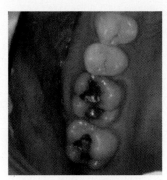

Photograph

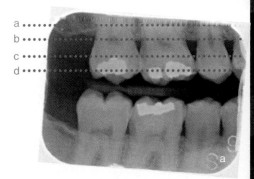

2D
Radiograph

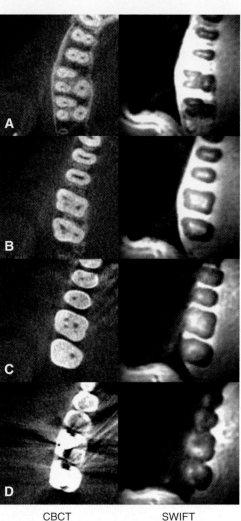

A

B

C

D

CBCT   SWIFT

FIGURE 14-20   4T SWIFT MR images of dentition. In these in vivo images, the four dotted lines drawn on the bitewing radiograph and labeled *a* through *d* indicate the location of the axial slices of the corresponding CBCT and SWIFT MR images. Note the lack of metallic artifact on the MR images compared with the CBCT image at level *d*. *(From Idiyatullin D, Corum C, Moeller S, et al: Dental magnetic resonance imaging: making the invisible visible, J Endod 37:745–752, 2011.)*

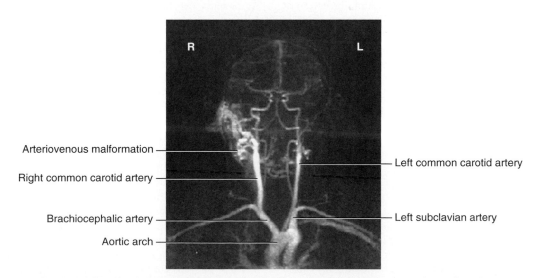

FIGURE 14-21   MR angiography of the head and neck. This image, made with gadolinium as a contrast agent, demonstrates an arteriovenous malformation in the region of the right face. Note the widened carotid artery and rich vasculature supply in the right midfacial region. This is a maximum intensity image made from a stack of individual slices. *(Image courtesy Dr. Susan White, UCLA School of Dentistry.)*

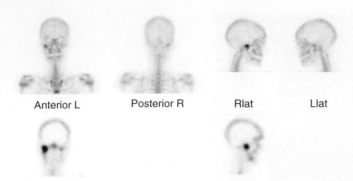

FIGURE 14-22 Radionuclide image with increased uptake of ^{99m}Tc-MDP in the region of the right TMJ. The planar images in the top row were captured with a gamma camera. The lower two tomographic images were captured with SPECT imaging.

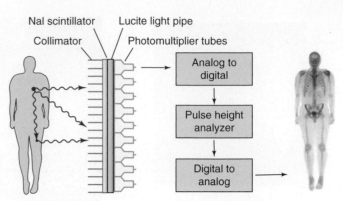

FIGURE 14-23 Gamma camera. The principal components of a gamma camera are a collimator to limit γ rays to rays perpendicular to the surface of the camera, a sodium iodide scintillator to absorb the γ rays and emit a flash of visible light, an acrylic (Lucite) light pipe to conduct the visible light flash, photomultiplier tubes to count the flashes of light and measure their energy, a pulse height analyzer to select only flashes from the administered radionuclide, and a monitor to display the resultant image. γ rays traveling parallel to the plates in the collimator pass through the collimator and contribute to the image. γ rays traveling obliquely are absorbed by the collimator and do not contribute to the image. The photon resulting from Compton scattering in the leg is rejected by the pulse height analyzer and does not contribute to the image. This image is an anterior view of a patient after intravenous injection of ^{99m}Tc-MDP.

GAMMA CAMERA

Gamma cameras (also called Anger cameras and scintillation cameras) are the most common means of forming an image (Fig. 14-23). These cameras capture photons and convert them to light and then to a voltage signal. This signal is reconstructed to a planar image that shows the distribution of the radionuclide in the patient. The first part of the gamma camera is a collimator. It absorbs γ rays that do not travel parallel to the plates, improving image resolution. The γ rays that pass through the collimator strike a scintillation crystal. This crystal, often made of sodium iodide with trace amounts of thallium, fluoresces when it absorbs γ rays. These flashes of light are detected by an array of photomultiplier tubes coupled to the crystal with light pipes. The photomultiplier tubes capture the flash and amplify the signal. The size of the signal is proportional to the energy of the absorbed photon. The signals from the photomultiplier tubes go through an analog-to-digital converter and then to a pulse height analyzer. This device detects the intensity of the signal, and thus the energy of the incident absorbed photons, and uses only photons from the radionuclide when forming the final image. Many of the γ rays released from the radionuclide in the patient undergo Compton absorption at some distant site and result in a new scattered photon. If these scattered, lower energy photons pass through the collimator of the gamma camera, they may degrade image resolution. However, these scattered photons are detected by the pulse height analyzer and are rejected so that they do not contribute to the image. Gamma cameras have a spatial resolution of 3 to 5 mm. Use of a scintillation crystal for acquisition of data for image formation has led to the labeling of this technique as scintigraphy.

SINGLE PHOTON EMISSION COMPUTED TOMOGRAPHIC IMAGING

SPECT imaging is a method of acquiring tomographic slices through a patient (Fig. 14-24). Most gamma cameras have SPECT imaging capability. In this technique, either a single or a multiple gamma camera is rotated 360 degrees around the patient. Image acquisition takes about 30 to 45 minutes. The acquired data are processed by filtered back-projection and, more recently, iterative reconstruction algorithms, to form numerous contiguous axial slices, similar to CT imaging by x ray. These data can be used to construct multiplanar images of the study area (see Fig. 14-24, C). Tomography enhances contrast and removes superimposed activity. SPECT images have been fused with CT images more recently

to improve identification of the location of the radionuclide (see Fig. 14-24, E).

Applications

The most common use of nuclear medicine in the maxillofacial region is to investigate abnormal metabolic bone activity, for instance, in assessing growth activity in cases of condylar hyperplasia and presence of metastatic lesions. Traditionally, a combination of ^{99m}Tc MDP and gallium citrate was used to help diagnose osteomyelitis, but CT imaging is now used more frequently. SPECT images are used to assess mandibular growth in patients with asymmetry and extent of bisphosphonate-induced osteonecrosis in the jaws (Fig. 14-25) and provide prognostic information for patients with cancer and osteonecrosis of the jaws.

POSITRON EMISSION TOMOGRAPHIC IMAGING

PET imaging is a more advanced imaging modality in nuclear medicine. PET imaging, which is reported to have a sensitivity nearly 100 times that of a gamma camera, relies on positron-emitting radionuclides generated in a cyclotron. The utility of PET imaging is based not only on its sensitivity but also on the fact that the most commonly used radionuclides (^{11}C, ^{13}N, ^{15}O, ^{18}F) are isotopes of elements that occur naturally in organic molecules. Although fluorine does not technically fit into this category, it is a chemical substitute for hydrogen. These radionuclides are used as is or, more commonly, incorporated into a radiopharmaceutical such as glucose or amino acids by use of a medical cyclotron. After the radiopharmaceutical is injected into the patient, the isotope distributes within the body tissue according to the carrier molecule and emits a positron. This positron interacts with a free electron and mutual annihilation occurs, resulting in the production of two 551-keV photons emitted at 180 degrees to each other. The PET scanner consists of a ring of many detectors in a circle around the patient (Fig. 14-26). The detector crystals are often made of bismuth germinate. Electronically coupled opposing detectors simultaneously identify the pair of γ photons using coincidence detection

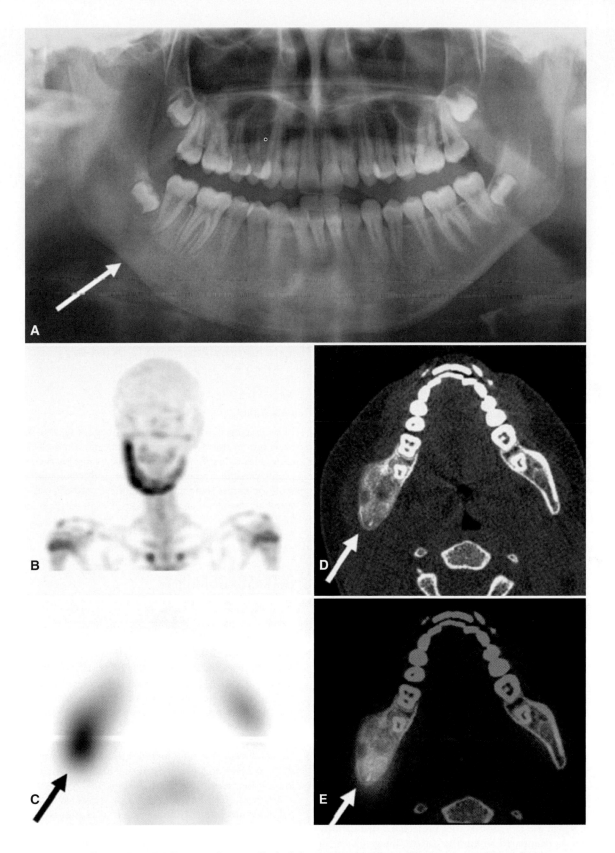

FIGURE 14-24 SPECT/CT imaging of a 14-year-old girl with chronic osteomyelitis of the mandible. **A,** Panoramic view demonstrating expansion and sclerosis of the right mandible *(arrow)*. **B,** Planar radionuclide image showing uptake throughout the mandible and especially on the right side. **C,** SPECT axial image showing increased activity in the posterior regions of both sides of the mandible and especially on the right side *(arrow)*. **D,** CT axial image at the same level as the image in **C**. Note periosteal expansion and lytic areas in the right mandible *(arrow)*. **E,** SPECT/CT fusion image demonstrating the area of greatest activity in the right mandible *(arrow)*. *(Modified from Strobel K, Merwald M, Huellner MW, et al: [Importance of SPECT/CT for resolving diseases of the jaw] [in German]. Radiologe 52:638–645, 2012.)*

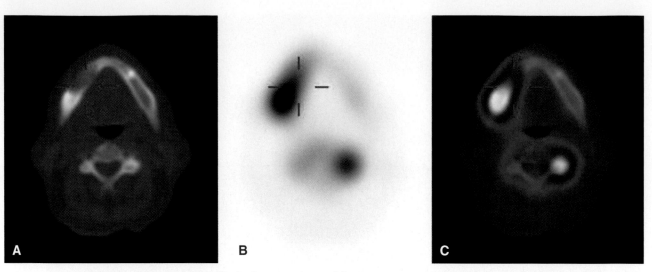

FIGURE 14-25 SPECT image of bisphosphonate osteonecrosis of the jaw in a woman with breast cancer treated with zoledronic acid for 2 years because of a metastatic lesion to C2. **A,** Axial CT image demonstrating bisphosphonate-associated osteonecrosis of the jaw (BRONJ) in the left mandible that is mostly lytic but also sclerotic more posteriorly. **B,** SPECT image showing extensive deposition of ^{99m}Tc pertechnetate in the left body of the mandible and region of right articular surface of C2. **C,** Fusion image demonstrating isotope uptake most extensive in the sclerotic (posterior) portion of the BRONJ lesion and in the sclerotic metastatic lesion in C2. *(Images courtesy Dott.ssa Franca Dore, Azienda Ospedaliero-Universitaria Trieste.)*

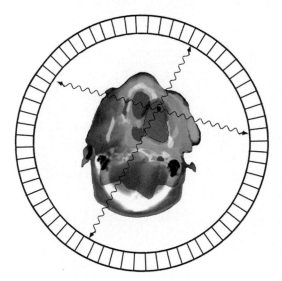

FIGURE 14-26 PET scanner consists of a ring of detectors that measure pairs of 511 keV γ rays traveling in opposite directions from positron annihilation. Each pair is recorded simultaneously; thus, the location of the radionuclide can be determined as the intersection of the pairs of detectors recording simultaneous events. The location of the common source of the radionuclide is readily determined as the intersection of the flight paths of the γ rays.

circuits that measure events within 10 to 20 ns. Thus, the annihilation event is known to have occurred along the line joining the two detectors. Raw PET scan data consist of many of these coincidence lines, which are reorganized into projections that identify where isotope is concentrated within the patient. Image quality in PET scans has been improved in recent years using time-of-flight techniques. The time-of-flight methods measure the slight difference in the arrival times of the two γ photons at the detectors and use this information to determine the location of positron annihilation along the path. The spatial resolution of a PET scanner is about 5 mm.

Applications

PET imaging is useful in skeletal imaging for assessing primary bone tumors, locating metastases in bone, and detecting osteomyelitis. Fluorodeoxyglucose (FDG) is a radiopharmaceutical commonly used for studying glucose use in the brain and heart and to look for cancer metastases. PET images are often fused with CT scans to facilitate anatomic localization of radionuclide (Fig. 14-27). The PET/CT combination has been shown to be quite helpful in staging and treatment planning of squamous cell carcinoma in the head and neck.

ULTRASONOGRAPHY

Sonography is a technique based on sound waves that acquires images in real time without the use of ionizing radiation. The phenomenon perceived as sound is the result of periodic changes in the pressure of air against the eardrum. The periodicity of these changes ranges from 1500 to 20,000 Hz. By definition, ultrasound has a periodicity greater than 20 kHz, which is greater than the audible range. Diagnostic ultrasonography (or sonography), the clinical application of ultrasound, uses vibratory frequencies in the range of 1 to 20 MHz.

Scanners used for sonography generate electrical impulses that are converted into ultra-high-frequency sound waves by a transducer, a device that can convert one form of energy into another—in this case, electrical energy into sonic energy. The most important component of the transducer is a thin piezoelectric crystal or material made up of a great number of dipoles arranged in a geometric pattern. A dipole may be thought of as a distorted molecule that appears to have a positive charge on one end and a negative charge on the other. The most widely used piezoelectric material is lead zirconate titanate. The electrical impulse generated by the scanner causes the dipoles in the crystal to realign themselves with the electric field and to change the crystal's thickness suddenly. This abrupt change begins a series of vibrations that produce the sound waves that are transmitted into the tissues being examined.

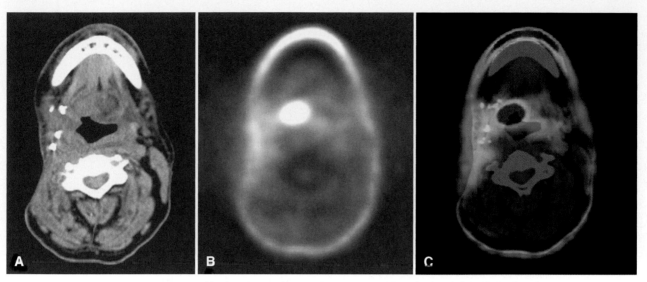

FIGURE 14-27 PET scan and fused PET/CT scan. This patient has a known recurrent carcinoma at the base of the tongue. **A,** Soft tissue algorithm CT image at the level of the inferior border of the mandible. The four metallic objects on the patient's right side posterior to the mandible represent vascular clips from prior surgery. **B,** FDG-PET scan showing an oval-shaped region of high metabolic activity of tumor at the right tongue base. The FDG activity in the anterior mandible is related to low-level metabolic activity in the vicinity of a reconstruction plate. **C,** Fused images **A** and **B** demonstrating the region of high metabolic activity superimposed on the CT anatomy. The intensity of the FDG activity has been color-coded with red being the highest intensity and purple being the lowest. Images were acquired on a combined PET/CT scanner. *(Courtesy Dr. Todd W. Stultz, Cleveland Clinic, OH.)*

The transducer emitting ultrasound is held against the body part being examined. The ultrasonic beam passes through or interacts with tissues of different acoustic impedance. Sonic waves that reflect (echo) toward the transducer cause a change in the thickness of the piezoelectric crystal, which produces an electrical signal that is amplified, processed, and ultimately displayed as an image on a monitor. Typically, the transducer serves as both a transmitter and a receiver. Current techniques permit echoes to be processed at a sufficiently rapid rate to allow perception of motion; this is referred to as **real-time imaging**.

The ultrasound signal transmitted into a patient is attenuated by a combination of absorption, reflection, refraction, and diffusion. The higher the frequency of the sound waves, the higher the image resolution, but the less the penetration of the sound through soft tissue. The fraction of the beam that is reflected to the transducer depends on the acoustic impedance of the tissue, which is a product of its density (and the velocity of sound through it) and the beam's angle of incidence. Because of its acoustic impedance, a tissue has a characteristic internal echo pattern. Consequently, not only can changes in echo patterns distinguish between different tissues and boundaries, but they also can be correlated with pathologic changes within a tissue. Tissues that do not produce signals, such as fluid-filled cysts, are said to be **anechoic** and appear black. Tissues that produce a weak signal are **hypoechoic**, whereas tissues that produce intense signals, such as ligaments, skin, or needles or catheters, are **hyperechoic** and appear bright. Thus, interpretation of sonograms relies on knowledge of both the physical properties of ultrasound and the anatomy of the tissues being scanned.

Ultrasonography is used in the head and neck region for evaluation of neoplasms in the thyroid, parathyroid, salivary glands, or lymph nodes; stones in salivary glands or ducts; Sjögren's syndrome, and the vessels of the neck, including the carotid artery for atherosclerotic plaques (Figs. 14-28 and 14-29). Ultrasonography is

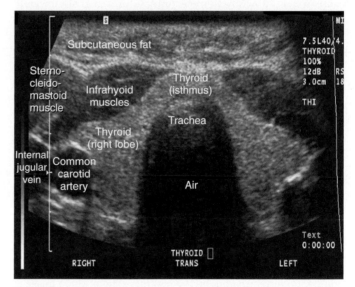

FIGURE 14-28 Ultrasound examination (transverse section) of a healthy thyroid gland. This image shows glandular, muscular, adipose, and vascular tissues because of the different acoustic impedance of these tissues. *(Courtesy Dr. Christos Angelopoulos, Columbia University, College of Dental Medicine, NY.)*

also used to guide fine-needle aspiration in the neck. More recent advances include three-dimensional imaging to allow multiplanar reformatting, surface renderings (e.g., of a fetal face), and color Doppler sonography for evaluation of blood flow.

CONVENTIONAL TOMOGRAPHY

Conventional tomography is a radiographic technique, usually using film, designed to image a slice or plane of tissue. This

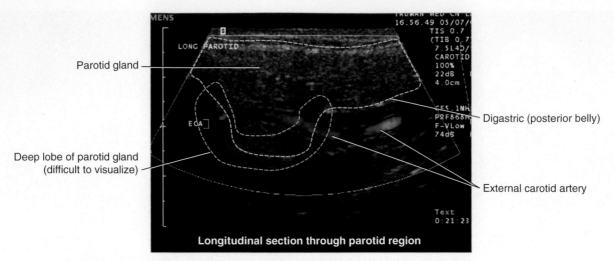

Longitudinal section through parotid region

Parotid gland

Deep lobe of parotid gland (difficult to visualize)

Digastric (posterior belly)

External carotid artery

FIGURE 14-29 Doppler ultrasound examination. Longitudinal section through the parotid gland, including the deep lobe, and posterior belly of digastric muscle. With Doppler ultrasound, the transducer records small changes in the direction of blood flow. In this image, the external carotid artery is coded red where blood flows toward the transducer and blue where it moves away from the transducer. *(Courtesy Dr. Christos Angelopoulos, Columbia University, College of Dental Medicine, NY.)*

imaging is accomplished by blurring the images of structures lying outside the plane of interest through the process of motion "unsharpness." Since the introduction of CT imaging, MR imaging, and cone-beam imaging, which have superior contrast resolution, film-based tomography has been used less frequently. When conventional tomography is used in dentistry, it is applied primarily to high-contrast anatomy, such as that encountered in TMJ and dental implant imaging.

Conventional tomography uses an x-ray tube and radiographic film rigidly connected and capable of moving about a fixed axis or fulcrum (Fig. 14-30). The examination begins with the x-ray tube and film positioned on opposite sides of the fulcrum, which is located within the body's plane of interest (focal plane). As the exposure begins, the tube and film move in opposite directions simultaneously through a mechanical linkage. With this synchronous movement of tube and film, the images of objects located within the focal plane (at the fulcrum) remain in fixed positions on the radiographic film throughout the length of tube and film travel and are clearly imaged. The images of objects located outside the focal plane have continuously changing positions on the film; as a result, the images of these objects are blurred beyond recognition by motion unsharpness. The resulting zone of sharp image is called the tomographic layer. Blurring of overlying structures is greatest (and the tomographic layer the thinnest) under the following circumstances:

- Overlying structures lie far from the focal plane.
- The focal plane lies far from the film.
- The long axis of the structure to be blurred is oriented perpendicular to the direction of tube travel.
- The distance of tube travel is large.

There are at least five types of tomographic movement: linear, circular, elliptic, hypocycloidal, and spiral (Fig. 14-31). Mechanically, the simplest tomographic motion is linear. More complex movements, such as circular, elliptic, hypocycloidal, and spiral, produce images without streaking artifacts common to the linear movements. Many of the more expensive panoramic units are capable of making tomographic sections of the jaws (Fig. 14-32).

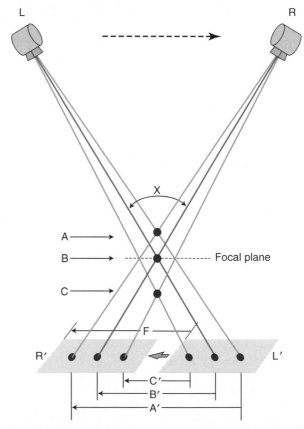

FIGURE 14-30 Tomographic techniques. As the x-ray tube moves from left to right, the film moves in the opposite direction. In this figure, points *A* and *C* lie outside the focal plane (the plane that contains the fulcrum), whereas object *B* lies at the center of tube/film movement. Only objects that lie in the focal plane (i.e., *B*) remain in sharp focus because the image of *B* moves exactly the same distance (*B'*) as the film travels (*F*), and thus its image remains stationary on the film. The image of point *A* moves more than the film (distance *A'*) and the image of point *C* moves less than the film (distance *C'*); therefore, the images of both are blurred. *X* is the tomographic angle. The greater the tomographic angle, the thinner the tomographic layer.

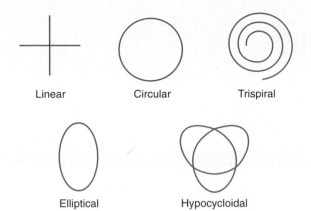

Linear	Circular	Trispiral

Elliptical	Hypocycloidal

FIGURE 14-31 Tomographic movements. Linear movements, either vertical or horizontal, are mechanically simple but result in streaking artifacts. More complex motions result in fewer streaking artifacts and sharper images.

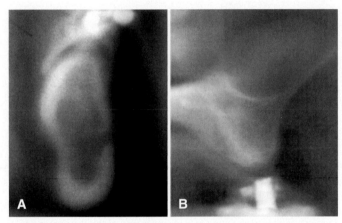

FIGURE 14-32 Linear tomographic images made by panoramic unit. **A,** Mandibular tomogram in the region of the mental foramen. **B,** Maxillary tomogram in the premolar region acquired with an Orthopantomograph OP 100 panoramic unit (Instrumentarium Dental, Tuusula, Finland). Note the dome-shaped opacity in the floor of the maxillary sinus consistent with a mucous retention phenomenon. (**B,** Courtesy Brad Potter, DDS, Augusta, GA.)

BIBLIOGRAPHY

Computed Tomography

Bononmo L, Foley D, Imhof H, et al: *Multidetector computed tomography technology: advances in imaging techniques*, London, 2003, Royal Society of Medicine Press.

Bushberg JT, Seibert JA, Leidholdt EM Jr, et al: *The essential physics of medical imaging*, ed 3, Baltimore, 2012, Lippincott Williams & Wilkins.

Buzug TM: *Computed tomography: from photon statistics to modern cone-beam CT*, Berlin, 2008, Springer.

Fishman EK, Jeffrey RB Jr: *Multidetector CT: principles, techniques, and clinical applications*, Philadelphia, 2004, Lippincott Williams & Wilkins.

Kalender W: *Computed tomography: fundamentals, systems technology, image quality, applications*, ed 2, Erlangen, 2005, Publicis Corporate Publishing.

Knollmann F, Coakley FV: *Multislice CT: principles and protocols*, Philadelphia, 2006, Saunders.

Marchal G, Vogl TJ, Heiken JP, et al: *Multidetector-row computed tomography*, Milan, 2005, Springer.

Magnetic Resonance Imaging

Blink EJ: An easy introduction to basic MRI physics for anyone who does not have a degree in physics: http://mri-physics.net/.

Bushberg JT, Seibert JA, Leidholdt EM Jr, et al: *The essential physics of medical imaging*, ed 3, Baltimore, 2012, Lippincott Williams & Wilkins.

Bushong SC: *Magnetic resonance imaging: physical and biological principles*, ed 3, St Louis, 2003, Mosby.

Elison JM, Leggitt VL, Thomson M, et al: Influence of common orthodontic appliances on the diagnostic quality of cranial magnetic resonance images, *Am J Orthod Dentofacial Orthop* 134:563–572, 2008.

Idiyatullin D, Corum C, Moeller S, et al: Dental magnetic resonance imaging: making the invisible visible, *J Endod* 37:745–752, 2011.

Kendi AT, Khariwala SS, Zhang J, et al: Transformation in mandibular imaging with sweep imaging with fourier transform magnetic resonance imaging, *Arch Otolaryngol Head Neck Surg* 137:916–919, 2011.

Patel A, Bhavra GS, O'Neill JR: MRI scanning and orthodontics, *J Orthod* 33:246–249, 2006.

Tutton LM, Goddard PR: MRI of the teeth, *Br J Radiol* 75:552–562, 2002.

Weishaupt D, Koechli DC, Marincek B: *How does MRI work? An introduction to the physics and function of magnetic resonance imaging*, ed 2, Berlin, 2008, Springer.

Westbrook C, Roth CK, Talbot J: *MRI in practice*, ed 4, Oxford, 2011, Wiley-Blackwell.

Nuclear Medicine

Christian P, Waterstram-Rich KM: *Nuclear medicine and PET/CT: technology and techniques*, ed 7, St Louis, 2011, Mosby.

Dore F, Filippi L, Biasotto M, et al: Bone scintigraphy and SPECT/CT of bisphosphonate-induced osteonecrosis of the jaw, *J Nucl Med* 50:30–35, 2009.

Hutton BF: Recent advances in iterative reconstruction for clinical SPECT/PET and CT, *Acta Oncol* 50:851–858, 2011.

Krasny A, Krasny N, Prescher A: Anatomic variations of neural canal structures of the mandible observed by 3-tesla magnetic resonance imaging, *J Comput Assist Tomogr* 36:150–153, 2012.

Lois C, Jakoby BW, Long MJ, et al: An assessment of the impact of incorporating time-of-flight information into clinical PET/CT imaging, *J Nucl Med* 51:237–245, 2010.

Mettler FA, Guiberteau MJ: *Essentials of nuclear medicine*, ed 6, Philadelphia, 2012, Saunders.

Schiepers C: *Diagnostic nuclear medicine*, ed 2, Berlin, 2006, Springer.

Sharp PF, Gemmell HG, Murray AD: *Practical nuclear medicine*, ed 3, London, 2005, Springer-Verlag.

Van den Wyngaert T, Huizing MT, Fossion E, et al: Prognostic value of bone scintigraphy in cancer patients with osteonecrosis of the jaw, *Clin Nucl Med* 36:17–20, 2011.

Wilson MA: *Nuclear medicine*, Philadelphia, 1998, Lippincott-Raven.

Ultrasound

Emshoff R, Bertram S, Strobl H: Ultrasonographic cross-sectional characteristics of muscles of the head and neck, *Oral Surg Oral Med Oral Pathol Oral Radiol Endod* 87:93–106, 1999.

Goldman LW, Fowlkes JB, editors: *Categorical course in diagnostic radiology physics: CT and US cross-sectional imaging*, Oak Brook, IL, 2000, RSNA Publications.

Kremkau FW: *Sonography: principles and instruments*, ed 8, St Louis, 2010, Saunders.

Middleton WD, Kurtz AB, Hertzberg BA: *Ultrasound: the requisites*, ed 2, St Louis, 2004, Mosby.

Rumack CM, Wilson SR, Charboneau JW, et al: *Diagnostic ultrasound*, ed 4, Philadelphia, 2011, Mosby.

Shimizu M, Okamura K, Yoshiura K, et al: Sonographic diagnostic criteria for screening Sjögren's syndrome, *Oral Surg Oral Med Oral Pathol Oral Radiol Endod* 102:85–93, 2006.

Tempkin B: *Ultrasound scanning: principles and protocols*, ed 3, St Louis, 2009, Saunders.

15 Quality Assurance and Infection Control

OUTLINE

A quality assurance program in radiology is a series of procedures designed to ensure optimal and consistent operation of each component in the imaging chain. When all components are functioning properly, the result is consistently high-quality radiographs made with low exposure to patients and office personnel.

The goal of an infection control program in radiology is to avoid cross-contamination among patients and between patients and the dental staff in the course of imaging.

RADIOGRAPHIC QUALITY ASSURANCE

Because radiographs are indispensable for patient diagnosis, the dentist must ensure that optimal exposure and film processing conditions are maintained. To reach this goal, a quality assurance program includes evaluation of the performance of x-ray machines, manual and automatic film processing procedures, image receptors, and viewing conditions. Optimization of all steps in the imaging chain results in the most diagnostic images and the lowest exposure for patients. Examples of common faults in digital sensor handling are provided in Chapter 4, and problems with film processing are presented in Chapter 5. To minimize these problems, it is best if one individual is given the responsibility for implementing the quality assurance program and for taking corrective action when indicated. Most of these tasks refer to film processing. Using digital sensors greatly simplifies these tasks. Most of these steps are quickly accomplished, yet they can have a significant influence on radiographic quality (Box 15-1).

DAILY TASKS

Several tasks should be performed daily to ensure excellent radiographs.

Compare Film Radiographs with Reference Film

One of the most common causes of poor film radiographs is poor processing in the darkroom, in particular, the use of depleted solutions. A simple and effective means for constant monitoring of the quality of images produced in an office is to check daily films against a reference film. Soon after film processing solutions are replaced, a patient film that has been properly exposed and

processed with exact time-temperature technique is mounted on a corner of the viewbox. This image, with optimal density and contrast, serves as a reference for the radiographs made in the following days and weeks (Fig. 15-1). All subsequent images should be compared with this reference film.

Comparison of daily images with the reference film may reveal problems before they interfere with the diagnostic quality of the images. When a problem is identified, it is important to determine the probable source and to take corrective action. For instance, if the processing solutions have become depleted, the resultant radiographs are light and have reduced contrast. Both developer and fixer should be changed when degradation of the image quality is evident. Light images may also result from cold solutions or insufficient developing time. Dark images may be caused by excessive developing time, developer that is too warm, or light leaks.

There are two methods that are more accurate than a reference film but require additional equipment and more time to perform. These are use of a sensitometer and densitometer and the use of a step wedge.

Sensitometer and Densitometer

The most accurate and rigorous method of testing film processing solutions is to use a sensitometer and densitometer. A sensitometer exposes film to a calibrated light pattern. After processing, a densitometer is used to measure the optical density of each step in the test pattern of the film exposed by the sensitometer. A change in the density readings from day to day indicates a problem in the darkroom.

Enter Findings in Retake Log

Another simple and effective means of reducing the number of faulty radiographs is to keep a retake log. All errors for images that must be reexposed are recorded. This process quickly reveals the source of recurring problems.

Replenish Processing Solutions

At the beginning of each work day, the levels of the processing solutions should be checked and replenished if necessary. The developer is replenished with fresh developing solution, and the fixer is replenished with fresh fixing solution.

BOX 15-1 Schedule of Radiographic Quality Assurance Procedures

DAILY

- Check processing by comparing radiographs with reference film, step wedge, or sensitometry and densitometry
- Enter causes of retakes in a log
- Replenish processing solutions
- Check temperature of processing solutions
- Run larger roller transport clean-up film through automatic processor

WEEKLY

- Replace processing solutions
- Clean processing equipment
- Clean viewboxes
- Review retake log

MONTHLY

- Examine photostimulable phosphor plates for scratches
- Check darkroom safelighting and for light leaks
- Clean intensifying screens
- Rotate film stock
- Check exposure charts
- Inspect leaded aprons and thyroid collars for damage such as cracks or tears

YEARLY

- Verify digital sensors with quality assurance apparatus
- Calibrate x-ray machine

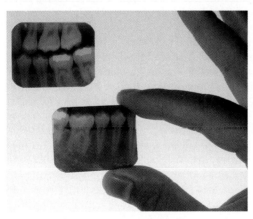

FIGURE 15-1 Radiographs should be checked daily against a reference film made with fresh solutions. As processing solutions become exhausted, the daily images become increasingly light and lose contrast. When these changes are apparent, both the developer and the fixer should be changed.

Check Temperature of Processing Solutions

At the beginning of each work day, the temperature of the processing solutions should be checked. The solutions must reach the optimal temperature before use—68°F (20°C) for manual processing and 82°F (28°C) for heated automatic processors. The instructions accompanying the film and processor verify the optimal temperature. Unheated automatic processors should be located away from windows or heaters that may cause their temperature to vary during the day. Proper temperature regulation is required for accurate time-temperature processing.

WEEKLY TASKS

Replace Processing Solutions

How frequently processing solutions are replaced depends primarily on the rate of use of the solutions but also on the size of tanks, whether a cover is used, and the temperature of the solutions. In most offices, the solutions should be changed weekly or every other week. The results of the step-wedge test help determine the proper frequency.

Clean Processing Equipment

Regular cleaning of the processing equipment is necessary for optimal operation. The solution tanks of manual and automatic processing equipment should be cleaned when the solutions are changed. The rollers of automatic film processors should be cleaned weekly according to the manufacturer's instructions. After cleaning, the tanks and rollers should be rinsed twice as long as the manufacturer recommends to prevent the cleaner from interfering with the action of the film processing solutions.

Clean Viewboxes

Viewboxes should be cleaned weekly to remove any particles or defects that may interfere with film interpretation.

Review Retake Log

The retake record should be reviewed weekly to identify any recurring problems with film processing conditions or operator technique. This information can be used to educate staff or to initiate corrective actions.

MONTHLY TASKS

Photostimulable Phosphor Plates

Photostimulable phosphor (PSP) plates may become scratched in the course of use. These scratches may be seen as light streaks on processed images (see Fig. 4-22, *A*). Plates should be inspected monthly for such defects and removed from service when such defects are found.

Check Darkroom Safelighting

Film becomes fogged in the darkroom because of inappropriate safelight filters, excessive exposure to safelights, and stray light from other sources. These films are dark, show low contrast, and have a muddy gray appearance. The darkroom should be inspected monthly to assess the integrity of the safelights (preferably GBX-2 filters with 15-watt bulbs). The glass filter should be intact, with no cracks. To check for light leaks in a darkroom, all lights are turned off; the individual allows his or her vision to accommodate to the dark and checks for light leaks, especially around doors and vents. Light leaks should be marked with chalk or masking tape. Weather stripping is useful for sealing light leaks under doors.

Clean Intensifying Screens

All intensifying screens in panoramic and cephalometric film cassettes should be cleaned monthly. The presence of scratches or debris results in recurring light areas on the resultant images. The foam supporting the screens must be intact and capable of holding both screens closely against the film. If close contact between the film and screens is not maintained, the image loses sharpness.

Rotate Film Stock

Dental x-ray film is quite stable when it is properly handled. X-ray film should be stored in a cool, dry facility away from a radiation source. Stock should be rotated when new film is received so that old film does not accumulate in storage. The oldest film always should be used first but never after its expiration date.

Check Exposure Charts

Each month, inspection should be done of exposure tables listing the proper peak kilovoltage (kVp), milliamperes (mA), and exposure times for making radiographs of each region of the oral cavity that are posted by each x-ray machine (Fig. 15-2). One should verify that the information is legible and accurate. These tables help ensure that all operators use the appropriate exposure factors. Typically, the mA is fixed at its highest setting; the kVp is fixed, usually at 70 kVp; and the exposure time is varied to account for patient size and location of the area of interest in the mouth.

Exposure times are initially determined empirically. In the case of PSP plates and digital sensors, one should start by using the exposure times suggested by the manufacturer. Exposure times are slowly and systematically reduced to the point that image degradation is noticed. With film, careful time-temperature processing (described in Chapter 5) must be used with fresh solutions during this initial determination of exposure times.

Check Leaded Aprons and Collars

Leaded aprons and collars should be visually inspected for evidence of cracking. A fluoroscopic examination performed by a qualified individual can confirm any cracks in the lead shielding. These items should be replaced as necessary. Cracking is usually caused by folding the shields when not in use. It can be minimized by hanging the aprons from a hook or draping them over a handrail.

YEARLY TASKS

Digital Sensors

Digital sensors and PSP plates should also be checked yearly for signs of image degradation. Failing sensors may reveal loss of sensitivity, contrast resolution, or spatial resolution. Phantoms designed for this purpose are available to aid in such testing (Fig. 15-3).

Calibrate X-Ray Machine

When a new x-ray machine is purchased, state regulations require that it be installed by a qualified expert. When in use, x-ray machines are generally quite stable, and only rarely is a malfunction of the machine the cause of poor radiographs. X-ray machines need to be calibrated annually only, unless a specific problem is identified or substantive repair is necessary that may affect operation. Usually, dental service companies or health physicists should make these machine measurements because of the specialized equipment and knowledge required. The following parameters should be measured:

1. X-ray output. A radiation dosimeter should be used to measure the intensity and reproducibility of radiation output (Fig. 15-4). Acceptable values are shown in Figure 3-3.
2. Collimation and beam alignment. The field diameter for dental intraoral x-ray machines should be no greater than $2\frac{3}{4}$ inches. The tip of the position-indicating device (PID), or aiming cylinder, should be closely aligned with the x-ray beam. For panoramic machines, the beam exiting the patient should not be larger than the film slit holding the film cassette; this may be tested by taping dental films in front of and behind the slit. A pin stick should be made through both films to allow subsequent realignment. Both films are exposed, processed, and realigned. The exposure to the film in front of the slit should be comparable in size to the film exposure behind the slit. Service is required if the front film exposure is larger than or not well oriented with the film exposure behind the slit.
3. Beam energy. The kVp or half-value layer (HVL) of the beam should be measured to ensure that the beam has sufficient energy for film exposure without excessive soft tissue dosage. Measurement of kVp requires specialized equipment. It should be accurate within 5 kVp. Measurement of HVL requires a dosimeter. The HVL should be at least 1.5 mm aluminum (Al) at 70 kVp and 2.5 mm Al at 90 kVp.
4. Timer. Electrical pulse counters count the number of pulses generated by an x-ray machine during a preset time interval. The timer should be accurate and reproducible.
5. mA. The linearity of the mA control should be verified if two or more mA settings are available on the machine. An exposure using the usual adult bitewing setting is made. The mA is then reduced to the lower value, and another exposure time is selected, ensuring that the product of the mA and time in seconds (impulses) is the same as for the adult bitewing. For example, if the machine has 10-mA and 15-mA settings, and 15 mA and 24 impulses are used for adult bitewings, one should select 15 mA and 24 impulses for the first exposure and measure the dose. A second exposure is made at 10 mA and 36 impulses, and the dose is measured. The dose at each exposure

X-Ray Machine: (Brand name)
Location: (Room)
mA: 15
kVP: 70
Sensor: (Brand name)

Projection	Exposure time	
	Seconds	Impulses
Adult periapicals		
Incisors	0.25	15
Premolars	0.30	18
Molars	0.35	21
Occlusal	0.40	24
Adult bitewings		
Premolar	0.30	18
Molar	0.35	21
Edentulous periapicals		
Incisors	0.20	12
Premolars	0.25	15
Molars	0.30	18
Occlusal	0.35	21
Children		
Anterior periapicals	0.25	15
Posterior periapicals	0.25	15
Bitewing	0.25	15
Occlusal	0.30	18

FIGURE 15-2 Sample wall chart showing identification information for x-ray machine, sensor or film type, mA and kVp settings, and appropriate exposure times for various anatomic locations and patient sizes. The optimal exposure times must be determined empirically in each office because they vary with the machine settings used, source-to-skin distance, and other factors.

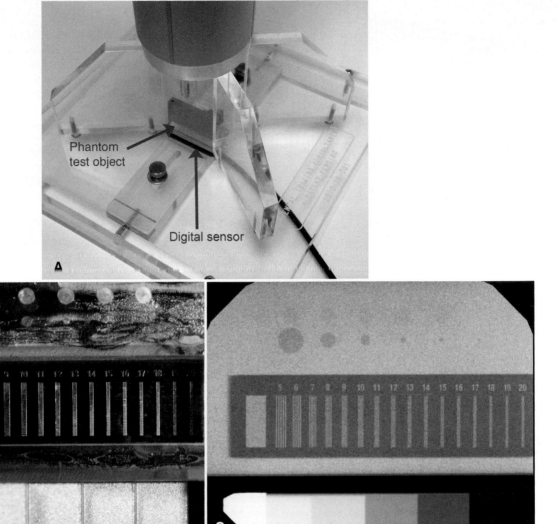

FIGURE 15-3 Phantom for measuring image quality performance of digital dental x-ray systems. **A,** Plastic stand allows positioning of the aiming tube of the x-ray machine over the test device, which is positioned over the digital sensor. **B,** Test device contains, from the top, two rows of wells of varying diameter and depth in an acrylic background for measuring contrast detail, an etched pattern of slits in a metallic background for measuring the spatial resolution in line pairs per millimeter, and a calibrated step wedge for measuring dose response. **C,** Resulting image. *(Images courtesy Dr. Peter K. Mah: www.dentalimagingconsultants.com.)*

combination should be the same ($15 \times 24 = 10 \times 36$). A discrepancy implies nonlinearity in the mA control or a fault in the timer. The step wedge described previously may also be used in place of the dosimeter. In this case, the density of each step of each image should be the same.

6. Tube head stability. The tube head should be stable when placed around the patient's head, and it should not drift during the exposure. When the tube head is unstable, service is necessary to adjust the suspension mechanism.

7. Focal spot size. Measure the size of the focal spot because it may become enlarged with excessive heat buildup within an x-ray machine. An enlarged focal spot contributes to geometric fuzziness in the resultant image. A specialized piece of equipment is required for this test.

INFECTION CONTROL

Dental personnel and patients are at increased risk for acquiring tuberculosis, herpes viruses, upper respiratory infections, and hepatitis strains A through E. After the recognition of acquired immunodeficiency syndrome (AIDS) in the 1980s, rigorous hygienic procedures were introduced in dental offices. The primary goal of infection control procedures is to prevent cross-contamination and disease transmission from patient to staff, from staff to patient, and from patient to patient. The potential for cross-contamination in dental radiography is great. In the course of making radiographs, an operator's hands become contaminated by contact with a patient's mouth and saliva-contaminated films and film holders. The operator also must adjust the x-ray tube head and x-ray

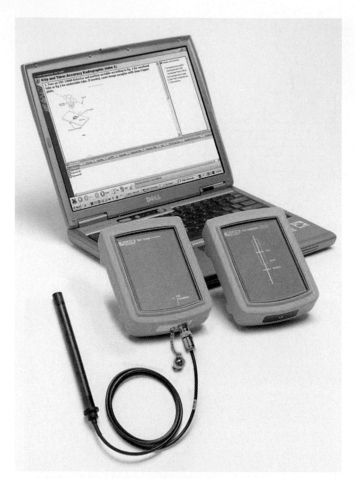

FIGURE 15-4 Device for measuring exposure output of an x-ray machine. The probe on the left is intended to be included in a phantom to measure cone-beam computed tomographic exposure. The aiming cylinder of an intraoral dental x-ray machine may be positioned over the center of the device on the right, and an exposure may be made. These units measure average and maximum kVp, dose, dose rate, HVL, and exposure time in seconds or pulses. *(Image courtesy Fluke Biomedical: www.flukebiomedical.com.)*

BOX 15-2   Key Steps in Radiographic Infection Control

- Apply standard precautions
  - Wear gloves during all radiographic procedures
  - Disinfect and cover x-ray machine, working surfaces, chair, and apron
  - Sterilize nondisposable instruments
  - Use barrier-protected film (sensor) or disposable container
  - Prevent contamination of processing equipment

---

machine control panel settings to make the exposure. These actions lead to the possibility of cross-contamination. Cross-contamination also may occur when an operator handles digital sensors or opens film packets to process the films in the darkroom. The procedures described in the following sections minimize or eliminate such cross-contamination (Box 15-2). Each dental office or practice should have a written policy describing its infection control practices. It is best if one individual in a practice, usually the dentist, assumes responsibility for implementing these procedures. This person also educates other members of the practice.

STANDARD PRECAUTIONS

Standard precautions (sometimes called universal precautions) are infection control practices designed to protect workers from exposure to diseases spread by blood and certain body fluids including saliva. Under standard precautions, all human blood and saliva are treated as if known to be infectious for human immunodeficiency virus (HIV) and hepatitis B virus. Accordingly, the means used to protect against cross-contamination are used for all individuals. The American Dental Association (ADA) and the U.S. Centers for Disease Control and Prevention (CDC) stress the use of standard precautions because many patients are unaware that they are carriers of infectious disease or choose not to reveal this information.

Wear Gloves during All Radiographic Procedures

Gloves are a critical factor in preventing contamination between a patient and staff member. After the patient is seated, the practitioner should wash his or her hands and put on disposable gloves in sight of the patient if the operatory arrangement permits. The practitioner should always wear gloves when making radiographs or handling contaminated film packets or associated materials such as cotton rolls and film-holding instruments or when removing barrier protections from surfaces and radiographic equipment. Staff should also wear personal protective equipment such as eyewear, a mask, or face shield if exposure to bodily fluids is anticipated.

Disinfect and Cover Clinical Contact Surfaces

Clinical contact surfaces are surfaces that might be touched by gloved hands or instruments that go into the mouth. These include the x-ray machine and control panel, chair-side computer, beam alignment device, dental chair and headrest, leaded apron, thyroid collar, and surfaces on which film is placed. The CDC classifies these as noncritical items. These are objects that may come in contact with saliva, blood, or intact skin but not oral mucous membranes. The goal of preventing cross-contamination is addressed in part by disinfecting all such surfaces and by using barriers to isolate equipment from direct contact. Barriers made of clear plastic wrap should be changed when damaged and routinely after each patient.

Barriers should cover working surfaces that were previously cleaned and disinfected. Barriers protect the underlying surface from becoming contaminated. An effective barrier for the countertops and x-ray control console is plastic wrap, which may be conveniently stored in a butcher's paper dispenser mounted on a wall. When covering the x-ray control console, the operator should be sure to include the exposure switch and the exposure time control if they are integral parts of the unit (Fig. 15-5). An x-ray exposure switch that is separate from the console should be covered with a sandwich bag or food storage bag or wrapped with plastic wrap.

The dental chair headrest, headrest adjustments, and chair back may be easily covered with a plastic bag (Fig. 15-6). The x-ray tube head, PID, and yoke should be covered while they are still wet with disinfectant with a barrier to stop any dripping (Fig. 15-7). The bag should be secured by tying a knot in the open end or by placing a heavy rubber band over the x-ray tube head just proximal to the swivel. Also, the leaded apron should be cleaned, disinfected, and covered between patients because it is frequently contaminated with saliva as the result of handling (readjusting its position) during a radiographic procedure. The apron should be suspended on a heavy coat hanger to permit turning front to back.

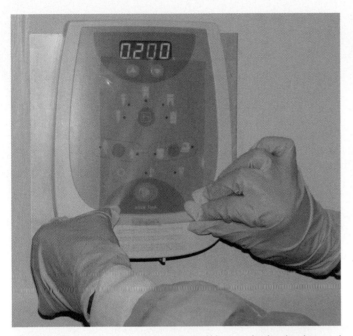

FIGURE 15-5 The exposure control console should be covered with a clean barrier and changed after every patient.

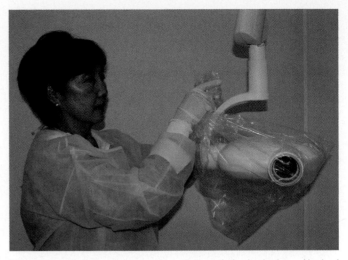

FIGURE 15-7 A plastic bag is slipped over the x-ray tube head with a large rubber band just proximal to the swivel or tic ends, as shown here. The plastic is pulled tight over the PID and secured with a light rubber band slipped over the PID and placed next to the head.

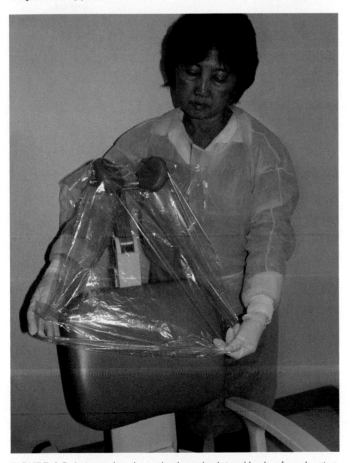

FIGURE 15-6 A new plastic bag is placed over the chair and headrest for each patient.

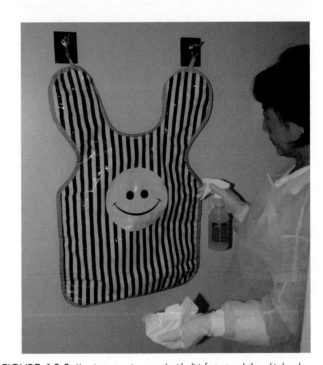

FIGURE 15-8 Hanging apron is sprayed with disinfectant and then dried and covered with a garment bag.

It should be sprayed with a detergent-containing disinfectant and then wiped and covered with the same type of plastic garment bag used for the x-ray head and chair back (Fig. 15-8). Charts should be kept away from sources of contamination and not handled during the radiographic examination.

Although barriers greatly aid infection control, they do not replace the need for effective surface cleaning and disinfection. Experience has demonstrated that failure of mechanical barriers is common during the daily activity of treatment. It is advantageous and reassuring to the operator to know that whenever this happens, the surfaces that may become accidentally exposed are clean and disinfected. Any surface that may be contaminated should be surface disinfected. Operators should avoid touching walls and other surfaces with contaminated gloves. Good surface disinfectants include iodophors, chlorines, and synthetic phenolic compounds. Although the ADA does not recommend specific chemical disinfectants and sterilants, it does suggest that when dentists use a chemical agent for disinfection or sterilization, the agent should be an Environmental Protection Agency (EPA)–registered hospital disinfectant of low to intermediate activity. The agent should also be tuberculocidal–an effective killer of tuberculosis–and capable of preventing other infectious diseases, including hepatitis B virus and HIV.

Panoramic and cephalometric equipment should receive the same maintenance for decontamination and disinfection as other equipment. Panoramic bite-blocks, chin rest, and patient handgrips should be cleaned with detergent-iodine disinfectant and covered with a plastic bag. Disposable bite-blocks may be used. The head-positioning guides, control panel, and exposure switch should be carefully wiped with a paper towel that is well moistened with disinfectant. The radiographer should wear disposable gloves while positioning and exposing the patient. The gloves should be removed before the cassette is removed from the machine for processing because the cassette and film remain extraoral and should not be handled with contaminated disposable gloves. Cephalostat ear posts, ear post brackets, and forehead support or nasion pointer should be cleaned and disinfected with iodine-detergent disinfectant. These may then also be covered in plastic.

After patient exposures are completed, the barriers should be removed, and contaminated working surfaces (including surfaces in the darkroom) and the apron should be sprayed with disinfectant and wiped as described previously. The barriers should be replaced in preparation for the next patient.

Sterilize Nondisposable Instruments

Film-holding instruments are classified by the CDC as semicritical items–instruments that are not used to penetrate soft tissue or bone but do come in contact with the oral mucous membrane. It is best to use film-holding instruments that are heat sterilizable. After using, these instruments, disassemble the aiming ring, support arm, and bite-block. Each instrument should be cleaned with hot water and soap to remove saliva and debris. The cleaned components are then loaded into plastic or paper pouches and sterilized with steam under pressure (autoclave). After sterilization, the instruments should be kept in pouches for storage and subsequent transport to the radiography area. When the instruments are taken to the radiography area, it is good technique to keep them in the pouch until immediately before use. After use, instruments should be replaced in the pouch to reinforce cleanliness in the area. The same sterilization pouch should be used to transport the contaminated instruments back to the cleaning and sterilizing room.

Use Barriers with Digital Sensors

Sensors for digital imaging cannot be sterilized, so it is important to use a barrier to protect them from contamination when placed in the patient's mouth (Fig. 15-9). Typically, the manufacturers of these sensors recommend the use of plastic barrier sheaths. The supplemental use of latex finger cots provides significant added protection and is recommended for routine use when using digital sensors. Because such barriers may fail, the sensors should be cleaned and disinfected with an EPA-registered, intermediate-level hospital disinfectant after every patient. The manufacturer of such equipment should be consulted for the proper disinfectant. PSP sensors are placed in disposable plastic bags with a folded seal for use in the mouth. Because the entire plastic bag goes into the mouth with PSP sensors, these plates possibly can become contaminated with saliva when removed from the plastic bags for processing. This contamination could lead to cross-contamination of other plates and the processing equipment. To minimize this problem, PSP plates should be disinfected between patients using a method recommended by the manufacturer.

Use Barrier-Protected Film (Sensor) or Disposable Container

Film should be obtained in advance from a central source. To prevent contamination of bulk supplies of film, they should be dispensed in procedure quantities. The required number of films for a full-mouth or interproximal series should be prepackaged in coin envelopes or paper cups in the central preparation room. These envelopes of films should be dispensed with the film-holding instruments. For unanticipated occasions in which an unusual number of films are required, a small container of films can be on hand in the central preparation and sterilizing room. No one wearing contaminated gloves should retrieve a film from this supply. Films should be dispensed only by staff members with clean hands or wearing clean gloves.

Film packets may be prepackaged in a plastic envelope (Fig. 15-10), which protects the film from contact with saliva and blood

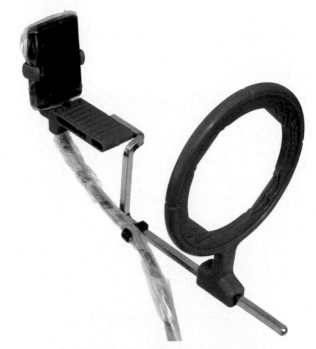

FIGURE 15-9 Film-holding instrument with barrier wrapping to protect sensor and cord from saliva. *(Image courtesy Dentsply Rinn: www.rinncorp.com.)*

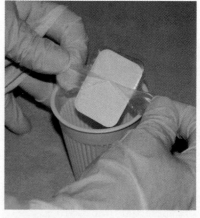

FIGURE 15-10 Dental film with a plastic barrier to protect film from contact with saliva. During opening, the plastic is removed and the clean film is allowed to drop into a container.

during exposure. Barrier-protected film fits in most film-holding instruments. An attractive feature of the protective envelopes is the ease with which they may be opened and the film extracted. For best results, the packet should be immersed in a disinfectant after the films have been exposed in the patient's mouth. Then the packet should be dried and opened, allowing the film to drop out. The barrier envelopes can be conveniently opened in a lighted area, the film can be dropped onto a clean work area or into a clean paper or plastic cup, and the film can be transferred to the daylight loader or darkroom for processing.

If barrier-protected film is not used, the exposed film should be placed in a disposable container for later transport to the darkroom for processing. Paper film packets are exposed to saliva and possibly blood during exposure in the patient's mouth. To prevent saliva from seeping into a paper film packet, a paper towel should be placed beside the container for exposed films. The practitioner should use this towel to wipe each film as it is removed from the patient's mouth and before it is placed with the other exposed films. This problem may also be avoided by using film packaged in vinyl.

Prevent Contamination of Processing Equipment

After all film exposures are made, the operator should remove his or her gloves and take the container of contaminated films to the darkroom. The goal in the darkroom is to break the infection chain so that only clean films are placed into processing solutions. Two towels should be placed on the darkroom working surface. The container of contaminated films should be placed on one of these towels. After the exposed film is removed from its packet, it should be placed on the second towel. The film packaging is discarded on the first towel with the container.

The procedure to remove film from a packet without touching (contaminating) is simple. Figure 15-11 illustrates the method for opening a contaminated film packet while wearing contaminated gloves without touching the film. The practitioner dons a clean pair of gloves, picks up the film packet by the color-coded end, and pulls the tab upward and away from the packet to reveal the black paper tab wrapped over the end of the film. Holding the film over a cup, the practitioner carefully grasps the black paper tab that wraps the film and pulls the film from the packet. When the film is pulled from the packet, it falls from the paper wrapping into the cup. The paper wrapper may need to be shaken lightly to cause the film to fall free. The packaging materials should be placed on the first paper towel. After all films are opened, the practitioner gathers the contaminated packaging and container and discards them along with the contaminated gloves. The clean films are processed in the usual manner. It is not necessary to wear gloves when handling processed films, film mounts, or patient charts.

An alternative procedure when exposing films in vinyl packaging is to place the exposed film, still in the protective plastic envelope, in an approved disinfecting solution when it is removed from the mouth and after wiping it with a paper towel. It should remain in the disinfectant after the exposure of the last film for the recommended time. Immersion for 30 seconds in a 5.25% solution of sodium hypochlorite is effective.

Automatic film processors with daylight loaders present a special problem because of the risk for contaminating the sleeves with contaminated gloves or film packets. One approach is to clean the films by immersion in a disinfectant, with or without a plastic envelope, as previously described. With this method, the operator cleans the films, puts on clean gloves, and takes only cleaned film packets into the daylight loader. An alternative approach is to open

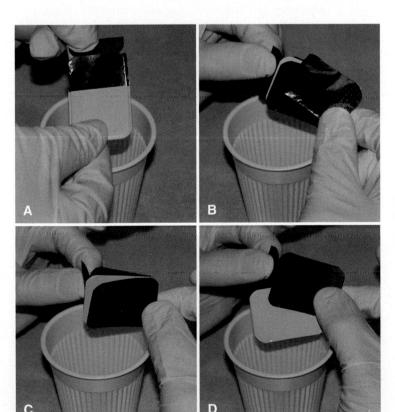

FIGURE 15-11 Method for removing films from packet without touching them with contaminated gloves. **A,** Packet tab is opened, and lead foil and black interleaf paper are slid from wrapping **B,** Foil is rotated away from black paper and discarded. **C,** Paper wrapping is opened. **D,** Film is allowed to fall into a clean cup.

the top of the loader, place a clean barrier on the bottom, and insert the cup of exposed film packets into a clean cup. The operator closes the top, puts on clean gloves, pushes his or her hands through the sleeve, and opens the film packets, allowing the film to drop into the clean cup. After all film packets have been opened, the contaminated gloves are removed, the films are loaded into the developer, and hands are removed. The top of the loader may be removed, and the contaminated materials are then removed.

BIBLIOGRAPHY

Quality Assurance

American Dental Association Council on Scientific Affairs: The use of dental radiographs: update and recommendations, *J Am Dent Assoc* 137:1304–1312, 2006.

American Dental Association Council on Scientific Affairs: Dental radiographic examinations: recommendations for patient selection and limiting radiation exposure. Revised 2012: http://www.ada.org/sections/professionalResources/pdfs/Dental_Radiographic_Examinations_2012.pdf.

Goren AD, Lundeen RC, Deahl ST II, et al: Updated quality assurance self-assessment exercise in intraoral and panoramic radiography, American Academy of Oral and Maxillofacial Radiology, Radiology Practice Committee, *Oral Surg Oral Med Oral Pathol Oral Radiol Endod* 89:369–374, 2000.

Kodak Dental Radiography Series: *Quality assurance in dental radiography*, N-416, Rochester, NY, 1998, Eastman Kodak.

Mah P, McDavid WD, Dove SB: Quality assurance phantom for digital dental imaging, *Oral Surg Oral Med Oral Pathol Oral Radiol Endod* 112:632–639, 2011.

Michel R, Zimmerman TL: Basic radiation protection considerations in dental practice, *Health Phys* 77:S81–S83, 1999.

National Council for Radiation Protection and Measurements: *Radiation protection in dentistry*, NCRP Report No. 145, Bethesda, MD, 2003, National Council on Radiation Protection and Measurement.

National Radiological Protection Board: Guidance notes for dental practitioners on the safe use of x-ray equipment (2001): www.nrpb.org.uk.

Quality control recommendations for diagnostic radiography, Volume 1, Dental facilities, CRCPD Publication 01-4, July 2001.

Infection Control

American Academy of Oral and Maxillofacial Radiology infection control guidelines for dental radiographic procedures, *Oral Surg Oral Med Oral Pathol* 73:248–249, 1992.

American Dental Association Council on Scientific Affairs and American Dental Association Council on Dental Practice: Infection control recommendations for the dental office and the dental laboratory, *J Am Dent Assoc* 127:672–680, 1996.

Bartoloni JA, Chariton DG, Flint DJ: Infection control practices in dental radiology, *Gen Dent* 51:264–271, 2003.

Hubar JS, Gardiner DM: Infection control procedures used in conjunction with computed dental radiography, *Int J Comput Dent* 3:259–267, 2000.

Kalathingal S, Youngpeter A, Minton J, et al: An evaluation of microbiologic contamination on a phosphor plate system: is weekly gas sterilization enough? *Oral Surg Oral Med Oral Pathol Oral Radiol Endod* 109:457–462, 2010.

Kohn WG, Collins AS, Cleveland JL, et al; Centers for Disease Control and Prevention: Guidelines for infection control in dental health-care settings–2003, *MMWR Morb Mortal Wkly Rep* 52(RR-17):1–61, 2003.

MacDonald DS, Waterfield JD: Infection control in digital intraoral radiography: evaluation of microbiological contamination of photostimulable phosphor plates in barrier envelopes, *J Can Dent Assoc* 77:b93, 2011.

Miller CH, Palenik CJ: *Infection control and management of hazardous materials for the dental team*, ed 4, St Louis, 2009, Mosby.

Palenik CJ: Infection control practices for dental radiography, *Dent Today* 23:52–55, 2004.

Rutala WA, Weber DJ; Healthcare Infection Control Practices Advisory Committee (HICPAC): *Guideline for disinfection and sterilization in healthcare facilities*, Atlanta, GA, 2008, Department of Health and Human Services, Centers for Disease Control and Prevention.

Thomas LP, Abramovitch K: Infection control for dental radiographic procedures, *Tex Dent J* 122:184–188, 2005.

U.S. Department of Labor, Occupational Safety and Health Administration: Occupational exposure to bloodborne pathogens, needlestick and other sharp injuries, final rule, *Fed Reg* 66:5317–5325, 2001.

Prescribing Diagnostic Imaging

Sharon L. Brooks

OUTLINE

The decision to prescribe diagnostic images should be based on the individual needs of the patient. In this chapter, the term diagnostic images includes conventional (film-based) radiographs as well as any digital image format produced by x rays. Likewise, the commonly used term radiograph is not restricted to images produced on film, but rather it also includes common intraoral and extraoral digital images.

Patient imaging needs are determined by findings from the dental history and clinical examination and modified by patient age and general health. Diagnostic imaging is necessary when the history and clinical examination have not provided enough information for complete evaluation of a patient's condition and formulation of an appropriate treatment plan. Patients should be exposed to x rays only when, in the dentist's judgment, it is reasonably likely that the patient would benefit by the discovery of clinically useful information in the resultant image.

ROLE OF RADIOGRAPHS IN DISEASE DETECTION AND MONITORING

The goal of dental care is to preserve and improve patients' oral health, while minimizing other health-related risks. Although the diagnostic information provided by diagnostic imaging may be of definite benefit to the patient, the radiologic examination does carry the potential for harm from exposure to ionizing radiation. One of the most effective means of reducing possible harm is to avoid making radiographs that would not contribute information pertinent to patient care. The judgment that underlies the decision to make a radiologic examination centers on several factors, including the following:

- Prevalence of the diseases that may be detected radiographically in the oral cavity
- Ability of the clinician to detect these diseases clinically and in diagnostic images

- Consequences of undetected and untreated disease
- Impact of asymptomatic, anatomic, and pathologic variations detected in the image on patient treatment, including the need for follow-up
- Impact of anatomic variations on dental treatment planning for conditions such as dental implants, extractions, and orthodontic treatment

As a general principle, diagnostic imaging is indicated when a reasonable probability exists that it would provide valuable information about a disease that is not evident clinically. Conversely, radiographs are not indicated when they are unlikely to yield information contributing to patient care. Information derived from the image considered to be clinically useful includes data that are valuable in detecting disease, in monitoring the progression of known diseases, and in planning dental treatment.

For many clinical situations, it is not readily apparent to the practitioner whether diagnostic images have a reasonable probability of providing valuable information. In these situations, the practitioner must use clinical judgment after weighing the patient factors to decide whether imaging is indicated.

The philosophy of prescribing images only when there is a high probability of obtaining clinically useful information has been advocated by all the organizations responsible for developing or endorsing guidelines for ordering diagnostic imaging. However, many dentists use radiographs as a screening tool, simply to see "what's there," without having a specific suspicion of disease arising from the dental history or clinical examination. There are probably numerous reasons for this use of radiographs. Some dentists think that they have not provided an adequate service to their patients if they cannot assure them that they have searched diligently for disease with all reasonable diagnostic methods, including diagnostic images. They may state that having complete information, regardless of whether it affects the treatment plan, is of such benefit that it outweighs the risk of the radiation exposure. Other dentists raise medicolegal issues, stating fear of lawsuits if they fail to detect disease. Others express concern about the effect on the efficiency of the dental office of the extended examinations required for prescribing diagnostic images on the basis of signs and symptoms. The next few paragraphs address these concerns.

In contrast to dentistry, screening imaging is rarely used in medicine with the exception of mammography for women older than a certain age or with increased risk factors for breast cancer, and there is controversy over whether even this type of examination should be used as frequently as it is today. Breast cancer is a relatively common yet serious disease that should be detected early, before the cancer becomes large enough to be found clinically. However, diseases of the jaws (with the exceptions of caries and periapical and periodontal disease) are rare and concentrated in certain ages, sexes, and ethnicities. These diseases are unlikely to be discovered on routine screening radiographs before they have produced signs or symptoms that could be found with a thorough clinical examination and history. Periodontal disease can be diagnosed clinically, although diagnostic images are used to determine the extent of bone loss and the presence of other factors that may affect prognosis. Periapical disease is usually associated with extensive restorations or caries that can be detected clinically. However, dental caries on proximal surfaces may not be detectable on clinical examination until it has reached an advanced stage; thus, this is one occult disease for which screening radiographs are considered appropriate. Regarding the threat of lawsuits for failure to diagnose, dentists who follow guidelines on the use of diagnostic imaging developed or endorsed by authoritative bodies that help establish the standard of care should have no concerns. Although lawsuits can be filed for many reasons, it is unlikely that they will be successful if it can be shown that the practitioner did a thorough clinical examination and history and carefully considered the guidelines when determining whether to order diagnostic imaging.

Some dentists set up their practices so that new patients are automatically seen first by the dental hygienist, who takes a predetermined set of diagnostic images at the first appointment, before the dentist sees the patient. Although this may make efficient use of the dentist's time, it is contrary to the recommendations of the American Dental Association (ADA) that the selection of number and type of radiographs should be based on the findings of the clinical examination. Performing a thorough examination before ordering images should not be an insurmountable obstacle for an efficient dental practice.

Regarding the issue of cost versus benefit of diagnostic images, there is little risk of harm for any individual patient from one set of images, even if no important diagnostic information is revealed. However, there is a large societal cost, both in terms of health care dollars and radiation risk, if millions of dental patients receive unproductive examinations, as would happen if routine screening were widespread. In addition, there is a growing concern among the public and the medical profession about the increasing use of ionizing radiation in health care in general and the risks it poses to the public.

Our philosophy is that the prescription of diagnostic imaging should be based on the need for diagnostic information for patients on a case-by-case basis. The next section discusses some of the clinical situations that may call for a radiologic examination.

CARIES

Dental caries is the most common dental disease, affecting people of all ages. Although the caries prevalence rates of developed countries have been decreasing since the 1970s, probably partially as a result of the widespread use of fluoride, increasing numbers of older adults are maintaining their teeth throughout their lifetimes, leaving them at risk for developing both coronal and root caries. In addition, caries prevalence is not uniformly distributed throughout the population, with children of lower socioeconomic background having a higher rate of untreated caries than other children.

Although occlusal, buccal, and lingual carious lesions are reasonably easy to detect clinically, interproximal caries and caries associated with existing restorations are much more difficult to detect with a clinical examination only (see Chapter 18). Studies have repeatedly demonstrated that clinicians using intraoral images detect caries not evident clinically, both in enamel and in dentin. Although a radiologic examination is very important for diagnosis of dental caries, the optimal frequency for such an examination should be based on mitigating features, such as the patient's age, medical condition, diet, oral hygiene practices, oral health status, and the nature of the caries process itself.

Carious lesions demonstrate one of three behaviors: (1) progression, (2) arrest, or (3) regression. Only about 50% of lesions progress beyond the initial, just-detectable defect, and in most instances the lesions demonstrate a slow rate of progression through enamel (months to years). Mechanisms are also in use to enhance remineralization of early enamel lesions. However, the rate of caries progression is significantly faster in deciduous enamel than in permanent enamel, and patients vary widely in their rates of formation of caries and in their rates of caries progression.

Because the presence of caries cannot be determined with confidence by clinical examination alone, it is necessary to expose patients periodically through bitewing radiographs to monitor dental caries. The length of the exposure intervals varies considerably because of different patient circumstances. For most patients in good physical health with adequate oral hygiene, an infrequent radiologic examination is needed to monitor dental caries. However, if the patient history and clinical examination suggest that the individual has a relatively high caries experience, shorter intervals allow careful monitoring of disease.

PERIODONTAL DISEASES

Some form of periodontal disease affects most people at some point during their lives, gingivitis more often in younger individuals and periodontitis more commonly in older adults. Periodontal diseases are responsible for a substantial portion of all teeth lost. A consensus exists among practitioners that radiologic examinations play an important role in the evaluation of patients with periodontal disease after the disease is initially detected on clinical examination (see Chapter 19). In addition to providing a picture of the extent of alveolar bone support for the dentition, radiologic examinations help demonstrate local factors that complicate the disease, including the presence of gingival irritants such as calculus and faulty restorations. Occasionally, the length and morphologic features of roots, visible on periapical radiographs, are crucial factors in the prognosis of the disease. These observations suggest that when clinical evidence exists of periodontal disease other than nonspecific gingivitis, it is appropriate to make intraoral images, generally a combination of periapical and bitewing images, to help establish the severity of the disease. Follow-up images after therapy is complete help the clinician monitor the progression of disease and determine whether the destruction of alveolar bone has been halted.

PERIAPICAL INFLAMMATORY DISEASE

When a patient presents with a toothache, deep caries, or a large or deep restoration, the likelihood of an inflammatory lesion of pulpal origin occurring at the apex of the tooth increases. Usually the clinical examination combined with a periapical radiograph is sufficient to make the diagnosis and plan the treatment, endodontic therapy, or extraction. However, in cases with complex root canal anatomy, evidence of failed endodontic treatment, intraoperative or postoperative complications, or situations where the periapical view does not provide adequate information, a limited-volume, high-resolution cone-beam computed tomographic (CBCT) examination might be useful.

DENTAL ANOMALIES

Abnormal formation of teeth may be manifested as deviations in number, size, and composition. These abnormalities in dental development occur more frequently and are more likely to have a serious impact in the permanent dentition than in the primary dentition. The most frequently encountered anomalies are the presence of supernumerary teeth, usually mesiodens, or developmentally absent teeth, usually second premolars (see Chapter 31).

Only a few anomalies exist for which orthodontic treatment or surgical correction or modification must start at an early age. When the dentist suspects an abnormality requiring treatment, diagnostic images to confirm and localize it are not required until the time when the treatment is most appropriate. For example, a panoramic examination of a 5-year-old child to determine the presence or absence of permanent teeth may be poorly timed. Although the examination provides evidence that one or more second premolars or lateral incisors are developmentally missing, this information usually does not influence the current treatment plan. When examination for dental anomalies is appropriate, both the radiation dose and the anticipated diagnostic benefit should be considered. Projections that best demonstrate the required diagnostic information should be selected. A panoramic image of the lower face is usually best for observing the presence or absence of teeth in all quadrants, although a periapical or occlusal radiograph is sufficient for an examination limited to one area.

GROWTH AND DEVELOPMENT AND DENTAL MALOCCLUSION

Children and adolescents are often examined to assess the growth and development of the teeth and jaws. This assessment considers the relationship of one jaw to the other and to the soft tissues. An examination of occlusion, growth, and development requires an individualized radiologic examination that may include periapical radiographs or a panoramic view to supplement other images ordered to assess dental disease. In addition, a patient of any age group who is being considered for orthodontic treatment may need other images, such as lateral or posteroanterior cephalometric, occlusal, carpal index (wrist), or temporomandibular joint (TMJ) images, depending on the clinical findings (Fig. 16-1). CBCT imaging is being used increasingly frequently for orthodontic evaluation to provide three-dimensional information about jaw relationships and to substitute for multiple other imaging examinations (see Chapters 11 and 12). At the present time, it is unclear which patients would benefit from CBCT imaging in terms of treatment considerations. There is adequate information in the literature to demonstrate the value of CBCT imaging in the evaluation and treatment of impacted teeth but less information on

other conditions of interest in orthodontics. The American Association of Orthodontists and the American Academy of Oral and Maxillofacial Radiology more recently developed a joint position statement on the use of CBCT imaging in orthodontics. Broadly, the statement recommends using CBCT imaging only when justified by individual need and the clinical question cannot be answered by using lower dose conventional imaging. Dose-reduction protocols should be used when possible. CBCT imaging is also used in some cases of impacted mandibular third molars when the relationship of the inferior alveolar nerve to the root apex is unclear with conventional images.

The dentist who is the primary provider of orthodontic treatment should select the number and type of images needed. The needs of each patient should be considered individually. Selecting the appropriate images should allow a maximal diagnostic yield with a minimal radiation exposure after consideration of the clinical examination, the study of plaster models and photographs, and the optimal time to initiate treatment.

OCCULT DISEASE

Occult disease refers to disease that presents no clinical signs or symptoms. Occult diseases in the jaws include a combination of dental and intraosseous findings. Dental findings may include incipient carious lesions, resorbed or dilacerated roots, and hypercementosis. Intraosseous findings include osteosclerosis, unerupted teeth, periapical disease, and a wide variety of cysts and benign and malignant tumors (see Chapters 20 to 26). Small carious lesions, resorption of root structure, and bony lesions may go unnoticed until signs and symptoms develop.

Although the consequences of some occult diseases may be quite serious, most serious diseases are rare. Often a historical or clinical sign or symptom of intraosseous disease suggests its presence. For instance, an unusual contour of bone or an absent third molar, not explained by a history of extraction, suggests the possibility of an impaction with the potential for an associated dentigerous cyst. Although patient history and clinical signs and symptoms do not always accurately predict dental and intraosseous findings, most of these true occult diseases are not clinically relevant, or they are so rare that except for caries as described previously the dentist need not obtain a radiologic examination of the jaws solely to screen for them in dentate individuals in the absence of unusual clinical signs or symptoms. Caries is an exception because of its much higher prevalence than other occult diseases.

There is a considerable difference of opinion regarding whether asymptomatic edentulous patients seen for routine denture construction should have screening images taken to look for occult disease. Several studies have demonstrated a relatively large number of findings in diagnostic images of edentulous patients, including retained root tips and areas of sclerotic bone, but almost all these findings required no treatment and did not affect the outcome of care. For that reason, some experts recommend no images of edentulous patients if the clinical examination is negative for signs and symptoms of disease. Others think that screening radiographs of these patients are of value. As the standard of care for completely or partially edentulous patients moves toward dental implants rather than removable prosthetics, imaging to assess the quantity and quality of bone available for implants is gaining in importance.

There has been increasing interest in the last few years in using panoramic images to screen patients for the presence of calcified atheromas in the bifurcation of the carotid artery, a finding that may indicate an increased risk for the development of a

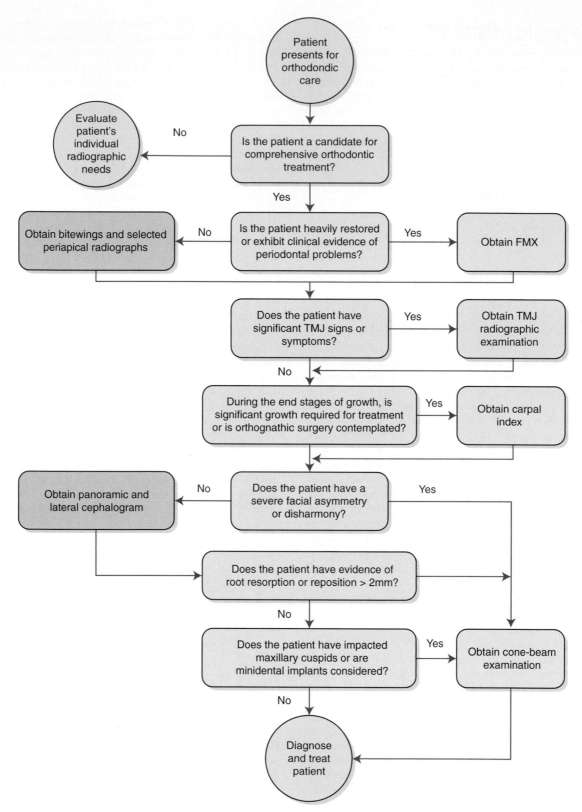

FIGURE 16-1 Example of a clinical algorithm to order radiographs for orthodontic patients. Selected radiographs are ordered after the dentist's consideration of the patient's history and clinical characteristics. *FMX,* Full-mouth examination; *TMJ,* temporomandibular joint. *(Modified from White SC, Pae E-K: Patient and image selection criteria for cone-beam imaging, Semin Orthod 15:19–28, 2009.)*

cerebrovascular accident (stroke). However, the value of this finding has been questioned more recently because a noncalcified vulnerable plaque, which is not visible on panoramic radiographs, may put the patient at more risk for stroke than a more stable calcified plaque. Nevertheless, the general consensus at this time is that panoramic images made for dental purposes should be evaluated for this calcification, particularly in patients older than 55 years, but that these images should not be made simply to screen for atheromas without other dental indications. (See Chapter 28 for more details.)

JAW DISEASE

Imaging of known jaw lesions, such as fibro-osseous diseases or neoplastic diseases, before biopsy and definitive treatment, is also important for appropriate management of the patient. For small lesions of the jaws, periapical or panoramic radiographs may be enough as long as the lesion can be seen in its entirety. If clinical evidence of swelling exists, some type of radiograph at 90 degrees to the original plane (often an occlusal image) should be made to determine whether there is expansion of the jaw or perforation of the buccal or lingual cortical bone. If lesions are too large to fit on standard dental radiographs, extend into the maxillary sinus or other portions of the head outside the jaws, or are suspected to be malignant, additional imaging such as medical computed tomographic (CT) imaging or CBCT imaging is appropriate before biopsy (see Chapters 11 to 14). Both of these types of images can provide excellent bone detail, but if there is a suspicion that the lesion may involve the surrounding soft tissue, medical CT imaging should be used instead of CBCT imaging because it can provide images of the soft tissue. These types of imaging can define the extent of the lesion, indicate an appropriate biopsy site, suggest an operative approach, and provide information about the nature of the lesion. If the lesion is not based in bone but in the adjacent soft tissue, magnetic resonance (MR) imaging, which has superior contrast resolution of soft tissue, should be used. In the initial steps of the investigation, referral to an oral and maxillofacial radiologist to order and report on the most appropriate diagnostic imaging before the biopsy procedure is reasonable.

TEMPOROMANDIBULAR JOINT

Many types of diseases affect the TMJ, including congenital and developmental malformations of the mandible and cranial bones; acquired disorders such as disk displacement, neoplasms, fractures, and dislocations; inflammatory diseases that produce capsulitis or synovitis; and arthritides of various types, including rheumatoid arthritis and osteoarthritis. The goal of TMJ imaging, similar to that for imaging other body parts, should be to obtain new information that would influence patient care. Radiologic examination may not be needed for all patients with signs and symptoms referable to the TMJ region, particularly if no treatment is contemplated (see Chapter 27). The decision regarding whether and how to image the joints should depend on the results of the history and clinical findings, the clinical diagnosis, degree of diagnostic certainty required, and results of prior examinations as well as the tentative treatment plan and expected outcome.

The cost of the examination and the radiation dose should also influence the decision if more than one type of examination can provide the desired information. For example, information about the status of the osseous tissues can be obtained from panoramic radiographs, medical CT imaging, or CBCT imaging. For investigation of the soft tissue joint components, such as the disk, and for viewing the surrounding soft tissues, MR imaging is used. MR imaging is not capable of providing the detailed images of osseous structures as seen with CBCT imaging. The subtlety of the expected findings and the amount of detail required should be considered when selecting the examination to perform. However, according to the International Consortium on Diagnosis of Temporomandibular Disorders, the only imaging technique with adequate validity to diagnose degenerative joint disease is CT imaging. If soft tissue information such as disk position is necessary for patient care, MR imaging is appropriate.

IMPLANTS

Use of osseointegrated implants, metal screws that are inserted into the mandible or maxilla, is an increasingly common method of replacing missing teeth. Prosthetic appliances are affixed to the screws after a period of healing. Preoperative planning is crucial to ensure success of the implants. The dentist must evaluate the adequacy of the height and thickness of bone for the desired implant; the quality of the bone, including the relative proportion of medullary and cortical bone; the location of anatomic structures such as the mandibular canal or maxillary sinus; and the presence of structural abnormalities such as undercuts that may affect placement or angulation of the implant (see Chapter 33).

Standard periapical and panoramic images can supply information regarding the vertical dimensions of the bone in the proposed implant site. However, some type of cross-sectional imaging, preferably CBCT imaging, is recommended before implant placement for visualization of important anatomic landmarks, determination of size and path of insertion of implant, and evaluation of the adequacy of the bone for anchorage of the implant. There is also increasing use of implant planning software and preparation of surgical drilling guides, which require the three-dimensional data from medical CT imaging or CBCT imaging. Postoperative evaluation of implants may be needed later on to judge healing, assess complete seating of fixtures, and ensure continued health of the surrounding bone.

PARANASAL SINUSES

Because dentists are not usually the primary providers of treatment for acute or chronic sinus disease, the necessity to perform sinus imaging may be limited in general dental practice. However, because sinus disease can manifest as pain in the maxillary teeth and because periapical inflammation of maxillary molars and premolars can also lead to changes in the mucosa of the maxillary sinus, circumstances occur in which the dentist needs to obtain an image of the maxillary sinus. Another reason to image this area is to assess the need for bone augmentation or sinus lift before implant placement in the posterior maxilla. Periapical and panoramic radiographs demonstrate the floor of the maxillary sinus well, but visualization of other walls requires additional imaging techniques, such as occipitomental (Waters) view, CBCT imaging, or medical CT imaging. For the investigation of diseases of the maxillary sinus, referral to an oral and maxillofacial radiologist would be a reasonable step (see Chapter 26).

TRAUMA

Patients who have sustained trauma to the oral region may visit a dentist for evaluation and management of the injuries. For proper management, it is important to determine the full extent of the injuries. Periapical or panoramic views are helpful for evaluation of fractures of the teeth. If a suspected root fracture is not visible on a periapical radiograph, a second image made with a different angulation may be helpful. A fracture that is not perpendicular to the beam may not be detectable unless root resorption is present. Occasionally, limited-volume, high-resolution CBCT imaging may provide important information about tooth fractures, although artifacts owing to the presence of metallic restorations or dense root canal fillings may obscure a fracture. Thus, a tooth with a history of trauma should be monitored and evaluated radiologically on a periodic basis, even if the original image is negative.

Fractures of the mandible frequently can be detected with panoramic radiographs, supplemented by images at 90 degrees, such as a posteroanterior or reverse-Towne view (see Chapter 30) or occlusal view. Trauma to the maxilla and midface requires medical CT imaging or CBCT imaging for a thorough evaluation. Affected patients are more likely to report to a hospital emergency department than to a general dental office. The hospital may have a standard protocol for trauma cases. Ideally, the clinician responsible for managing care determines the appropriate diagnostic images for the specific case.

RADIOLOGIC EXAMINATIONS

After concluding that a patient requires a diagnostic image, the dentist should consider which examination is most appropriate to meet all the patient's diagnostic and treatment planning needs. Various image projections are available. When choosing a projection, the dentist should consider the anatomic relationships, the size of the field, and the radiation dose from each view. Table 16-1 summarizes common types of radiologic examinations for general dental patients and factors to consider in choosing the most appropriate one. For example, a panoramic image provides broad area coverage with moderate resolution. Intraoral images give more detailed information but a significantly higher radiation dose per unit area exposed. The clinician must use clinical judgment to weigh these factors. Examples of all these image types can be found in previous chapters.

INTRAORAL IMAGES

Intraoral images are examinations made by placing the x-ray film or digital imaging receptor within the patient's mouth during the exposure. These exposures offer the dentist a high-detail view of the teeth and bone in the area exposed. Such views are most appropriate for revealing caries and periodontal and periapical disease in a localized region. A complete-mouth or full-mouth examination consists of periapical views of all the tooth-bearing regions as well as interproximal views (see Chapter 7).

Periapical Views

Periapical views show all of a tooth and the surrounding bone and are very useful for revealing caries and periodontal and periapical disease. These views may be made of a specific tooth or region or as part of a full-mouth examination.

Interproximal Views

Interproximal views (bitewings) show the coronal aspects of both the maxillary and the mandibular dentition in a region as well as the surrounding crestal bone. These views are most useful for revealing proximal caries and evaluating the height of the alveolar bony crest. They can be made in either the anterior or the posterior region of the mouth.

Occlusal Views

Occlusal views are intraoral images in which the film or digital image receptor is positioned in the occlusal plane. They are often used in lieu of periapical views in children because the small size of the patient's mouth limits the film or receptor placement. In

TABLE 16-1 Dental Radiographic Examinations and Their Properties

Type of Examination	Coverage	Resolution	Relative Exposure*	Detectable Disease
INTRAORAL RADIOGRAPHS				
Periapical	Limited	High	1	Caries, periodontal disease, occult disease
Bitewings	Limited	High	10	Caries, periodontal bone level
Full-mouth periapical	Limited	High	14–17	Caries, periodontal disease, dental anomalies, occult disease
Occlusal	Moderate	High	2.5	Dental anomalies, occult disease, salivary stones, expansion of jaw
EXTRAORAL RADIOGRAPHS				
Panoramic	Broad	Moderate	1–2	Dental anomalies, occult disease, extensive caries, periodontal disease, periapical disease, TMJ
Film tomography/slice	Moderate	Moderate	0.2–0.6	TMJ, implant site assessment
CBCT imaging	Broad	Moderate to high	4–42	Implant, TMJ, craniofacial relationships, dental anomalies, extent of disease, fracture
CT/head imaging	Broad	High	25–800	Extent of craniofacial disease, fracture, implants
MR imaging	Broad	Moderate	—	Soft tissue disease, TMJ
Skull	Broad	Moderate	30	Fracture, anatomic relation, jaw disease

Note. The relative exposures assume use of F-speed film and rectangular collimation for periapical films, round collimation for bitewings and occlusal views, and rare-earth screens for panoramic examinations. With D-speed film, the intraoral values are more than doubled compared with F-speed film, and with round collimation the periapical values increase by 2.5 times compared with rectangular collimation. *CBCT,* cone-beam computed tomography; *CT,* computed tomography; *MR,* magnetic resonance; *TMJ,* temporomandibular joint.

*From Frederiksen N, Benson B, Sokolowski T: Effective dose and risk assessment from computed tomography of the maxillofacial complex, *Dentomaxillofac Radiol* 24:55–58, 1995; Scaf G, Lurie AG, Mosier KM, et al: Dosimetry and cost of imaging osseointegrated implants with film-based and computed tomography, *Oral Surg Oral Med Oral Pathol Oral Radiol Endod* 83:41–48, 1997; White SC: 1992 assessment of radiation risks from dental radiology, *Dentomaxillofac Radiol* 21:118–126, 1992; Ludlow JB, Davies-Ludlow LE, Brooks SL, et al: Dosimetry of 3 CBCT devices for oral and maxillofacial radiology: CB Mercuray, NewTom 3G and i-CAT, *Dentomaxillofac Radiol* 35:219–226, 2006.

adults, occlusal images may supplement periapical views, providing visualization of a greater area of teeth and bone, and can provide a right-angle view. They are useful for demonstrating impacted or abnormally placed maxillary anterior teeth or visualizing the region of a palatal cleft. Occlusal views may also demonstrate buccal or lingual expansion of bone or presence of a sialolith in the submandibular duct.

EXTRAORAL IMAGES

Extraoral images are examinations made of the orofacial region by use of imaging receptors located outside the mouth. The relationships among patient position, receptor location, and beam direction vary depending on the specific information desired. The standard technique for making several extraoral images is discussed in Chapter 9. Only the panoramic image is described here because it has common use as a radiologic examination for general dental patients.

Panoramic Images

Panoramic images provide a broad view of the jaws, teeth, maxillary sinuses, nasal fossa, and TMJs (see Chapter 10). They show which teeth are present, the relative state of development, the presence or absence of dental abnormalities, and many traumatic and pathologic lesions in bone. Panoramic images are the technique of choice for initial examinations of edentulous patients. Because this system is an extraoral technique and sometimes uses intensifying screens and because the image receptor and x-ray tube are in motion during the patient exposure, the resolution of the images is less than with intraoral images (see Chapter 10). Increasingly, panoramic radiographs are made with digital sensors rather than film. Panoramic images are also susceptible to artifacts from improper patient positioning that negatively affect the image. Consequently, this system is generally considered inadequate for independent diagnosis of caries, root abnormalities, and periapical changes.

In most dental patients, oral disease involving the teeth or jaw bones lies within the area imaged by periapical images. Therefore, when a full-mouth set of radiographs is available, a panoramic examination is usually redundant because it does not add information that alters the treatment plan. However, situations may exist in which a panoramic image may be preferred over a periapical examination, such as for assessing growth and development in a child or adolescent. Panoramic views are most useful when the required field of view is large but the need for high resolution is of less importance. However, the image quality of digital panoramic examinations is frequently higher than their film counterparts, and thus in many cases a digital panoramic image, supplemented with bitewings, may be preferred over periapical images. Although the selection of a radiologic examination should be based on the extent of the expected information it is likely to provide, the relatively low dose of radiation from the panoramic examination should also be a qualifying factor.

Advanced Imaging Procedures

Various advanced imaging procedures, such as medical CT imaging, CBCT imaging, MR imaging, ultrasonography, and nuclear medicine scans, may be required in specific diagnostic situations. These techniques are discussed in Chapter 14, although in general the dentist should refer the patient to an oral and maxillofacial radiologist or a medical imaging center for these procedures rather than performing them in the dental office.

As more dentists acquire CBCT units for their office, questions will arise about the most appropriate use of this technology. Position statements on the use of CBCT imaging in endodontics and implant dentistry have been developed. The ADA has also developed basic guidelines on the use of CBCT imaging in general in dentistry. In all of these documents, there is a single basic theme: this technology should be used only when the three-dimensional information provided would be of direct benefit in the diagnosis and treatment of the patient's condition because the radiation dose is generally higher than with conventional imaging. The higher radiation dose is particularly of concern when imaging children, who are more sensitive to the effects of radiation than are adults.

GUIDELINES FOR ORDERING DIAGNOSTIC IMAGING

The ADA has issued the following guidelines recommending which images (radiographs) to make and how often to repeat them:
- Make radiographs only after a clinical examination and only when there is an expectation that the diagnostic yield would affect patient care.
- Order only images that directly benefit the patient in terms of diagnosis or treatment plan.
- Use the least amount of radiation exposure necessary to generate an acceptable view of the imaged area.

PREVIOUS DIAGNOSTIC IMAGES

Most patients have been seen previously by a dentist and have already had radiographs made. These images are helpful regardless of when they were exposed. If they are relatively recent, they may be adequate to the diagnostic problem at hand. Even if they were made so long ago that they are not likely to reflect the current status of the patient, they may still prove useful. These previous images may demonstrate whether a condition has worsened, has remained unchanged, or has shown healing, such as in the progression of caries or periodontal disease.

ADMINISTRATIVE IMAGES

Administrative images are images made for reasons other than diagnosis, including images made for an insurance company or for an examining board. The authors think that it is appropriate to expose patients only when it benefits their health care. Most administrative images do not serve such an objective. This recommendation is often not adhered to in practice, and dentists are left to sort out the most appropriate criteria to use in their practices.

USE OF GUIDELINES TO ORDER DENTAL DIAGNOSTIC IMAGES

At any time, patients generally have a combination of diseases that the clinician must consider. Therefore, guidelines specify not only which examinations to order but also which specific patient factors influence the number and type of images to order.

A panel of individuals was convened in the mid-1980s at the request of a branch of the U.S. Food and Drug Administration (FDA) to develop a set of guidelines for the making of dental radiographs. The panel addressed the topic of appropriate images for an adequate evaluation of a new or recall asymptomatic patient seeking general dental care. The guidelines were updated in 2004 to reflect changes in technology and to address situations not considered in the first document, and they were updated again in 2012 (Table 16-2). However, there was no change in philosophy between the original and current guidelines.

The guidelines describe circumstances (patient age, medical and dental history, and physical signs) that suggest the need for diagnostic images. These circumstances are called selection criteria. The guidelines also suggest the types of examinations most likely to benefit the patient in terms of yielding diagnostic information. They recommend that images not be made unless some expectation exists that they would provide evidence of diseases that would affect the treatment plan. The ADA was an equal partner with the FDA in the revision of the guidelines and recommends their use.

These guidelines also form the basis of the recommendations in this chapter. Use of the guidelines can help optimize patient care, minimize the total diagnostic radiation burden, and responsibly allocate health care resources. However, the practitioner, who is the only one who knows the patient's dental history and susceptibility to oral disease, must make the ultimate decision on whether to order images, using the guidelines as a resource, not as a standard of care or a regulation.

Central to the guidelines is the idea that dentists should expose patients to radiation only when they reasonably expect that the resulting diagnostic image would benefit patient care. Two situations mandate a need for radiology: some clinical evidence of an abnormality that requires further evaluation for a complete assessment or a high probability of disease that warrants a screening examination.

Selection criteria for images are signs or symptoms found in the patient history or clinical examination that suggest that a radiologic examination would yield clinically useful information. A key concept in the use of selection criteria is recognition of the need to consider each patient individually. Prescription of diagnostic images should be decided on an individual basis according to the patient's demonstrated need.

The guidelines include a description of clinical situations in which images are likely to contribute to the diagnosis, treatment, or prognosis. Two examples highlight the differences between ordering images for dental diseases with clinical signs and symptoms and dental diseases with no clinical indicators but high prevalences. In the first situation, a patient has a hard swelling in the premolar region of the mandible with expansion of the buccal and lingual cortical plates. The clinical sign of swelling alerts the dentist to the need for a diagnostic image to determine the nature of the abnormality causing the swelling.

An example of the second situation is a patient who comes seeking general dental care after not having seen a dentist for many years. Even without clinical evidence of caries, bitewings are indicated because of the prevalence of dental caries in the population. Because this patient has not had interproximal radiographs for many years, it is reasonable to assume that the patient may benefit from the examination by the detection of interproximal caries. Although no clinical signs exist that predict the presence of early caries, the dentist relies on clinical knowledge of the prevalence of caries to decide that this radiograph has a reasonable probability of finding disease.

Without some specific indication, it is inappropriate to expose the patient "just to see if there is something there." The major exception to this rule is the use of interproximal images for caries when no clinical signs exist of early lesions. The probability of finding occult disease in a patient with all permanent teeth erupted and no clinical or historical evidence of abnormality or risk factors is so low that making a periapical or panoramic survey just to look for such disease is not indicated.

PATIENT EXAMINATION

The ordering of diagnostic images requires a reasonable expectation that they would provide information that would contribute to solving the diagnostic problem at hand. The first step is a careful examination of the patient, including transillumination of the anterior teeth to evaluate for interproximal decay. The clinical examination provides indications regarding the nature and extent of the radiologic examination appropriate to the situation.

A team of dentists tested the ability of the original ADA guidelines to reduce the number of intraoral images, while still offering adequate diagnostic information. This testing of the use of selection criteria demonstrated that a small but significant number of findings were not 100% covered in the anterior region if only posterior interproximal and selected periapical images were used. The testing suggested that anterior interproximal or anterior periapical images are also indicated to detect interproximal caries and periodontal disease in the anterior region, specifically for patients with high levels of dental disease. A panoramic radiograph could be made in place of the periapical images to supplement the posterior bitewings if the totality of the disease expected indicates a broad area of coverage and fine detail is not required.

In the ADA/FDA guidelines, patients are classified by stage of dental development, by whether they are being evaluated for the first time (without previous documentation) or being reevaluated during a recall visit, and by an estimate of their risk for having dental caries or periodontal disease. A footnote to Table 16-2 also outlines some other clinical findings that indicate when diagnostic images are likely to contribute to a complete description of the asymptomatic patient.

Applying these guidelines to the specific circumstances with each patient requires clinical judgment and an amalgamation of knowledge, experience, and concern. Clinical judgment is also required to recognize situations that are *not* described by the guidelines but in which patients would need diagnostic images nonetheless.

Initial Visit

The guidelines recommend that a child with primary dentition who is cooperative and has closed posterior contacts have only interproximal views to examine for caries. Additional periapical or occlusal views are recommended only in the case of clinically evident diseases or specific historical or clinical indications such as those listed at the footnote of Table 16-2. Patients without evidence of disease and with open proximal contacts may not require a radiologic examination at this time.

For radiologic examination of a new patient in the transitional dentition, after eruption of the first permanent tooth, the guidelines recommend interproximal views to assess for dental caries and a panoramic radiograph or selected periapical or occlusal views to evaluate growth and development, this being a time when management of dental anomalies might begin.

The guidelines group adolescents and dentate adults together to identify the kind and extent of appropriate radiologic examination. The guidelines recommend that these patients receive an individualized examination consisting of interproximal views and panoramic or periapical views selected on the basis of specific historical or clinical indications. The presence of generalized dental disease often indicates the need for a full-mouth examination. Alternatively, the presence of only a few localized

| TABLE 16-2 | American Dental Association Recommendations for Prescribing Dental Radiographs* |

Type of Encounter	PATIENT AGE AND DENTAL DEVELOPMENTAL STAGE	
	Child with Primary Dentition (before Eruption of First Permanent Tooth)	Child with Transitional Dentition (after Eruption of First Permanent Tooth)
New patient* being evaluated for oral diseases	Individualized radiographic exam consisting of selected periapical/occlusal views and/or posterior bitewings if proximal surfaces cannot be visualized or probed. Patients without evidence of disease and with open proximal contacts may not require a radiographic examination at this time	Individualized radiographic exam consisting of posterior bitewings with panoramic exam or posterior bitewings and selected periapical images
Recall patient* with clinical caries or at increased risk for caries[†]	Posterior bitewing exam at 6- to 12-mo intervals if proximal surfaces cannot be examined visually or with a probe	
Recall patient* with no clinical caries and not at increased risk of developing caries[†]	Posterior bitewing examination at 12- to 24-mo intervals if proximal surfaces cannot be examined visually or with a probe	
Recall patient* with periodontal disease	Clinical judgment as to the need for and type of radiographic images for the evaluation of periodontal disease. Imaging may consist of, but is not limited to, selected bitewing and/or periapical images of areas in which periodontal disease (other than nonspecific gingivitis) can be demonstrated clinically	
Patient (new and recall) for monitoring of dentofacial growth and development and/or assessment of dental/skeletal relationships	Clinical judgment as to need for and type of radiographic images for evaluation and/or monitoring of dentofacial growth and development or assessment of dental and skeletal relationships	
Patient with other circumstances, including, but not limited to, proposed or existing implants, other dental and craniofacial pathosis, restorative/endodontic needs, treated periodontal disease, and caries remineralization	Clinical judgment as to need for and type of radiographic images for evaluation and/or monitoring of these conditions	

PATIENT AGE AND DENTAL DEVELOPMENTAL STAGE		
Adolescent with Permanent Dentition (before Eruption of Third Molars)	Adult, Dentate or Partially Edentulous	Adult, Edentulous
Individualized radiographic exam consisting of posterior bitewings with panoramic exam or posterior bitewings and selected periapical images; full-mouth intraoral radiographic exam is preferred when patient has clinical evidence of generalized dental disease or a history of extensive dental treatment		Individualized radiographic exam, based on clinical signs and symptoms
Posterior bitewing exam at 6- to 12-mo intervals if proximal surfaces cannot be examined visually or with a probe	Posterior bitewing examination at 6- to 18-mo intervals	Not applicable
Posterior bitewing exam at 18- to 36-mo intervals	Posterior bitewing exam at 24- to 36-mo intervals	Not applicable
Clinical judgment as to the need for and type of radiographic images for the evaluation of periodontal disease. Imaging may consist of, but is not limited to, selected bitewing and/or periapical images of areas in which periodontal disease (other than nonspecific gingivitis) can be demonstrated clinically		Not applicable
Clinical judgment as to need for and type of radiographic images for evaluation and/or monitoring of dentofacial growth and development or assessment of dental and skeletal relationships. Panoramic or periapical exam to assess developing third molars	Usually not indicated for monitoring of growth and development. Clinical judgment as to the need for and type of radiographic images for evaluation of dental and skeletal relationships	
Clinical judgment as to need for and type of radiographic images for evaluation and/or monitoring of these conditions		

Note. The recommendations in this table are subject to clinical judgment and may not apply to every patient. They are to be used by dentists only after reviewing the patient's health history and completing a clinical examination. Because every precaution should be taken to minimize radiation exposure, protective thyroid collars and aprons should be used whenever possible.

*Clinical situations for which radiographs may be indicated, but are not limited to, include the following: *positive historical findings*—previous periodontal or endodontic treatment, history of pain or trauma, familial history of dental anomalies, postoperative evaluation of healing, remineralization monitoring, presence of implants, previous implant pathoses, or evaluation for implant placement; *positive clinical signs/symptoms*—clinical evidence of periodontal disease, large or deep restorations, deep carious lesions, mal-posed or clinically impacted teeth, swelling, evidence of dental/facial trauma, mobility of teeth, sinus tract ("fistula"), clinically suspected sinus pathosis, growth abnormalities, oral involvement in known or suspected systemic disease, positive neurologic findings in the head and neck, evidence of foreign objects, pain and/or dysfunction of TMJ, facial asymmetry, abutment teeth for fixed or removable partial prosthesis, unexplained bleeding, unexplained sensitivity of teeth, unusual eruption, spacing or migration of teeth, unusual tooth morphology, calcification or color, unexplained absence of teeth, clinical dental erosion, or peri-implantitis.

[†]Factors increasing risk for caries may be assessed using the ADA Caries Risk Assessment forms (0-6 years old) and (>6 years old): http://www.ada.org.

Adapted from the U.S. Department of Health and Human Services, Public Health Service, Food and Drug Administration; and American Dental Association, Council on Dental Benefit Programs, Council on Scientific Affairs.

abnormalities or diseases suggests that a more limited examination consisting of interproximal and selected periapical views may suffice. In circumstances with no evidence of current or past dental disease, only interproximal views may be necessary for caries examination.

For an edentulous patient presenting for prosthetic treatment, an individualized examination that is based on clinical signs and symptoms should be performed. This may include a panoramic image or selected periapical or occlusal views, with some type of cross-sectional examination if dental implants are being considered.

Recall Visit

Patients who are returning after initial care require careful examination before determining the need for diagnostic images. As at the initial examination, selected periapical views should be obtained if any of the historical or clinical signs or symptoms listed in the footnote to Table 16-2 are present and need further evaluation.

The guidelines recommend interproximal radiographs for recall patients to detect interproximal caries. The optimal frequency for these views depends on the age of the patient and the probability of finding this disease. If the patient has clinically demonstrable caries or the presence of high-risk factors for caries (poor diet, poor oral hygiene, and others that can be assessed via the ADA Caries Risk Assessment forms: *http://www.ada.org*), bitewings are exposed at fairly frequent intervals (6 to 12 months for children and adolescents and 6 to 18 months for adults) until no carious lesions are clinically evident. The recommended intervals are longer for individuals not at high risk for caries: 12 to 24 months for a child, 18 to 36 months for an adolescent, and 24 to 36 months for an adult. Individuals can change risk category, going from high to low risk or the reverse.

Clinical judgment about need for and type of radiologic examination should be used for other circumstances, such as evaluating the status of periodontal disease, monitoring growth and development, and endodontic or restorative considerations. The interproximal examination may be supplemented by a panoramic, selected periapical or occlusal, or advanced imaging examination, depending on the patient's specific needs.

A radiologic examination may be required in many other situations, such as for patients contemplating orthodontic or implant treatment or patients with intraosseous lesions. The goal should be to obtain the necessary diagnostic information with the minimal radiation dose and financial cost, which can be substantial for advanced imaging procedures such as MR imaging. The dentist should determine specifically what type of information is needed and the most appropriate technique for obtaining it. An example of a clinical algorithm for ordering diagnostic images before orthodontic treatment is shown in Figure 16-1, using guidelines endorsed by the American Academy of Orthodontics. Because guidelines for ordering diagnostic images for other situations are not as well developed, the dentist must rely on clinical judgment.

SPECIAL CONSIDERATIONS

Pregnancy

Occasionally, it is desirable to obtain diagnostic images of a pregnant patient. The x-ray beam is largely confined to the head and neck region in dental x-ray examinations; fetal exposure is only about 1 μGy for a full-mouth examination. This exposure is quite small compared with that received normally from natural background sources. Because the use of radiologic procedures in all patients is predicated on there being a diagnostic need for them, the guidelines apply to pregnant patients as well as patients who are not pregnant. However, the ADA recommends the use of protective thyroid collars and aprons during dental radiography for all patients as well as the use of all other dose-limiting techniques, following the principle of ALARA (*A*s *L*ow *A*s *R*easonably *A*chievable).

Radiation Therapy

Patients with a malignancy in the oral cavity or perioral region often receive radiation therapy for their disease. Some oral tissues receive 50 Gy or more. Although such patients are often apprehensive about receiving additional exposure, dental exposure is insignificant compared with what they have already received. The average skin dose from an intraoral radiograph is approximately 3 mGy, less if faster film or digital imaging is used. Patients who have received radiation therapy may have radiation-induced xerostomia and are at a high risk for development of radiation caries, which may produce serious consequences if extractions are needed in the future. Patients who have had radiation therapy to the oral cavity should be carefully followed up because they are at special risk for dental disease.

EXAMPLES OF USE OF THE GUIDELINES

Consider the ways in which the guidelines can be applied to different clinical situations:

- The first visit of a 5-year-old boy to a dental office. A careful clinical examination reveals that the patient is cooperative and that the posterior teeth are in contact. Posterior bitewings are recommended to detect caries. If all of this patient's teeth are present, no evidence exists of decay, a reasonably good diet is being observed, and the parent seems well motivated to promote good oral hygiene, no further radiologic examination is required at this time. Images for the detection of developmental abnormalities are not in order at this age because a complete appraisal cannot be made at age 5 years. Even if it could be made, it is too early to initiate treatment for such abnormalities.
- A 25-year-old woman receiving a 6-month checkup after her last treatment for a fractured incisor. No caries is evident on interproximal images made 6 months ago; currently no clinical signs suggest caries, and the patient does not have high-risk factors for caries. No evidence exists of periodontal disease or other remarkable signs or symptoms in general or associated with the recently fractured tooth. As long as the fractured incisor shows normal vitality testing, no radiographs are recommended for this patient. If the incisor is nonvital, a periapical view of this tooth should be exposed.
- A 45-year-old man returning to the dentist's office after 1 year. At his last visit, two three-surface amalgam restorations were placed on premolars, and root canal therapy was performed on number 30. The patient has a 5-mm pocket in the buccal furcation of number 3 but no other evidence of periodontal disease. The guidelines recommend that this patient receive interproximal images to see whether he still has active caries and periapical views of numbers 3 and 30 to evaluate the extent of the periodontal disease and periapical disease, respectively.
- A 65-year-old woman coming to the office for the first time. No previous diagnostic images are available. The patient has a history of root canal therapy in two teeth, although she does

not know which teeth were treated. Clinical examination reveals multiple carious teeth, multiple missing teeth, and pockets of more than 3 mm involving most of the remaining teeth. The guidelines recommend a full-mouth examination, including interproximal images, for this patient because of the high probability of finding caries, periodontal disease, and periapical disease.

BIBLIOGRAPHY

Guidelines for Ordering Radiographs

American Association of Endodontists, American Academy of Oral and Maxillofacial Radiology: Use of cone-beam computed tomography in endodontics. Joint position statement of the American Association of Endodontists and the American Academy of Oral and Maxillofacial Radiology, *Oral Surg Oral Med Oral Pathol Oral Radiol Endod* 111:234–237, 2011.

American Academy of Oral and Maxillofacial Radiology: Clinical recommendations regarding use of cone beam computed tomography in orthodontic treatment. *Oral Surg Oral Med Oral Pathol Oral Radiol* 116(2):238–257, 2013.

American Dental Association Council on Scientific Affairs: Dental radiographic examinations: recommendations for patient selection and limiting radiation exposure. Revised 2012: http://www.ada.org/sections/professionalResources/pdfs/Dental_Radiographic_Examinations_2012.pdf.

American Dental Association Council on Scientific Affairs: The use of cone-beam computed tomography in dentistry. An advisory statement from the American Dental Association Council on Scientific Affairs, *J Am Dent Assoc* 143:899–902, 2012.

Atchison KA, Luke LS, White SC: An algorithm for ordering pretreatment orthodontic radiographs, *Am J Orthod Dentofac Orthop* 102:29–44, 1992.

Atchison KA, White SC, Flack VF, et al: Assessing the FDA guidelines for ordering dental radiographs, *J Am Dent Assoc* 126:1372–1383, 1995.

Bohay RN, Stephens RG, Kogon SL: A study of the impact of screening or selective radiography on the treatment and post delivery outcome for edentulous patients, *Oral Surg Oral Med Oral Pathol Oral Radiol Endod* 86:353–359, 1998.

Brooks SL: A study of selection criteria for intraoral dental radiography, *Oral Surg Oral Med Oral Pathol* 62:234–239, 1986.

Brooks SL, Brand JW, Gibbs SI, et al: Imaging of the temporomandibular joint: a position paper of the American Academy of Oral and Maxillofacial Radiology, *Oral Surg Oral Med Oral Pathol Oral Radiol Endod* 83:609–618, 1997.

European Commission: Radiation protection 136, European guidelines on radiation protection in dental radiology: the safe use of radiographs in dental practice, 2004: http://ec.europa.eu/energy/nuclear/radioprotection/publication/doc/136_en.pdf. Accessed July 2, 2012.

Rushton VE, Horner K, Worthington HV: Routine panoramic radiography of new adult patients in general dental practice: relevance of diagnostic yield to treatment and identification of radiographic selection criteria, *Oral Surg Oral Med Oral Pathol Oral Radiol Endod* 93:488–495, 2002.

SEDENTEXCT Guidelines: Guidelines on CBCT for dental and maxillofacial radiology: http://www.sedentexct.eu. Accessed July 2, 2012.

Tyndall DA, Price JB, Tetradis S, et al: Position statement of the American Academy of Oral and Maxillofacial Radiology on selection criteria for the use of radiology in dental implantology with emphasis on cone beam computed tomography, *Oral Surg Oral Med Oral Pathol Oral Radiol* 113:817–826, 2012.

U.S. Department of Health and Human Services, Public Health Service, Food and Drug Administration, and American Dental Association, Council on Dental Benefit Programs, Council on Scientific Affairs: The selection of patients for dental radiographic examinations, revised ed (2012): http://www.fda.gov/Radiation-EmittingProducts/RadiationEmittingProductsandProcedures/MedicalImaging/MedicalX-Rays/ucm116504.htm.

White SC, Heslop EW, Hollender LG, et al: Parameters of radiologic care: an official report of the American Academy of Oral and Maxillofacial Radiology, *Oral Surg Oral Med Oral Pathol Oral Radiol Endod* 91:498–511, 2001.

Disease Detection

Atchison KA, White SC, Flack VF, et al: Efficacy of the FDA selection criteria for radiographic assessment of the periodontium, *J Dent Res* 74:1424–1432, 1995.

Atieh MA: Diagnostic accuracy of panoramic radiographs in determining the relationship between the inferior alveolar nerve and mandibular third molar, *J Oral Maxillofac Surg* 68:74–82, 2010.

Corbet EF, Ho DK, Lai SM: Radiographs in periodontal disease and management, *Austral Dent J* 54(Suppl 1):S27–S43, 2009.

Devereux L, Moles D, Cunningham SJ, et al: How important are lateral cephalometric radiographs in orthodontic treatment planning? *Am J Orthod Dentofac Orthop* 139:e175–e181, 2011

Friedlander AH, Freymiller EG: Detection of radiation-accelerated atherosclerosis of the carotid artery by panoramic radiography: a new opportunity for dentists, *J Am Dent Assoc* 134:1361–1365, 2003.

Jindal SK, Sheikh S, Kulkarni S, et al: Significance of pre-treatment panoramic radiographic assessment of edentulous patients—a survey, *Med Oral Patol Oral Cir Bucal* 16:e600–606, 2011.

Madden RP, Hodges JS, Salmen CW, et al: Utility of panoramic radiographs in detecting cervical calcified carotid atheroma, *Oral Surg Oral Med Oral Pathol Oral Radiol Endod* 103:543–548, 2007.

Masood F, Robinson W, Beavers KS, et al: Findings from panoramic radiographs of the edentulous population and review of the literature, *Quintessence Int* 38:e298–e305, 2007.

Moles DR, Downer MC: Optimum bitewing examination recall intervals assessed by computer simulation, *Commun Dent Health* 17:14–19, 2000.

Mupparapu M, Kim IH: Calcified carotid artery atheroma and stroke: a systematic review, *J Am Dent Assoc* 138:483–492, 2007.

Reddy MS, Geurs NC, Jeffcoat RL, et al: Periodontal disease progression, *J Periodontol* 71:1583–1590, 2000.

Schiffman E, Ohrbach R, Truelove E, et al: Diagnostic criteria for temporomandibular disorders (DC/TMD) for clinical and research applications. Recommendations of the International RDC/TMD Consortium Network and the Orofacial Pain Special Interest Group, *J Orofac Pain* [In press].

Senel B, Kamburoglu K, Ucok O, et al: Diagnostic accuracy of different imaging modalities in detection of proximal caries, *Dentomaxillofac Radiol* 39:501–511, 2010.

White SC, Atchison KA, Hewlett ER, et al: Efficacy of FDA guidelines for ordering radiographs for caries detection, *Oral Surg Oral Med Oral Pathol* 77:531–540, 1994.

White SC, Atchison KA, Hewlett ER, et al: Clinical and historical predictors of dental caries on radiographs, *Dentomaxillofac Radiol* 24:121–127, 1995.

Yoon SJ, Yoon W, Kim OS, et al: Diagnostic accuracy of panoramic radiographs in the detection of calcified carotid arteries, *Dentomaxillofac Radiol* 37:104–108, 2008.

Radiation Dosage and Effects

Claus EB, Calvocoressi L, Bondy ML, et al: Dental x-rays and risk of meningioma, *Cancer* 118(18):4530–4537, 2012. See also Tetradis, et al. below.

Goske MJ, Applegate KE, Boylan J, et al: The "Image Gently" campaign: increasing CT radiation dose awareness through a national education and awareness program, *Pediatr Radiol* 38:265–269, 2008.

Ludlow IB, Davies-Ludlow LE, Brooks SL, et al: Dosimetry of 3 CBCT devices for oral and maxillofacial radiology: CB Mercuray, NewTom 3G and i-CAT, *Dentomaxillofac Radiol* 35:219–226, 2006.

Ludlow JB, Davies-Ludloe LE, White SC: Patient risk to common dental radiographic exams: the impact of 2007 ICRP recommendations regarding dose calculation, *J Am Dent Assoc* 139:1237–1243, 2008.

Ludlow JB, Ivanovic M: Comparative dosimetry of dental CBCT devices and 64 row CT for oral and maxillofacial radiology, *Oral Surg Oral Med Oral Pathol Oral Radiol Endod* 106:930–938, 2008.

Tetradis S, White SC, Service SK: Dental X-Rays and Risk of Meningioma; the Jury is Still Out, *The journal of evidence-based dental practice* 12(3):174–177, 2012.

White SC, Mallya SM: Update on the biological effects of ionizing radiation, relative dose factors, and radiation hygiene, *Aust Dent J* 57(Suppl 1):2–8, 2012.

Principles of Radiographic Interpretation

Mariam Baghdady

OUTLINE

D entists are expected to have basic skills in interpreting any intraoral or extraoral images that might be used in dental practice. This ability requires the mastery of two identifiable and nonseparable components of visual diagnosis: perception, the ability to recognize abnormal patterns in the image, and cognition, the interpretation of these abnormal patterns to arrive at a diagnosis. This chapter provides an overview of diagnostic reasoning in oral radiology. It also provides an analytic framework to aid in the interpretation of diagnostic images. This framework will equip the reader with a systematic method of image analysis.

ADEQUATE DIAGNOSTIC IMAGES

Any method of image analysis is limited by the information contained in the available diagnostic images. Ensuring that there are an adequate number of images of diagnostic quality that display the region of interest in its entirety is an essential first step. When using plain or projection images, multiple images at slightly different projection angles and images exposed at right angles to one another often provide significant additional information. When appropriate, the use of advanced forms of diagnostic imaging can also provide valuable diagnostic information (see Chapter 16).

VISUAL SEARCH STRATEGIES

The ability to find and identify abnormal patterns in the diagnostic image first involves a visual search of the entire image. An ability to recognize an abnormal pattern requires an in-depth knowledge of the variations of appearances of normal anatomy. This is especially true in searching panoramic images. It is likely that experienced radiologists use a free search pattern when analyzing a diagnostic image. However, more recent research has shown that

the employment of a systematic search strategy by novice clinicians improves their ability to detect abnormalities in panoramic images. A systematic search strategy involves the identification of a list of normal anatomic structures that would be contained within the image. In a panoramic image, this strategy might involve identifying the posterior border of the maxilla, the floor of the sinus, the zygomatic process of the maxilla, and the orbital rim. In a periapical image, the list might include crown, root structure, pulp and pulp canal, periodontal membrane space, and lamina dura. In a data set of cone-beam computed tomographic (CBCT) images, the normal anatomy would be inspected through the whole image volume using axial, coronal, and sagittal image slices. When faced with a complex appearance of anatomic structures, having a systematic search strategy enables the novice clinician to search the complete image in a meaningful and more successful fashion. When an abnormality has been detected in an image, the clinician must focus on formulating an interpretation of the abnormality.

DIAGNOSTIC REASONING IN ORAL RADIOLOGY

Clinical reasoning in diagnostic oral radiology can be considered unique in that the initial task requires the clinician to engage in a complex perceptual phase that involves differentiating normal and abnormal anatomic structures on two-dimensional images that represent three-dimensional structures. After the search process, if a finding is deemed abnormal, the clinician forms a mental three-dimensional image of the abnormality that includes the precise location, size, internal structure, and how the abnormality affects the surrounding normal structures. This complex perceptual step is a method of identifying features of the abnormality used to arrive at a plausible diagnosis.

A common method for a novice clinician is to memorize specific features of each type of abnormality and then attempt to use this information to interpret images. This approach has been shown to be ineffective in correct interpretation of radiographic abnormalities. However, it has been found that understanding the basic disease mechanism underlying the changes that each type of abnormality can render in the diagnostic image is more effective in enhancing a clinician's diagnostic accuracy. The terms "disease mechanism" and "basic science" are used to represent the pathophysiologic basis of abnormalities at the cellular, tissue, and biochemical levels. More recent research suggests that the understanding of disease mechanisms plays an essential role in enhancing diagnostic accuracy in novice clinicians. Basic science knowledge apparently creates a coherent mental representation of diagnostic categories and their features. According to this theory, basic sciences may assist in "true understanding" of the diagnostic entities by creating coherent mental representations of different disease categories. Hence, when clinicians understand why certain features occur, they are able to make the diagnosis that "makes sense," rather than simply focusing on feature counting and rote memory. Also, more recent research shows that teaching disease mechanisms and radiographic features in an integrated fashion produced novice clinicians with higher diagnostic accuracy than novice clinicians who were taught in a segregated manner.

Worth, a pioneer in diagnostic oral radiology, stated, "Radiographic appearances are governed by anatomic and physiologic changes in the presence of disease processes. Radiologic diagnosis is founded on knowledge of these alterations, the prerequisite being awareness of disease mechanisms."

ANALYSIS OF ABNORMAL FINDINGS

There are two main forms of diagnostic processing described in radiology; the first is the analytic or systematic strategy. This approach relies on a step-by-step analysis of all the imaging features of an abnormal finding so that a diagnosis can be made based on these findings (Fig. 17-1). This analytic process is believed to reduce bias and premature closure of the decision-making process.

The second form, a nonanalytic strategy, assumes that simply viewing an abnormal finding automatically leads to a holistic diagnostic hypothesis, which is followed by a deliberate search for features that support the initial hypothesis. The nonanalytic approach suggests that the clinician makes an automatic decision regarding the diagnosis without thorough feature analysis of the image. For example, expert radiologists may rely on pattern recognition as a nonanalytic diagnostic strategy.

There is some empirical evidence that nonanalytic reasoning can be successfully employed by novice clinicians. However, critics of teaching novices to rely on nonanalytic processing argue that the success of this diagnostic strategy is limited by the novice's minimal experience and the varied appearances of both normal anatomy and pathologic disorders in images.

Although these two processes are viewed as separate mechanisms, research provides evidence that they are complementary and should not be viewed as being mutually exclusive. Students learning oral radiology could potentially benefit from specific training in the use of combined analytic and nonanalytic diagnostic strategies.

An analytic tool for the analysis of abnormal findings is presented in the next section. The main function of this tool is to collect all the available imaging characteristics of the abnormal finding. Once the information is assembled, it is useful in the diagnostic process.

As the imaging characteristics are being collected, it is important to integrate the disease mechanism underlying these characteristics when possible. For instance, Figure 17-2 depicts the maturation of periapical osseous dysplasia (periapical cemental dysplasia). At the first stage (Fig. 17-2, *A*), the periapical bone is resorbed and replaced with fibrous tissue, and therefore it appears radiolucent in the image. In a later maturation stage, this abnormality produces amorphous bone in the center (Fig. 17-2, *B*), resulting in a radiopaque mass in the center surrounded by a soft tissue radiolucent rim. Knowledge of the disease mechanism allows for the correct diagnosis of a lesion of periapical osseous dysplasia in an unusual location in the maxilla and after the associated tooth has been extracted (Fig. 17-2, *C*).

FIGURE 17-1 Diagram illustrating the diagnostic process in oral radiology. The learning strategy phase represents the stage at which a novice learns about disease categories. The diagnostic strategy phase demonstrates the diagnostic techniques used by the clinician when faced with an abnormality.

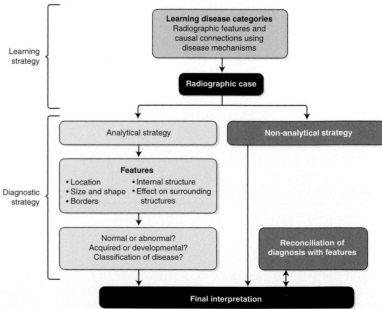

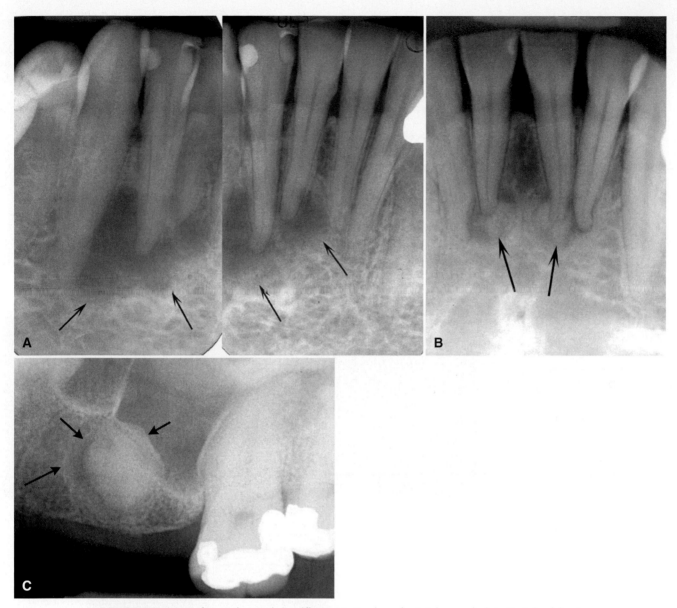

FIGURE 17-2 Series of periapical images showing different maturation phases of periapical osseous dysplasia. **A,** Early radiolucent phase after periapical bone has been resorbed and replaced with fibrous tissue *(arrows).* **B,** Late maturation phase showing central amorphous bone (radiopaque) surrounded by a soft tissue margin *(arrows).* **C,** Mature phase of periapical osseous dysplasia in an unusual location and after the associated tooth has been extracted.

ANALYTIC OR SYSTEMATIC STRATEGY

STEP 1: LOCALIZE ABNORMALITY

Localized or Generalized

The anatomic location and limits of the abnormality should be described. This information aids in starting to select various disease categories. If an abnormal appearance affects all the osseous structures of the maxillofacial region, generalized disease mechanisms, such as metabolic or endocrine abnormalities of bone, are considered. If the abnormality is localized, one considers whether it is unilateral or bilateral. Variations of normal anatomy are more commonly bilateral. For instance, a bilateral mandibular radiolucency may indicate normal anatomy, such as extensive submandibular gland fossa. Abnormal conditions are more commonly unilateral. For instance, fibrous dysplasia commonly is unilateral.

This is not to say that localized pathologic lesions cannot occur bilaterally in the maxillofacial region. A few abnormalities, such as Paget's disease and cherubism, are always seen bilaterally in the jaws. Also, when cherubism involves the mandible, the first region to be involved is in the midramus region, and this is the mechanism behind the anterior displacement of molars (Fig. 17-3).

Position in the Jaws

Identifying the exact location of the lesion in the maxillofacial complex aids the diagnostic process in two ways: (1) it determines the epicenter and (2) some lesions tend to be found in specific locations.

Determining the epicenter of the lesion or the point of origin assists in indicating the tissue types that compose the abnormality in question. The epicenter can be estimated on the basis of the assumption that the abnormality grew equally in every direction.

This estimation may become less accurate with very large lesions or lesions with ill-defined boundaries. Following are a few examples of relating the epicenter of the lesion to the tissue of origin:

- If the epicenter is coronal to a tooth, the lesion probably is composed of odontogenic epithelium (Fig. 17-4).
- If it is above the inferior alveolar nerve canal (IAC), the likelihood is greater that it is composed of odontogenic tissue (Fig. 17-5).
- If the epicenter is below the IAC, it is unlikely to be odontogenic in origin (Fig. 17-6).
- If it originates within the IAC, the tissue of origin probably is neural or vascular in nature (Fig. 17-7).

- The probability of cartilaginous lesions and osteochondromas occurring is greater in the condylar region.
- If the epicenter is within the maxillary antrum, the lesion is not of odontogenic tissue, as opposed to a lesion that has grown into the antrum from the alveolar process of the maxilla (Fig. 17-8).

The other reason to establish the exact location of the lesion is that particular abnormalities tend to be found in very specific locations. Following are a few examples of this observation:

- The epicenters of central giant cell granulomas commonly are located anterior to the first molars in the mandible and anterior to the cuspid in the maxilla in young patients.

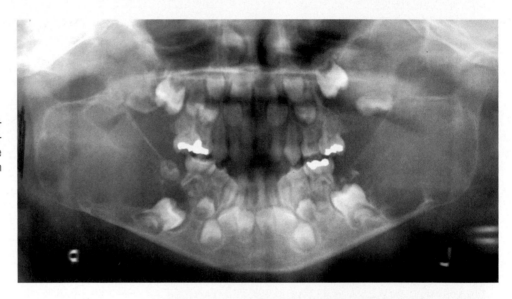

FIGURE 17-3 This lesion, cherubism, is bilateral, manifesting in both the left and the right mandibular rami. Because the origin of the lesion is in the midramus region, the mandibular molars have been displaced anteriorly on both sides.

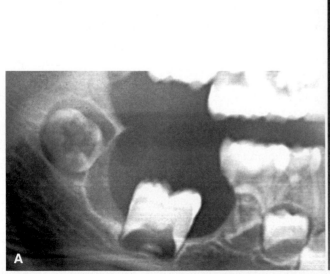

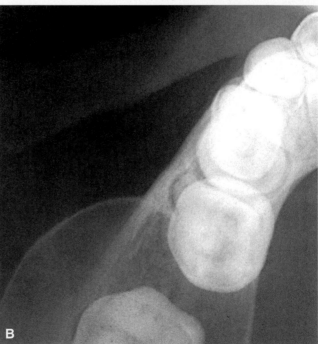

FIGURE 17-4 **A**, Cropped panoramic image of a lesion where the epicenter is coronal to the unerupted mandibular first molar. **B**, Occlusal projection providing a right-angle view of the same lesion.

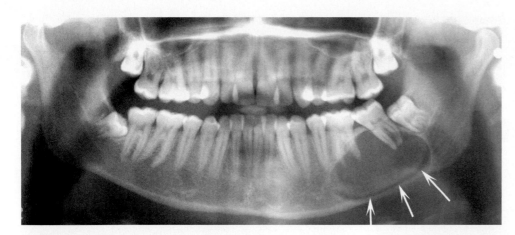

FIGURE 17-5 Panoramic image revealing a cystic ameloblastoma within the body of the left mandible. The inferior alveolar nerve canal has been displaced inferiorly to the inferior cortex *(arrows)*, indicating that the lesion started superior to the canal.

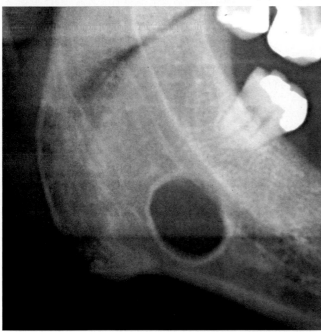

FIGURE 17-6 Cropped panoramic image displaying a lesion (developmental salivary gland defect) below the inferior alveolar canal and thus unlikely to be of odontogenic origin.

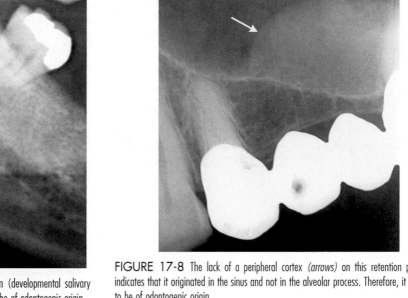

FIGURE 17-8 The lack of a peripheral cortex *(arrows)* on this retention pseudocyst indicates that it originated in the sinus and not in the alveolar process. Therefore, it is unlikely to be of odontogenic origin.

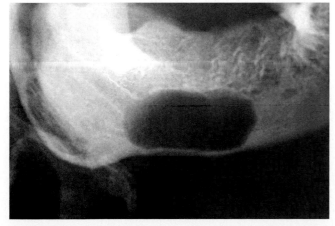

FIGURE 17-7 Lateral oblique view of the mandible revealing a lesion within the inferior alveolar canal. The smooth fusiform expansion of the canal indicates a neural lesion.

- Osteomyelitis occurs in the mandible and rarely in the maxilla.
- Periapical osseous dysplasia (periapical cemental dysplasia) occurs in the periapical region of teeth (see Fig. 17-2).

Single or Multifocal

Establishing whether an abnormality is solitary or multifocal aids in understanding the disease mechanism of the abnormality. Additionally, the list of possible multifocal abnormalities in the jaws is relatively short. Examples of lesions that can be multifocal in the jaws are periapical cemental dysplasia, keratocystic odontogenic tumors, metastatic lesions, multiple myeloma (Fig. 17-9), and leukemic infiltrates. Exceptions to all these points may occur occasionally. However, these criteria may serve as a guide to an accurate interpretation.

Size

Finally, the size of the lesion is considered. There are very few size restrictions for a particular lesion, but the size may aid in the

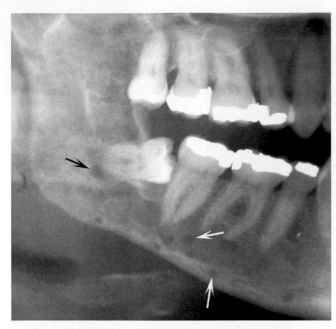

FIGURE 17-9 Cropped panoramic film revealing several small, punched-out lesions of multiple myeloma (a few are indicated by *arrows*) involving the body and ramus of the mandible.

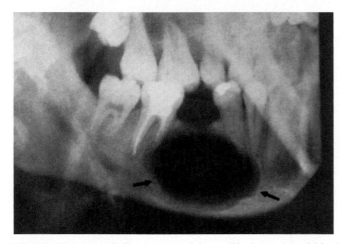

FIGURE 17-10 Lateral oblique projection of the mandible showing the well-defined border (*arrows*) of a residual cyst.

differential diagnosis. For instance, when differentiating between a dentigerous cyst and a hyperplastic follicle surrounding the coronal portion of a tooth, size may be considered a determining factor. Because dentigerous cysts have growth potential, they are often much larger than a hyperplastic follicle.

STEP 2: ASSESS PERIPHERY AND SHAPE

One should study the periphery of the lesion. Is the periphery well defined or ill defined? If an imaginary pencil can be used to draw confidently the limits of the lesion, the margin is well defined (Fig. 17-10). The clinician should not become concerned if some small regions are ill defined; these may be due to the shape or direction of the x-ray beam at that particular location. A well-defined lesion is one in which most of the periphery is well defined. In contrast, it is difficult to draw an exact delineation around most of an

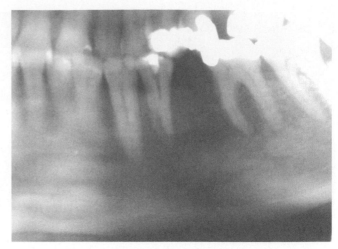

FIGURE 17-11 Cropped panoramic image showing the poorly defined border of a malignant neoplasm that has destroyed bone between the first molar and the first bicuspid.

ill-defined periphery (Fig. 17-11). The periphery can also have a dimension or a zone of transition. For instance, a thin radiopaque line or cortex at the periphery would represent a narrow zone of transition, as opposed to a thick sclerotic border, which would represent a relatively thick zone of transition. Further analysis of these two types of peripheries or borders can help define the nature of the lesion.

Well-Defined Borders

Punched-Out Border. A punched-out border is one that has a sharp boundary or a very narrow zone of transition in which no bone reaction is apparent immediately adjacent to the abnormality; this is analogous to punching a hole in a radiograph with a paper punch. The border of the resulting hole is well defined, and the surrounding bone has a normal appearance up to the edge of the hole. This type of border sometimes is seen in multiple myeloma (see Fig. 17-9).

Corticated Border. A corticated margin is a thin, fairly uniform radiopaque line of reactive bone at the periphery of a lesion. This is commonly seen with cysts and benign slow-growing tumors (see Fig. 17-4).

Sclerotic Margin. A sclerotic margin represents a wider zone of transition made up of a thick radiopaque border of reactive bone that usually is not uniform in width. This margin may be seen with periapical osseous dysplasia and may indicate a very slow rate of growth or the potential for the lesion to stimulate the production of surrounding bone (see Fig. 17-2).

Soft Tissue Capsule. A radiopaque lesion may have a soft tissue capsule, which is indicated by the presence of a radiolucent line at the periphery. This soft tissue capsule may be seen in conjunction with a corticated periphery, as is observed with odontomas and cementoblastomas (Figs. 17-12 and 17-13).

Ill-Defined Borders

Blending Border. A blending border is a gradual, often wide zone of transition between the adjacent normal bone trabeculae and the abnormal-appearing trabeculae of the lesion. The focus of this observation is on the trabeculae and not on the radiolucent marrow

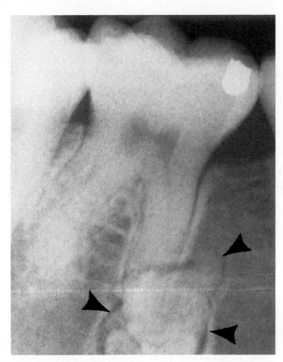

FIGURE 17-12 Thin, radiolucent periphery indicating a soft tissue capsule positioned between the internal radiopaque structure of this odontoma and the radiopaque outer cortical boundary (arrows).

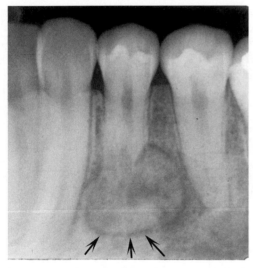

FIGURE 17-13 Periapical image revealing a radiopaque mass associated with the root of the first bicuspid. The prominent radiolucent periphery (arrows) is characteristic of a soft tissue capsule of this benign cementoblastoma.

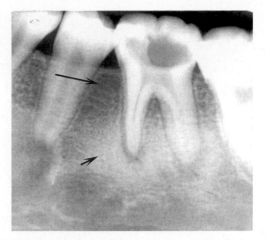

FIGURE 17-14 Periapical image shows a gradual transition from the dense trabeculae of sclerosing osteitis (short arrow) to the normal trabecular pattern near the crest of the alveolar process (long arrow). This is an example of an ill-defined, blending border.

spaces. Examples of conditions with this type of margin are sclerosing osteitis (Fig. 17-14) and fibrous dysplasia.

Invasive Border.   An ill-defined invasive border appears as an area of radiolucency with few or no trabeculae representing bone destruction just behind and at the leading margin of the lesion and usually has a wide zone of transition (Fig. 17-15). In contrast to the blending border, the focus of this observation is on the enlarging radiolucency at the expense of bone trabeculae. These borders have also been described as permeative because the lesion grows around existing trabeculae, producing radiolucent, finger-like, or bay-type extensions at the periphery. This growth may result in enlargement of the marrow spaces at the periphery (Fig. 17-16). Invasive borders are usually associated with rapid growth and can be seen with malignant lesions.

Shape

The lesion may have a particular shape, or it may be irregular. Two examples follow:

- A circular or fluid-filled shape, similar to an inflated balloon, is characteristic of a cyst. It can also be described as hydraulic (see Fig. 17-4).
- A scalloped shape is a series of contiguous arcs or semicircles that may reflect the mechanism of growth (Fig. 17-17). This shape may be seen in cysts (e.g., keratocystic odontogenic tumors), cystlike lesions (e.g., simple bone cysts), and some tumors. Occasionally, a lesion with a scalloped periphery is referred to as multilocular; however, the term multilocular is reserved for the description of the internal structure in this text.

STEP 3: ANALYZE INTERNAL STRUCTURE

The internal appearance of a lesion can be classified into one of three basic categories: totally radiolucent, totally radiopaque, or mixed radiolucent and radiopaque (mixed density). A totally radiolucent interior is common in cysts (see Fig. 17-4, A), and a totally radiopaque interior is observed in osteomas. The mixed density internal structure is seen as the presence of calcified structures (white) against a radiolucent (black) backdrop. A challenging aspect of this analysis may be the decision concerning whether a perceived calcified structure is in the internal aspect of the lesion or resides on either side of it; this is difficult to determine by using two-dimensional images representing three-dimensional structures. The shape, size, pattern, and density of the calcified structure should be examined. For example, bone can be identified by the presence of trabeculae. Also, the degree of radiopacity may help. For instance, enamel is more radiopaque than bone. Following is a list of most radiolucent to most radiopaque material seen in plain radiographs:

- Air, fat, and gas
- Fluid

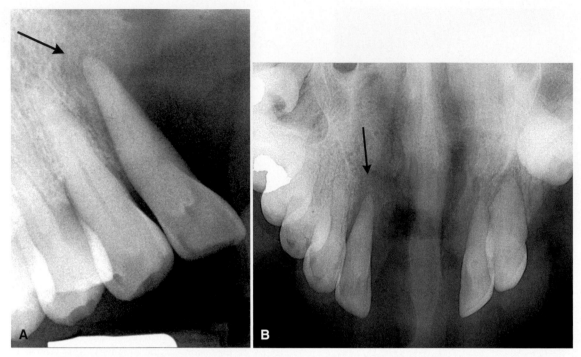

FIGURE 17-15 Periapical **(A)** and occlusal **(B)** images revealing a squamous cell carcinoma in the anterior maxilla. The invasive margin extends beyond the lateral incisor *(arrow)*, and the radiolucent region with no apparent trabeculae represents bone destruction behind this margin.

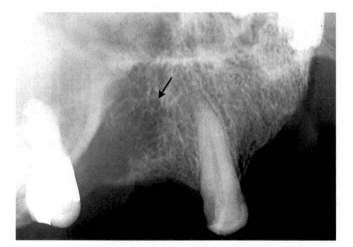

FIGURE 17-16 Lateral occlusal view of a lesion revealing an ill-defined periphery with enlargement of the small marrow spaces at the margin *(arrow)*. This is characteristic of a malignant neoplasm, in this case a lymphoma.

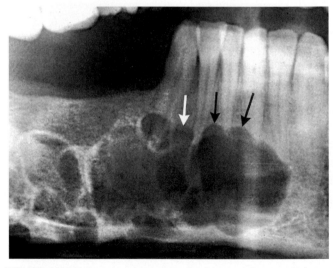

FIGURE 17-17 Cropped panoramic image of an odontogenic keratocyst displaying a scalloped border, especially around the apex of the associated teeth *(arrows)*.

- Soft tissue
- Bone marrow
- Trabecular bone
- Cortical bone and dentin
- Enamel
- Metal

This list is useful, but the amount of the tissue or material in the area can affect the degree of radiolucency or radiopacity. For example, a large amount of cortical bone may be as radiopaque as enamel.

The following section describes possible internal structures that may be seen in mixed density lesions

Abnormal Trabecular Patterns

Abnormal bone may have various trabecular patterns different from normal bone. These variations result from a difference in the number, length, width, and orientation of the trabeculae. For instance, in fibrous dysplasia, the trabeculae usually are greater in number, shorter, and not aligned in response to applied stress to the bone but are randomly oriented, resulting in patterns described as an orange-peel or a ground-glass appearance (Fig. 17-18). Another example is the stimulation of new bone formation on existing trabeculae in response to inflammation. The result is thick trabeculae, giving the area a more radiopaque appearance (see Fig. 17-14).

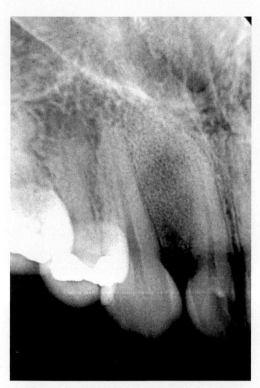

FIGURE 17-18 Periapical image of a small lesion of fibrous dysplasia between the lateral incisor and cuspid demonstrates a change in bone pattern. A greater number of trabeculae per unit area are present, and the trabeculae are small and thin and randomly oriented in an orange-peel pattern.

Internal Septation

Septations within a lesion represent bone that has been organized into long strands or walls within the lesion. If these septa appear to divide the internal structure into at least two compartments, the term multilocular is used to describe the lesion. The origin of this internal bone may be trapped bone, such as in ameloblastomas, or reactive bone, such as in giant cell granulomas, or the bone may be manufactured by the lesion, such as in ossifying fibromas. The length, width, and orientation of the septa should be assessed. The appearance of the septa also informs the observer about the nature and pathology of the lesion. For instance, curved, coarse septa may be seen in ameloblastoma giving the internal pattern a multilocular, "soap bubble" appearance. This pattern reflects the cystic formations at the histologic level within the ameloblastoma as these cystic regions remodel the trapped bone into curved shapes (Fig. 17-19, A and B). This pattern also may be observed sometimes in odontogenic keratocysts. Another example of internal septation is seen in giant cell granulomas. These bony septa are reactive bone formation and in some cases represent poorly calcified osteoid and appear as low density and wispy or granular septations in the image. Odontogenic myxomas also exhibit internal septation. In some cases, this tumor contains a few straight, thin septa.

Dystrophic Calcification

Dystrophic calcification is calcification that occurs in damaged soft tissue. It is most commonly seen in calcified lymph nodes that appear as dense, cauliflower-like masses in the soft tissue. In chronically inflamed cysts, the calcification may have a very delicate, particulate appearance without a recognizable pattern.

Amorphous Bone

This type of dystrophic bone has a homogeneous, dense, amorphous structure and sometimes is organized into round or oval shapes (see Fig. 17-2).

Tooth Structure

Tooth structure usually can be identified by the organization into enamel, dentin, and pulp chambers. Also, the internal density is equivalent to the density of tooth structure and greater than the density of the surrounding bone (see Fig. 17-12).

STEP 4: ANALYZE EFFECTS OF LESION ON SURROUNDING STRUCTURES

Evaluating the effects of the lesion on surrounding structures allows the observer to infer its behavior. The behavior may aid in identification of the disease. However, knowledge of the mechanisms of various diseases is required. For instance, inflammatory disease, as is seen in periapical osteitis, can stimulate bone resorption or formation. Bone formation may occur on the surface of existing trabeculae, resulting in thick trabeculae, which is reflected in the trabecular pattern and in an overall increase in the radiopacity of the bone (see Fig. 17-14). A space-occupying lesion, such as a cyst, slowly creates its own space by displacing teeth and other surrounding structures (see Fig. 17-4). The following sections give examples of effects on surrounding structures and the conclusions that may be inferred from the behavior of the lesions.

Teeth, Lamina Dura, and Periodontal Membrane Space

Displacement of teeth is seen more commonly with slower growing, space-occupying lesions. The direction of tooth displacement is significant. Lesions with an epicenter above the crown of a tooth (i.e., follicular cysts and occasionally odontomas) displace the tooth apically (see Fig. 17-4, A). Because cherubism originates and grows in the mandibular ramus, it has a propensity to push molars in an anterior direction (see Fig. 17-3). Some lesions (e.g., lymphoma, leukemia, Langerhans' cell histiocytosis) grow in the papilla of developing teeth and may push the developing tooth in a coronal direction (Fig. 17-20).

Resorption of teeth usually occurs with a more chronic or slowly growing process (see Fig. 17-4, A). It may also result from chronic inflammation. Although tooth resorption is more commonly related to benign processes, malignant tumors occasionally resorb teeth.

Widening of the periodontal membrane space may be seen with many different kinds of abnormalities. It is important to observe whether the widening is uniform or irregular and whether the lamina dura is still present. For instance, orthodontic movement of teeth results in widening of the periodontal membrane space, but the lamina dura remains intact. Malignant lesions can quickly grow down the ligament space, resulting in an irregular widening and destruction of the lamina dura (Fig. 17-21).

Surrounding Bone Reaction

Some abnormalities can stimulate a peripheral bone reaction. An example is the peripheral cortex of a cyst or sclerotic border of periapical osseous dysplasia as described in the analysis of periphery. The corticated border of a cyst is not actually part of the cyst but is a bone reaction. Identification of peripheral bone formation provides a behavioral characteristic that suggests that the abnormality has the ability to stimulate an osteoblastic reaction. An

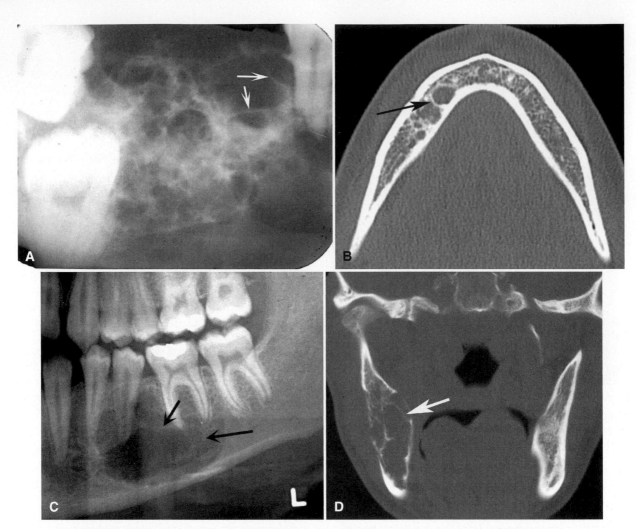

FIGURE 17-19 **A,** Periapical image of an ameloblastoma. The multilocular pattern created by septa *(arrows)* divides the internal structure into small, soap bubble—like compartments. **B,** Axial CT image of an ameloblastoma has typically curved septa *(arrow).* **C,** Cropped panoramic image of a giant cell granuloma with low-density granular septations *(arrows).* **D,** Coronal CT image of a myxoma has typically straight septa *(arrow).*

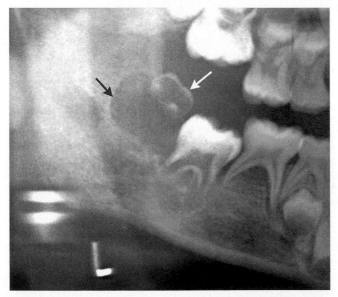

FIGURE 17-20 Leukemic infiltration of the mandible showing coronal displacement of the developing second molar *(white arrow)* from the remnants of its crypt *(black arrow).* There is a lack of a lamina dura around the apex of the first molar and widening of the periodontal ligament space around the second deciduous molar.

inflammatory lesion, such as periapical rarefying osteitis, can stimulate a sclerotic bone reaction (see Fig. 17-14); some metastatic malignant tumors such as prostate and breast metastatic lesions can stimulate an osteoblastic reaction.

Inferior Alveolar Nerve Canal and Mental Foramen

Changes to the inferior alveolar nerve canal can be characteristic to specific disease processes. Superior displacement of the inferior alveolar canal is strongly associated with fibrous dysplasia. Widening of the inferior alveolar canal with the maintenance of a cortical boundary may indicate the presence of a benign lesion of vascular or neural origin within the canal (see Fig. 17-7). Irregular widening with cortical destruction may indicate the presence of a malignant neoplasm growing down the length of the canal.

Outer Cortical Bone and Periosteal Reactions

The cortical boundaries of bone may remodel in response to the growth of a lesion within the maxilla or mandible. A slowly growing lesion may allow time for the outer periosteum to manufacture new bone so that the resulting expanded bone appears to have maintained an outer cortical plate (see Fig. 17-4, *B*). A rapidly growing lesion outstrips the ability of the periosteum to respond, and the cortical plate may be missing (Fig. 17-22). The remodeled external shape of the mandible or maxilla can provide information

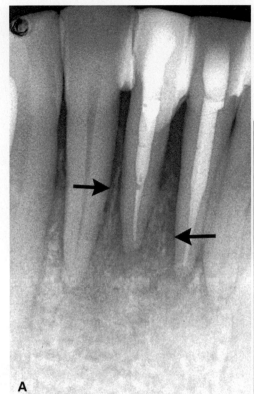
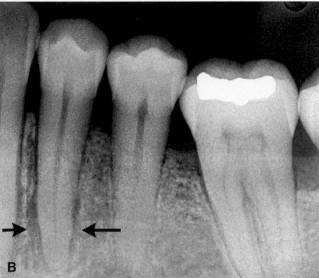

FIGURE 17-21 **A** and **B,** Periapical films revealing a malignant lymphoma that has invaded the mandible. There is irregular widening of the periodontal ligament spaces *(arrows).*

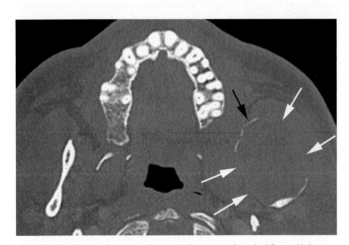

FIGURE 17-22 Axial CT image of an ameloblastoma involving the left mandibular ramus shows significant expansion of the ramus with some periosteal bone formation *(black arrow)* but with many regions of no periosteal bone formation *(white arrows),* which likely reflects a fast rate of expansion by the ameloblastoma.

on the growth pattern of the entity. For instance, a tumor such as ossifying fibroma often has a concentric growth pattern, whereas a bone dysplasia such as fibrous dysplasia enlarges the bone with a growth pattern that is along the bone without an obvious epicenter (Fig. 17-23).

Exudate from an inflammatory lesion can lift the periosteum off the surface of the cortical bone stimulating the osteoblasts of the periosteum to lay down new bone (Fig. 17-24). When this process occurs more than once, an onion-skin type of pattern can be seen. This pattern is most commonly seen in inflammatory

lesions and more rarely in tumors such as leukemia and Langerhans' cell histiocytosis. Other examples of patterns of reactive periosteal bone formation include a spiculated new bone formed at right angles to the outer cortical plate, which is seen with metastatic lesions of the prostate gland or in a radiating pattern of spiculated bone seen in osteogenic sarcoma (Fig. 17-25) or a hemangioma.

STEP 5: FORMULATE INTERPRETATION

The preceding steps enable the observer to collect all the radiographic findings analytically in an organized fashion. (Box 17-1 presents the process in abbreviated form.) Now the significance of each observation must be determined. The ability to give more significance to some observations over others comes with experience; this is also seen in a nonanalytic approach. After an initial diagnosis has been reached, ambiguities are resolved either by searching for more features or by putting more weight on one feature or the other. For instance, in the analysis of a hypothetical lesion, the observations of tooth movement, tooth resorption, and an invasive destructive border are made. The effects on the teeth in this example may indicate a benign process; however, the invasive border and bone destruction are more important characteristics and indicate a malignant process. In the analytic approach (see Fig. 17-1), all these accumulated characteristics are used to make a diagnostic decision. A diagnostic algorithm such as shown in Figure 17-26 can aid in this decision-making process. Following this algorithm, the observer makes decisions regarding which general category the entity fits into and then proceeds to smaller, more specific categories. This is not an infallible method because any algorithm occasionally may fail because lesions sometimes do not behave as expected.

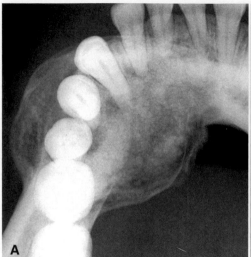
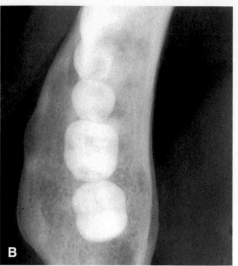

FIGURE 17-23 **A,** Occlusal image of an ossifying fibroma. The concentric expansion of the mandible is characteristic of a benign tumor. **B,** Occlusal image of fibrous dysplasia with mild expansion of the mandible but without an obvious epicenter as it causes expansion along the mandible.

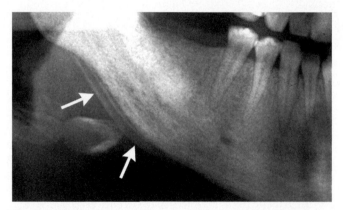

FIGURE 17-24 Panoramic image of osteomyelitis revealing at least two layers of new bone *(arrows)* produced by the periosteum at the inferior aspect of the mandible.

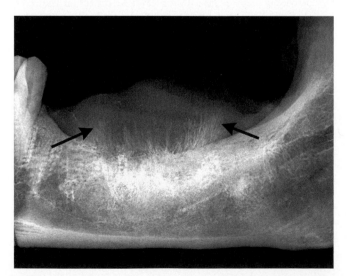

FIGURE 17-25 Specimen radiograph of a resected mandible with an osteosarcoma. Note the fine linear spicules of bone at the superior margin of the alveolar process *(arrows).*

BOX 17-1   Analysis of Intraosseous Lesions

STEP 1: LOCALIZE ABNORMALITY
- Anatomic position (epicenter)
- Localized or generalized
- Unilateral or bilateral
- Single or multifocal

STEP 2: ASSESS PERIPHERY AND SHAPE
Periphery
- Well defined
  - Punched-out
  - Corticated
  - Sclerotic
  - Soft tissue capsule
- Ill defined
  - Blending
  - Invasive

Shape
- Circular
- Scalloped
- Irregular

STEP 3: ANALYZE INTERNAL STRUCTURE
- Totally radiolucent
- Totally radiopaque
- Mixed (describe pattern)

STEP 4: ANALYZE EFFECTS OF LESION ON SURROUNDING STRUCTURES
- Teeth, lamina dura, periodontal membrane space
- Inferior alveolar nerve canal and mental foramen
- Maxillary antrum
- Surrounding bone density and trabecular pattern
- Outer cortical bone and periosteal reactions

STEP 5: FORMULATE INTERPRETATION

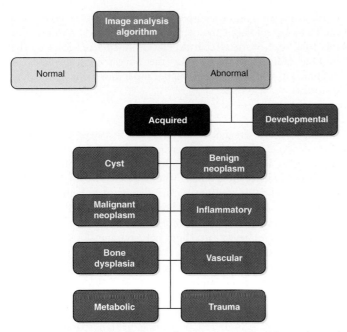

FIGURE 17-26 Algorithm representing the diagnostic process that follows evaluation of the radiographic features of an abnormality.

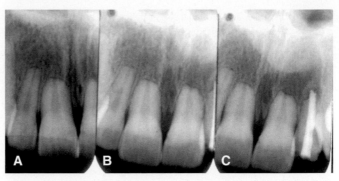

FIGURE 17-27 **A-C,** Periapical films revealing external resorption of the maxillary incisors, which is an acquired abnormality because of the presence of the wide pulp chambers at the apex of the roots of the teeth.

Decision 1: Normal or Abnormal

The clinician should determine whether the structure of interest is a variation of normal or represents an abnormality. This is a crucial decision because variations of normal do not require treatment or further investigation. However, as previously stated, to be proficient in the interpretation of diagnostic images, the clinician needs an in-depth knowledge of the various appearances of normal anatomy.

Decision 2: Developmental or Acquired

If the area of interest is abnormal, the next step is to decide whether the radiographic characteristics (location, periphery, shape, internal structure, and effects on surrounding structures) indicate that the region of interest represents a developmental abnormality or an acquired change. For instance, the observation that a tooth has an abnormally short root leads to the pertinent question, "Did the tooth develop a short root, or was the root at one time of normal length and has become shorter?" If the answer is the latter, the process must be external root resorption—an acquired abnormality. If the tooth merely developed a short root, the pulp canal should not be visible to the very end of the root because of normal apexification. In contrast, external root resorption may shorten the root, but the canal remains visible to the end of the root (Fig. 17-27).

Decision 3: Disease Classification

If the abnormality is acquired, the next step is to select the most likely disease category of the acquired abnormality. The disease category can be established through observing the features and how they reflect a particular disease mechanism. The categories may include cysts, benign tumors, malignant tumors, inflammatory lesions, bone dysplasias (fibro-osseous lesions), vascular abnormalities, metabolic diseases, or physical changes such as fractures. The following chapters describe the characteristic radiographic findings based on the disease mechanisms of these abnormalities. The analysis should strive at least to narrow the interpretation to one of these disease categories; this directs the next course of action for continued investigation, referral, and treatment. This is a good time to bring the clinical information, such as patient history and clinical signs and symptoms, into the decision-making process. When possible, considering this information at the end helps avoid the problem of doing an incomplete search of the images or trying to make the radiographic characteristics fit a preconceived diagnosis.

Decision 4: Ways to Proceed

After analyzing the images, the clinician must decide in what way to proceed. This decision may require further imaging, treatment, biopsy, or observation of the abnormality (watchful waiting). For example, if the lesion fits in the malignant category, the patient first should be referred to an oral and maxillofacial radiologist to complete the diagnostic imaging to stage the lesion and select the biopsy site and then should be referred to a surgeon for biopsy and treatment. Periapical osseous dysplasia may not require any further investigation or treatment. In other cases, a period of watchful waiting, followed by reexamination in a few months, may be indicated if the abnormality appears benign and no clear need for immediate treatment exists.

With advanced training or experience in diagnostic imaging, the clinician may be able to name one specific abnormality or at least make a short list of entities from one of the divisions of acquired abnormalities. When analyzing diagnostic images, it is advisable to create a formal report for the purposes of documentation and communication with other clinicians.

WRITING A DIAGNOSTIC IMAGING REPORT

The radiographic report can be subdivided into the following subsections.

PATIENT AND GENERAL INFORMATION

This section appears at the beginning and contains the following information: address of the radiology clinic; the date of the dictation; the referring clinician's name and clinic or address; and the patient's name, age, sex, and any numeric identification such as a clinic or medical registration number.

IMAGING PROCEDURE

This section gives a list of the imaging procedures provided along with the date of the examination. An example could be the following: panoramic and intraoral maxillary standard occlusal images plus axial and coronal CT images of the mandible with administration of contrast material made on February 20, 2012.

CLINICAL INFORMATION

This is an optional section that includes pertinent clinical information regarding the patient provided by the referring clinician or the clinician dictating the report if a clinical examination was made before the radiologic examination. The clinical information should remain brief and summarize the information pertaining to the lesion in question. For example: mass in floor of mouth, possible ranula, and patient has a history of lymphoma.

FINDINGS

This section comprises an objective detailed list of observations made from the diagnostic images. This can follow the previously presented step-by-step analysis of the extent of the lesion, periphery and shape, internal structure, and effects on surrounding structures. This section does not include an interpretation.

INTERPRETATION

This section is shorter and provides an interpretation for the preceding observations. The clinician should endeavor to provide a definitive interpretation. When this is not possible, a short list of conditions or a differential diagnosis (in order of likelihood) is acceptable. In some situations, advice regarding additional studies, when required, and treatment may be included. Lastly, the name and signature of the clinician composing the report is included.

SELF-TEST

To practice the analytic technique presented, the reader should examine Figure 17-4, *A* and *B,* and write down all observations and the results of the diagnostic algorithm before reading the following section.

DESCRIPTION

Location

The abnormality is singular and unilateral, and the epicenter lies coronal to the mandibular first molar.

Periphery and Shape

The lesion has a well-defined cortical boundary and a spherical or round shape. The periphery also attaches to the cementoenamel junction.

Internal Structure

The internal structure is totally radiolucent.

Effects

This lesion has displaced the first molar in an apical direction, which reinforces the decision that the origin was coronal to this

tooth. Also, the lesion has displaced the second molar distally and the second premolar in an anterior direction. Apical resorption of the distal root of the second deciduous molar has occurred. The occlusal radiograph reveals that the buccal cortical plate has expanded in a smooth, curved shape, and a thin cortical boundary still exists.

Analysis

Making all the observations is an important first step; the following is an analysis built on these observations. To accomplish this next step, further knowledge of pathologic conditions and a certain amount of practice are required. The first objective is to select the correct category of diseases (e.g., inflammatory, benign tumor, cyst); at this point, the clinician should try not to let all the names of specific diseases be overwhelming.

These images reveal an abnormal appearance. The coronal location of the lesion suggests that the tissue making up this abnormality probably is derived from a component of the dental follicle. The effects on the surrounding structures indicate that this abnormality is acquired. The displacement and resorption of teeth, intact peripheral cortex, curved shape, and radiolucent internal structure all indicate a slow-growing, benign, space-occupying lesion, most likely in the cyst category. Odontogenic tumors, such as an ameloblastic fibroma, may be considered but are less likely because of the shape. The most common type of cyst in a follicular location is a dentigerous cyst. Odontogenic keratocysts occasionally are seen in this location, but the tooth resorption and degree of expansion are not characteristic of that pathologic condition. Therefore, the final interpretation is a follicular cyst, with odontogenic keratocyst and ameloblastic fibroma as possibilities in the differential diagnosis but less likely. Treatment usually is indicated for follicular cysts, and the patient should be referred for surgical consultation.

BIBLIOGRAPHY

Baghdady M, Carnahan H, Lam E, et al: The integration of basic sciences and clinical sciences in oral radiology, *J Dent Educ* 2013 (in press).

Baghdady M, Pharoah M, Regehr G, et al: The role of basic sciences in diagnostic oral radiology, *J Dent Educ* 73:1187–1193, 2009.

Eva KW, Hatala RM, LeBlanc VR, et al: Teaching from the clinical reasoning literature: combined reasoning strategies help novice diagnosticians overcome misleading information, *Med Educ* 41: 1152–1158, 2007.

Woods N: Science is fundamental: the role of biomedical knowledge in clinical reasoning, *Med Educ* 41:1173–1177, 2007.

Worth HM: *Principles and practice of oral radiologic interpretation,* Chicago, 1972, Year Book Medical Publishers.

Dental Caries

Ann Wenzel

OUTLINE

DISEASE MECHANISM

Caries is a multifactorial disease with interaction among three factors: (1) the tooth, (2) the microflora, and (3) the diet. If not disturbed, bacteria accumulate at specific tooth sites to form what is known as bacterial plaque or biofilm. The development of caries requires both the presence of bacteria and a diet containing fermentable carbohydrates. Caries is an infectious disease; because it is the lactic acid produced by bacteria from the fermentation of carbohydrates that causes the dissolution, or demineralization, of the dental hard tissues. The *Streptococcus mutans* group plays a central role in demineralization. In the initial stages of the disease, bacteria are located on the tooth surface. It is only after severe demineralization or cavity formation has occurred that bacteria penetrate into the hard tissues. The demineralized area in the tooth surface, called the carious lesion, is not the disease but a reflection of continuing or past microbial activity in the biofilm.

The initial carious lesion is a subsurface loss of mineral in the outer tooth surface. It appears clinically as a chalky white spot (indicating present activity) or an opaque or dark, brownish spot (indicating past activity). A lesion beneath active bacterial plaque will progress, slowly or quickly, but if the biofilm is removed or disturbed, the lesion will arrest. However, an arrested lesion may become reactive and progress any time there is activity in the biofilm. Alternatively, remineralization in the outermost parts of an arrested lesion can occur, such as after the use of fluorides. Caries is an ever-dynamic process.

The rate and extent of mineral loss depend on many factors. Mineral loss occurs faster in an active lesion when intercrystalline voids form. Demineralization may extend well into dentin before a breakdown of the outer surface (cavitation) occurs, resulting in a clinically visible cavity. With lesion progression and no intervention, demineralization may progress through the enamel and the dentin and eventually into the pulp and may destroy the tooth (Fig. 18-1).

ROLE OF RADIOGRAPHY IN DETECTION OF CARIOUS LESIONS

Radiography is useful for detecting carious lesions because the caries process causes demineralization of enamel and dentin. The lesion is seen in a diagnostic image as a radiolucent (darker) zone because the demineralized area of the tooth does not absorb as many x-ray photons as the unaffected portion.

Radiography is a valuable supplement to a thorough clinical examination of the teeth for detecting caries lesions. A careful clinical examination assessing the carious activity on the tooth surface may be possible for smooth surfaces and to some extent for occlusal surfaces. However, when the surface is clinically intact (i.e., no breakdown leading to cavitation has occurred), even the most meticulous examination may fail to reveal demineralizations beneath the surface, including occlusal surfaces. Clinical access to proximal tooth surfaces in contact is limited. Numerous clinical studies have shown that a radiologic examination can reveal carious lesions that would otherwise remain undetected both in occlusal and in proximal surfaces.

The lesion detected in the diagnostic image is merely a result of the bacterial activity, past or present, on the tooth surface, and radiography cannot reveal whether the lesion is arrested or active. An old inactive lesion would still appear as a demineralized "scar" in the hard tissues (Fig. 18-2). The reason is that remineralization takes place only in its outermost surface because mineral-containing solutions from saliva cannot diffuse into the body of the lesion. Because the image mirrors only the current extent of demineralization, one radiograph alone cannot distinguish between an active and an arrested lesion. Only a second image taken at a later time can reveal whether the disease was active.

There has been a dramatic decline in the prevalence of caries in Western countries in recent decades, leaving a smaller fraction of the population with rapidly progressing carious lesions. Therefore, the interval between examinations should be customized for

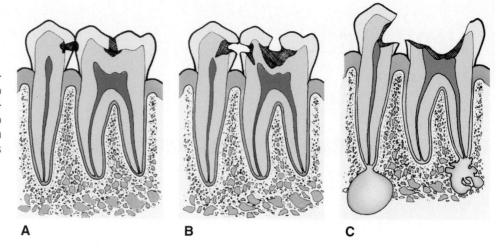

FIGURE 18-1 **A,** Proximal and occlusal demineralization penetrating through tooth enamel and into the dentin. **B,** Proximal and occlusal tissue demineralization and cavitation nearing the pulp chamber of two vital teeth. **C,** Severe demineralization and cavitation reaching the pulp chamber resulting in two nonvital pulps and periapical inflammatory disease.

A   B   C

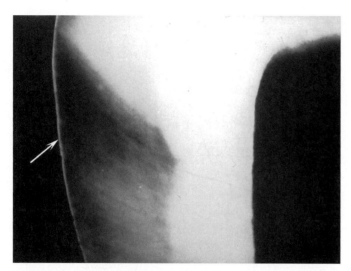

FIGURE 18-2 Microradiograph of an inactive carious lesion *(dark region)* halfway through enamel with an intact, well-mineralized surface *(arrow).* The inner dark area represents dentin.

each patient on the basis of the perceived caries activity and susceptibility. For caries-free individuals, the interval may be lengthened, whereas the interval should be shorter for individuals with active caries. When a decision is made to monitor a lesion, factors such as oral hygiene, fluoride exposure, saliva flow, diet, caries history, extent of restorative care, and age should be considered in determining the time interval between radiologic examinations (see Chapter 16).

EXAMINATION WITH CONVENTIONAL INTRAORAL FILM

The bitewing projection is the most useful image for detecting carious lesions (see Chapter 7). The use of a film holder with a beam-aiming device reduces the number of overlapping contact points and improves image quality, minimizing interpretation errors. Periapical images are useful primarily for detecting changes in the periapical bone. Use of a paralleling technique for obtaining periapical images increases the value of this projection in detecting carious lesions of both anterior and posterior teeth, especially with heavily restored teeth.

Traditionally, No. 2 "adult" films are used for a bitewing examination from the age of approximately 7 to 8 years onward. When it is necessary to examine all the contact surfaces from the cuspid to the most distal molar, one or two bitewing images per side are required, depending on the number of teeth that are present (Fig. 18-3). The use of a single No. 3 film often results in overlapping contact points and "cone-cut" images and is not recommended. In small children, No. 0 or "child" film may be used instead of No. 2 film (Fig. 18-4).

Conventional radiographs used to detect carious lesions should be mounted in frames with dark borders and interpreted with use of a light box with sufficient luminance and a magnifying viewer. Figure 18-5 shows a series of radiographs showing early lesions with and without magnification.

EXAMINATION WITH DIGITAL INTRAORAL RECEPTORS

Digital image receptors may replace film for intraoral radiography. Two different methods are available: (1) solid-state sensors (charge-coupled device (CCD) and complementary metal oxide semiconductor technology (CMOS)) with a cord that connects the receptor to the computer or without a cord (signal is transferred by radio wave) and (2) storage phosphors (photostimulable phosphor plates (PSP) that use a filmlike plate that is processed (scanned) after exposure (see Chapter 4). The holders available for bitewing examinations with phosphor plates appear similar to those for film; universal sensor holders are also available. However, there may be some problems when solid-state sensors are used for bitewing examinations. First, the surface area of the sensor is smaller than the surface area of a No. 2 film, resulting in the display of fewer interproximal tooth surfaces per bitewing image than with film. Second, the stiffness and increased thickness of these sensors create more discomfort for the patient and may result in more projection errors and retakes. When digital bitewing images are used, they should be displayed on a quality monitor in their full resolution for interpretation and viewed in a room with subdued light.

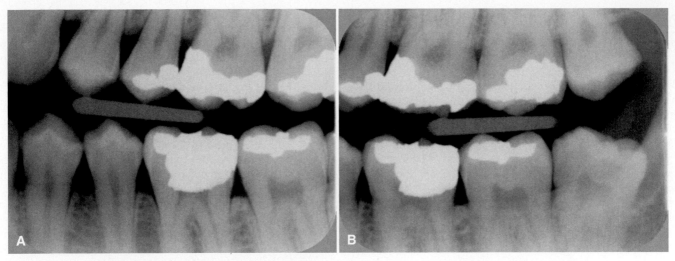

FIGURE 18-3 Two bitewing images from the patient's left side covering the surfaces from the distal surface of the canine to the distal surface of the most posterior molar.

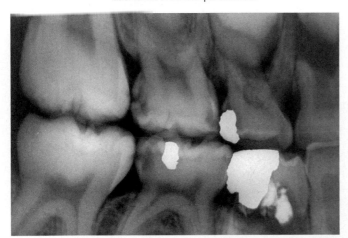

FIGURE 18-4 Bitewing image of the mixed dentition demonstrates dentinal carious lesions involving the mesial and distal surfaces of the second deciduous molars and small enamel lesions in the mesial surfaces of the first permanent molars. An extensive lesion involves the crown and root structure of the mandibular first deciduous molar.

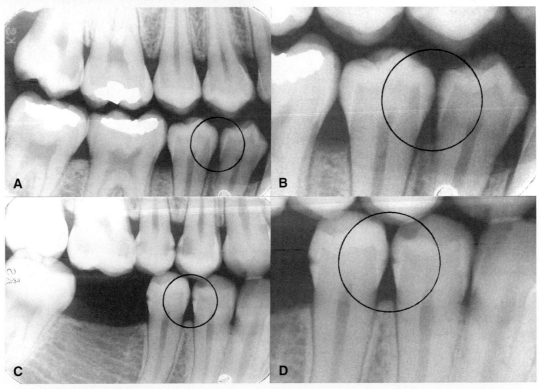

FIGURE 18-5 A–D, Examples of the use of image magnification to detect enamel carious lesions in premolars. A and C are not magnified. B and D are magnified.

DETECTION OF CARIOUS LESIONS

PROXIMAL SURFACES

Typical Appearance

The shape of the early radiolucent lesion in the enamel is classically a triangle with its broad base at the tooth surface (see Fig. 18-5) spreading along the enamel rods, but other appearances are common, such as a "notch," a dot, a band, or one or more thin lines (Fig. 18-6). When the demineralizing front reaches the dentinoenamel junction (DEJ), it spreads along the junction, frequently forming the base of a second triangle with apex directed toward the pulp chamber (Fig. 18-7). This triangle typically has a wider base than in the enamel and progresses toward the pulp along the direction of the dentinal tubules. More irregular shapes of demineralization may be seen.

Lesions involving proximal surfaces are most commonly found in the area between the contact point and the free gingival margin (Fig. 18-8). The fact that this type of lesion does not start below the gingival margin helps distinguish a carious lesion from cervical burnout. Close attention should be paid to intact proximal surfaces adjacent to a tooth surface with a restoration because occasionally this surface is inadvertently damaged during the restorative procedure and is at greater risk for caries (Fig. 18-9).

Because the proximal surfaces of posterior teeth are often broad, the loss of small amounts of mineral from incipient lesions and the advancing front of active lesions are often difficult to detect in the image. Lesions confined to enamel may not be evident until approximately 30% to 40% demineralization has occurred. For this reason, the actual depth of penetration of a carious lesion is often deeper than seen in the image.

False Interpretations

Even experienced dentists often do not agree on the presence or absence of carious lesions when examining the same set of images, especially when the lesions are limited to the enamel. Occasionally, a carious lesion may be incorrectly detected when the tooth surface is actually unaffected (a false-positive outcome). Various morphologic phenomena, such as pits and fissures, cervical burnout, and Mach band effect, and dental anomalies, such as hypoplastic pits and concavities produced by wear, can mimic the appearance of a carious lesion (Fig. 18-10). In cases where the demineralization is not yet visible in the image, failure to detect the lesion is a false-negative outcome (Fig. 18-11). Also, overlapping contact points in the radiographic image may obscure a lesion (Fig. 18-12). Approximately half of all proximal lesions in enamel cannot be detected by diagnostic imaging. The possibility of false-positive diagnoses of small lesions, combined with the knowledge that

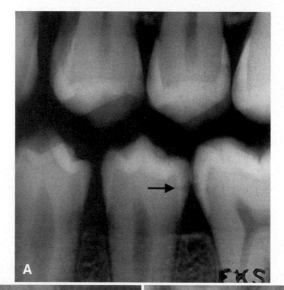

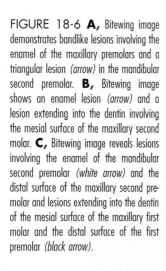

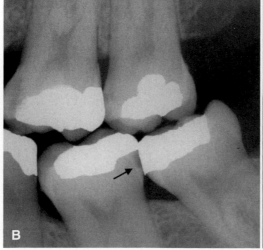

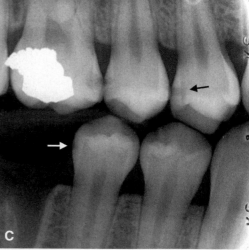

FIGURE 18-6 **A,** Bitewing image demonstrates bandlike lesions involving the enamel of the maxillary premolars and a triangular lesion (arrow) in the mandibular second premolar. **B,** Bitewing image shows an enamel lesion (arrow) and a lesion extending into the dentin involving the mesial surface of the maxillary second molar. **C,** Bitewing image reveals lesions involving the enamel of the mandibular second premolar (white arrow) and the distal surface of the maxillary second premolar and lesions extending into the dentin of the mesial surface of the maxillary first molar and the distal surface of the first premolar (black arrow).

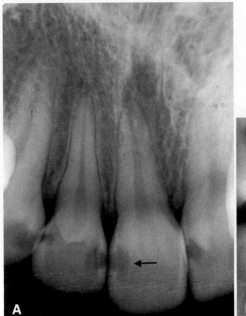
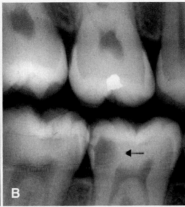
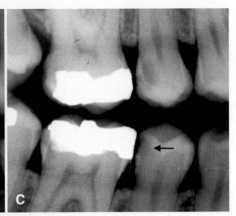

FIGURE 18-7 **A,** Periapical image demonstrates several proximal carious lesions that have extended into the dentin. The lesions extend along the DEJ to involve a greater amount of dentin than enamel *(arrow)*. **B,** Bitewing image demonstrates an extensive proximal carious lesion involving the distal aspect of the mandibular first molar *(arrow)*. The pulp horn has been reduced as a result of the formation of tertiary (irritation) dentin. **C,** Bitewing image shows two lesions involving the dentin in the distal surfaces of the second premolars; one lesion has resulted in cavitation *(arrow)*.

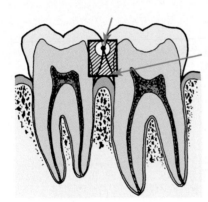

FIGURE 18-8 Proximal caries-susceptible zone. This region extends from the contact point *(upper arrow)* down to the height of the free gingival margin *(lower arrow)*. It increases with recession of the alveolar bone and gingival tissues.

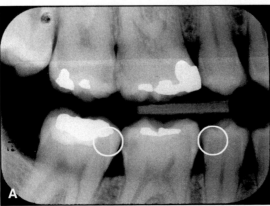
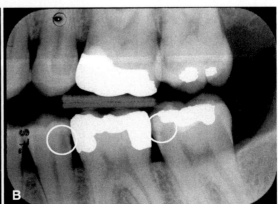

FIGURE 18-9 **A** and **B,** Pair of bitewing images. Dentinal lesions *(circles)* have developed in surfaces adjacent to a restored surface in the patient's left side but not in the same surfaces of the teeth in the right side.

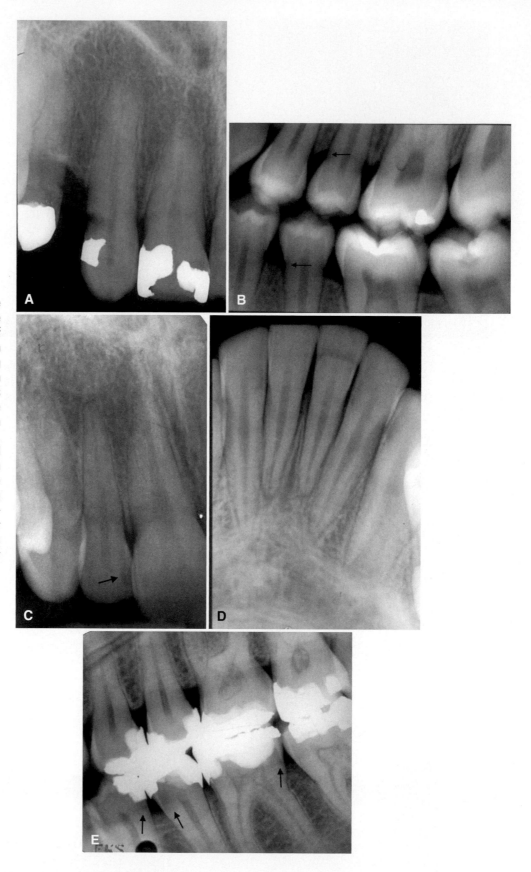

FIGURE 18-10 **A,** Periapical image reveals a radiolucent region similar in appearance to a carious lesion in the distal cervical aspect of the maxillary cuspid, which is caused by abrasion from a clasp from a partial denture. **B,** Bitewing image shows cervical burnout *(arrows),* which can mimic carious lesions. **C,** Periapical image shows a small concavity in the mesial surface of the lateral incisor, which creates a radiolucent region similar in appearance to a carious lesion *(arrow).* **D,** Periapical image shows a band of enamel hypoplasia involving the left central incisor, which produces a linear radiolucent region that may be misinterpreted as a carious lesion. **E,** Bitewing image shows the overlapping shadow of the alveolar process, which creates a Mach band effect *(arrows)* resulting in apparent radiolucent regions in the crowns of the premolars and first molar that may mimic carious lesions.

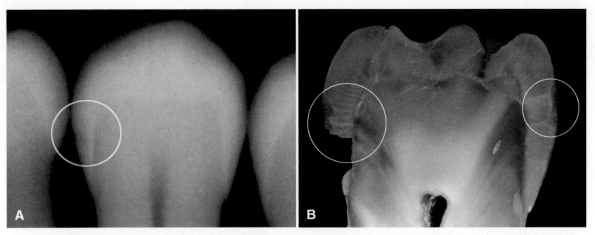

FIGURE 18-11 **A,** Radiograph of an extracted tooth with a lesion just into dentin in the left side *(circle)* but no visible lesion in the right side. **B,** The same tooth after sectioning assessed under a microscope reveals lesions in both sides; the lesion in the right side is only in enamel. Enamel in the left side has broken off during sectioning.

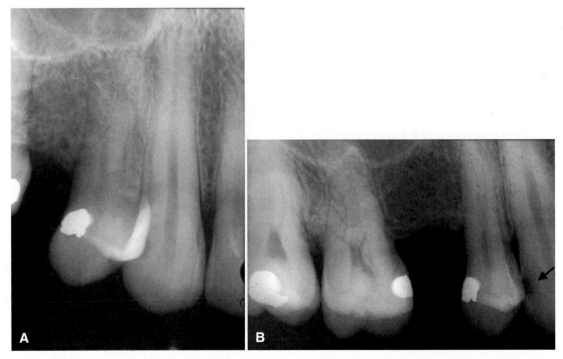

FIGURE 18-12 **A,** Periapical image in which a proximal carious lesion involving the distal surface of the cuspid is not apparent. **B,** Periapical image in which change in the horizontal orientation of the x-ray beam has separated the overlapping images of the opposing surfaces of the premolar and cuspid, revealing the presence of the lesion *(arrow).*

caries progresses slowly in most individuals, argues for a conservative approach to operative treatment. A lesion extending into the dentin in the radiograph may be easier to detect with greater agreement among experienced observers. Occasionally, the demineralization in the enamel is not obvious, and a dentinal lesion is overlooked (see Fig. 18-6, *A,* distal surface of the maxillary second premolar, and Fig. 18-6, *B,* mesial surface of the maxillary second molar).

Lesions with and without Clinical Cavitation

Potentially, a progressing proximal lesion may be arrested if cavitation has not developed. If cavitation has occurred, the lesion will always be active because the bacteria that colonize within the cavity cannot be removed. The presence of cavitation cannot be accurately determined in the diagnostic image, although the greater the depth of the lesion in the image, the greater the likelihood of cavitation. Because extensive demineralization must occur before the surface breaks down, the percentage of enamel lesions with surface cavitation is very small. Approximately half of lesions that are just into dentin have surface cavitation. The deeper the lesion has penetrated into dentin, the more likely it is cavitated, and dentinal lesions extending more than halfway to the pulp will most likely be cavitated. Temporarily separating proximal surfaces with orthodontic elastics or springs may allow direct inspection to determine whether there is cavitation. This method is easier in children than adults. An advanced imaging method, cone-beam computed tomographic imaging (see Chapter 11), is very accurate in determining whether or not a cavity exists in a proximal tooth surface; however, because of the much larger radiation burden and extensive resources that this method demands, it is not recommended for routine use to detect caries lesion cavitation. However, a cone-beam computed tomographic examination performed for another diagnostic reason should be assessed also for proximal surface cavities in teeth without restorations.

Treatment Considerations

Operative treatment is usually not indicated for lesions detected in enamel, and the dentist and the patient may arrest lesion progression with conservative intervention. However, cavitated lesions require operative treatment. For dentinal lesions, the decision whether to provide operative treatment is individualized for each patient. In cases where it is decided to monitor the lesion, a follow-up radiograph should be taken to evaluate whether the lesion has arrested or is progressing. The interval between radiologic examinations should be determined individually, taking into account previous caries history, age, and the site of the lesion because the progression rate differs highly among the various tooth surfaces. Care should be taken to reproduce the same image geometry in follow-up images by using standardized film holders to provide a means of accurate comparison of depth of the lesion. When digital images are made with reproducible geometry, they can be superimposed, and the information in the one image can be subtracted from the other, resulting in a subtraction image that displays the changes that have occurred between the two examinations (Fig. 18-13).

Progression of a lesion indicates the need for operative therapy. With highly motivated patients who clean the surface and with topical fluoride treatment, more than half of shallow dentinal lesions can be arrested, avoiding restorative therapy.

OCCLUSAL SURFACES

Typical Appearance

Carious lesions in children and adolescents most often occur on occlusal surfaces of posterior teeth. The demineralization process originates in enamel pits and fissures where the biofilm develops. The lesion spreads along the enamel rods and, if undisturbed, penetrates to the DEJ, where it may be seen as a thin radiolucent line between enamel and dentin. The classic appearance of lesions extending into the dentin is a broad-based, bowl-shaped, radiolucent zone, often beneath a fissure, with little or no apparent changes in the enamel. The deeper the occlusal lesion, the easier it is to detect on the image (Fig. 18-14).

Occlusal lesions commonly start in the sides of a fissure wall rather than at the base and then tend to penetrate nearly

perpendicularly toward the DEJ. Early lesions appear clinically as chalky white; older lesions may be seen as yellow, brown, or black discolorations of the occlusal fissures. Finding such discolored fissures in a clinically intact occlusal surface suggests that a radiologic examination is indicated to determine whether a carious lesion has penetrated beyond the DEJ. If the lesion has not crossed the DEJ, it may not be visible in the image.

False Interpretations

Pitfalls in the interpretation of dentinal occlusal lesions include superimposition of the image of the buccal pit with or without an associated carious lesion or a nonmetal restoration, which may simulate an occlusal lesion or a deep occlusal fissure. Direct clinical inspection of the tooth most often eliminates any such confusion.

When an occlusal lesion is confined to enamel, the surrounding enamel often obscures the lesion. As the carious process progresses, a radiolucent line extends along the DEJ. As the lesion extends into the dentin, the margin between the carious and noncarious dentin is diffuse and may obscure the fine radiolucent line at the DEJ. Therefore, false-positive detection rates may be as high as false-negative detection rates for shallow lesions. A false-negative outcome may not represent a severe mistake because in most cases the process progresses slowly, and the lesion is detected at a later time. A false-positive outcome may result in a sound surface being irreversibly damaged. Also, when there is a sharply defined density difference, such as between enamel and dentin, there may appear to be a more radiolucent region immediately adjacent to the enamel. This is an optical illusion referred to as the Mach band (see Fig. 18-10, E). The Mach band can contribute to the number of false-positive interpretations; therefore, when there are no clinical signs of a lesion, it would be reasonable to observe these cases and withhold operative treatment.

Cavitation and Treatment Considerations

As an occlusal lesion spreads through the dentin, it undermines the enamel, and eventually masticatory forces cause cavitation. When the cavitation is visible on clinical inspection, it is usually an indication that the lesion is already well into dentin, and if information regarding extent relative to the pulp chamber is needed, a radiologic examination is required. Without cavitation, fissure discoloration may indicate the need for radiologic examination. A dentinal lesion without clinically apparent cavitation but with a radiolucent extension well into dentin indicates that the carious lesion has passed the DEJ (see Fig. 18-14) and requires operative treatment.

RAMPANT CARIES

Severe, rapidly progressing carious destruction of teeth is usually termed rampant caries and can be seen in children with poor

FIGURE 18-13 Subtraction image made from two bitewing images taken with a 2-year interval. The contours of four maxillary teeth can be seen. Between the two examinations, a filling was placed *(rectangle)*, a new deep dentinal lesion has developed *(large circle)*, and a lesion has progressed from enamel into dentin *(small circle)*.

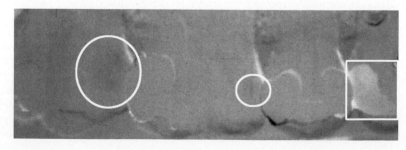

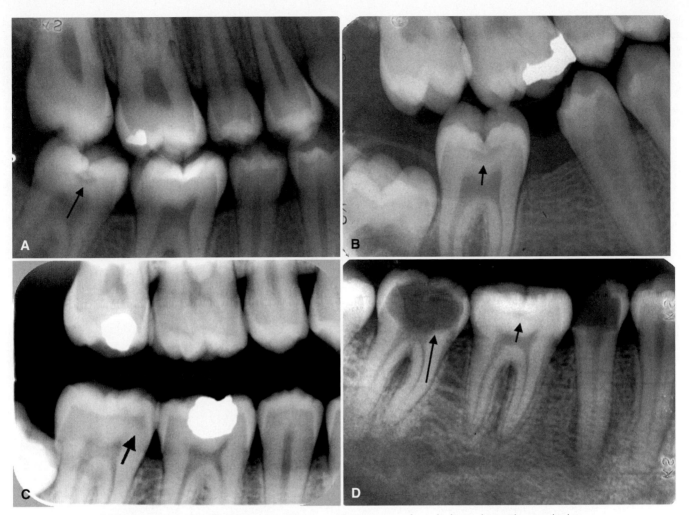

FIGURE 18-14 **A** and **B**, Bitewing images demonstrate a classic appearance of an occlusal carious lesion with a triangular shape in the enamel with the base oriented to the DEJ *(arrows)*. **C**, Bitewing image is not as clear, but there is an ill-defined radiolucent region under the occlusal enamel surface *(arrow)*. **D**, Periapical image shows there is a subtle occlusal lesion in the first molar *(short arrow)* and an extensive cavitated lesion in the second molar *(long arrow)*.

dietary and oral hygiene habits (see Fig. 18-4). However, this condition is becoming increasingly rare because of widespread availability of fluoride in water supplements and topical application and enlightened practices of good nutrition and hygiene. Rampant caries may also be seen in people with xerostomia. Radiographs of individuals with rampant caries demonstrate severe (advanced) tooth destruction, especially of the mandibular anterior teeth.

BUCCAL AND LINGUAL SURFACES

Buccal and lingual carious lesions often occur in enamel pits and fissures of teeth. When small, these lesions are usually round; as they enlarge, they become elliptic or semilunar. They demonstrate sharp, well-defined borders.

It may be difficult to differentiate between buccal and lingual carious lesions on a radiograph. When viewing buccal or lingual lesions, the clinician should look for a uniform noncarious region of enamel surrounding the apparent radiolucency (Fig. 18-15). This well-defined circular area represents parallel noncarious enamel rods surrounding the buccal or palatal lesion. However, occlusal

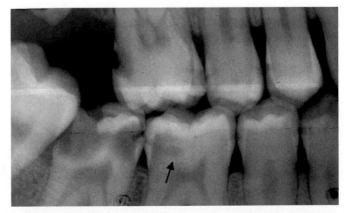

FIGURE 18-15 Bitewing image reveals the presence of a small buccal lesion *(arrow)* involving the mandibular first molar. Note the presence of 12 proximal carious lesions. Also, the abnormal position of the mandibular third molar created an enhanced site for plaque accumulation, resulting in an extensive carious lesion involving the second molar.

lesions ordinarily are more extensive than lingual or buccal caries, and their outline is not as well defined. Clinical evaluation with visual and tactile methods is usually the definitive method to detect buccal or lingual lesions.

ROOT SURFACES

Root surface lesions involve both cementum and dentin and are associated with gingival recession. The exposed cementum is relatively soft and usually only 20 to 50 μm thick near the cementoenamel junction, so it rapidly degrades by attrition, abrasion, and erosion. Root surface caries should be detected clinically, and most often radiographs are not needed for diagnosis. In proximal root surfaces, radiologic examination may reveal lesions that have gone undetected (Fig. 18-16).

A pitfall in the detection of root lesions is that a surface may appear to be carious as a result of the cervical burnout

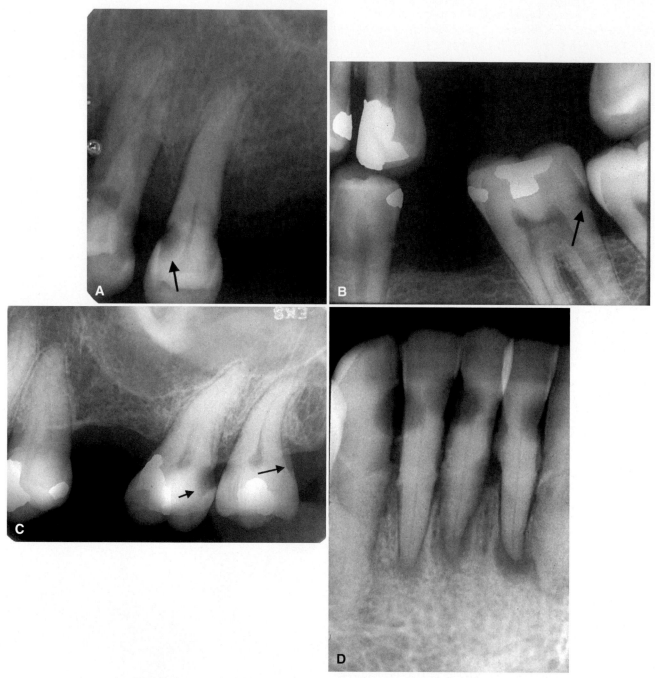

FIGURE 18-16 **A,** Periapical image shows root surface carious lesions involving the distal aspect of the first premolar and the mesial and distal aspect of the second premolar. The lesion undermines the enamel surface *(arrow).* **B,** Bitewing image reveals a root surface lesion involving the distal cervical region of the second molar *(arrow)*; this location is due in part to the low third molar contact point on the distal surface, the result of abnormal mesial tipping of both molars. **C,** Periapical image shows a carious lesion in the distal root surface of the maxillary second molar *(short arrow)* and an example of cervical burnout *(long arrow).* The sharp line from overlapping roots delineates radiolucent cervical burnout. **D,** Periapical image demonstrates multiple root lesions involving the mandibular incisors. Note the associated periapical inflammatory lesions.

phenomenon (see Figs. 18-10, *B*, and 18-16, *C*). The true carious lesion may be distinguished from the intact surface primarily by the absence of an image of the root edge and by the appearance of a diffuse rounded inner border where the tooth substance has been lost.

ASSOCIATED WITH DENTAL RESTORATIONS

A carious lesion developing at the margin of an existing restoration may be termed secondary or recurrent caries. However, a lesion developing in a restored surface is most frequently a new primary demineralization, either because of faulty shaping or inadequate extension of the restoration leading to plaque accumulation (Fig. 18-17). These lesions should be treated as any new carious lesion. It is important not to confuse secondary or recurrent caries with residual caries, which is carious tissue that remains if the original lesion is not completely removed. In situations where the radiographic lesion is very close to the pulp, carious dentin may be left on purpose during operative treatment. Medication that stimulates the development of tertiary dentin is placed in the cavity (indirect pulp capping). After some months, the remaining carious dentin is removed, and a permanent filling is placed.

A lesion next to a restoration may be obscured by the radiopaque image of the restoration. Thus, two radiographic views made at different horizontal or vertical angulations of the central ray can be helpful where there are multiple radiopaque restorations. Also, the detection of secondary carious lesions depends on a careful clinical examination. Recurrent lesions at the mesiogingival and distogingival margins are most frequently detected in the image.

Restorative materials vary in their appearance in the image depending on thickness, density, atomic number, and the x-ray beam energy used to make the image. Some materials can be confused with caries. Older calcium-hydroxide liners without barium, lead, or zinc (added to lend radiopacity) appear radiolucent and may resemble recurrent or residual caries. Despite the calcium present, the relatively large proportion of low-atomic-number material in calcium hydroxide causes its radiodensity to be similar to a carious lesion. Older composite, plastic, or silicate restorations also may simulate lesions. However, it is often possible to identify and differentiate these radiolucent materials from carious lesions by their well-defined and smooth outline reflecting the preparation or from their radiopaque liners (Fig. 18-18).

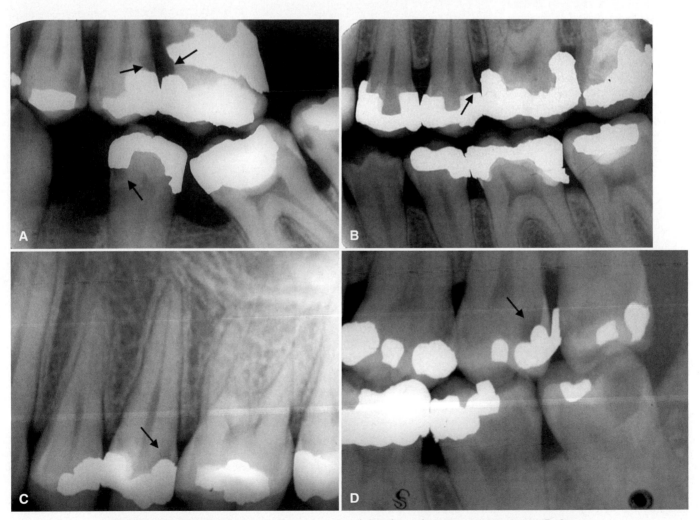

FIGURE 18-17 A, Bitewing image reveals several interproximal carious lesions; three are recurrent caries *(arrows).* **B,** Bitewing image demonstrates recurrent carious lesion in the distal surface of the maxillary second premolar *(arrow).* Note the overhang to the restoration placed on the mesial surface of the first molar. **C,** Periapical image reveals a recurrent carious lesion *(arrow)* involving the distal surface of the second premolar. **D,** There is an overhang to the restoration on the distal aspect of this maxillary second molar and an associated recurrent carious lesion *(arrow).*

FIGURE 18-18 **A,** Periapical image shows radiolucent restorations placed in the mesial and distal surfaces of the lateral incisor and mesial surface of the cuspid. The well-defined margins are useful to differentiate from carious lesions. **B,** Periapical image in which the radiopaque liner *(arrow)* on the internal aspect of the restoration placed on the distal surface of the central incisor is useful to differentiate from a carious lesion. Note the sharp margins of the restoration placed in the mesial surface of the lateral incisor. **C,** Periapical image demonstrates four radiolucent restorations and one carious lesion. The carious lesion involves the distal surface of the lateral incisor. The diffuse margin of the lesion is in contrast to the well-defined margins of the restorations. **D,** Periapical image shows a recurrent carious lesion *(arrow)* involving the distal surface of the central incisor in contact with the radiolucent restoration. Note the diffuse ill-defined margin of the lesion compared with the well-defined margin of the restoration.

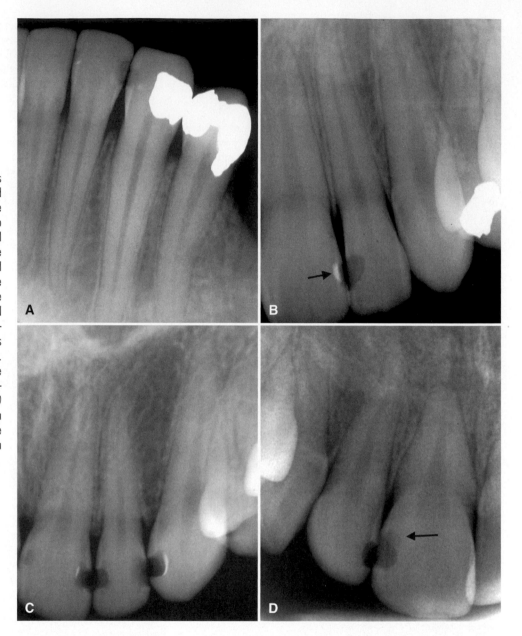

THERAPY AFTER RADIATION

Patients who have received therapeutic radiation to the head and neck may have a loss of salivary gland function, leading to xerostomia (dry mouth) and a change in the bacterial flora and possibly intrinsic change to the tooth structure. Untreated, this condition induces rampant destruction of the teeth, termed radiation caries (see Chapter 2). Typically, the destruction begins at the cervical region and may aggressively encircle the tooth, causing the entire crown to be lost, with only root fragments remaining in the jaws. The radiographic appearance of radiation caries is characteristic: radiolucent shadows appearing at the necks of teeth, most obvious on the mesial and distal aspects. Variations in the depth of destruction may be present, but generally there is uniformity within a given region of the mouth. Figure 18-19 shows examples of radiation caries in patients with xerostomia after therapeutic radiation for cancer of the head and neck. Use of topical fluorides as remineralizing solutions and meticulous oral hygiene can markedly reduce the radiation damage to teeth resulting from xerostomia.

ALTERNATIVE DIAGNOSTIC TOOLS TO DETECT DENTAL CARIES

Other methods have been developed in addition to clinical inspection and radiography to detect carious lesions. These include quantitative light-induced fluorescence, laser light fiberoptic transillumination (FOTI), electrical conductance measurements (ECM), and ultrasonography. Quantitative light-induced fluorescence may be used to quantify mineral loss on smooth surfaces, whereas FOTI and ECM have been applied on occlusal surfaces. FOTI and ECM operate by displaying a value that provides quantitative information on the depth of the lesion. None of these methods can unequivocally distinguish between enamel and dentin lesions or between shallow and deep dentin lesions. FOTI has been used primarily for proximal surfaces but may also be applied to occlusal surfaces. FOTI is less sensitive than radiography for distinguishing shallow and deep lesions. ECM is better than FOTI in identifying occlusal caries in young children. There is little evidence at the

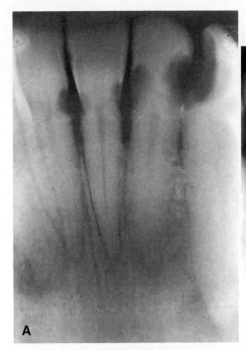
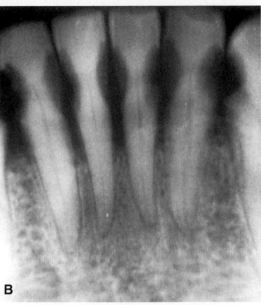

FIGURE 18-19 **A** and **B,** Two periapical images reveal multiple carious lesions that occurred after therapeutic radiation exposure. The lesions start in the region of the cementoenamel junction.

present time that these methods are used in place of traditional diagnostic methods in the clinic.

TREATMENT CONSIDERATIONS

Carious lesions in enamel require interceptive treatment but rarely operative treatment. The detection of small areas of demineralization in the image requires a decision as to whether these represent active or inactive arrested lesions. When the lesion appears to be limited to enamel, the probability of cavitation is low, and the prospect of arresting or reversing the caries process is good. Also, if the lesion extends just into the dentin, treatment should include a means to stop the microbiologic activity and possibly reverse the demineralization process. Treatment of such lesions may include reductions in sugar intake; proper oral hygiene to reduce bacteria; and use of topical fluorides to inhibit microbiologic activity, retard demineralization, and promote remineralization of the outermost parts of the lesion. This approach may be successful if the surface of the tooth is not cavitated and a follow-up radiograph shows no progression of the lesion. However, when the surface of a lesion is cavitated or follow-up images reveal progression of the lesion in dentin, a restoration is usually required. Cavitated carious lesions require removal of the infected tissues, possibly stepwise over a period for extensive lesions, and restoration of the tooth to form and function.

BIBLIOGRAPHY

Fejerskov O, Kidd EAM: *Dental caries: the disease and its clinical management,* ed 2, Munksgaard, 2008, Blackwell.

Kidd EAM, Fejerskov O: What constitutes dental caries? Histopathology of carious enamel and dentin related to the action of cariogenic biofilms, *J Dent Res* 83(Spec Issue C):C35–C38, 2004.

NIH Consensus Development Conference on Diagnosis and Management of Dental Caries Throughout Life. Bethesda, MD, March 26–28, 2001. Conference papers, *J Dent Educ* 65:935–1179, 2001.

Pitts NB, Stamm JW: International Consensus Workshop on Caries Clinical Trials (ICW-CCT). Final consensus statements: agreeing where the evidence leads, *J Dent Res* 83(Spec Issue C):C125–C128, 2004.

Selwitz RH, Ismail AI, Pitts NB: Dental caries, *Lancet* 369:51–59, 2007.

SUGGESTED READINGS

Radiographic Caries Detection

Bahrami G, Hagstrøm C, Wenzel A: Bitewing examination with four digital receptors, *Dentomaxillofac Radiol* 32:317–321, 2003.

Haiter-Neto F, Wenzel A, Gotfredsen E: Diagnostic accuracy of cone beam computed tomography scans compared with intraoral image modalities for detection of caries lesions, *Dentomaxillofac Radiol* 37:18–22, 2008.

Hellén-Halme K, Petersson A, Nilsson M: Effect of ambient light and monitor brightness and contrast settings on the detection of approximal caries in digital radiographs: an in vitro study, *Dentomaxillofac Radiol* 37:380–384, 2008.

Hintze H, Wenzel A: A two-film versus a four-film bite-wing examination for caries diagnosis in adults, *Caries Res* 33:380–396, 1999.

Hintze H, Wenzel A, Danielsen B: Behaviour of approximal carious lesions assessed by clinical examination after tooth separation and radiography: a 2.5-year longitudinal study in young adults, *Caries Res* 33:415–422, 1999.

Isidor S, Faaborg-Andersen M, Hintze H, et al: Effect of monitor display on detection of approximal caries lesions in digital radiographs, *Dentomaxillofac Radiol* 38:537–541, 2009.

Lunder N, von der Fehr FR: Approximal cavitation related to bite-wing image and caries activity in adolescents, *Caries Res* 30:143–147, 1996.

Mejáre I: Bitewing examination to detect caries in children and adolescents—when and how often? *Dent Update* 32:588–590, 593–594, 596–597, 2005.

Mejáre I, Stenlund H, Zelezny-Holmlund C: Caries incidence and lesions progression from adolescence to young adulthood: a prospective 15-year cohort study in Sweden, *Caries Res* 38:130–141, 2004.

Mjör IA, Toffenetti F: Secondary caries: a literature review with case reports, *Quintessence Int* 31:165–179, 2000.

Nyvad B, Fejerskov O: Assessing the stage of caries lesion activity on the basis of clinical and microbiological examination, *Community Dent Oral Epidemiol* 25:69–75, 1997.

Nyvad B, Machiulskiene V, Baelum V: Reliability of a new caries diagnostic system differentiating between active and inactive caries lesions, *Caries Res* 33:252–260, 1999.

Petersson GH, Bratthall D: The caries decline: a review of reviews, *Eur J Oral Sci* 104:436–443, 1996.

Poorterman JHG, Weerheijm KL, Groen HJ, et al: Clinical and radiographic judgement of occlusal caries in adolescents, *Eur J Oral Sci* 108:93–98, 2000.

Qvist V, Johannesen L, Bruun M: Progression of approximal caries in relation to iatrogenic preparation damage, *J Dent Res* 71:1370–1373, 1992.

Ratledge DK, Kidd EA, Beighton D: A clinical and microbiological study of approximal carious lesions, 1: the relationship between cavitation, radiographic lesion depth, the site specific gingival index and the level of infection of the dentine, *Caries Res* 35:3–7, 2001.

Wenzel A: A review of dentists' use of digital radiography and caries diagnosis with digital systems, *Dentomaxillofac Radiol* 35:307–314, 2006.

Wenzel A, Anthonisen PN, Juul MB: Reproducibility in the assessment of caries lesion behaviour: a comparison between conventional film and subtraction radiography, *Caries Res* 34:214–218, 2000.

Wenzel A, Haiter-Neto F, Gotfredsen E: Risk factors for a false positive test outcome in diagnosis of caries in approximal surfaces: impact of radiographic modality and observer characteristics, *Caries Res* 41:170–176, 2007.

Wenzel A, Hirsch E, Christensen JH, et al: Detection of cavitated approximal surfaces using cone beam CT and intraoral receptors, *Dentomaxillofac Radiol* 42:39458105, 2013.

Young SM, Lee JT, Hodges RJ, et al: A comparative study of high-resolution cone beam computed tomography and charge-coupled device sensors for detecting caries, *Dentomaxillofac Radiol* 38:445–451, 2009.

Treatment Decision

Bader JD, Shugars DA: What do we know about how dentists make caries-related treatment decisions? *Community Dent Oral Epidemiol* 25:97–103, 1997.

Bader JD, Shugars DA: The evidence supporting alternative management strategies for early occlusal caries and suspected occlusal dentinal caries, *J Evid Based Dent Pract* 6:91–100, 2006.

Bjorndal L, Kidd EA: The treatment of deep dentine caries lesions, *Dent Update* 32:402–404, 407–410, 413, 2005.

Pitts NB: Diagnostic tools and measurements–impact on appropriate care, *Community Dent Oral Epidemiol* 25:24–35, 1997.

Pitts NB: Are we ready to move from operative to non-operative/ preventive treatment of dental caries in clinical practice? *Caries Res* 38:294–304, 2004.

Ricketts DN, Kidd EA, Innés N, et al: Complete or ultraconservative removal of decayed tissue in unfilled teeth, *Cochrane Database Syst Rev* (3):CD003808, 2006.

Rimmer PA, Pitts NB: Temporary elective tooth separation as a diagnostic aid in general dental practice, *Br Dent J* 169:87–92, 1990.

Periodontal Diseases

Susanne Perschbacher

OUTLINE

DISEASE MECHANISM

Several distinct yet related disorders of the periodontium are collectively known as periodontal diseases. Periodontal diseases are a set of conditions characterized by an inflammatory host response in the periodontal tissues that may lead to localized or generalized alterations in the soft tissues around the teeth, loss of supporting bone, and ultimately loss of the teeth. Periodontal diseases are broadly classified as gingival diseases and periodontitis. Gingival diseases may be dental plaque-induced or non–plaque-induced. Bacterial plaque-associated gingivitis is much more common than non–plaque-induced inflammatory diseases affecting the gingiva, such as viral or fungal infections, mucocutaneous and allergic conditions, and traumatic injuries. Gingivitis manifests as inflammation of the soft tissue surrounding the teeth with gingival swelling, edema, and erythema.

Periodontitis is classified, primarily by the clinical presentation, as chronic, aggressive, and periodontitis as a manifestation of a systemic disease. Other, less common types of periodontal conditions include necrotizing periodontal diseases, periodontal abscesses, and periodontitis associated with endodontic lesions. Periodontitis is distinguished from gingivitis by the clinically detectable destruction of host tissues seen as the loss of soft tissue attachment and supporting bone of the involved teeth. Although periodontitis is always preceded by gingivitis, gingivitis does not always progress to periodontitis.

Dental plaque, which varies greatly in its bacterial composition, plays a primary role in the initiation of periodontitis. Periodontitis-implicated plaque bacteria species, predominantly gram-negative rods and spirochetes, have the ability to colonize on the tooth and root surfaces, spread into the region between the root and the gingival margin, and invade the surrounding tissue in some cases. These bacteria are capable of causing damage to the host tissue either directly, through the release of toxins, or, more significantly, indirectly, by stimulating a host inflammatory reaction. As part of the host response, the release of inflammatory mediators, especially from neutrophils, is responsible for much of the injury to the surrounding soft tissue and stimulation of osteoclastic bone resorption. The resulting inflammatory response causes loss of, and apical migration of, the epithelial attachment, resulting in pocket formation and further enhancing bacterial colonization.

The clinical manifestations of this interplay between bacterial plaque and the host tissues are clinical signs of inflammation. Gingivitis, seen as gingival swelling, edema, and erythema, is the most common first clinical sign. Progression to periodontitis is manifested with pocket formation, the universal presentation of this disease. Other clinical signs include bleeding, purulent exudate, edema, resorption of the alveolar crest, and tooth mobility. Rather than a steady continuous progression from mild to moderate to severe, periodontitis often progresses in bursts. There are cyclic periods of active inflammation and tissue destruction followed by healing and quiescent phases (often years) of no appreciable change. The extent of disease activity is best measured by longitudinal probing of periodontal attachment level. The relative duration of the destructive and quiescent phases depends on the form of periodontitis, the nature of the bacterial pathogens, and the host response. Host factors, such as systemic disease, age, genetic predisposition, immune system status, occlusal trauma, and stress, influence the onset and progression of the disease. Spontaneous remission of the destructive process may occur. The disease usually is painless, and most patients are unaware of its presence. Various forms of therapy are effective, including oral hygiene, scaling, and surgical treatment.

Individuals more prone to periodontal disease include smokers; older individuals; and individuals with poor education, neglected dental care, previous periodontal destruction, and systemic diseases such as diabetes or infection with human immunodeficiency virus (HIV).

The prevalence of periodontal disease in the U.S. population depends on the method of assessment and the threshold used. If loss of attachment by the formation of pockets measuring greater than 4 mm is used, the prevalence is about 23%. The incidence of adult periodontitis increases with age. The prevalence of aggressive periodontitis is less than 1%. Also, it appears that the prevalence of periodontal disease in the United States has declined in the last 30 years, but this may change with an increasing elderly population and an increase in retention of teeth.

ASSESSMENT OF PERIODONTAL DISEASE

CONTRIBUTIONS OF DIAGNOSTIC IMAGES

Radiographs play an integral role in the assessment of periodontal disease. They provide unique information about the status of the periodontium and a permanent record of the condition of the bone throughout the course of the disease. Diagnostic images aid the clinician in identifying the extent of destruction of alveolar bone, local contributing factors, and features of the periodontium that influence the prognosis. These images also help in the assessment of the clinical crown-to-root ratio, an important factor that is affected by periodontal bone loss and that influences the prognosis of the tooth and any planned prosthesis. Important features related to periodontal status that may be identified in diagnostic images are listed in Box 19-1.

The clinical and radiologic examinations are complementary. The clinical examination should include periodontal probing, a gingival index, mobility charting, and an evaluation of the amount of attached gingiva. Features that are not well delineated by diagnostic images are most apparent clinically, and features that radiographs best demonstrate are difficult to identify and evaluate clinically. Images are an adjunct to the diagnostic process. Although images can demonstrate advanced periodontal lesions well, other equally important changes in the periodontium may not be seen. Therefore, a complete diagnosis of periodontal disease requires insight from a clinical examination of the patient combined with evidence displayed in the diagnostic image.

LIMITATIONS OF INTRAORAL IMAGES

Intraoral images (bitewing and periapical projections) may provide an incomplete presentation of the status of the periodontium. They have the following limitations:

---

1. These images provide a two-dimensional view of three-dimensional structures. Because the image fails to reveal the three-dimensional nature of the anatomy, bony defects overlapped by higher bony walls may be hidden. Also, because of overlapping tooth structure, only the interproximal bone is seen clearly. However, subtle decrease in the apparent density of the root structure (appears more radiolucent) may indicate bone loss on the buccal or lingual aspect of the tooth. Use of multiple images made at different angulations, as in a full-mouth set, allows the viewer to use the buccal object rule to obtain three-dimensional information, such as whether cortical plate loss has occurred on the buccal or lingual aspects.
2. These images typically show less severe bone destruction than is actually present. The earliest (incipient) mild destructive lesions in bone do not cause a sufficient change in density to be detectable.
3. These images do not demonstrate the soft tissue-to-hard tissue relationships and thus provide no information about the depth of soft tissue pockets.
4. Bone level is often measured from the cementoenamel junction (CEJ); however, this reference point is not valid in situations where there is overeruption or where there is passive eruption in patients with severe attrition.

For these reasons, although diagnostic images play an invaluable role in diagnosis and treatment planning, their use must be supplemented by careful clinical examination.

TECHNICAL PROCEDURES

The usefulness of intraoral images in the evaluation of periodontal disease can be improved by making images with high technical quality. Interproximal (bitewing), in some cases vertical bitewing, and periapical radiographs are useful for evaluating the periodontium. This material is covered in greater detail in the chapters on projection geometry and intraoral radiographic technique (see Chapters 6 and 7), but the features that are particularly important for imaging the alveolar bone are emphasized here.

Image Receptor Placement and Beam Alignment

The image receptor should be placed parallel with the long axis of the teeth or as near to this ideal position as the size and structure of the mouth permit. The x-ray beam is directed perpendicular to the long axis of the tooth and the plane of the image receptor. These measures result in the best undistorted images of the teeth and periodontal tissues. Interproximal (bitewing) images more accurately record the distance between the CEJ and the crest of the interradicular alveolar bone because the beam is oriented at right angles to the long axis of the teeth with interproximal views, providing an accurate view of the relationship of the height of the alveolar bone to the roots. Periapical views, especially in the posterior maxilla, may present a distorted view of the relationship between the teeth and the height of the alveolar bone because the presence of the hard palate often requires the x-ray tube to be oriented slightly downward toward the posterior teeth to capture the apices of these teeth on the image. In this circumstance, the level of the buccal alveolar bone may be projected near or above the level of the lingual CEJ, making the bone height appear greater than it actually is.

The teeth are depicted in their correct positions relative to the alveolar process when there is (1) no overlapping of the proximal contacts between crowns, (2) no overlapping of roots of adjacent

---

teeth, and (3) overlapping of the buccal and lingual cusps of molars.

In cases where standard interproximal images cannot depict the alveolar crest because of the extent of bone loss, the use of vertical interproximal (vertical bitewing) images may be advantageous. This method uses No. 2 image receptors in a vertical orientation and can be used to cover the molar, premolar, canine, and midline regions. These views can produce the ideal geometry of the interproximal views, while still demonstrating the alveolar bone level when there has been moderate or severe bone loss. Panoramic images are not recommended for evaluation of periodontal disease because the distortion and poor image detail of panoramic views tend to lead the clinician to underestimate minor marginal bone destruction and overestimate major destruction.

For radiography of the alveolar bone, a beam energy of 70 to 80 kVp should be used. Images that are slightly light are more useful for examining cortical margins of bone. A properly collimated beam reduces scattered radiation and improves image contrast.

Special Considerations and Techniques

The dentist must determine the optimal frequency of radiographic examination for patients with periodontal disease. Radiographs of all diseased areas must be available at the beginning of periodontal therapy to aid in diagnosis and allow treatment planning. The extent of continued disease activity, which can be determined clinically, should dictate the frequency of subsequent radiographic examinations.

Computers and image-processing techniques have been used to enhance images to achieve improved detection of alveolar bone loss associated with periodontal disease. The most widely used of these techniques is subtraction radiography (see Chapter 4). The advantage of this method is that it allows better detection of small amounts of bone loss between images made at different times than may be achieved by visual inspection. However, image subtraction is difficult to use because the images must be made with the same orientation of the primary x-ray beam, bone, and image receptor at each examination, which is difficult to accomplish in general practice. The more recent introduction of software programs that can correct for some discrepancies in positioning and alignment in sequential digital images makes subtraction techniques more forgiving. Nonetheless, this diagnostic technique remains primarily a research tool.

Cone-Beam Computed Tomographic Imaging

Current research does not support the use of cone-beam computed tomographic (CBCT) imaging for routine periodontal assessment because it does not offer a significant advantage over conventional imaging techniques when the additional cost and radiation dose are considered. However, the three-dimensional imaging provided by CBCT imaging may allow better visualization of some bony defects that are not well depicted on conventional images. For example, CBCT imaging permits more complete assessment of the architecture of complex vertical defects and craters, furcations, and buccal and lingual plate loss, which are often not seen clearly on interproximal or periapical radiographs (Fig. 19-1). Therefore, CBCT imaging, particularly small-volume and high-resolution scans, may have a role in guiding management of selected lesions, especially when surgery is being considered. The utility of CBCT imaging can be limited by streaking artifacts caused by metallic restorations, which may obscure the details of the bony architecture being examined.

APPEARANCE OF NORMAL ANATOMY

The normal alveolar bone that supports the dentition has a characteristic appearance. A thin layer of opaque cortical bone often covers the alveolar crest. The height of the crest lies at a level approximately 0.5 to 2.0 mm below the level of the CEJs of adjacent teeth. Between posterior teeth, the alveolar crest is parallel to a line connecting adjacent CEJs (Fig. 19-2). Between anterior teeth, the alveolar crest usually is pointed and may have a well-defined cortex (Fig. 19-3). A well-mineralized cortical outline of the alveolar crest indicates the absence of periodontitis activity. However, lack of a well-mineralized alveolar crest may be found in patients with or without periodontitis.

The alveolar crest is continuous with the lamina dura of adjacent teeth. In the absence of disease, this bony junction between the alveolar crest and lamina dura of posterior teeth forms a sharp angle next to the tooth root. The periodontal ligament (PDL) space is often slightly wider around the cervical portion of the tooth root, especially in adolescents with erupting teeth. In this situation, if the lamina dura still forms a sharp, well-defined angle with the alveolar crest, the condition is a variant of normal and is not an indication of disease. The buccal-lingual thickness of alveolar crests varies widely, and it may be very thin coronally. This may appear in a two-dimensional image as an increase in radiolucency toward the crest. These sorts of variations in density alone are not an indication of disease and may be a variation of normal.

Because gingivitis is an inflammatory condition confined to the gingiva, there are no significant changes to the underlying bone, and therefore the appearance of the bone in a diagnostic image is normal.

IMAGING FEATURES OF PERIODONTAL DISEASE

For all types of periodontal disease, the changes seen in diagnostic images reflect changes seen with any inflammatory disease of bone. These changes can be divided into changes in the morphology of the supporting alveolar bone and changes to the internal density and trabecular pattern. Changes in morphology become apparent as a result of loss of the interproximal crestal bone and bone overlapping the buccal or lingual aspects of the tooth roots. Changes to the internal aspect of the alveolar bone reflect either a reduction or an increase in bone structure or a mixture of both. A reduction is seen as an increase in radiolucency because of a decrease in number and density of existing trabeculae. An increase in bone is seen as an increase in radiopacity (sclerosis) as the result of an increase primarily in the thickness, density, and number of trabeculae. Similar to all inflammatory lesions of bone, periodontal disease usually has a combination of bone loss and bone formation or sclerosis. However, acute early lesions predominantly display bone loss, whereas chronic lesions have a greater component of bone sclerosis. The following patterns of bone loss may be seen in the diagnostic image as the result of periodontitis.

CHANGES IN MORPHOLOGY OF ALVEOLAR BONE
Early Bone Changes
Early periodontitis appears as areas of localized erosion of the interproximal alveolar bone crest (Fig. 19-4). The anterior regions show blunting of the alveolar crests and slight loss of alveolar bone height. The posterior regions may also show a loss of the normally sharp angle between the lamina dura and alveolar crest. In early periodontal disease, this angle may lose its normal cortical surface (margin) and appear rounded off, having an irregular and diffuse

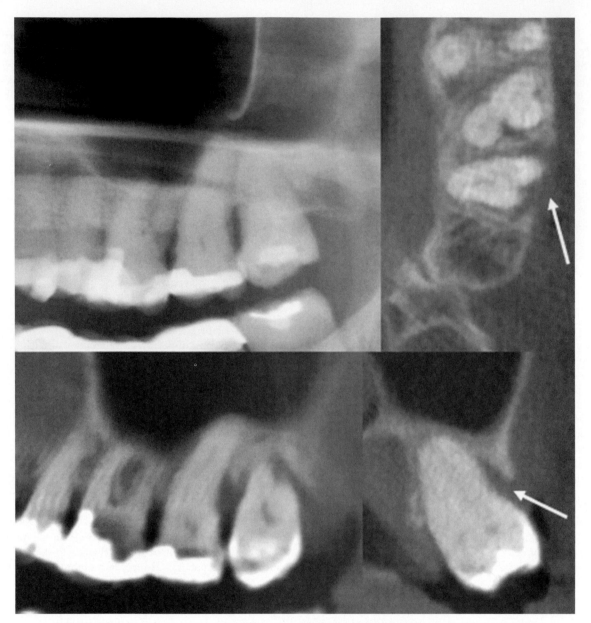

FIGURE 19-1 Cropped panoramic image *(top left)* demonstrates moderate bone loss between the second and third molars. Axial *(top right)*, coronal *(bottom right)*, and parasagittal *(bottom left)* CBCT images demonstrate the bone defects in this region more clearly. Periodontal bone loss around the buccal surface of the third molar is well visualized *(arrows)*, which could not be appreciated on the panoramic image.

border. Even if only slight changes are apparent, the disease process may not be of recent onset because significant loss of attachment must be present for 6 to 8 months before evidence of bone loss appears in an image. Also, variations in angle of projection of the x-ray beam can cause a slight change in the apparent height of the alveolar bone. Small regions of bone loss on the buccal or lingual aspects of the teeth are much more difficult to detect.

A mild lesion does not always develop into a more severe lesion later; however, if the periodontitis progresses, the destruction of alveolar bone extends beyond early changes in the alveolar crest and may induce a variety of defects in the morphology of the alveolar crest. These patterns of bone loss have been divided into horizontal bone loss, vertical (angular) defects, interdental craters, buccal or lingual cortical plate loss, and furcation involvement of multirooted teeth. The presence and severity of these bone defects

may vary among patients and within a patient. The intraoral image is valuable in showing the extent and morphology of residual bone, but complete assessment of bone loss and the diagnosis and staging of periodontitis requires integration of the radiologic information with the results of a clinical examination.

Horizontal Bone Loss

Horizontal bone loss describes the appearance of loss in height of the alveolar bone where the crest is still horizontal (i.e., parallel to an imagined line joining the CEJs of adjacent teeth) but is positioned apically more than a couple of millimeters from the CEJs. Horizontal bone loss may be mild, moderate, or severe, depending on its extent. Mild bone loss may be defined as loss of 20%, or approximately 1 to 2 mm, of the normal supporting bone height, and moderate loss is loss of between 20%, or approximately 2 mm,

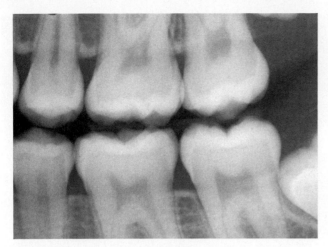

FIGURE 19-2 The normal alveolar crest lies 0.5 to 2.0 mm below the adjacent CEJs and forms a sharp angle with the lamina dura of the adjacent tooth. The crests may not always appear with a well-defined outer cortex.

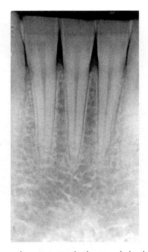

FIGURE 19-3 Between the anterior teeth, the normal alveolar crest is pointed and well corticated, coming to within 0.5 to 2.0 mm of the adjacent CEJs.

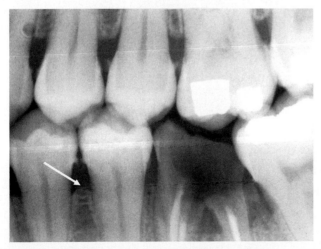

FIGURE 19-4 Initial periodontal disease is seen as a loss of cortical density and a rounding of the junction between the alveolar crest and the lamina dura (arrow). Note also the more pronounced bone loss around the mandibular first molar and the generalized interproximal calculus.

and 50% of the supporting bone height. Severe loss is anything beyond this point. Normal crestal bone height can be up to 2 mm from the CEJ, and therefore assessment of the quantity of bone loss must be considered from this point and not from the CEJ itself. Care must also be taken in using the CEJ as a reference point in cases of overeruption and severe attrition (Fig. 19-5). With overeruption, the alveolar bone will not necessarily remodel to keep a normal relationship to the CEJ, and the situation is similar in passive eruption, which may accompany severe attrition. Although in this case bone loss is not due to periodontitis, there still may be loss of attachment, which could be of clinical significance.

In horizontal bone loss, the crest of the buccal and lingual cortical plates and the intervening interdental bone have been resorbed (Fig. 19-6). The extent of bone loss evident at a single examination does not indicate the current activity of the disease. For example, a patient who previously had generalized periodontal disease and subsequent successful therapy will likely always show bone loss, but the bone level may remain stable. Reformation of the cortication of the alveolar crests is a good indicator of stabilization of the periodontium.

Vertical Bone Defects

A vertical (or angular) osseous defect is a bony lesion that is localized to a single tooth, although an individual may have multiple vertical osseous defects. These defects develop when bone loss progresses down the root of the tooth, resulting in deepening of the clinical periodontal pocket. This manifests as a vertical deformity within the alveolus that extends apically along the root of the affected tooth from the alveolar crest. The outline of the remaining alveolar bone typically displays an oblique angulation to an imaginary line connecting the CEJ of the affected tooth to the neighboring tooth. In its early form, a vertical defect appears as abnormal widening of the PDL space at the alveolar crest (Fig. 19-7, A). The vertical defect is described as three-walled (surrounded by three bony walls) when both buccal and lingual cortical plates remain; it is described as two-walled when one of these plates has been resorbed and as one-walled when both plates have been lost (Fig. 19-7, B). The distinctions among these groups are important in designing the treatment plan.

Vertical defects often are difficult or impossible to recognize on a radiograph because one or both of the cortical bony plates remain superimposed over the defect. Visualization of the depth of pockets may be aided by inserting a gutta-percha point before making the intraoral image. The point appears to follow the defect because gutta-percha is relatively inflexible and radiopaque (Fig. 19-8). Clinical and surgical inspections are the best means of determining the number of remaining bony walls. CBCT imaging may also help to characterize the defect more clearly (Fig. 19-9).

Interdental Craters

The interproximal crater is a two-walled, troughlike depression that forms in the crest of the interdental bone between adjacent teeth. The buccal and lingual outer cortical walls of the interproximal bone extend further coronally than the cancellous bone between them, which has been resorbed. In the image this appears as a bandlike or irregular region of bone with less density at the crest, immediately adjacent to the more dense normal bone apical to the base of the crater (Fig. 19-10). These defects are more common in the posterior segments, likely as a result of the broader buccal-lingual dimension of the alveolar crest in these regions.

FIGURE 19-5 **A,** This maxillary second bicuspid is overerupted; the etiology of the low bone level *(arrow)* relative to the CEJ is not necessarily the result of periodontal disease. **B,** An example of passive eruption related to severe attrition resulting in the apparent increase in the distance from the CEJ to the bone height *(arrows)* cannot be attributed to periodontal disease. However, the resultant change in bone level relative to the CEJ still may be clinically significant.

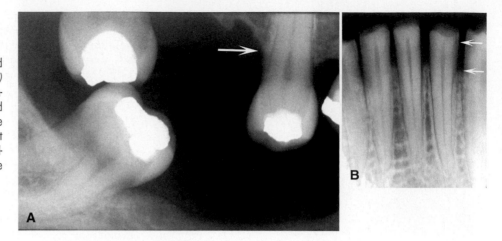

FIGURE 19-6 Horizontal bone loss is seen in the anterior region **(A)** and the posterior region **(B)** as a loss of the buccal and lingual cortical plates and interdental alveolar bone.

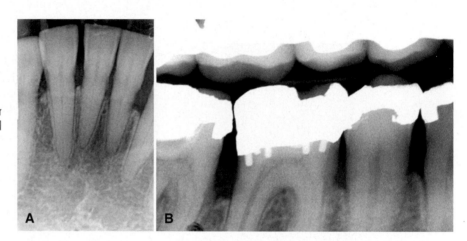

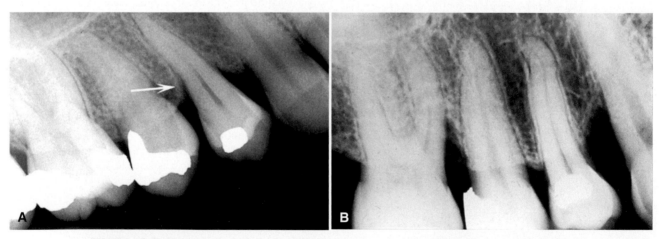

FIGURE 19-7 **A,** Example of a developing vertical defect; note the abnormal widening of the PDL space *(arrow).* **B,** Maxillary periapical image reveals two examples of more severe vertical defects affecting the mesial surface of the first molar and the distal surface of the canine.

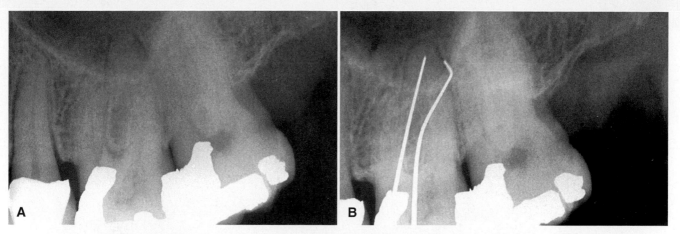

FIGURE 19-8 Gutta-percha may be used to visualize the depth of infrabony defects. **A,** Radiograph fails to show the osseous defect without the use of the gutta-percha points. **B,** Radiograph reveals an osseous defect extending to the region of the apex. *(Courtesy H. Takei, DDS, Los Angeles, CA.)*

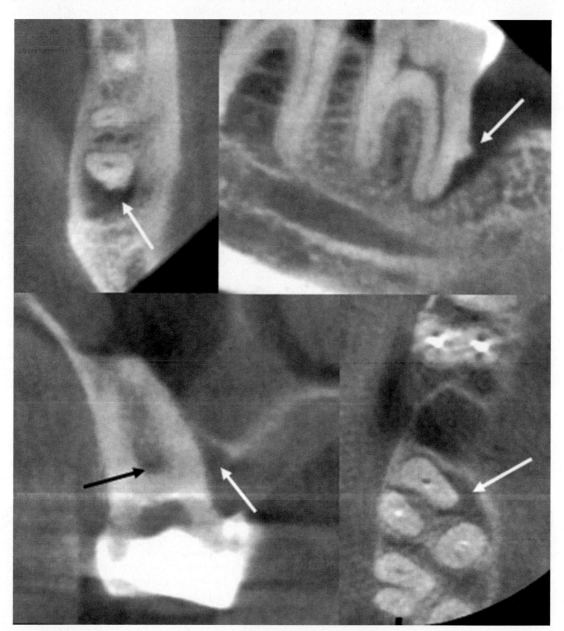

FIGURE 19-9 CBCT sections demonstrating details of the architecture of two three-walled vertical defects *(white arrows)*. Axial *(upper left)* and parasagittal *(upper right)* reconstructions show a deep vertical defect on the distal surface of the mandibular left second molar. Calculus is seen on the root surface. Coronal *(lower left)* and axial *(lower right)* images of another case show a three-walled defect on the palatal aspect of the mesiobuccal root of a maxillary molar. Early furcation involvement is also detected on this tooth *(black arrow)*.

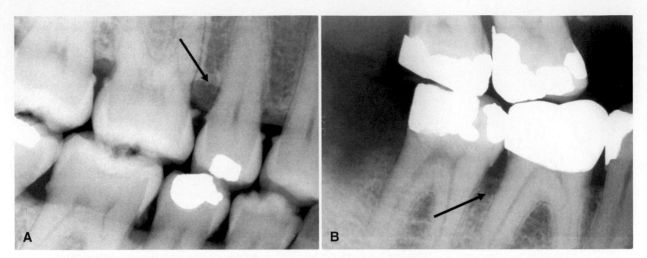

FIGURE 19-10 Interproximal craters, existing as defects between the buccal and lingual cortical plates, seen as a radiolucent band **(A)** or trough **(B)** apical to the level of the crestal edges. The *arrows* indicate the base of the craters.

Buccal or Lingual Cortical Plate Loss

The buccal or lingual cortical plate adjacent to the teeth may resorb. Loss of a cortical plate may occur alone or with another type of bone loss, such as horizontal bone loss. This type of loss is indicated by an increase in the radiolucency of the root of the tooth near the alveolar crest. The shape seen usually is a semicircular shadow with the apex of the radiolucency directed apically in relation to the tooth (Fig. 19-11). Lack of bone loss at the interproximal region of the tooth may make this kind of defect difficult to detect.

Osseous Deformities in the Furcations of Multirooted Teeth

Progressive periodontal disease and its associated bone loss may extend into the furcations of multirooted teeth. As bone resorption extends down the side of a multirooted tooth, eliminating the bone covering the root, it can reach the level of the furcation and beyond. Widening of the PDL space at the apex of the interradicular bony crest of the furcation is strong evidence that the periodontal disease process involves the furcation (Fig. 19-12, *A*). If sufficient bone loss has occurred on the lingual and buccal aspects of a mandibular molar furcation, the radiolucent image of the lesion becomes prominent (Fig. 19-12, *B*). The bony defect may also involve only the buccal or lingual cortical plate and extend under the roof of the furcation. In such a case, if the defect does not extend through to the other cortical plate, it appears more irregular and radiolucent than the adjacent normal bone. By use of the buccal object rule with images made at different angulations, it may be possible to determine whether the buccal or the lingual cortical plate has been resorbed.

If the crestal bone is below the furcation but the disease process has not extended into the interradicular bone, the width of the periodontal membrane space appears normal. Also, the septal bone may appear more radiolucent but otherwise be normal. In the mandible, the external oblique ridge may mask furcation involvement of the third molars. Convergent roots may also obscure furcation defects in maxillary and mandibular second and third molars.

The loss of interradicular bone in the furcation of a maxillary molar may originate from the buccal, mesial, or distal surface of the tooth. The most common route for furcation involvement of the maxillary permanent first molar is from the mesial side. The

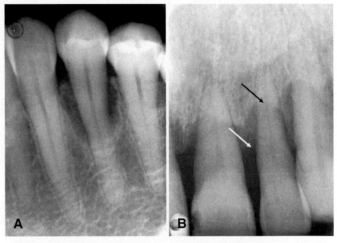

FIGURE 19-11 A, Loss of the lingual alveolar crest adjacent to this mandibular first bicuspid without associated interproximal bone loss. **B,** Loss of the buccal cortical bone adjacent to the maxillary central and lateral incisors. The *black arrow* indicates the level of the buccal alveolar crest, which demonstrates more profound loss relative to the lingual alveolar crest *(white arrow)*.

image of furcation involvement is not as sharply defined around maxillary molars as around mandibular molars because the palatal root is superimposed on the defect (Fig. 19-12, *C*). However, this pattern of bone destruction occasionally is prominent and appears as an inverted "J" shadow with the hook of the "J" extending into the trifurcation (Fig. 19-12, *D*) or as a radiolucent triangle superimposed over the roots of the involved tooth with its apex pointing toward the furcation.

Definitive diagnosis of complex furcation deformities requires careful clinical examination and sometimes surgical exploration. Intraoral images are an important tool in identifying potentially involved sites as well as providing information about root morphology and length, which is of significance to treatment planning and prognosis. CBCT imaging can also be used to confirm involvement of a tooth and allow more detailed characterization of osseous furcation defects in cases where this information is required for improved treatment planning.

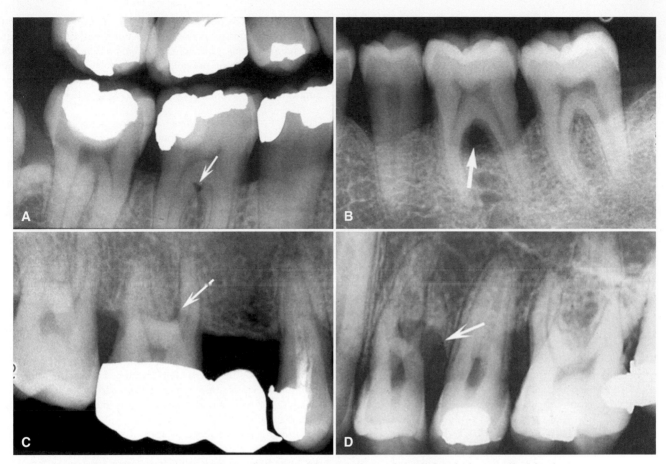

FIGURE 19-12 **A,** periapical image revealing very early furcation involvement of a mandibular molar characterized by slight widening of the PDL space in the furcation region *(arrow)*. **B,** Periapical image revealing a profound radiolucent lesion within the furcation region *(arrow)* resulting from loss of bone in the furcation region and the buccal and lingual cortical plates. **C,** Angulation of this periapical view of a maxillary first molar projected the palatal root away from the trifurcation region revealing early widening of the furcation PDL space *(arrow)*. **D,** Example of an inverted "J" shadow *(arrow)* resulting from bone destruction extending into the trifurcation region of a three-rooted maxillary first bicuspid.

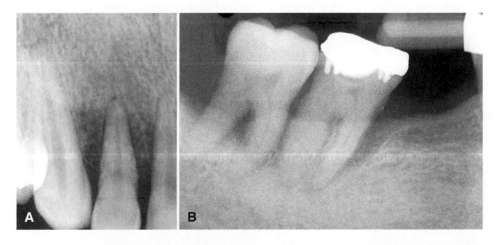

FIGURE 19-13 **A,** Example of a primarily radiolucent reaction around this maxillary lateral incisor. The trabeculae toward the alveolar crest on the mesial and distal aspect of the tooth are barely perceptible, and the marrow spaces are enlarged. **B,** Periapical film revealing a predominantly sclerotic bone reaction resulting from the periodontal disease involving the mandibular molars. The trabeculae are thickened, and the marrow spaces are barely perceptible.

CHANGES TO INTERNAL DENSITY AND TRABECULAR PATTERN OF BONE

As with all other inflammatory lesions, the periodontal lesion may stimulate a reaction in the surrounding bone. The peripheral bone may appear more radiolucent or more sclerotic (radiopaque) or more commonly with a mixture of these patterns. Very rarely, no apparent change is seen in the surrounding bone. A radiolucent change reflects loss of density and number of trabeculae. The trabeculae appear very faint, which is more commonly seen in early or acute lesions (Fig. 19-13, *A*). If the trabeculae are sufficiently decalcified, they may not appear in the image even though they are still present; this accounts for the apparent reformation of bone in some cases where the acute inflammation resolves with successful treatment and the trabeculae remineralize. The sclerotic bone reaction appears radiopaque because of deposition of bone on existing trabeculae at the expense of the marrow, resulting in thicker trabeculae that may eventually be so dense as to appear as an amorphous radiopaque mass (Fig. 19-13, *B*). This sclerotic reaction may extend some distance from the periodontal lesion, sometimes to the inferior aspect of the mandible. Usually the surrounding bone reaction is a mixture of both bone loss and sclerosis.

Inflammatory products from a periodontal lesion can extend through the cortex of the floor of the maxillary sinus to cause a regional mucositis (Fig. 19-14). In rare cases, a periosteal reaction might be seen on the buccal or lingual aspect of the alveolar process.

OTHER PATTERNS OF PERIODONTAL BONE LOSS

Periodontal Abscess

A periodontal abscess is a rapidly progressing, destructive lesion that usually originates in a deep soft tissue pocket. It occurs when the coronal portion of the pocket becomes occluded or when foreign material becomes lodged between a tooth and the gingiva. Clinically, pain and swelling and sometimes a draining sinus are present in the region. If the lesion is acute, there may be no visible changes in the image. If the lesion persists, a radiolucent region appears, often superimposed over the root of a tooth. The radiolucency may be a rounded area of rarefaction, and a bridge of bone may be present over the coronal aspect of the lesion, separating it from the crest of the alveolar ridge (Fig. 19-15). After treatment, some of the lost bone may regenerate.

Aggressive Periodontitis

Disease Mechanism. Aggressive periodontitis refers to periodontal disease of an aggressive and rapid nature that usually occurs in patients younger than 30 years. The severity of the disease appears to be an exuberant reaction to a minimum amount of plaque accumulation and may result in early tooth loss. The term "aggressive periodontitis" has replaced the term "early-onset periodontitis." Aggressive periodontitis is subclassified into localized

aggressive periodontitis and generalized aggressive periodontitis. The cause of aggressive periodontitis is unknown; however, specific bacterial pathogens, especially *Actinobacillus actinomycetemcomitans*; functional defects of polymorphonuclear leukocytes; exuberant immune responses; and inheritable genetic factors have been implicated.

Clinical Presentation. Localized aggressive periodontitis is associated with attachment loss involving the incisors and first molars. In this form, the amount of bone loss correlates with the time of tooth eruption, in that the teeth that erupt first (incisors and first molars) have the most bone loss. This disease usually commences around puberty, and the bone loss is rapid—up to three to four times the rate seen in chronic periodontitis. There are usually few signs of soft tissue inflammation or plaque accumulation despite the presence of deep bony pockets. Often the patient presents with drifting and mobile incisors and early loss of first molars.

Generalized aggressive periodontitis can involve a variable number of teeth, from at least three to all of the dentition, and by definition is not confined to the first molars and incisors. This rapidly progressing disease usually affects individuals younger than 30 years. The gingiva may appear normal as in the localized form or may have an exuberant inflammatory response. If there is a history of premature loss of deciduous teeth and the permanent teeth are rapidly lost soon after erupting, a possible diagnosis of Papillon-Lefèvre syndrome might be considered. This syndrome is usually seen with an associated hyperkeratosis of palmar and plantar surfaces.

Estimates of prevalence of aggressive periodontitis are 0.53% and 0.13% for the localized and generalized forms, respectively, in the United States. Black individuals are affected more commonly than whites with both the localized and the generalized forms. Black men are more commonly affected with localized disease than black women, whereas white women are more likely than white men to have localized disease.

Imaging Features. The radiographic appearance of the bone loss in localized aggressive periodontitis typically consists of deep vertical defects (Fig. 19-16). Maxillary teeth are involved slightly more often than mandibular teeth, and strong left-right symmetry is common. The generalized form of aggressive periodontitis can involve several teeth or all the dentition, and the rapid bone loss may be of the vertical or horizontal pattern.

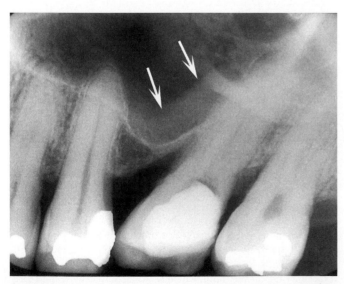

FIGURE 19-14 Periapical film revealing a localized mucositis within the maxillary sinus *(arrows)* immediately adjacent to a vertical periodontal defect.

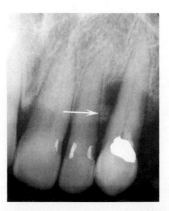

FIGURE 19-15 Example of a periodontal abscess related to the maxillary canine; note the well-defined area of bone loss over the midroot region of the tooth and extending in a mesial direction toward the lateral incisor. There appears to be a layer of bone *(arrow)* separating the area of bone destruction from the crest of the alveolar process.

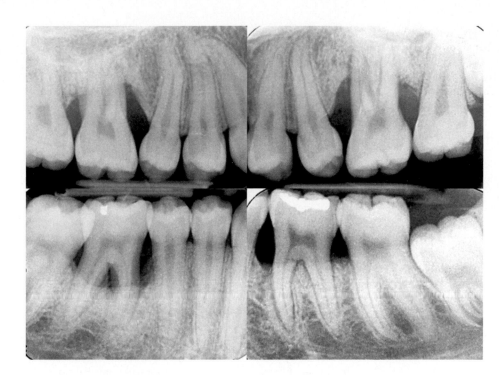

FIGURE 19-16 Typical vertical bone loss in localized aggressive periodontitis. Note the bone loss is confined to the region of the first molars. *(Courtesy T. D. Charbeneau, DDS, Dallas, TX.)*

Treatment.   Early identification and treatment of aggressive periodontitis is important because of the rapid progression of this condition and the associated tooth loss. Response to conventional periodontal therapy is unpredictable but is more likely to be successful when initiated earlier. Treatment consists of scaling, curettage, and administration of antibiotics and may include surgical and regenerative therapies.

DENTAL CONDITIONS ASSOCIATED WITH PERIODONTAL DISEASES

Various changes in the dentition and its supporting structures that have been associated with and potentially can exacerbate periodontal disease may be evident in diagnostic images. These conditions, including occlusal trauma and tooth mobility, open contacts, and local irritating factors such as overhanging and faulty restorations and calculus, should be identified as part of a complete clinical and radiologic assessment.

OCCLUSAL TRAUMA

Traumatic occlusion causes degenerative changes in response to occlusal pressures that are greater than the physiologic tolerances of the tooth's supporting tissues. These changes occur either as a result of maladaptation in response to excessive occlusal force on teeth or by normal occlusal forces on a periodontium already compromised by bone loss. In addition to clinical signs and symptoms such as increased mobility, wear facets, unusual response to percussion, and a history of contributing habits, there are associated findings in the images, including widening of the PDL space, thickening of the lamina dura, bone loss, and an increase in the number and size of trabeculae. Other sequelae of traumatic occlusion include hypercementosis and root fractures. Traumatic occlusion alone does not cause gingivitis or periodontitis, affect the epithelial attachment, or lead to pocket formation, but in the presence of preexisting periodontitis bone loss may be accelerated.

Traumatic occlusion can be definitively diagnosed only by clinical evaluation and not by the imaging findings alone.

TOOTH MOBILITY

Widening of the PDL space suggests tooth mobility, which may result from occlusal trauma or a lack of bone support arising from advanced bone loss. If the affected tooth has a single root, the socket may develop an hourglass shape. If the tooth is multirooted, it may show widening of the PDL space at the apices and in the region of the furcation. These changes result when the tooth moves about an axis of rotation at some midpoint on the roots. In addition, the image of the lamina dura may appear broad and hazy and show increased density.

OPEN CONTACTS

When the mesial and distal surfaces of adjacent teeth do not touch, the patient has an open contact. This condition may be dangerous to the periodontium because of the potential for food debris to become trapped in the region. Trapped food particles may damage the soft tissue and induce an inflammatory response and contribute to the development of localized periodontal disease. Open contacts are associated with periodontal disease more than closed contacts. Similar potential situations in which periodontal disease may develop are discrepancies in the height of two adjacent marginal ridges or tipped teeth (Fig. 19-17). Abnormal tooth alignment does not cause periodontal disease but provides an environment where the disease may develop as a result of difficulty in maintaining adequate oral hygiene.

LOCAL IRRITATING FACTORS

Other local factors that are apparent in an image may provide an environment where periodontal disease may develop or may aggravate existing periodontal disease. For instance, calculus deposits (Fig. 19-18) can prevent effective cleansing of a sulcus and lead to enhanced plaque formation and the progression of periodontal disease. Calculus is most commonly seen on the mandibular incisors but may be localized to any surface or generalized throughout the dentition. Defective restorations with overhanging or poorly contoured margins can also lead to the accumulation of plaque owing to difficulty in cleaning around them, thus providing an environment where periodontal disease may develop (Fig. 19-19).

EVALUATION OF PERIODONTAL THERAPY

Occasionally, signs of successful treatment of periodontal disease are visible in the posttreatment images. Reformation of the interproximal cortex (Fig. 19-20) and the sharp line angle between the cortex and lamina dura is a good indicator of stabilization of the disease, although this sign is not seen in all patients. The relatively radiolucent margins of bone that were undergoing active resorption before treatment may become more sclerotic (radiopaque) after successful therapy. In some cases, there may have been considerable mineral loss of the cancellous bone (appearing radiolucent) so that the bone is not apparent in the image. Successful

treatment may result in remineralization, causing the bone to become visible in the image, giving the false impression that bone has actually grown into periodontal defects. In many cases, there are no apparent changes in the images after successful treatment. Also, intraoral images do not disclose the therapeutic elimination of soft tissue periodontal pockets; therefore, healing is best assessed by clinical evaluation.

Sequential images made with different beam angulations may give the false impression that bone has grown into the periodontal defects. Therefore, in a longitudinal study, effort should be given to duplicate the image geometry as well as using ideal exposure and processing variables. For instance, too high an x-ray exposure or too long a developing time increases the density of the image (more black), and thin bone such as the alveolar crest may not be apparent, giving the false impression that the bone has been resorbed. Alternatively, light images may give the false impression of bone growth.

DIFFERENTIAL DIAGNOSIS

Most cases of bone loss around teeth are caused by periodontal diseases. This fact can make the clinician less sensitive to other diseases with similar manifestations that should always be considered in the differential diagnosis. Occasionally, more serious diseases are missed or recognized late. The most likely clinical sign of disease other than periodontal disease is the presence of one or a few adjacent loose teeth when the rest of the mouth shows no signs of periodontal disease. Suspicion should be heightened if the bone destruction does not have the pattern or morphology normally associated with periodontal disease. Periodontal disease originates in the gingival sulcus at the alveolar crest and progresses along the periodontium, against the affected tooth. Thus, bone loss caused by periodontal disease, such as vertical defects, should appear larger at the coronal aspect and less severe at the leading edge apically; this differs from other diseases, which may destroy the supporting bone in a more widespread, or invasive, pattern.

Squamous cell carcinoma of the alveolar process may mimic the appearance of periodontal disease and is occasionally treated as such, resulting in a delay in diagnosis and treatment (Fig. 19-21, *A*). This malignancy may display characteristics in the image that suggest its true nature, such as extensive bone destruction of a localized region, beyond the periodontium, or invasive characteristics (see Chapter 24). Irregular widening of the PDL space along

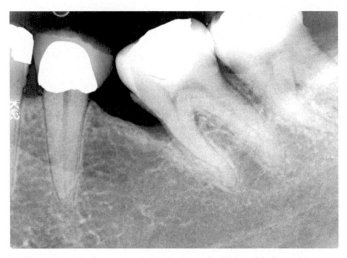

FIGURE 19-17 The second molar has tipped mesially after loss of the first molar, creating an abnormal tooth alignment that was difficult for the patient to maintain and leading to localized periodontal disease. Note the calculus on the mesial surface of the second molar. The crown on the second premolar was constructed with an enlarged distal contour to stop further tipping of the molar.

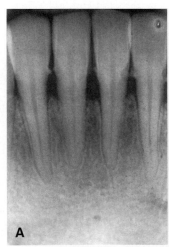
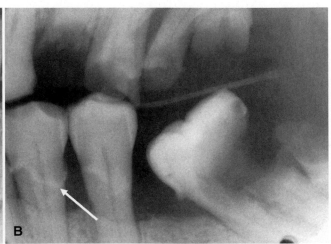

FIGURE 19-18 Calculus may be seen as small angular radiopaque deposits projecting between interproximal surfaces of the teeth (**A**) or as radiopaque bands across the roots representing circumferential accumulation (*arrow* in **B**).

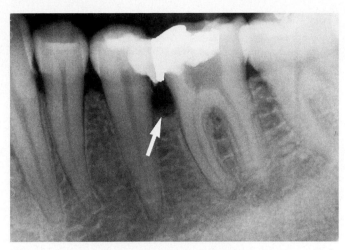

FIGURE 19-19 These overhanging restorations provided an environment suitable for plaque accumulation and subsequent localized periodontal bone loss *(arrow)*.

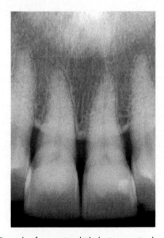

FIGURE 19-20 Example of a case in which the interproximal cortex of the alveolar crest has reformed after successful periodontal therapy.

its entire length, with a ragged periphery and destruction of the lamina dura, is suggestive of infiltration by a carcinoma, rather than periodontal disease. In some cases, squamous cell carcinoma may mimic periodontal disease, and only the clinical characteristics of the lesion and the failure to respond to treatment indicate the presence of malignancy.

Any lesion of bone destruction that has ill-defined borders and a lack of peripheral bone response (sclerosis) should be viewed with suspicion. Another disease to be considered is Langerhans' cell histiocytosis (Fig. 19-21, *B*). Often this disease may manifest as single or multiple regions of bone destruction around the roots of teeth, similar to periodontal disease. The condition may appear similar to localized aggressive periodontitis except that the bone destruction does not correlate with the time of tooth eruption, as is seen in periodontitis. Also, in histiocytosis, the epicenter of the bone destruction is in the midroot region rather than at the crest, which may give early lesions an "ice cream scoop" appearance, with the alveolar crest less resorbed or even intact (see Chapter 23).

CONDITIONS THAT AFFECT PERIODONTAL DISEASE

Although these conditions do not cause periodontal disease, they can influence its course by interfering with the body's natural defenses against irritants or limiting its capacity to repair. Although any systemic disease may have some influence on other body systems, only a few appear to influence the periodontium and outcome of periodontal treatment. These include diabetes mellitus, hematologic disorders (e.g., monocytic conditions and less often myelogenous leukemia, neutropenia, hemophilia and nonhemophilic polycythemia vera), genetic and hereditary disturbances (e.g., Papillon-Lefèvre syndrome, Down syndrome, hypophosphatemia, Chédiak-Higashi syndrome), hormonal changes (e.g., puberty, pregnancy, menopause), and stress.

DIABETES MELLITUS

Diabetes mellitus is the most common and important systemic disease to influence the onset and course of periodontal disease. Uncontrolled diabetes may result in protein breakdown, degenerative vascular changes, lowered resistance to infection, and increased

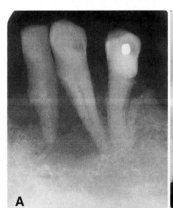
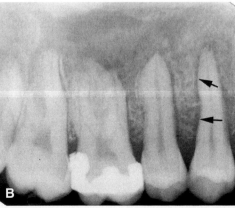
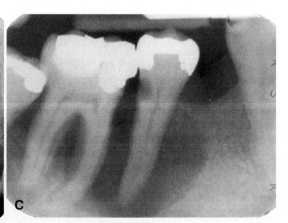

FIGURE 19-21 **A,** Periapical film of a case of squamous cell carcinoma of the alveolar process of the mandible; note the irregular bone destruction. **B,** Periapical film of a malignant tumor extending from the maxillary sinus into the alveolar process and invading the PDL space of the adjacent teeth; note the irregular widening *(arrows)*. **C,** Periapical film of Langerhans' cell histiocytosis demonstrating an alveolar lesion with bone destruction; note that the epicenter would be at the midroot region instead of the alveolar crest, as seen in periodontal disease.

severity of infections. Consequently, patients with uncontrolled diabetes are more disposed to the development of periodontal disease than individuals with normal glucose metabolism. Patients with uncontrolled diabetes and periodontal disease also show more severe and rapid alveolar bone resorption and are more prone to the development of periodontal abscesses. In patients whose diabetes is under control, periodontal disease responds normally to traditional treatment.

ACQUIRED IMMUNODEFICIENCY SYNDROME

The incidence and severity of periodontal disease is high in patients with acquired immunodeficiency syndrome (AIDS). In these individuals, the disease process is characterized by a rapid progression that leads to bone sequestration and loss of several teeth. These patients may not respond to standard periodontal therapy.

RADIATION THERAPY

High-dose irradiation to the oral tissues as a treatment for malignant conditions may have a detrimental effect on the periodontium. Radiation therapy to the jaws results in bone that is hypovascular, hypocellular, and hypoxic. This bone may be less able to remodel and be more susceptible to infections, resulting in rapid bone loss that is indistinguishable from the radiographic characteristics of periodontal disease. Teeth that have been exposed to high-dose radiation fields have been shown to demonstrate greater recession, attachment loss, and mobility than teeth in the same mouth that were not within the field.

BIBLIOGRAPHY

Clinical Characteristics of Periodontal Diseases

Armitage GC: Periodontal diseases: diagnosis, *Ann Periodontol* 1:37–215, 1996.

Herrera C, González I, Sanz M: The periodontal abscess (I): clinical and microbiological findings, *J Clin Periodontol* 27:387–394, 2000.

Newman MG, Takei HH, Klokkevold PR, et al: *Carranza's clinical periodontology*, Philadelphia, 2006, Saunders.

Walsh TF, al-Kohail OS, Fosam EB: The relationship of bone loss observed on panoramic radiographs with clinical periodontal screening, *J Clin Periodontol* 24:153–157, 1997.

Epidemiology

Melvin WL, Sandifer JB, Gray JL: The prevalence and sex ratio of juvenile periodontitis in a young racially mixed population, *J Periodontol* 62:330–334, 1991.

Papapanou PN: Periodontal diseases: epidemiology, *Ann Periodontol* 1:1–36, 1996.

Position paper: epidemiology of periodontal diseases. American Academy of Periodontology, *J Periodontol* 67:935–945, 1996.

Etiology

Bimstein E, Garcia-Godoy F: The significance of age, proximal caries, gingival inflammation, probing depths, and the loss of lamina dura in the diagnosis of alveolar bone loss in the primary molars, *ASDC J Dent Child* 61:125–128, 1994.

Page RC, Offenbacher S, Schroeder HE, et al: Advances in the pathogenesis of periodontitis: summary of developments, clinical implications and future directions, *Periodontol 2000* 14:216–248, 1997.

Salvi GE, Lawrence HP, Offenbacher S, et al: Influence of risk factors on the pathogenesis of periodontitis, *Periodontol 2000* 14:173, 1997.

Schwartz Z, Goultschin J, Dean DD, et al: Mechanisms of alveolar bone destruction in periodontitis, *Periodontol 2000* 14:158, 1997.

Van Dyke TE, Serhan CN: Resolution of inflammation: a new paradigm for the pathogenesis of periodontal diseases, *J Dent Res* 82:82–90, 2003.

Radiographic Manifestations

Gutteridge DL: The use of radiographic techniques in the diagnosis and management of periodontal diseases, *Dentomaxillofac Radiol* 24:107–113, 1995.

Jeffcoat MK, Wang IC, Reddy MS: Radiographic diagnosis in periodontics, *Periodontol 2000* 7:54–68, 1995.

Khocht A, Zohn H, Deasy M, et al: Screening for periodontal disease: radiographs vs PSR, *J Am Dent Assoc* 127:749–756, 1996.

Koral SM, Howell TH, Jeffcoat MK: Alveolar bone loss due to open interproximal contacts in periodontal disease, *J Periodontol* 52:447–450, 1981.

Mann J, Pettigrew J, Beideman R, et al: Investigation of the relationship between clinically detected loss of attachment and radiographic changes in early periodontal disease, *J Clin Periodontol* 12:247–253, 1985.

Nielsen IM, Glavind L, Karring T: Interproximal periodontal intrabony defects: prevalence, localization, and etiological factors, *J Clin Periodontol* 7:187–198, 1980.

Rams TE, Listgarten MA, Slots J: Utility of radiographic crestal lamina dura for predicting periodontitis disease activity, *J Clin Periodontol* 21:571–576, 1994.

Waite IM, Furniss JS, Wong WM: Relationship between clinical periodontal condition and the radiological appearance at first molar sites in adolescents: a 3-year study, *J Clin Periodontol* 21:155–160, 1994.

Aggressive Periodontitis

Albandar JM, Brown LJ, Löe H: Dental caries and tooth loss in adolescents with early onset periodontitis, *J Periodontol* 67:960–967, 1996.

Albandar JM, Brown LJ, Löe H: Clinical features of early onset periodontitis, *J Am Dent Assoc* 128:1393–1399, 1997.

Brown LJ, Albandar JM, Brunelle JA, et al: Early onset periodontitis: progression of attachment loss during 6 years, *J Periodontol* 67:968–975, 1996.

Loe H, Brown LJ: Early onset periodontitis in the United States of America, *J Periodontol* 62:608–616, 1991,

Page RC, Altman LC, Ebersole JL, et al: Rapidly progressive periodontitis: a distinct clinical condition, *J Periodontol* 54:197–209, 1983.

Radiographic Technique

Bragger I: Radiographic diagnosis of periodontal disease progression, *Curr Opin Periodontol* 3:59–67, 1996.

Gröndahl K, Gröndahl HG, Webber RL, et al: Influence of variations in projection geometry on the detectability of periodontal bone lesions: a comparison between subtraction radiography and conventional radiographic technique, *J Clin Periodontol* 11:411–420, 1984.

Pepelassi EA, Diamanti-Kipioti A: Selection of the most accurate method of conventional radiography for the assessment of periodontal osseous destruction, *J Clin Periodontol* 24:557–567, 1997.

Reed B, Polson A: Relationships between bitewing and periapical radiographs in assessing crestal alveolar bone levels, *J Periodontol* 55:22–27, 1984.

Subtraction Radiography

Eickholz P, Hausmann E: Evidence for healing of periodontal defects 5 years after conventional and regenerative therapy: digital subtraction and bone level measurements, *J Clin Periodontol* 29:922–928, 2002.

Cone-Beam Computed Tomographic Imaging

Mol A, Balasundaram A: In vitro cone beam computed tomography imaging of periodontal bone, *Dentomaxillofac Radiol* 37:319–324, 2008.

Vandenberghe B, Jacobs R, Yang J: Detection of periodontal bone loss using digital intraoral and cone beam computed tomography images: an in vitro assessment of bony and/or infrabony defects, *Dentomaxillofac Radiol* 37:252–260, 2008.

Walter C, Weiger R, Zitzmann NU: Accuracy of three-dimensional imaging in assessing maxillary molar furcation involvement, *J Clin Periodontol* 37:436–441, 2010.

Occlusal Trauma

Burgett FG: Trauma from occlusion: periodontal concerns, *Dent Clin North Am* 39:301–311, 1995.

Wank GS, Kroll YJ: Occlusal trauma: an evaluation of its relationship to periodontal prostheses, *Dent Clin North Am* 25:511–532, 1981.

Systemic Disease

Emrich LJ, Shlossman M, Genco RJ: Periodontal disease in non-insulin-dependent diabetes mellitus, *J Periodontol* 62:123–131, 1991.

Epstein JB, Lunn R, Le N, et al: Periodontal attachment loss in patients after head and neck radiation therapy, *Oral Surg Oral Med Oral Pathol Oral Radiol Endod* 86:673–677, 1998.

Farzim I, Edalat M: Periodontosis with hyperkeratosis palmaris and plantaris (the Papillon-Lefèvre syndrome): a case report, *J Periodontol* 45:316–318, 1974.

Nelson RG, Schlossman M, Budding LM, et al: Periodontal diseases and NIDDM in Pima Indians, *Diabetes Care* 13:836–840, 1990.

Rateitschak-Plüss EM, Schroeder HE: History of periodontitis in a child with Papillon-Lefèvre syndrome: a case report, *J Periodontol* 55:35–46, 1984.

Winkler JR, Grassi M, Murray PA: Clinical description and etiology of HIV-associated periodontal disease. In Robinson PB, Greenspan JS, editors: *Prospectus on oral manifestations of AIDS*, Littleton, MA, 1988, PSG Publishing.

Inflammatory Disease

Linda Lee

DISEASE MECHANISM

Inflammatory lesions are the most common pathologic condition of the jaws. The jaws are unique from other bones of the body in that the presence of teeth creates a direct pathway for infectious and inflammatory agents to invade bone by means of caries and periodontal disease. The body responds to chemical, physical, or microbiologic injury with inflammation. The inflammatory response destroys or walls off the injurious stimulus and sets up an environment for repair of the damaged tissue.

Under normal conditions, bone metabolism represents a balance of osteoclastic bone resorption and osteoblastic bone production. This is a complex, interdependent relationship in which osteoblasts mediate the resorptive activity of the osteoclasts. Mediators of inflammation (cytokines, prostaglandins, and many growth factors) tip this balance to favor either bone resorption or bone formation. For the purposes of this chapter, all inflammatory conditions of bone, regardless of the specific etiology, are considered to represent a spectrum or continuum of conditions with different clinical features (e.g., site, severity, duration).

When the initial source of inflammation is a necrotic pulp and the bony lesion is restricted to the region of the tooth, the condition is called a periapical inflammatory lesion. When the infection spreads in the bone marrow and is no longer contained to the vicinity of the tooth root apex, it is called osteomyelitis. Another source of inflammatory lesions in bone is extension of inflammation into bone from the overlying soft tissues; this type of lesion includes periodontal lesions (see Chapter 19) and pericoronitis, an inflammation that arises in the tissues surrounding the crown of a partially erupted tooth. The names of the various inflammatory lesions tend to describe their clinical and imaging presentations and behavior; however, all have the same underlying disease mechanism, including a common response of the bone to the injury.

GENERAL CLINICAL FEATURES

The four cardinal signs of inflammation—redness, swelling, heat, and pain—may be observed in varying degrees with inflammation of the jaws. Acute lesions are lesions of recent onset. The onset typically is rapid, and these lesions cause pronounced pain, often accompanied by fever and swelling. Chronic lesions have a prolonged course with a longer insidious onset and pain that is less intense. Fever may be intermittent and low grade, and swelling may occur gradually. Some chronic, low-grade infections may not produce any significant clinical symptoms.

GENERAL IMAGING FEATURES

LOCATION

With periapical inflammatory lesions, which are pathologic conditions of the pulp, the epicenter typically is located at the apex of a tooth. However, lesions of pulpal origin also may be located anywhere along the root surface because of accessory canals or perforations caused by root canal therapy or root fractures. Periodontal lesions have an epicenter that is located at the alveolar crest. If periodontal bone loss is severe, the bone inflammatory changes may extend to the root furcation level or to the root apex. Osteomyelitis, a diffuse, uncontained inflammation of the bone, most commonly is found in the posterior mandible. The maxilla rarely is involved.

PERIPHERY

Most often the periphery is ill defined, with a gradual blending of normal trabecular pattern into a sclerotic pattern, or the normal trabecular pattern may gradually fade into a radiolucent region of bone loss.

INTERNAL STRUCTURE

The internal structure of inflammatory lesions presents a spectrum of appearances. Cancellous bone may respond to an insult by tipping the bone metabolic balance either in favor of resorption (giving the area a radiolucent appearance) or in favor of bone formation (resulting in a radiopaque or sclerotic appearance). Usually there is a combination of these two reactions. The radiolucent regions may show no evidence of previous trabeculation or a very faint pattern of trabeculation. The increased radiopacity is caused by an increase in bone formation on existing trabeculae. Radiographically, these trabeculae appear thicker and more numerous, replacing marrow spaces. In acute disease, resorption typically predominates; with chronic disease, excessive bone formation leads to an overall radiopaque, sclerotic appearance. In cases of osteomyelitis, careful examination of the x-ray images may reveal sequestra, which appear as ill-defined areas of radiolucency containing a radiopaque island of nonvital bone.

EFFECTS ON SURROUNDING STRUCTURES

The effects of inflammation on surrounding cancellous bone include stimulation of bone formation, resulting in a sclerotic pattern, or bone resorption, resulting in radiolucency. The periodontal ligament space (PDL) involved in the lesion is widened; this widening is greatest at the source of the inflammation. For example, with periapical lesions, the widening is greatest around the apical region of the root; the widening is greatest at the alveolar crest in periodontal disease. With chronic infections, root resorption may occur, and cortical boundaries may be resorbed. The periosteal component of bone, whether on the surface of the jaws or lining the floor of the maxillary sinus, also responds to inflammation. The periosteum contains a layer of pluripotential lining cells that, under the right conditions, differentiate into osteoblasts and lay down new bone. Inflammatory exudate from infection within the bone can penetrate the cortex, lift up the periosteum from the surface of the bone, and stimulate the periosteum to produce new bone. Because inflammatory exudate is a fluid, the periosteum is lifted from the surface of bone in a manner that positions the periosteum almost parallel to the surface of the bone; thus, the layer of new bone is almost parallel to the bone surface.

PERIAPICAL INFLAMMATORY LESIONS

SYNONYMS

Periapical inflammatory lesions have been called acute apical periodontitis, chronic apical periodontitis, periapical abscess, and periapical granuloma. Radiolucent presentations have been called rarefying osteitis, whereas radiopaque presentations have been called sclerosing osteitis, condensing osteitis, and focal sclerosing osteitis. Chapter 21 discusses periapical cysts of inflammatory origin (radicular cysts).

DISEASE MECHANISM

A periapical inflammatory lesion is defined as a local response of the bone around the apex of a tooth that occurs as a result of necrosis of the pulp or through destruction of the periapical tissues by extensive periodontal disease (Fig. 20-1). The pulpal necrosis may occur as a result of pulpal invasion of bacteria through caries or trauma. In Figure 20-1, the periapical inflammatory lesion is characterized by apical periodontitis, an inflammatory process that may histologically represent either a periapical abscess or a periapical granuloma. Toxic metabolites from the necrotic pulp exit the root apex to incite an inflammatory reaction in the periapical periodontal ligament and surrounding bone (apical periodontitis).

This reaction is characterized histologically by an inflammatory infiltrate composed predominantly of lymphocytes mixed with polymorphonuclear neutrophils. Depending on the severity of the response, the neutrophils may collect to form pus, resulting in an apical abscess. This result is categorized as acute inflammation. Alternatively, in an attempt to heal from apical periodontitis, the body stimulates the formation of granulation tissue mixed with a chronic inflammatory infiltrate composed predominantly of lymphocytes, plasma cells, and histiocytes, giving rise to periapical granuloma. Entrapped epithelium (the rests of Malassez) may proliferate to form a radicular or apical cyst. Acute exacerbations of the chronic lesions may occur intermittently.

If the surrounding bone marrow becomes involved with the inflammatory reaction through the spread of pyogenic organisms (bacteria that stimulate an inflammatory response), the localized periapical abscess may transform into osteomyelitis. The exact point at which a periapical inflammatory lesion becomes osteomyelitis is not easily determined or defined. The size of the area of inflammation is not as important as the severity of the reaction. However, considering the size of the lesion, periapical inflammatory lesions usually involve only the local bone adjacent to the apex of the tooth, whereas osteomyelitis involves a larger volume of bone. Periapical lesions occasionally may be large, but the epicenter of the lesion remains in the vicinity of the tooth apex. If the periapical lesion extends farther, so that the lesion no longer is centered on the tooth apex, osteomyelitis may be considered as a possible diagnosis. The distinction between periapical inflammation and osteomyelitis can be made if sequestra are detected in x-ray images. Progression from periapical inflammation to osteomyelitis is relatively rare, and other factors play a role in its development, such as a decrease in the host defenses and an increase in the virulence of pathogenic microorganisms.

CLINICAL FEATURES

The symptoms of periapical inflammatory lesions can range across a broad spectrum, from being asymptomatic to an occasional toothache to severe pain with or without facial swelling, fever, and lymphadenopathy. A periapical abscess usually manifests with severe pain, mobility, and sometimes elevation of the involved tooth, swelling, and tenderness to percussion. Palpation of the apical region elicits pain. Spontaneous drainage into the oral cavity through a fistula (parulis) may relieve the acute pain. In rare cases, a dental abscess may manifest with systemic symptoms (e.g., fever, facial swelling, lymphadenopathy) along with pain. The acute lesion may evolve into a chronic one (periapical granuloma or cyst), which may be asymptomatic except for intermittent flare-ups of "toothache" pain, which mark the acute exacerbation of the chronic lesion. Patients often give a history of intermittent pain. The associated tooth may be asymptomatic, or it may be mobile or sensitive to percussion. More often, however, the periapical lesion arises in the chronic form de novo; in this case, it may be asymptomatic. The clinical presentation does not necessarily correlate with the histologic or imaging findings.

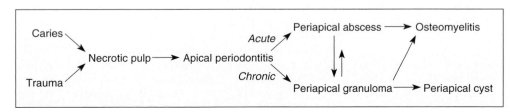

FIGURE 20-1 Interrelationship of possible results of periapical inflammation.

IMAGING FEATURES

The features of periapical inflammatory lesions vary depending on the time course of the lesion. Because very early lesions may not show any changes in the image, diagnosis of these lesions relies solely on the clinical symptoms (Fig. 20-2). More chronic lesions may show lytic (radiolucent) or sclerotic (radiopaque) changes, or both.

Location

In most cases, the epicenter of periapical inflammatory lesions is found at the apex of the involved tooth (Fig. 20-3). The lesion usually starts within the apical portion of the periodontal ligament space. Less often, such lesions are centered about another region of the tooth root; this may occur because of accessory pulpal canals, perforation of the root structure from instrumentation of the pulp canal, and root fracture.

Periphery

In most instances, the periphery of periapical inflammatory lesions is ill defined, showing a gradual transition from the surrounding normal trabecular pattern into the abnormal bone pattern of the lesion (Fig. 20-4; see Fig. 20-3, *C*). Rarely, the periphery may be

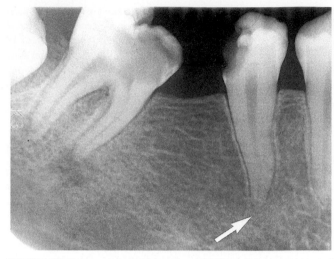

FIGURE 20-2 Very early lesion involving the pulp of the second bicuspid without significant change in the periapical bone *(arrow)*. In contrast, note the loss of the lamina dura and periapical bone at the apex of the mesial root of the second molar. Also note the subtle halo of sclerotic bone reaction around this apical radiolucency.

FIGURE 20-3 Periapical inflammatory lesions associated with a mandibular first molar **(A)** and a maxillary lateral incisor **(B)**. In both cases, the epicenter of bone destruction is located at the apex of the root. Also, note gradual widening of the periodontal membrane space *(arrow)* characteristic of an inflammatory lesion. **C,** Periapical image of sclerosing osteitis related to the first molar shows a gradual transition from thick and numerous trabeculae *(short arrow)* to a normal trabecular pattern *(long arrow)*.

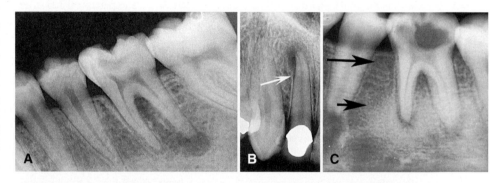

FIGURE 20-4 Examples of a mixture of rarefying and sclerosing osteitis. Note the similarity of the pattern, comprising a radiolucent region at the apex of the tooth surrounded by a radiopaque reaction of sclerotic dense bone.

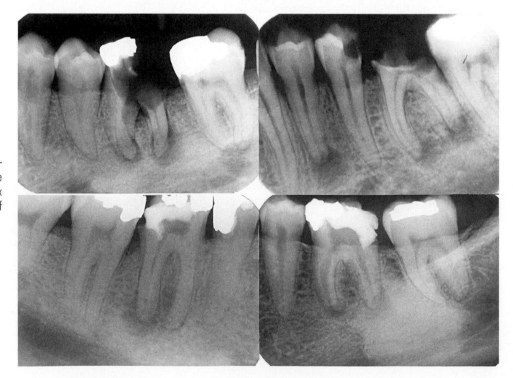

well defined, with a sharp transition zone and an appearance suggesting a cortical boundary.

Internal Structure

Early periapical inflammatory lesions may show no apparent change in the normal bone pattern. The earliest detectable change is loss of bone density, which usually results in widening of the periodontal ligament space at the apex of the tooth and later involves a larger diameter of surrounding bone. At this early stage, no evidence may be seen of a sclerotic bone reaction (see Fig. 20-2). Later in the evolution of the disease, a mixture of sclerosis and rarefaction (loss of bone giving a radiolucent appearance) of normal bone occurs (see Fig. 20-4). The percentage of these two bone reactions varies. When most of the lesion consists of increased bone formation, the term *periapical sclerosing osteitis* is used (Fig. 20-5), and when most of the lesion is undergoing bone resorption, the term *periapical rarefying osteitis* is used (see Fig. 20-3, *A*). The area of greatest bone resorption usually is centered on the apex of the tooth, with the sclerotic pattern located at the periphery. The radiolucent regions may be bereft of any bone structure or may have a faint outline of trabeculae. Close inspection of sclerotic regions reveals thicker than normal trabeculae and sometimes an increase in the number of trabeculae per unit area. In chronic cases, the new bone formation may result in a very dense sclerotic region of bone, obscuring individual trabeculae. Occasionally, the lesion may appear to be composed entirely of sclerotic bone (sclerosing osteitis), but usually some evidence exists of widening of the apical portion of the periodontal membrane space (see Fig. 20-5).

Effects on Surrounding Structures

As mentioned previously, periapical inflammatory lesions may stimulate either the resorption of bone or the manufacture of new bone. The lamina dura around the apex of the tooth usually is lost. The sclerotic reaction of the cancellous bone may be limited to a small region around the tooth apex or may be extensive in some cases. In rare instances in the mandible, the sclerotic reaction may extend to the inferior cortex. In chronic cases, external resorption

of the apical region of the root may occur. If the lesion is long-standing, the pulp canal may appear wider than adjacent teeth. This is a result of the death of odontoblasts and subsequent cessation of the formation of secondary dentin, which occurs naturally with time to diminish the caliber of the pulp canal slowly.

Nearby cortical boundaries may be destroyed, such as a segment of the floor of the maxillary antrum, the floor of the nasal fossa, or the buccal or lingual plates of the alveolar process immediately adjacent to the root apex. These lesions are capable of producing an inflammatory periosteal reaction, most notably in the adjacent floor of the maxillary antrum. This usually results in a thin layer of new bone produced by the inflamed periosteum within the maxillary antrum, sometimes referred to as a "halo shadow" (Fig. 20-6). A regional mucositis may be present within the adjacent segment of the maxillary antrum. Periosteal reaction may also occur on the buccal or lingual surfaces of the alveolar process and in rare cases on the inferior aspect of the mandible.

DIFFERENTIAL DIAGNOSIS

The two types of lesions that most often must be differentiated from periapical inflammatory lesions are periapical osseous dysplasia (POD) and a dense bone island (DBI) (enostosis, osteosclerosis) at the apex of a tooth. In the early radiolucent phase of POD, the imaging characteristics may not reliably differentiate this lesion from a periapical inflammatory lesion (Fig. 20-7). The diagnosis may rely solely on the clinical examination, including a test of tooth vitality. With long-standing periapical inflammatory lesions, the pulp chamber of the involved tooth may be wider than the adjacent teeth. More mature POD lesions may show evidence of a dense, radiopaque structure within the radiolucency, which helps in the differential diagnosis. Also, a common site for POD is associated with the apical region of the mandibular anterior teeth. External root resorption is more common with inflammatory lesions than with POD. When a DBI is centered on the root apex, it may mimic an inflammatory lesion. However, the periodontal ligament space around the apex of the tooth has a normal uniform width (Fig. 20-8). Also, the periphery of a DBI usually is well defined and does not blend gradually with surrounding trabeculae.

Small, radiolucent periapical lesions with a well-defined periphery simulating a cortex may be either periapical granulomas or cysts (radicular cysts). Differentiation may be impossible unless other characteristics of a cyst, such as displacement of adjacent structures and expansion of the outer cortical boundaries of the jaw, are present. Lesions larger than 1 cm in diameter usually are radicular cysts. If the patient has had endodontic treatment or apical surgery, a periapical radiolucency may remain that may look like periapical rarefying osteitis (Fig. 20-9). In either case, the destroyed bone may not be replaced with normal-appearing bone but with dense fibrous scar tissue. The differential diagnosis cannot be made on radiologic grounds alone; thus, the clinical signs and symptoms must take precedence.

In rare cases, metastatic lesions and malignancies such as leukemia may grow in the periapical segment of the periodontal membrane space. Close inspection of the surrounding bone may reveal other small regions of malignant bone destruction.

MANAGEMENT

Standard dental treatment of periapical lesions includes root canal therapy or extraction with the intention of eliminating the necrotic material in the root canal and the source of inflammation. If left untreated, the tooth may become asymptomatic because of

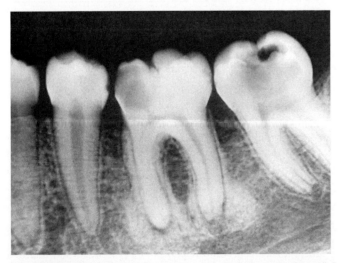

FIGURE 20-5 Periapical sclerosing osteitis associated with the first molar. This is called a sclerosing lesion because most of the lesion is bone formation, resulting in a very radiopaque density. Note, however, the small region of bone loss next to the root apex and the widening of the periodontal membrane space.

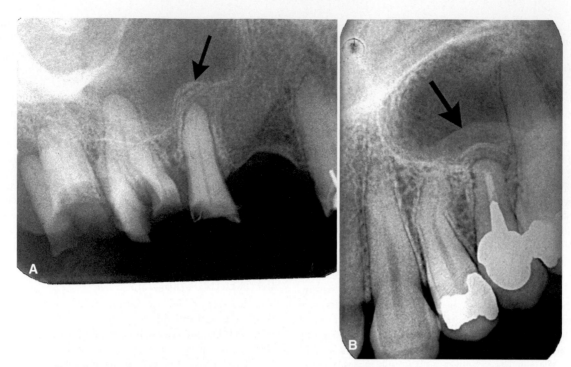

FIGURE 20-6 Periostitis resulting in bone formation emanating from the floor of the maxillary antrum that arises from apical inflammatory lesions. **A,** Laminated type of periosteal bone formation *(arrow)*. **B,** Periostitis and mucositis. Mucositis is characterized by a slight radiopaque band *(arrow)* next to periosteal bone formation.

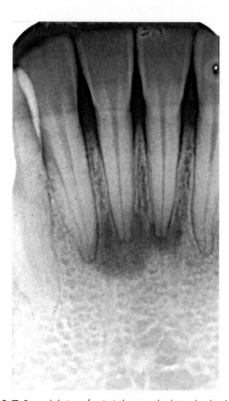

FIGURE 20-7 Two early lesions of periapical osseous dysplasia related to the apical region of the mandibular central incisors; note the similarity to apical rarefying osteitis.

drainage established through the carious lesion or a parulis. However, the possibility always exists that the lesion will spread to involve a larger area of bone, resulting in osteomyelitis, or into the surrounding soft tissue, which may result in a space infection or cellulitis.

Post–Endodontic Treatment Complications

Recurrence or persistent inflammatory lesions after endodontic treatment can occur. Possible etiologies include inadequate root canal filling, instrumentation perforation of the outer root surface, unusual morphology of the root canal, unusual accessory canal, or root fracture. The application of high-resolution, small field-of-view cone-beam computed tomographic (CBCT) images has been very useful in the determination of the etiology of these complications (Fig. 20-10).

OSTEOMYELITIS

DISEASE MECHANISM

Osteomyelitis is an inflammation of bone. The inflammatory process may spread through the bone to involve the marrow, cortex, cancellous portion, and periosteum. In the jaws, pyogenic organisms that reach the bone marrow from abscessed teeth or postsurgical infection usually cause osteomyelitis. However, in some instances, no source of infection can be identified, and hematogenous spread is presumed to be the origin. In some patients, no infectious organisms can be identified, possibly because of previous antibiotic therapy or inadequate methods of bacterial isolation. Bacterial colonies also may be present in small, isolated pockets of bone that may be missed during sampling.

In patients with osteomyelitis, the bacteria and their products stimulate an inflammatory reaction in bone, causing resorption of the endosteal surface of the cortical bone. This resorption may progress through the cortical bone to the outer periosteum. In young patients, in whom the periosteum is more loosely attached to the outer cortex of bone than it is in adults, the periosteum is lifted up by inflammatory exudate, and new bone is laid down. This periosteal reaction is a characteristic, but not pathognomonic, feature of osteomyelitis. The hallmark of osteomyelitis is the

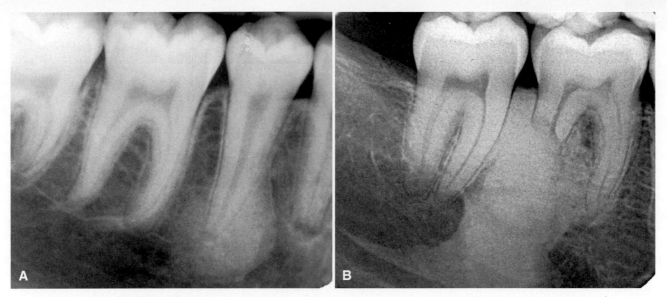

FIGURE 20-8 DBI (enostosis) in periapical positions. **A,** DBI around the apex of a second bicuspid. The periodontal membrane space is uniform in width. **B,** DBI associated with apical root resorption of a vital tooth. The most common site of DBI and root resorption is the mesial or distal root of mandibular first molars.

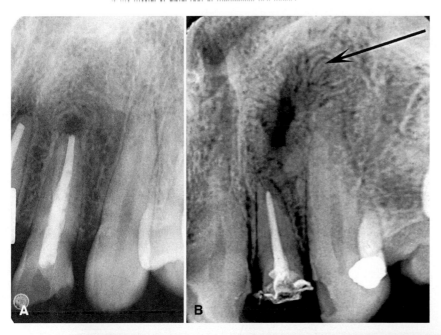

FIGURE 20-9 **A,** Radiolucent apical scar after successful end-odontic treatment. **B,** Healing periapical inflammatory lesion *(arrow)* associated with the apical region of a maxillary lateral incisor. Note the radiating, spokelike pattern of new bone forming from the periphery of the lesion.

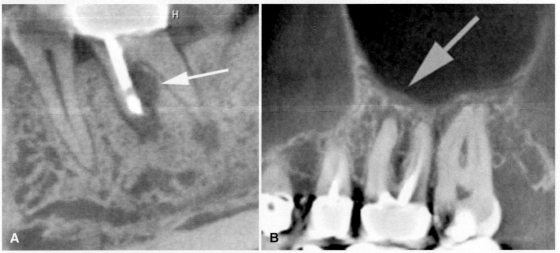

FIGURE 20-10 **A,** Sagittal cone-beam CT image showing perforation of the distal surface of the mesial root of the first mandibular molar. Note the bone resorption extending into the furcation region *(arrow)* and the surrounding sclerotic bone reaction. **B,** Sagittal cone-beam CT image revealing an area of periapical rarefying osteitis related to the mesial root of the left maxillary first molar and a secondary mucositis within the adjacent sinus *(arrow)* secondary to a missed canal that was not filled during endodontic therapy.

development of sequestra. A sequestrum is a segment of bone that has become necrotic because of ischemic injury caused by the inflammatory process.

Numerous forms of osteomyelitis have been described. For the sake of simplicity, they are grouped into two major phases here, acute and chronic, with the recognition that these represent two ends of a continuum without a definite separating boundary in the process of bone inflammation. Other forms of osteomyelitis have been described as separate and distinct clinicopathologic entities with unique imaging features. These are Garré's osteomyelitis and diffuse sclerosing osteomyelitis. We consider them as part of the same continuum. Garré's osteomyelitis is an exuberant periosteal response to inflammation. Diffuse sclerosing osteomyelitis is a chronic form of osteomyelitis with a pronounced sclerotic response. All these variations of osteomyelitis have the same underlying process of the bone's response to inflammation. The features expressed by each subtype represent only variations in the type and degree of bone reaction.

Osteomyelitis may resolve spontaneously or with appropriate antibiotic intervention. However, if the condition is not treated or is treated inadequately, the infection may persist and continue to spread and become chronic in about 20% of patients. Some chronic systemic diseases, immunosuppressive states, and disorders of decreased vascularity may predispose an individual to the development of osteomyelitis. For example, osteopetrosis, sickle cell anemia, and acquired immunodeficiency syndrome (AIDS) have been documented as underlying factors in the development of osteomyelitis.

ACUTE PHASE

Synonyms

Acute suppurative osteomyelitis, pyogenic osteomyelitis, subacute suppurative osteomyelitis, Garré's osteomyelitis, proliferative periostitis, and periostitis ossificans are synonyms for the acute phase of osteomyelitis.

Disease Mechanism

The acute phase of osteomyelitis is caused by infection that has spread to the bone marrow. With this condition, the medullary spaces of the bone contain an inflammatory infiltrate consisting predominantly of neutrophils and, to a lesser extent, mononuclear cells. In the jaws, the most common source of infection is a periapical lesion from a nonvital tooth. Infection also can occur as a result of trauma or hematogenous spread.

The changes described by Garré may accompany acute osteomyelitis. It is thought that the inflammatory exudate spreads subperiosteally, elevating the periosteum and stimulating formation of new bone. This condition is more common in younger individuals because the periosteum is loosely attached to the bone surface in younger people and has greater osteogenic potential.

Clinical Features

The acute phase of osteomyelitis can affect people of all ages, and it has a strong male predilection. It is much more common in the mandible than in the maxilla, possibly because of the poorer vascular supply to the mandible. The typical signs and symptoms of acute osteomyelitis are rapid onset, pain, swelling of the adjacent soft tissues, fever, lymphadenopathy, and leukocytosis. The associated teeth may be mobile and sensitive to percussion. Purulent drainage also may be present. Paresthesia of the lower lip in the third division of the fifth cranial nerve distribution may occur.

Imaging Examination

In addition to a complete examination with plain images (panoramic, intraoral periapical, and occlusal images), the following additional modalities may be used. A two-phase nuclear medicine study composed of a technetium bone scan followed by a gallium citrate scan may help to confirm the diagnosis. With inflammatory lesions, a positive result on the technetium scan indicates increased bone metabolic activity, and a positive result on the gallium scan in the same location indicates an inflammatory cell infiltrate. Either Multidetector computed tomography (MDCT) or CBCT imaging is the imaging method of choice. CT imaging reveals more bone surface for detecting periosteal new bone and is the best imaging method for detecting sequestra (Fig. 20-11). Magnetic resonance imaging (MRI) with T2-weighted images to display abnormal bone marrow edema has also been used.

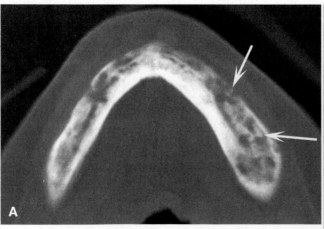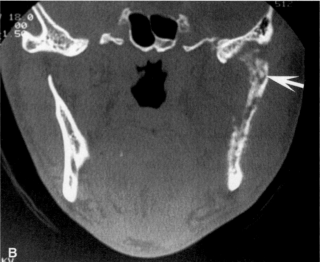

FIGURE 20-11   CT images of multiple sequestra. **A,** Axial image (bone window) revealing multiple sequestra *(arrows)*. **B,** Coronal image (bone window) demonstrating a sequestrum *(arrow)* in two different cases of chronic osteomyelitis.

Imaging Features

Very early in the disease, no changes may be identifiable. The bone may be filled with inflammatory exudate and inflammatory cells and may show no change in the diagnostic image.

Location.   The most common location is the posterior body of the mandible. The maxilla is a rare site.

Periphery.   Acute osteomyelitis most often presents an ill-defined periphery with a gradual transition to normal trabeculae.

Internal Structure.   The first evidence of the acute form of osteomyelitis is a slight decrease in the density of the involved bone, with a loss of sharpness of the existing trabeculae. The bone resorption becomes more profound in time, resulting in an area of radiolucency in one focal area or in scattered regions throughout the involved bone (Fig. 20-12). Later, the appearance of sclerotic

regions becomes apparent. Sequestra may be present but usually are more apparent and numerous in chronic forms (Fig. 20-13). Sequestra can be identified by closely inspecting a region of bone resorption (radiolucency) for an island of bone. This island of nonvital bone may vary in size from a small dot (smaller sequestra usually are seen in young patients) to larger segments of radiopaque bone.

Effects on Surrounding Structures.   Acute osteomyelitis can stimulate either bone resorption or bone formation. Portions of cortical bone may be resorbed. An inflammatory exudate can lift the periosteum and stimulate bone formation. In the diagnostic image, this appears as a thin, faint, radiopaque line adjacent to and almost parallel or slightly convex to the surface of the bone. A radiolucent band separates this periosteal new bone from the bone surface (Fig. 20-14). As the lesion develops into a more chronic phase, cyclic and periodic acute exacerbations may produce more inflammatory exudate, which lifts the periosteum even further from the bone

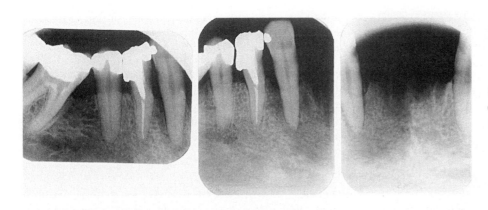

FIGURE 20-12 Acute osteomyelitis involving the body of the right mandible, with initial blurring of bony trabeculae. *(Courtesy Lars Hollender, DDS, PhD, Seattle, WA.)*

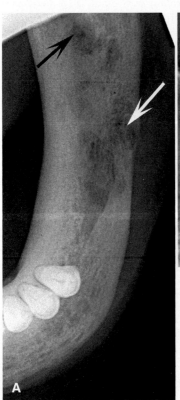

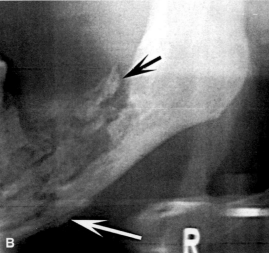

FIGURE 20-13 Examples of sequestra. **A,** Occlusal film demonstrates small sequestra as radiopaque islands of bone in radiolucent regions in the chronic phase of osteomyelitis *(arrows)*. **B,** Panoramic film reveals large sequestra *(black arrow)* and a periosteal reaction at the inferior border of the mandible in a case of chronic osteomyelitis *(white arrow)*.

surface and stimulates the periosteum to form a second layer of bone. This layer of bone is detected in the image as a second radiopaque line almost parallel to the first and separated from it by a radiolucent band. This process may continue and may result in several lines (an onion-skin appearance), and eventually a massive amount of new bone may be formed. This condition is referred to as proliferative periostitis and is seen more often in children (Fig. 20-15). The effects on the teeth and lamina dura may be the same as the effects described for periapical inflammatory lesions.

Differential Diagnosis

The differential diagnosis of the acute phase of osteomyelitis may include fibrous dysplasia, especially in children. Aside from the clinical signs of acute infection, the most useful radiographic characteristic to distinguish osteomyelitis from fibrous dysplasia is the way the enlargement of the bone occurs. The new bone that

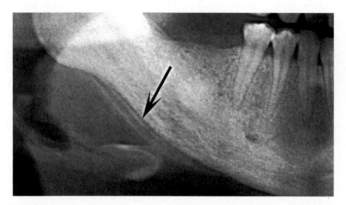

FIGURE 20-14 Osteomyelitis of the mandible with a periosteal reaction located at the inferior cortex. Note the radiolucent line *(arrow)* between the inferior cortex of the mandible and the first layer of periosteal new bone. A second radiolucent line separates the second layer of new bone from the first layer.

enlarges the jaws in osteomyelitis is laid down by the periosteum and is on the outside of the outer cortical plate. In fibrous dysplasia, the new bone is manufactured on the inside of the mandible; the outer cortex, which may be thinned, is on the outside and contains the lesion. This point of differentiation is important because the histologic appearance of a biopsy specimen of new periosteal bone in osteomyelitis may be similar to that of fibrous dysplasia, and the condition may be reported as such.

Malignant neoplasia (e.g., osteosarcoma, squamous cell carcinoma) that invades the mandible at times may be difficult to differentiate from the acute phase of osteomyelitis, especially if the malignancy has been secondarily infected via an oral ulcer; this may result in a mixture of inflammatory and malignant radiographic characteristics. If part of the inflammatory periosteal bone has been destroyed, the possibility of a malignant neoplasm should be considered. The differential diagnosis may include other lesions that can cause bone destruction and may stimulate a periosteal reaction that is similar to that seen in inflammatory lesions. Langerhans' cell histiocytosis causes lytic ill-defined bone destruction and often results in the formation of periosteal reactive new bone. This lesion rarely stimulates a sclerotic bone reaction such as that seen in osteomyelitis. Leukemia and lymphoma may stimulate a similar periosteal reaction.

Management

As with all inflammatory lesions of the jaws, removal of the source of inflammation is the primary goal of therapy. Removal of a tooth or root canal therapy may be indicated. Antimicrobial treatment is the mainstay of treatment of acute osteomyelitis, along with surgical incision and drainage.

CHRONIC PHASE

Synonyms

Chronic diffuse sclerosing osteomyelitis, chronic nonsuppurative osteomyelitis, chronic osteomyelitis with proliferative periostitis, and Garré's chronic nonsuppurative sclerosing osteitis are synonyms for the chronic phase of osteomyelitis.

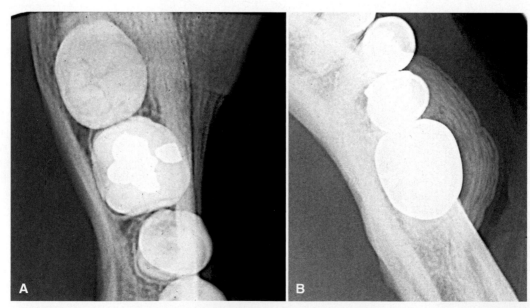

FIGURE 20-15 **A** and **B,** Proliferative periostitis resulting from inflammatory lesions. Note the multiple layers of new bone on the buccal aspect of the mandible, resulting in an onion-skin appearance.

Disease Mechanism

The chronic phase of osteomyelitis may be a sequela of inadequately treated acute osteomyelitis, or it may arise de novo. Diffuse sclerosing osteomyelitis refers to chronic osteomyelitis in which the balance in bone metabolism is tipped toward increased bone formation, subsequently producing a sclerotic bone pattern in the image. The symptoms of the chronic form generally are less severe and have a longer history than the symptoms of the acute form. They include intermittent, recurrent episodes of swelling, pain, fever, and lymphadenopathy. As with the acute form, paresthesia and drainage with sinus formation also may occur. In some cases, pain may be limited to the advancing front of the osteomyelitis, or the patient may have little or no pain. Histologically, a chronic inflammatory infiltrate may be seen within the medullary spaces of bone; however, this may be quite sparse, with only fibrosis of the marrow seen with scattered regions of inflammation. At this stage of the disease, the offending etiologic agent rarely is found because culture results usually are negative. If left untreated, osteomyelitis can spread and involve both sides of the mandible. Further spread into the temporomandibular joint may cause septic arthritis. Ear infections and infection of the mastoid air cells also may develop.

Chronic osteomyelitis as illustrated here is similar to the bone lesions described in chronic recurrent multifocal osteomyelitis (CRMO) and osteomyelitis of the SAPHO syndrome (synovitis [inflammatory arthritis], acne [pustulosa], pustulosis [psoriasis, palmoplantar pustulosis], hyperostosis [acquired], and osteitis [osteomyelitis]) with respect to the imaging findings, lack of microbiologic findings, and clinical features such as intermittent recurrent pain and swelling of the involved bone. CRMO is a condition that often occurs symmetrically in the long bones in children. It is characterized by pain of the affected bone with or without swelling and has been described as a nonpurulent osteomyelitis with negative microbiologic cultures. The imaging features are identical to chronic osteomyelitis as described here. Treatment has consisted of systemic steroids, nonsteroidal antiinflammatory drugs (NSAIDs), and bisphosphonates therapy because antibiotic and surgical therapy have not been effective treatment. Chronic osteomyelitis of the jaw in children not having a clear etiology may be a unifocal variant of CRMO.

The imaging features of the bone lesions of SAPHO syndrome are similar, if not identical, to the features of chronic osteomyelitis but may be more extensive (see Fig. 20-18). These lesions are refractory to antibiotic therapy, responding to antiinflammatory agents such as steroids and NSAIDs. Some experts consider both CRMO and SAPHO syndrome to be chronic nonbacterial osteomyelitis syndromes with CRMO being at the severe end of the spectrum. CRMO occurs in a younger age group, and SAPHO syndrome occurs in adults. The imaging features of the jaw lesions of chronic osteomyelitis can be identical to the features of these two conditions.

Imaging Examination

If chronic osteomyelitis is suspected from the clinical examination, in addition to a complete series of plain films, either CBCT or MDCT imaging is the imaging method of choice. CT imaging is important because of its ability to demonstrate sequestra (see Fig. 20-11) and periosteal new bone formation, and it allows accurate staging of the disease. This staging is important for future assessment of healing. MRI is not as useful because of the lack of bone marrow edema in the chronic phase; however, it may be useful during acute exacerbation of the disease. Scintigraphy using bone scans, gallium, or labeled white blood cell scans is not particularly useful for differential diagnosis. Bone scans indicate increased bone formation, which is nonspecific, and often gallium scans (which highlight inflammatory cells) are not positive because of a very low population of inflammatory cells. The amount of bone activity assessed with bone scans with single photon emission computed tomography (SPECT) has been used to monitor healing (see Fig. 14-23). There are also reports of the use of positron emission tomography to detect a high cellular metabolic rate in tissues, but this type of imaging is nonspecific.

Imaging Features

Location. As in the acute phase of osteomyelitis, the most common site is the posterior mandible.

Periphery. The periphery may be better defined than in the acute phase, but it is still difficult to determine the exact extent of chronic osteomyelitis. Usually a gradual transition is seen between the normal surrounding trabecular pattern and the dense granular pattern characteristic of this disease. When the disease is active and is spreading through bone, the periphery may be more radiolucent and have poorly defined borders.

Internal Structure. The internal structure comprises regions of greater and lesser radiopacity compared with surrounding normal bone. Most of the lesion usually is composed of the more radiopaque or sclerotic bone pattern (Fig. 20-16). In older, more chronic lesions, the internal bone density can be exceedingly radiopaque and equivalent to cortical bone. In these cases, no obvious regions of radiolucency may be seen. In other cases, small regions of radiolucency may be scattered throughout the radiopaque bone. A close inspection of the radiolucent regions may reveal an island of bone or sequestrum within the center (Fig. 20-17). Often the sequestrum appears more radiopaque than the surrounding bone. Detection may require illumination of the radiolucent regions of the film with an intense light source. CT is superior for revealing the internal structure and sequestra, especially in cases with very dense sclerotic bone. The bone pattern usually is very granular, obscuring individual bone trabeculae. A similar appearance can be seen in cases of SAPHO syndrome (Fig. 20-18).

Effects on Surrounding Structures. Chronic osteomyelitis often stimulates the formation of periosteal new bone, which is seen radiographically as a single radiopaque line or a series of radiopaque lines (similar to onion skin) parallel to the surface of the cortical bone. Over time, the radiolucent strip that separates this new bone from the outer cortical bone surface may be filled in with granular sclerotic bone. When this occurs, it may be impossible to identify the original cortex, which makes it difficult to determine whether the new bone is derived from the periosteum. After a considerable amount of time, the outer contour of the mandible also may be altered, assuming an abnormal shape, and the girth of the mandible may be much larger than on the unaffected side. The roots of teeth may undergo external resorption, and the lamina dura may become less apparent as it blends with the surrounding granular sclerotic bone. If a tooth is nonvital, the periodontal ligament space usually is enlarged in the apical region. In patients with extensive chronic osteomyelitis, the disease may slowly spread to the mandibular condyle and into the joint, resulting in a septic arthritis. Further spread may involve the inner ear and mastoid air cells. Chronic lesions may develop a draining

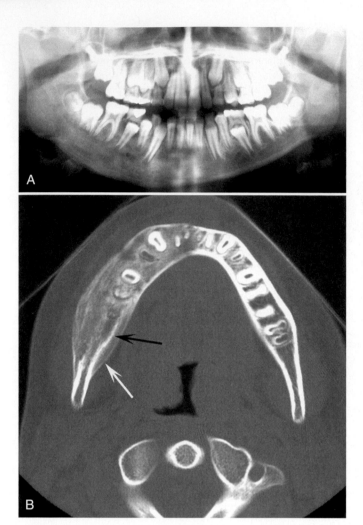

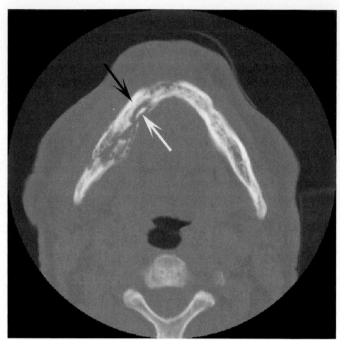

FIGURE 20-17 Axial CT image using bone window of chronic osteomyelitis with a mixture of increased bone density *(black arrow)*, areas of radiolucency or low attenuation, and presence of sequestra *(white arrow)*.

FIGURE 20-16 Chronic osteomyelitis. **A,** Panoramic film demonstrates chronic osteomyelitis of the right mandible; note the increase in density and size of the right mandible compared with the left side. **B,** Axial CT image using bone window of the mandible of the same case. Note the increase in bone density, increase in width of the mandible, new periosteal bone formation *(white arrow)*, and evidence of the original cortex *(black arrow)*.

fistula, which may appear as a well-defined break in the outer cortex or in the periosteal new bone (Fig. 20-19).

Differential Diagnosis

Very sclerotic, radiopaque chronic lesions of osteomyelitis may be difficult to differentiate from fibrous dysplasia, Paget's disease of bone, and osteosarcoma. In children, osteomyelitis with a proliferative periosteal response may be misinterpreted as fibrous dysplasia (see "Differential Diagnosis" under the Acute Phase section of Osteomyelitis). Differentiation of the chronic form of osteomyelitis may be even more difficult if considerable remodeling and loss of a distinct original cortex have occurred. In these cases, inspection of the bone surface at the most peripheral part of the lesion may reveal subtle evidence of periosteal new bone formation. The presence of sequestra indicates osteomyelitis. Paget's disease affects the entire mandible, which is rare in osteomyelitis. Periosteal new bone formation and sequestra are not seen in Paget's disease. Dense, granular bone may be seen in some forms of osteosarcoma, but usually evidence of bone destruction is found. A characteristic spiculated (sunray-like) periosteal response also may be seen. As mentioned in the section on acute osteomyelitis, other entities, such as Langerhans' cell histiocytosis, leukemia, and

lymphoma, may stimulate a similar periosteal response, but these usually produce evidence of bone destruction characteristic of malignant tumors. The imaging method of choice for aiding in the differential diagnosis is either CBCT or MDCT imaging because of its ability to reveal sequestra and periosteal new bone.

Management

Chronic osteomyelitis tends to be more difficult to eradicate than the acute form. In cases involving an extreme osteoblastic response (very sclerotic mandible), the subsequent lack of an adequate blood supply may work against healing. Hyperbaric oxygen therapy and creative modes of long-term antibiotic delivery have been used with limited success. Surgical intervention, which may include sequestrectomy, decortication, or resection, often is necessary. The probability of successful treatment, especially when using long-term antibiotic therapy with decortication, is greater in the first 2 decades of life. If cultures are negative, antibiotic therapy is not effective. It may be that the inflammatory response has become the main disease process, and antiinflammatory agents such as steroids and NSAIDs are more effective. More recently, the use of bisphosphonate therapy has provided some therapeutic success.

RADIATION-INDUCED CHANGES TO THE JAWS
DISEASE MECHANISM

Therapeutic radiation, usually given for treatment of a malignancy of the head and neck region, damages the cellular elements of bone tissue by immediate or delayed cell death, cellular injury with recovery, arrested cellular division, or abnormal repair. The maturity and type of bone and the dose of radiation are factors that affect how the bone responds to this injury. When immature bone is irradiated, growth retardation occurs; the amount is related to the radiation dose and the stage of bone growth—the earlier the stage, the greater the effect. Radiation damage to mature bone is

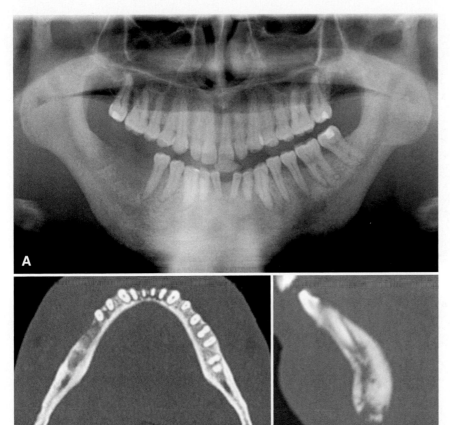

FIGURE 20-18 Case of SAPHO syndrome in which both the wrist and the mandible were involved. **A,** Panoramic image showing diffuse sclerotic bone reaction, bone resorption of the inferior aspect of the body of the mandible, and widening of the periodontal ligament spaces around most teeth. **B,** Axial CT image showing the mostly sclerotic bone reaction with some regions of bone resorption. **C,** Sagittal CT image of the anterior body of the mandible showing resorption of the inferior cortex and a sequestrum *(arrow).*

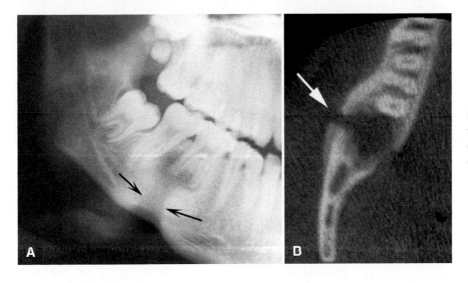

FIGURE 20-19 **A,** Fistulous tract extending inferiorly from the apex of the first molar through the inferior cortex of the mandible *(arrows).* **B,** Axial cone-beam CT image of a fistulous tract extending through the buccal cortical plate *(arrow).*

also likely dose dependent and can affect the osteoblasts resulting in a decrease in matrix formation and stimulation of osteoclastic bone resorption. Alternatively, in some regions, osteoblasts are stimulated to form bone, possibly as an attempt at healing. Also the radiation can damage the fine blood vessels, and this can result in bone that is hypocellular and hypovascular. The lack of sufficient vascularity results in a hypoxic environment in which adequate healing of bone is compromised. Differentiation should be made between postradiation changes and osteoradionecrosis. By definition, osteoradionecrosis signifies bone necrosis or death. Therapeutic radiation exposure can cause bone damage and

changes without necrosis, although it is possible that such changes may make the bone more susceptible to necrosis, especially after surgical intervention.

IMAGING FEATURES

The regions most frequently affected by radiation therapy are the posterior mandible followed by the posterior maxilla. Because of the proximity of these parts of the jaws to nearby malignant tumors, they receive a relatively large radiation exposure. After radiation therapy, no visible changes may be apparent in the images, or the changes observed are similar to changes seen in

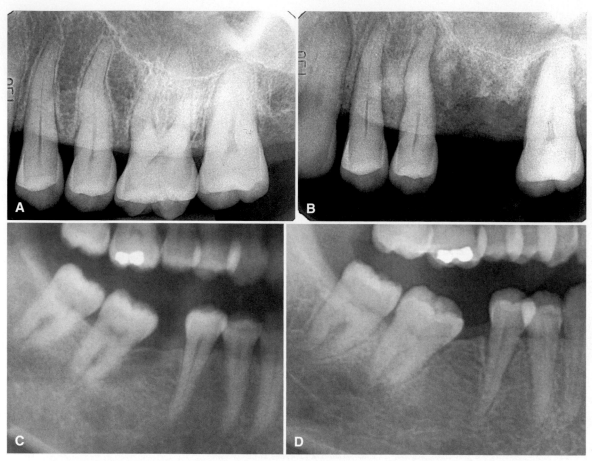

FIGURE 20-20 Changes in the maxilla after therapeutic radiation exposure. Periapical films were taken before radiotherapy **(A)** and within 6 months of receiving the radiation **(B)**. Note the combination of bone sclerosis and profound bone destruction around the teeth and alveolar crest and widening of the periodontal membrane space. In another case, cropped panoramic image **(C)** taken before radiation and image **(D)** taken after radiation demonstrating widening of the periodontal membrane spaces.

inflammatory diseases of bone. The ill-defined periphery and the irregular and ill-defined regions of bone resorption and sclerosis of the internal structure are the same as in osteomyelitis (see previous description).

However, more characteristic changes can occur after therapeutic radiation exposure. In the alveolar process of the jaws, the most frequently occurring change is an irregular widening of the whole periodontal ligament space around the involved teeth (Fig. 20-20). A more recent study showed that greater than 50% of patients who have received therapeutic radiation therapy to the jaws exhibit widening of the periodontal ligament space (PDL). Most cases are detected by 2 years after radiation, and the widening of the PDL was more significant with doses to the mandible greater than 45 Gy. Other changes included resorption of the alveolar crest, similar to periodontal disease bone loss (see Fig. 20-20, *B*).

There may be prominent bone resorption in nonalveolar regions of the jaws exposed to therapeutic radiation. For example, in the maxilla, parts of the osseous structure, such as cortical borders of the sinus, simply disappear (Fig. 20-21). An early change seen in the outer cortical plate of the mandible is a sharply defined region of bone resorption (Fig. 20-22).

DIFFERENTIAL DIAGNOSIS

Radiation-induced widening of the periodontal ligament space must be distinguished from periapical inflammatory lesions of the teeth to avoid unnecessary endodontic or surgical therapy. In periapical inflammatory disease, the widest part of the periodontal ligament space is at the apex, and in periodontal disease, it is at the alveolar crest; the irregular widening of the entire periodontal ligament space seen after radiation exposure has no specific epicenter. Vitality testing and thorough clinical examination are important to avoid unnecessary treatment. Radiation-induced periodontal bone like loss is difficult to differentiate from conventional periodontal disease. The regions of bone sclerosis and resorption may be very similar to inflammatory diseases of the jaws.

OSTEORADIONECROSIS

DISEASE MECHANISM

Radiation-induced damage to bone may result in bone death; this is likely related to doses greater than 50 Gy. Histologically, bone necrosis is defined by the absence of osteocytes within the lacunae. Bone necrosis occurs more commonly in the mandible than the maxilla, which may be related to the vascular supply of the mandible. Often the mucosal covering is lost, and the necrotic bone becomes exposed to the oral environment. It is likely that bone with radiation-induced changes is susceptible to becoming necrotic from infection, dental extraction, or denture trauma. The necrotic bone is also susceptible to pathologic fractures. Secondary infection is common, further exacerbating the inflammatory reaction.

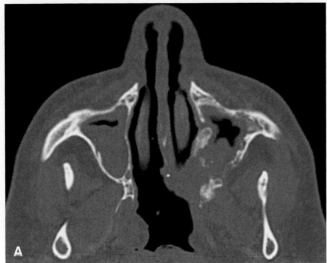

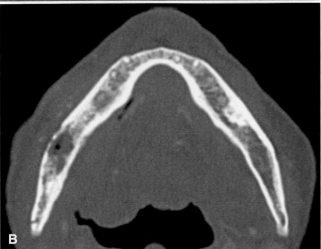

FIGURE 20-21 Postradiation changes. **A,** Axial CT image. Note the resorption of the posterior maxilla. **B,** Axial CT image showing a mixture of sclerosis and resorption in the mandible.

CLINICAL FEATURES

Osteoradionecrosis is characterized by the presence of exposed bone for at least 3 months occurring at any time after the delivery of radiation therapy (Fig. 20-23). This exposed bone may completely sequestrate, often leading to the exposure of more bone. The posterior mandible is affected more often than the anterior portion likely because it is frequently in the direct field of the radiation treatment owing to the proximity of primary tumors and metastatic lesions in lymph nodes being treated. Pathologic fracture also may occur. Pain may or may not be present. Intense pain may occur, with intermittent swelling and drainage extraorally. However, many patients feel no pain with bone exposure.

RADIOLOGIC EXAMINATION

The prescription of diagnostic imaging would be the same as used for chronic phase osteomyelitis, with CT imaging being the imaging modality of choice.

IMAGING FEATURES

Changes to the appearance of bone are the same as seen with osteomyelitis and radiation-induced changes (see preceding descriptions) and often with prominent bone sclerosis. However, the radiologic identification of osteoradionecrosis relies on the identification of dead bone in the form of sequestra. Bone sequestra are seen more commonly in the mandible, and often the sequestra seen are segments of detached cortical bone (Fig. 20-24). In contrast to osteomyelitis, there is no periosteal bone reaction in most cases. The presence of a pathologic fracture (Fig. 20-25) is suggestive of osteoradionecrosis. The presence of osteoradionecrosis cannot always be diagnosed from the diagnostic image, and often clinically obvious signs of exposed necrotic bone may not have significant changes in the panoramic image. In these cases, CT imaging is required.

DIFFERENTIAL DIAGNOSIS

Bone resorption, stimulated by high levels of irradiation, may simulate bone destruction from a malignant neoplasm, especially

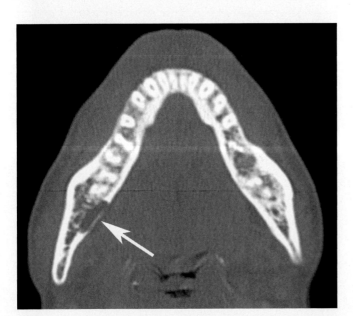

FIGURE 20-22 Axial CT image showing a well-defined region of cortical bone resorption *(arrow)*, an early change in therapeutic radiation exposure.

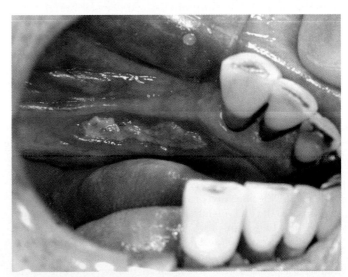

FIGURE 20-23 Clinically exposed necrotic bone in the lingual cortical region of the mandibular premolar region of the alveolar process.

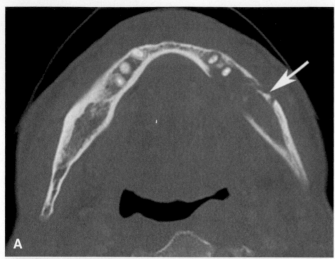

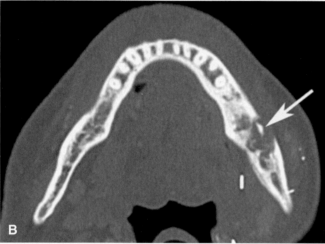

FIGURE 20-24 Examples of osteoradionecrosis. **A,** Axial CT image showing extensive bone resorption and the presence of a sequestrum *(arrow).* **B,** Axial CT image showing more prominent sclerotic bone reaction and sequestrum *(arrow).* In both examples, the sequestra represent detached segments of the former outer cortical bone.

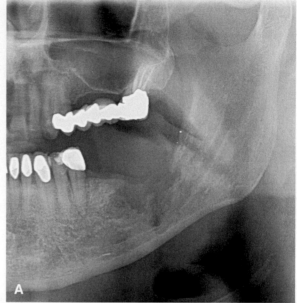

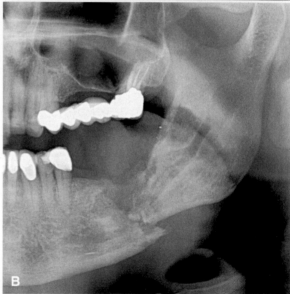

FIGURE 20-25 **A,** Cropped panoramic image of a patient with bone resorption secondary to therapeutic radiation exposure. **B,** Development of a pathologic fracture in the same patient after 3 months.

in the maxilla. For this reason, the detection of a recurrence of the malignant neoplasm (usually squamous cell carcinoma) in the presence of osteoradionecrosis may be very difficult. If recurrence is suspected, CT and MRI may be used to detect an associated soft tissue mass. Differentiation from other sclerotic lesions, as in chronic osteomyelitis, is less difficult because of the history of radiation therapy.

MANAGEMENT

Treatment of osteoradionecrosis at the present time is unsatisfactory. Decortication with sequestrectomy and hyperbaric oxygen with antibiotics have been used with limited success because of poor healing after surgery. Conservative approaches with the aim to maintain the integrity of the lower border of the mandible, keeping the site free of infection and the patient free of pain, may in the long-term prove more successful. The incidence of osteoradionecrosis has declined because of the use of intensity modulated radiotherapy and preventive therapy. Removal of teeth that have significant periodontal disease or have a poor prognosis before radiation treatment and excellent oral and denture hygiene are the mainstays of preventive treatment.

BISPHOSPHONATE-RELATED OSTEONECROSIS OF THE JAWS

DISEASE MECHANISM

Bisphosphonates are potent synthetic analogs of pyrophosphates that act to inhibit osteoclasts and reduce bone metabolism. These drugs have become important in the treatment of the bone lesions of multiple myeloma, hypercalcemia of malignancy, metastatic bone tumors, and osteoporosis. A complication of intraoral exposure of necrotic bone has been described more recently in patients receiving these medications. The bone exposure occurs more commonly in patients receiving the more potent aminobisphosphonates intravenously and after an invasive dental surgical procedure, such as extraction, periodontal or endodontic surgery, or implant placement. Bisphosphonate-related osteonecrosis has now been well-documented, although the pathogenesis remains unclear.

CLINICAL FEATURES

Clinically, patients typically have an area of exposed bone after an invasive dental surgical procedure. However, cases related to denture trauma and spontaneous cases have occurred (Fig. 20-26). Ulceration of palatal tori resulting in bone exposure is most likely the result of trauma. The most common areas affected are the posterior mandible (60%) and the maxilla (40%), or both (9%) may be affected. The incidence of bone exposure is difficult to determine, but more recent studies suggest that approximately 3% of patients receiving these drugs have exposed bone. The areas may be asymptomatic, or patients may present with pain and swelling.

IMAGING FEATURES

A spectrum of radiographic findings may or may not correlate well with the clinical symptoms. More often than not, there are no specific imaging findings with the clinically exposed bone. In other cases, the changes seen are indistinguishable from osteoradionecrosis or chronic osteomyelitis with the presence of sequestra (Fig. 20-27). Other reported findings include an increase in bone

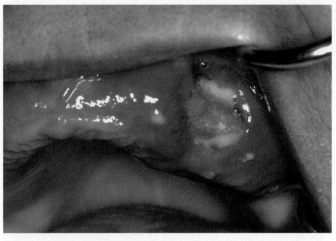

FIGURE 20-26 Bisphosphonate-related exposed necrotic bone involving the buccal aspect of a maxillary edentulous ridge in the premolar region.

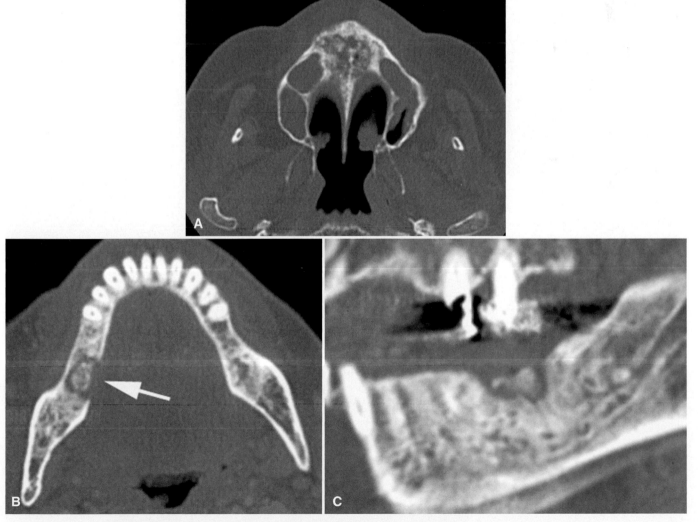

FIGURE 20-27 **A,** Axial CT image of a patient with bisphosphonate-related osteonecrosis. Note several sequestra in the anterior palate. Axial **(B)** and sagittal **(C)** CT images of oral bisphosphonate-related necrosis. *Arrow* **(B)** points to large sequestrum.

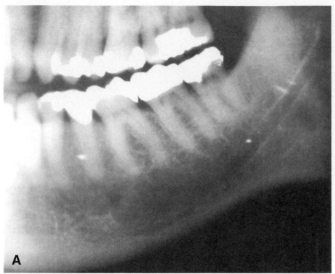

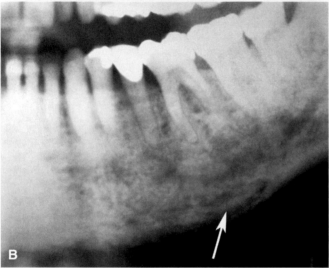

FIGURE 20-28 Two cropped panoramic images **(A** and **B)** of the same patient taken 1 year apart demonstrate a developing sclerotic bone pattern with a sequestra (arrow) related to bisphosphonate therapy.

sclerosis (Fig. 20-28), widening of the periodontal membrane space, and thickening of the lamina dura (Fig. 20-29).

MANAGEMENT

Treatment of bisphosphonate-related bone exposure is unsatisfactory. Surgical intervention and hyperbaric oxygen therapy have not been consistently successful. The mainstay of therapy is preventive in nature. Patients who are scheduled to be administered the potent aminobisphosphonates intravenously should have a dental examination to remove potential and real sources of infection to obviate the need for invasive dental procedures in the future. The situation is complicated further by the fact that the half-life of these drugs in bone can be very long (estimated at approximately 12 years). Once bone is exposed, treatment is aimed at controlling the symptoms of pain and infection with antibiotic mouth rinses and systemic antibiotic therapy.

DIAGNOSTIC IMAGING OF SOFT TISSUE INFECTIONS

Diagnostic imaging may be used to confirm the presence and extent of soft tissue infections. MRI and CT imaging may be used to differentiate soft tissue neoplasia from inflammatory lesions. T2 or T1 MRI can be used with gadolinium and fat suppression to detect the presence of soft tissue edema. CT imaging usually is used with intravenous contrast medium. The CT image characteristics that suggest the presence of soft tissue inflammation include abnormal fascial planes, thickening of the overlying skin and adjacent muscles, streaking of the fat planes, and abnormal collections of gas in the soft tissue (Fig. 20-30). Over time, the contrast between soft tissue planes may disappear, and the presence of an abscess may become evident as a well-defined region of low density surrounded by a wide border of contrast-enhanced (more radiopaque) tissue. Lymphadenopathy resulting from infections such as tuberculosis of the head and neck may be visualized on MR and CT images (Fig. 20-31).

FIGURE 20-29 Two cropped panoramic images **(A** and **B)** of the same patient taken 7 years apart reveal thickening of the lamina dura around the teeth.

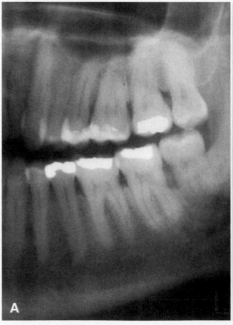

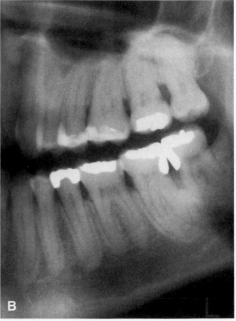

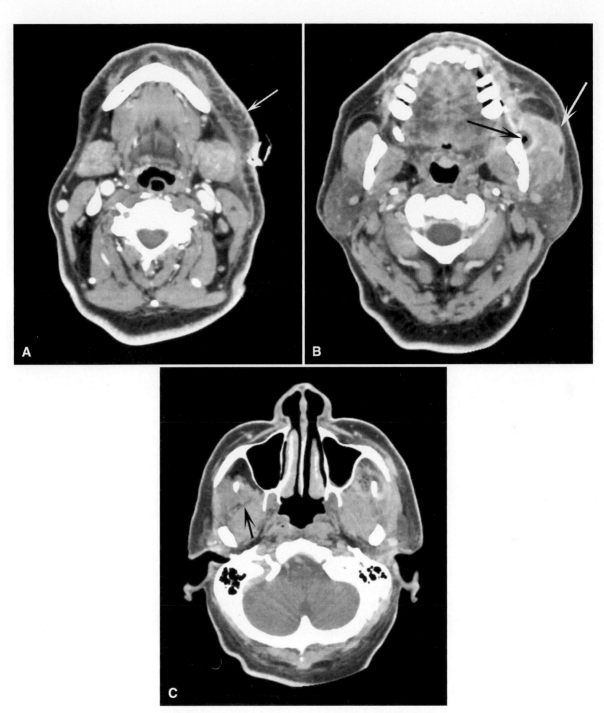

FIGURE 20-30 Three axial CT images, using a contrast medium, of a soft tissue infection. **A,** Streaking (reticulation pattern) of the fat planes and thickening of the skin *(arrow).* **B,** Thickening of the masseter muscle *(white arrow)* and a radiolucent pocket of gas *(black arrow).* **C,** Loss of distinctive soft tissue planes; for example, individual muscles defined by fat planes (the lateral border of the normal lateral pterygoid muscle *[arrow]* is not apparent on the opposite affected side). *(Courtesy Stuart White, DDS, Los Angeles, CA.)*

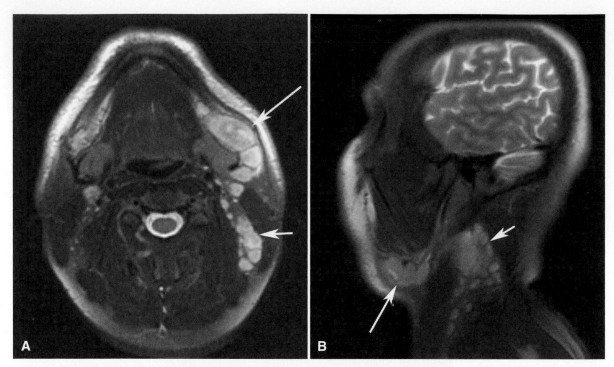

FIGURE 20-31 Axial T2-weighted **(A)** and sagittal T2-weighted **(B)** MR images of a patient with tuberculosis with significant lymphadenopathy involving the submandibular lymph nodes *(long arrows)* and level II nodes *(short arrows)*.

PERICORONITIS

SYNONYM

Operculitis is a synonym for pericoronitis.

DISEASE MECHANISM

The term pericoronitis refers to inflammation of the tissues surrounding the crown of a partially erupted tooth. This condition is seen most often in association with the mandibular third molars in young adults. The gingiva surrounding the erupted portion of the crown becomes inflamed when food or microbial debris become trapped under the soft tissue. The gingiva subsequently becomes swollen and may become secondarily traumatized by the opposing occlusion. This inflammation may extend into the bone surrounding the crown of the tooth.

CLINICAL FEATURES

Patients with pericoronitis typically complain of pain and swelling. Trismus is a common presentation when the partially erupted tooth is a lower third molar, and usually pain is felt on occlusion. An ulcerated operculum is usually the source of the pain. Pericoronitis can affect patients of any age or sex but is most commonly seen during the time of eruption of the third molars in young adults.

IMAGING FEATURES

The imaging features of pericoronitis can range from no changes when the inflammatory lesion is confined to the soft tissues to localized rarefaction and sclerosis to osteomyelitis in the most severe cases.

Location

When bone changes are associated with pericoronitis, they are centered on the follicular space or the portion of the crown still embedded in bone or in close proximity to bone. The mandibular third molar region is the most common location.

Periphery

The periphery of pericoronitis is ill defined, with a gradual transition of the normal trabecular pattern into a sclerotic region.

Internal Structure

The internal structure of bone adjacent to the pericoronitis most often is sclerotic with thick trabeculae. An area of bone loss or radiolucency immediately adjacent to the crown that enlarges the follicular space may be seen (Fig. 20-32). If this lesion spreads considerably, the internal pattern becomes consistent with osteomyelitis (see the next section).

Effects on Surrounding Structures

As with periapical inflammatory lesions, pericoronitis may cause the typical changes of sclerosis and rarefaction of surrounding bone. In extensive cases, evidence of periosteal new bone formation may be seen at the inferior cortex, the posterior border of the ramus, and along the coronoid notch of the mandible.

DIFFERENTIAL DIAGNOSIS

The differential diagnosis of pericoronitis includes other mixed-density or sclerotic lesions that can exist adjacent to the crown of a partially erupted third molar. These include DBI and fibrous dysplasia. The clinical symptoms indicative of an inflammatory lesion usually exclude these conditions. Neoplasms to be considered include the sclerotic form of osteosarcoma and, in older patients, squamous cell carcinoma. The occurrence of squamous cell carcinoma in the midst of a preexisting inflammatory lesion may be difficult to identify. Features characteristic of malignant neoplasia, such as profound cortical bone destruction and invasion, help with the diagnosis.

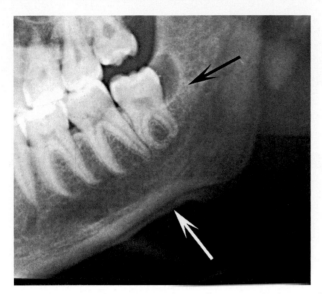

FIGURE 20-32 Cropped panoramic view of a case of pericoronitis related to a partially erupted third molar. Note the sclerotic bone reaction adjacent to the follicular cortex *(black arrow)* and the periosteal reaction *(white arrow)*.

MANAGEMENT

The aim of treatment of pericoronitis is removal of the partially erupted tooth. However, in the acute phase, when trismus may prevent adequate access, antibiotic therapy and reduction in occlusion of the opposing tooth should relieve symptoms until definitive treatment is provided.

BIBLIOGRAPHY

Periapical Inflammatory Lesions

Heersche JNM: Bone cells and bone turnover: the basis for pathogenesis. In Tam CS, Heersche JNM, Murray TM, editors: *Metabolic bone disease: cellular and tissue mechanisms*, Boca Raton, FL, 1989, CRC Press.
Stern MH, Dreizen S, Mackler BF, et al: Quantitative analysis of cellular composition of human periapical granuloma, *J Endocrinol* 7:117–122, 1981.

Pericoronitis

Blakey GH, White RP Jr, Offenbacher S, et al: Clinical/biological outcomes of treatment for pericoronitis, *J Oral Maxillofac Surg* 54:1150–1160, 1996.

Osteomyelitis

Becker W: Imaging osteomyelitis and the diabetic foot, *Q J Nucl Med* 43:9–20, 1999.
Compeyrot-Lacassagne S, Rosenberg AM, Babyn P, et al: Pamidronate treatment of chronic noninfectious inflammatory lesions of the mandible in children, *J Rheumatol* 34:1585–1589, 2007.
Guhlmann A, Brecht-Krauss D, Suger G, et al: Chronic osteomyelitis: detection with FDG PET and correlation with histopathologic findings, *Radiology* 2006:749–754, 2006.
Ledermann HP, Kaim A, Bongartz G, et al: Pitfalls and limitations of magnetic resonance imaging in chronic posttraumatic osteomyelitis, *Eur Radiol* 10:1815–1823, 2000.

Monsour PAK, Dalton JB: Chronic recurrent multifocal osteomyelitis involving the mandible: case reports and review of the literature, *Dentomaxillofac Radiol* 39:184–190, 2010.
Morrison WB, Schweitzer ME, Batte WG, et al: Osteomyelitis of the foot: relative importance of primary and secondary MR imaging signs, *Radiology* 207:625–632, 1998.
Nordin U, Wannfors K, Colque-Navarro P, et al: Antibody response in patients with osteomyelitis of the mandible, *Oral Surg Oral Med Oral Pathol Oral Radiol Endod* 79:429, 1995.
Orpe EC, Lee L, Pharoah MJ: A radiological analysis of chronic sclerosing osteomyelitis of the mandible, *Dentomaxillofac Radiol* 25:125–129, 1996.
Petrikowski CG, Pharoah MJ, Lee L, et al: Radiographic differentiation of osteogenic sarcoma, osteomyelitis, and fibrous dysplasia of the jaws, *Oral Surg Oral Med Oral Pathol Oral Radiol Endod* 80:744–750, 1995.
Suei Y, Taguchi A, Tanimoto K: Diagnostic points and possible origin of osteomyelitis in synovitis, acne, pustulosis, hyperostosis and osteitis (SAPHO) syndrome: a radiographic study of 77 mandibular osteomyelitis cases, *Rheumatology* 42:1398–1403, 2003.
Suei Y, Tanimoto K, Taguchi A, et al: Possible identity of diffuse sclerosing osteomyelitis and chronic recurrent multifocal osteomyelitis: one entity or two? *Oral Med Oral Pathol Oral Radiol Endod* 80:401–408, 1995.
Van Merkesteyn JP, Groot RH, Bras J, et al: Diffuse sclerosing osteomyelitis of the mandible: clinical radiographic and histologic findings in twenty seven patients, *J Oral Maxillofac Surg* 46:825–829, 1988.
Wannfors K, Hammarström L: Infectious foci in chronic osteomyelitis of the jaws, *Int J Oral Surg* 14:493–503, 1985.
Wood RE, Nortjé CJ, Grotepass F, et al: Periostitis ossificans versus Garré's osteomyelitis, Part I: what did Garré really say? *Oral Surg Oral Med Oral Pathol* 65:773–777, 1988.

Radiation-Induced Changes to Bone

Becker M, Schroth G, Zbären P, et al: Long-term changes induced by high dose irradiation of the head and neck region: imaging findings, *Radiographics* 17:5–26, 1997.
Williams HJ, Davies AM: The effect of x-rays on bone: a pictorial review, *Eur Radiol* 16:619–633, 2006.

Osteoradionecrosis

Chan KC: *Jaw bone changes on panoramic imaging after head and neck radiotherapy*, M.Sc. thesis, 2012, University of Toronto.
Curi MM, Dib LL: Osteoradionecrosis of the jaws: a retrospective study of the background factors and treatment in 104 cases, *J Oral Maxillofac Surg* 55:540–544, 1997.
Hermans R, Fossion E, Ioannides C, et al: CT findings in osteoradionecrosis of the mandible, *Skeletal Radiol* 25:31–36, 1996.
Marx RE: Osteoradionecrosis: a new concept of its pathophysiology, *J Oral Maxillofac Surg* 41:283–288, 1983.
Wong JK, Wood RE, McLean M: Conservative management of osteoradionecrosis, *Oral Surg Oral Med Oral Pathol Oral Radiol Endod* 84:16–21, 1997.

Bisphosphonate-Related Osteonecrosis

Jadu F, Lee L, Pharoah M, et al: A retrospective study assessing the incidence, risk factors and comorbidities of pamidronate-related necrosis of the jaws in multiple myeloma patients, *Ann Oncol* 18:2015–2019, 2007.
Woo SB, Hellstein J, Kalmar JR: Narrative [corrected] review: bisphosphonates and osteonecrosis of the jaws, *Ann Intern Med* 144:753–761, 2006.

DISEASE MECHANISM

A cyst is a pathologic cavity filled with fluid, lined by epithelium, and surrounded by a definite connective tissue wall. Cysts occur more often in the jaws than in any other bone because most cysts originate from the numerous rests of odontogenic epithelium that remain after tooth formation. The cystic fluid either is secreted by the cells lining the cavity or is derived from the surrounding tissue fluid. The cyst has a spherical or round shape based on accumulation of fluid within the cavity. Without resistance, for example, within an air space such as the maxillary sinus, the cyst grows in a concentric fashion resulting in a spherical shape, but when growing within bone, its shape is influenced by the resistance of adjacent hard tissue. For instance, a water-filled balloon develops a flat side when placed on a table top; similarly, a cyst reaching a thick segment of cortical bone may develop a flat side.

CLINICAL FEATURES

The most common clinical features are swelling and lack of pain (unless the cyst becomes secondarily infected or is related to a nonvital tooth). Cysts are often associated with unerupted teeth, especially third molars.

IMAGING FEATURES

LOCATION

Cysts may occur centrally (within bone) in any location in the maxilla or mandible but are rare in the condyle and coronoid process. Odontogenic cysts are found most often in the tooth-bearing regions. In the mandible, they originate above the inferior alveolar nerve canal. Odontogenic cysts may grow into the maxillary sinus. Some nonodontogenic cysts also originate within the antrum (see Chapter 26). A few cysts arise in the soft tissues of the orofacial region.

PERIPHERY

Cysts that originate in bone usually have a periphery that is well defined and corticated (characterized by a fairly uniform, thin, radiopaque line). However, a secondary infection or a chronic state can change this appearance into a thicker, more sclerotic boundary or make the cortex less apparent.

SHAPE

Cysts usually are round or oval, resembling a fluid-filled balloon. Some cysts may have a scalloped boundary.

INTERNAL STRUCTURE

Cysts often are totally radiolucent. However, long-standing cysts may have dystrophic calcification, which can give the internal aspect a sparse, particulate appearance. Some cysts have septa, which produce multiple loculations separated by these bony walls or septa. Cysts that have a scalloped periphery may appear to have internal septa. Occasionally, bony ridges produced by the peripheral scalloping are positioned so that their image overlaps the internal aspect of the cyst, giving the false impression of internal septa.

EFFECTS ON SURROUNDING STRUCTURE

Cysts grow slowly, sometimes causing displacement and resorption of teeth. The resorbing root often has a sharp, curved border. Cysts can expand the mandible, usually in a smooth, curved manner, and change the buccal or lingual cortical plate into a thin cortical boundary. Cysts may displace the inferior alveolar nerve canal in an inferior direction or expand into the maxillary antrum, maintaining a thin layer of bone separating the internal aspect of the cyst from the antrum.

ODONTOGENIC CYSTS

RADICULAR CYST

Synonyms

Synonyms for radicular cyst include periapical cyst, apical peri-odontal cyst, and dental cyst.

Disease Mechanism

A radicular cyst is a cyst that most likely results when rests of epithelial cells (Malassez) in the periodontal ligament are stimulated to proliferate and undergo cystic degeneration by inflammatory products from a nonvital tooth. This cyst is thought to grow by osmotic pressure.

Clinical Features

Radicular cysts are the most common type of cyst in the jaws. They arise from nonvital teeth (i.e., teeth that have necrotic pulps because of extensive caries, large restorations, or previous trauma). Radicular cysts often produce no symptoms unless secondary infection occurs. A cyst that becomes large may cause swelling. On palpation, the swelling may feel bony and hard if the cortex is intact, crepitant as the bone thins, and rubbery and fluctuant if the outer cortex is perforated. The incidence of radicular cysts is greater in the third to sixth decades and shows a slight male predominance.

Imaging Features

Location.   In most cases, the epicenter of a radicular cyst is located approximately at the apex of a nonvital tooth (Fig. 21-1). It occasionally appears on the mesial or distal surface of a tooth root at the opening of an accessory canal or infrequently in a deep peri-odontal pocket. Most radicular cysts (60%) are found in the maxilla, especially around incisors and canines. Because of the distal inclination of the root, cysts that arise from the maxillary lateral incisor may expand into or invaginate the antrum. Radicular cysts may also form in relation to a nonvital deciduous molar and be positioned buccal to the developing bicuspid.

Periphery and Shape.   The periphery usually has a well-defined cortical border (Fig. 21-2). If the cyst becomes secondarily infected, the inflammatory reaction of the surrounding bone may result in loss of this cortex (see Fig. 21-1, *B*) or alteration of the cortex into a more sclerotic border. The outline of a radicular cyst usually is curved or circular, unless it is influenced by surrounding structures such as cortical boundaries.

Internal Structure.   In most cases, the internal structure of radicular cysts is radiolucent. Occasionally, dystrophic calcification may develop in long-standing cysts, appearing as sparsely distributed, small particulate radiopacities.

Effects on Surrounding Structures.   If a radicular cyst is large, displacement and resorption of the roots of adjacent teeth may occur. The resorption pattern may have a curved outline. In rare cases, the cyst may resorb the roots of the related nonvital tooth. The cyst may invaginate the sinus, but there typically is evidence of a cortical boundary between the contents of the cyst and the sinus cavity (see Fig. 21-2, *B*). The outer cortical plates of the maxilla or mandible may expand in a curved or circular shape (Fig. 21-3). Cysts may displace the mandibular alveolar nerve canal in an inferior direction.

Differential Diagnosis

Differentiation of a small radicular cyst from an apical granuloma or a periapical pocket cyst may be difficult or impossible in some cases. A round shape, a well-defined cortical border, and a size greater than 2 cm in diameter are more characteristic of a cyst. Other periapical radiolucencies to consider are an early stage of periapical osseous (cemental) dysplasia and an apical scar or a surgical defect because normal bone may never fill in the defect completely in such cases. The patient's history helps with the differentiation. Radicular cysts that originate from the maxillary lateral incisor and are positioned between the roots of the lateral incisor and the cuspid may be difficult to differentiate from a keratocystic odontogenic tumor (KOT), also known as odontogenic keratocyst, or a lateral periodontal cyst. The vitality of the involved tooth should be tested. A nonvital tooth may have a larger pulp chamber than neighboring teeth because of the lack of secondary dentin, which normally forms with time in the pulp chamber and canal of a vital tooth (see Fig. 21-1).

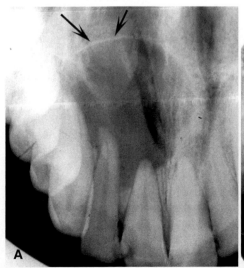
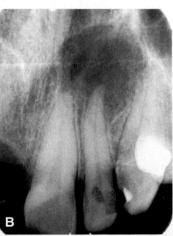

FIGURE 21-1 Radicular cysts. **A,** Note the epicenter is apical to the lateral incisor and the presence of a peripheral cortex *(arrows)*. **B,** Note the lack of a well-defined peripheral cortex because this cyst was secondarily infected. Also note the root canal of the lateral incisor is abnormally wide and it is visible at the root apex.

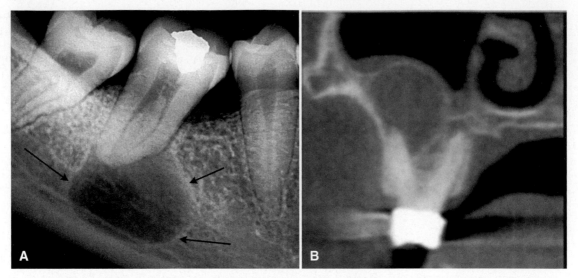

FIGURE 21-2 **A,** Periapical film of a radicular cyst reveals a lesion with a well-defined cortical boundary *(arrows).* The presence of the inferior cortex of the mandible has influenced the circular shape of the cyst. **B,** Coronal cone-beam CT image of a radicular cyst related to the buccal root of a maxillary molar. Note the circular shape of the cyst as it invaginates the maxillary sinus. *(Courtesy Dr. Bernard Friedland, Harvard University.)*

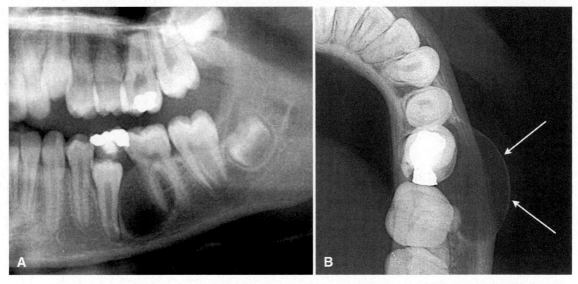

FIGURE 21-3 **A** and **B,** Two images of a radicular cyst originating from a nonvital deciduous second molar show expansion of the buccal cortical plate to a circular or hydraulic shape *(arrows in* **B***)* and displacement of the adjacent permanent teeth.

A large radicular cyst that has invaginated the maxillary antrum may collapse and start filling in with new bone (Fig. 21-4). With biopsy, the histologic analysis may result in an erroneous diagnosis of ossifying fibroma or a benign fibro-osseous lesion. Radiographically, the important feature is that the new bone always forms first at the periphery of the cyst wall and grows toward the center as the cyst shrinks; this is a different pattern of bone formation than is seen with benign bone-forming lesions.

Management

Treatment of a tooth with a radicular cyst may include extraction, endodontic therapy, and apical surgery. Treatment of a large radicular cyst usually involves surgical removal or marsupialization. The radiographic appearance of the periapical area of an endodontically treated tooth should be checked periodically to ensure that normal healing is occurring (Fig. 21-5). Characteristically, new bone grows into the defect from the periphery, sometimes resulting in a radiating pattern resembling the spokes of a wheel. However, in a few cases, normal bone may not completely fill the defect, especially if there was a secondary infection or a considerable amount of bone destruction, including the buccal and lingual cortical plates. Recurrence of a radicular cyst is unlikely if it has been removed completely.

RESIDUAL CYST

Disease Mechanism

A residual cyst is a cyst that remains after incomplete removal of the original cyst. The term residual is used most often for a

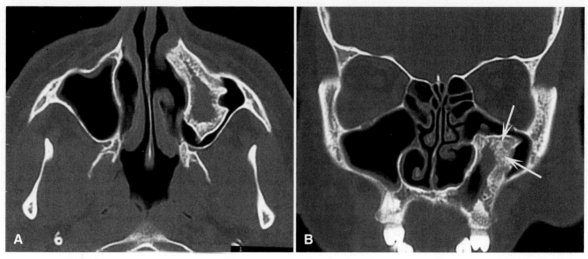

FIGURE 21-4 Axial (**A**) and coronal (**B**) CT images with use of a bone algorithm of a collapsing radicular cyst within the sinus. Note the unusual shape and the fact that new bone is being formed from the periphery (*arrows* in **B**) toward the center. *(Courtesy Drs. S. Ahing and T. Blight, University of Manitoba.)*

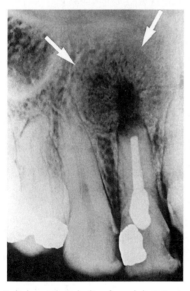

FIGURE 21-5 Radicular cyst that is healing after endodontic treatment. *Arrows* show the original outline of the cyst; the new bone grows toward the center from the periphery.

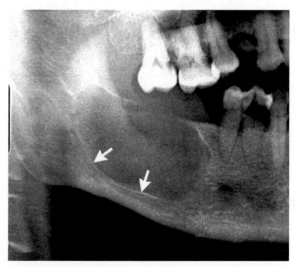

FIGURE 21-6 The epicenter of this infected residual cyst is above the inferior alveolar nerve canal and has displaced the canal in an inferior direction *(arrows)*. The cortical boundary is not continuous around the whole cyst.

radicular cyst that may be left behind, most commonly after extraction of a tooth.

Clinical Features

A residual cyst usually is asymptomatic and often is discovered on radiographic examination of an edentulous area. However, there may be some expansion of the jaw or pain in the case of secondary infection.

Imaging Features

Location. Residual cysts occur in both jaws, although they are found slightly more often in the mandible. The epicenter is positioned in the former periapical region of the involved and missing tooth. In the mandible, the epicenter is always above the inferior alveolar nerve canal (Fig. 21-6).

Periphery and Shape. A residual cyst has a cortical margin, unless it becomes secondarily infected. Its shape is oval or circular.

Internal Structure. The internal aspect of a residual cyst typically is radiolucent. Dystrophic calcifications may be present in long-standing cysts.

Effects on Surrounding Structures. Residual cysts can cause displacement or resorption of teeth, or they may cause expansion of the outer cortical plates of the jaws. The cyst may invaginate into the maxillary antrum or depress the inferior alveolar nerve canal.

Differential Diagnosis

Without the patient's history and previous radiographs, clinicians may have difficulty determining whether a solitary cyst in the jaws is a residual cyst. Other examples of common solitary cysts include KOTs. A residual cyst has greater potential for expansion compared with a KOT. The epicenter of a Stafne developmental salivary gland defect is located below the mandibular canal (and thus is unlikely to be odontogenic in nature).

Management

The treatment for residual cysts is surgical removal or marsupialization, or both if the cyst is large.

DENTIGEROUS CYST

Synonym

Follicular cyst is a synonym for dentigerous cyst.

Disease Mechanism

A dentigerous cyst is a cyst that forms around the crown of an unerupted tooth. It begins when fluid accumulates in the layers of reduced enamel epithelium or between the epithelium and the crown of the unerupted tooth. This lesion is usually classified as a developmental cyst, but some evidence suggests that in a few cases inflammation may be the etiology. An eruption cyst is the soft tissue counterpart of a dentigerous cyst.

Clinical Features

Dentigerous cysts are the second most common type of cyst in the jaws. They develop around the crown of an unerupted or supernumerary tooth. The clinical examination reveals a missing tooth or teeth and possibly a hard swelling, occasionally resulting in facial asymmetry. The patient typically has no pain or discomfort. Dentigerous cysts around supernumerary teeth account for about 5% of all dentigerous cysts, most developing around a mesiodens in the anterior maxilla.

Imaging Features

Location. The epicenter of a dentigerous cyst is found just above the crown of the involved tooth, most commonly a mandibular or maxillary third molar or a maxillary canine (Fig. 21-7). An important diagnostic point is that this cyst attaches at the cementoenamel junction. Some dentigerous cysts are eccentric, developing from the lateral aspect of the follicle so that they occupy an area beside the crown instead of above the crown (see Fig. 21-7, D). Cysts related to maxillary third molars often grow into the maxillary antrum and may become quite large before they are discovered. Cysts attached to the crown of mandibular molars may extend a considerable distance into the ramus.

Periphery and Shape. Dentigerous cysts typically have a well-defined cortex with a curved or circular outline. If infection is present, the cortex may be missing.

Internal Structure. The internal aspect is completely radiolucent except for the crown of the involved tooth.

Effects on Surrounding Structures. A dentigerous cyst has a propensity to displace and resorb adjacent teeth (Fig. 21-8; see Fig. 21-7). It commonly displaces the associated tooth in an apical direction (Fig. 21-9). The degree of displacement may be considerable. For instance, maxillary third molars or cuspids may be pushed to the floor of the orbit (see Fig. 21-8), and mandibular third molars may be moved to the condylar or coronoid regions or to the inferior cortex of the mandible. The floor of the maxillary antrum may be displaced as the cyst invaginates the antrum, or a cyst may displace the inferior alveolar nerve canal in an inferior direction (Fig. 21-10). This slow-growing cyst often expands the outer cortical boundary of the involved jaw. As in the case with radicular cysts, dentigerous cysts that invaginate the sinus can drain and collapse with new bone formation at the periphery (see Fig. 21-10, C and D).

Differential Diagnosis

Because the histopathologic appearance of the lining epithelium is not specific, the diagnosis relies on the radiographic and surgical observation of the attachment of the cyst to the cementoenamel junction. However, histopathologic examination must always be done to eliminate other possible lesions in this location.

One of the most difficult differential diagnoses to make is between a small dentigerous cyst and a hyperplastic follicle. A cyst should be considered with any evidence of tooth displacement or considerable expansion of the involved bone. The size of the normal follicular space is 2 to 3 mm. If the follicular space exceeds 5 mm, a dentigerous cyst is more likely. If uncertainty remains, the region should be reexamined in 4 to 6 months to detect any increase in size or any influence on surrounding structures characteristic of cysts.

The differential diagnosis of a dentigerous cyst also may include a KOT, an ameloblastic fibroma, and a cystic ameloblastoma. A KOT does not expand the bone to the same degree as a dentigerous cyst, is less likely to resorb teeth, and may attach further apically on the root instead of at the cementoenamel junction. It may be impossible to differentiate a small ameloblastic fibroma or cystic ameloblastoma from a dentigerous cyst if there is no internal structure. Other rare lesions that may have a similar pericoronal appearance are adenomatoid odontogenic tumors and calcified odontogenic cysts, both of which can surround the crown and root of the involved tooth. Evidence of a radiopaque internal structure is sometimes found in these two lesions. Occasionally, a radicular cyst at the apex of a primary tooth surrounds the crown of the developing permanent tooth positioned apical to it, giving the false impression of a dentigerous cyst associated with the permanent tooth. This occurs most often with the mandibular deciduous molars and the developing bicuspids. In these cases, the clinician should look for extensive caries or large restorations in a primary tooth, an etiology that would support a diagnosis of a radicular cyst.

Management

Dentigerous cysts are treated by surgical removal, which may include the tooth as well. Large cysts may be treated by marsupialization before removal. The cyst lining should be submitted for histologic examination because ameloblastomas have been reported to occur there. In addition, squamous cell carcinoma and mucoepidermoid carcinoma have been reported to arise from the cyst lining of chronically infected cysts.

BUCCAL BIFURCATION CYST

Synonyms

Synonyms for buccal bifurcation cyst (BBC) include mandibular infected buccal cyst, paradental cyst, and inflammatory paradental cyst.

Disease Mechanism

BBCs probably derive from the epithelial cell rests in the periodontal membrane of the buccal bifurcation of mandibular molars. The histopathologic characteristics of the lining are not distinctive. The etiology of proliferation is unknown; one theory holds that

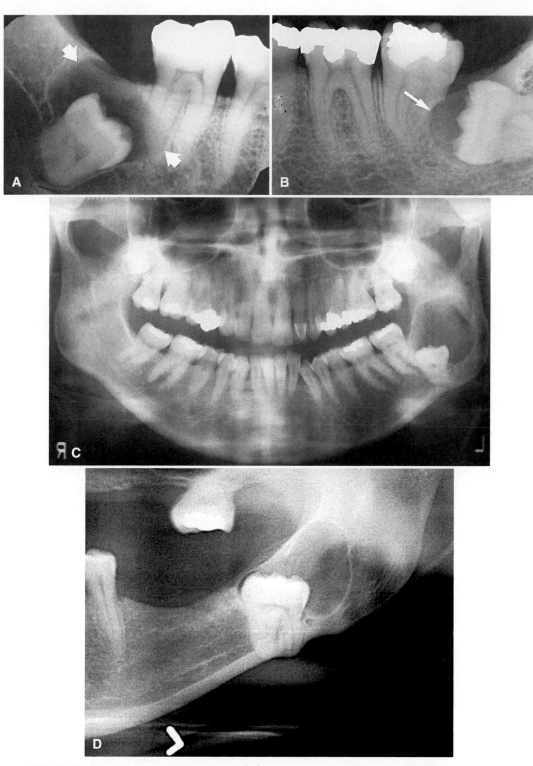

FIGURE 21-7 Dentigerous cysts. **A,** Cyst that surrounds the crown of a third molar *(arrows)*. **B,** The cyst has caused resorption of the distal root of the second molar *(arrow)*. **C,** Cyst that involves the ramus of the mandible. **D,** Dentigerous cyst that is expanding distally from the involved third molar.

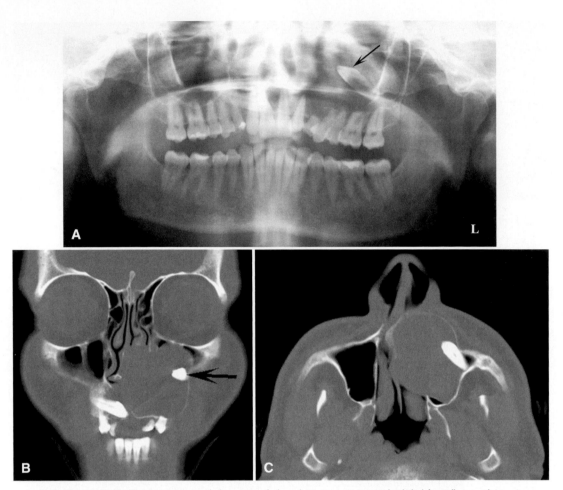

FIGURE 21-8 **A,** Panoramic image reveals the presence of a large dentigerous cyst associated with the left maxillary cuspid *(arrow),* which has been displaced. Note the displacement and resorption of other teeth in the left maxilla. **B** and **C,** Coronal and axial CT images of the same case show superior-lateral displacement of the cuspid, expansion of the anterior wall of the maxilla, and expansion of the cyst into the nasal fossa.

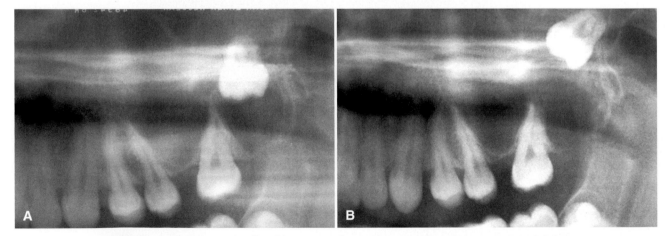

FIGURE 21-9 **A** and **B,** Panoramic films of the same case taken several years apart demonstrate superior-posterior displacement of a maxillary third molar by a dentigerous cyst.

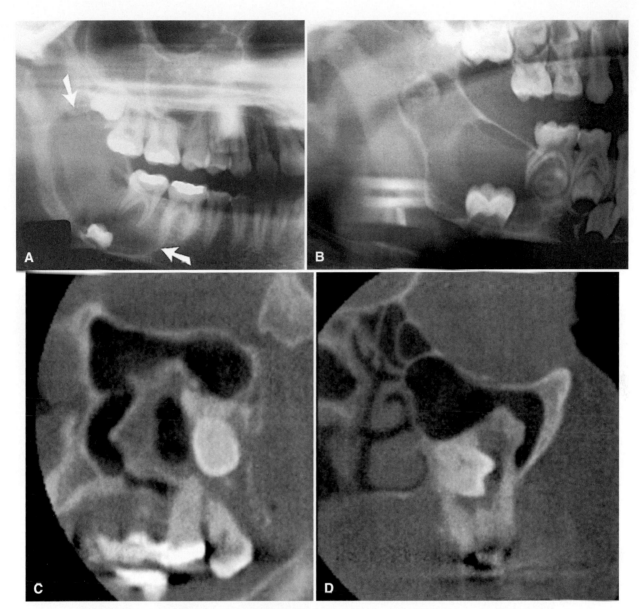

FIGURE 21-10 Dentigerous cysts displacing teeth. **A,** The third molar has been displaced to the inferior cortex. **B,** The developing second molar has been displaced into the ramus by a cyst associated with the first molar. Axial **(C)** and coronal **(D)** CT images with bone algorithm reveal a maxillary third molar displaced into the space occupied by the maxillary antrum; note the presence of a cortex between the cyst and the antrum.

inflammation is the stimulus, but inflammation is not always present. The World Health Organization includes these cysts under inflammatory cysts.

It is possible that the paradental cyst of the third molar and the BBC (associated with first and second molars) are the same entity. The BBC is certainly a distinct clinical entity. An associated enamel extension into the furcation region of third molars with paradental cysts has not been documented with molars involved in a BBC. Also, the inflammatory component associated with paradental cysts is not always present with BBCs.

Clinical Features

A common sign is the lack of or a delay in eruption of a mandibular first or second molar. On clinical examination, the molar may be missing, or the lingual cusp tips may be abnormally protruding through the mucosa, higher than the position of the buccal cusps. The first molar is involved more frequently than the second molar. The teeth are vital. A hard swelling may occur buccal to the involved molar, and if it is secondarily infected, the patient has pain. The age of detection is younger, within the first 2 decades for a BBC, rather than the third decade with a paradental cyst of the third molar.

Imaging Features

Location.   A BBC is most commonly located in association with a mandibular first molar followed by the second molar. The cyst occasionally is bilateral. It is always located in the buccal furcation of the affected molar (Fig. 21-11). On periapical and panoramic films, the lesion may appear to be centered a little distal to the furcation of the involved tooth.

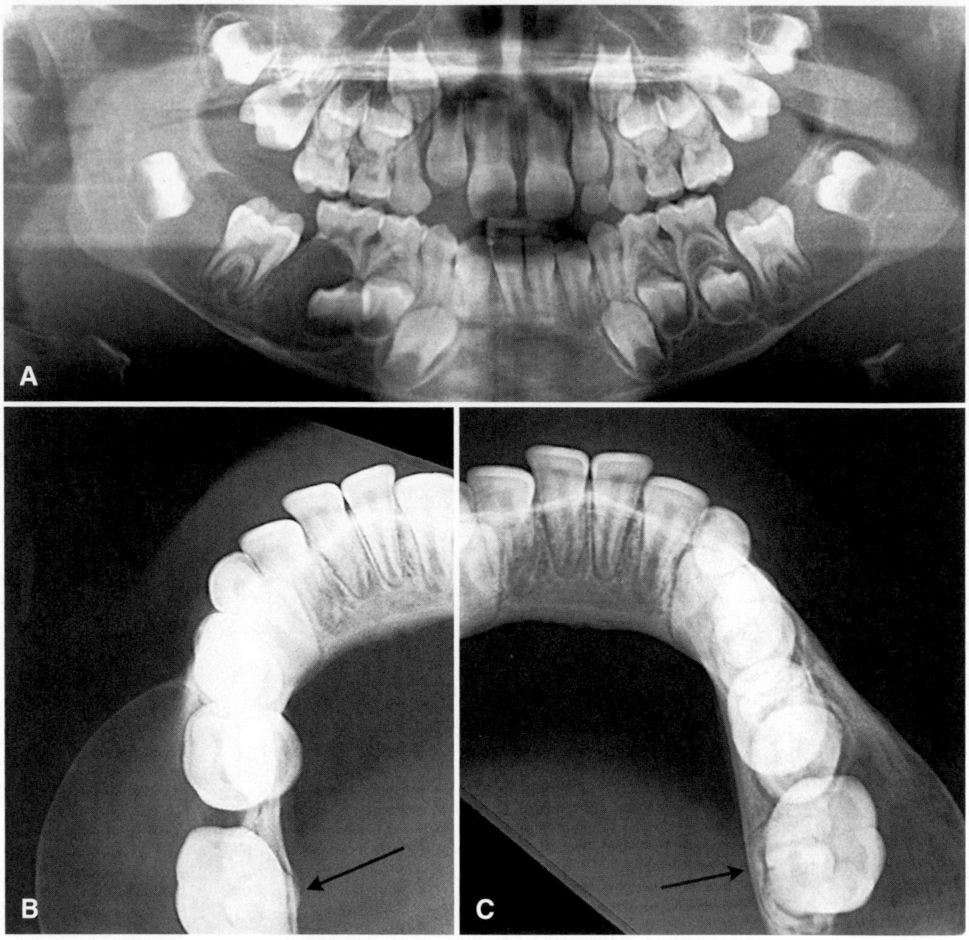

FIGURE 21-11 Bilateral BBCs. **A,** Panoramic image shows cysts related to the mandibular first molars. The occlusal surface of each tooth has been tipped in relation to the other teeth, and adjacent teeth have been displaced. **B** and **C,** Occlusal films of the same case. Note the smooth curved expansion of the buccal cortex and the displacement of the roots of the first molars into the lingual cortical plate *(arrows).*

Periphery and Shape.

In some cases, the periphery is not readily apparent, and the lesion may be a very subtle radiolucent region superimposed over the image of the roots of the molar. In other cases, the lesion has a circular shape with a well-defined cortical border. Some cysts can become quite large before they are detected.

Internal Structure.

The internal structure is radiolucent.

Effects on Surrounding Structures.

The most striking diagnostic characteristic of a BBC is the tipping of the involved molar so that the root tips are pushed into the lingual cortical plate of the mandible (see Fig. 21-11, *B* and *C*) and the occlusal surface is tipped toward the buccal aspect of the mandible (see Fig. 21-11, *A*). This accounts for the lingual cusp tips being positioned higher than the buccal tips. This tipping may be detected in a panoramic or periapical film if the image of the occlusal surface of the affected tooth is apparent and the unaffected teeth are not. The best diagnostic film is the cross-sectional (standard) mandibular occlusal projection, which demonstrates the abnormal position of the tooth roots. If the cyst is large enough, it may displace and resorb the adjacent teeth and cause a considerable amount of smooth expansion of the buccal cortical plate. If the cyst is secondarily infected, periosteal new bone formation is seen on the buccal cortex adjacent to the involved tooth (Fig. 21-12).

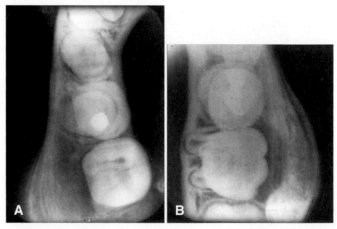

FIGURE 21-12 **A** and **B,** Occlusal views of two examples of BBCs that have been secondarily infected. Note the laminated periosteal new bone formation on the buccal aspect of the first molars and the abnormal position of the roots of the first molar in **B**. *(Courtesy Dr. Doug Stoneman, University of Toronto.)*

Differential Diagnosis

Diagnosis of a BBC relies entirely on clinical and radiographic information. The major differential diagnoses include lesions that could elicit an inflammatory periosteal response on the buccal aspect of mandibular molars, such as a periodontal abscess or

Langerhans' cell histiocytosis (see Fig. 21-12). The fact that only a BBC tilts the molar as described helps to differentiate it from other lesions. A dentigerous cyst is also in the differential diagnosis. However, the epicenter of a dentigerous cyst is different because a BBC starts near the bifurcation region of the tooth and does not surround the crown, as does a dentigerous cyst.

Management

A BBC usually is removed by conservative curettage, although some cases have resolved without intervention. The involved molar should not be removed. BBCs do not recur.

KERATOCYSTIC ODONTOGENIC TUMOR

Synonyms

Synonyms for KOT include odontogenic keratocyst and primordial cyst.

Disease Mechanism

The World Health Organization has reclassified this cystic lesion into a unicystic or multicystic odontogenic tumor on the basis of the tumor-like characteristics of the lining epithelium. Because the gross and radiographic appearance of KOT is cystic in nature, this neoplasm is presented in this chapter. In contrast to most cysts, which are thought to grow solely by osmotic pressure, the epithelium in a KOT appears to have innate growth potential, consistent with a benign tumor. This difference in the mechanism of growth gives a KOT a different radiographic appearance from cysts. The epithelial lining is distinctive also because it is keratinized (hence the name) and thin (four to eight cells thick). Occasionally, budlike proliferations of epithelium grow from the basal layer into the adjacent connective tissue wall. Also, islands of epithelium in the wall may give rise to satellite microcysts. The inside of the cyst often contains a viscous or cheesy material derived from the epithelial lining.

Clinical Features

KOTs account for about one tenth of all cystic lesions in the jaws. Although they occur in a wide age range, most develop during the second and third decades, with a slight male predominance. The cysts sometimes form around an unerupted tooth. KOTs usually have no symptoms, although mild swelling may occur. Pain may occur with secondary infection. Aspiration may reveal a thick, yellow, cheesy material (keratin). In contrast to cysts, KOTs have a high propensity for recurrence, possibly because of small satellite cysts or fragments of epithelium left behind after surgical removal of the cyst.

Imaging Features

Location. The most common location of KOTs is the posterior body of the mandible (90% occur posterior to the canines) and ramus (>50%) (Fig. 21-13). The epicenter is located superior to the inferior alveolar nerve canal. This type of cyst occasionally has the same pericoronal position as, and is indistinguishable from, a dentigerous cyst (see Fig. 21-13, *B*).

Periphery and Shape. As with cysts, KOTs usually show evidence of a cortical border, unless they have become secondarily infected. The cyst may have a smooth, round or oval shape identical to that of other cysts, or it may have a scalloped outline (a series of contiguous arcs) (see Figs. 21-13 and 21-15, *C*).

Internal Structure. The internal structure is most commonly radiolucent. The presence of internal keratin does not increase the radiopacity. In some cases, curved internal septa may be present, giving the lesion a multilocular appearance (Fig. 21-14, *A*; see Fig. 21-13).

Effects on Surrounding Structures. An important characteristic of the KOT is its propensity to grow along the internal aspect of the jaws, causing minimal expansion of the cortical plates (Fig. 21-15). This growth with minimal expansion occurs throughout the body mandible except for the upper ramus and coronoid process, where considerable expansion may occur (see Fig. 21-14, *C*). Occasionally, the expansion of large lesions may exceed the ability of the periosteum to form new bone, allowing the cystic wall to contact soft tissue peripheral to the outer cortex of the

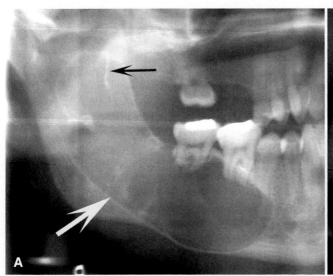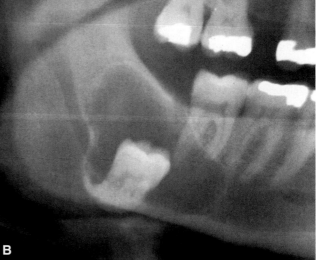

FIGURE 21-13 A, In this panoramic image, a large KOT occupies the ramus and body of the mandible. Note septa *(black arrow)*, inferiorly displaced mandibular canal *(white arrow)*, and root resorption. **B,** Keratocyst has a pericoronal position relative to the impacted third molar, and the distal margin has a scalloped shape.

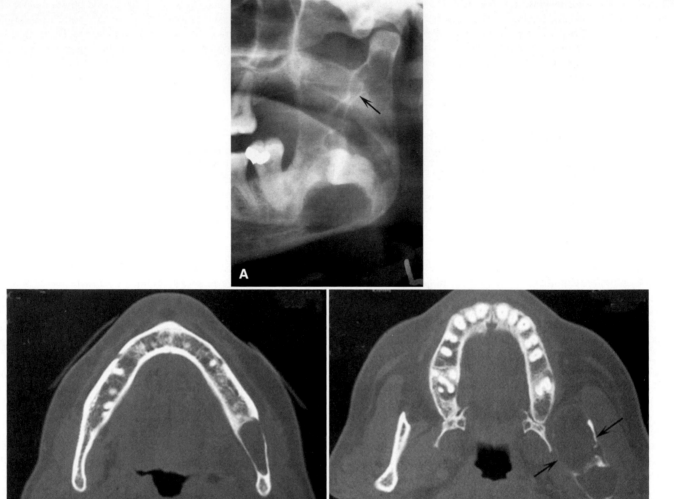

FIGURE 21-14 **A,** Cropped panoramic image of a KOT occupying the mandibular ramus; note the septa *(arrow).* **B** and **C,** Two axial CT images with bone algorithm of the same case demonstrate very little expansion in the body **(B)** but significant expansion in the upper ramus *(arrows* in **C).**

mandible (Fig. 21-16). The relatively slight expansion common with these lesions probably contributes to their late detection, which occasionally allows them to reach a large size. KOTs occasionally displace and resorb teeth, but to a slightly lesser degree than dentigerous cysts. The inferior alveolar nerve canal may be displaced inferiorly. In the maxilla, this cyst can invaginate and occupy the entire maxillary antrum.

Differential Diagnosis

When in a pericoronal position, a KOT may be indistinguishable from a dentigerous cyst. The lesion is likely to be a KOT if the cystic outline is connected to the tooth at a point apical to the cementoenamel junction or if no expansion of the cortical plates has occurred. Also, although KOTs can develop occlusal to developing teeth, often the follicle of the involved tooth is not enlarged as in dentigerous cysts. The typical scalloped margin and multilocular appearance of the KOT may resemble an ameloblastoma, but the latter has a greater propensity to expand. Occasionally, large lateral periodontal cysts, especially in the maxilla, have a growth pattern similar to a KOT that causes minimum bone

expansion. A KOT may show some similarity to an odontogenic myxoma, especially in the characteristics of mild expansion and multilocular appearance. A simple bone cyst (SBC) often has a scalloped margin and minimal bone expansion, similar to a KOT; however, the margins of an SBC usually are more delicate and often difficult to detect. If several KOTs are found (which occurs in 4% to 5% of cases), these tumors may constitute part of a basal cell nevus syndrome.

Management

If a KOT is suspected, referral to a radiologist for a complete radiologic examination is advisable. Because this tumor has a propensity to recur, an accurate determination of the extent and location of any cortical perforations with soft tissue extension is best achieved with computed tomographic (CT) imaging. In the case of multiple cysts and the possibility of basal cell nevus syndrome, a thorough radiologic examination that includes a CT scan is required. This examination allows accurate determination of the number of cysts and other osseous characteristics that confirm the diagnosis.

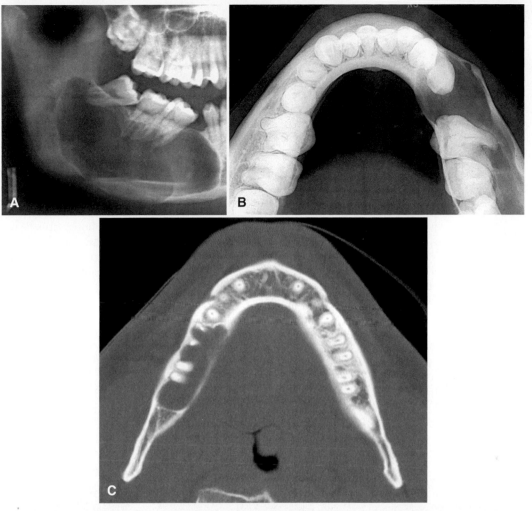

FIGURE 21-15 **A** and **B,** Large KOT occupying most of the right body and ramus of the mandible. Despite the large size, the buccal and lingual cortical plates of the mandible have been expanded only slightly, as can be seen in the occlusal film **(B)**. **C,** KOT within the body of the mandible. Note the lack of expansion and the cyst scalloping between the roots of the teeth.

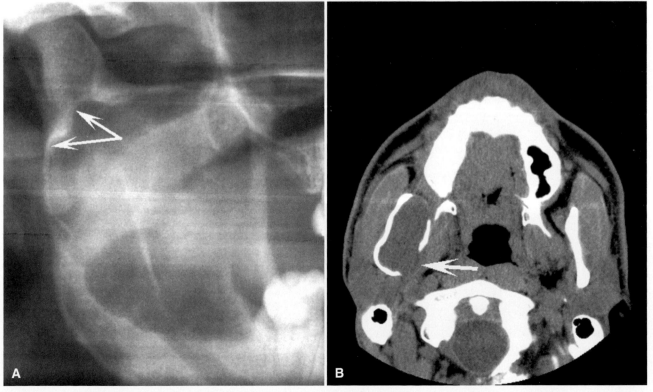

FIGURE 21-16 **A,** Cropped panoramic image reveals a large KOT occupying most of the ramus; note the scalloping margin *(arrows)*. **B,** Axial CT image with soft tissue window of the same case shows perforation of the medial cortex and contact with the medial pterygoid muscle *(arrow)*.

Surgical treatment may vary and can include resection, curettage, or marsupialization to reduce the size of large lesions before surgical excision. More attention usually is devoted to complete removal of the cystic walls to reduce the chance of recurrence. After surgical treatment, it is important to make periodic posttreatment clinical and radiographic examinations to detect any recurrence. Recurrent lesions usually develop within the first 5 years but may occur as late as 10 years.

BASAL CELL NEVUS SYNDROME

Synonyms

Synonyms for basal cell nevus syndrome include nevoid basal cell carcinoma syndrome and Gorlin-Goltz syndrome.

Disease Mechanism

The term basal cell nevus syndrome comprises numerous abnormalities, including multiple nevoid basal cell carcinomas of the skin, skeletal abnormalities, central nervous system abnormalities, eye abnormalities, and multiple KOTs. It is inherited as an autosomal dominant trait with variable expressivity.

Clinical Features

Basal cell nevus syndrome starts to appear early in life, usually after 5 years of age and before 30 years of age, with the development of KOTs within the jaws and skin basal cell carcinomas. Typically, multiple KOTs appear in multiple quadrants and earlier in life than solitary KOTs. The recurrence rate of KOTs in this syndrome appears to be higher than with the solitary variety. A thorough radiologic examination including CT imaging is required to detect all the jaw lesions. The skin lesions are small, flattened, flesh-colored or brown papules that can occur anywhere on the body but are especially prominent on the face, neck, and trunk. Occasionally, basal cell carcinomas form later in life than the jaw lesions or not at all. Skeletal anomalies include bifid rib (most common) and other costal abnormalities, such as agenesis, deformity, and synostosis of the ribs; kyphoscoliosis; vertebral fusion; polydactyly; shortening of the metacarpals; temporal and temporoparietal bossing; minor hypertelorism; and mild prognathism. Calcification of the falx cerebri and other parts of the dura occur early in life.

Imaging Features

Location. The location is the same as that of solitary KOTs, as described previously. Multiple KOTs may develop bilaterally and can vary in size from 1 mm to several centimeters in diameter (Fig. 21-17).

Other Imaging Features. The reader should refer to the preceding description of the imaging features of KOTs. In addition, a

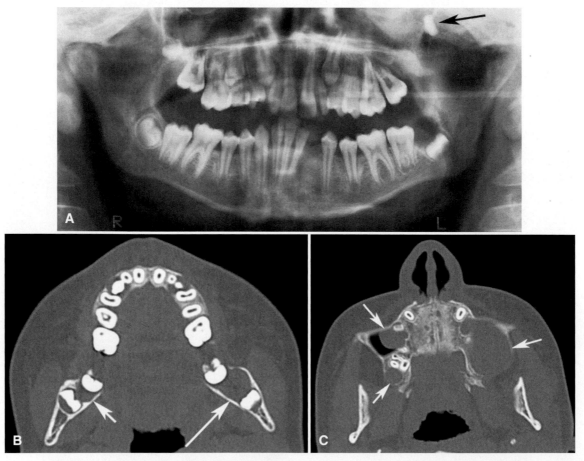

FIGURE 21-17 **A,** Panoramic image of a case of basal cell nevus syndrome. Note the small KOT related to the unerupted left mandibular third molar and a large KOT within the left maxilla that has displaced the left maxillary third molar *(arrow)*. **B,** Axial CT image of the same case. Note the small mandibular KOT *(long arrow)* seen in the panoramic image and another small KOT *(short arrow)* in the right mandible that is not seen in the panoramic film. **C,** Another axial CT image from the same case reveals the large KOT in the left maxilla and two other KOTs *(arrows)* not readily apparent in the panoramic image.

radiopaque line of the calcified falx cerebri may be prominent on the posteroanterior skull projection. Occasionally, this calcification may appear laminated.

Differential Diagnosis

The presence of a cortical boundary and other cystic characteristics differentiates basal cell nevus syndrome from other abnormalities characterized by multiple radiolucencies (e.g., multiple myeloma). Cherubism appears as bilateral multilocular lesions but usually has significant jaw expansion, which is not characteristic of basal cell nevus syndrome. Also, cherubism pushes posterior teeth in an anterior direction, a distinctive characteristic. Occasionally, patients with multiple dentigerous cysts may show some similarities, but dentigerous cysts are more expansile.

Management

KOTs are treated more aggressively than other solitary KOTs because there appears to be an even greater propensity for recurrence. It is reasonable to examine the patient yearly for new and recurrent cysts. A panoramic film may not be an adequate screening film (see Fig. 21-17), and therefore CT imaging is the modality of preference. Referral for genetic counseling may be appropriate.

LATERAL PERIODONTAL CYST

Disease Mechanism

Lateral periodontal cysts are thought to arise from epithelial rests in periodontium lateral to the tooth root. This condition usually is unicystic, but it may appear as a cluster of small cysts, a condition referred to as botryoid odontogenic cysts. It has been postulated that a lateral periodontal cyst is the intrabony counterpart of the gingival cyst in an adult.

Clinical Features

The lesions usually are asymptomatic and less than 1 cm in diameter. The disorder has no apparent sexual predilection, and the age distribution extends from the second to the ninth decades (mean age is about 50 years). If these cysts become secondarily infected, they mimic a lateral periodontal abscess.

Imaging Features

Location.   Of lateral periodontal cysts, 50% to 75% develop in the mandible, mostly in a region extending from the lateral incisor to the second premolar (Fig. 21-18). Most cysts are small, but occasionally these cysts can attain a considerable size (see Fig. 21-18, *B*).

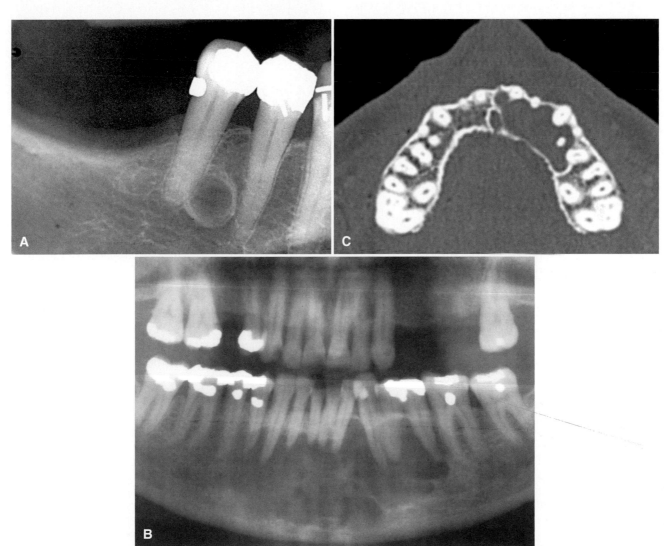

FIGURE 21-18 **A,** Lateral periodontal cyst in the mandibular premolar region. Note the classic well-defined cortical border. **B,** Cropped panoramic image with a large lateral periodontal cyst crossing the midline of the mandible. **C,** Axial CT bone window image of a large lateral periodontal cyst causing minimal expansion of the maxilla.

These cysts can appear in the maxilla, especially between the lateral incisor and the cuspid.

Periphery and Shape.   A lateral periodontal cyst appears as a well-defined radiolucency with a prominent cortical boundary and a round or oval shape. Rare large cysts have a more irregular shape.

Internal Structure.   The internal aspect usually is radiolucent. The botryoid variety may have a multilocular appearance, although this aspect is related more to the histologic appearance.

Effects on Surrounding Structures.   Small cysts may efface the lamina dura of the adjacent root. Large cysts can displace adjacent teeth. Occasionally, large cysts have a similar growth pattern to KOTs with minimum expansion of the involved bone (see Fig. 21-18, *C*).

Differential Diagnosis

Because the location and radiographic appearance of a lateral periodontal cyst are similar in other conditions, the following lesions should be included in the differential diagnosis: small KOT, mental foramen, small neurofibroma, and radicular cyst at the foramen of a lateral (accessory) pulp canal. The multiple (botryoid) cysts with a multilocular appearance may resemble a small ameloblastoma.

Management

Lateral periodontal cysts usually do not require sophisticated imaging because of their small size. Excisional biopsy or simple enucleation is the treatment of choice because these cysts do not tend to recur.

GLANDULAR ODONTOGENIC CYST

Synonym

Sialo-odontogenic cyst is a synonym for glandular odontogenic cyst.

Disease Mechanism

Glandular odontogenic cyst is a rare cyst derived from odontogenic epithelium with a spectrum of characteristics including salivary gland features such as mucus-producing cells. Some authors hypothesize a relationship to a central mucoepidermoid carcinoma.

Clinical Features

There is a slight female predominance with mean age ranging from 46 to 50 years. This cyst has an aggressive behavior and a tendency to recur after surgery.

Imaging Features

Location.   This cyst occurs more commonly in the mandible and most often in the anterior mandible and in the maxilla, commonly the globulomaxillary region.

Periphery and Shape.   There is usually a cortical boundary that may be smooth or scalloped.

Internal Structure.   Both unilocular and multilocular appearances (Fig. 21-19) of this cyst have been reported.

Effects on Surrounding Structures.   Expansion of the outer cortical plates of the jaws with regions of perforation through the cortex has been reported. Displacement of teeth is a common feature.

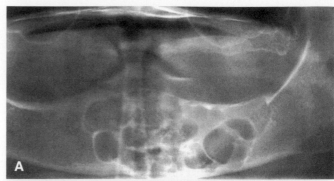

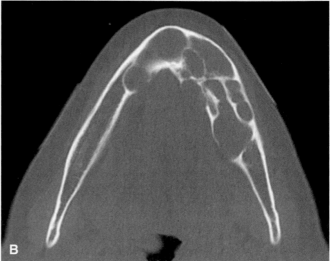

FIGURE 21-19 **A,** Cropped panoramic image of a glandular odontogenic cyst with a multilocular appearance very similar to an ameloblastoma. **B,** Axial CT image detailing the multilocular internal cystic structure.

Differential Diagnosis

This cyst can appear identical to an ameloblastoma and in some cases may be similar to a KOT. Similar multilocular appearances have been associated with central mucoepidermoid carcinomas.

Treatment

Because of the high rate of recurrence with conservative treatments such as enucleation, more aggressive treatment, including resection, may be considered. Treated cases should be followed with periodic radiographic examinations to assess for recurrence.

CALCIFYING CYSTIC ODONTOGENIC TUMOR

Synonyms

Synonyms for calcifying cystic odontogenic tumor (CCOT) include calcifying odontogenic cyst, calcifying epithelial odontogenic cyst, dentinogenic ghost cell tumor, and Gorlin's cyst.

Disease Mechanism

The World Health Organization now categorizes this entity as a tumor. CCOTs are uncommon, slow-growing, benign lesions. They occupy a spectrum ranging from a cyst to an odontogenic tumor, with characteristics of a cyst alone or sometimes characteristics of a solid neoplasm (epithelial proliferation and a tendency to continue growing). This lesion may manufacture calcified tissue identified as dysplastic dentin, and in some instances the lesion is associated with an odontoma. This lesion also sometimes contains a more solid component that gives it an appearance resembling an ameloblastoma, although it does not behave like one.

Clinical Features

CCOTs have a wide age distribution that peaks at 10 to 19 years of age, with a mean age of 36 years. A second incidence peak occurs during the seventh decade. Clinically, the lesion usually appears as a slow-growing, painless swelling of the jaw. Occasionally, the patient complains of pain. In some cases, the expanding lesion may destroy the cortical plate, and the cystic mass may become palpable as it extends into the soft tissue. The patient may report a discharge from such advanced lesions. Aspiration often yields a viscous, granular, yellow fluid.

Imaging Features

Location. At least 75% of CCOTs occur in bone, with a nearly equal distribution between the jaws. Most (75%) occur anterior to the first molar, especially associated with cuspids and incisors, where the cyst sometimes manifests as a pericoronal radiolucency.

Periphery and Shape. The periphery can vary from well defined and corticated with a curved, cystlike shape to ill defined and irregular.

Internal Structure. The internal aspect can vary in appearance. It may be completely radiolucent; it may show evidence of small foci of calcified material that appear as white flecks or small smooth pebbles; or it may show even larger, solid, amorphous masses (Fig. 21-20). In rare cases, the lesion may appear multilocular.

Effects on Surrounding Structures. In 20% to 50% of cases, this tumor is associated with a tooth (most commonly a cuspid) and impedes its eruption. Displacement of teeth and resorption of roots may occur. Perforation of the cortical plate may be seen radiographically with enlarging lesions.

Differential Diagnosis

When no internal calcifications are evident and this lesion has a pericoronal position, it may be indistinguishable from a dentigerous cyst. Other lesions that have internal calcifications to be considered include an adenomatoid odontogenic tumor, ameloblastic fibro-odontoma, and calcifying epithelial odontogenic tumor. The common location for the CCOT is not common for either the fibro-odontoma or the calcifying epithelial odontogenic tumor. Finally, long-standing cysts may have dystrophic calcification, giving a similar appearance.

Management

This tumor can be treated with enucleation and curettage. Because clinicians generally have little experience with the more solid neoplastic variants, it is wise to follow treatment with periodic radiographic evaluations for recurrence.

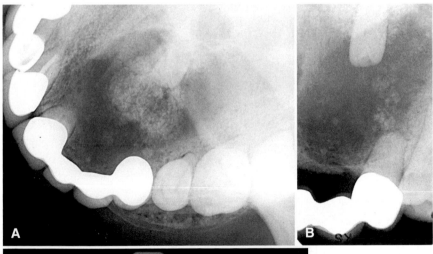

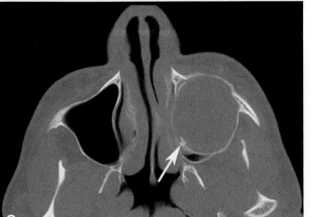

FIGURE 21-20 **A** and **B,** CCOT related to the lateral incisor. Note the well-defined corticated border, internal calcifications, and resorption of part of the root of the central incisor. **C,** Axial CT image of a large CCOT invaginating into the maxillary sinus. Note the small calcifications along the posterior border *(arrow)*.

NONODONTOGENIC CYSTS

NASOPALATINE DUCT CYST

Synonyms

Nasopalatine canal cyst, incisive canal cyst, nasopalatine cyst, median palatine cyst, and median anterior maxillary cyst are synonyms for nasopalatine duct cyst.

Definition

The nasopalatine canal usually contains remnants of the nasopalatine duct, a primitive organ of smell, and the nasopalatine vessels and nerves. A cyst occasionally forms in the nasopalatine canal when these embryonic epithelial remnants of the nasopalatine duct undergo proliferation and cystic degeneration.

Clinical Features

Nasopalatine duct cysts account for about 10% of jaw cysts. The age distribution is broad, with most cases being discovered in the fourth through sixth decades. The incidence is three times higher in males. Most of these cysts are asymptomatic or cause such minor symptoms that they are tolerated for long periods. The most frequent complaint is a small, well-defined swelling just posterior to the palatine papilla. This swelling usually is fluctuant and blue if the cyst is near the surface. The deeper nasopalatine duct cyst is covered by normal-appearing mucosa, unless it is ulcerated from masticatory trauma. If the cyst expands, it may penetrate the labial plate and produce a swelling below the maxillary labial frenum or to one side. The lesion also may bulge into the nasal cavity and distort the nasal septum. Pressure from the cyst on the adjacent nasopalatine nerves that occupy the same canal may cause a burning sensation or numbness over the palatal mucosa. In some cases, cystic fluid may drain into the oral cavity through a sinus tract or a remnant of the nasopalatine duct. The patient usually detects the fluid and reports a salty taste.

Imaging Features

Location.   Most nasopalatine duct cysts are found in the nasopalatine foramen or canal. However, if this cyst extends posteriorly to involve the hard palate (Fig. 21-21), it often is referred to as a median palatal cyst (Fig. 21-22). If it expands anteriorly between the central incisors, destroying or expanding the labial plate of bone and causing the teeth to diverge, it sometimes is referred to as a median anterior maxillary cyst. This cyst may not always be positioned symmetrically.

Periphery and Shape.   The periphery usually is well defined and corticated and is circular or oval in shape. The shadow of the nasal spine sometimes is superimposed on the cyst, giving it a heart shape.

Internal Structure.   Most nasopalatine duct cysts are totally radiolucent. Some rare cysts may have internal dystrophic

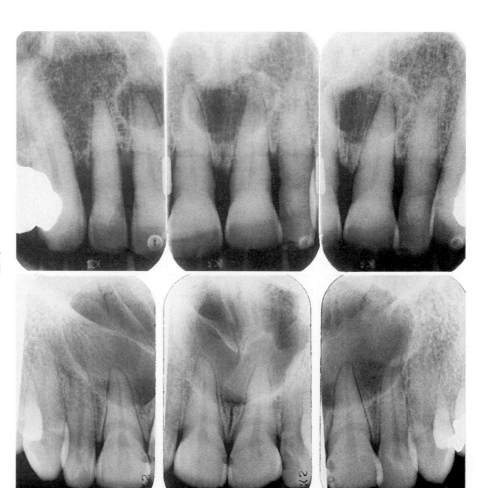

FIGURE 21-21 Two examples of nasopalatine duct cysts. Note the uniform periodontal membrane space around all the apices.

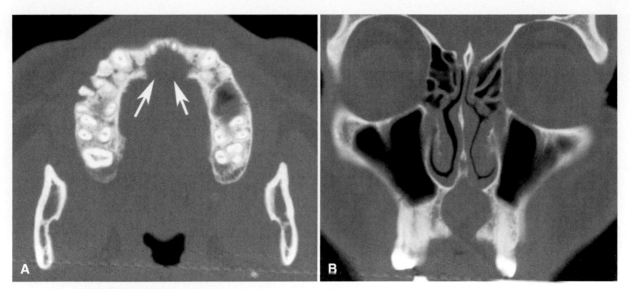

FIGURE 21-22 **A,** Axial CT image of a nasopalatine duct cyst positioned palatal to both maxillary central incisors *(arrows).* **B,** Coronal CT image of the same case.

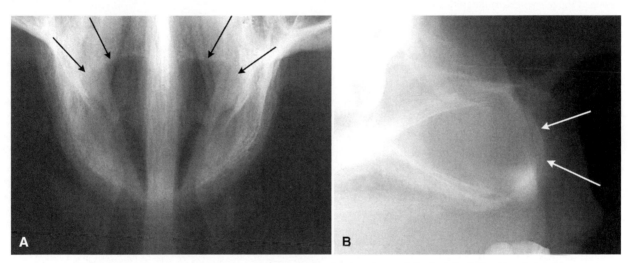

FIGURE 21-23 A nasopalatine canal cyst viewed from two perspectives *(arrows):* a standard occlusal view **(A)** and from the lateral aspect **(B)**, which is created by placing the film outside the mouth against the cheek and directing the x-ray beam at a tangent to the labial surface of the central incisors.

calcifications, which may appear as ill-defined, amorphous, scattered radiopacities.

Effects on Surrounding Structures.

Most commonly, this cyst causes the roots of the central incisors to diverge, and occasionally root resorption occurs. Seen from a lateral perspective, the cyst may expand the labial cortex and the palatal cortex (Fig. 21-23). The floor of the nasal fossa may be displaced in a superior direction.

Differential Diagnosis

The most common differential diagnosis is a large incisive foramen. A foramen larger than 6 mm may simulate the appearance of a cyst. However, a clinical examination should reveal the expansion characteristic of a cyst and other changes that occur with a space-occupying lesion, such as displacement of teeth. A lateral view of the anterior maxilla, with an occlusal film held outside the mouth and against the cheek, also can help in the differential diagnosis,

as can a cross-sectional (standard) occlusal view. If doubt still exists, comparison with previous images may be useful, aspiration may be attempted, or another image may be made in 6 months to 1 year to assess any change in size. A radicular cyst or granuloma associated with a central incisor is similar in appearance to an asymmetric nasopalatine cyst. The presence or absence of the lamina dura and enlargement of the periodontal ligament space around the apex of the central incisor indicate an inflammatory lesion. A vitality test of the central incisor may be useful. A second periapical view taken at a different horizontal angulation should show an altered position of the image of a nasopalatine duct cyst, whereas a radicular cyst should remain centered about the apex of the central incisor.

Management

The appropriate treatment for a nasopalatine cyst is enucleation, preferably from the palate to avoid the nasopalatine nerve. If the

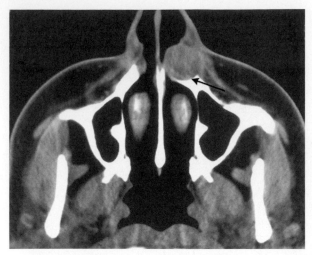

FIGURE 21-24 Nasolabial cyst shown in an axial CT image with a soft tissue algorithm. Note the well-defined periphery and the erosion of the labial aspect of the alveolar process (arrow).

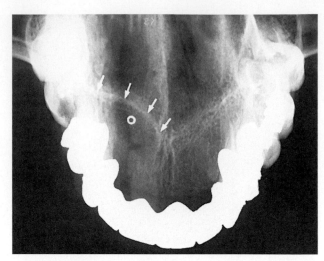

FIGURE 21-25 Occlusal view of a nasolabial cyst. Radiograph shows erosion of the alveolar bone (o) and elevation of the floor of the nasal fossa (arrows). (From Chinellato LE, Damante JH: Contribution of radiographs to the diagnosis of naso-alveolar cyst. Oral Surg Oral Med Oral Pathol 58:729-735, 1984.)

cyst is large and the danger exists of devitalizing the tooth or creating a naso-oral or antro-oral fistula, the surgeon may elect to perform marsupialization.

NASOLABIAL CYST

Synonym

A synonym for nasolabial cyst is nasoalveolar cyst.

Disease Mechanism

The exact origin of nasolabial cysts is unknown. They may be fissural cysts arising from the epithelial rests in fusion lines of the globular, lateral nasal, and maxillary processes. Alternatively, the source of the epithelium may be from the embryonic nasolacrimal duct, which initially lies on the bone surface.

Clinical Features

When this rare lesion is small, it may produce a very subtle, unilateral swelling of the nasolabial fold and may elicit pain or discomfort. When large, it may bulge into the floor of the nasal cavity, causing some obstruction, flaring of the alae, distortion of the nostrils, and fullness of the upper lip. If infected, it may drain into the nasal cavity. It usually is unilateral, but bilateral lesions have occurred. Age at detection ranges from 12 to 75 years, with a mean age of 44 years. About 75% of these lesions occur in females.

Imaging Features

Location. Nasolabial cysts are primarily soft tissue lesions located adjacent to the alveolar process above the apices of the incisors. Because this is a soft tissue lesion, plain radiographs may not show any detectable changes. The investigation could include either CT imaging or magnetic resonance imaging, both of which can provide an image of soft tissues (Fig. 21-24).

Periphery and Shape. Thin axial CT images with use of the soft tissue algorithm with contrast medium reveal a circular or oval lesion with slight soft tissue enhancement of the periphery.

Internal Structure. In CT images with the soft tissue algorithm, the internal aspect appears homogeneous and relatively radiolucent compared with the surrounding soft tissues.

Effects on Surrounding Structures. Occasionally, a cyst causes erosion of the underlying bone (Fig. 21-25), producing an increased radiolucency of the alveolar process beneath the cyst and apical to the incisors. Also, the usual outline of the inferior border of the nasal fossa may become distorted, resulting in a posterior bowing of this margin.

Differential Diagnosis

The swelling caused by an infected nasolabial cyst may simulate an acute dentoalveolar abscess. It is important to establish the vitality of the adjacent teeth. This cyst may also resemble a nasal furuncle if it pushes upward into the floor of the nasal cavity. A large mucous extravasation cyst or a cystic salivary adenoma should also be considered in the differential diagnosis of an uninfected nasolabial cyst.

Management

The nasolabial cyst should be excised through an intraoral approach. These cysts do not tend to recur.

CYSTS ORIGINATING IN SOFT TISSUES

The following four cysts may be encountered in the soft tissues adjacent to the maxillofacial region.

THYROGLOSSAL DUCT CYST

Disease Mechanism

Thyroglossal duct cyst develops from epithelial remnants of the thyroglossal duct, which at one point during development of the thyroid gland extends from the foramen cecum in the midline of the dorsal surface of the tongue to the isthmus of the thyroid gland. This cyst is the most common congenital cyst and midline mass of the head and neck.

Clinical Features

The cyst manifests as a slow-growing, painless mass, unless secondarily infected, in the midline of the neck. Most are detected in the first 2 decades of life. Most occur at the level of or below the hyoid bone, but cysts can occur above the hyoid bone to the tongue.

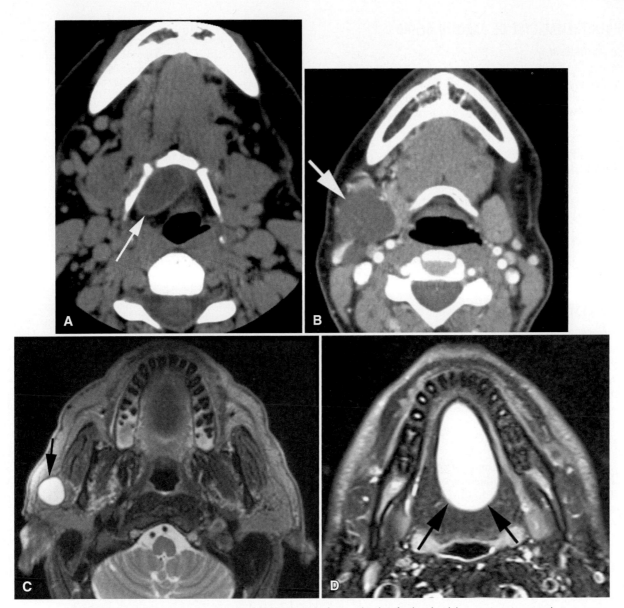

FIGURE 21-26 Four soft tissue cysts. **A,** Axial CT scan using soft tissue algorithm of a thyroglossal duct cyst *(arrow)* positioned inside the hyoid bone. Note the cystic shape and homogeneous low attenuation of the internal structure. **B,** Axial CT scan using soft tissue algorithm of a branchial cleft cyst *(arrow)* positioned just below the angle of the mandible and displacing the submandibular salivary gland medially. **C,** Axial MR image using T2 weighting of a lymphoepithelial cyst *(arrow)* positioned in the right parotid gland. Note the homogeneous high signal (white) internal structure indicating fluid. **D,** Axial MR image using T2 weighting of a dermoid cyst *(arrows)* in the floor of the mouth.

Imaging Features

The periphery is usually well defined and has a curved outline characteristic of a cyst, but the shape is influenced by the impingement of surrounding structures. The internal structure on CT images is homogeneous and low attenuation equivalent to fluid (Fig. 21-26, *A*). Many of the cysts have a relationship with the hyoid bone and can occur anterior, posterior, superior, or inferior to the hyoid bone.

BRANCHIAL CLEFT CYST

Disease Mechanism

The etiology for these cysts is controversial but seems to be related to remnants of the first to fourth fetal branchial arches. The cyst wall is usually composed of stratified squamous cell lining with some lymphoid tissue elements.

Clinical Features

These cysts occur in the lateral aspect of the neck and anterior to the sternocleidomastoid muscle. If related to the first branchial arch, it may have a preauricular position inferior to behind the angle of the mandible and sometimes related to the parotid gland. This cyst usually manifests as a slow-growing, painless (unless secondarily infected) fluctuant swelling in the second and third decades of life.

Imaging Features

As described for thyroglossal cysts, the shape and internal image density are cystlike (Fig. 21-26, *B*). The lateral position differentiates it from a thyroglossal cyst. When associated with the parotid gland, it may be difficult to differentiate from a lymphoepithelial cyst.

LYMPHOEPITHELIAL CYST OF PAROTID GLAND

Disease Mechanism

This cyst was once called a branchial cyst, but because of differences in development compared with a branchial cleft cyst, some authors believe this cyst is not of branchial origin. Commonly positioned within the parotid gland, the histologic appearance is very similar to a branchial cleft cyst.

Clinical Features

The mean age of the appearance of this cyst is the fifth decade with a slight female propensity. It usually manifests as a slow-growing enlargement in the parotid gland region. Some cysts appear to be related to human immunodeficiency virus infections.

Imaging Features

Most commonly, this cyst has a circular cystic shape with an internal density of fluid, and it is usually located within the parotid gland (Fig. 21-26, *C*).

DERMOID CYST

Disease Mechanism

Dermoid cysts are a cystic form of a teratoma thought to be derived from trapped embryonic cells that are totipotential. The resulting cysts are lined with epidermis and cutaneous appendages and filled with keratin or sebaceous material (and in rare cases with bone, teeth, muscle, or hair, in which case they are properly called teratomas).

Clinical Features

Dermoid cysts usually become clinically apparent between 12 and 25 years of age and usually manifest as a slow, painless swelling. About 10% or less arise in the head and neck with the orbital region most common, and only 1% to 2% develop in the oral cavity. Of these, about 25% occur in the floor of the mouth and on the tongue. When located in the neck or floor of the mouth, these cysts may interfere with breathing, speaking, and eating. On palpation, cysts may be fluctuant or doughy, according to their contents.

Imaging Features

Dermoid cysts are well defined with a cystic shape. Occasionally, the internal aspect may be uniformly low attenuation equivalent to fluid or may have a soft tissue multilocular appearance (Fig. 21-26, *D*). If teeth or bone form in the cyst, their radiopaque images, with characteristic shapes and densities, are apparent on the radiograph.

Differential Diagnosis

Lesions that are clinically similar to dermoid cysts are ranula (unilateral or bilateral blockage of Wharton's ducts), thyroglossal duct cysts, cystic hygromas, and branchial cleft cysts.

FORMER CYSTS

It has become clear over time that some names used to describe distinct entities are no longer valid. These names include primordial cysts (now recognized largely to be KOTs), median palatal cysts (now recognized as a variant of the nasopalatine duct cyst), and median mandibular and globulomaxillary cysts (because the theory of entrapment of epithelium is no longer accepted). Globulomaxillary cysts are now recognized to be radicular or lateral periodontal cysts or KOTs.

CYSTLIKE LESIONS

SBCs are included in this chapter because of their historic classification and because the characteristics and behavior seen in diagnostic imaging are cystic in nature. However, these lesions are not true cysts.

SIMPLE BONE CYST

Synonyms

Synonyms for SBC are traumatic bone cyst, hemorrhagic bone cyst, extravasation cyst, progressive bone cavity, solitary bone cyst, and unicameral bone cyst.

Disease Mechanism

An SBC is a cavity within bone that is lined with connective tissue. It may be empty, or it may contain fluid. However, because it has no epithelial lining, it is not a true cyst. The etiology of SBCs is unknown, although they may be a localized aberration in normal bone remodeling or metabolism. This theory is supported indirectly by the fact that these bony cavities often occur inside lesions of cemento-osseous dysplasia and fibrous dysplasia. No evidence exists to support a traumatic cause.

Clinical Features

SBCs are very common. Most occur in the first 2 decades of life, with a mean age of 17 years. The lesion shows a male predominance of approximately 2:1. Multiple SBCs can develop, especially when the disorder occurs with cemento-osseous dysplasia. The occurrence of SBCs in cemento-osseous dysplasia is seen in an older population, with a mean age of 42 years, and with a female predominance of 4:1. SBCs are asymptomatic in most cases, but occasionally pain or tenderness may be present, especially if the cyst has become secondarily infected. Expansion of the mandible or tooth movement is possible but unusual. The teeth in the affected region usually are vital. Most SBCs are discovered by chance, during radiographic examinations, and for this reason they can become quite large. There is no significant incidence of pathologic fractures. Aspiration usually produces only a few milliliters of straw-colored or serosanguineous fluid.

Imaging Features

Location. Almost all SBCs are found in the mandible (Fig. 21-27); in rare cases, they develop in the maxilla. The lesion can occur anywhere in the mandible but is seen most often in the ramus and posterior mandible in older patients. SBCs also frequently occur with cemento-osseous and fibrous dysplasia.

Periphery and Shape. The margin may vary from a well-defined, delicate cortex to an ill-defined border without a cortex that blends into the surrounding bone. The boundary usually is better defined in the alveolar process around the teeth than in the inferior aspect of the body of the mandible. The shape most often is smooth and curved, similar to a cyst, with an oval or scalloped border. The lesion often scallops between the roots of the teeth (see Fig. 21-27).

Internal Structure. The internal structure is totally radiolucent; it may occasionally appear multilocular, although the lesion does not usually contain true septa. This appearance is the result of pronounced scalloping of the endosteal surface of either the buccal or the lingual plates (Fig. 21-28). The ridges of bone produced by the scalloping give the appearance of septa on a lateral view of the mandible.

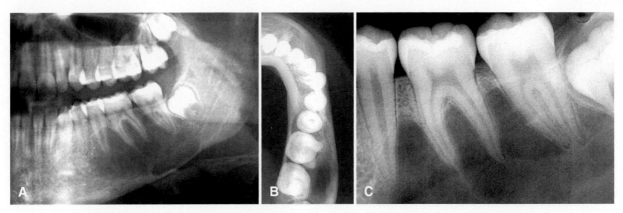

FIGURE 21-27 Panoramic film **(A)**, occlusal film **(B)**, and periapical film **(C)** demonstrating SBC. The occlusal film shows that no expansion has occurred in the buccal or lingual cortical plates. Except for the superior border, the borders are ill defined; the lesion has scalloped around the teeth, and the inferior border of the mandible is thinned, but the lamina dura is still present.

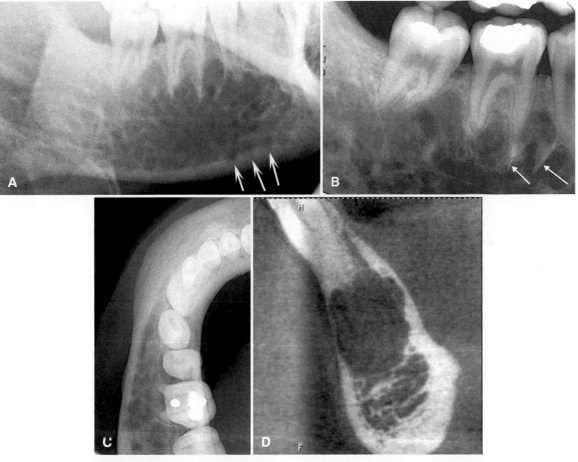

FIGURE 21-28 Lateral oblique **(A)**, periapical **(B)**, and occlusal **(C)** views of SBC. The SBC has a multilocular appearance in the lateral oblique view of the mandible **(A)**. The periapical view appears to show internal septa **(B)** (arrows) because of the scalloping of the endosteal surface of the cortical plates, as seen in the inferior cortex in **A** (arrows), and of the endosteal surface of the buccal cortex in the occlusal view **(C)**. **D,** Cone-beam CT sagittal image of a different SBC in the anterior mandible. Note the scalloping of the endosteal surface of the lingual cortex and lack of peripheral cortex.

Effects on Surrounding Structures.   In most cases, these lesions have no effect on the surrounding teeth, although rare cases of tooth displacement and resorption have been documented. Often the lesion involves all the bone around the roots of the teeth but leaves the lamina dura intact or only partly disrupted (Fig. 21-29).

Similarly, the sparing of the cortical boundary of the crypt around a developing tooth is characteristic. As previously mentioned, these lesions have a propensity to scallop the endosteal surface of the outer cortex of the mandible. SBCs also have a tendency to grow along the long axis of the bone, causing minimal expansion

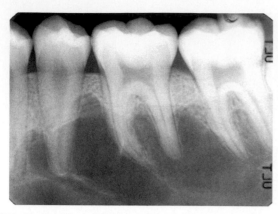

FIGURE 21-29 SBC in which the lamina dura is maintained on most root surfaces involved with the lesion except for the mesial surface of the distal root tip of the first molar.

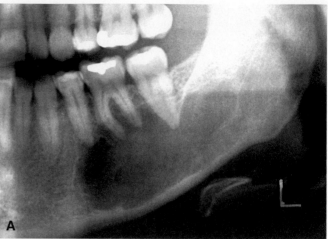

A

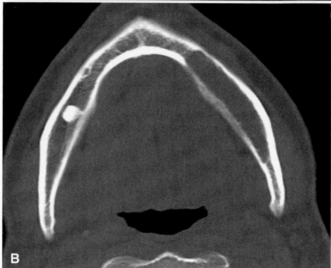

B

FIGURE 21-30 **A** and **B,** SBC extending from the first bicuspid posteriorly to the base of the ramus and occupying most of the mandible. Considering the extent of the lesion, very little expansion of the buccal or lingual cortical plates has occurred, as can be seen in the axial CT image **(B)** with bone algorithm.

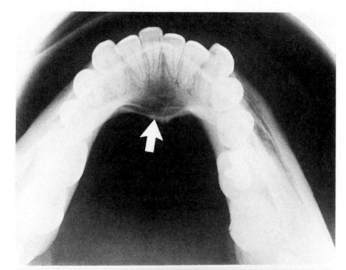

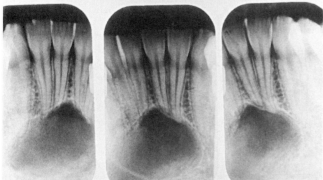

FIGURE 21-31 SBC *(arrow)* positioned in the anterior of the mandible. The superior aspect of the peripheral cortex is better defined than the inferior border, and evidence exists of some expansion of the mandible's lingual cortex, which may be due in part to muscle attachment at the genial tubercles.

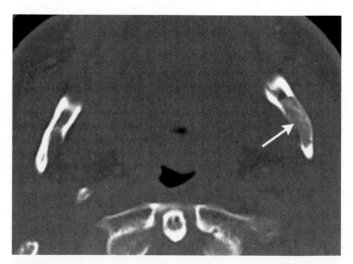

FIGURE 21-32 Axial CT image with a bone algorithm displaying a small SBC in the process of healing *(arrow)*. Note the fine internal granular bone and very slight expansion of the ramus.

(Fig. 21-30). However, expansion of the involved bone can occur and is more common with larger lesions (Fig. 21-31).

Differential Diagnosis

SBCs may have an appearance similar to that of a true cyst, especially a KOT. This is because KOTs tend to grow along bone with very little expansion and often have scalloped borders similar to those of an SBC. However, KOTs usually have a more definite cortical boundary, resorb and displace teeth, and occur in an older age group. Because the SBC may remove bone around teeth without affecting the teeth, there may be a tendency to include a malignant lesion in the differential diagnosis. However, maintenance of some lamina dura and the lack of an invasive periphery and bone destruction should be enough to remove this category of diseases from consideration.

The diagnosis relies primarily on radiographic and surgical observations because the histopathologic aspects are not characteristic. These lesions occasionally heal spontaneously. A biopsy and analysis of a healing cyst may falsely indicate the presence of an ossifying fibroma or fibrous dysplasia because of the formation of new immature bone (Fig. 21-32).

Management

The customary treatment is a conservative opening into the lesion and careful curettage of the lining; this usually initiates bleeding and subsequent healing. Spontaneous healing has been reported. Periodic follow-up radiographic examinations are advisable, especially if the patient declines treatment. These lesions can recur, but it is rare.

BIBLIOGRAPHY

Shear M: Cysts of the jaws: recent advances, *J Oral Pathol* 14:43–59, 1985.

Shear M: Developmental odontogenic cysts: an update, *J Oral Pathol Med* 23:1–11, 1994.

Odontogenic Cysts

Radicular Cyst

Stockdale CR, Chandler NP: The nature of the periapical lesion: a review of 1108 cases, *J Dent* 16:123–129, 1988.

Syrjänen S, Tammisalo E, Lilja R, et al: Radiological interpretation of the periapical cysts and granulomas, *Dentomaxillofac Radiol* 11:89–92, 1982.

Toller PA: Origin and growth of cysts of the jaws, *Ann R Coll Surg Engl* 40:306–336, 1967.

Wood RE, Nortjé CJ, Padayachee A, et al: Radicular cysts of primary teeth mimicking premolar dentigerous cysts: report of three cases, *ASDC J Dent Child* 55:288–290, 1988.

Residual Cyst

High AS, Hirschmann PN: Age changes in residual cysts, *J Oral Pathol* 15:524–528, 1986.

Schwimmer AM, Aydin F, Morrison SN: Squamous cell carcinoma arising in residual odontogenic cyst: report of a case and review of literature, *Oral Surg Oral Med Oral Pathol* 72:218–221, 1991.

Dentigerous Cyst

Daley TD, Wysocki GP: The small dentigerous cyst, *Oral Surg Oral Med Oral Pathol Oral Radiol Endod* 79:77–81, 1995.

Lustmann J, Bodner L: Dentigerous cysts associated with supernumerary teeth, *Int J Oral Maxillofac Surg* 17:100–102, 1988.

Main DM: Follicular cysts of mandibular third molar teeth: radiological evaluation of enlargement, *Dentomaxillofac Radiol* 18:156–159, 1989.

Maxymiw WG, Wood RE: Carcinoma arising in a dentigerous cyst: a case report and review of the literature, *J Oral Maxillofac Surg* 49:639–643, 1991.

Buccal Bifurcation Cyst

Bohay RN, Weinberg S: The paradental cyst of the mandibular permanent first molar: report of a bilateral case, *J Dent Child* 59:361–365, 1992.

Packota GV, Hall JM, Lanigan DT, et al: Paradental cysts on mandibular first molars in children: report of five cases, *Dentomaxillofac Radiol* 19:126–132, 1990.

Philipsen HP, Reichert PA, Ogawa I, et al: The inflammatory paradental cyst: a critical review of 342 from a literature survey, including 17 new cases from the author's files, *J Oral Pathol Med* 33:147–155, 2004.

Shear M: *Cysts of the oral regions*, Bristol, UK, 1976, John Wright & Sons.

Stoneman DW, Worth HM: The mandibular infected buccal cyst–molar area, *Dent Radiogr Photogr* 56:1–14, 1983.

Keratocystic Odontogenic Tumor

Barnes L: *World Health Organization classification of tumours: pathology and genetics: head and neck tumours*, Lyon, 2005, IARC Press.

Brannon RB: The odontogenic keratocyst: a clinicopathological study of 312 cases. I: clinical features, *Oral Surg Oral Med Oral Pathol* 42:54–72, 1976.

Kakarantza-Angelopoulou E, Nicolatou O: Odontogenic keratocysts: clinicopathologic study of 87 cases, *J Oral Maxillofac Surg* 48:593–599, 1990.

Myoung H, Hong SP, Hong SD, et al: Odontogenic keratocyst: review of 256 cases for recurrence and clinicopathologic parameters, *Oral Surg Oral Med Oral Pathol Oral Radiol Endod* 91:328–333, 2001.

Shear M: The aggressive nature of the odontogenic keratocyst: is it a benign cystic neoplasm, II: proliferation and genetic studies, *Oral Oncol* 38:323–331, 2002.

Basal Cell Nevus Syndrome

Donatsky O, Hjörting-Hansen E, Philipsen HP, et al: Clinical, radiographic, and histologic features of the basal cell nevus syndrome, *Int J Oral Surg* 5:19–28, 1976.

Evans DC, Farndon PA, Burnell LD, et al: The incidence of Gorlin syndrome in 173 consecutive cases of medulloblastoma, *Br J Cancer* 64:959–961, 1991.

Gorlin RJ: Nevoid basal cell carcinoma syndrome, *Medicine* 66:98–113, 1987.

Lam EWN, Lee L, Perschbacher SE, et al: The occurrence of keratocystic odontogenic tumours in nevoid basal cell carcinoma syndrome, *Dentomaxillofac Radiol* 38:475–479, 2009.

Lateral Periodontal Cyst

Shear M, Pindborg JJ: Microscopic features of the lateral periodontal cyst, *Scand J Dent Res* 83:103–110, 1975.

Weathers DR, Waldron CA: Unusual multilocular cysts of the jaws (botryoid odontogenic cysts), *Oral Surg Oral Med Oral Pathol* 36:235–241, 1973.

Wysocki GP, Brannon RB, Gardner DG, et al: Histogenesis of the lateral periodontal cyst and the gingival cyst of the adult, *Oral Surg Oral Med Oral Pathol* 50:327–334, 1980.

Glandular Odontogenic Cyst

Koppang HS, Johannessen S, Haugen LK, et al: Glandular odontogenic cyst: report of two cases and literature review of 45 previously reported cases, *J Oral Pathol Med* 27:455–462, 1998.

Noffke C, Raubenheimer EJ: The glandular odontogenic cyst: clinical and radiologic features: review of the literature and report of nine cases, *Dentomaxillofac Radiol* 31:333–338, 2002.

Calcifying Cystic Odontogenic Tumor

Johnson A III, Fletcher M, Gold L, et al: Calcifying odontogenic cyst: a clinicopathologic study of 57 cases with immunohistochemical evaluation for cytokeratin, *J Oral Maxillofac Surg* 55:679–683, 1997.

Moleri AB, Moreira LC, Carvalho JJ: Comparative morphology of 7 new cases of calcifying odontogenic cysts, *J Oral Maxillofac Surg* 60:689–696, 2002.

Yoshiura K, Tabata O, Miwa K, et al: Computed tomographic features of calcifying odontogenic cysts, *Dentomaxillofac Radiol* 27:12–16, 1998.

Nonodontogenic Cysts

Nasopalatine Duct Cyst

Elliott KA, Franzese CB, Pitman KT: Diagnosis and surgical management of nasopalatine duct cysts, *Laryngoscope* 114:1336–1340, 2004.

Mraiwa RJ, Jacobs R, Van Cleynenbreugel J, et al: The nasopalatine duct cyst revisited using 2D and 3D CT imaging, *Dentomaxillofac Radiol* 33:396–402, 2004.

Swanson KS, Kaugars GE, Gunsolley JC: Nasopalatine duct cyst: an analysis of 334 cases, *J Oral Maxillofac Surg* 49:268–271, 1991.

Nasolabial Cyst

Choi JH, Cho JH, Kang HJ, et al: Nasolabial cysts: a retrospective analysis of 18 cases, *Ear Nose Throat J* 81:94–96, 2002.

Yuen H, Julian CY, Samuel CL: Nasolabial cysts: clinical features, diagnosis and treatment, *Br J Oral Maxillofac Surg* 45:293–297, 2007.

Soft Tissue Cysts

Thyroglossal Duct Cyst

Ahuja AT, Wong KT, King AD, et al: Imaging for thyroglossal duct cyst: the bare essentials, *Clin Radiol* 60:141–148, 2005.

Branchial Cleft Cyst

Glosser JW, Pires CA, Feinberg SE: Branchial cleft or cervical lymphoepithelial cysts: etiology and management, *J Am Dent Assoc* 134:81–86, 2003.

Lymphoepithelial Cyst

Wu L, Cheng J, Maruyama S, et al: Lymphoepithelial cyst of the parotid gland: its possible histopathogenesis based on clinicopathologic analysis of 64 cases, *Hum Pathol* 40:683–692, 2009.

Dermoid Cyst

Pryor SG, Lewis JE, Weaver AL, et al: Pediatric dermoid cysts of the head and neck, *Otolaryngol Head Neck Surg* 132:938–942, 2005.

Seward GR: Dermoid cysts of the floor of the mouth, *Br J Oral Surg* 3:36–47, 1965.

Cystlike Lesions

Simple Bone Cyst

Damante JH, Da S, Guerra EN, et al: Spontaneous resolution of simple bone cysts, *Dentomaxillofac Radiol* 31:182–186, 2002.

Kaugars GE, Cale AE: Traumatic bone cyst, *Oral Surg Oral Med Oral Pathol* 63:318–324, 1987.

Perdigao AF, Silva EC, Sakurai E, et al: Idiopathic bone cavity: a clinical, radiographic and histological study, *Br J Oral Maxillofac Surg* 41:407–409, 2003.

Saito Y, Hoshina Y, Nagamine T, et al: Simple bone cyst: a clinical and histopathologic study of fifteen cases, *Oral Surg Oral Med Oral Pathol* 74:487–491, 1992.

Sapp PJ, Stark ML: Self-healing traumatic bone cysts, *Oral Surg Oral Med Oral Pathol* 69:597–602, 1990.

Benign Tumors

DISEASE MECHANISM

A benign tumor represents a new uncoordinated growth that generally has the following characteristics. Benign tumors are slowly growing and spread by direct extension and not by metastases. They tend to resemble the tissue of origin histologically. For example, an ameloblastoma, a tumor thought to be derived from odontogenic epithelium, often is composed of cells that resemble ameloblasts. It is thought that benign tumors have unlimited growth potential. Hamartomas often are included in the category of benign tumors. However, hamartomas are overgrowths of disorganized normal tissue that have a limited growth potential. For example, an odontoma is a hamartoma of dental tissue (disorganized enamel, dentin, and pulp tissues) derived from the dental follicle that stops growing at approximately the same time as other normal dental tissues. Included in this chapter are hyperplasias. Hyperplasia refers to a growth formed by an increase in the number of cells of a tissue but differs from a hamartoma in that the tissue is in a normal arrangement. Hyperplasia is generally thought to be a reaction to a stimulus, such as inflammation. Therefore, hyperplasias have limited growth potential and tend to regress when the stimulus is removed.

CLINICAL FEATURES

Benign tumors typically have an insidious onset and grow slowly. These tumors usually are painless, do not metastasize, and are not life-threatening unless they interfere with a vital organ by direct extension.

Benign tumors are usually detected clinically by enlargement of the jaws or are found during a radiographic examination. Sometimes the radiologic examination is performed to try to discover the reason for the lack of development of a tooth.

RADIOLOGIC EXAMINATION

Once the clinician has made a preliminary diagnosis of the presence of a tumor, a full radiologic examination should be performed to document the extent and characteristics of the lesion. This examination may entail further images, such as panoramic, intraoral, or occlusal images. For central bone lesions, the addition of computed tomographic (CT) imaging is essential for assessing the three-dimensional characteristics of the entity. If the lesion originates in soft tissue or has extended from bone into the surrounding soft tissue, magnetic resonance imaging (MRI) may be required.

A thorough radiologic examination provides information regarding the extent of the lesion. On one hand, sometimes the characteristics are so specific that a preliminary diagnosis of the type of benign tumor can be made. On the other hand, the imaging characteristics of the lesion may fail to indicate the type of tumor. A thorough workup also indicates the most favorable biopsy site. In most cases, the radiologic examination should be completed before the biopsy procedure.

IMAGING FEATURES

The following general features suggest the presence of a benign neoplasm.

LOCATION

Because many tumors have a specific anatomic predilection, the location of a particular neoplasm is important in establishing the differential diagnosis. For example, odontogenic lesions occur in the alveolar processes above the inferior alveolar nerve canal, where tooth formation occurs. Vascular and neural lesions may originate inside the mandibular canal, arising from the neurovascular tissues. Cartilaginous tumors occur in jaw locations where residual cartilaginous cells lie, such as around the mandibular condyle.

PERIPHERY AND SHAPE

Benign tumors enlarge slowly by formation of additional internal tissue and, as a result, the borders of benign tumors appear relatively smooth, well defined, and sometimes corticated. If the tumor produces a calcified product, such as abnormal tooth material or abnormal bone, the most mature part of the tumor is in the central region with the most immature aspect at the periphery. Sometimes a radiolucent band of soft tissue or capsule results at the periphery where the calcified product has not yet formed; this band separates the more mature internal radiopaque portion from the surrounding normal bone.

INTERNAL STRUCTURE

The internal structure may be completely radiolucent or radiopaque or may be a mixture of radiolucent and radiopaque tissues. If the lesion contains radiopaque elements, these structures usually represent residual bone, reactive bone formation, or a calcified material that is being produced by the tumor. Curved septa that are characteristic in ameloblastoma represent residual bone trapped inside the tumor that has remodeled into curved septa by internal cystic structures. An ameloblastoma does not produce bone. An osteoblastoma often has an internal granular radiopaque pattern produced by the abnormal bone that is actually being manufactured by the tumor. Often the internal pattern is characteristic for specific types of tumors and may help with the diagnosis. A totally radiolucent internal structure is not as useful as an aid to the diagnosis.

EFFECTS ON SURROUNDING STRUCTURES

The manner in which a tumor affects adjacent tissues may suggest a benign behavior. For example, a benign tumor exerts pressure on neighboring structures, resulting in the displacement of teeth or bony cortices. If the growth is slow enough, there is adequate time for the outer cortex to remodel in response to the pressure, resulting in an appearance that the cortex has been displaced by the tumor (Fig. 22-1). This appearance is caused by simultaneous resorption of bone along the inner surface (endosteal) of the cortex and deposition of bone along the outer cortical surface by the periosteum (Fig. 22-2). Through this remodeling process, the cortex maintains its integrity and resists perforation, although faster growing tumors may exceed this process resulting in perforation of the cortex. Benign tumors may also cause bodily displacement of nearby teeth (Fig. 22-3). The movement of teeth adjacent to benign tumors is slow because these lesions grow slowly.

The roots of teeth may be resorbed by either benign or malignant tumors, but root resorption more commonly is associated with benign processes. The benign tumors especially likely to resorb roots are ameloblastomas, ossifying fibromas, and central giant cell granulomas. Benign tumors tend to resorb the adjacent root surfaces in a smooth fashion. Bone dysplasias such as fibrous dysplasia do not usually resorb teeth. When root resorption is associated with malignant tumors, the resorption is usually in smaller quantities causing thinning of the root into a "spiked" shape.

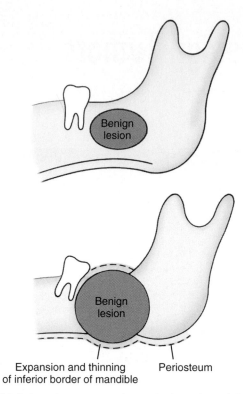

FIGURE 22-1 Benign lesions growing in bone tend to be round or oval. They grow by displacing adjacent tissues.

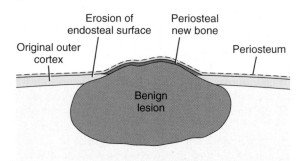

FIGURE 22-2 The host bone of a benign tumor may expand as a result of outward remodeling of its cortical borders. As the benign tumor extends toward the periphery of the bone, the periosteum lays down new bone along the outer cortex, maintaining the integrity of the cortex.

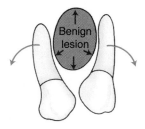

FIGURE 22-3 A benign lesion usually grows slowly, causing displacement of adjacent teeth.

HYPERPLASIAS

DISEASE MECHANISM

Bony hyperplasias are included in this chapter but are not considered tumors because of the normal arrangement of the tissue and limited growth potential; in some cases, this growth is in response to a stimulus. Bony hyperplasias are growths of normal new bone that sometimes occur in characteristic locations. In dentistry, the terms exostosis and hyperostosis are both used to describe a bony growth that occurs on the surface of normal bone. In the medical literature, the term exostosis often is used for a surface bony growth with a cartilage cap (osteochondroma). Therefore, the term hyperostosis may be preferred to avoid confusion.

TORUS PALATINUS

Synonym

A synonym for torus palatinus is palatine torus.

Disease Mechanism

Torus palatinus is a bony protuberance (hyperostosis) that occurs in the middle third of the midline of the hard palate.

Clinical Features

Torus palatinus, the most common hyperostosis, occurs in about 20% of the population, although various studies have shown marked differences in racial groups. It develops about twice as often in women as in men and more often in Native Americans, Eskimos, and Norwegians. Although it may be discovered at any age, it is rare in children. It usually begins developing in young adults before 30 years of age and is thought to arise through interplay of genetic and environmental factors. The base of the bony nodule extends along the central portion of the hard palate,

and the bulk reaches downward into the oral cavity. The size and shape of a torus palatinus can vary, and these lesions have been described as flat, lobulated, nodular, or mushroom-like (Fig. 22-4, *A*). Normal mucosa covers the bony mass and may appear pale and sometimes ulcerated when traumatized. Patients often are unaware of this hyperplasia, and patients who do discover it may insist that it occurred suddenly and has been growing rapidly.

Imaging Features

Location.   On maxillary periapical or panoramic images, a torus palatinus appears as a dense radiopaque shadow below and attached to the hard palate. It may be superimposed over the apical areas of the maxillary teeth, especially if the torus has developed in the middle or anterior regions of the palate. The image of a palatal torus may project over the roots of the maxillary molars (Fig. 22-4, *B*), but this image usually moves in its position relative to the roots of the teeth if another film is taken with a different horizontal or vertical angulation of the central ray (Fig. 22-5).

Periphery and Shape.   The border of the radiopaque shadow usually is well defined and may have a convex or a lobulated outline (Fig. 22-6).

Internal Structure.   The internal aspect is homogeneously radiopaque.

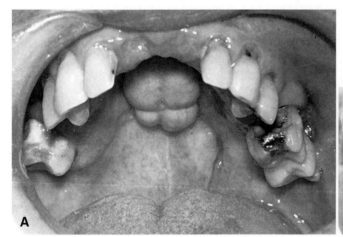
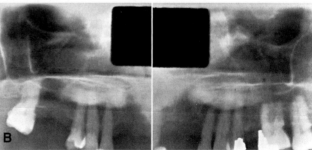

FIGURE 22-4 **A,** Clinical photograph of torus palatinus. **B,** Panoramic image shows the radiopaque shadow of torus palatinus above the maxillary premolars and canine. *(Courtesy Ronald Baker, DDS, Chapel Hill, NC.)*

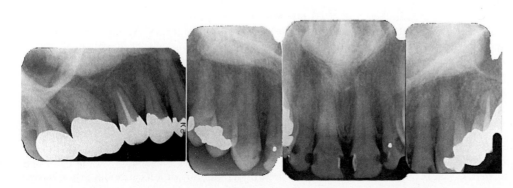

FIGURE   22-5 Maxillary periapical images show a radiopaque area with the well-defined borders of torus palatinus.

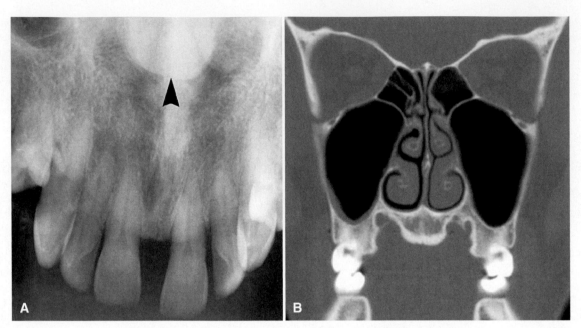

FIGURE 22-6 **A,** Torus palatinus *(arrowhead)* on an occlusal image. **B,** Coronal CT image.

Treatment

A torus palatinus usually does not require treatment, although removal may be necessary if a maxillary denture is to be made.

TORUS MANDIBULARIS

Synonym

A synonym for torus mandibularis is mandibular torus.

Disease Mechanism

Torus mandibularis is a hyperostosis that protrudes from the lingual aspect of the mandibular alveolar process, usually near the premolar teeth.

Clinical Features

Tori occur less often on the lingual surface of the mandible than on the palate, with the former occurring in about 8% of the population. These tori develop singly or multiply, unilaterally or bilaterally (usually bilaterally), and most often in the premolar region. The size also varies, ranging from an outgrowth that is just palpable to one that contacts a torus on the opposite side. In contrast to torus palatinus, torus mandibularis develops later, being first discovered in middle-aged adults. However, it has the same gender predilection as torus palatinus. In women, the occurrence of torus mandibularis correlates with that of torus palatinus, but this apparently is not the case in men. As with torus palatinus, torus mandibularis may occur more often in individuals of Asian ancestry.

Genetic and environmental factors seem to be involved in the development of torus mandibularis, but masticatory stress is reported as an essential factor underlying its formation. The high prevalence among Eskimos and other subarctic peoples who make extraordinary chewing demands on their teeth seems to support this suggestion. Also, a patient with a torus mandibularis has, on average, more teeth present than a patient without a torus.

Imaging Features

Location.   Recognition of mandibular tori relies on their appearance and location. Their presence bilaterally reinforces this impression, although they can occur unilaterally. On mandibular periapical images, a torus mandibularis appears as a radiopaque shadow, usually superimposed on the roots of premolars and molars and occasionally over a canine or incisor. It usually is superimposed over about three teeth.

Periphery.   Mandibular tori are sharply demarcated anteriorly on periapical images and are less dense and less well defined as they extend posteriorly (Fig. 22-7). There is no margin between the periphery of the torus and the surface of the mandible because the torus is continuous with the mandibular cortex.

Internal Structure.   On occlusal images, a mandibular torus appears as radiopaque and homogeneous (Fig. 22-8).

Treatment

A torus mandibularis usually does not require treatment, although removal may be necessary if a mandibular denture is planned.

HYPEROSTOSIS

Synonym

Exostosis is a synonym for hyperostosis. In the dental literature, the terms hyperostosis and exostosis are equivalent, but in the medical literature the term exostosis is often used as an equivalent term for osteochondroma, which is different from the entity hyperostosis.

Disease Mechanism

In addition to tori, other hyperostoses or exostoses may occur at other sites in the jaws. These are usually small regions of osseous hyperplasia of cortical bone and occasionally internal cancellous bone and usually occur on the surface of the alveolar process.

Clinical Features

Hyperostoses may develop most commonly on the buccal surface of the maxillary alveolar process, usually in the canine or molar area. They may also occur on the palatal surface or crest and less commonly on the mandibular alveolar process. Occasionally, they grow on the crest under a pontic of a fixed bridge. They are less

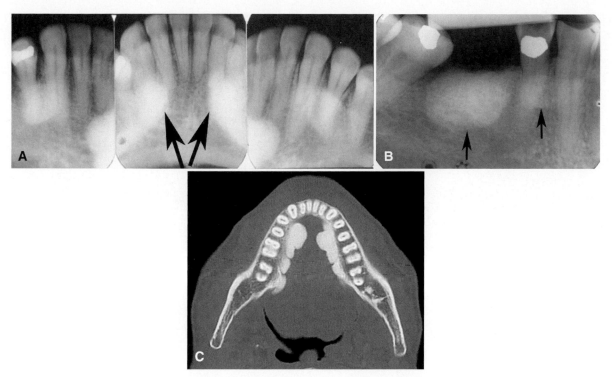

FIGURE 22-7 **A** and **B,** Mandibular tori usually are seen as dense radiopacities *(arrows).* **C,** Axial CT image with bilateral mandibular tori.

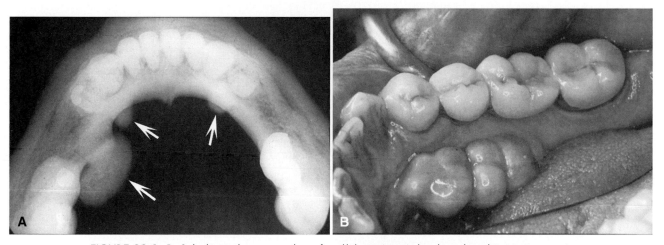

FIGURE 22-8 **A,** Occlusal image shows an unusual case of mandibular tori *(arrows)* where the number and size are not symmetric between the sides. **B,** Clinical picture of a different case. The tori extend from the region of the cuspid to the first molar. (**B,** *Courtesy Dr. Bernard Friedland, Harvard University.)*

common than mandibular or palatine tori, may attain a large size, and may be solitary or multiple. They are nodular, pedunculated, or flat prominences on the surface of the bone. They are covered with a normal mucosa and are bony hard on palpation. Published studies suggest a male predominance and an increase in frequency with age. As with the tori described previously, they appear to be more prevalent in Native Americans.

Imaging Features

Location.   The maxillary alveolar process is the most common location, and usually the image overlaps the roots of the adjacent teeth.

Periphery.   The periphery of a hyperostosis is usually well defined and smoothly contoured with a curved border (Fig. 22-9). However, some may have poorly defined borders that blend into the surrounding normal bone.

Internal Structure.   The internal aspect of a hyperostosis usually is homogeneous and radiopaque. Although large hyperostoses can have an internal cancellous bone pattern, they most often consist only of cortical bone.

Treatment

Hyperostoses usually do not require treatment.

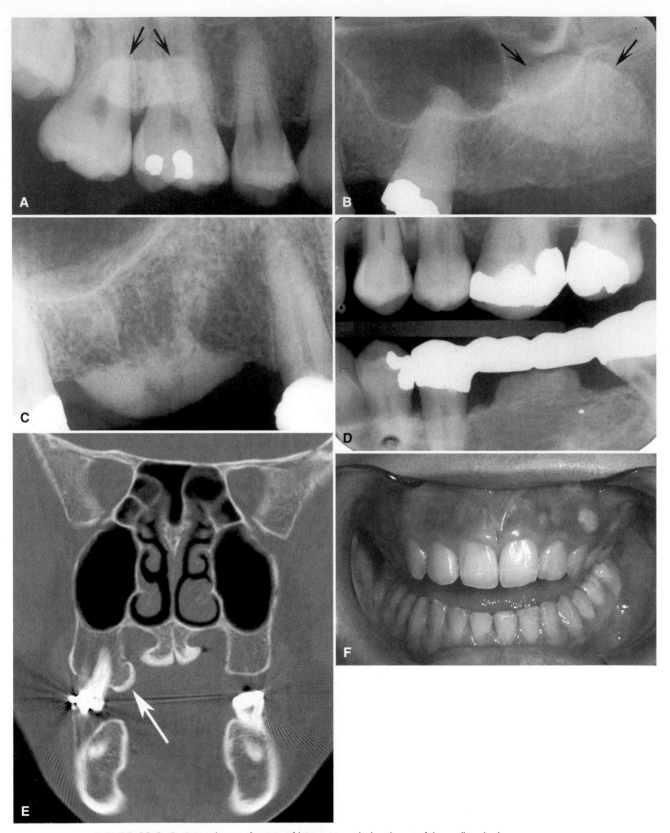

FIGURE 22-9 **A,** Periapical image of a region of hyperostosis on the buccal aspect of the maxillary alveolar process, seen as a region of slight increase in radiopacity overlapping the roots of the molars *(arrows).* **B,** Another example of hyperostosis overlapping an edentulous ridge. **C,** Hyperostosis on the crest of the alveolar ridge. **D,** Hyperostosis under a bridge pontic. **E,** Coronal CT image of hyperostosis located on the palatal aspect of the right maxillary alveolar process. Note the presence of a maxillary torus. **F,** Clinical photograph of a small hyperostosis occurring on the labial surface of the maxillary alveolar ridge.

DENSE BONE ISLAND

Synonyms

Enostosis and periapical idiopathic osteosclerosis are synonyms for dense bone island (DBI).

Disease Mechanism

DBIs are the internal counterparts of exostoses. They are localized growths of compact bone that develop within the cancellous bone.

Clinical Features

DBIs are asymptomatic.

Imaging Features

Location.   DBIs are more common in the mandible than in the maxilla. They occur most often in the premolar-molar area (Fig. 22-10), although their existence does not correlate with the presence or absence of teeth.

Periphery.   The periphery is usually well defined but occasionally blends with the trabeculae of the surrounding bone. There is no trace of a radiolucent margin or capsule as the radiopaque DBI abuts directly against normal bone.

Internal Structure.   The internal aspect of DBIs usually is uniformly radiopaque without any characteristic pattern, but sometimes there may be patches of more radiolucent areas depending on form and thickness.

Effects on Surrounding Structures.   Rarely, a DBI is located periapical to a tooth root and is associated with external root resorption (see Fig. 22-10, C). The tooth most often involved is the mandibular first molar. In all circumstances, the tooth is vital, and the root resorption appears to be self-limiting. In very rare cases, DBIs can inhibit the eruption of a tooth and even displace a tooth.

Differential Diagnosis

Several radiopaque entities must be considered in forming a differential diagnosis. Periapical osseous dysplasia (POD) can be differentiated by the presence of its radiolucent periphery. When a DBI is located at the root apex, it may resemble periapical sclerosing osteitis. However, in periapical osteitis, there is an associated widening of the periapical portion of the periodontal membrane space. Also, periapical osteitis should be centered on the root apex of the tooth and extend in a more symmetric form in every direction. Finally, an inflammatory lesion may have an apparent etiology, such as a large restoration or carious lesion. There may be some similarity to hypercementosis or a benign cementoblastoma, but in both cases there should be a soft tissue (radiolucent) capsule at the periphery. DBIs are often static but may increase in size, especially when there is active growth of the jaws. If five or more DBIs are present, familial adenomatous polyposis (e.g., Gardner's syndrome) should be considered.

Treatment

DBI does not require treatment. If multiple DBIs are present, the patient's family history should be reviewed for incidences of cancer of the intestine.

BENIGN TUMORS

Benign neoplasias are separated into two major groups: (1) odontogenic tumors and (2) nonodontogenic tumors.

ODONTOGENIC TUMORS

DISEASE MECHANISM

Odontogenic tumors arise from the tissues of the odontogenic apparatus. According to the World Health Organization (WHO), these tumors can be classified into three categories depending on the type of tissue that makes up each tumor: (1) tumors composed of odontogenic epithelium, (2) mixed tumors composed of both odontogenic epithelium and odontogenic ectomesenchyme (connective tissue), and (3) tumors composed of primarily ectomesenchyme. Odontogenic tumors account for 1.3% to 15% of all oral tumors. Benign jaw tumors are presented in this chapter according to their tissues of origin. This format should assist the reader in learning to correlate the radiographic appearance of tumors with the underlying pathologic basis of the disease process.

ODONTOGENIC EPITHELIAL TUMORS

Ameloblastoma

Synonyms.   Synonyms for ameloblastoma include adamantinoma, adamantoblastoma, and epithelial odontoma.

Disease Mechanism.   Ameloblastoma, a true neoplasm of odontogenic epithelium, is a persistent and locally invasive tumor; it has aggressive but benign growth characteristics. Ameloblastomas are by far the most common odontogenic tumor. Ameloblastoma is an aggressive neoplasm that arises from remnants of the dental lamina and dental organ (odontogenic epithelium). Malignant forms of this neoplasm exist, and these are discussed in Chapter 24. Ameloblastomas may be divided into solid/multicystic type, unicystic type, and desmoplastic type. The unicystic variant may develop as a single entity or may form from the epithelial lining of a dentigerous cyst; this is called a mural (within the wall) ameloblastoma. The existence of peripheral (soft tissue location) forms of this neoplasm is well documented.

Clinical Features.   There is a slight predilection for this lesion to occur in men, and it develops more often in African Americans. Although it may be found in young children (3 years) and in individuals older than 80 years, most patients are between 20 and 50 years of age, with the average age at discovery about 40 years.

Ameloblastomas grow slowly, and few, if any, symptoms occur in the early stages. The tumor is frequently discovered during a routine dental examination. Usually the patient eventually notices gradually increasing facial asymmetry. Swelling of the cheek, gingiva, or hard palate has been reported as the chief complaint in 95% of untreated maxillary ameloblastomas. The mucosa over the mass is normal, but teeth in the involved region may be displaced and become mobile. In most cases, patients with ameloblastomas do not have pain, paresthesia, fistula, ulcer formation, or tooth mobility. As the tumor enlarges, palpation may elicit a bony hard sensation or crepitus as the bone thins. If the lesion destroys overlying bone, the swelling may feel firm or fluctuant. As it grows, this tumor can cause bony expansion and sometimes erosion through the adjacent cortical plate with subsequent invasion of the adjacent soft tissues.

An untreated tumor may grow to a great size and is more of a concern in the maxilla, where it can extend into vital structures and reach into the cranial base. Tumors that develop in the maxilla may extend into the paranasal sinuses, orbit, nasopharynx, or vital structures at the base of the skull. Recurrence rates are higher in older patients and in patients with multilocular lesions. As seen with other jaw tumors, local recurrence, whether detected

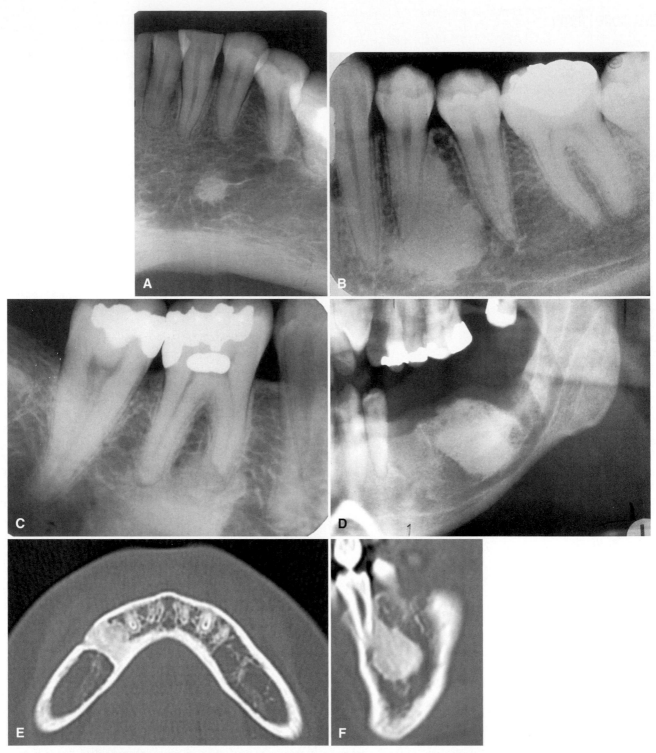

FIGURE 22-10 **A,** Small DBI apical to the first bicuspid. Note the lack of a soft tissue capsule. Also, some of the surrounding trabeculae appear to merge into the radiopaque mass. **B,** Larger DBI between the bicuspids. Note the normal-appearing periodontal membrane space. **C,** DBI apical to the first molar causing external root resorption of the mesial root. **D,** Large DBI occupying the body of the left mandible. **E** and **F,** Axial and sagittal CT images of DBI. Note the sharp margin without any soft tissue capsule.

radiographically or histologically, may have a more aggressive character than the original tumor.

Imaging Features

Location.   Most ameloblastomas (80%) develop in the molar-ramus region of the mandible, but they may extend to the symphyseal area. Most lesions that occur in the maxilla are in the third molar area and extend into the maxillary sinus and nasal floor. In either jaw, this tumor can originate in an occlusal position to a developing tooth (Fig. 22-11).

Periphery.   An ameloblastoma is usually well defined and frequently delineated by a cortical border. The border is often curved,

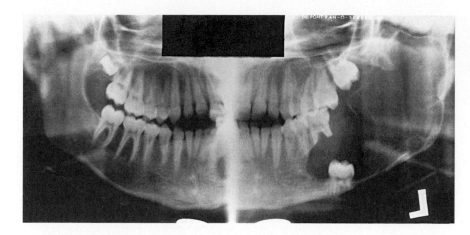

FIGURE 22-11 Unicystic ameloblastoma developing occlusal to the left second mandibular molar causing expansion of the mandibular body and ramus to the sigmoid notch and condylar neck as well as inferior displacement of the mandibular second molar and root resorption of the alveolar left first molar. *(Courtesy E. J. Burkes, DDS, Chapel Hill, NC.)*

and in small lesions the border and shape may be indistinguishable from a cyst (Fig. 22-12). The periphery of lesions in the maxilla is usually more ill defined.

Internal Structure. The internal structure varies from totally radiolucent (see Fig. 22-11) to mixed with the presence of bony septa creating internal compartments. These septa can be straight but are more commonly coarse and curved and originate from normal bone that has been trapped within the tumor. Because this tumor frequently has internal cystic components, these septa are often remodeled into curved shapes providing honeycomb (numerous small compartments or loculations) or soap bubble (larger compartments of variable size) patterns (see Fig. 22-12). Generally, the loculations are larger in the posterior mandible and smaller in the anterior mandible. In the desmoplastic variety, the internal structure can be composed of very irregular sclerotic bone resembling a bone dysplasia or bone-forming tumor (Fig. 22-13).

Effects on Surrounding Structures. There is a pronounced tendency for ameloblastomas to cause extensive root resorption (Fig. 22-14). Tooth displacement is common. Because a common point of origin is occlusal to a tooth, some teeth may be displaced apically. An occlusal radiograph may demonstrate cystlike expansion and thinning of an adjacent cortical plate leaving a thin "eggshell" of bone (Fig. 22-15). CT images often reveal regions of perforation of the expanded cortical plate owing to the inability of the production of periosteal new bone to keep up with the rate of growth of the expanding ameloblastoma (Fig. 22-16). Unicystic types of ameloblastoma may cause extreme expansion of the mandibular ramus, and often the anterior border of the ramus is no longer visible in the panoramic image (Fig. 22-17).

Recurrent Ameloblastoma. Ameloblastomas may recur when the initial surgical procedure inadequately removes the entire tumor. Recurrent tumor has a characteristic appearance of multiple small cystlike structures with very coarse sclerotic cortical margins (Fig. 22-18) and sometimes separated by normal bone.

Additional Imaging. If a preliminary diagnosis of ameloblastoma is made, multidetector CT (MDCT) imaging is highly recommended. MDCT imaging not only can confirm the diagnosis but also accurately demonstrates the anatomic extent of the tumor (see Fig. 22-16). In this regard, MDCT imaging has an advantage over cone-beam CT imaging in that it can display soft tissue structures (soft tissue algorithm) and can detect perforation of the outer cortex and invasion into the surrounding soft tissues. If soft tissue

invasion is extensive, an MRI can provide superior images of the nature and extent of the invasion. CT examination is essential in the postsurgical follow-up assessment of ameloblastoma.

Differential Diagnosis. Small unilocular ameloblastomas that are located around the crown of an unerupted tooth often cannot be differentiated from a dentigerous cyst. Because the appearance of the internal bony septa is important for the identification of ameloblastoma, other types of lesions that also have internal septa, such as odontogenic keratocyst, giant cell granuloma, odontogenic myxoma, and ossifying fibroma, may have a similar appearance. An odontogenic keratocyst may contain curved septa, but usually the keratocyst tends to grow along the bone without marked expansion, which is characteristic of ameloblastomas. Giant cell granulomas occur in a younger age group and have more granular or wispy ill-defined septa. Odontogenic myxomas may have similar-appearing septa; however, there are usually one or two thin sharp, straight septa, which is characteristic of the myxoma. The presence of even one such septum may indicate a myxoma. Also, myxomas are not as expansile as ameloblastomas and tend to grow along the bone. The septa in ossifying fibroma are usually wide, granular, and ill defined, and often there are small, irregular trabeculae.

Treatment. The most common treatment is surgical resection. The surgical procedure should take into account the tendency of the neoplasm to invade adjacent bone beyond its apparent radiographic margins. MDCT imaging and MRI are useful in determining the exact extent of the tumor. If the ameloblastoma is relatively small, it may be removed completely by an intraoral approach, and larger lesions may require resection of the jaw. The maxilla is usually treated more aggressively because of the tendency of ameloblastoma to invade adjacent vital structures. Radiation therapy may be used for inoperable tumors, especially tumors in the posterior maxilla.

Calcifying Epithelial Odontogenic Tumor

Synonyms. Synonyms for calcifying epithelial odontogenic tumor (CEOT) include Pindborg tumor and ameloblastoma of unusual type with calcification.

Disease Mechanism. CEOTs are rare neoplasms. They account for about 1% of odontogenic tumors. These tumors usually are located within bone and produce a mineralized substance within

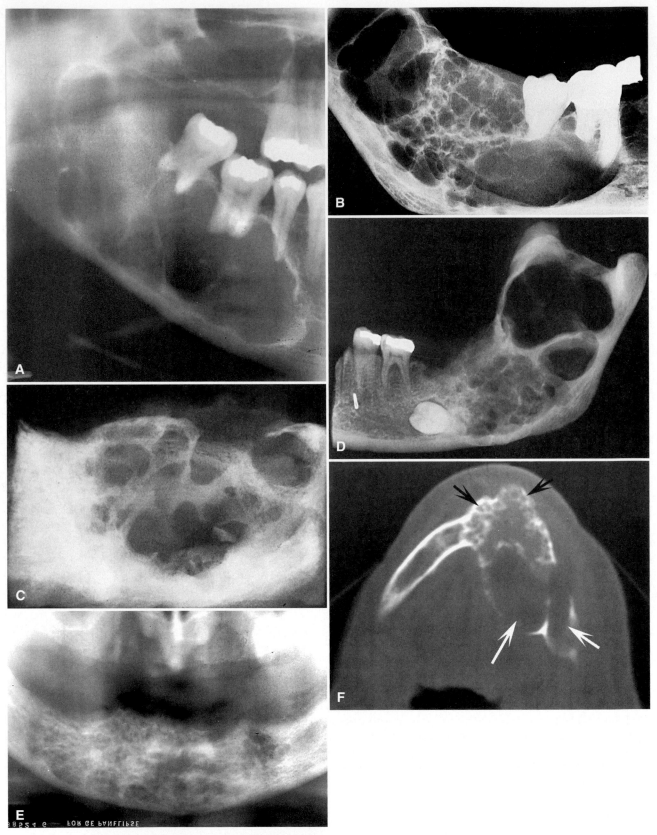

FIGURE 22-12 Multilocular ameloblastomas. **A,** Large lesion in the mandibular body and ramus shows only a few straight septa. **B,** Lateral radiograph of a resected mandibular specimen containing a multilocular ameloblastoma. Note the coarse, curved septa. **C,** Another surgical specimen of an ameloblastoma. **D,** Large multilocular lesion in the right mandibular ramus. **E,** Cropped panoramic image showing small loculations that are more common in the anterior mandible. **F,** Axial CT image using bone algorithm shows a large ameloblastoma. Note the smaller loculations in the anterior mandible *(black arrows)* and the larger loculations in the posterior mandible *(white arrows).*

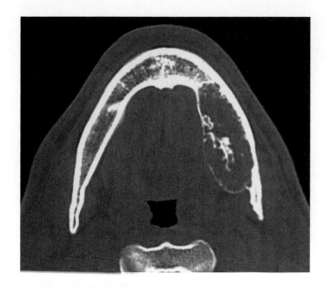

FIGURE 22-13 Example of the desmoplastic type of ameloblastoma. Note the internal irregular bone formation on this axial CT image.

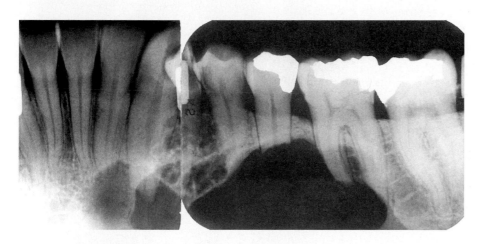

FIGURE 22-14 Root resorption of the premolars and canine adjacent to a radiolucent ameloblastoma in the left mandible.

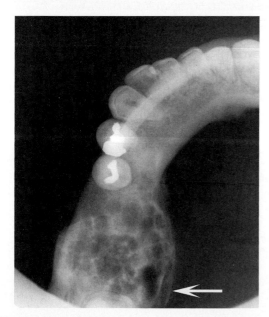

FIGURE 22-15 Occlusal film demonstrating expansion of the lingual cortex with maintenance of a thin outer shell of bone (arrow).

amyloid-like material and contain strands or sheets of polyhedral epithelial cells in fibrous stroma.

Clinical Features. A CEOT is less aggressive than an ameloblastoma and is found in about the same age group. Rarely this tumor may have an extraosseous location. The neoplasm is more common in men, and patients range in age from 8 to 92 years, with an average age of about 42 years (average age is considerably younger in men and older in women). Jaw expansion is a regular feature and usually the only symptom. Palpation of the swelling reveals a hard tumor.

Imaging Features

Location. Similar to ameloblastomas, CEOTs have a definite predilection for the mandible, with a ratio of at least 2 : 1, and most develop in the premolar-molar area, with a 52% association with an unerupted or impacted tooth. In about half of cases, radiographs taken early in the development of these tumors reveal a radiolucent area around the crown of a mature, unerupted tooth.

Periphery. The border may have a well-defined cystlike cortex. In some tumors, the boundary may be irregular and ill defined.

Internal Structure. The internal aspect may appear unilocular or multilocular with numerous scattered, radiopaque foci of varying

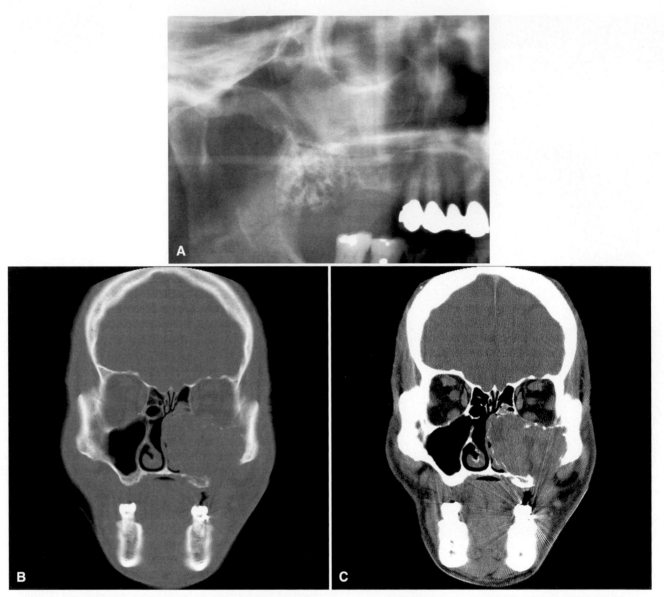

FIGURE 22-16 **A,** Cropped panoramic image of an ameloblastoma involving the left maxilla. Note the multilocular appearance in the tuberosity region. It is impossible to determine the extent of the lesion with the panoramic film. **B** and **C,** The same coronal CT image slices using both bone and soft tissue algorithms of the same case. Note the aggressive nature of the tumor as it has grown into the sinus and nasal fossa and perforated the lateral cortical plate of the maxilla.

size and density. Some radiopaque elements may have a crescent shape or a doughnut shape with a radiolucent center. The most characteristic and diagnostic finding is the appearance of radiopacities close to the crown of the embedded tooth (Fig. 22-19). In addition, small, thin, opaque trabeculae may cross the radiolucency in many directions.

Effects on Surrounding Structures.   CEOTs may displace a developing tooth or prevent its eruption. Associated expansion of the jaw with maintenance of a cortical boundary may also occur.

Differential Diagnosis.   Lesions with a completely radiolucent internal structure may mimic dentigerous cysts or ameloblastomas. Other lesions with radiopaque foci, including adenomatoid odontogenic tumor, ameloblastic fibro-odontoma, and calcifying odontogenic cyst, may have similar appearances. However, the prominent location of the CEOT and the age of the patient help in the differential diagnosis.

Treatment.   The treatment of a CEOT is more conservative than treatment of an ameloblastoma, with local resection.

MIXED ODONTOGENIC TUMORS

Odontoma

Synonyms.   Compound odontoma, compound composite odontoma, complex odontoma, complex composite odontoma, odontogenic hamartoma, calcified mixed odontoma, and cystic odontoma are synonyms for odontoma.

Disease Mechanism.   The term odontoma is used to identify a tumor that is characterized by the production of mature enamel,

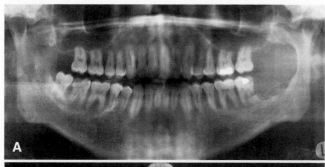

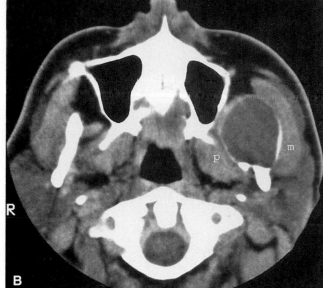

dentin, cementum, and pulp tissue. These components are seen in various states of histodifferentiation and morphodifferentiation. Because of its limited and slow growth and well-differentiated tooth tissue, this lesion is considered to be a hamartoma and not a true tumor.

The structural relationship of the component tissues may vary from nondescript masses of dental tissue referred to as a complex odontoma to multiple well-formed teeth (denticles) of a compound odontoma. A dilated odontoma has been described as another type of odontoma; however, this is a single structure that actually may be the most severe expression of a dens in dentes.

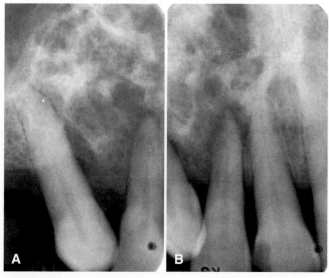

FIGURE 22-17 **A,** Panoramic film of a unicystic ameloblastoma occupying the left mandibular ramus. Note the absence of the anterior border of the ramus. **B,** Axial CT image using soft tissue algorithm shows significant expansion toward the masseter *(m)* and lateral pterygoid *(p)* muscles.

FIGURE 22-18 **A** and **B,** Periapical films of a recurrent ameloblastoma of the right maxilla. Note the sclerotic margins of the small cystic lesions.

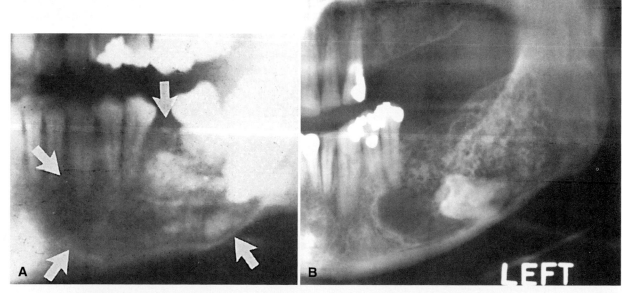

FIGURE 22-19 **A,** Calcifying odontogenic tumor or Pindborg tumor *(arrows).* **B,** The tumor appears as a mixed radiolucent-radiopaque lesion associated with an unerupted tooth. (**A,** *Courtesy M. Gornitsky, DDS, Montreal, Canada.* **B,** *Courtesy Dr. D. Lanigan, University of Saskatchewan.)*

Clinical Features.   Odontomas are the most common odontogenic tumor. They often interfere with the eruption of permanent teeth (Fig. 22-20). The lesion shows no gender predilection, and most begin forming while the normal dentition is developing. Odontomas develop and mature while the corresponding teeth are forming and cease development when the associated teeth complete development. Most odontomas occur in the second decade of life and many times are found during investigation of delayed eruption of adjacent teeth or retained primary teeth. In rare cases, odontomas are associated with primary teeth. They persist if left untreated, although they do not continue to increase in size and may be detected later in life. Compound odontomas are about twice as

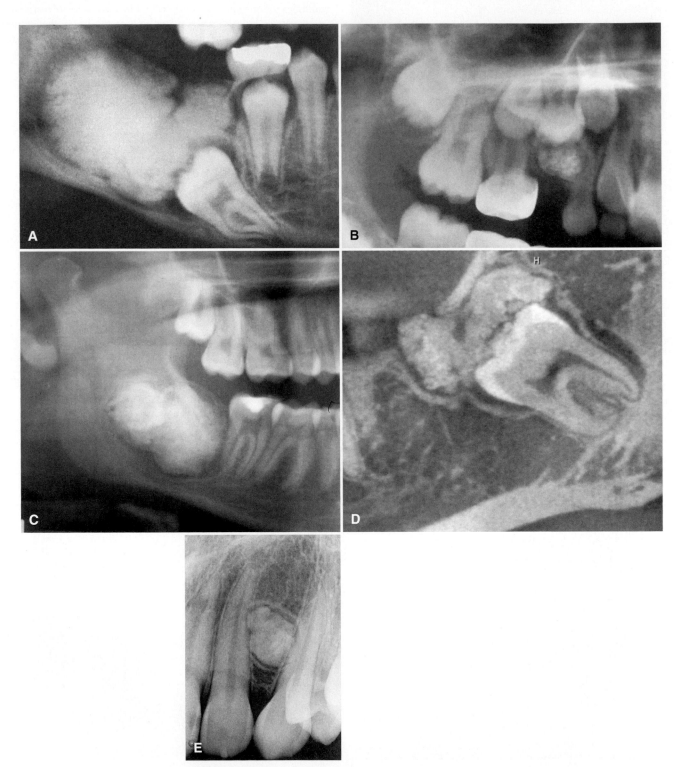

FIGURE 22-20 A series of complex odontomas. **A-C,** Cropped panoramic images. **D,** Sagittal cone-beam CT image. **E,** Periapical image. In all these examples note the toothlike density of calcified internal structure, thin radiolucent capsule, and interference with the eruption of associated teeth.

common as the complex type. Although the compound variety forms equally between men and women, 60% of complex odontomas occur in women. In rare circumstances, a compound odontoma may erupt into the oral cavity of a child.

Imaging Features

Location.   More of the compound type (62%) occurs in the anterior maxilla in association with the crown of an unerupted canine. In contrast, 70% of complex odontomas are found in the mandibular first and second molar area.

Periphery.   The borders of odontomas are well defined and may be smooth or irregular. These lesions have a cortical border, and immediately inside and adjacent to the cortical border is a soft tissue capsule.

Internal Structure.   The contents of these lesions are largely radiopaque. Compound odontomas have a number of toothlike structures or denticles that look like deformed teeth (Fig. 22-21). Complex odontomas contain an irregular mass of calcified tissue (see Fig. 22-20). The degree of radiopacity is equivalent to or exceeds adjacent tooth structure and may vary in the degree of radiopacity from one region to another, reflecting variations in amount and type of hard tissue that has been formed. A dilated odontoma has a single calcified structure with a more radiolucent central portion that has an overall form similar to a doughnut (Fig. 22-22).

Effects on Surrounding Structures.   Odontomas can interfere with the normal eruption of teeth. Most odontomas (70%) are associated with abnormalities, such as impaction, malpositioning, diastema, aplasia, malformation, and devitalization of adjacent teeth. Large complex odontomas may cause expansion of the jaw with maintenance of the cortical boundary.

Differential Diagnosis.   A toothlike appearance of the radiopaque structures within a well-defined lesion leads to easy recognition of a compound odontoma. Complex odontomas differ from ossifying fibromas by their tendency to associate with unerupted molar teeth and because they usually are more radiopaque than ossifying fibromas. Odontomas may also develop in much younger patients than ossifying fibromas. Periapical osseous dysplasia (periapical cemental dysplasia) may resemble complex odontomas but are usually multiple and centered on the periapical region of teeth. However, the differential diagnosis may be more difficult if the

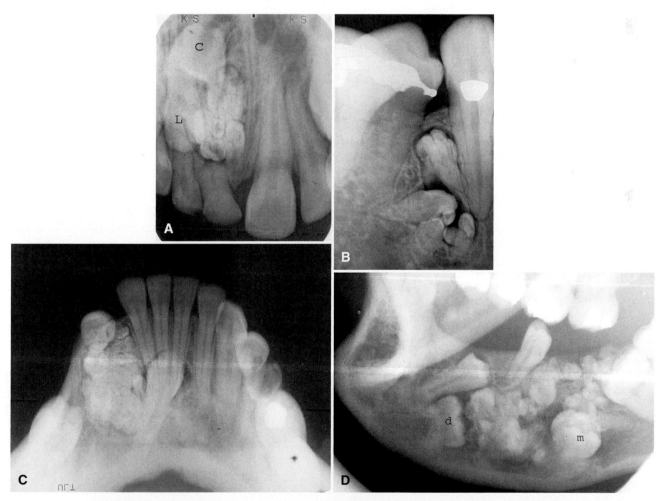

FIGURE 22-21 Examples of compound odontomas. Note the numerous internal components and the radiolucent capsule. **A,** Compound odontoma in the anterior maxilla, which has interfered with the eruption of the central incisor (C) and the lateral incisor (L). **B,** Compound odontoma within the mandible. **C,** Compound odontoma within the anterior mandible interfering with the eruption of the cuspid. **D,** Compound odontoma within the mandible interfering with the eruption of the first premolar, deciduous molar (d), and first molar (m).

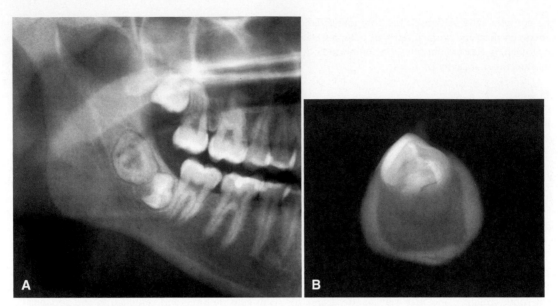

FIGURE 22-22 **A,** Cropped panoramic image demonstrating a dilated odontoma positioned immediately distal to the unerupted third molar. **B,** Radiograph of a specimen. Part of the odontoma resembles a tooth crown.

osseous dysplastic lesion is solitary and located in an edentulous region of the jaws. The periphery of osseous dysplasia usually has a wider, uneven sclerotic border, whereas odontomas have a well-defined cortical border, and usually the soft tissue capsule is more uniform and better defined with odontomas compared with osseous dysplasia. DBIs, although radiopaque, do not have a soft tissue capsule, as is seen with odontomas.

Treatment.   Complex and compound odontomas are usually removed by simple excision. They do not recur and are not locally invasive.

Ameloblastic Fibroma

Synonyms.   Synonyms for ameloblastic fibroma include soft odontoma, soft mixed odontoma, mixed odontogenic tumor, fibroadamantoblastoma, and granular cell ameloblastic fibroma.

Disease Mechanism.   Ameloblastic fibromas are benign, mixed odontogenic tumors. They constitute a neoplastic proliferation of odontogenic epithelium as well as the primitive mesenchymal components resembling the dental papilla. Enamel, dentin, and cementum are not formed in this tumor.

Clinical Features.   The behavior of ameloblastic fibromas is completely benign. There is not complete agreement regarding sex predilection. Most of these tumors occur between 5 and 20 years of age, during the period of tooth formation, with an average age of about 15 years. They usually produce a painless, slow-growing expansion and displacement of the involved teeth (Fig. 22-23). Although the most common symptom is swelling or occlusal pain, the tumor may be discovered on a routine dental radiograph. It may be associated with a missing tooth.

Imaging Features
Location.   Ameloblastic fibromas usually develop in the premolar-molar area of the mandible. In some cases, the tumor may involve the ramus and extend forward to the premolar-molar area. A common location is near the crest of the alveolar process

(Fig. 22-24) or in a follicular relationship with an unerupted tooth (located occlusal to the tooth), or it may arise in an area where a tooth failed to develop.

Periphery.   The borders of an ameloblastic fibroma are well defined and often corticated in a manner similar to that of a cyst.

Internal Structure.   An ameloblastic fibroma is more commonly unilocular (totally radiolucent) (Fig. 22-25) but may be multilocular with indistinct curved septa (see Fig. 22-23).

Effects on Surrounding Structures.   If the lesion is large, there may be expansion with an intact cortical plate. The associated tooth or teeth may be inhibited from normal eruption or may be displaced in an apical direction.

Differential Diagnosis.   A common difficulty occurs in differentiating a small tumor with a follicular relationship to an unerupted tooth from a small dentigerous cyst or a hyperplastic follicle. The radiologic features may not allow the differentiation between these three entities. This tumor may have similar features to an ameloblastoma; however, ameloblastic fibroma occurs at an earlier age, and the septa in an ameloblastoma are more defined and coarse. The septa in ameloblastic fibroma are infrequent and often very fine. Giant cell granulomas may appear multilocular, but these tumors usually have an epicenter anterior to the first molar in young patients, and the septa are characteristically granular and ill defined. Odontogenic myxomas can appear multilocular, but usually a few sharp straight septa can be identified, which are not characteristic of ameloblastic fibromas, and myxomas usually occur in an older age group.

Treatment.   Ameloblastic fibromas are benign, and the rate of recurrence is low. A conservative surgical approach, including enucleation and mechanical curettage of the surrounding bone, is reported to be successful for these cases.

Ameloblastic Fibro-Odontoma
Disease Mechanism.   An ameloblastic fibro-odontoma is a mixed tumor with all the elements of an ameloblastic fibroma but with scattered collections of enamel and dentin. Some authorities

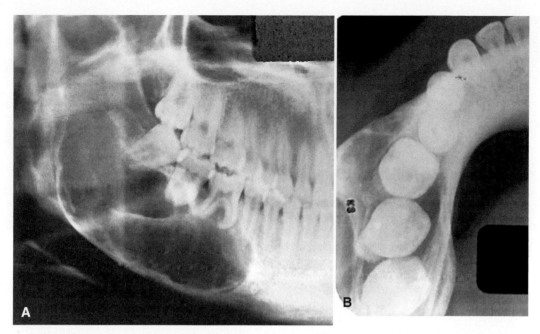

FIGURE 22-23 Ameloblastic fibroma in the body and ramus of the right mandible. **A,** Panoramic radiograph. **B,** Occlusal radiograph showing mediolateral expansion of the mandible.

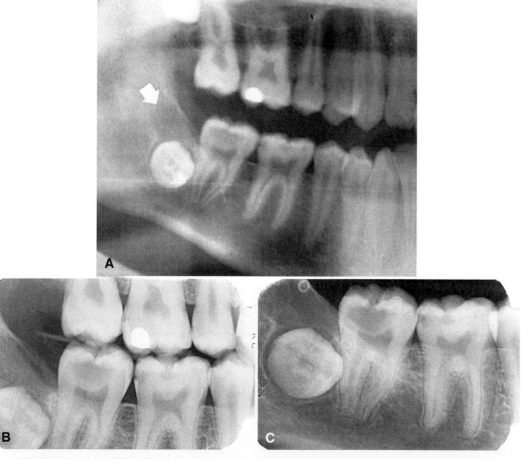

FIGURE 22-24 Ameloblastic fibroma. **A,** Ameloblastic fibroma seen as a radiolucency above the unerupted third molar *(arrow)*. **B,** Bitewing radiograph of the same lesion. **C,** Periapical radiograph. *(Courtesy G. Sanders, DDS, La Crosse, WI.)*

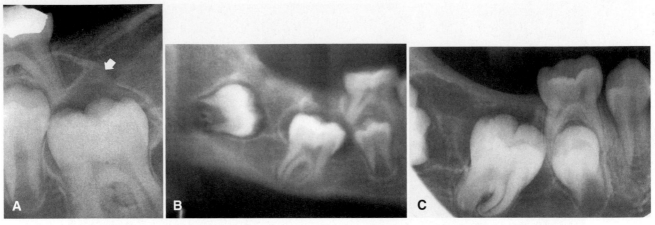

FIGURE 22-25 **A,** Ameloblastic fibroma appearing as a unilocular outgrowth of the follicle of the unerupted first permanent molar. **B,** Cropped panoramic image. **C,** Periapical film illustrating an ameloblastic fibroma associated with the crowns of the first and second molars.

consider an ameloblastic fibro-odontoma to be an early stage of a developing odontoma; however, there is compelling evidence that ameloblastic fibro-odontoma is a separate entity and has a more neoplastic behavior than odontoma. There are probably some lesions that are incorrectly identified as an ameloblastic fibro-odontoma and are really a developing odontoma.

Clinical Features.   The clinical features are similar to odontomas, often associated with a missing tooth or tooth that has failed to erupt. Occasionally, this tumor takes the position of a missing tooth. This tumor appears during the same age range as odontomas and ameloblastic fibromas with no particular sex predilection.

Imaging Features
Location.   Most cases occur in the posterior aspect of the mandible. The epicenter of the lesion is usually occlusal to a developing tooth or toward the alveolar crest.

Periphery.   This tumor is usually well defined and sometimes corticated.

Internal Structure.   The internal structure is mixed with most of the lesion being radiolucent. Small lesions may appear as enlarged follicles with only one or two small, discrete radiopacities. Larger lesions may have a more extensive calcified internal structure (Fig. 22-26). In some cases, these small calcifications have a round shape with a radiopaque enamel-like margin giving a shape similar to a small doughnut, and some may appear as small deformed teeth. Most often an associated impacted tooth is present.

Differential Diagnosis.   If calcification is not detected, this tumor cannot be differentiated from an ameloblastic fibroma. Differentiation from a developing odontoma may be difficult, but generally these tumors have a greater soft tissue component (radiolucent) than an odontoma. It may be argued that given time the amount of hard tissue will increase; however, the distribution of hard tissue is different. A complex odontoma, which shares a common location, usually has one mass of disorganized tissue in the center, whereas the ameloblastic fibro-odontoma usually has multiple scattered mature small pieces of dental hard tissue. Although the compound odontoma has multiple denticles, the posterior mandible is a rare location, and the organization of the tooth material in ameloblastic fibro-odontomes is never organized enough to

resemble a tooth. Lastly, the ameloblastic fibro-odontomas do not occur early enough compared with odontomas to be considered a precursor.

Treatment.   Usually conservative enucleation is used, although recurrence has been reported.

Adenomatoid Odontogenic Tumor
Synonyms.   Adenoameloblastoma and ameloblastic adenomatoid tumor are synonyms for adenomatoid odontogenic tumor.

Disease Mechanism.   Adenomatoid odontogenic tumors are uncommon, nonaggressive tumors of odontogenic epithelium and have a variety of patterns mixed with mature connective tissue stroma. The origin of adenomatoid odontogenic tumors may be from enamel organ epithelium and is classified as a mixed tumor because it contains connective tissue stroma and sometimes calcifications that have been interpreted as enamel-like or dentinoid material. Adenomatoid odontogenic tumors account for 3% of all oral tumors. Both central and peripheral tumors occur. The central tumors are divided into the follicular type (tumors associated with the crown of an embedded tooth) and the extrafollicular type (tumors with no embedded tooth). Approximately 73% of central lesions are the follicular type.

Clinical Features.   Adenomatoid odontogenic tumors occur in the age range of 5 to 50 years; however, about 70% occur in the second decade, with an average age of 16 years. The tumor has a 2:1 female predilection. The follicular type is diagnosed earlier than the extrafollicular type, probably because the failure of the associated tooth to erupt is noted. The tumor is slow growing and manifests as a gradually enlarging, painless swelling or asymmetry, often associated with a missing tooth.

Imaging Features
Location.   At least 75% of adenomatoid odontogenic tumors occur in the maxilla (Fig. 22-27). The incisor-canine-premolar region and especially the cuspid region is the usual area involved in both jaws. It occurs more commonly in the maxilla. This tumor may have a follicular relationship with an impacted tooth; however, it often does not attach at the cementoenamel junction

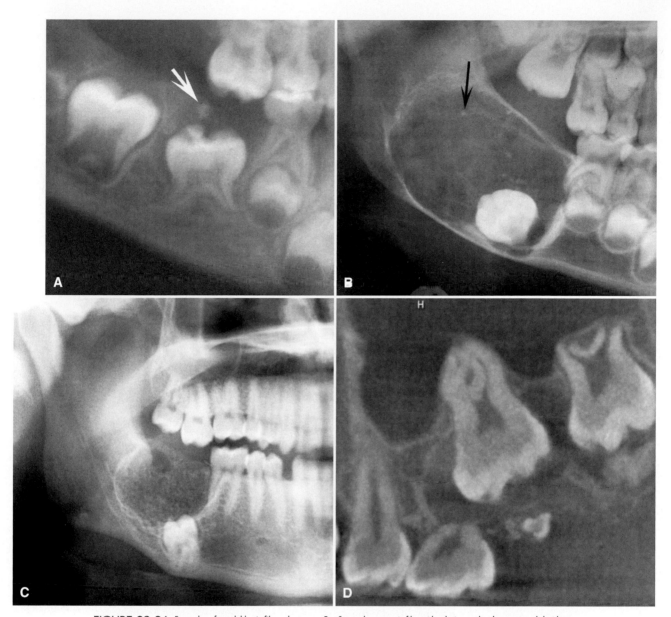

FIGURE 22-26 Examples of ameloblastic fibro-odontoma, **A,** Cropped panoramic film with a lesion occlusal to a second deciduous molar. The lesion is ill-defined and radiolucent except for two small radiopacities *(arrow).* **B,** Cropped panoramic image of a well-defined radiolucent lesion with only a few scattered radiopacities. **C,** Cropped panoramic image of a lesion with numerous radiopacities. **D,** Sagittal cone-beam CT image of an ameloblastic fibroma impeding the eruption of the first and second maxillary molars. Note the radiopacities with toothlike density occlusal to both teeth.

but surrounds a greater part of the tooth, most often a canine (Fig. 22-28).

Periphery.   The usual appearance is a well-defined corticated or sclerotic border.

Internal Structure.   Internal radiopaque foci develop in about two thirds of cases. One tumor may be completely radiolucent, another may contain faint radiopaque foci (see Fig. 22-28), and some may show dense clusters of ill-defined radiopacities; occasionally, the calcifications are small and with well-defined borders, similar to a cluster of small pebbles (see Fig. 22-28, *B*). Intraoral radiographs may be required to demonstrate the calcifications within the lesion, which may not be seen on panoramic radiographs. Microscopic studies have verified that the size, number, and density of small radiopacities in the central radiolucency of the lesion vary from tumor to tumor and seem to increase with age.

Effects on Surrounding Structures.   As the tumor enlarges, adjacent teeth are displaced. Root resorption is rare. This lesion also may inhibit eruption of an involved tooth. Although some expansion of the jaw may occur, the outer cortex is maintained.

Differential Diagnosis.   When this tumor is completely radiolucent and has a follicular relationship with an impacted tooth, the differentiation from a follicular cyst or a pericoronal odontogenic keratocyst may be difficult. If the attachment of the radiolucent lesion is more apical than the cementoenamel junction, a follicular cyst can be discounted; however, this would not exclude

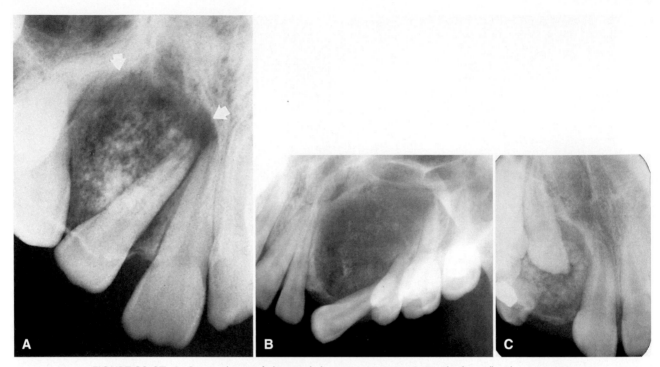

FIGURE 22-27 **A-C,** Intraoral images of adenomatoid odontogenic tumor *(arrows, Fig. A)* within the maxilla with various amounts of calcification, some of which have a pebble-like shape. (**A,** *Courtesy R. Howell, DDS, Morgantown, WV.*)

FIGURE 22-28 Adenomatoid odontogenic tumor within the mandible. **A,** Cropped panoramic image with no apparent internal calcifications. **B,** Cropped cone-beam CT image of a tumor related to the first premolar. Note the pebble-like calcifications distal to the premolar. *(Courtesy of Dr. Milan Madhavji, Toronto, Canada.)*

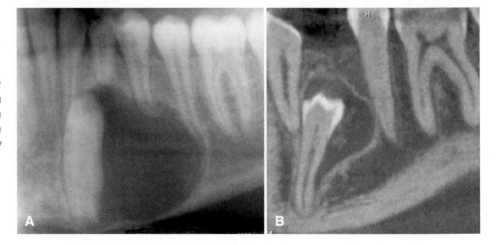

an odontogenic keratocyst. If there is a calcified product (radiopacities) in this tumor, other lesions with calcifications might be entertained in the differential diagnosis. The maxillary and mandibular anterior regions are also common sites for calcifying odontogenic cysts. It may be impossible to differentiate the extrafollicular type of adenomatoid odontogenic tumor from a calcifying odontogenic cyst. Ameloblastic fibro-odontoma and CEOT occur more commonly in the posterior mandible.

Treatment. Conservative surgical excision is adequate because the tumor is not locally invasive, is well encapsulated, and is separated easily from the bone. The theory that adenomatoid odontogenic tumors are hamartomas is supported by the innocuous behavior of the lesion because, as with odontomas, adenomatoid odontogenic tumors stop developing about the time tooth structures complete their growth. The recurrence rate is 0.2%.

MESENCHYMAL TUMORS

Odontogenic Myxoma

Synonyms. Synonyms for odontogenic myxoma include myxoma, myxofibroma, and fibromyxoma.

Disease Mechanism. Odontogenic myxomas are uncommon, accounting for only 3% to 6% of odontogenic tumors. They are benign, intraosseous neoplasms that arise from odontogenic ectomesenchyme and resemble the mesenchymal portion of the dental papilla. These myxomas are not encapsulated and tend to infiltrate the surrounding cancellous bone but do not metastasize. They have a loose, gelatinous consistency and show microscopic characteristics similar to those of soft tissue myxomas of the extremities. Odontogenic myxomas develop only in the bones of the facial skeleton. The theory that this lesion develops from odontogenic rather than nonodontogenic ectomesenchyme is supported by the fact that it appears only in the jaws, and in some cases odontogenic epithelium can be detected microscopically.

Clinical Features.

If odontogenic myxomas have a gender predilection, they favor females slightly. Although the lesion can occur at any age, more than half arise in individuals between 10 and 30 years; it rarely occurs before age 10 or after age 50. It grows slowly and may or may not cause pain. It causes swelling eventually and may grow quite large if left untreated. It may also invade the maxillary sinus. Recurrence rates of 25% have been reported. This high rate may be explained by the lack of encapsulation of the tumor, its poorly defined boundaries, and the extension of nests or pockets of myxoid (jelly-like) tumor into trabecular spaces, where they are difficult to detect and remove surgically.

Imaging Features

Location. Myxomas more commonly affect the mandible by a margin of 3 : 1. In the mandible, these tumors occur in the premolar and molar areas and only rarely in the ramus and condyle (non–tooth-bearing areas). Myxomas in the maxilla usually involve the alveolar process in the premolar and molar regions and the zygomatic process.

Periphery. The lesion usually is well defined, and it may have a corticated margin but most often is poorly defined, especially in the maxilla.

Internal Structure. When it occurs pericoronally with an impacted tooth, an odontogenic myxoma may have a cystlike, unilocular outline, although most have a mixed radiolucent-radiopaque internal pattern. Residual bone trapped within the tumor remodels into curved and straight, coarse or fine septa. The presence of these septa gives the tumor a multilocular appearance. A characteristic septum identified with this tumor is a straight, thin, etched septum (Fig. 22-29). These septa have been described as making a tennis racket–like or stepladder-like pattern, but this pattern is rarely seen. In reality, most septa are curved and coarse, but the finding of one or two of these straight septa helps in the identification of this tumor (Fig. 22-30).

Effects on Surrounding Structures. When growing in a tooth-bearing area, an odontogenic myxoma displaces and loosens teeth but

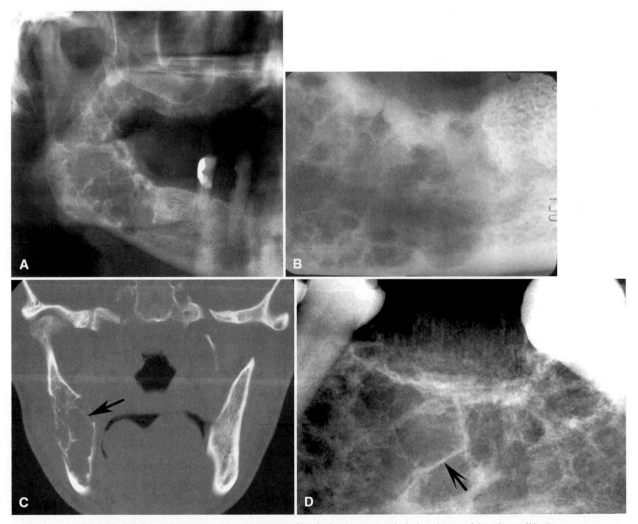

FIGURE 22-29 Odontogenic myxoma. **A,** Panoramic film of a large myxoma in the body and ramus of the right mandible. **B,** Periapical view. **C,** Coronal CT image. Notice the presence of a few straight septa, especially visible on the CT image *(arrow)*. The CT image also shows some modest expansion considering the overall size of the tumor. **D,** Periapical view of a different lesion. Note the one straight sharp septum *(arrow)*.

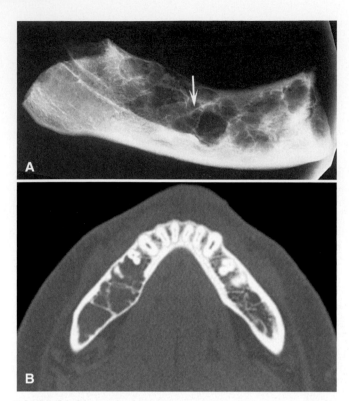

FIGURE 22-30 **A,** Film of a surgical specimen of an odontogenic myxoma. Note the sharp straight septum *(arrow).* **B,** Axial CT image with some straight septa.

rarely causes resorption of teeth. The lesion also frequently scallops between the roots of adjacent teeth similar to a simple bone cyst. This tumor has a tendency to grow along the involved bone without the same amount of expansion seen with other benign tumors; however, when achieving a large size, there may be considerable expansion.

Additional Imaging.   CT imaging and in particular MRI can help in establishing the intraosseous extent of the tumor and guide the surgeon in planning the resection margins. The high tissue signal characteristic of this tumor on T2-weighted MR images is particularly useful in establishing tumor extent and the presence of a recurrent tumor (Fig. 22-31).

Differential Diagnosis.   Because odontogenic myxomas most often have a multilocular internal pattern, the differential diagnosis should include other multilocular lesions, such as ameloblastomas, central giant cell granulomas, and central hemangiomas. The finding of characteristic thin straight septa with less than expected bone expansion is very useful in the differential diagnosis. Occasionally, a small area of expansion with straight septa may be projected over an intact outer bony cortex and give a spiculated appearance seen in osteogenic sarcomas (see Fig. 22-29, D). Careful inspection of this area of expansion reveals a thin but intact outer cortex that would not be seen in osteogenic sarcoma. An odontogenic fibroma occasionally has the same radiographic characteristics and cannot be reliably differentiated from a myxoma.

Treatment.   Odontogenic myxomas are treated by resection with a generous amount of surrounding bone to ensure removal of

myxomatous tumor that infiltrates the adjacent marrow spaces. With appropriate treatment, the prognosis is good.

Benign Cementoblastoma

Synonyms.   Cementoblastoma and true cementoma are synonyms for benign cementoblastoma.

Disease Mechanism.   Benign cementoblastomas are slow-growing, mesenchymal neoplasms composed principally of cementum-like tissue. The tumor manifests as a bulbous growth around and attached to the apex of a tooth root. Its histologic characteristics are identical to osteoblastomas, and some authors consider cementoblastomas to be osteoblastomas and, as a consequence, classify these as bone tumors. The tumor most often develops with permanent teeth but in rare cases occurs with primary teeth.

Clinical Features.   Although statistical data suggest that benign cementoblastomas are uncommon, they occur more often than published accounts indicate. The lesion is more common in males than females, and ages of reported patients range from 12 to 65 years, although most patients are relatively young. There is no racial predilection. The tumor usually is a solitary lesion that is slow growing but that may eventually displace teeth. The involved tooth is vital and often painful. The pain seems to vary from patient to patient and can be relieved by antiinflammatory drugs.

Imaging Features

Location.   Benign cementoblastomas occur more often in the mandible (78%) and form most commonly on the roots of a premolar or first molar (90%).

Periphery.   The lesion is a well-defined radiopacity with a cortical border and a well-defined radiolucent band just inside the cortical border.

Internal Structure.   Benign cementoblastomas are mixed radiolucent-radiopaque lesions in which most of the internal structure is radiopaque. The resulting pattern may be amorphous or may have a wheel spoke pattern (Fig. 22-32). The density of the cemental mass usually obscures the outline of the enveloped root. This central radiopaque mass as mentioned is surrounded by a radiolucent band indicating that the tumor is maturing from the central aspect to the periphery.

Effects on Surrounding Structures.   If the root outline is apparent, in most cases various amounts of external resorption can be seen. If large enough, this tumor can cause expansion of the mandible and in some cases there is a perforation through the outer cortical plate without periosteal reaction.

Differential Diagnosis.   The most common lesion to simulate this appearance is a solitary lesion of periapical osseous dysplasia. The differential diagnosis may be difficult in some cases, and the presence or absence of symptoms or observation of the lesion over a period of time may be required. Generally, the radiolucent band around the benign cementoblastoma is usually better defined and uniform than with osseous dysplasia. Also, owing to the pattern of growth of the cementoblastomas, the overall shape is more uniform and circular than the more irregular undulating outline of cemental dysplasia. Other lesions that may be included in the differential diagnosis are periapical sclerosing osteitis, DBI, and hypercementosis. However, periapical sclerosing osteitis and DBIs do not have a soft tissue capsule, as does benign cementoblastoma. Hypercementosis should be surrounded by a

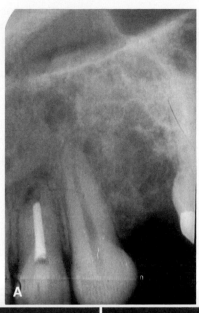

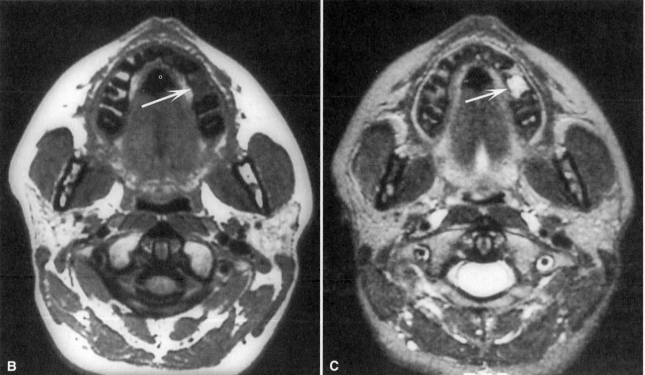

FIGURE 22-31 **A,** Periapical film obtained to investigate a possible recurrence of an odontogenic myxoma in the alveolar process between the cuspid and the first molar after treatment by surgical curettage. **B,** Axial MR image using T1 weighting shows a low signal (black) from the segment of the alveolar process between the cuspid and molar. **C,** Axial MR image of the same image slice as **B** but using T2 weighting resulting in a high signal (white) from the same alveolar segment, which is characteristic of an odontogenic myxoma and confirming the presence of a recurrence.

periodontal membrane space, which is usually thinner than the soft tissue capsule of the benign cementoblastoma, and there is no root resorption or jaw expansion with hypercementosis.

Treatment.   Benign cementoblastomas are apparently self-limiting and rarely recur after enucleation. Simple excision and extraction of the associated tooth are sufficient treatment. In some cases, the tumor may be amputated from the tooth, which is treated endodontically.

Central Odontogenic Fibroma

Synonyms.   Synonyms for central odontogenic fibroma include simple odontogenic fibroma and odontogenic fibroma (WHO type).

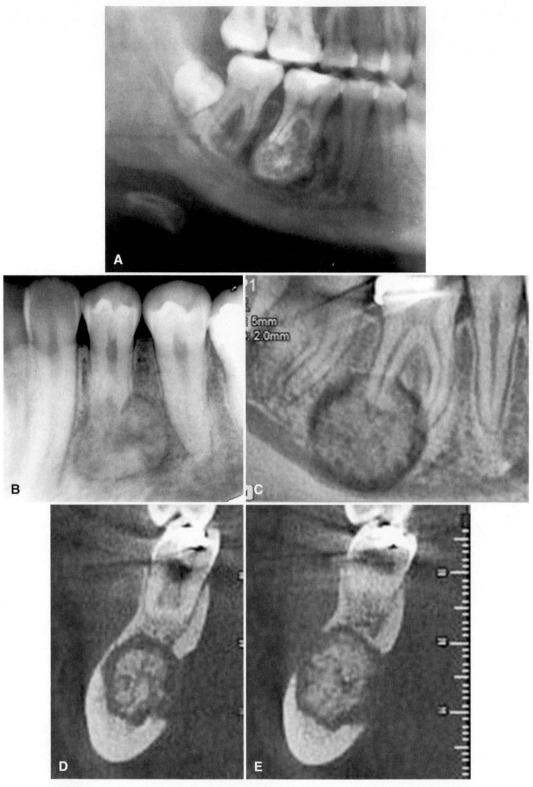

FIGURE 22-32 Cementoblastoma. **A,** Portion of a panoramic radiograph showing a large, bulbous, radiopaque mass attached to the roots of the mandibular right first molar. A radiolucent band can be seen surrounding the mass, and root resorption of the molar roots has occurred. **B,** Periapical radiograph of a lesion associated with a bicuspid. **C-E,** Panoramic and cross-sectional cone-beam CT images of a cementoblastoma related to the roots of a mandibular first molar. There is perforation of the buccal and lingual cortical plates without evidence of periosteal bone formation. (**A** and **B,** Courtesy B. Pynn, Canada; **C-E,** courtesy Dr. Mohammad Amintavakoli, Shahid Beheshti University, Tehran, Iran.)

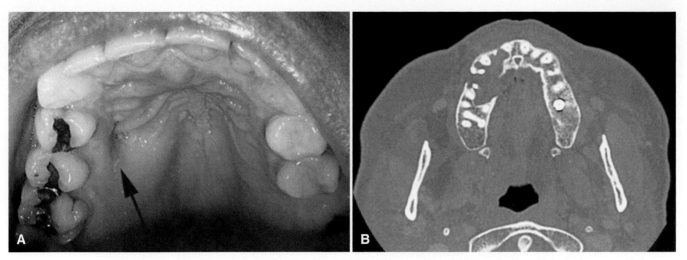

FIGURE 22-33 **A,** Clinical picture of an odontogenic fibroma of the maxilla demonstrating a cleft *(arrow)* in the palatal mucosa. **B,** Axial CT image of the same case showing loss of both the buccal and the palatal cortical plates without extension into the surrounding tissues and resorption of bone around the roots of the maxillary teeth with displacement or root resorption.

Disease Mechanism.   Central odontogenic fibromas are rare neoplasms that sometimes are divided into two types according to histologic appearance: (1) the simple type, which contains mature fibrous tissue with sparsely scattered odontogenic epithelial rests; and (2) the WHO type, which is more cellular, has more epithelial rests and may contain calcifications that resemble dysplastic dentin, cementum, or osteoid. One theory is that these types merely represent a spectrum and that odontogenic myxoma may be a part of this range.

Clinical Features.   Most cases of central odontogenic fibromas occur between the ages of 11 and 39 years. The neoplasm shows a definite female preponderance, with a reported ratio of 2.2:1. Affected patients may be asymptomatic or may have swelling and mobility of the teeth. An unusual and distinctive feature of some maxillary cases is a cleft or depression in the palatal mucosa where expansion by the tumor would be expected (Fig. 22-33, *A*).

Imaging Features
Location.   Central odontogenic fibromas occur slightly more often in the mandible. The prevalent site is the molar-premolar region in the mandible and anterior to the first molar in the maxilla.
Periphery.   The periphery usually is well defined.
Internal Structure.   Smaller lesions usually are unilocular, and larger lesions have a multilocular pattern. The internal septa may be fine and straight, as in odontogenic myxomas, or may be granular, resembling septa seen in giant cell granulomas. Some lesions are totally radiolucent, whereas unorganized internal calcification has been reported in others.
Effects on Surrounding Structures.   A central odontogenic fibroma may cause expansion with maintenance of a thin cortical boundary or occasionally can grow along the bone with minimum expansion similar to an odontogenic myxoma. Tooth displacement is common, and root resorption has been reported. Some maxillary lesions have a distinctive behavior of resorbing the bone around teeth without tooth displacement or resorption and without expansion of the alveolar process (Fig. 22-33, *B*).

Differential Diagnosis.   The histologic features may resemble those of a central (originating in bone) desmoplastic fibroma if no epithelial rests are apparent. Desmoplastic fibromas are more aggressive and tend to break through the peripheral cortex and invade surrounding soft tissue. The septa in desmoplastic fibroma are very thick, straight, and angular. If thin, straight septa are present in the odontogenic fibroma, it may be impossible to differentiate this neoplasm from an odontogenic myxoma on radiographic criteria alone. If granular septa are present, the appearance may be identical to a giant cell granuloma.

Treatment.   Central odontogenic fibromas are treated with simple excision. These lesions have a very low recurrence rate.

NONODONTOGENIC BENIGN TUMORS
BENIGN TUMORS OF NEURAL ORIGIN
Neurilemoma
Synonym.   Schwannoma is a synonym for neurilemoma.

Disease Mechanism.   A central neurilemoma is a tumor of neuroectodermal origin, arising from Schwann's cells that make up the inner layer covering the peripheral nerves. Although rare, it is the most common intraosseous nerve tumor. This tumor has practically no potential for malignant transformation.

Clinical Features.   Neurilemomas grow slowly, can occur at any age (but most commonly arise in the second and third decades), and occur with equal frequency in males and females. The mandible and sacrum are the most common sites. These lesions cause few symptoms other than those related to the location and size of the tumor. The usual complaint is swelling. Although pain is uncommon unless the tumor encroaches on adjacent nerves, paresthesia may arise, especially with lesions originating in the inferior alveolar canal. Pain, when present, usually develops at the site of the tumor; if paresthesia occurs, it is felt anterior to the tumor.

Imaging Features

Location. Neurilemomas most often involve the mandible, with less than 1 in 10 cases occurring in the maxilla. The tumor most often is located within an expanded inferior alveolar nerve canal posterior to the mental foramen (Fig. 22-34).

Periphery. In keeping with the slow growth rate, the margins of these tumors are well defined and usually corticated as they expand the cortical walls of the inferior alveolar canal. Small lesions may appear cystlike but more commonly are fusiform in shape as the tumor expands the canal.

Internal Structure. The internal structure is uniformly radiolucent. When lesions have a scalloping outline, this may give a false impression of a multilocular pattern.

Effects on Surrounding Structures. If the tumor reaches either the mandibular foramen or the mental foramen, it can cause enlargement of the foramen. Expansion of the inferior alveolar canal is slow, and the outer cortex of the canal is maintained and the expansion of the canal is usually localized with a definite epicenter unless the lesion is large. The expanding tumor may cause root resorption of adjacent teeth (Fig. 22-34).

Differential Diagnosis. Because neurilemomas most commonly originate within the inferior alveolar canal, vascular lesions, such as hemangioma or arteriovenous (A-V) fistula, should be considered. However, neurilemomas have a distinct epicenter, whereas vascular lesions usually cause more of a uniform widening of the whole canal, do not have an obvious epicenter, and usually change the course of the canal, most commonly to a serpiginous shape. Only neural tumors and vascular lesions originate within the inferior alveolar canal, but malignant lesions that grow down and enlarge the canal should be in the differential diagnosis. With a malignant lesion, the appearance is different with an irregular widening and destruction of the cortical boundaries of the canal.

Treatment. Excision is usually the treatment of choice. These lesions generally do not recur if completely removed. A capsule usually is present, facilitating surgical removal, although occasionally preservation of the nerve may not be possible. However, periodic examination is indicated to check for recurrence.

Neuroma

Synonyms. Amputation neuroma and traumatic neuroma are synonyms for neuroma.

Disease Mechanism. Despite its name, a neuroma is not a neoplasm. Rather, it is an overgrowth of severed nerve fibers attempting to regenerate with abnormal proliferation of scar tissue after a fracture involving a peripheral nerve. As a result, the proliferating nerve forms a disorganized collection of nerve fibers composed of varying proportions of axons, perineural connective tissue, Schwann's cells, and scar tissue. The original nerve damage may be the result of mechanical or chemical irritation of the nerve caused by fracture, orthognathic surgery, removal of a tumor or cyst, extrusion of endodontic cement, dental implants, or tooth extraction.

Clinical Features. Central neuromas are slow-growing, reactive hyperplasias that seldom become large, rarely exceeding 1 cm in diameter. They may cause various symptoms, including severe pain resulting from pressure applied as the tangled mass enlarges in its bony cavity or as the result of external trauma. The patient may have reflex neuralgia, with pain referred to the eyes, face, and head.

Imaging Features. The imaging features of a neuroma relate to the extent and shape of the proliferating mass of neural tissue.

Location. The most common location is the mental foramen, followed by the anterior maxilla and the posterior mandible.

Periphery. Neuromas usually have well-defined, corticated borders. They may occur in various shapes, depending on the amount of resistance to expansion offered by the surrounding bone. In the mandible, the tumor usually forms in the mandibular canal.

Internal Structure. The internal structure is totally radiolucent.

Effects on Surrounding Structures. Some expansion of the inferior alveolar nerve canal may occur.

Differential Diagnosis. It is impossible to differentiate this lesion from other benign neural tumors.

Treatment. Treatment is recommended because neuromas tend to continue to enlarge. They also may cause pain. Regardless of the type of injury that precipitates development of the neuroma, recurrence is uncommon after simple excision.

Neurofibroma

Synonym. Neurinoma is a synonym for neurofibroma.

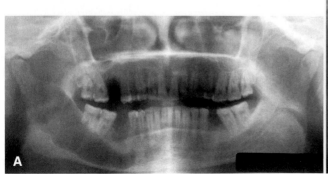
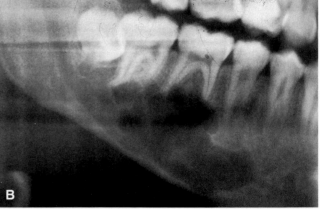

FIGURE 22-34 **A,** Panoramic film of a large neurilemoma expanding all of the inferior alveolar nerve canal from the mandibular to the mental foramen. **B,** Cropped panoramic image of a smaller tumor.

Disease Mechanism.   Neurofibromas are moderately firm, benign, well-circumscribed tumors caused by proliferation of Schwann's cells in a disorderly pattern that includes portions of nerve fibers, such as peripheral nerves, axons, and connective tissue of the sheath of Schwann. As neurofibromas grow, they incorporate axons. In contrast, neurilemomas are composed entirely of Schwann's cells and grow by displacing axons.

Clinical Features.   The central lesion of a neurofibroma may be the same as the multiple lesions that develop in von Recklinghausen's disease. Central lesions also may occur in von Recklinghausen's disease but are rare. Neurofibromas can occur at any age but usually are found in young patients. Neurofibromas associated with the mandibular nerve may produce pain or paresthesia. Neurofibromas also may expand and perforate the cortex, causing swelling that is hard or firm to palpation.

Imaging Features

   Location.   Central neurofibromas may occur in the mandibular canal, in the cancellous bone, and below the periosteum.

   Periphery.   As with neurilemomas, the margins of the radiolucency in neurofibromas usually are sharply defined and may be corticated. However, despite the benign nature and slow growth of the neurofibroma, some of these lesions have indistinct margins.

   Internal Structure.   The tumors usually appear unilocular but occasionally may have a multilocular appearance.

   Effects on Surrounding Structures.   A neurofibroma of the inferior dental nerve shows a fusiform enlargement of the canal (Fig. 22-35).

Differential Diagnosis.   Differentiation from other types of neural lesions may be impossible. This tumor can be differentiated from vascular lesions because the expansion of the canal is in a fusiform shape, whereas vascular lesions enlarge the whole canal and alter its path.

Treatment.   Solitary central lesions that have been excised seldom recur. However, it is wise to reexamine the area periodically because these tumors are not encapsulated, and some undergo malignant change.

Neurofibromatosis

Synonym.   A synonym for neurofibromatosis is von Recklinghausen's disease.

Disease Mechanism.   Neurofibromatosis is a syndrome consisting of café au lait spots on the skin; multiple peripheral nerve tumors; and various other dysplastic abnormalities of the skin, nervous system, bones, endocrine organs, and blood vessels. The two major classifications are neurofibromatosis 1 (NF1), a generalized form, and NF2, a central form. Oral lesions may occur as part of NF1 or may be solitary and are called segmental or forme fruste manifestations (Fig. 22-36). More recent observations of abnormal fat tissue in close association with changes in the osseous structure of the mandible support the theory that a mesodermal dysplasia is part of the spectrum of changes that may be observed in NF1 lesions.

Clinical Features.   Neurofibromatosis is one of the most common genetic diseases, occurring in 1:3000 births and present in about 30 people per 10,000. The peripheral nerve tumors are of two types, schwannomas and neurofibromas. Some manifestations are congenital, but most appear gradually during childhood and adult life. Café au lait spots become larger and more numerous with age; most patients eventually have more than six spots larger than 1.5 cm in diameter. Other skin lesions include freckles; soft, pedunculated, cutaneous neurofibromas; and firm, subcutaneous neurofibromas.

Imaging Features.   The morphologic changes in the jaws with neurofibromatosis can be characteristic. These changes include the following alterations in the shape of the mandible: enlargement of the coronoid notch in either or both the horizontal and the vertical dimensions; an obtuse angle between the body and the ramus; deformity of the condylar head; lengthening of the condylar neck; and lateral bowing and thinning of the ramus, as seen in basal skull views (see Fig. 22-35). Changes in mandibular morphology can continue to increase in severity through the second decade. Other radiographic changes include enlargement of the mandibular canal and mental and mandibular foramina and an increased incidence

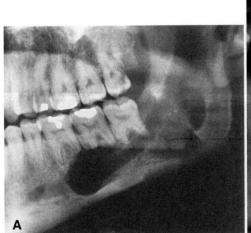
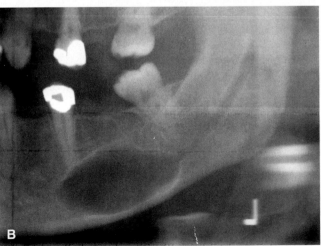

FIGURE 22-35 Neurofibroma. **A,** Portion of a panoramic radiograph shows a neurofibroma forming in the mandibular body along the path of the mandibular canal. **B,** Cropped panoramic image of a neurofibroma within the body of the left mandible. Note the fusiform shape as the tumor expands the canal.

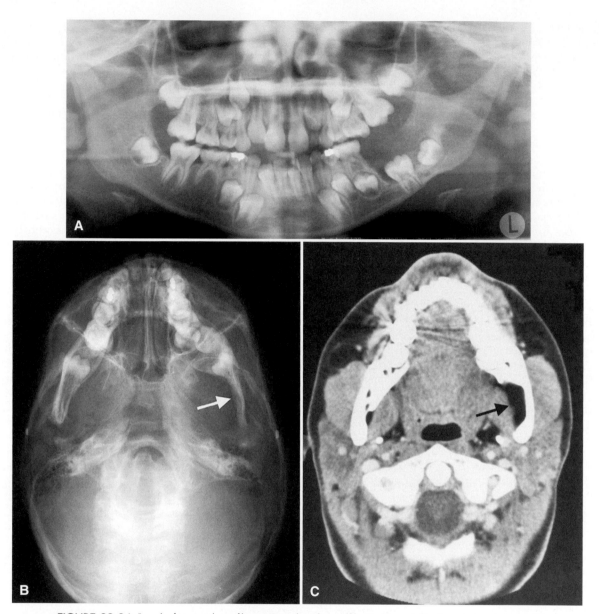

FIGURE 22-36 Example of segmental neurofibromatosis involving the mandible. **A,** Panoramic film demonstrates enlargement of the left coronoid notch, enlargement of the mandibular foramen, and interference of the eruption of the first and second molars. **B,** Basal skull view of the same case reveals thinning and bowing of the ramus in a lateral direction *(arrow)*. **C,** CT axial image using soft tissue algorithm shows fatty tissue adjacent to the abnormal ramus *(arrow)*.

of branched mandibular canal. Erosive changes to the outer contour of the mandible and interference with normal eruption of the molars also may occur. Abnormal accumulations of fatty tissue within deformities of the mandible have been observed in images produced by MDCT imaging (see Fig. 22-36, *C*).

Treatment.   Most patients live a normal life with few or no symptoms. Small cutaneous and subcutaneous neurofibromas can be removed if they are painful, but large plexiform neurofibromas should be left alone. Malignant conversion of these lesions has occurred in rare cases.

MESODERMAL TUMORS

Osteoma
Disease Mechanism.   Osteomas can form from membranous bones of the skull and face. The cause of a slow-growing osteoma is

obscure, but the tumor may arise from cartilage or embryonal periosteum. It is unclear whether osteomas are benign neoplasms or hamartomas. This lesion may be solitary or multiple, occurring on a single bone or on numerous bones. Osteomas originate from the periosteum and may occur either externally or within the paranasal sinuses (Fig. 22-37). It is more common in the frontal and ethmoid sinuses than in the maxillary sinuses (see Chapter 27). Structurally, osteomas can be divided into three types: (1) lesions composed of compact bone (ivory), (2) lesions composed of cancellous bone, and (3) lesions composed of a combination of compact and cancellous bone.

Clinical Features.   Osteomas can occur at any age but most frequently are found in individuals older than 40 years. The only symptom of a developing osteoma is the asymmetry caused by a bony, hard swelling on the jaw. The swelling is painless until its size or position interferes with function. The osteomas are attached to the cortex of the jaw by a pedicle or along a wide base. The mucosa covering the tumor is normal in color and freely movable. Cortical-type osteomas develop more often in men, whereas women have the highest incidence of the cancellous type. Although most osteomas are small, some may become large enough to cause severe damage, especially osteomas that develop in the frontoethmoid region.

Imaging Features

Location.   The mandible is more commonly involved than the maxilla. This entity is found most frequently on the posterior aspect of the mandible commonly on the lingual side of the ramus or on the inferior mandibular border below the molars (Fig. 22-38). Other locations include the condylar and coronoid regions. The mandibular lesion may be exophytic, extending outward into adjacent soft tissues (Fig. 22-39). Osteomas also occur in the paranasal sinuses, especially the frontal sinus.

Periphery.   Osteomas have well-defined borders.

Internal Structure.   Osteomas composed solely of compact bone are uniformly radiopaque; osteomas containing cancellous bone show evidence of internal trabecular structure.

Effects on Surrounding Structures.   Large lesions can displace adjacent soft tissues, such as muscles, and cause dysfunction. In some

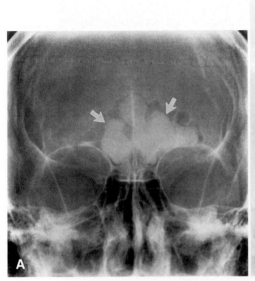
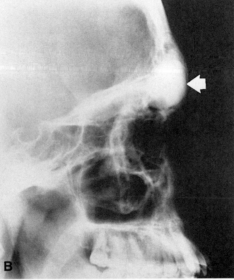

FIGURE 22-37 Osteoma in the frontal sinus. **A,** Caldwell view shows a large, amorphous mass in the frontal sinus *(arrows)*. **B,** Lateral view shows an osteoma occupying most of the space in the sinus *(arrow)*. *(Courtesy G. Himadi, DDS, Chapel Hill, NC.)*

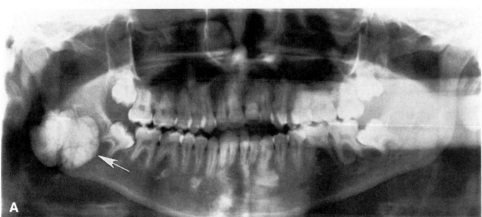
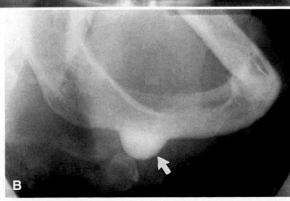

FIGURE 22-38 Osteoma. **A,** Panoramic radiograph shows an osteoma in the right mandibular angle region *(arrow)*. **B,** Oblique lateral jaw radiograph shows a solid radiopaque osteoma attached to the inferior border of the mandible *(arrow)*. (**A,** *From Matteson SR, et al: Semin Adv Oral Radiol Dent Radiol Photogr 57:1, 1985.)*

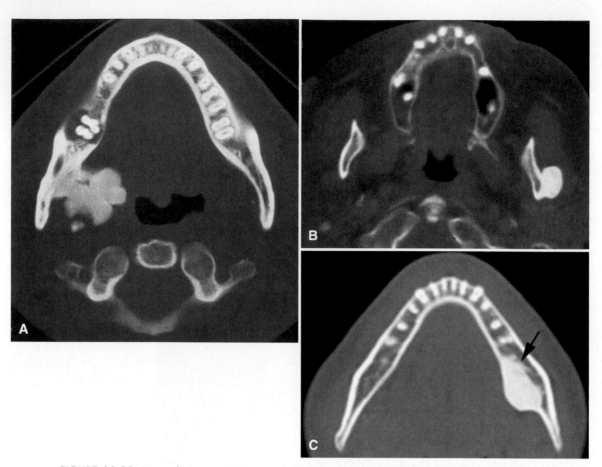

FIGURE 22-39 CT scans of osteomas. **A,** Osteoma on the lingual side of the mandibular ramus. **B,** Osteoma on the lateral side of the mandibular ramus. **C,** Osteoma on the lingual side of the mandibular body with the formation of adjacent dense bone within the mandible *(arrow)*.

cases, there is a sclerotic bone reaction within the cancellous portion of the parent bone and adjacent to the base of the osteomas. The appearance of this sclerotic bone is identical to a DBI (see Fig. 22-39, *C*).

Differential Diagnosis.   Usually the appearance is characteristic and does not present a problem with diagnosis. However, osteomas involving the condylar head can be difficult to differentiate from osteochondromas, osteophytes, or condylar hyperplasia, and osteomas involving the coronoid process may be similar to osteochondromas. A small osteoma may be similar in appearance to a torus or a large hyperostosis (exostosis).

Treatment.   Unless the osteoma interferes with normal function or presents a cosmetic problem, this lesion may not require treatment. In such cases, the osteoma should be kept under observation. Resection of osteomas is possible and may be difficult if the osteoma is of the cortical (ivory) type.

Gardner's Syndrome

Synonym.   A synonym for Gardner's syndrome is familial adenomatous polyposis.

Disease Mechanism.   Familial adenomatous polyposis is an inherited disorder resulting in the growth of multiple polyps in the colon. These polyps can become malignant at an average age of 39 in the classic form or at an average age of 59 years in the attenuated form. Gardner's syndrome is a type of familial adenomatous polyposis in which there are additional growths outside the colon. This syndrome is characterized by multiple osteomas, multiple DBIs (enostosis), epidermoid cysts, subcutaneous desmoid tumors, and multiple polyps of the small and large intestine. Also, dental abnormalities include an increased frequency of supernumerary and impacted teeth and odontomas. The associated osteomas appear during the second decade. They are most common in the frontal bone, mandible, maxilla, and sphenoid bones (Fig. 22-40). Because osteomas and enostosis often develop before intestinal polyps, early recognition of the syndrome may be a lifesaving event. Occasionally, osteomas may not be present but the presence of five or more DBIs may indicate a familial multiple polyposis syndrome (Fig. 22-41). Multiple unerupted supernumerary and permanent teeth in both jaws also occur with Gardner's syndrome. Multiple osteomas may occur as isolated findings in the absence of the diseases associated with Gardner's syndrome.

Treatment.   Generally, the removal of osteomas is unnecessary unless the tumors interfere with normal function or present a cosmetic concern. It is most important to recognize the relationship of multiple osteomas and multiple DBIs with familial adenomatous polyposis for early diagnosis. A family history of intestinal

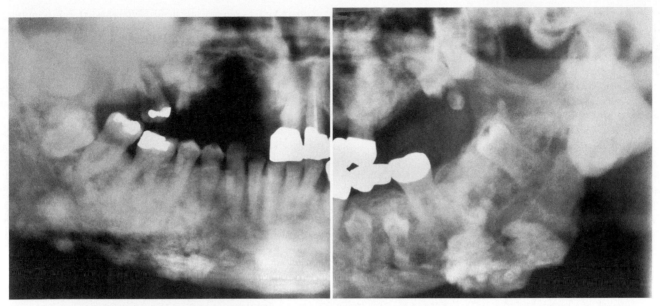

FIGURE 22-40 Osteoma with Gardner's syndrome. Panoramic radiograph shows several osteomas and DBIs throughout both jaws. Note the impacted mandibular left second premolars.

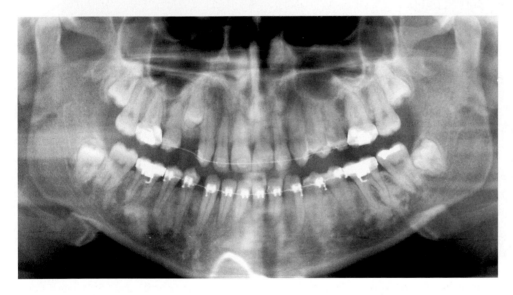

FIGURE 22-41 Panoramic film of a patient with familial multiple polyposis syndrome. Note the multiple DBIs throughout the jaws; one has interfered with the eruption of the maxillary right first bicuspid.

cancer may also help. These patients should be referred to their family physician for examination for intestinal polyposis and treatment.

Central Hemangioma

Disease Mechanism.   A hemangioma is a proliferation of blood vessels creating a mass that resembles a neoplasm, although in many cases it is actually a hamartoma. Hemangiomas can occur anywhere in the body but are most frequently noticed on the skin and subcutaneous tissues. The central (intraosseous) type most often is found in the vertebrae and skull and rarely in the jaws. The lesions may be developmental or traumatic in origin.

Clinical Features.   Hemangiomas are more prevalent in females than males with a ratio of 2:1. This tumor occurs most commonly in the first decade but may occur later in life. Enlargement is slow, producing a nontender expansion of the jaw that occurs over several months or years. The swelling may or may not be painful, is not tender, and usually is bony hard. Pain, if present, probably is the throbbing type. Some tumors may be compressible or pulsate, and a bruit may be detected on auscultation. Anesthesia of the skin supplied by the mental nerve may occur. The lesion may cause loosening and migration of teeth in the affected area. Bleeding may occur from the gingiva around the neck of the affected teeth. These teeth may demonstrate rebound mobility; that is, when depressed into their sockets, they rebound to their original position within several minutes because of the pressure of the vascular network around the tooth. Aspiration with a syringe produces arterial blood that may be under considerable pressure.

Imaging Features

Location.   Hemangiomas affect the mandible about twice as often as the maxilla. In the mandible, the most common site is the posterior body and ramus and within the inferior alveolar canal.

Periphery.   In some instances, the periphery is well defined and corticated; in other cases, it may be ill defined and even simulate the appearance of a malignant tumor. This variation probably is related to the amount of residual bone present around the blood vessels. The formation of linear spicules of bone emanating from the surface of the bone in a sun-ray–like appearance can occur when the hemangioma breaks through the outer cortex and displaces the periosteum (Fig. 22-42).

Internal Structure.   When there is residual bone trapped around the blood vessels, the result may be a multilocular appearance. Small radiolucent locules may resemble enlarged marrow spaces surrounded by coarse, dense, and well-defined trabeculae (Fig. 22-43). These internal trabeculae may produce a honeycomb pattern composed of small circular radiolucent spaces that represent blood vessels that are oriented in the same direction of the x-ray beam. When the inferior alveolar canal is involved, the whole canal is increased in width and often the normal path of the canal is altered into a serpiginous shape sometimes creating a multilocular appearance (Fig. 22-44). Some lesions may be totally radiolucent. When the hemangioma involves soft tissue, the formation of phlebolith (small areas of calcification or concretions found in a vein with slow blood flow) may occur within surrounding soft tissues (Fig. 22-45). They develop from thrombi that become organized and mineralized and consist of calcium phosphate and calcium carbonate.

Effects on Surrounding Structures.   The roots of teeth in the region of the vascular lesion often are resorbed or displaced. When the lesion involves the inferior alveolar nerve canal, the canal can be enlarged along its entire length, and its shape may be changed to a serpiginous path. The mandibular and mental foramen may be enlarged. Hemangiomas can influence the growth of bone and teeth. The involved bone may be enlarged and have coarse, internal trabeculae. Also, developing teeth may be larger and erupt

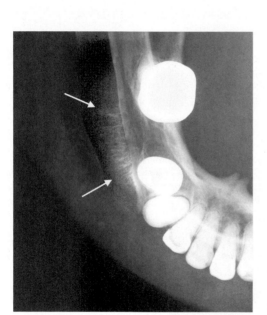

FIGURE 22-42 Occlusal film of a case of a central hemangioma of the mandible with adjacent spiculation *(arrows)*, which has a very similar appearance to the spiculation seen in osteogenic sarcoma.

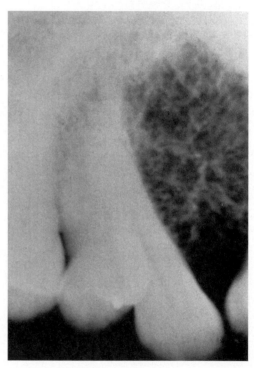

FIGURE 22-43 Hemangioma in the anterior maxilla shows a coarse trabecular pattern. *(Courtesy E. J. Burkes, DDS, Chapel Hill, NC.)*

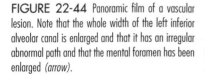

FIGURE 22-44 Panoramic film of a vascular lesion. Note that the whole width of the left inferior alveolar canal is enlarged and that it has an irregular abnormal path and that the mental foramen has been enlarged *(arrow)*.

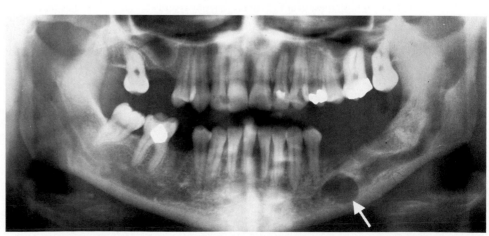

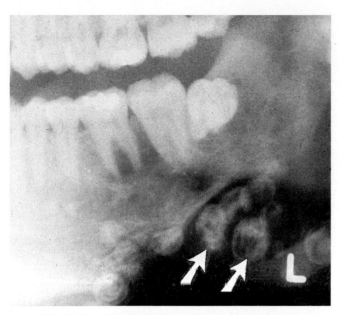

FIGURE 22-45 Soft tissue hemangioma with phleboliths *(arrows)*.

earlier when in an intimate relationship with a hemangioma (Fig. 22-46). Further diagnostic imaging to document better the distribution and degree of involvement of the osseous and soft tissues of the maxillofacial region should include modalities such as conventional angiography and MR angiography.

Differential Diagnosis. Hemangiomas should be considered in the differential diagnosis of multilocular lesions involving the body of the ramus and body of the mandible. Demonstration of involvement of the inferior alveolar canal is an important indicator of a vascular lesion. In most cases, soft tissue changes suggest a vascular lesion. When a hemangioma produces a sun-ray, spiculated bone pattern at its periphery, the appearance may be difficult to differentiate from an osteogenic sarcoma (see Fig. 22-42).

Treatment. Central hemangiomas should be treated without delay because trauma that disrupts the integrity of the affected jaw may result in lethal exsanguination. Specifically, embolization (introduction of inert materials into the lesion by a vascular route), surgery (en bloc resection with ligation of the external carotid artery), and sclerosing techniques have been used singly or together.

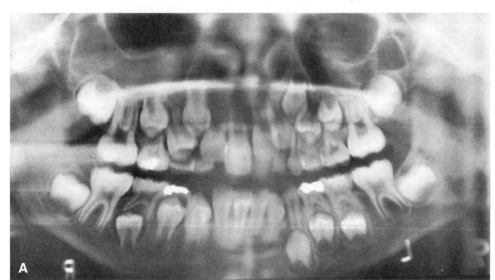

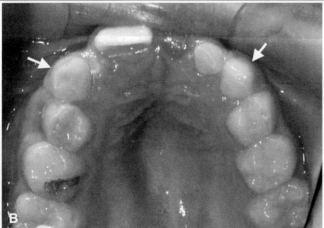

FIGURE 22-46 **A,** Panoramic film demonstrates the effect of a soft tissue hemangioma on the developing dentition. The root development and eruption of the right cuspids and bicuspids are significantly advanced compared with the left side. **B,** Occlusal photograph from the same case. Note the difference in size of the maxillary deciduous cuspids.

Arteriovenous Fistula

Synonyms.   Synonyms for A-V fistula include A-V defect, A-V shunt, A-V aneurysm, and A-V malformation.

Disease Mechanism.   An A-V fistula is not a tumor but a direct communication between an artery and a vein that bypasses the intervening capillary bed. It usually results from trauma but in rare instances may be a developmental anomaly. An A-V fistula can occur anywhere in the body, in soft tissue, in the alveolar process, and centrally in the jaw. The head and neck are the most common sites.

Clinical Features.   The clinical appearance of a central A-V aneurysm can vary considerably, depending on the extent of bone or soft tissue involvement. The lesion may expand bone, and a mass may be present in the extraosseous soft tissue. The soft tissue swelling may have a purple discoloration. Palpation or auscultation of the swelling may reveal a pulse. Alternatively, neither the bone nor the soft tissue may be expanded, and no pulse may be clinically apparent. Aspiration produces blood. Recognition of the hemorrhagic nature of these lesions is of utmost importance because extraction of an associated tooth may be immediately followed by life-threatening bleeding.

Imaging Features
   Location.   These lesions most commonly develop in the ramus and retromolar area of the mandible and involve the mandibular canal.
   Periphery.   The margins usually are well defined and corticated.
   Internal Structure.   A tortuous path of an enlarged vessel in bone may give a multilocular appearance. Otherwise, the lesion is radiolucent.
   Effects on Surrounding Structures.   Both central lesions and lesions in adjacent soft tissue can erode bone, resulting in well-defined (cystlike) lesions in the bone. Changes in the inferior alveolar canal may occur, as described in the preceding section on hemangiomas.

Additional Imaging.   MDCT imaging with injection of contrast material is a useful method for aiding the differential diagnosis of any vascular lesion and other neoplasms of the jaws (Fig. 22-47). MR angiography is now being used routinely to document the size, extent, and vessels involved with the vascular lesion. Angiography, a radiographic procedure performed by injecting a radiopaque contrast agent into the blood vessels and making images, provides the same information and is usually used when interventional therapy is planned in conjunction with the angiography (Fig. 22-48).

Differential Diagnosis.   Occasionally, the imaging appearance is not specific for A-V aneurysm. The differential diagnosis is similar to hemangiomas and includes multilocular lesions. However, association with the inferior alveolar canal is important in differentiation.

Treatment.   An A-V aneurysm is treated surgically.

Osteoblastoma

Synonym.   Giant osteoid osteoma is a synonym for osteoblastoma.

Disease Mechanism.   An osteoblastoma is an uncommon, benign tumor of osteoblasts with areas of osteoid and immature bone. This tumor occurs most often in the spine of a young person. Agreement apparently is increasing that if osteoblastomas and osteoid osteomas are different lesions; they differ only in size and morphologic and histologic features. The osteoid trabeculae in an osteoblastoma generally are larger (broader and longer, with wider trabecular spaces) than those in an osteoid osteoma. An osteoblastoma is usually less painful, and it has more osteoclasts. In addition, benign osteoblastomas are considered more aggressive lesions. On the level of their ultrastructures, the two lesions essentially are similar or at least closely related.

Clinical Features.   Both osteoblastomas and osteoid osteomas are rare in the jaws. The male-to-female ratio is 2 : 1, although some studies indicate a higher female occurrence, and the average age is 17 years, with most lesions occurring in the second and third decades of life. Clinically, patients often report pain and swelling of the affected region; however, the pain is more severe in osteoid osteomas and is often relieved by salicylates.

Imaging Features
   Location.   Osteoblastomas are found both in the tooth-bearing regions and commonly around the temporomandibular joint (within the condyle or the temporal bone).
   Periphery.   The borders may be diffuse or may show some sign of a cortex. Lesions often have a soft tissue capsule around the periphery indicating that this tumor is more mature in the central regions where there is evidence of abnormal bone (Fig. 22-49).
   Internal Structure.   The internal structure may be entirely radiolucent in early developing tumors or may show varying degrees of calcific material. The internal calcification may take the form of fine granular bone trabeculae.
   Effects on Surrounding Structures.   Osteoblastomas can expand bone, but usually a thin outer cortex is maintained. This lesion may invaginate the maxillary sinus or the middle cranial fossa.

Differential Diagnosis.   An important differential diagnosis may be a well-defined osteogenic sarcoma because the histologic appearance may be very similar. The differentiation may rely on the benign features of the osteoblastoma as revealed in the diagnostic images. Osteoblastomas do not normally break through cortical boundaries and invade surrounding soft tissue. Osteoid osteomas are usually smaller and have an associated sclerotic bone reaction at the periphery. Sometimes the appearance of an osteoblastoma may be similar to a large area of cemental dysplasia. Both have a soft tissue capsule but the osteoblastoma behaves more aggressively like a tumor.

Treatment.   Osteoblastomas are treated with curettage or local excision. Recurrences have been described, and in a few cases the differentiation from a low-grade osteosarcoma may be difficult.

Osteoid Osteoma

Disease Mechanism.   An osteoid osteoma is a benign tumor that is extremely rare in the jaws. Its true nature is unknown, but some investigators think it is a variant of osteoblastoma. The tumor has an oval or round, tumor-like core usually only about 1 cm in diameter, although some may reach 5 or 6 cm. This core consists of osteoid and newly formed trabeculae within highly vascularized, osteogenic connective tissue. The tumor usually develops within the outer cortex but may form within the cancellous bone. There

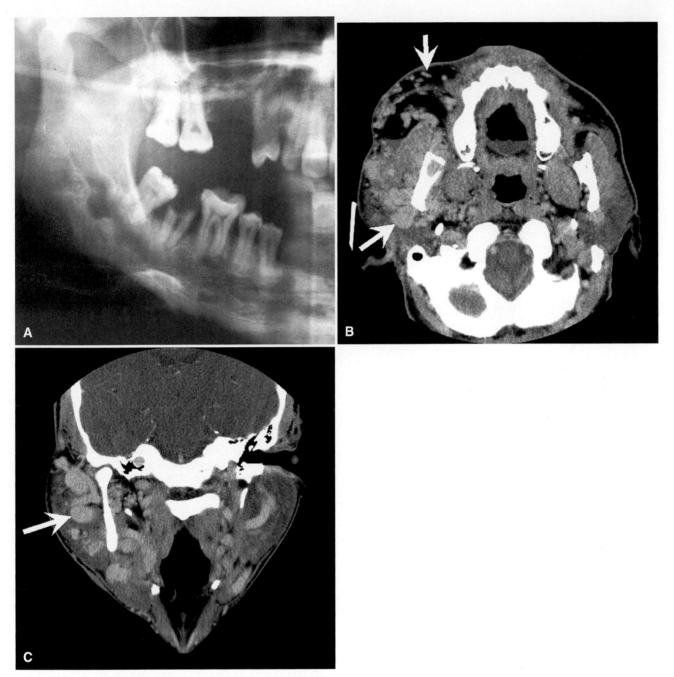

FIGURE 22-47 A, Panoramic film of a patient with an A-V malformation. Note the enlarged and irregular inferior alveolar canal. **B** and **C,** Axial and coronal CT images using soft tissue algorithm obtained after administration of intravascular contrast medium, which causes the blood vessels to be more radiopaque *(arrows).*

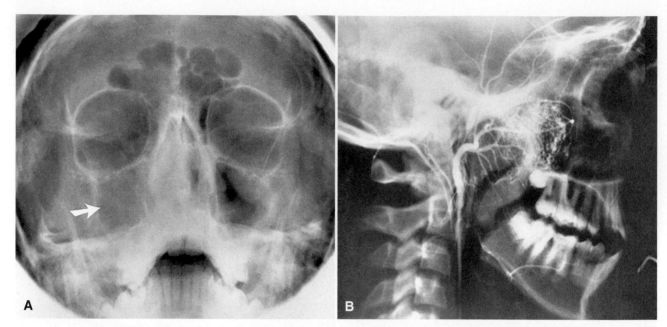

FIGURE 22-48 Vascular lesion in the right maxillary sinus. **A,** Waters' radiograph shows the opacified maxillary antrum *(arrow)*. **B,** Note the tumor vascularization on this angiogram. A radiopaque dye has been injected into the vasculature to enhance visualization. *(Courtesy G. Himadi, DDS, Chapel Hill, NC.)*

is a sclerotic bone reaction around the periphery, often thinner in lesions within the cancellous bone.

Clinical Features.   Osteoid osteomas occur most often in young people, usually males between the ages of 10 and 25 years. They seldom occur before age 4 years or after age 40. This condition affects at least twice as many males as females. Most of the lesions occur in the femur and tibia; the jaws are rarely involved. Severe pain in the bone that can be relieved by antiinflammatory drugs is characteristic. In addition, the soft tissue over the involved bony area may be swollen and tender.

Imaging Features
   Location.   The lesion is most common in the cortex of the limb bones and spine. In the jaws osteoid osteomas are more common in the body of the mandible.
   Periphery.   The margins are well defined by a rim of sclerotic bone (Fig. 22-50).
   Internal Structure.   The internal aspect of young lesions is composed of a small ovoid or round radiolucent area (core). In more mature lesions, the central radiolucency may have radiopaque foci representing abnormal bone.
   Effects on Surrounding Structures.   As previously mentioned, this tumor can stimulate a sclerotic bone reaction and cause thickening of the outer cortex by stimulating periosteal new bone formation.

Differential Diagnosis.   Osteoid osteomas are extremely rare in the jaws. A clinician who suspects that a sclerotic lesion is an osteoid osteoma should also consider sclerosing osteitis, cemento-ossifying fibroma, benign cementoblastoma, and cemental dysplasia. The presence of a central radiolucency usually eliminates enostosis or osteosclerosis. Scintigraphy using a bone scan helps in the differential diagnosis by revealing considerable vascularity in the blood pool phase and a very high comparative bone metabolism.

Treatment.   Complete excision currently is the recommended treatment because it often relieves the pain and cures the disease. A new, more conservative treatment involving radiofrequency thermoablation is obtaining success rates of 76% to 100%. Although spontaneous remission can occur in some cases, the data are insufficient for identifying such cases in advance.

Ossifying Fibroma
Synonyms.   Synonyms for ossifying fibroma include cemento-ossifying fibroma, cementifying fibroma, and juvenile aggressive ossifying fibroma.

Disease Mechanism.   This bone tumor consists of highly cellular, fibrous tissue that contains varying amounts of abnormal bone. Previously, acellular amorphous calcified material contained within some lesions was defined as cementum or cementum-like; however, it now seems likely that this represents abnormal amorphous bone. Therefore, there is no cogent rationale for using the term cementum or cementum-like tissue. Other internal regions of this tumor can have irregular trabeculae of woven or lamellar bone. The resulting internal pattern may be very similar to or indistinguishable from fibrous dysplasia. One distinguishing feature that may be present is a soft tissue capsule at the periphery not seen in fibrous dysplasia.
   Juvenile ossifying fibroma is a very aggressive form of ossifying fibroma that occurs in the first 2 decades of life. Although the histopathologic definition of this entity is controversial, the radiologic appearance has similarities to that of ossifying fibroma but may be much more expansile.

Clinical Features.   The clinical features of ossifying fibroma can vary from indolent to aggressive behavior. Ossifying fibroma can occur at any age but usually is found in young adults. Females are affected more often than males. The disease usually is asymptomatic at the time of discovery. Occasionally, facial asymmetry

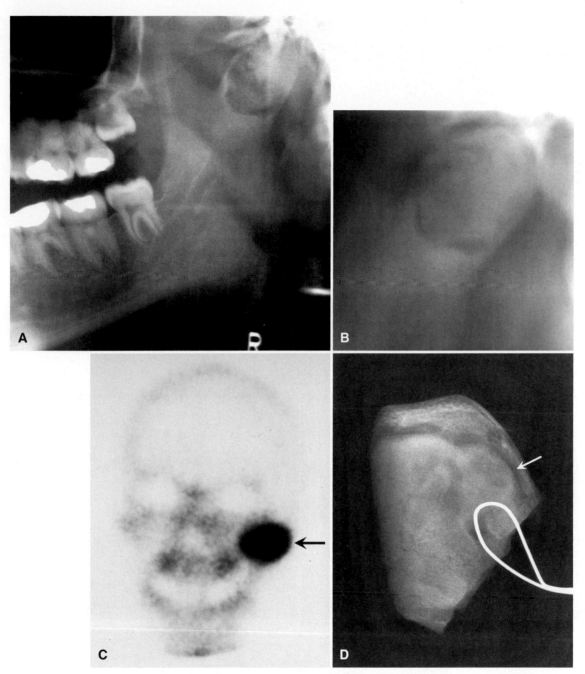

FIGURE 22-49 A, Cropped panoramic film of an osteoblastoma occupying the left condyle. Note the enlargement of the condyle and presence of a soft tissue capsule surrounding an internal structure of granular bone. **B,** Tomograph of the left condyle. **C,** Technetium bone scan demonstrates increased bone activity in the left condyle *(arrow)*. **D,** Radiograph of the surgical specimen. Note the internal granular bone surrounded by a soft tissue capsule *(arrow)*.

develops. Displacement of the teeth may be an early clinical feature, although most lesions are discovered during routine dental examinations. In cases of juvenile ossifying fibroma, rapid growth may occur in a young patient, resulting in deformity of the involved jaw.

Imaging Features

Location. Ossifying fibroma appears almost exclusively in the facial bones and most commonly in the mandible, typically inferior to the premolars and molars and superior to the inferior alveolar canal. In the maxilla, it occurs most often in the canine fossa and zygomatic arch area.

Periphery. The borders are usually well defined. A thin, radiolucent line, representing a fibrous capsule, may separate it from surrounding bone (Fig. 22-51). Sometimes the bone next to the lesion develops a sclerotic border.

Internal Structure. The internal structure is a mixed radiolucent-radiopaque density with a pattern that depends on the amount and form of the manufactured calcified material. In some instances, the internal structure may appear almost totally radiolucent with

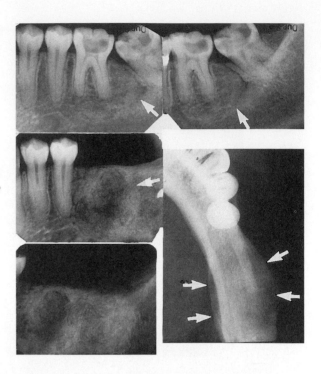

FIGURE 22-50 Osteoid osteoma *(single arrow)* appears as a mixed radiolucent-radiopaque lesion in the molar region. The lesion has caused expansion of the buccal and lingual cortex of the mandible *(multiple arrows)*. *(Courtesy A. Shawkat, DDS, Radcliff, KY.)*

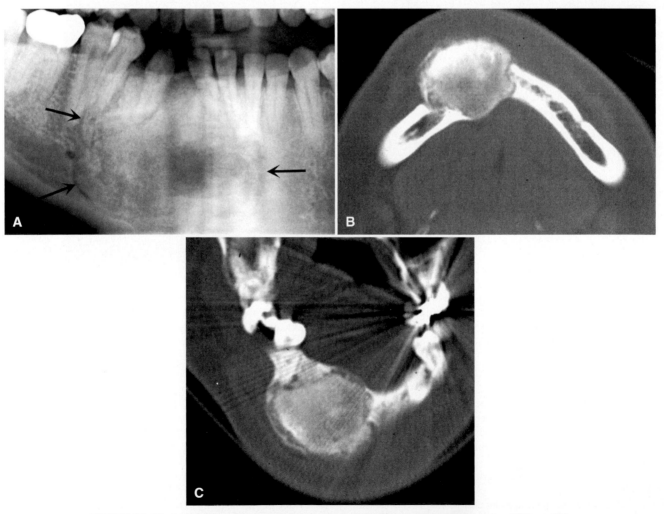

FIGURE 22-51 Ossifying fibroma depicted on a panoramic film *(arrows)* **(A)**, axial CT image **(B)**, and coronal CT image **(C)**. Note the homogeneous, radiopaque internal structure of amorphous bone and the radiolucent band at the periphery.

just a hint of calcified material. In the type that contains mainly abnormal trabeculae of bone, the pattern may be similar to that seen in fibrous dysplasia, or a wispy (similar to stretched tufts of cotton) or flocculent (similar to large, heavy snowflakes) pattern may be seen (Fig. 22-52). Lesions that produce more amorphous bone may contain solid, homogeneously radiopaque regions that do not have any intrinsic pattern (see Fig. 22-51).

Effects on Surrounding Structures.   Ossifying fibroma can be distinguished from the previously mentioned bone dysplasias by its tumor-like behavior; this is reflected in the growth of the lesion, which tends to be concentric within the medullary part of the bone with outward expansion approximately equal in all directions. This growth can result in displacement of teeth or of the inferior alveolar canal and expansion of the outer cortical plates of bone. A significant point is that the outer cortical plate, although displaced and thinned, remains intact. Ossifying fibroma can grow into and occupy the entire maxillary sinus (Fig. 22-53), expanding its walls outward; however, a bony partition always exists between the internal aspect of the remaining sinus and the tumor. The lamina dura of involved teeth usually is missing, and resorption of teeth may occur.

Differential Diagnosis.   The differential diagnosis of ossifying fibroma includes lesions with a mixed radiolucent-radiopaque internal structure. The differentiation from fibrous dysplasia can be very difficult. The boundaries of ossifying fibroma usually are better defined, and these lesions occasionally have a soft tissue capsule and cortex, whereas fibrous dysplasia usually blends in with surrounding bone. The internal structure of fibrous dysplasia lesions in the maxilla may be more homogeneous and show less variation. Both types of lesions can displace teeth, but ossifying fibroma displaces from a specific point or epicenter. Fibrous dysplasia rarely resorbs teeth. The expansion of the jaws associated with ossifying fibroma is more concentric about a definite epicenter, but fibrous dysplasia enlarges the bone while distorting the overall shape to a smaller degree; in other words, the expanded bone still resembles normal morphology.

Great difficulty may arise in differentiating ossifying fibroma from fibrous dysplasia when the lesion involves the maxillary antrum. Fibrous dysplasia usually displaces the lateral wall of the maxilla into the maxillary antrum, maintaining the outer shape of the wall, whereas an ossifying fibroma has a more convex shape as it extends into the maxillary antrum (see Fig. 22-53; also see Chapter 23). Also, fibrous dysplasia may change the bone around the teeth without displacing the teeth from an obvious epicenter of a concentrically growing benign tumor. The importance of this differentiation lies in the treatment, which is resection for an ossifying fibroma and observation for fibrous dysplasia.

The differential diagnosis of the type of ossifying fibroma that produces a mainly homogeneous amorphous bone from periapical osseous dysplasia (POD) may be difficult, especially with large single lesions of POD. However, POD is often multifocal, whereas ossifying fibroma is not. Also, the presence of a simple bone cyst is a characteristic of either florid osseous dysplasia or POD but not ossifying fibroma. Ossifying fibroma behaves in a more tumor-like fashion, with the displacement of teeth and concentric expansion. A wide sclerotic border is more characteristic of the slow-growing cemental dysplasia as well as undulating expansion.

Other lesions to be considered include those that have internal calcifications similar to the pattern seen in ossifying fibroma. These include giant cell granuloma, calcifying odontogenic cysts, calcifying epithelial odontogenic (Pindborg), and adenomatoid odontogenic tumors.

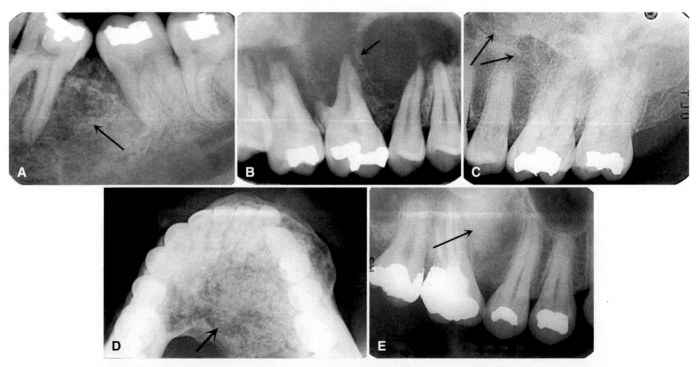

FIGURE 22-52 Various bone patterns seen in ossifying fibroma. **A,** Wispy trabecular pattern *(arrow)*. **B,** Most of this pattern is radiolucent with a few wispy trabeculae *(arrow)*. **C,** Fibrous dysplasia granular-like pattern *(arrows)*. **D,** Flocculent pattern with larger tufts of bone formation *(arrow)*. **E,** Solid, radiopaque, cementum-like pattern *(arrow)*.

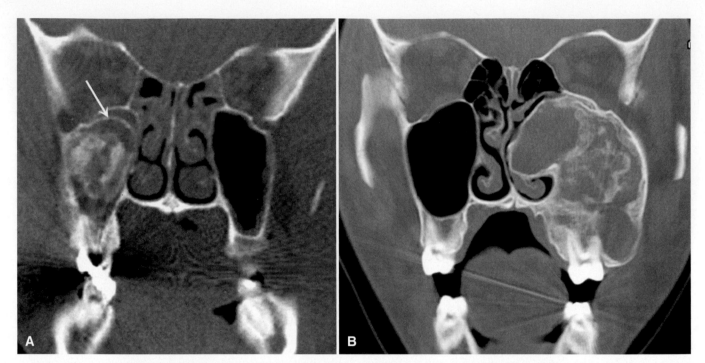

FIGURE 22-53 Large ossifying fibromas involving the maxilla. **A,** Coronal CT image of a lesion invaginating the maxillary antrum. In contrast to in fibrous dysplasia, the peripheral border of the lesion *(arrow)* does not parallel the original shape of the antrum. **B,** Coronal CT scan of a larger lesion expanding the maxilla, occupying all of the maxillary antrum, and extending into the nasal fossa.

Occasionally, the diagnosis of osteogenic sarcoma is considered. However, characteristics suggesting a malignant lesion should be seen, such as cortical bone destruction and invasion into the surrounding soft tissues and along the periodontal ligament space.

Management. The prognosis of ossifying fibroma is favorable with surgical enucleation or resection. Large lesions require a detailed determination of the extent of the lesion, which can be obtained with CT imaging. Even if the lesion has reached appreciable size, it usually can be separated from the surrounding tissue and completely removed. Recurrence after removal is unlikely.

Desmoplastic Fibroma of Bone

Synonym. A synonym for desmoplastic fibroma of bone is aggressive fibromatosis; this is usually reserved for tumors that originate in soft tissue.

Disease Mechanism. A desmoplastic fibroma of bone is an aggressive, infiltrative neoplasm that produces abundant collagen fibers. It is composed of fibroblast-like cells that have ovoid or elongated nuclei in abundant collagen fibers. The lack of pleomorphism of the cells is important.

Clinical Features. Patients usually complain of facial swelling, pain (in rare cases), and sometimes dysfunction, especially when the neoplasm is close to the joint. The lesion occurs most often in the first 2 decades of life, with a mean reported age of 14 years. Although it originates in bone, the tumor may invade the surrounding soft tissue extensively. It also may occur as part of Gardner's syndrome.

Imaging Features

Location. Desmoplastic fibromas of bone may occur in the mandible or maxilla, but the most common site is the ramus and posterior mandible.

Periphery. The periphery most often is ill defined and has an invasive characteristic commonly seen in malignant tumors.

Internal Structure. The internal aspect may be totally radiolucent, especially when the lesion is small. Larger lesions appear to be multilocular with very coarse, thick septa. These wide septa may be straight or may have an irregular shape (Fig. 22-54). On T1-weighted MRI, the internal structure has a low signal, which helps in determining intraosseous extent because of the contrast with the high signal from the bone marrow.

Effects on Surrounding Structures. Desmoplastic fibromas of bone can expand bone and often break through the outer cortex, invading the surrounding soft tissue. Usually CT scan or MRI is required to determine the exact soft tissue extent of the lesion.

Differential Diagnosis. Distinguishing this neoplasm from a fibrosarcoma may be difficult during the histologic examination. The appearance may not be helpful because a desmoplastic fibroma often has the appearance of a malignant neoplasm. However, the presence of coarse, irregular, and sometimes straight septa may help support the correct diagnosis. The appearance of these septa also helps differentiate the lesion from other multilocular tumors. Very small lesions may resemble simple bone cysts.

Treatment. Resection of this neoplasm with adequate margins is recommended because of its high recurrence rate. Patients who have been treated for the condition should be followed closely with frequent radiologic examinations.

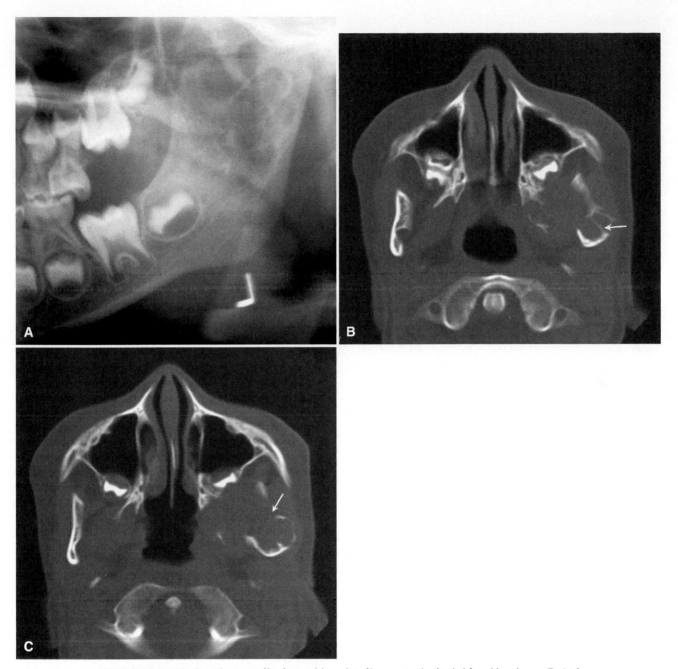

FIGURE 22-54 **A,** Cropped panoramic film of a central desmoplastic fibroma centered within the left condyle and ramus. **B,** Axial CT image using bone algorithm reveals thick straight septa *(arrows)*. **C,** CT image at a higher level reveals that the tumor has broken through the anterior cortex of the condylar head.

BIBLIOGRAPHY

Barnes L, Eveson JW, Reichart P, et al: Odontogenic tumors. In *World Health Organization Classification of Tumours. Pathology and genetics of head and neck tumours,* Lyon, 2005, IARC Press.

Daley TD, Wysocki GP, Pringle GA: Relative incidence of odontogenic tumors and oral and jaw cysts in a Canadian population, *Oral Surg Oral Med Oral Pathol* 77:276–280, 1994.

Hoffman S, Jacoway JR, Krolls SO: Intraosseous and parosteal tumors of the jaws. In *Atlas of tumor pathology, series 2, fascicle 24,* Washington, DC, 1987, Armed Forces Institute of Pathology.

Regezi JA, Kerr DA, Courtney RM: Odontogenic tumors: an analysis of 706 cases, *J Oral Surg* 36:771–778, 1978.

Unni KK: *Dahlin's bone tumors: general aspects and data on 11,087 cases,* ed 5, Philadelphia, 1996, Lippincott-Raven.

Torus Palatinus

Eggan S, Natvig B, Gåsemyr J: Variation in torus palatinus prevalence in Norway, *Scand J Dent Res* 102:54–59, 1994.

Gorsky M, Raviv M, Kfir E, et al: Prevalence of torus palatinus in a population of young and old Israelis, *Arch Oral Biol* 41:623–625, 1996.

Haugen LK: Palatine and mandibular tori: a morphologic study in the current Norwegian population, *Acta Odontol Scand* 50:65–77, 1992.

Torus Mandibularis

Eggen S, Natvig B: Concurrence of torus mandibularis and torus palatinus, *Scand J Dent Res* 102:60–63, 1994.

Hyperostosis

Jainkittivong A, Langlais RP: Buccal and palatal exostosis: prevalence and concurrence with tori, *Oral Surg Oral Med Oral Pathol Oral Radiol Endod* 90:48–53, 2000.

Enostosis

McDonnel D: Dense bone island: a review of 107 patients, *Oral Surg Oral Med Oral Pathol* 76:124–128, 1993.

Petrikowski GC, Peters E: Longitudinal radiographic assessment of dense bone islands of the jaws, *Oral Surg Oral Med Oral Pathol Oral Radiol Endod* 83:627–634, 1997.

Ameloblastoma

Atkinson CH, Harwood AR, Cummings BJ: Ameloblastoma of the jaw: a reappraisal of the role of megavoltage irradiation, *Cancer* 53:869–873, 1984.

Kim S, Jang HS: Ameloblastoma: a clinical, radiographic, and histopathologic analysis of 71 cases, *Oral Surg Oral Med Oral Pathol Oral Radiol Endod* 91:649–253, 2001.

Effiom OA, Odukoya O: Desmoplastic ameloblastoma: analysis of 17 Nigerian cases, *Oral Surg Oral Med Oral Pathol Oral Radiol Endod* 111:e27–e31, 2011.

Ueta E, Yoneda K, Ohno A, et al: Intraosseous carcinoma arising from mandibular ameloblastoma with progressive invasion and pulmonary metastasis, *Int J Oral Maxillofac Surg* 25:370–372, 1996.

Weissman JL, Snyderman CH, Yousem SA, et al: Ameloblastoma of the maxilla: CT and MR appearance, *AJNR Am J Neuroradiol* 14:223–226, 1993.

Adenomatoid Odontogenic Tumor

Dare A, Yamaguchi A, Yoshiki S, et al: Limitation of panoramic radiography in diagnosing adenomatoid odontogenic tumors, *Oral Surg Oral Med Oral Pathol* 77:662–668, 1994.

Hicks MJ, Flaitz CM, Batsakis JG: Pathology consultation: adenomatoid and calcifying epithelial odontogenic tumors, *Ann Otol Rhinol Laryngol* 102:159, 1993.

Philipsen HP, Reichart PA: Adenomatoid odontogenic tumor: facts and figures, *Oral Oncol* 35:125–131, 1998.

Calcifying Epithelial Odontogenic Tumor

Franklin CD, Pindborg JJ: The calcifying epithelial odontogenic tumor: a review and analysis of 113 cases, *Oral Surg Oral Med Oral Pathol* 42:753–765, 1976.

Kaplan I, Buckner A, Caleron S, et al: Radiological and clinical features of calcifying epithelial odontogenic tumor, *Dentomaxillofac Radiol* 30:22–28, 2001.

Piñtino B, Fernández-Alba J, Garcia-Rozado A, et al: Calcifying epithelial odontogenic (Pindborg) tumor: a series of 4 distinctive cases and review of the literature, *J Oral Maxillofac Surg* 63:1361–1368, 2005.

Compound Odontoma

Haishima K, Haishima H, Yamada Y, et al: Compound odontomes associated with impacted maxillary primary central incisors: report of 2 cases, *Int J Pediatr Dent* 4:251–256, 1994.

Kaugars GE, Miller ME, Abbey LM: Odontomas, *Oral Surg Oral Med Oral Pathol* 67:172–176, 1989.

Nik-Hussein NN, Majid ZA: Erupted compound odontoma, *Ann Dent* 52:9–11, 1993.

Ameloblastic Fibroma

Dallera P, Bertoni F, Marchetti C, et al: Ameloblastic fibroma: a follow-up of six cases, *Int J Oral Maxillofac Surg* 25:199–202, 1996.

Trodahl JN: Ameloblastic fibroma: a survey of cases from the Armed Forces Institute of Pathology, *Oral Surg Oral Med Oral Pathol* 33:547–558, 1972.

Odontogenic Myxoma

Cohen MA, Mendelsohn DB: CT and MR imaging of myxofibroma of the jaws, *J Comput Assist Tomogr* 14:281–285, 1990.

Peltola J, Magnusson B, Happonen RP, et al: Odontogenic myxoma: a radiographic study of 21 tumours, *Br J Oral Maxillofac Surg* 32:298–302, 1994.

Simon EN, Merkx MA, Vuhahula E, et al: Odontogenic myxoma: a clinicopathological study of 33 cases, *Int J Oral Maxillofac Surg* 33:333–337, 2004.

Sumi Y, Miyaishi O, Ito K, et al: Magnetic resonance imaging of myxoma in the mandible: a case report, *Oral Surg Oral Med Oral Pathol Oral Radiol Endod* 90:671–676, 2000.

Benign Cementoblastoma

Brannon RB, Fowler CB, Carpenter WM, et al: Cementoblastoma: an innocuous neoplasm? A clinicopathological study of 44 cases and review of the literature with special emphasis on recurrence, *Oral Surg Oral Med Oral Pathol Oral Radiol Endod* 93:311–320, 2002.

Jelic JS, Loftus MJ, Miller AS, et al: Benign cementoblastoma: report of an unusual case and analysis of 14 additional cases, *J Oral Maxillofac Surg* 51:1033–1037, 1993.

Ruprecht A, Ross AS: Benign cementoblastoma (true cementoblastoma), *Dentomaxillofac Radiol* 12:31–33, 1983.

Central Odontogenic Fibroma

Brannon RB: Central odontogenic fibroma, myxoma (odontogenic myxoma, fibromyxoma) and central odontogenic granular cell tumor, *Oral Maxillofac Surg Clin North Am* 16:359, 2004.

Handlers JP, Abrams AM, Melrose RJ, et al: Central odontogenic fibroma: clinicopathologic features of 19 cases and review of the literature, *J Oral Maxillofac Surg* 49:46–54, 1991.

Kaffe I, Buchner A: Radiologic features of central odontogenic fibroma, *Oral Surg Oral Med Oral Pathol* 78:811–818, 1994.

Neurilemoma

Chi AC, Carey J, Muller S, et al: Intraosseous schwannoma of the mandible: case report and review of the literature, *Oral Surg Oral Med Oral Pathol Oral Radiol Endod* 96:54–65, 2003.

Minowa K, Sakakibara N, Yoshikawa K, et al: CT and MRI findings of intraosseous schwannoma of the mandible: a case report, *Dentomaxillofac Radiol* 36:113–116, 2007.

Hemangioma

Lund BA, Dahlin DC: Hemangiomas of the mandible and maxilla, *J Oral Surg* 22:234–242, 1964.

Fan X, Qiu W, Zhang Z, et al: Comparative study of clinical manifestation, plain-film radiography and computed tomographic scan in arteriovenous malformations of the jaws, *Oral Surg Oral Med Oral Pathol Oral Radiol Endod* 94:503–509, 2002.

Zlotogorski A, Buchner A, Kaffe I, et al: Radiological features of central haemangioma of the jaws, *Dentomaxillofac Radiol* 34:292–296, 2005.

Osteoma

Bilkay U, Erdem O, Ozek C, et al: Benign osteoma with Gardner syndrome: review of the literature and report of a case, *J Craniofac Surg* 15:506–509, 2004.

Earwaker J: Paranasal osteomas: a review of 46 cases, *Skeletal Radiol* 22:417–423, 1993.

Matteson S, Deahl ST, Alder ME, et al: Advanced imaging methods, *Crit Rev Oral Biol Med* 7:346–395, 1996.

Thakker NS, Evans DG, Horner K, et al: Florid oral manifestations in an atypical familial adenomatous polyposis family with late presentation of colorectal polyps, *J Oral Pathol Med* 25:459–462, 1996.

Neurofibromatosis

D'Ambrosio JA, Langlais RP, Young RS: Jaw and skull changes in neurofibromatosis, *Oral Surg Oral Med Oral Pathol* 66:391–396, 1988.

Lee L, Yan YH, Pharoah MJ: Radiographic features of the mandible in neurofibromatosis: a report of 10 cases and review of the literature, *Oral Surg Oral Med Oral Pathol Oral Radiol Endod* 81: 361–367, 1996.

Osteoblastoma

Alvares Capelozza AL, Gião Dezotti MS, Casati Alvares L, et al: Osteoblastoma of the mandible: systematic review of the literature and report of a case, *Dentomaxillofac Radiol* 34:1–8, 2005.

Jones AC, Prihoda TJ, Kacher JE, et al: Osteoblastoma of the maxilla and mandible: a report of 24 cases, review of the literature, and discussion of its relationship to osteoid osteoma of the jaws, *Oral Surg Oral Med Oral Pathol Oral Radiol Endod* 102:639–650, 2006.

Lucas DR, Unni KK, McLeod RA, et al: Osteoblastoma: clinicopathologic study of 306 cases, *Hum Pathol* 25:117–134, 1994.

Desmoplastic Fibroma of Bone

Hopkins KM, Huttula CS, Kahn MA, et al: Desmoplastic fibroma of the mandible: review and report of two cases, *J Oral Maxillofac Surg* 54:1249–1254, 1996.

Said-Al-Naief N, Fernandes R, Louis P, et al: Desmoplastic fibroma of the jaw: a case report and review of literature, *Oral Surg Oral Med Oral Pathol Oral Radiol Endod* 101:82–94, 2006.

This chapter discusses disorders of bone that do not easily fit into well-defined categories of disease.

BONE DYSPLASIAS

DISEASE MECHANISM

Bone dysplasias constitute a group of conditions in which normal bone is replaced with fibrous tissue containing abnormal bone. These lesions must be differentiated from tumors because the treatment is very different. Fibro-osseous lesion, originally a histopathologic term, is a commonly used term that includes the following bone dysplasias as well as neoplasms and other lesions of bone.

FIBROUS DYSPLASIA

Disease Mechanism

Fibrous dysplasia results from a localized change in normal bone metabolism that results in the replacement of all the components of cancellous bone by fibrous tissue containing varying amounts of abnormal-appearing bone. At the histologic level, the result is the appearance of numerous short, irregularly shaped trabeculae of woven bone. These trabeculae are not aligned in response to stress but rather have a random orientation. Compared with normal bone, there are more trabeculae per unit volume within the cancellous component of the involved bone. This histologic appearance is responsible for the abnormal internal trabecular pattern seen in diagnostic images. More recent research has found that mutations in the Gs alpha (GNAS1) gene on chromosome 20q13.32 can be detected in 93% of cases of fibrous dysplasia tested. Fibrous dysplasias may be solitary or multiple (Jaffe type) or may occur in another multiple form associated with McCune-Albright syndrome, which usually comprises polyostotic fibrous dysplasia, cutaneous pigmentation (café au lait spots), and hyperfunction of one or more of the endocrine glands.

Clinical Features

The solitary (monostotic) form of fibrous dysplasia, which accounts for 70% of all cases, is the type that most often involves the jaws. The most common sites (in order) are the ribs, femur, tibia, maxilla, and mandible. The multiple (polyostotic) form usually is found in children younger than 10 years, whereas monostotic disease typically is discovered in a slightly older age group. The lesions usually become static when skeletal growth stops, but proliferation may continue, particularly in the polyostotic form. The lesions may become active in pregnant women or with the use of oral contraceptives; abnormal growth may occur after surgical intervention in young patients. Studies of the sex distribution of fibrous dysplasia show no sexual predilection except for McCune-Albright syndrome, which affects females almost exclusively. Symptoms of the disease may be mild or absent. Monostotic fibrous dysplasia often is discovered as an incidental finding in diagnostic images. Patients with jaw involvement first may complain of unilateral facial swelling or an enlarging deformity of the alveolar process. Pain and pathologic fractures are rare. If extensive craniofacial lesions have impinged on nerve foramina, neurologic symptoms such as anosmia (loss of the sense of smell), deafness, or blindness may develop.

Imaging Features

Location. Fibrous dysplasia involves the maxilla almost twice as often as the mandible and occurs more frequently in the posterior aspect. Lesions more commonly are unilateral (Fig. 23-1) except for very rare extensive lesions of the maxillofacial region that are bilateral.

Periphery. The periphery of fibrous dysplasia lesions most commonly is ill defined, with a gradual blending of normal trabecular bone into an abnormal trabecular pattern. Occasionally, the boundary between normal bone and the lesion can appear sharp and even corticated, especially in young lesions (Fig. 23-2).

Internal Structure. The density and trabecular pattern of fibrous dysplasia lesions vary considerably. The variation is more pronounced in the mandible and more homogeneous in the maxilla. The internal aspect of bone may be more radiolucent, more radiopaque, or a mixture of these two variations compared with normal bone (see Fig. 23-1). The internal density is more radiopaque in the maxilla and the base of the skull. Early lesions may be more radiolucent (Fig. 23-3) than mature lesions and in rare cases may

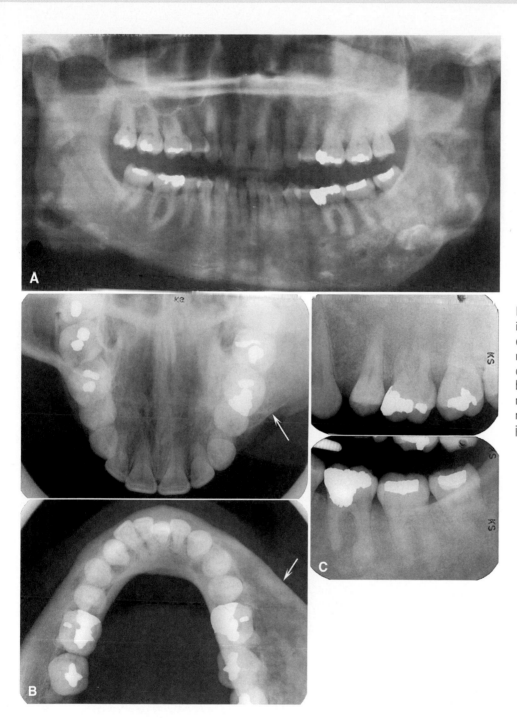

FIGURE 23-1 **A,** Unilateral fibrous dysplasia involving the left maxilla and mandible. **B,** Note the expansion of the lateral aspect of the maxilla and mandible *(arrows)* and the increased bone density caused by an increase in the number of internal trabeculae. **C,** Periapical films show a mixed radiolucent-radiopaque internal structure; however, the overall radiopacity is greater than on the right side of the jaws.

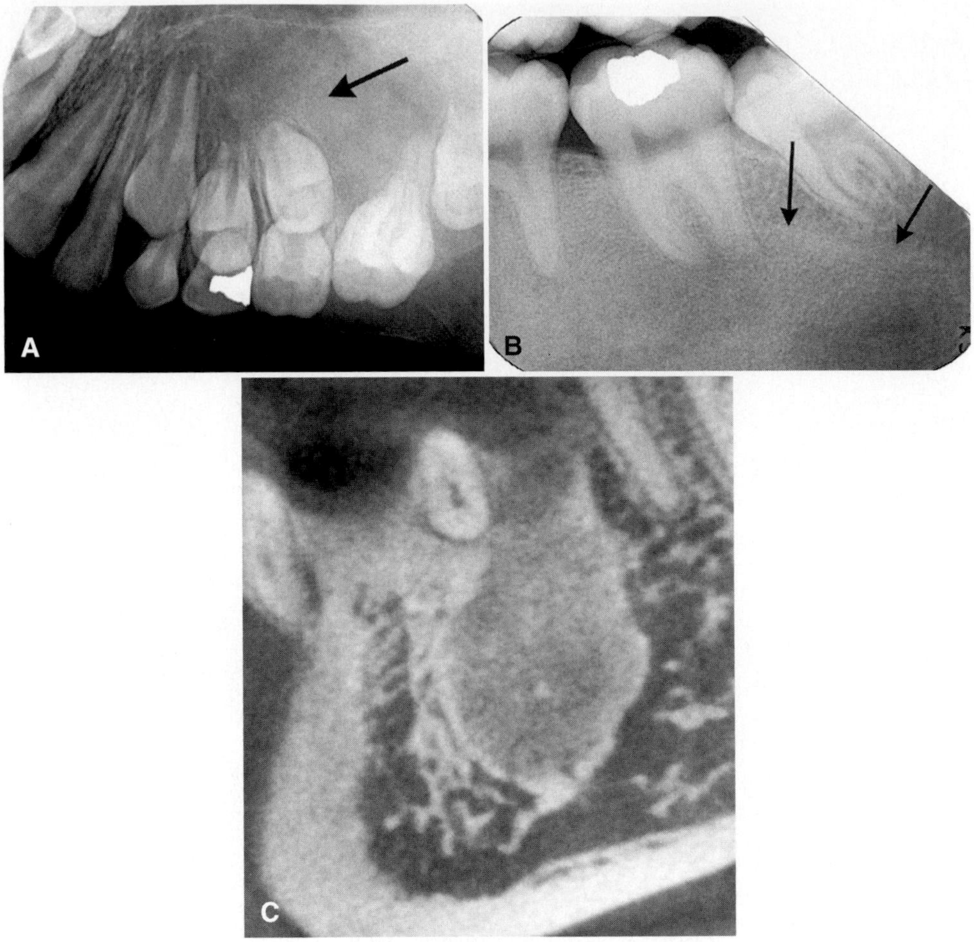

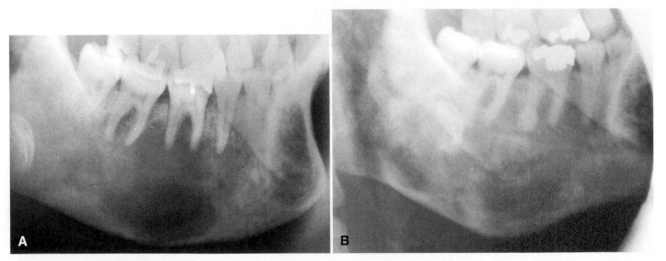

FIGURE 23-2 **A,** Fibrous dysplasia in the posterior maxilla, with an ill-defined anterior margin that blends into the normal bone pattern in the region of the unerupted cuspid. The internal pattern is granular *(arrow).* **B,** In contrast, the margin of this case of mandibular fibrous dysplasia has a well-defined, almost corticated margin *(arrows).* **C,** Sagittal cone-beam CT image of a small example of fibrous dysplasia. Note the cortical-like margin.

FIGURE 23-3 Fibrous dysplasia in the mandible. **A,** Early radiolucent stage. **B,** Same case 18 years later shows a more mature radiopaque appearance.

appear to have granular internal septa, giving the internal aspect a multilocular appearance.

The abnormal trabeculae usually are shorter, thinner, irregularly shaped, and more numerous than normal trabeculae. This creates a radiopaque pattern that can vary; it may have a granular appearance (or ground-glass appearance, resembling the small fragments of a shattered windshield), a pattern resembling the surface of an orange (peau d'orange), a wispy arrangement (cotton wool), or an amorphous, dense pattern (Fig. 23-4). A distinctive characteristic is the organization of the abnormal trabeculae into a swirling pattern similar to a fingerprint (Fig. 23-5). Occasionally, radiolucent regions resembling cysts may occur in mature lesions of

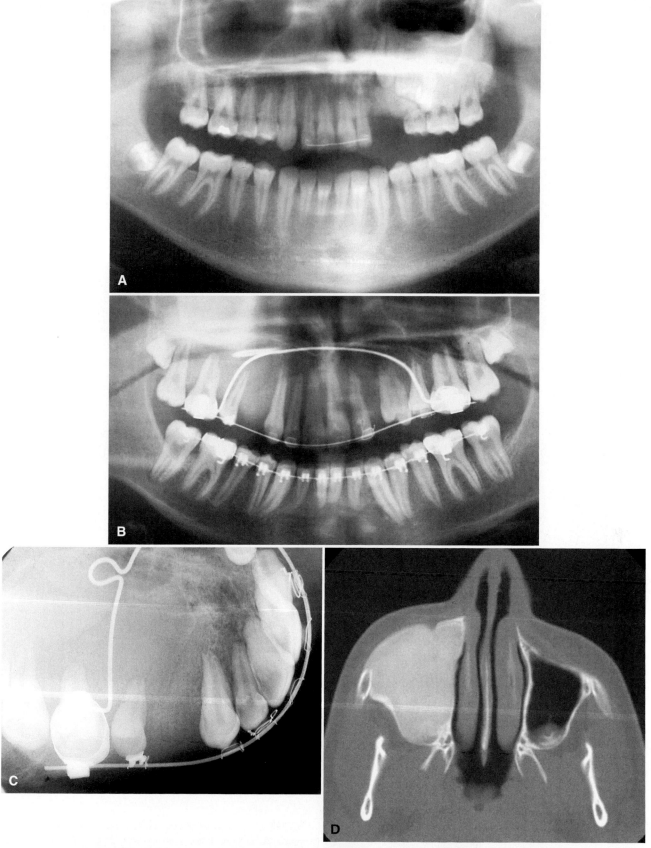

FIGURE 23-4 **A,** Very dense, amorphous pattern is seen in lesion of fibrous dysplasia involving the left maxilla and preventing the normal eruption of the cuspid and the bicuspids. **B-E,** Panoramic, occlusal, axial, and coronal CT images of an example of fibrous dysplasia with a homogeneous dense pattern, which occupies most of the right maxillary sinus.

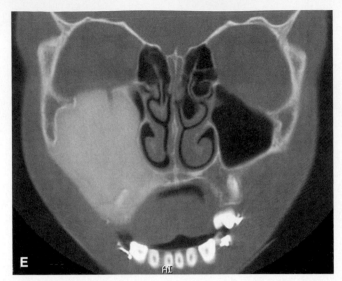

FIGURE 23-4, cont'd

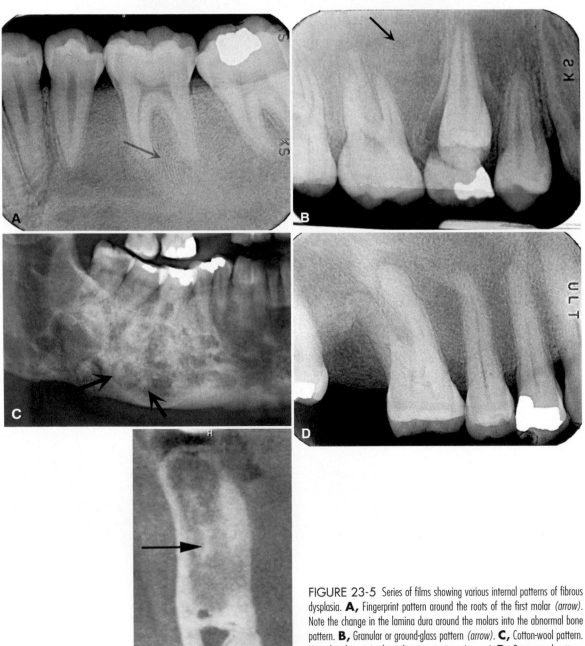

FIGURE 23-5 Series of films showing various internal patterns of fibrous dysplasia. **A,** Fingerprint pattern around the roots of the first molar *(arrow)*. Note the change in the lamina dura around the molars into the abnormal bone pattern. **B,** Granular or ground-glass pattern *(arrow)*. **C,** Cotton-wool pattern. Note the almost circular radiopaque regions *(arrows)*. **D,** Orange-peel pattern. **E,** Coronal cone-beam CT image shows a granular internal bone pattern with strands of more amorphous bone *(arrow)*.

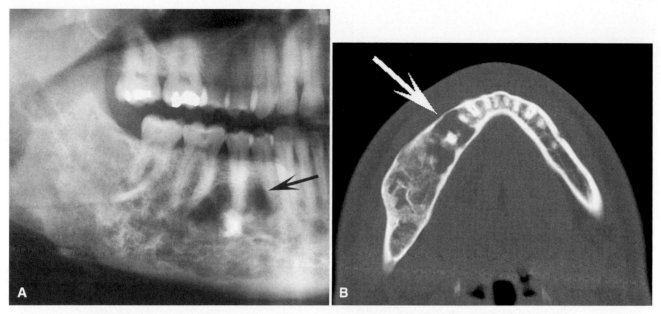

FIGURE 23-6 **A,** Cropped panoramic image of fibrous dysplasia of the mandible. There is a cystlike radiolucent lesion in the region of the bicuspids *(arrow).* **B,** Axial CT image using bone algorithm of the same case also reveals the same simple bonelike cyst *(arrow).*

fibrous dysplasia. These are bone cavities that are analogous to simple bone cysts and occur more commonly in mandibular lesions (Fig. 23-6).

Effects on Surrounding Structures. If the fibrous dysplasia lesion is small, it may have no effect on surrounding structures (subclinical variety). Effects on the involved bone may include expansion with maintenance of a thinned-outer cortex (Fig. 23-7). The expansion appears to affect the bone more evenly along its length rather than the more concentric expansion seen with benign tumors. Fibrous dysplasia may expand into the antrum by displacing its cortical boundary and subsequently occupying part or most of the maxillary sinus. Extension into the maxillary antrum usually occurs from the lateral wall, and the last section of the sinus to be involved usually is the most posterosuperior portion. Often the extension into the sinuses appears as a parallel thickening of the outer cortical border resulting in a residual antral air space, which still has approximately the normal anatomic shape of an antrum (Fig. 23-8). Cortical boundaries, such as the floor of the antrum, may be changed into the abnormal bone pattern. Often the bone surrounding the teeth is altered without affecting the dentition, and a distinct lamina dura disappears because this bone also is changed into the abnormal bone pattern (see Fig. 23-5). If the fibrous dysplasia increases the bone density, the periodontal ligament space may appear to be very narrow. Fibrous dysplasia can displace teeth or interfere with normal eruption, complicating orthodontic therapy. In rare cases, some root resorption may occur. Involved teeth may have hypercementosis. Fibrous dysplasia appears to be unique in its ability to displace the inferior alveolar nerve canal in a superior direction (see Fig. 23-8).

Differential Diagnosis

Other diseases can alter the bone pattern in a similar fashion. Metabolic bone diseases such as hyperparathyroidism may produce a similar pattern. However, these diseases are polyostotic, bilateral, and, in contrast to fibrous dysplasia, do not cause bone expansion.

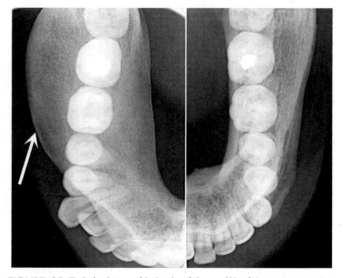

FIGURE 23-7 Occlusal views of both sides of the mandible of the same patient. Note the expansion of the right side of the mandible caused by fibrous dysplasia. The outer cortical plates have been displaced and thinned but are still intact *(arrow).*

Paget's disease may produce a similar pattern and may cause expansion, but it occurs in an older age group, and when it involves the mandible, the whole mandible is involved, in contrast to the unilateral tendency of fibrous dysplasia. Occasionally, periapical cemental dysplasia may show a similar bone pattern, but the distribution is different in that it often is bilateral, with an epicenter in the periapical region. Periapical cemental dysplasia also occurs in an older age group. With spontaneous healing of a simple bone cyst, the radiographic and histologic appearance of the new bone may be very similar to that of fibrous dysplasia.

Of paramount importance is the differentiation of osteomyelitis and osteogenic sarcoma because of both radiologic and

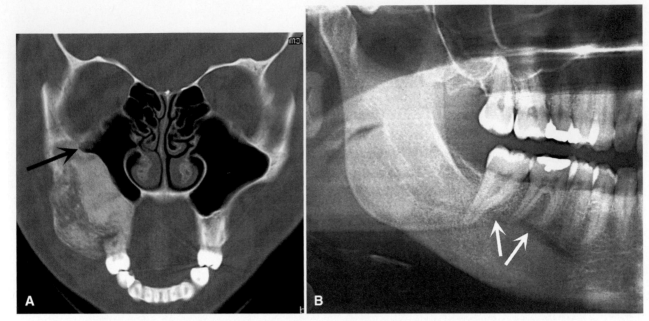

FIGURE 23-8 **A,** Coronal CT image using bone algorithm of a maxillary lesion of fibrous dysplasia. The lesion has caused the lateral wall of the maxilla to expand into the maxillary antrum. The shape of the lateral wall of the sinus has maintained the zygomatic recess *(arrow).* **B,** Mandibular fibrous dysplasia that has displaced the inferior alveolar nerve canal in a superior direction *(arrows).*

histologic similarities. Osteomyelitis may result in enlargement of the jaws, but the additional bone is generated by the periosteum; therefore, the new bone is laid down on the surface of the outer cortex, and close examination may reveal evidence of the original cortex within the expanded portion of the jaw. Fibrous dysplasia, in contrast, expands the internal aspect of bone, displacing and thinning the outer cortex so that the remaining cortex maintains its position at the outer surface of the bone. The identification of sequestra aids in the identification of osteomyelitis. Osteogenic sarcoma may produce a similar pattern but should show malignant radiologic features (see Chapter 24).

Some difficulty may arise in differentiating ossifying fibroma of the maxilla, especially the juvenile ossifying fibroma type. If the bone pattern is altered around the teeth without displacement of the teeth from one specific epicenter, the lesion probably is fibrous dysplasia. The shape of the bone expansion of fibrous dysplasia into the antrum reflects the original outer contour of the antral wall, which is different from the more convex extension of a neoplasm.

Management

In most cases, the radiographic characteristics of fibrous dysplasia and the clinical information are sufficient to allow the practitioner to make a diagnosis without a biopsy. There are reports of exaggerated growth from stimulation of a lesion during surgical intervention in young patients. A consultation with a dental radiologist is advisable. The radiologist may supplement the examination with computed tomographic (CT) imaging, which can give a more accurate, three-dimensional representation of the extent of the lesion and can serve as a precise baseline study for future comparisons. It is reasonable to continue occasional monitoring of the lesion or ask the patient to report any changes. With most lesions, growth is complete at skeletal maturation; orthodontic treatment and cosmetic surgery may be delayed until this time. Sarcomatous changes are unusual but

have been reported, especially if therapeutic radiation has been administered. In the case of female patients, hormonal changes from pregnancy or the use of oral contraceptives may stimulate growth or result in the development of lesions within the area of fibrous dysplasia, such as aneurysmal bone cysts (ABCs) or giant cell granulomas.

PERIAPICAL OSSEOUS DYSPLASIAS

It has been recognized more recently that it is impossible to identify cementum by either the histologic or the imaging appearance within these lesions and that this calcified material is likely amorphous bone. Therefore, the use of the term cementum should be discontinued. The term periapical osseous dysplasia (POD) has replaced periapical cemental dysplasia. This change in usage makes sense because it fits with the existing term florid osseous dysplasia (FOD), which is essentially the same disease but with a widespread involvement of the jaws.

Periapical Osseous Dysplasia

Synonyms. Periapical cemental dysplasia, periapical cemento-osseous dysplasia, cementoma, fibrocementoma, sclerosing cementoma, periapical osteofibrosis, periapical fibrous dysplasia, and periapical fibro-osteoma are synonyms for POD.

Disease Mechanism. POD is a localized change in normal bone metabolism that results in the resorption of normal cancellous bone and replacement with fibrous tissue and amorphous bone, abnormal bone trabeculae (similar to that seen in fibrous dysplasia), or a mixture of the two. Maturation phases correspond to the early phase, where the normal bone has been resorbed (radiolucent stage); developing phase, where abnormal bone is manufactured within the lesion (mixed radiolucent and radiopaque stage); and late or mature stage, where the internal structure is dominated by abnormal bone. By definition, the lesion is located near the apex of a tooth.

Clinical Features. POD is a common bone dysplasia that typically occurs in middle age; mean age is 39 years. It occurs nine times more often in females than in males and almost three times more often in blacks than in whites. It also frequently is seen in Asians. The involved teeth are vital, and the patient usually has no history of pain or sensitivity. The lesions usually come to light as an incidental finding during a periapical or panoramic imaging examination performed for other purposes. The lesions can become quite large, causing a notable expansion of the alveolar process, and may continue to enlarge slowly.

Imaging Features

Location. The epicenter of a POD lesion usually lies at the apex of a tooth (Fig. 23-9). In rare cases, the epicenter is slightly higher and over the apical third of the root. The condition has a predilection for the periapical bone of the mandibular anterior teeth, although any tooth can be involved, and in rare cases the maxillary teeth may be involved (Fig. 23-10). In most cases, the lesion is multiple and bilateral, but occasionally a solitary lesion arises. If the involved teeth have been extracted, this lesion can still develop, but the periapical location is less evident (Fig. 23-11). In these cases, the term osseous dysplasia may be more appropriate.

Periphery and Shape. In most cases, the periphery of a POD lesion is well defined. Often a radiolucent border of varying width is present, surrounded by a band of sclerotic bone that also can vary in width (Fig. 23-12). The sclerotic bone represents a reaction of the immediate surrounding bone. The lesion may be irregularly shaped or may have an overall round or oval shape centered over the apex of the tooth.

Internal Structure. The internal structure varies, depending on the maturity of the lesion. In the early stage, normal bone is resorbed and replaced with fibrous tissue that usually is continuous with the periodontal ligament (causing loss of the lamina dura). This appears as a radiolucency at the apex of the involved tooth (see Fig. 23-9).

In the mixed stage, radiopaque tissue appears in the radiolucent structure. This material usually is amorphous; has a round, oval, or irregular shape; and is composed of abnormal bone (see Fig. 23-12). Sometimes the amorphous bone forms a swirling pattern (Fig. 23-13). In some cases, the radiopaque material resembles the abnormal trabecular patterns seen in fibrous dysplasia (see Fig. 23-13).

In the mature stage, the internal aspect may be totally radiopaque without any obvious pattern. A thin, radiolucent margin usually can be seen at the periphery because this lesion matures from the center outward (Fig. 23-14). Occasionally, this radiolucent margin is not apparent, which makes the differential diagnosis more difficult. The internal structure may appear dramatically radiolucent if cavities resembling simple bone cysts form within the lesion (Fig. 23-15). In some cases, the simple bone cyst extends beyond the original margin of the cemental lesion.

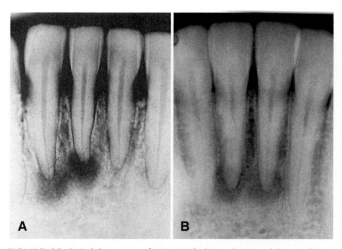

FIGURE 23-9　Radiolucent stage of POD. **A,** The lamina dura around the central incisor has been lost. **B,** The periodontal membrane space can still be seen around some of the teeth.

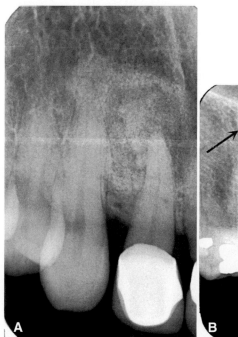

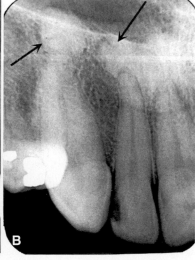

FIGURE 23-10　POD in the maxilla. **A,** Mixed lesion. **B,** Mature lesions (arrows).

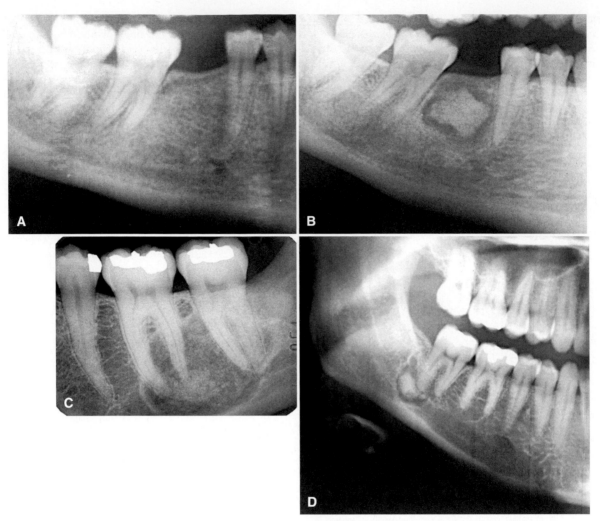

FIGURE 23-11 A and **B,** Portions of panoramic views of the same patient taken 3 years apart. Note development of a solitary lesion of POD in the apical region of the first molar extraction site. **C** and **D,** Solitary lesions in posterior mandible.

Effects on Surrounding Structures. The normal lamina dura of the teeth involved with the lesion is lost, making the periodontal ligament space either less apparent or appear wider (see Fig. 23-9). The tooth structure usually is not affected, although in rare cases some root resorption may occur. Also, hypercementosis occasionally occurs on the root of a tooth positioned within the lesion. Some lesions stimulate a sclerotic bone reaction from the surrounding bone. Small lesions do not cause expansion of the involved jaw. However, larger lesions may cause expansion of the jaw, an area that is always bordered by a thin, intact outer cortex similar to that seen in fibrous dysplasia. The expansion is usually undulating in shape. This lesion may elevate the floor of the maxillary antrum.

Differential Diagnosis. In early (radiolucent) POD lesions, the most important differential diagnosis is periapical rarefying osteitis. Occasionally, POD cannot be distinguished from this inflammatory lesion by radiographic characteristics alone. In these cases, the final diagnosis must rely on clinical information such as testing of the vitality of the involved tooth.

In the case of a solitary mature form of POD, the differential diagnosis may include a benign cementoblastoma, especially when periapical to the mandibular first molar. This tumor usually is

attached to the surface of the root, which may be partly resorbed. Also, the peripheral soft tissue capsule is better defined, and there may be a unique pattern to the internal structure, such as a radiating pattern. Expansion caused by the tumor is more concentric and less undulating than in POD. The presence or absence of clinical symptoms may help distinguish POD from benign cementoblastoma. Another lesion to consider is an odontoma. Odontomas often start occlusal to a tooth and prevent its eruption, but some odontomas may have a periapical position. The organization of the internal aspect into toothlike structures and the identification of enamel (very radiopaque) can help in the differential diagnosis. Also, the peripheral cortex and soft tissue capsule of an odontoma are more uniform in width and better defined than the periphery of POD. In mature POD lesions, the appearance may resemble a dense bone island. The finding of a radiolucent periphery, even if very slight, indicates a diagnosis of POD. Solitary lesions may be difficult to differentiate from a cemento-ossifying fibroma.

Management. The diagnosis of POD can be made on the basis of the appropriate radiologic and clinical characteristics. A possible complication of biopsy is secondary infection, which may occur

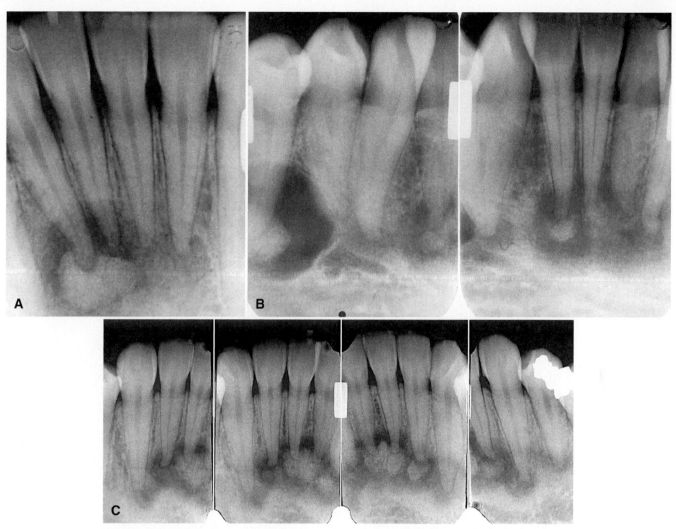

FIGURE 23-12 Mixed stage of POD. **A** and **B,** Radiopacity in the center of a radiolucent area. **C,** Multiple lesions. Note the band of sclerotic bone reaction at the periphery of the lesion.

in lesions that have abundant amorphous bone formation and poor vascularity. Treatment is not normally required. However, if the teeth have been removed and if considerable atrophy of the alveolar ridge has occurred, these segments of amorphous bone may reach the mucosal surface, much in the same way stones become exposed in old, worn concrete. These pieces of abnormal bone can perforate the mucosa when positioned under a denture, and the result is secondary infection. If this infection occurs, the pieces of amorphous bone may have to be removed surgically because they can act as sequestra in osteomyelitis.

Florid Osseous Dysplasia

Synonyms. Florid cemento-osseous dysplasia, gigantiform cementoma, and familial multiple cementomas are synonyms for FOD.

Disease Mechanism. FOD is a widespread form of POD. Normal cancellous bone is replaced with dense, acellular amorphous bone in a background of fibrous connective tissue. The lesion has a poor vascular supply, a condition that likely contributes to its susceptibility to infection. In some cases, a familial trend can be seen. No clear definition indicates when multiple regions of POD should be termed FOD. However, if POD is identified in three or four quadrants or is extensive throughout one jaw, it usually is considered to be FOD.

Clinical Features. Several key similarities exist between FOD and POD, including age, sex, and ethnicity of patients and comparable radiographic and histologic appearances. Most patients with FOD are female and middle-aged (mean age, 42 years), although the age range is broad. The condition shows a marked predilection for African Americans and Asians. A few documented cases appear to have a familial pattern. Often FOD produces no symptoms and is found incidentally during a radiographic examination. Occasionally, patients complain of low-grade intermittent, poorly localized pain in the affected bone, especially when a simple bone cyst has developed within the lesion. Extensive lesions often have an associated bony swelling. If the lesions become secondarily infected, features of osteomyelitis may develop, including mucosal ulceration, fistulous tracts with suppuration, and pain. Historically, FOD that was secondarily infected was diagnosed as chronic sclerosing osteomyelitis without the identification of the underlying bone dysplasia. A CT examination should be ordered to determine the extent of involvement with osteomyelitis. Teeth in the involved bone are vital unless other dental disease coincidentally affects them.

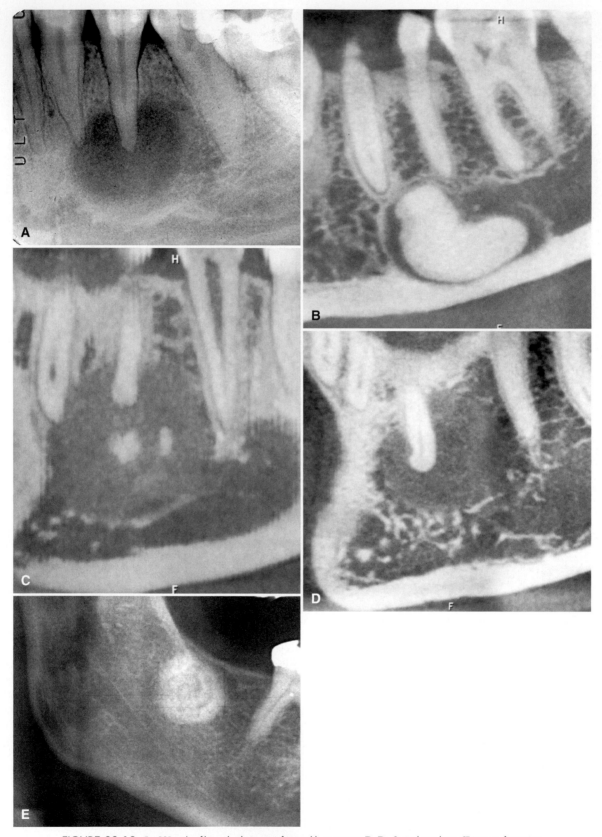

FIGURE 23-13 **A,** POD with a fibrous dysplasia type of internal bone pattern. **B-D,** Sagittal cone-beam CT images of variations of internal patterns, from homogeneous amorphous bone **(B)**, to a mix of fine granular bone with two foci of amorphous bone **(C)**, to totally granular fibrous dysplasia–like pattern **(D)**. **E,** Swirling internal pattern of cemental dysplasia.

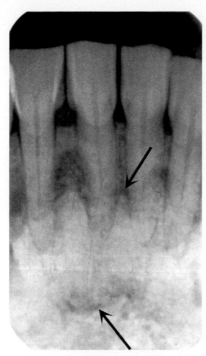

FIGURE 23-14 Mature stage of POD. Note the thin, radiolucent periphery (arrows).

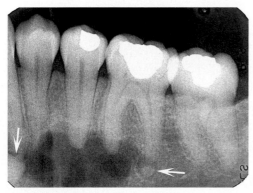

FIGURE 23-15 Simple bone cyst within an area of POD. Only a few regions of cementum-like tissue remain (arrows).

Imaging Features

Location. FOD lesions usually are bilateral and present in both jaws (Fig. 23-16). However, when they are present in only one jaw, the mandible is the more common location. The epicenter is apical to the teeth, within the alveolar process and usually posterior to the cuspid. In the mandible, lesions occur above the inferior alveolar canal.

Periphery. The periphery usually is well defined and has a sclerotic border that can vary in width, very similar to POD. The soft tissue capsule may not be apparent in mature lesions.

Internal Structure. The density of the internal structure can vary from an equal mixture of radiolucent and radiopaque regions to almost complete radiopacity. Some prominent radiolucent regions may be present, which usually represent the development of a simple bone cyst (Fig. 23-17). These cysts may enlarge with time even beyond the boundary of the lesion into the surrounding normal bone or may fill in with abnormal dysplastic cemento-osseous tissue. The radiopaque regions can vary from

small oval and circular regions (cotton-wool appearance) to large, irregular, amorphous areas of calcification. These calcified masses are similar in appearance to those seen in mature POD lesions and represent amorphous bone.

Effects on Surrounding Structures. Large FOD lesions can displace the inferior alveolar nerve canal in an inferior direction. FOD also can displace the floor of the antrum in a superior direction and can cause enlargement of the alveolar bone by displacement of the buccal and lingual cortical plates. The roots of associated teeth may have a considerable amount of hypercementosis, which may fuse with the abnormal surrounding foci of amorphous bone in the lesion. Extraction of these teeth may be difficult.

Differential Diagnosis. The fact that FOD is bilateral and centered in the alveolar process helps in the differentiation from other lesions. Paget's disease of bone may also show cotton-wool–type radiopaque regions with associated hypercementosis. However, Paget's disease affects the bone of the entire mandible, whereas FOD is centered above the inferior alveolar canal. Furthermore, Paget's disease often is polyostotic, involving other bones as well as the jaws. The well-defined nature of FOD, with its radiolucent periphery and surrounding sclerotic border, also is useful in making the differential diagnosis.

Another disease that may resemble FOD is chronic sclerosing osteomyelitis. Regions of cementum-like masses may appear similar to the sequestrum seen in osteomyelitis. This is not to be confused with a situation where FOD has become secondarily infected, resulting in osteomyelitis. The foci of amorphous bone that are secondarily infected have a wider and more profound radiolucent border (Fig. 23-18). CT imaging is essential for the diagnosis and to determine the extent of the osteomyelitis within the FOD.

Management. Under normal circumstances, FOD does not require treatment, although there is value in obtaining a panoramic film to establish the extent of the disease. In contrast to fibrous dysplasia, no age limit is apparent for the cessation of growth of FOD. Because of the propensity to develop secondary infections in FOD, the patient should be encouraged to maintain an effective oral hygiene program to avoid odontogenic infections. Also, if the teeth are extracted and severe atrophy of the alveolar process occurs, as in POD, the foci of amorphous bone emerge, and the pressure of the overlying denture may cause dehiscence in the mucosa, resulting in osteomyelitis. If osteomyelitis occurs, the avascular foci of amorphous bone become large sequestra. The osteomyelitis may spread slowly throughout the jaw from one region of FOD to another. It may be necessary to remove large areas of infected amorphous bone, leaving very little residual bone for prosthetic treatment.

OTHER LESIONS OF BONE
CENTRAL GIANT CELL GRANULOMA

Synonyms
Synonyms for central giant cell granuloma (CGCG) include giant cell reparative granuloma, giant cell lesion, and giant cell tumor.

Disease Mechanism
There is a debate as to whether CGCG is a reactive lesion to an as yet unknown stimulus or a neoplastic lesion. One theory suggests that the underlying mechanism is a neoplasm consisting

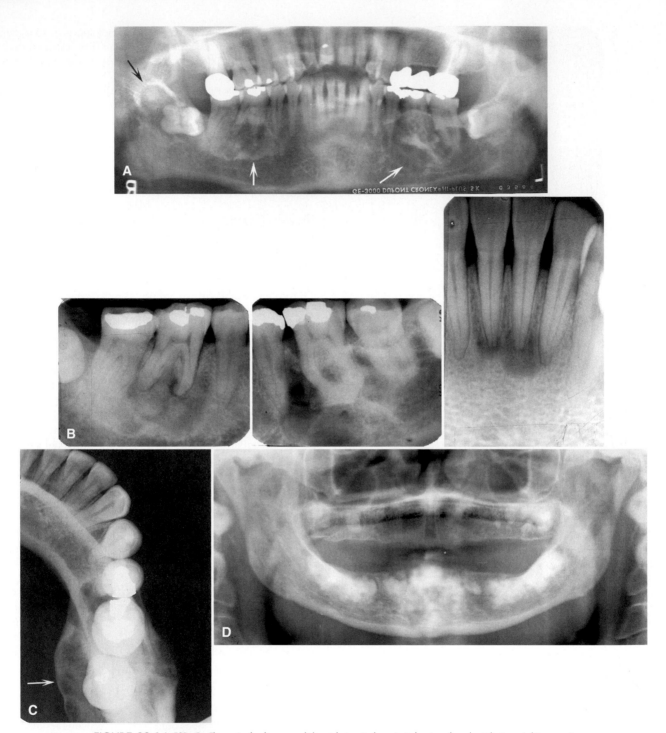

FIGURE 23-16 FOD. **A,** Three mixed radiopaque-radiolucent lesions in the periapical regions throughout the jaws *(white arrows).* Although the right third molar is horizontally impacted, the lesion still has a periapical relationship *(black arrow).* **B,** Composite of periapical films of the same case. Note the appearance of the lesions involving the mandibular incisors (not apparent in the panoramic film), which are identical to periapical cemental dysplasia. **C,** Occlusal film of the left mandibular lesion shows undulating expansion of the medial cortical plate *(arrow).* **D,** Panoramic film of a different case shows multiple, very mature, almost totally radiopaque lesions in edentulous jaws. The epicenter of all lesions is above the inferior alveolar canal.

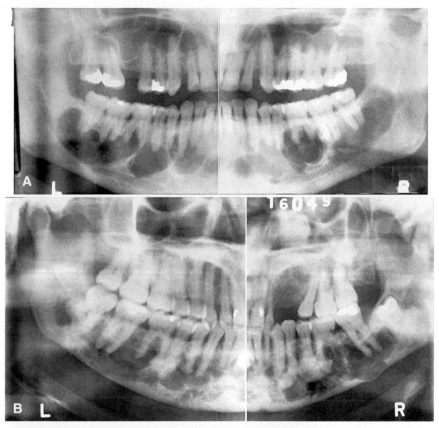

FIGURE 23-17 FOD associated with multiple simple bone cysts. **A,** Large cysts occupy most of the bone involved with FOD lesions. **B,** Another example of multiple simple bone cysts in lesions of FOD.

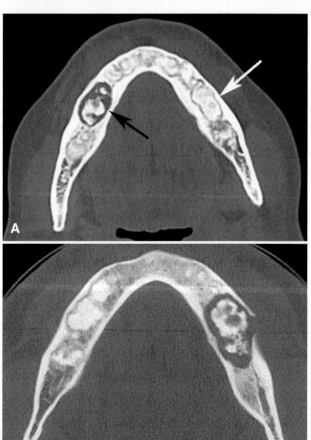

FIGURE 23-18 **A,** Axial CT image using bone algorithm of a case of FOD. Note the multiple foci of cemental dysplasia that are bordered by a soft tissue capsule *(white arrow)* and a cemental mass that has become secondarily infected with a wider, more pronounced radiolucent border *(black arrow).* **B,** Axial CT image of a different case of osteomyelitis caused by secondarily infected FOD. Note the break in the outer cortex where the lesion is draining into the surrounding soft tissues.

of osteoblast-like cells similar to giant cell tumors of bone. However, the imaging characteristics of the lesion are similar to characteristics of a benign tumor and occasionally maxillary lesions may have some aggressive malignant-type characteristics. The histologic appearance consists primarily of fibroblasts, numerous vascular channels, multinucleated giant cells, and macrophages. The relationship of giant cell tumor of bone to the giant cell granuloma is controversial and unclear.

Clinical Features

CGCG is a common lesion in the jaws that affects mostly adolescents and young adults; at least 60% of cases occur in individuals younger than 20 years old. The most common presenting sign of CGCG is painless swelling. Palpation of the suspect bone area may elicit tenderness, although the patient may complain of pain in a few cases. The overlying mucosa may have a purple color. Some of these lesions cause no symptoms and are found only on routine examination. The lesion usually grows slowly, although it may grow rapidly, creating the suspicion of a malignancy.

Imaging Features

Location. Lesions develop in the mandible twice as often as in the maxilla. In individuals in their first 2 decades, there is a tendency for the epicenter of the lesion to be anterior to the first molar in the mandible and anterior to the cuspid in the maxilla. However, in older individuals, this lesion can occur in greater frequency in the posterior aspect of the jaws.

Periphery. Because this neoplasm grows relatively slowly, it usually produces a well-defined radiographic margin in the mandible. In most cases, the periphery shows no evidence of cortication. Lesions in the maxilla may have ill-defined, almost malignant-appearing, borders.

Internal Structure. Some CGCG lesions show no evidence of internal structure (Fig. 23-19), especially small lesions. Other cases have

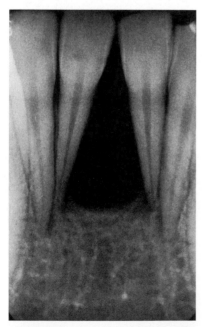

FIGURE 23-19 Periapical image of a giant cell granuloma in the anterior mandible with no evidence of internal structure.

a subtle granular pattern of calcification that may require a bright light source behind the film to enable visualization. Occasionally, this granular bone is organized into ill-defined, wispy septa (Fig. 23-20). If present, these granular septa are characteristic of this lesion, especially if they emanate at right angles from the periphery of the lesion. This characteristic is even stronger if a small indentation of the expanded cortical margin is seen at the point where this right-angle septum originates (Fig. 23-21). In some instances, the septa are better defined and divide the internal aspect into compartments, creating a multilocular appearance.

Effects on Surrounding Structures. Giant cell granulomas often displace and resorb teeth. The resorption of tooth roots is not a constant feature, but when it occurs, it may be profound and irregular in outline. The lamina dura of teeth within the lesion usually is missing. The inferior alveolar canal may be displaced in an inferior direction. This lesion has a strong propensity to expand the cortical boundaries of the mandible and maxilla. The expansion usually is uneven or undulating in nature, which may give the appearance of a double boundary when the expansion is viewed using occlusal film. The bone forming the border of the expanded mandible often has a granular texture compared with cortical bone (see Fig. 23-21, C). In some instances, the outer cortical plate of bone is destroyed instead of expanded; this occurs more often in the maxilla, where the cortical bone destruction may give the lesion a malignant appearance.

Differential Diagnosis

If the internal structure of the CGCG contains septa, the differential diagnosis may include ameloblastoma, odontogenic myxoma, and aneurysmal bone cyst (ABC). If a granular internal structure is present, ossifying fibroma may be considered. Useful characteristics for differentiating an ameloblastoma include the following: ameloblastomas tend to occur in an older age group and more often in the posterior mandible, and ameloblastomas have coarse, curved, well-defined trabeculae, whereas giant cell granulomas have wispy, ill-defined trabeculae, some of which are at right angles to the periphery. Odontogenic myxomas occur in an older age group, may have sharper and straighter septa, and do not have the same propensity to expand as giant cell granulomas. ABCs can appear identical radiographically to giant cell granulomas, especially in the appearance of the internal septa. However, ABCs are comparatively rare lesions that occur more often in the posterior aspect of the jaws and usually cause profound expansion.

A small CGCG lesion with a totally radiolucent internal structure may be similar in appearance to a cyst, especially a simple bone cyst. Evidence of displacement or resorption of the adjacent teeth or expansion of the outer cortical bone is more characteristic of a giant cell granuloma. The radiologic and histologic appearance of brown tumors of hyperparathyroidism may be identical to CGCG. Also the appearance may be identical to cherubism; however, the lesions in cherubism are multiple and have epicenters that are located in the most posterior aspect of the mandible and maxilla.

Management

If the lesion is in the maxilla, CT scans can be used to establish the exact extent and the involvement of surrounding structures, such as the maxillary antrum or nasal cavity. Also, CT imaging is required for large lesions, which pose the possibility of destruction of the outer cortical bone, to determine whether the adjacent soft

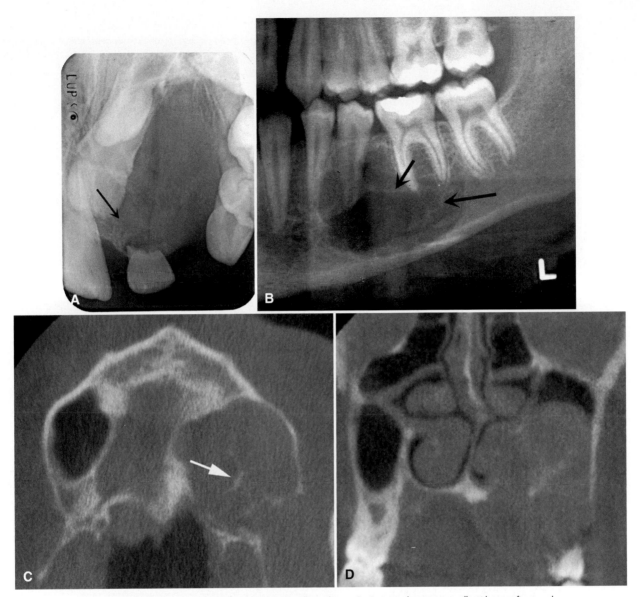

FIGURE 23-20 Various internal patterns seen in giant cell granulomas. **A,** Lesion in the anterior maxilla with a very fine granular pattern *(arrow).* **B,** Portion of a panoramic film showing wispy, ill-defined internal septa *(arrows).* **C** and **D,** Axial and coronal cone-beam CT images of a CGCG of the maxilla. Note the poorly calcified, barely visible internal septation *(arrow).*

tissue has been invaded. Occasionally, this lesion behaves very aggressively. If CGCG occurs after the second decade of life, hyperparathyroidism should be considered, and serum testing for elevated calcium or parathormone or full-body technetium bone scans can be ordered.

Treatment may include enucleation and curettage and resection of the jaw in some instances. The patient should be followed carefully to rule out recurrence, especially if conservative treatment is used. Recurrences are rare and are more common in the maxilla.

ANEURYSMAL BONE CYST

Disease Mechanism

An aneurysmal bone cyst (ABC) has been considered to be a reactive lesion of bone. However, several chromosomal translocations have been described more recently that all lead to activation of the *USP6* gene on chromosome 17p13, giving some credence to a neoplastic nature of this lesion. In diagnostic images, this lesion behaves similar to an aggressive benign tumor. This lesion is a proliferation of vascular spaces; fibroblasts; osteoclast-like cells; and reactive, poorly calcified woven bone. ABCs occasionally develop in association with other primary lesions, such as fibrous dysplasia, central hemangioma, giant cell granuloma, and osteosarcoma.

Clinical Features

More than 90% of reported jaw lesions have occurred in individuals younger than 30 years old. The condition appears to have a predilection for females. An ABC in the jaw usually manifests as a fairly rapid bony swelling (usually buccal or labial). Pain is an occasional complaint, and the involved area may be tender on palpation.

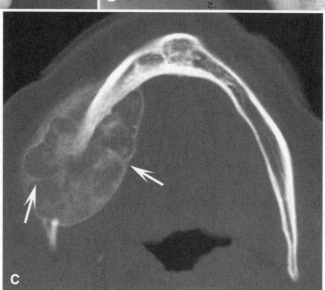

FIGURE 23-21 Characteristic expansion of the outer cortical plates caused by giant cell granulomas. **A** and **B,** Note the uneven expansion in **A** (arrow) and the indentation of the expansion with a right-angled septum in **B** (arrow). **C,** Axial CT image using bone algorithm reveals a giant cell granuloma within the mandible causing undulating expansion and containing two right-angled septa (arrows).

Imaging Features

Location. The mandible is involved more often than the maxilla (ratio of 3:2), and the molar and ramus regions are more involved than the anterior region (Fig. 23-22).

Periphery and Shape. The periphery usually is well defined, and the shape is circular or "hydraulic."

Internal Structure. Small initial lesions may show no evidence of an internal structure. Often the internal aspect has a multilocular appearance. The septa bear a striking resemblance to the wispy, ill-defined septa seen in giant cell granulomas (Fig. 23-23; see Fig. 23-22). Septa positioned at right angles to the outer expanded border are another similar finding. In CT soft tissue algorithm images, there may be more radiolucent regions, some of which have a roughly circular shape. These likely represent large vascular spaces.

Effects on Surrounding Structures. After an ABC becomes large, there is a strong propensity for extreme expansion of the outer cortical plates (see Figs. 23-22 and 23-23). This characteristic is more dramatic in these cysts than in most other lesions. ABCs can displace and resorb teeth.

Differential Diagnosis

The internal granular septa of ABCs resemble that of giant cell granulomas; the radiographic appearance of the two lesions may be identical. However, ABCs may expand to a greater degree, and they are more common in the posterior parts of the mandible. Ameloblastoma may be considered, but this lesion usually occurs in an older age group. ABCs may show a similarity to cherubism, which has giant cell–like features, but cherubism is a multifocal, bilateral disease.

The diagnosis is based on biopsy results. A hemorrhagic aspirate favors the diagnosis of ABC. A CT scan also is recommended to determine the extent of the lesion better.

Management

Surgical curettage and partial resection are the primary means of treatment. The recurrence rate ranges from 19% to about 50% after curettage, and approximately 11% after resection. Careful follow-up is needed.

CHERUBISM

Synonym

Familial fibrous dysplasia is a synonym for cherubism.

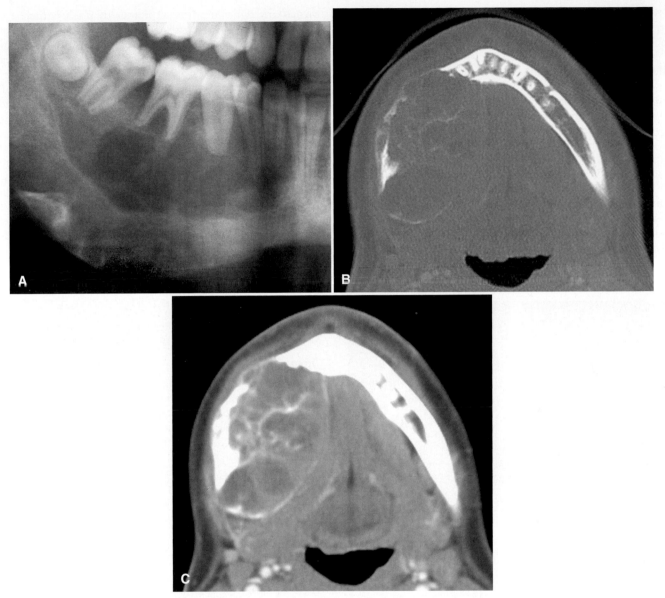

FIGURE 23-22 **A,** Cropped panoramic image of ABC occupying the body of the right mandible. **B,** Axial CT image at the same level of this case using bone algorithm. Note the wispy faint septa. **C,** Axial CT image at the same level using soft tissue algorithm. Note the low-attenuation regions of the internal structure representing fluid density.

Disease Mechanism

Cherubism is a rare, inherited autosomal dominant disease that causes bilateral enlargement of the jaws, giving the child a cherubic facial appearance. One mutation found was identified as *SH3BP2* on chromosome 4p16.3; however, there are likely other mutations involved. Rare unilateral lesions have been reported. The internal structure is indistinguishable from CGCG. The term familial fibrous dysplasia was a poor choice of early terminology because this lesion is not a bone dysplasia. The internal osseous tissue is not manufactured by this entity but is reactive bone as in giant cell granulomas. These lesions regress with age.

Clinical Features

Cherubism develops in early childhood between 2 and 6 years of age. The most common presenting sign is a painless, firm, bilateral enlargement of the lower face. Enlargement of the submandibular lymph nodes may occur, but no systemic abnormalities are involved. Because children's faces are chubby, mild cases may go undetected until the second decade. Profound swelling of the maxilla may result in stretching of the skin of the cheeks, which depresses the lower eyelids, exposing a thin line of sclera and causing an "eyes raised to heaven" appearance.

Imaging Features

Location. This lesion is bilateral and often affects both jaws. When present in only one jaw, the mandible is the most common location. The epicenter is always in the posterior aspect of the jaws, in the ramus of the mandible or the tuberosity of the maxilla (Fig. 23-24). The lesion grows in an anterior direction and in severe cases can extend almost to the midline.

Periphery. The periphery usually is well defined and in some instances corticated.

Internal Structure. The internal structure resembles CGCG, with fine, granular bone and wispy trabeculae forming a prominent multilocular pattern.

Effects on Surrounding Structures. Expansion of the cortical boundaries of the maxilla and mandible by cherubism can result in severe enlargement of the jaws. Maxillary lesions enlarge into the maxillary sinuses. Because the epicenter is in the posterior aspect of the jaws, the teeth are displaced in an anterior direction. The degree of displacement can be severe, and the tooth buds are destroyed with some lesions.

Differential Diagnosis

Although the radiographic appearance of cherubism may be similar to giant cell granuloma, the fact that cherubism is bilateral with an epicenter in the ramus should provide a clear differentiation. The differentiation of cherubism from fibrous dysplasia should not present any difficulties because fibrous dysplasia is more commonly a unilateral disease; also, the multilocular appearance and anterior displacement of teeth are more characteristic of cherubism. Cherubism may bear some similarity to multiple odontogenic keratocysts in basal cell nevus syndrome. The bilateral symmetry of cherubism, anterior displacement of teeth, and multilocular appearance are characteristics that help with the differential diagnosis.

Management

The distinctive radiographic features of cherubism may be more diagnostic than the histopathologic findings; therefore, the diagnosis can rely on the radiologic findings alone. Treatment can be delayed because the cystlike lesions usually become static and fill in with granular bone during adolescence and at the end of skeletal growth. After skeletal growth has stopped, conservative surgical procedures, if required, may be done for cosmetic problems. Surgery also may be required to uncover displaced teeth, and orthodontic treatment may be needed.

PAGET'S DISEASE

Synonym

Osteitis deformans is a synonym for Paget's disease.

Disease Mechanism

Paget's disease is a skeletal disorder and essentially a disease involving osteoclasts resulting in abnormal resorption and apposition of poor-quality osseous tissue in one or more bones. The disease may involve many bones simultaneously, but it is not a generalized skeletal disease. It is initiated by an intense wave of osteoclastic activity, with resorption of normal bone resulting in irregularly shaped resorption cavities. After a period of time, vigorous osteoblastic activity ensues, forming woven bone. Paget's disease is seen most frequently in Great Britain and Australia and less often in North America. This disease is an autosomal dominant trait with genetic heterogeneity and may involve paramyxoviral infection, but the etiology for the disease remains unclear.

Clinical Features

Paget's disease is primarily a disease of later middle and old age, having an incidence of about 3.5% of individuals older than 40 years of age. At age 65 years, the incidence of involvement in men is approximately twice that of women.

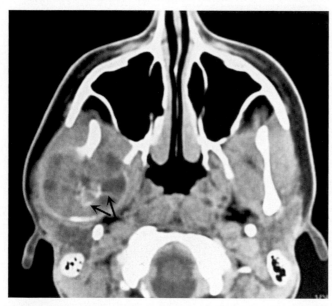

FIGURE 23-23 Axial CT image using a soft tissue algorithm demonstrates the presence of an ABC of the left mandibular condyle. Note the severe expansion and the wispy, ill-defined septa *(arrows).*

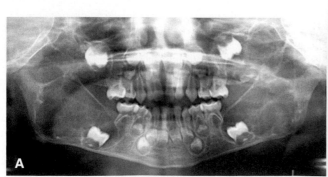
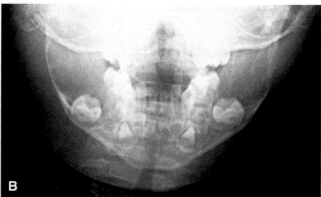

FIGURE 23-24 Cherubism. **A,** Panoramic image shows four lesions in the maxilla and mandible. The epicenters of the lesions are in the maxillary tuberosity and mandibular ramus; also note the anterior displacement of the unerupted maxillary first molars. The internal structure contains ill-defined septa. **B,** Portion of the posteroanterior skull view shows expansion of the mandible.

Affected bone is enlarged and commonly deformed because of the poor quality of bone formation, resulting in bowing of the legs, curvature of the spine, and enlargement of the skull. The jaws also enlarge when affected. Separation and movement of teeth may occur, causing malocclusion. Dentures may be tight or may fit poorly in edentulous patients.

Bone pain is an inconsistent symptom, most often directed toward the weight-bearing bones; facial or jaw pain is uncommon. Patients with Paget's disease may also have ill-defined neurologic pain as the result of bone impingement on foramina and nerve canals. Patients with Paget's disease often have severely elevated levels of serum alkaline phosphatase (greater than with any other disorder) during osteoblastic phases of the disease. These patients also often have high levels of hydroxyproline in the urine.

Imaging Features

Location. Paget's disease occurs most often in the pelvis, femur, skull, and vertebrae and infrequently in the jaws (Fig. 23-25). It affects the maxilla about twice as often as the mandible. Whenever the jaws are involved, the entire mandible or maxilla is always affected. Although this disease is bilateral, occasionally it affects only one maxilla, or the involvement may be significantly greater on one side.

Internal Structure. Generally, the appearance of the internal structure depends on the developmental stage of the disease. Paget's disease has three radiographic stages, although these often overlap in the clinical setting: (1) an early radiolucent resorptive stage; (2) a granular or ground-glass appearance second stage; and (3) a denser, more radiopaque appositional late stage. These stages are less apparent in the jaws.

The trabeculae are altered in number and shape. Most often they increase in number, but in the early stage they may decrease. The trabeculae may be long and may align themselves in a linear pattern (Fig. 23-26), which is more common in the mandible. They also may be short, with random orientation, and may have a granular pattern similar to that of fibrous dysplasia. A third pattern occurs when the trabeculae may be organized into rounded, radiopaque patches of abnormal bone, creating a cotton-wool appearance (Fig. 23-27).

The overall density of the jaws may decrease or increase, depending on the number of trabeculae. Often the disease produces areas of bone that appear radiolucent (commonly the alveolar process) and regions of increased density in one bone.

Effects on Surrounding Structures. Paget's disease always enlarges an affected bone to some extent, even in the early stage. Often the bone enlargement is impressive. Prominent pagetoid skull bones may swell to three or four times their normal thickness. In enlarged jaws, the outer cortex may be thinned but remains intact. The outer cortex may appear to be laminated in occlusal projections (see Fig. 23-26). When the maxilla is involved, the disease invariably involves the sinus floor. However, the air space usually is not diminished to a great extent. Cortical boundaries such as the sinus floor may be more granular and less apparent as sharp boundaries. The lamina dura may become less evident and may be altered into the abnormal bone pattern. Hypercementosis often develops on a few or most of the teeth in the involved jaw. This hypercementosis may be exuberant and irregular, which is characteristic of Paget's disease (Fig. 23-28). As previously mentioned, the teeth may become spaced or displaced in the enlarging jaw.

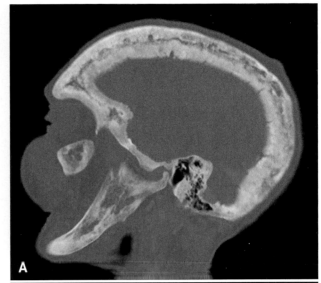
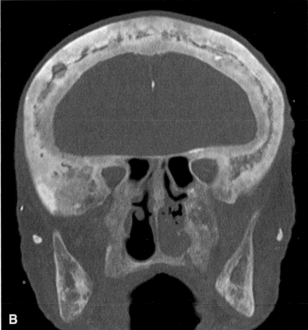

FIGURE 23-25 **A** and **B,** Axial and coronal bone algorithm CT images of a case of Paget's disease involving all of the cranial bones as well as the maxilla and mandible. Note increase in bone density and dimension between the internal and outer cortex of the skull. The coronal CT image **(B)** demonstrates enlargement of the mandibular ramus.

Differential Diagnosis

Paget's disease may appear similar to fibrous dysplasia. However, Paget's disease occurs in an older age group and is almost always bilateral. In the maxilla, fibrous dysplasia has a tendency to encroach on the antral air space, whereas Paget's disease does not. The linear trabeculae and cotton-wool appearance of Paget's disease are distinctive. FOD may have a cotton-wool pattern, but these lesions are centered above the inferior alveolar nerve canal and most commonly have a radiolucent capsule. The changes seen in FOD do not affect all of the jaw, in contrast to Paget's disease. The bone pattern in Paget's disease may show some similarities to the bone pattern in metabolic bone diseases, and both conditions may be bilateral. However, Paget's disease enlarges bone, and

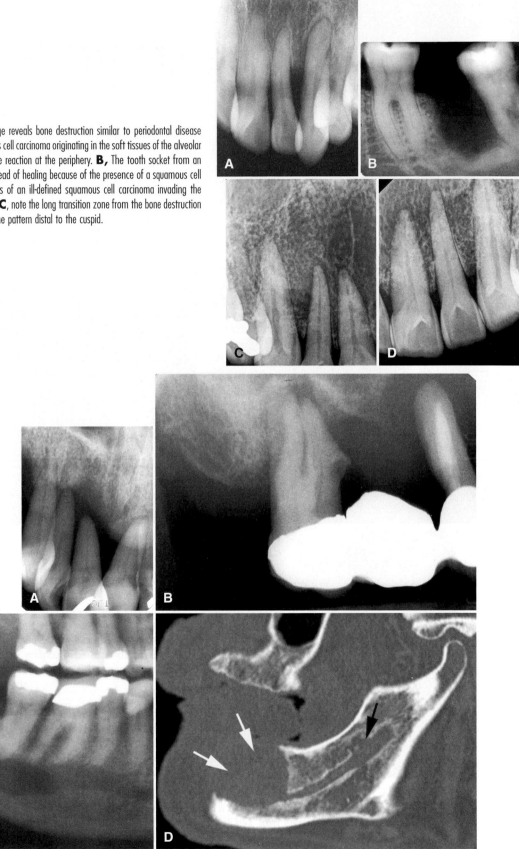

FIGURE 24-3 **A,** Periapical image reveals bone destruction similar to periodontal disease around the lateral incisor from a squamous cell carcinoma originating in the soft tissues of the alveolar process. Note the lack of a sclerotic bone reaction at the periphery. **B,** The tooth socket from an extracted second molar has enlarged instead of healing because of the presence of a squamous cell carcinoma. **C** and **D,** Periapical images of an ill-defined squamous cell carcinoma invading the alveolar process from the nasal cavity. In **C,** note the long transition zone from the bone destruction near the midline to the more normal bone pattern distal to the cuspid.

FIGURE 24-4 **A** and **B,** Periapical images of two cases of carcinoma of the alveolar process. Bone destruction around the tooth roots leaves the teeth bereft of any bone support. **C,** Cropped panoramic image of a carcinoma growing down the inferior alveolar canal shows the irregular width of the canal and destruction of its cortical borders. **D,** Sagittal CT image of another case of a carcinoma destroying the mandible in the region of the mental foramen *(white arrows)* and growing down the canal. Note the destruction of the peripheral cortex of the canal *(black arrow).*

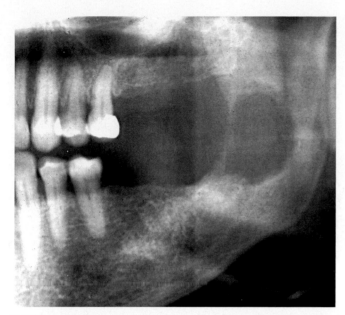

FIGURE 24-5 Primary intraosseous carcinoma in the left mandible exhibits no internal structure, a poorly defined periphery, and thinning of the overlying mandibular bone.

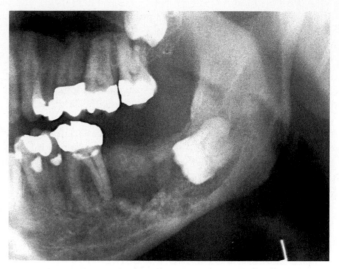

FIGURE 24-6 Carcinoma arising in a preexisting dentigerous cyst related to the mandibular left third molar shows absence of a cyst cortex, invasion into adjacent bone, and ill-defined borders.

Internal Structure.   The internal structure is wholly radiolucent with no evidence of bone production and very little residual bone left within the center of the lesion. If the lesion is small, overlying buccal or lingual plates may cast a shadow that may mimic the appearance of internal trabecular bone.

Effects on Surrounding Structures.   These lesions are capable of causing destruction of the antral or nasal floors, loss of the cortical outline of the mandibular neurovascular canal, and effacement of the lamina dura. Root resorption is unusual. Teeth that lose both lamina dura and supporting bone appear to be floating in space.

Differential Diagnosis

If the lesions are not aggressive and have a smooth border and radiolucent area, they may be mistaken for periapical cysts or granulomas. Alternatively, if lesions are not centered about the apex of a tooth, occasionally it is difficult to differentiate this condition from odontogenic cysts or tumors. If the border is obviously infiltrative with extensive bone destruction, a metastatic lesion must be excluded as well as multiple myeloma, fibrosarcoma, and carcinoma arising in a dental cyst. Examination of the oral cavity and especially the surface epithelium assists in differentiating this condition from surface squamous cell carcinoma.

Management.

Generally, these tumors are excised with their surrounding osseous structure in an en bloc resection. Radiation and chemotherapy may be used as adjunctive therapies.

SQUAMOUS CELL CARCINOMA ORIGINATING IN A CYST

Synonyms

Epidermoid cell carcinoma and carcinoma ex odontogenic cyst are synonyms for squamous cell carcinoma originating in a cyst.

Disease Mechanism

Squamous cell carcinoma arising in a preexisting dental cyst is uncommon and excludes invasion from surface epithelial carcinomas, metastatic tumors, and primary intraosseous carcinoma. They may arise from inflammatory periapical, residual, dentigerous, and keratocystic odontogenic tumors. Histologically, the lining squamous epithelium of the cyst gives rise to the malignant neoplasm.

Clinical Features

The most common presenting sign or symptom associated with this condition is pain. The pain may be characterized as dull and of several months' duration. Swelling is occasionally reported. Pathologic fracture, fistula formation, and regional lymphadenopathy may occur. If the upper jaw is involved, sinus pain or swelling may be present.

Imaging Features

Location.   This tumor may occur anywhere an odontogenic cyst is found—that is, the tooth-bearing portions of the jaws. Most cases occur in the mandible (Fig. 24-6), with a few cases reported in the anterior maxilla.

Periphery and Shape.   The radiologic picture of squamous cell carcinoma originating in a cyst mirrors the histologic findings. Because the lesion arises from a cyst, the shape is often round or ovoid. If it is a small lesion in a cyst wall, the periphery may be mostly well defined and even corticated. In this case, the radiographic differentiation from a normal cyst is impossible. As the malignant tissue progressively replaces cyst lining, the smooth border is lost or becomes ill-defined. The advanced lesion has an ill-defined, infiltrative periphery that lacks any cortication. Its shape becomes less "hydraulic" looking and more diffuse.

Internal Structure.   This lesion lacks any ability to produce bone. It is wholly radiolucent, perhaps more so than invasive surface carcinoma, owing to prior osteolysis from the cyst.

Effects on Surrounding Structures.   Carcinoma arising in dental cysts is capable of thinning and destroying the lamina dura of adjacent teeth or adjacent cortical boundaries, such as the inferior border of the jaw or floor of the nose. It can produce complete destruction of the alveolar process.

Differential Diagnosis

If a dental cyst is infected, it may lose its normal cortical boundary and appear ragged and identical to a malignant lesion arising in a preexisting cyst. However, inflamed cysts usually show a reactive peripheral sclerosis because of inflammatory products present in the cyst lumen. This sclerosis is not normally present in a cyst that has undergone malignant transformation. Nevertheless, the two may be difficult to differentiate radiologically, and cysts should always be submitted for histologic examination. Multiple myeloma may appear as a solitary lesion and may be difficult to distinguish, especially if it has a cystic well-defined shape. Metastatic disease may be similar, although it is commonly multifocal.

Management

The treatment of squamous cell carcinoma originating in a cyst is identical to the treatment described for primary intraosseous carcinoma.

SQUAMOUS CELL CARCINOMA ORIGINATING IN THE MAXILLARY SINUS

Disease Mechanism

Risk factors for developing squamous cell carcinoma originating in the mucosal lining of the maxillary sinus include chronic sinusitis, chemicals used in manufacturing such as volatile hydrocarbons, isopropyl oils, wood dust, and metals such as nickel and chromium.

Clinical Features

These malignancies occur most commonly in patients of African and Asian heritage. Men are affected more commonly than women. The initial signs may be very similar to inflammatory disease and may include recurrent sinusitis, nasal obstruction, epistaxis, sinus pain, and facial paresthesia (see Chapter 26).

Imaging Features

These lesions may manifest with opacification of the maxillary sinus with soft tissue and destruction of osseous structures bordering the maxillary sinus, such as posterior wall of the maxilla, zygomatic process of the maxilla, floor of the maxillary sinus, walls of the maxillary sinus, and the adjacent maxillary alveolar process (Fig. 24-7). An associated soft tissue mass may also project into the oral cavity.

CENTRAL MUCOEPIDERMOID CARCINOMA

Synonym

A synonym for central mucoepidermoid carcinoma is mucoepidermoid carcinoma.

Disease Mechanism

Central mucoepidermoid carcinoma is an epithelial tumor arising in bone, likely originating from pluripotential odontogenic epithelium or from a cyst lining. It is histologically indistinguishable from its soft tissue counterpart. The criteria for diagnosis of a central mucoepidermoid tumor are the presence of intact cortical plates, radiographic evidence of bone destruction, and typical histologic findings consistent with mucoepidermoid tumor. Additionally, the practitioner must exclude the possibility of an invasive overlying mucoepidermoid tumor or odontogenic tumor.

Clinical Features

In contrast to other malignant tumors of the jaws, the central mucoepidermoid tumor is more likely to mimic a benign tumor or cyst. The most common complaint is of a painless swelling. The swelling may have been present for months or years and has been reported to cause facial asymmetry. Occasionally, it may feel as if teeth have been moved, or a denture may no longer fit. Tenderness rather than severe pain may also be present. Paresthesia of the inferior alveolar nerve and spreading of the lesion to regional lymph nodes have been reported. In contrast to other oral malignancies, central mucoepidermoid tumor is more common in females than males.

Imaging Features

Location. The lesion is three to four times as common in the mandible as the maxilla, usually in the premolar and molar region with a few cases reported in the anterior mandible. The lesion most commonly occurs above the mandibular canal, similar to odontogenic tumors.

Periphery and Shape. Mucoepidermoid tumor manifests as a unilocular or multilocular expansile mass (Fig. 24-8). The border is most often well defined and well corticated and often crenated or undulating in nature, which is similar to benign odontogenic tumors. The peripheral cortication may be impressively thick, which belies its malignant nature. Rarely, the periphery is not corticated and has a more malignant appearance.

Internal Structure. The internal structure has features similar to a benign odontogenic tumor, such as a recurrent ameloblastoma. Lesions are often described as being multilocular or having either a soap bubble or a honeycomb internal structure, which is displayed as round radiolucent areas with or without thick or sclerotic bony peripheries. Also, there may be regions of amorphous sclerotic bone. This bone is not produced by the tumor but is merely remodeled residual bone.

Effects on Surrounding Structures. Mucoepidermoid tumor is capable of causing expansion of adjacent cortical plates, often with perforation and sometimes extension into the surrounding soft tissues. Similar to benign tumors, the mandibular canal may be depressed or pushed laterally or medially. Teeth remain largely unaffected by this disease, although adjacent lamina dura may be lost.

Differential Diagnosis

Some characteristics of this tumor may appear similar to a benign odontogenic tumor. Its malignant nature is revealed if there is expansion with perforation of the outer cortex with extension of the tumor into the surrounding soft tissues. The chief differential diagnosis is a recurrent ameloblastoma, with which it shares similarities in its peripheral and internal features. It may be impossible to differentiate the two. Odontogenic myxoma and central giant cell granuloma also may be confused with mucoepidermoid tumor, as may other odontogenic cysts or tumors.

Management

Mucoepidermoid carcinoma is treated surgically with en bloc resection encompassing a margin of adjacent normal bone. Neck dissection and postoperative radiation therapy may be required to control spread to lymph nodes.

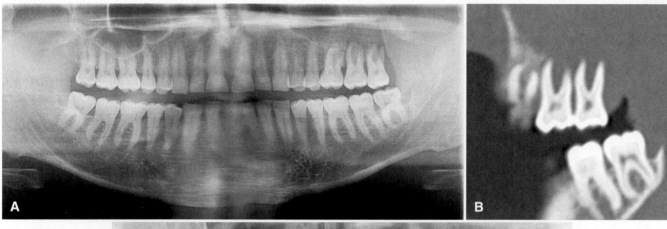

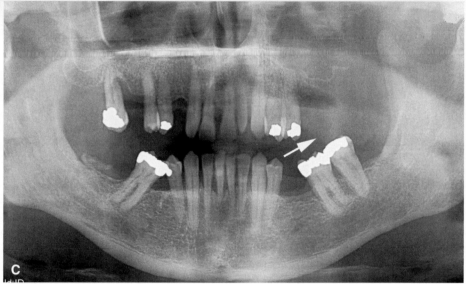

FIGURE 24-7 **A,** Panoramic image of a squamous cell carcinoma originating within the left maxillary sinus. There is destruction of the tuberosity, posterior floor of the sinus, posterior wall of the maxilla, and zygomatic process of the maxilla. **B,** Sagittal CT image shows destruction of bone around the molars and tuberosity region. **C,** Another sinus carcinoma with destruction of the left maxilla and presence of a soft tissue mass (arrow).

MALIGNANT AMELOBLASTOMA AND AMELOBLASTIC CARCINOMA

Disease Mechanism

Malignant ameloblastoma is defined as an ameloblastoma with typical benign histologic features that is deemed malignant because of its biologic behavior—that is, metastasis. The histologic features may not correlate with the clinical behavior. Ameloblastic carcinoma is an ameloblastoma exhibiting the histologic criteria of a malignant neoplasm, such as increased and abnormal mitosis and hyperchromatic, large, pleomorphic nuclei.

Clinical Features

Clinically, these lesions may behave as benign ameloblastomas, exhibiting a hard expansile mass of the jaw with displaced and perhaps loosened teeth and normal overlying mucosa. Tenderness of the overlying soft tissue has been reported. Metastatic spread may be to the cervical lymph nodes; lung or other viscera; and the skeleton, especially the spine. Local extension may occur into adjacent bones, connective tissue, or salivary glands. These tumors occur most commonly between the first and sixth decades of life and are more common in males than females.

Imaging Features

Location. These lesions are more common in the mandible than in the maxilla. Most occur in the premolar and molar region, where ameloblastoma is typically found.

Periphery and Shape. Similar to ameloblastoma, a well-defined border occurs with cortication, presence of crenations, or scalloping of the border. Malignant ameloblastoma may show some of the signs more commonly seen in malignant neoplasms—that is, loss of and subsequent breaching of the cortical boundary invading into the surrounding soft tissue.

Internal Structure. The lesions are either unilocular or, more commonly, multilocular, giving the appearance of a honeycomb or soap bubble pattern, as seen in benign ameloblastomas. Most of the septa are robust and thick (see Fig. 24-8, *C*).

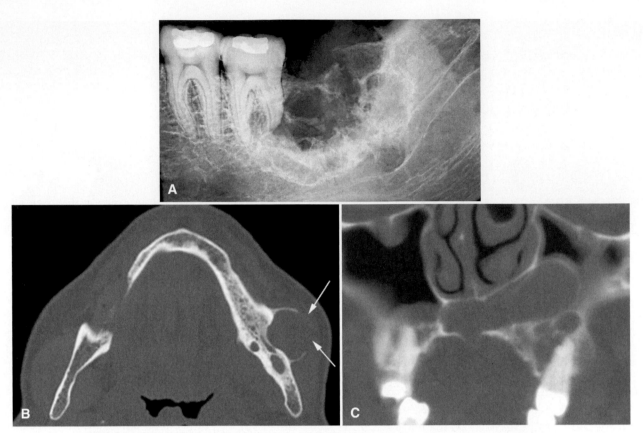

FIGURE 24-8 A, Multilocular radiolucency is characteristic of central mucoepidermoid carcinoma. This lesion has displaced the mandibular canal and destroyed the superior crest of the alveolar process and the distal supporting bone of the second molar. **B,** Axial CT image reveals multiple cystlike growths, some surrounded by sclerotic bone and expansion of the mandible with extension into the surrounding soft tissue *(arrow).* **C,** Coronal CT image of a maxillary mucoepidermoid carcinoma with a multilocular internal structure.

Effects on Surrounding Structures.   Teeth may be moved bodily by the tumor and may exhibit root resorption similar to a benign tumor. Bony borders may be effaced or breached, and as in benign ameloblastoma, the lesions may erode lamina dura and displace normal anatomic boundaries, such as the floor of the nose and maxillary sinus. The mandibular neurovascular canal may be displaced or eroded.

Differential Diagnosis

The differential diagnosis of this lesion should include benign ameloblastoma, odontogenic keratocyst, odontogenic myxoma, and central mucoepidermoid tumor, from which it may not be distinguishable radiologically. If the lesion is locally invasive and this is apparent radiologically, a diagnosis of carcinoma arising in a dental cyst should be entertained. If the patient is young and the location of the lesion is anterior to the second permanent molar, central giant cell granuloma may mimic some of its radiologic features. The final diagnosis often is the result of histologic evaluation or the detection of metastatic lesions.

Management

These lesions are most often treated with en bloc surgical resection. However, many may not be discovered to be malignant until the time of the first surgery or later. Because the histologic appearance of these lesions may mimic benign ameloblastoma, the initial treatment often is inadequate. In addition, the metastatic lesions may not appear for many months or years after treatment of the primary tumor, adding another reason for treatment failure.

METASTATIC TUMORS

SYNONYM

A synonym for metastatic tumors is secondary malignancy.

DISEASE MECHANISM

Metastatic tumors represent the establishment of new foci of malignant disease from a distant malignant tumor usually by way of the blood vessels. Metastatic lesions in the jaws usually arise from sites that are anatomically inferior to the clavicle. Metastatic lesions of the jaws usually occur when the distant primary lesion is already known, although occasionally the presence of a metastatic tumor may reveal the presence of a silent primary lesion. Jaw involvement accounts for less than 1% of metastatic malignancies found elsewhere, with most affecting the spine, pelvis, skull, ribs, and humerus. Most frequently the tumor is a type of carcinoma; the most common primary tumors are breast, lung, prostate, colon and rectum, kidney, thyroid, stomach, melanoma, testicle, bladder, ovarian, and cervical. In children, tumors include neuroblastoma, retinoblastoma, and Wilms' tumor. Metastatic carcinoma must be differentiated from the more common locally invading squamous carcinoma.

CLINICAL FEATURES

Women have almost twice the number of metastatic tumors as men. Metastatic disease is more common in patients in their fifth to seventh decade of life, and breast metastases outnumber all other types. Patients may complain of dental pain, numbness or paresthesia of the third branch of the trigeminal nerve, pathologic fracture of the jaw, or hemorrhage from the tumor site.

IMAGING FEATURES

Location

The posterior areas of the jaws are more commonly affected (Fig. 24-9), with the mandible being favored over the maxilla. The maxillary sinus may be the next most common site, followed by the anterior hard palate and mandibular condyle. Frequently, metastatic lesions of the mandible are bilateral (see Fig. 24-9, *B* and *C*). Also, lesions may be located in the periodontal ligament space (sometimes at the root apex), mimicking periapical and periodontal inflammatory disease, or in the papilla of a developing tooth.

Periphery and Shape

Metastatic lesions may be moderately well demarcated but have no cortication or encapsulation at their tumor margins; they also may have ill-defined invasive margins (see Fig. 24-9, *A*). The lesions are not usually round but polymorphous in shape. Both prostate

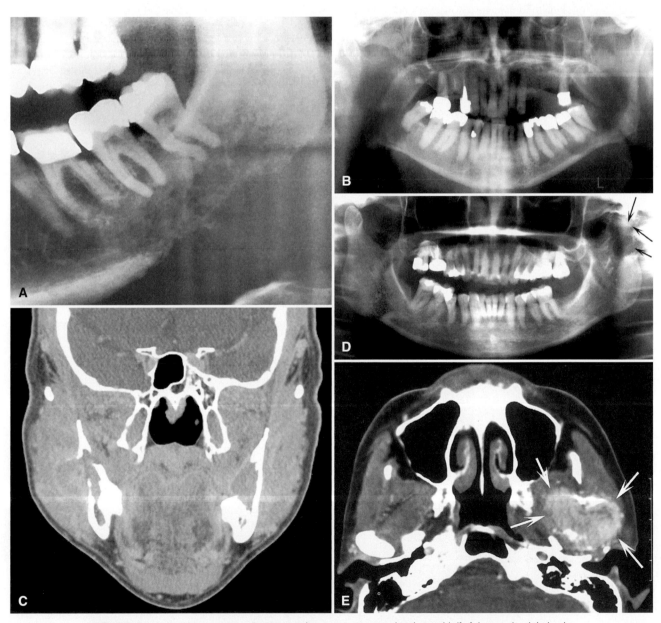

FIGURE 24-9 Metastatic carcinomas. **A,** Metastatic breast carcinoma surrounding the apical half of the second and third molar roots and extending inferiorly. It has destroyed the inferior border of the mandible. **B,** Bilateral metastatic lesions from the lung destroying the mandibular rami. **C,** Coronal CT image using soft tissue algorithm of the case shown in **B**. **D,** Destruction of the left mandibular condyle *(arrows)* from a thyroid metastatic lesion. **E,** Axial CT image using soft tissue algorithm of the case shown in **D** demonstrates invasion into surrounding soft tissue *(arrows)*.

and breast lesions may stimulate bone formation of the adjacent bone, which is sclerotic. The tumor may begin as a few zones of osseous destruction separated by normal bone. These small areas coalesce into a larger, ill-defined mass over time, and the jaw may become enlarged.

Internal Structure

Lesions are generally radiolucent, in which case the internal structure is a combination of residual normal trabecular bone in association with areas of bone lysis. If sclerotic metastases are present (i.e., prostate and breast), the normally ragged radiolucent area may appear as an area of patchy sclerosis, as the result of new bone formation (Fig. 24-10). The origin of this new bone is not the tumor but stimulation of surrounding normal bone. If the tumor is seeded in multiple regions of the jaw, the result is a multifocal appearance (multiple small radiolucent lesions) with normal bone between the foci. Significant dissemination of metastatic tumor may give the jaws a general radiolucent appearance or an appearance similar to osteopenia.

Effects on Surrounding Structures

Metastatic carcinomas may stimulate a periosteal reaction that usually takes the form of a spiculated pattern (prostate and neuroblastoma) (see Fig. 24-10). Typical of malignancy, the lesion effaces the lamina dura and can cause an irregular increase in the width of the periodontal ligament space. If the tumor has seeded in the papilla of a developing tooth, the cortices of the crypt may be totally or partially destroyed. Teeth may seem to be floating in a soft tissue mass and may be in an altered position because of loss of bony support. Extraction sockets may fail to heal and may increase in size. Resorption of teeth is rare (sometimes associated with multiple myeloma and chondrosarcoma); this is more common in benign lesions. The cortical bone of adjacent structures, such as the neurovascular canal, sinus, and nasal fossa, is destroyed. Occasionally, the tumor breaches the outer cortical plate of the jaws and extends into surrounding soft tissues or manifests as an intraoral mass (see Fig. 24-8, E).

DIFFERENTIAL DIAGNOSIS

In most cases, a known primary malignancy is present, and the diagnosis of metastasis is straightforward. Multiple myeloma may be confused with metastatic tumors; however, the border of multiple myeloma is usually better circumscribed than metastatic disease. When a lesion starts within the periodontal ligament space of a tooth, the appearance may be identical to that of a periapical inflammatory lesion. A point of differentiation is that the periodontal ligament space widening from inflammation is at its greatest width and centered about the apex of the root. In contrast, the malignant tumor usually causes irregular widening, which may extend up the side of the root. Odontogenic cysts, if secondarily infected, may have an ill-defined border giving a similar appearance to a metastatic lesion. Invasion of the jaws by primary tumors of the overlying epithelium, such as squamous cell carcinoma, may be indistinguishable from metastatic disease but can be differentiated by clinical examination.

MANAGEMENT

The presence of a metastatic tumor in the jaw indicates a poor prognosis. If metastatic disease is present, the patient usually dies within 1 to 2 years. If the appearance in the images is suspicious, an opinion from a dental radiologist should be sought, and tissue should be submitted for histologic analysis. Nuclear medicine may be employed to detect other metastatic lesions. Isolated malignant deposits, if symptomatic, may be treated with localized high-dose radiation treatment. On the rare occasion that the jaw is the first diagnosed site of malignant spread, it is imperative that the patient be referred quickly to an oncologist so that anticancer treatment can be delivered promptly. This treatment may take the form of

FIGURE 24-10 **A,** Partial panoramic image of prostate metastatic lesions involving the body and ramus of the body. Note the sclerotic bone reaction (arrows). **B,** Occlusal image of prostate lesions causing sclerosis and a spiculated periosteal reaction (arrows). **C** and **D,** Two periapical images of a metastatic lesion of breast carcinoma. Note the irregular widening of the periodontal membrane spaces and patchy sclerotic bone reaction, especially around the roots of the molars.

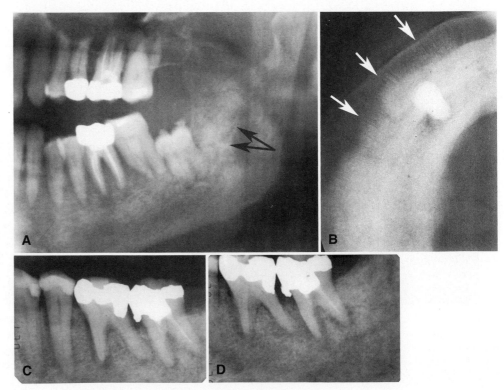

chemotherapy, radiation therapy, surgery, immunotherapy, or hormone treatment.

SARCOMAS

OSTEOSARCOMA

Synonym

Osteogenic sarcoma is a synonym for osteosarcoma.

Disease Mechanism

Osteosarcoma is a malignant neoplasm of bone in which osteoid is produced directly by malignant stroma as opposed to adjacent reactive bone formation. The three major histologic types are: (1) chondroblastic, (2) osteoblastic, and (3) fibroblastic osteosarcoma. The cause of osteosarcoma is unknown, but genetic mutation and viral causes have been suggested. It is also known to occur in association with Paget's disease and fibrous dysplasia after therapeutic irradiation.

Clinical Features

Osteosarcoma of the jaws is quite rare and accounts for approximately 7% of all osteosarcomas. The dentist may be the first health professional who observes tumors involving the jaws. The lesion occurs in all racial groups worldwide and in males twice as frequently as females. Jaw lesions typically occur with a peak in the fourth decade, about 10 years later on average than long bone lesions. The most commonly reported symptom or sign is swelling, which may be present 6 months before diagnosis; the swelling is usually rapid. Other indicators are pain, tenderness, erythema of overlying mucosa, ulceration, loose teeth, epistaxis, hemorrhage, nasal obstruction, exophthalmos, trismus, and blindness. Hypoesthesia has also been reported in cases involving neurovascular canals.

Imaging Features

Location. The mandible is more commonly affected than the maxilla. Although the lesion can occur in any part of either jaw, the posterior mandible, including the tooth-bearing region, angle, and vertical ramus, is most commonly affected. The posterior areas are also more commonly affected in the maxilla, with the most frequent sites being the alveolar ridge, antrum, and palate. The lesion may cross the midline.

Periphery and Shape. Osteosarcoma has an ill-defined border in most instances. When viewed against normal bone, the lesion can be either relatively radiolucent or radiopaque with no peripheral sclerosis or encapsulation. If the lesion involves the periosteum directly or by extension, one may see the typical "sunray" spicules or "hair-on-end" trabeculae (Fig. 24-11). This appearance occurs when the periosteum is displaced, partially destroyed, and disorganized. If the periosteum is elevated and maintains its osteogenic potential but is breached in the center, a Codman's triangle at the edges is formed (see Fig. 24-1, E). Even more rarely, laminar periosteal new bone may be present. In many cases, extension into surrounding soft tissues is prominent, and a soft tissue mass emanating from the bone is visible.

Internal Structure. Osteosarcoma may be entirely radiolucent, mixed radiolucent-radiopaque, or quite radiopaque. The internal osseous structure may take the appearance of granular-appearing or sclerotic-appearing bone, cotton balls, wisps, or honeycombed internal structures in areas with adjacent destruction of the preexisting osseous architecture. Whatever the resultant internal structure, the normal trabecular structure of the jaws is lost.

Effects on Surrounding Structures. Widening of the periodontal membrane is associated with osteosarcoma but is also seen in other malignancies (Fig. 24-12). The antral or nasal wall cortices may be lost in maxillary lesions. Mandibular lesions may destroy the cortex of the neurovascular canal and adjacent lamina dura. Alternatively, the neurovascular canal may be symmetrically widened and enlarged. Effects on the periosteum are discussed under the previous heading "Periphery and Shape."

Differential Diagnosis. If internal structure of abnormal bone is minimal or absent, fibrosarcoma or metastatic carcinoma may appear similar to osteosarcoma. If osseous structure is visible, the practitioner should also consider chondrosarcoma. If spiculated periosteal new bone is present, prostate and breast metastases should be considered. A comprehensive physical examination and laboratory tests assist in determining if the lesion is primary or metastatic. Benign tumors such as ossifying fibroma and bone dysplasias such as fibrous dysplasia are better demarcated; are more uniform in internal structure; and lack invasive, destructive characteristics. The histopathology of a biopsy specimen of osteosarcoma may be interpreted as a benign fibro-osseous lesion, and the correct diagnosis in these cases relies on the imaging characteristics alone. Ewing's sarcoma, solitary plasmacytoma, and osteomyelitis share some of the radiographic characteristics of osteosarcoma. Osteosarcoma is generally not associated with signs of infection.

Management. The management of osteosarcoma is resection with a large border of adjacent normal bone. Such resection may be possible in orthopedic cases but may be complicated by the presence of important adjacent anatomic structures in the head and neck. Generally, radiation therapy and chemotherapy are used only for controlling metastatic spread or for palliation.

CHONDROSARCOMA

Synonym

Chondrogenic sarcoma is a synonym for chondrosarcoma.

Disease Mechanism

Chondrosarcoma is a malignant tumor of mesenchymal origin that produces cartilage. There are several histologic subtypes that develop most commonly in the craniofacial region, including clear cell, dedifferentiated, myxoid, and mesenchymal forms. These tumors may occur centrally within bone, on the periphery of bone, or, less commonly, in soft tissue. Some form directly from malignant mesenchymal cells, and some form from preexisting cartilaginous lesions. In the case of the latter, they are termed secondary chondrosarcomas.

Clinical Features

Generally, these tumors occur at any age, although they are more common in adults (mean age, 47 years). They affect males and females equally. A patient with chondrosarcoma may have a firm or hard mass of relatively long duration. Enlargement of these lesions may cause pain, headache, and deformity. Less frequent signs and symptoms include hemorrhage from tumor or from the necks of the teeth, sensory nerve deficits, proptosis, and visual disturbances. The tumors invariably are covered with

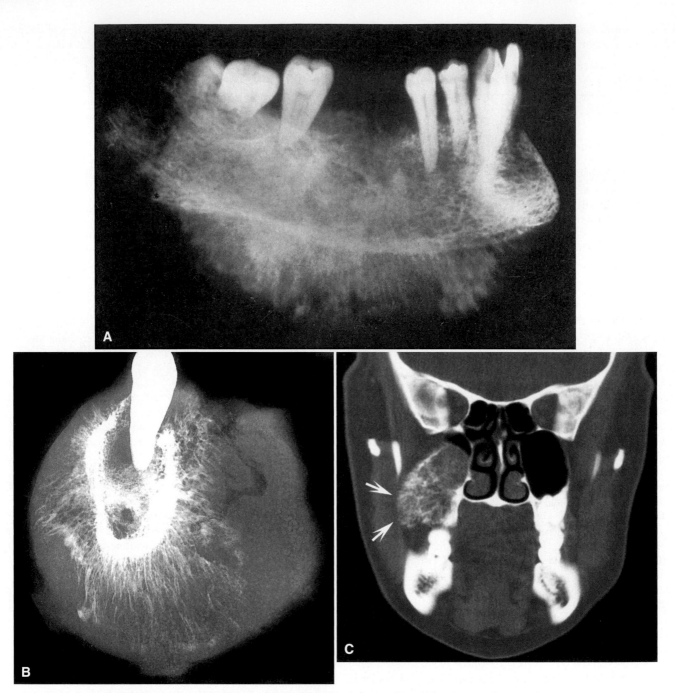

FIGURE 24-11 A and **B,** Radiographs of a resected mandible of a 25-year-old man with osteosarcoma, showing sunray spicules. **C,** Coronal CT image of an osteosarcoma of the maxilla. Note the spiculated bone formation extending laterally from the maxilla *(arrows).*

normal overlying skin or mucosa unless secondarily ulcerated. If chondrosarcoma occurs in or near the temporomandibular joint region, trismus or abnormal joint function may result.

Imaging Features

Location.   Chondrosarcomas are unusual in the facial bones, accounting for about 10% of all cases. They occur in the mandible and maxilla with equal frequency. Maxillary lesions typically occur in the anterior region in areas where cartilaginous tissues may be present in the maxilla. Mandibular lesions occur in the coronoid process, condylar head and neck (see Fig. 24-13, *B* and *C*), and occasionally the symphyseal region.

Periphery and Shape.   Chondrosarcomas are slow-growing tumors, and their radiologic signs may be misleading and benign in nature. The lesions are generally round, ovoid, or lobulated. Their borders are generally well defined and at times corticated; at other times melding with adjacent normal bone occurs. Occasionally, peripheral periosteal new bone may be present perpendicular to the original cortex, giving the so-called sunray or

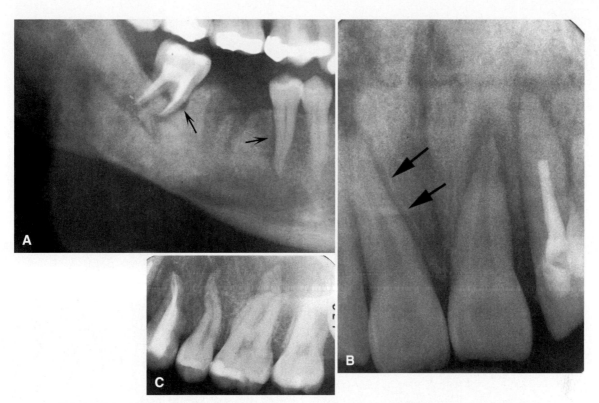

FIGURE 24-12 **A,** Cropped panoramic image shows an osteosarcoma occupying the body of the right mandible. Note the widened ligament spaces *(arrows)* and that the density of the mandible in the first molar region is greater than normal because of abnormal bone formation from the tumor. **B** and **C,** Periapical images of another case of osteosarcoma show irregular widening of the periodontal membrane space of the teeth of the left maxilla and extending to the right maxilla where the ligament space of the left central incisor is widened *(arrows)*.

hair-on-end appearance. Uncommonly, these lesions are ill defined and invasive. Aggressive lesions such as these have infiltrative, ill-defined, and noncorticated borders.

Internal Structure.   Chondrosarcomas usually exhibit some form of calcification within their center, giving them a mixed radiolucent-radiopaque appearance. This mixture sometimes takes the form of moth-eaten bone alternating with islands of residual bone unaffected by tumor. Lesions are rarely completely radiolucent. The central radiopaque structure has been described as "flocculent," implying snowlike features. This diffuse calcification may be superimposed on a bony background that resembles granular or ground-glass–appearing abnormal bone (Fig. 24-13, *A*). Careful examination of these areas of flocculence may reveal a central radiolucent nidus, which is probably cartilage surrounded by calcification. The result is rounded or speckled areas of calcification.

Effects on Surrounding Structures.   Chondrosarcoma, being relatively slow growing, often expands normal cortical boundaries rather than rapidly destroying them. In mandibular cases, the inferior border or alveolar process may be grossly expanded, while still maintaining its cortical covering. Maxillary lesions may push the walls of the maxillary sinus or nasal fossa and impinge on the infratemporal fossa. Lesions of the condyle cause its expansion and perhaps remodeling of the corresponding articular fossa and eminence. If lesions occur in the articular disk region, a widened joint space may be present with corresponding remodeling of the condylar neck. Erosion of the articular fossa may

also occur. If lesions occur near teeth, root resorption and tooth displacement may occur, as may widening of the periodontal membrane space.

Differential Diagnosis.   Osteosarcoma is often indistinguishable from chondrosarcoma in diagnostic images. Although the typical calcifications of chondrosarcoma may be absent from osteosarcoma, the two share many other radiologic features. Fibrous dysplasia may have a similar internal pattern, although the internal calcification of chondrosarcomas represents calcified cartilage. Generally, the periphery of fibrous dysplasia is better defined without signs of bone destruction, and its margin with adjacent teeth differs from chondrosarcoma. For instance, fibrous dysplasia alters the bone pattern up to and including the lamina dura, leaving a normal or thin periodontal ligament space. Because chondrosarcomas may be slow growing and displace teeth and other surrounding structures, these characteristics may be misinterpreted as benign features.

Management.   The management of chondrosarcoma is surgical. Radiation therapy and chemotherapy generally have no role to play. Patients with chondrosarcomas have a relatively good 5-year survival rate, but 10-year survival is poor.

EWING'S SARCOMA

Synonyms

Synonyms for Ewing's sarcoma include endothelial myeloma and round cell sarcoma.

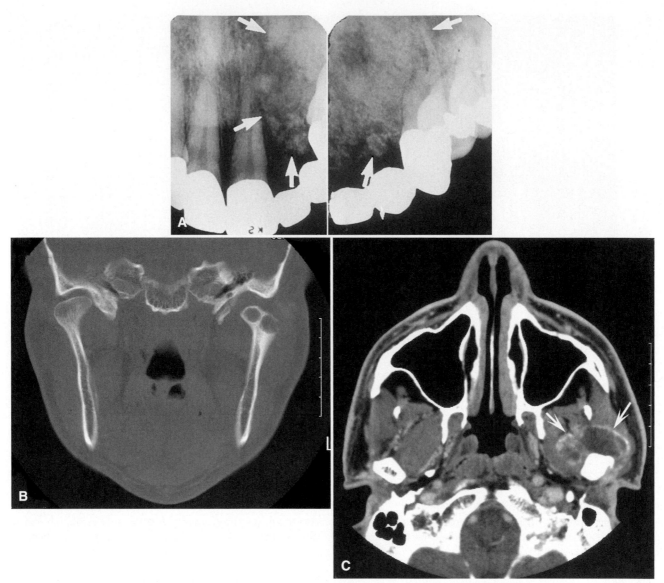

FIGURE 24-13 **A,** Chondrosarcoma of the anterior maxilla, with irregular calcification in the internal structure of the tumor *(arrows).* **B,** Coronal CT image using bone algorithm of a chondrosarcoma involving the mandibular condyle (note the two areas of bone destruction). **C,** Axial CT scan using soft tissue algorithm demonstrating the soft tissue extent of the lesion *(arrows)* and sparse calcifications. (**A,** *Courtesy L. Hollender, DDS, Seattle, WA.)*

Disease Mechanism

Ewing's sarcoma is a small round cell tumor that appears to have a common origin with primitive neuroectodermal tumors. It is a tumor of long bones and is relatively rare in the jaws. Lesions arise in the medullary portion of the bone and spread to the endosteal and later periosteal surfaces.

Clinical Features

Ewing's sarcoma is most common in the second decade of life; most patients are between 5 and 30 years old. Males are twice as likely to have the disease as females. In addition, multicentric lesions have been reported. Other reported findings at the time of presentation include, in descending frequency, swelling, pain, loose teeth, paresthesia, exophthalmos, ptosis, epistaxis, ulceration, shifted teeth, trismus, and sinusitis. Cervical lymphadenopathy has also been reported.

Imaging Features

Location.   Mandibular cases outnumber maxillary cases by about 2:1, with the highest frequency found in posterior areas in both jaws. Generally, the lesions develop within the marrow space first and then extend to involve overlying cortical plates. This neoplasm rarely occurs in the jaws.

Periphery and Shape.   Ewing's sarcoma is a radiolucency that is poorly demarcated and never corticated. Its advancing edge destroys bone in an uneven fashion, resulting in a ragged border. The lesions are usually solitary and may cause pathologic fracture with adjacent radiographically visible soft tissue masses (Fig. 24-14). They may be round or ovoid but generally have no typical shape.

Internal Structure.   Ewing's sarcoma is a destructive process with little induction of bone formation. Because it commences on

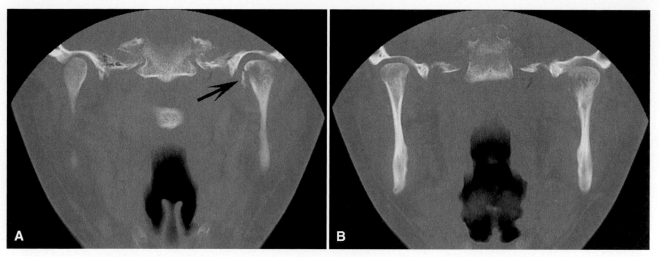

FIGURE 24-14 **A** and **B,** Coronal CT images using bone algorithm demonstrate Ewing's sarcoma involving the left mandibular condyle. Note the irregular margins, destruction of the medial cortex of the condyle, and a small pathologic fracture *(arrow).*

the internal aspect of the bone and involves the endosteal and periosteal surfaces later in its course, it is usually entirely radiolucent.

Effects on Surrounding Structures.   Ewing's sarcoma may stimulate the periosteum to produce new bone; this is usually the result of gross disturbances to the overlying periosteum and takes the form of Codman's triangle or "sunray" or "hair-on-end" spiculation. Laminar periosteal new bone formation has been reported to occur but is not a common feature of active Ewing's sarcoma lesions of the jaws. Adjacent normal structures, such as the mandibular neurovascular canal, inferior border of the mandible, and alveolar cortical plates, may be effaced. If the lesion abuts teeth or tooth follicles, the cortices of these structures are destroyed. This tumor does not characteristically cause root resorption, although it does destroy the supporting bone of adjacent teeth.

Differential Diagnosis

Inflammatory or infectious lesions such as osteomyelitis of the jaw may share some of the radiographic features of Ewing's sarcoma. Although both lesions are radiolucent, osteomyelitis is likely to have demonstrable sequestra present within the confines of the lesion, whereas Ewing's sarcoma does not. Inflammatory lesions contain some sign of reactive bone formation, resulting in a sclerotic bone pattern internally or at the periphery and differ in the associated periosteal bone formation.

Eosinophilic granuloma of the jaw is also a destructive process, which occurs in the same part of the bone. It is associated with laminar periosteal bone reaction, whereas Ewing's sarcoma in the jaws is not associated with laminar periosteal bone reaction. Other central primary malignancies of bone, such as osteosarcoma, chondrosarcoma, and fibrosarcoma, may be difficult to differentiate from this condition.

Management

Too few cases of maxillofacial Ewing's sarcoma are available at any single treatment center for any specific treatment policy to have been adopted. Surgery, radiation therapy, and chemotherapy may be used alone or in combination.

FIBROSARCOMA
Disease Mechanism

Fibrosarcoma is a neoplasm composed of malignant fibroblasts that produce collagen and elastin. The etiology is unknown, although it may arise secondarily in tissues that have received therapeutic levels of radiation.

Clinical Features

These lesions occur equally in males and females with a mean age in the fourth decade. The usual presenting symptom is a mass that is slowly to rapidly enlarging. The mass may be within bone, in which case it usually is accompanied by pain. Peripheral lesions or lesions exiting from bone may invade local soft tissues, causing a bulky, clinically obvious lesion. If central or peripheral lesions reach a large size, pathologic fracture may occur. If fibrosarcomas involve the course of peripheral nerves, sensory neural abnormalities may occur. Overlying mucosa, although initially normal, may become erythematous or ulcerated. Involvement of the temporomandibular joint or paramandibular musculature is often accompanied by trismus.

Imaging Features

Location.   Most cases of fibrosarcoma of the jaws occur in the mandible, with the greatest number of these occurring in the premolar and molar region.

Periphery and Shape.   Fibrosarcomas have ill-defined borders that are best described as ragged (Fig. 24-15). They are poorly demarcated, are noncorticated, and lack any semblance of a capsule. These tumors are generally shaped in a fashion that suggests that they have grown along a bone, and so they tend to be elongated through the marrow space. The radiographic border may underestimate the extent of the tumor because these lesions typically are infiltrative. If soft tissue lesions occur adjacent to bone, they may cause a saucer-like depression in the underlying bone or invade it as would a squamous cell carcinoma. Finally, sclerosis may occur in the adjacent normal bone whether the fibrosarcoma is peripheral to bone or central.

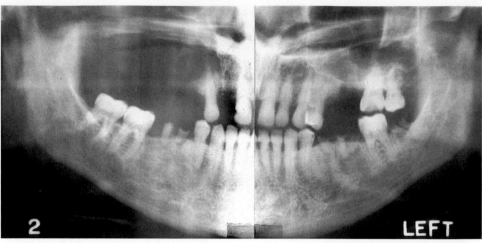

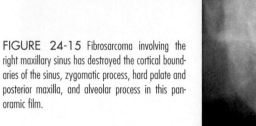

FIGURE 24-15 Fibrosarcoma involving the right maxillary sinus has destroyed the cortical boundaries of the sinus, zygomatic process, hard palate and posterior maxilla, and alveolar process in this panoramic film.

Internal Structure.   Fibrosarcomas have little internal structure. In most cases, the lesions are entirely radiolucent. If the lesions have been present for some time and are not overly aggressive, either residual jawbone or reactive osseous bone formation occurs.

Effects on Surrounding Structures.   The most common effect on adjacent structures is destruction. In the mandible, the alveolar process, inferior border of the jaw, and cortices of the neurovascular canal are lost. In the maxilla, the inferior floor of the maxillary sinus, posterior wall of the maxilla, and nasal floor can be destroyed. In either jaw, lamina dura and follicular cortices are obliterated. Destruction of the outer cortical plate is usually accompanied by a protruding soft tissue mass. Root resorption is uncommon. Teeth are more likely to be grossly displaced and lose their support bone so that they appear to be floating in space. In addition, widening of the periodontal membrane space occurs with this tumor, as in other malignancies. Periosteal reaction is uncommon; however, if the lesion disrupts the periosteum, a Codman's triangle or "sunray" spiculation may be evident.

Differential Diagnosis

This solitary, ragged radiolucency with little internal structure is difficult to differentiate from other central malignancies. If the lesion does not cause enlargement of the jaw, the practitioner must rule out metastatic carcinoma, multiple myeloma, and primary or secondary intraosseous carcinoma. Another possibility is a grossly infected dental cyst, although these usually show some degree of induced peripheral sclerosis in adjacent bone. If a fibrosarcoma exhibits enlargement of the affected jaw with an associated soft tissue mass, other sarcomas such as chondrosarcoma and osteosarcoma (both usually have internal structure) and a central desmoplastic fibroma should be ruled out. Ewing's sarcoma and radiolucent osteosarcomas may not be distinguishable from this tumor. Finally, peripheral invasive squamous cell carcinoma shares some of these radiologic features, but its ulcerative surface features differentiate it from fibrosarcoma, which usually lacks these.

Management

The management of fibrosarcoma is chiefly surgical. A wide margin of adjacent normal bone is taken if anatomically possible. Radiation therapy and chemotherapy are usually palliative treatments.

MALIGNANCIES OF THE HEMATOPOIETIC SYSTEM
MULTIPLE MYELOMA
Synonyms
Synonyms for multiple myeloma include myeloma, plasma cell myeloma, and plasmacytoma.

Disease Mechanism
Multiple myeloma is a malignant neoplasm of plasma cells (derived from B lymphocytes). These cells accumulate in bone marrow and interfere with normal hematopoiesis. It is the most common malignancy of bone in adults. Single lesions are called plasmacytoma, and multiple lesions are termed multiple myeloma.

Clinical Features
Multiple myeloma is a fatal systemic malignancy. A patient with multiple myeloma is usually between 35 and 70 years old (mean age, 60 years). The patient may complain of fatigue, weight loss, fever, bone pain, and anemia, although the typical presenting feature is low back pain. Secondary signs include amyloidosis and hypercalcemia; in half of all patients, characteristic Bence Jones protein is present in the urine, which causes the urine to be foamy. The disease is more common in men. When this clonal cellular proliferation occurs, these cells occupy first cancellous and later cortical bone, replacing the normally radiopaque bone with areas of radiolucency.

Orally, patients may complain of dental pain, swelling, hemorrhage, paresthesia, and dysesthesia, or they may have no complaints. The number of patients with demonstrable radiologic findings in the jaws at the time of diagnosis is relatively small.

Imaging Features
Location.   Multiple myeloma (Fig. 24-16) is seen more frequently in the mandible than the maxilla but is uncommon in either. Publications reveal a wide variation in the incidence of jaw lesions in patients with multiple myeloma. In the mandible, lesions of the posterior body, ramus, and condyle are common. Maxillary lesions usually appear in posterior sites.

Periphery and Shape.   The periphery of multiple myeloma lesions is well defined but not corticated; it lacks any sign of bone reaction

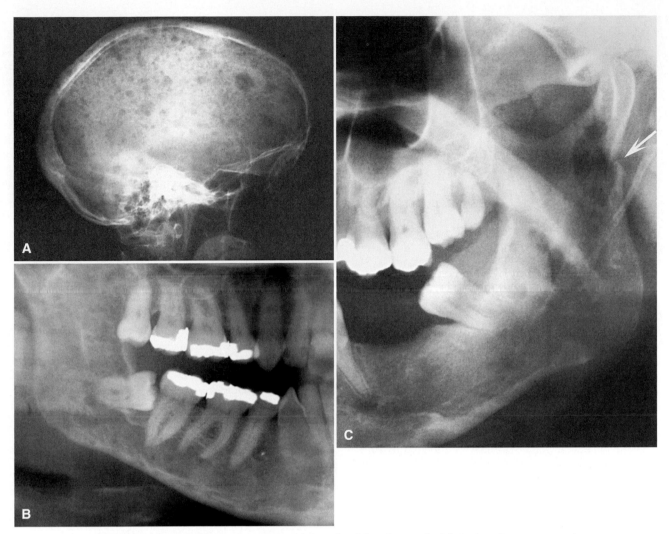

FIGURE 24-16 **A,** Multiple myeloma, seen as multiple circular radiolucent lesions in the skull. **B,** Cropped panoramic image of a different case shows multiple small lesions of multiple myeloma present through the body and ramus of the mandible. **C,** Cropped panoramic image shows a solitary lesion in the condylar neck region and a pathologic fracture *(arrow)*.

(Fig. 24-17). The lesions have been described as appearing "punched out." However, many appear ragged and even infiltrative. Some lesions have an oval or cystic shape. Untreated or aggressive areas of destruction may become confluent, giving the appearance of multilocularity. If the lesion is located in the periapical periodontal ligament space, it may have a border similar to that seen in inflammatory or infectious periapical disease. Lesions may be difficult to detect in the image if there is osteoporosis secondary to kidney disease. However, often there may be a scalloped erosion of the endosteal surface of the inferior cortex of the mandible. Soft tissue lesions have been reported in the jaws and nasopharynx.

Internal Structure.   No internal structure is visible; these lesions are totally radiolucent. Occasionally islands of residual bone, yet unaffected by tumor, give the appearance of the presence of new trabecular bone within the mass.

Effects on Surrounding Structures.   If a good deal of bone mineral is lost, teeth may appear to be "too opaque" and may stand out conspicuously from their osteopenic background. In rare cases, there may be irregular root resorption. Lamina dura and follicles

of impacted teeth may lose their typical corticated surrounding bone in a manner analogous to that seen in hyperparathyroidism. The same may be said of the mandibular neurovascular canal, which, although usually visible, loses its cortical boundary in whole or in part. These changes are profound when there is associated renal disease. Mandibular lesions may cause thinning of the lower border of the mandible or endosteal scalloping. Any cortical boundary may be effaced if lesions involve them. Periosteal reaction is uncommon, but if present, it takes the form of a single radiopaque line or, more rarely, a "sunray" appearance.

Differential Diagnosis.

The most likely disease to be mistaken for multiple myeloma is the radiolucent form of metastatic carcinoma. Knowledge of a prior malignancy in a patient may help differentiate multiple myeloma from metastatic carcinoma. Severe osteomyelitis may yield a radiologic picture similar to multiple myeloma; however, a visible cause for it usually exists. In addition, inflammatory lesions and infections generally cause sclerosis in adjacent bone, which multiple myeloma does not. Simple bone cysts may be bilateral in the mandible and may be mistaken for multiple myeloma. They

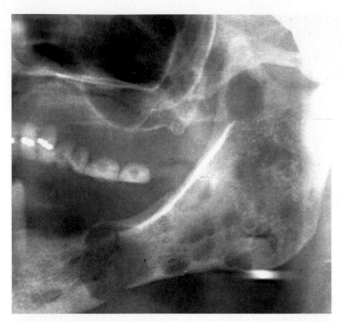

FIGURE 24-17 Cropped panoramic image depicting multiple areas of well-defined bone destruction lacking any cortical boundary. The lesions are multiple, separate, and appear to be "punched out," typical of changes seen in multiple myeloma. *(Courtesy G. Petrikowski, DDS, Toronto, Ontario, Canada.)*

are usually corticated in part and characteristically interdigitate between the roots of the teeth in a much younger population. Generalized radiolucency of the jaws may be caused by hyperparathyroidism but is differentiated based on abnormal blood chemistry. However, brown tumors of hyperparathyroidism, if present with generalized radiolucency of the jaws and similar symptoms, can readily be confused with multiple myeloma. Other metabolic diseases, such as Gaucher's disease or oxalosis, may cause many changes similar to multiple myeloma that are observed on dental radiographs.

Management

Multiple myeloma is usually treated with chemotherapy with or without autologous or allogeneic bone marrow transplantation. Radiation therapy may be used for treatment of symptomatic osseous lesions when palliation is required.

NON-HODGKIN'S LYMPHOMA

Synonyms

Synonyms for non-Hodgkin's lymphoma include malignant lymphoma and lymphosarcoma.

Disease Mechanism

Non-Hodgkin's lymphoma is a malignant tumor of cells normally resident in the lymphatic system. These cells include lymphocytes at various levels of maturation. In general, lymphomas occur within lymph nodes; however, extranodal sites, such as bone, skin, gastrointestinal mucosa, tonsils, and Waldeyer's ring, can be involved. The term non-Hodgkin's lymphoma describes a family of heterogeneous tumors of varying type and severity. The classification of these diseases is difficult, and numerous means exist of subdividing these tumors. The current working formulation for clinical usage classifies tumors based on their histologic appearance into low-grade, intermediate-grade, or high-grade tumors, with the last being the most aggressive.

Clinical Features

Non-Hodgkin's lymphoma occurs in all age groups but is rare in patients in the first decade of life. The maxillary sinus, palate, tonsillar area, and bone may be sites of primary or secondary lymphoma spread. Lesions occurring outside lymph nodes in the head and neck may be present in one of five cases. Patients may feel unwell, experiencing night sweats, pruritus, and weight loss. Palpable painless swelling, lymphadenopathy, and sensorineural deficits may accompany isolated lesions of the jaws. Lesions present for some time may cause pain and ulceration. Teeth resident in a lymphoma may become mobile, as the supporting bone is lost.

Imaging Features

Location.   Most non-Hodgkin's lymphomas of the head and neck occur in the lymph nodes. Non-Hodgkin's lymphoma that is extranodal is likely to affect the maxillary sinus, posterior mandible, and maxillary regions. A few cases have originated within the inferior alveolar nerve canal.

Periphery and Shape.   Most non-Hodgkin's lymphomas initially take the shape and form of the host bone. If these lesions are untreated, they are capable of causing destruction of the overlying cortex (Fig. 24-18). They may appear rounded or multiloculated and lack a defining outer cortex. The borders generally are ill defined and invasive. Occasionally, lymphoma appears as multiple areas of destruction, which likely appear as finger-like extensions of malignant tumor cells in a buccal or lingual direction. Visible lesions occurring in the maxillary sinus or nasopharynx have a smooth periphery.

Internal Structure.   The internal structure of lymphoma is almost always entirely radiolucent. It is rare to see reactive bone formation. Occasionally, patchy radiopacity may be present, but this is rare.

Effects on Surrounding Structures.   In maxillary sinus lesions, the antral walls may be effaced, and a soft tissue mass may be visible radiographically, either internally within the sinus or external to the maxillary sinus. Lesions involving the mandible destroy the cortex of the neurovascular canal. This tumor has a propensity to grow in the periodontal ligament space of mature teeth (Fig. 24-19). The cortex of the crypts of developing teeth may be lost when the lymphoma is located in the developing papilla, and the involved teeth may be displaced in an occlusal direction and exfoliated. Periosteal reaction is uncommon but may take the form of laminated or spiculated bone formation. With the advent of soft tissue imaging with MRI, it has become apparent that this tumor has a habit of growing along soft tissue spaces (fat layers) and along the surface of bone.

Differential Diagnosis

Multiple myeloma and metastatic carcinoma are easily confused with non-Hodgkin's lymphoma of the jaws. However, Ewing's sarcoma and Langerhans' histiocytosis, although also capable of producing the same effects, occur in a slightly younger age group. Osteolytic osteosarcoma and any of the central squamous cell carcinomas may not be distinguishable radiographically from non-Hodgkin's lymphoma. Squamous cell carcinoma arising in the maxillary sinus may be difficult to differentiate from lymphoma of the maxillary sinus. Other lesions that can displace developing

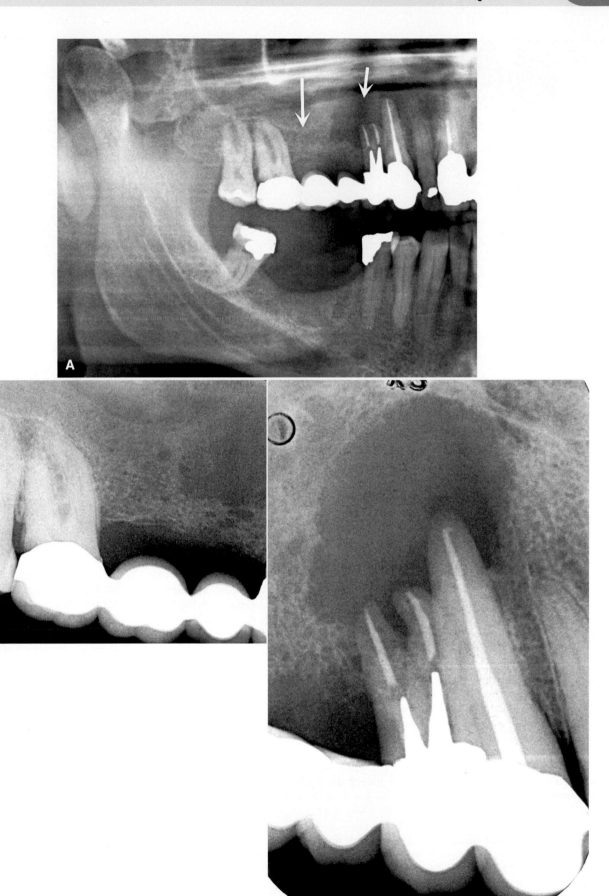

FIGURE 24-18 **A,** Panoramic image revealing a malignant lymphoma invading the right maxilla. Note the ill-defined bone destruction and loss of the anterior aspect of the floor of the maxillary antrum *(arrows).* **B,** Intraoral radiographs also show ill-defined bone destruction and the lack of any bone reaction or formation.

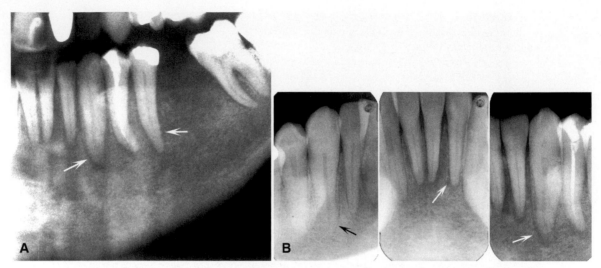

FIGURE 24-19 **A,** Cropped panoramic image reveals an ill-defined lymphoma invading the left body of the mandible. Note the irregular widening of the periodontal ligament spaces *(arrows)*. **B,** Intraoral films of the same case demonstrate widened periodontal ligament spaces *(white arrows)* compared with the normal periodontal ligament space of the right mandibular cuspid *(black arrow)*.

teeth in an occlusal direction include leukemia and Langerhans' histiocytosis. Differentiation from apical rarefying osteitis may be difficult; however, careful inspection of the radiographic film may reveal the presence of an infiltrative border and adjacent bone destruction.

Management

The management of extranodal or isolated nodal disease is radiation therapy with or without concomitant chemotherapy. Treatment depends on histologic variants and the location and extent of disease.

BURKITT'S LYMPHOMA

Synonym

A synonym for Burkitt's lymphoma is African jaw lymphoma.

Disease Mechanism

Burkitt's lymphoma is a high-grade B-cell lymphoma that differs from other B-cell lymphomas with respect to its histologic appearance and clinical behavior. It was first described by Denis Burkitt in East Africa as African jaw lymphoma.

Two separate forms of the disease have been described: (1) the endemic African Burkitt's lymphoma and (2) the American form. The latter is not characterized by jaw involvement (although it occurs), but has involvement of abdominal viscera. African Burkitt's lymphoma affects young children, whereas American Burkitt's lymphoma affects adolescents and young adults. Cases of endemic and nonendemic Burkitt's tumor have been described throughout the world.

Clinical Features

The disease affects more males than females. Clinically, the hallmark of this tumor is rapidity of growth with a tumor doubling time of less than 24 hours. It may involve children 2 years old and adults in their seventh decade, although it is primarily a disease of youth. Jaw tumors are rapidly growing and cause facial deformity very early in their course. They are capable of blocking nasal passages, displacing orbital contents, causing gross facial swelling, and eroding through skin. These rapidly growing tumors are more characteristic of African Burkitt's lymphoma than the American form and cause pain and paresthesia. Teeth may become loosened rapidly, and alveolar bone may become grossly distended. Paresthesia of the inferior alveolar nerve or other sensory facial nerves is common.

Imaging Features

Location. Extranodal disease is the norm in Burkitt's tumor. African cases may involve one jaw or both the maxilla and the mandible and affect the posterior parts of the jaws. By contrast, American cases may not involve the facial bones but are more likely to affect the abdominal viscera and testes.

Periphery and Shape. The lesions may begin as multiple, ill-defined, noncorticated radiolucencies, which later coalesce into larger, ill-defined radiolucencies with an expansile periphery. They are of no specific shape, although they expand rapidly and have been likened to a balloon. This expansion breaches its outer cortical limits, causing gross balloon-like expansion with thinning of adjacent structures and production of a soft tissue tumor mass adjacent to the osseous lesion. Lesions that abut the orbital contents or the maxillary sinus may show a smooth surface soft tissue mass radiologically.

Internal Structure. Burkitt's lymphoma does not produce bone and rarely induces production of reactive bone within its center. For this reason, the lesions are radiolucent in almost all cases. It is particularly radiolucent in the jaw of a child.

Effects on Surrounding Structures. Erupted teeth in the area of Burkitt's tumor are grossly displaced, as are developing tooth crypts. Tumor cells within the crypt may displace the developing tooth bud to one side of its crypt. A tumor that is located apical to a developing tooth may cause it to be displaced such that it appears to erupt with little if any root formation. After tumor involvement of the developing dental structures occurs, root development ceases. Lamina dura of teeth in the area is destroyed, and cortical boundaries, such as the maxillary sinus, nasal floor, orbital walls, and inferior border of the mandible, are thinned and later destroyed. The cortex of the inferior alveolar canal is lost, although it is difficult to see in the normal pediatric patient in any case. If periosteum is involved, the border may show "sunray" spiculation, although this is rare. Cases that involve the orbit displace the orbital contents, seen both clinically and radiologically.

Differential Diagnosis

Metastatic neuroblastoma and Ewing's tumor may cause similar changes clinically and radiologically. Osteolytic osteosarcoma can grow rapidly and may be indistinguishable from Burkitt's tumor on clinical and radiologic grounds. Cherubism has more internal structure, does not breach bony borders, is bilateral, and grows much more slowly. Finally, non-Hodgkin's lymphoma must be considered, although it occurs in a much older age group in most cases.

Management

Burkitt's tumor is treated with chemotherapy. Chemotherapy regimens vary according to geographic locale, but the tumor is exquisitely sensitive to combinations of chemotherapeutic agents.

LEUKEMIA

Synonyms

Synonyms for leukemia include acute myelogenous leukemia, acute lymphoblastic leukemia, chronic myelogenous leukemia, and chronic lymphocytic leukemia.

Disease Mechanism

Leukemia is a malignant tumor of hematopoietic stem cells. These malignant cells displace normal bone marrow constituents and spill out into the peripheral blood. They are subdivided into acute leukemias and chronic leukemias and further subdivided by the cell of origin. Acute leukemias occur with a bimodal age distribution, with very young patients and very old patients being the most commonly affected. Most cases of leukemia are associated with nonrandom chromosomal abnormalities.

Clinical Features

A patient with chronic leukemia may have no presenting signs or complaints. Patients with acute leukemia generally feel unwell with weakness and bone pain. They may exhibit pallor, spontaneous hemorrhage, hepatomegaly, splenomegaly, lymphadenopathy, and fever. Oral symptoms are generally absent but if present include loose teeth, petechiae, ulceration, and boggy enlarged gingiva.

Imaging Features

Radiologic signs associated with chronic leukemia are comparatively rare.

Location. Leukemia affects the entire body because it is a malignancy of bone marrow, which discharges malignant cells into circulating blood. Manifestations in the jaws may be seen more often in areas of developing teeth. Frequently, leukemia may be localized around the periapical region of a tooth, giving the appearance of a rarefying osteitis. Involvement of jaws in adults is rare.

Periphery and Shape. Leukemia must be considered a systemic malignancy, and its oral radiologic features may be present bilaterally as ill-defined patchy radiolucent areas. With time and lack of treatment, these patchy areas may coalesce to form larger areas of ill-defined radiolucent regions of bone (Fig. 24-20). The teeth may appear to stand out conspicuously from their surrounding osteopenic bone.

Internal Structure. The internal structure of leukemia is characterized by patchy areas of radiolucency and generalized radiolucency of the bone. Rarely, granular bone may be seen within these lesions. Occasionally, foci of leukemic cells may be present as a mass that may behave like a localized malignant tumor. These lesions are called chloromas and are rare in the jaws.

Effects on Surrounding Structures. Leukemia does not cause expansion of bone, although occasionally a single layer of periosteal new bone may be seen in association with this disease; this is uncommon in chronic leukemia. Developing teeth in their crypts and teeth undergoing eruption may be displaced in an occlusal direction (Fig. 24-21) or into the oral cavity before root development. Less commonly, developing teeth may be displaced from their normal position. The result of this is premature loss of teeth. The lamina dura and cortical outlines of follicles may be effaced. If

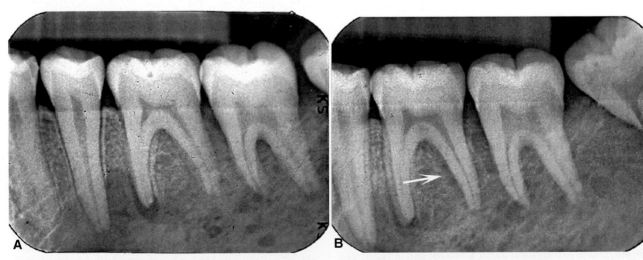

FIGURE 24-20 **A** and **B,** Periapical radiographs of the left mandible demonstrate multifocal areas of bone destruction and widening of portions of the periodontal ligament space *(arrow)* characteristic of infiltration of the mandible with leukemia.

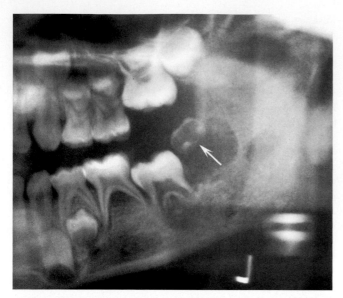

FIGURE 24-21 Cropped panoramic film demonstrates occlusal displacement of the developing mandibular second molar out of its follicle (arrow).

lesions affect the periodontal structures, the crestal bone may be lost.

Differential Diagnosis

Generally, a medical diagnosis has been reached by the time oral radiologic signs of leukemia are present. However, the development of radiologic changes may be the first indication of the relapse of treatment. Occasionally, lymphoma or neuroblastoma may mimic some of the features of destruction seen in leukemia. A metabolic disorder may be considered in cases in which generalized rarefaction of bone is seen. These conditions all are excluded based on blood testing. With apical lesions, careful examination of the involved tooth clinically and radiologically typically shows no apparent cause for rarefying osteitis.

Management

The management of leukemia is primarily through a combination of chemotherapy with or without allogeneic or autologous bone marrow transplantation. Some chronic leukemias are managed with low-dose chemotherapy.

DENTAL RADIOLOGY FOR CANCER SURVIVORS

Patients who have survived cancer require dental treatment just as any other patient. For a cancer survivor, dental radiologic examination may be more important than for a healthy patient receiving a routine examination. Some patients who have received a full course of radiation therapy are concerned about the additional exposure from a dental radiographic examination. However, this is not a valid concern because the small dose associated with dental imaging examinations is negligible compared with the radiation dose received from cancer therapy.

A patient treated for head and neck malignancy with radiation therapy, even with today's advanced radiotherapeutic methods, is prone to develop postradiation dental caries and osteoradionecrosis. Careful clinical examination and a thorough dental radiologic examination may be required periodically to ensure that the remaining dentition and periodontal apparatus is in good shape.

Radiation caries occurs in many patients and appears clinically different from typical dental caries. If untreated, these carious teeth become nonvital and may cause infection in the underlying jaw. If they require extraction, healing can be expected to be slow, and osteoradionecrosis occasionally may result. Also, bisphosphonates are used with some cancer therapy as in multiple myeloma. Changes seen with either radiation therapy or bisphosphonate therapy may mimic odontogenic inflammatory disease and should be differentiated to avoid unnecessary treatment and secondary osteonecrosis (see Chapter 20).

The role of radiology in these patients is not restricted to examination of the teeth and supporting structures. Equally important is monitoring of the outcome of treatment and specifically the examination of dental radiographs for evidence of tumor recurrence, development of metastases, and osteonecrosis.

BIBLIOGRAPHY

Squamous Cell Carcinoma

Brown JS, Lowe D, Kalavrezos N, et al: Patterns of invasion and routes of tumor entry into the mandible by oral squamous cell carcinoma, *Head Neck* 24:370–383, 2002.

Casiglia J, Woo SB: A comprehensive review of oral cancer, *Gen Dent* 49:72–82, 2001.

Carter RL: Patterns and mechanisms of spread of squamous carcinomas of the oral cavity, *Clin Otolaryngol* 15:185–191, 1990.

McGregor AD, MacDonald D: Routes of entry of squamous cell carcinoma to the mandible, *Head Neck Surg* 10:294–301, 1988.

O'Brien CJ, Carter RL, Soo KC, et al: Invasions of the mandible by squamous carcinomas of the oral cavity and oropharynx, *Head Neck Surg* 8:247–256, 1986.

Rao LP, Das SR, Mathews A, et al: Mandibular invasion in oral squamous cell carcinoma: investigation by clinical examination and orthopantomogram, *Int J Oral Maxillofac Surg* 33:454–457, 2004.

Stambuk H, Karimi HE, Lee N, et al: Oral cavity and oropharynx tumors, *Radiol Clin North Am* 45:1–20, 2007.

Squamous Cell Carcinoma Originating in Bone

Ariji E, Ozeki S, Yonetsu K, et al: Central squamous cell carcinoma of the mandible: computed tomographic findings, *Oral Surg Oral Med Oral Pathol* 77:541–548, 1994.

Elzay RP: Primary intra-osseous carcinoma of the jaws, *Oral Surg Oral Med Oral Pathol* 54:299–303, 1982.

Lin YJ, Chen CH, Wang WC, et al: Primary intraosseous carcinoma of the mandible, *Dentomaxillofac Radiol* 34:112–116, 2005.

Suei Y, Tanimoto K, Taguchi A, et al: Primary intra-osseous carcinoma: review of the literature and diagnostic criteria, *J Oral Maxillofac Surg* 52:580–583, 1994.

Squamous Cell Carcinoma Originating in a Cyst

Cavalcanti MGP, Veltrini VC, Ruprecht A, et al: Squamous-cell carcinoma arising from an odontogenic cyst–the importance of computed tomography in the diagnosis of malignancy, *Oral Surg Oral Med Oral Pathol Oral Radiol Endod* 100:365–368, 2005.

Dabbs DJ, Schweitzer RJ, Schweitzer LE, et al: Squamous cell carcinoma arising in recurrent odontogenic keratocyst, *Head Neck* 16:375–378, 1994.

Eversole LR, Sabre WR, Lovin S: Aggressive growth and neoplastic potential of odontogenic cysts, *Cancer* 35:270–282, 1975.

Kaffe I, Ardekian L, Peled M, et al: Radiological features of primary intra-osseous carcinoma of the jaws: analysis of the literature and report of a new case, *Dentomaxillofac Radiol* 27:209–214, 1998.

van der Wal KGH, de Visscher JGAM, Eggink HF: Squamous cell carcinoma arising in a residual cyst, *Int J Oral Maxillofac Surg* 23:350–352, 1993.

Mucoepidermoid Carcinoma

Chan KC, Pharoah M, Lee L, et al: Intraosseous mucoepidermoid carcinoma: a review of diagnostic imaging features of four jaw cases, *Dentomaxillofac Radiol* 42:20110162, 2013.

Inagaki M, Yuasa K, Nakayama E, et al: Mucoepidermoid carcinoma in the mandible, *Oral Surg Oral Med Oral Pathol Oral Radiol Endod* 85:613–618, 1998.

Johnson B, Velez I: Central mucoepidermoid carcinoma with an atypical radiographic appearance, *Oral Surg Oral Med Oral Path Oral Radiol Endod* 1056:e51–e53, 2008.

Raut D, Khedkar S: Primary intraosseous mucoepidermoid carcinoma of the maxilla: a case report and review of the literature, *Dentomaxillofac Radiol* 38:163–168, 2009.

Strick MJ, Kelly C, Soames JV, et al: Malignant tumors of the minor salivary glands—a 20 year review, *Br J Plast Surg* 57:624–631, 2004.

Malignant Ameloblastoma and Ameloblastic Carcinoma

Ameerally P, McGurk M, Shaheen O: Atypical ameloblastoma: report of three cases and review of the literature, *Br J Oral Maxillofac Surg* 34:235–239, 1996.

Buff SJ, Chen JT, Ravin CC, et al: Pulmonary metastasis from ameloblastoma of the mandible: report of a case and review of the literature, *J Oral Surg* 38:374–376, 1980.

Slootweg PJ, Muller H: Malignant ameloblastoma or amelo-blastic carcinoma, *Oral Surg Oral Med Oral Pathol* 57:168–176, 1984.

Suomalainen A, Hietanen J, Robinson S, et al: Ameloblastic carcinoma of the mandible resembling odontogenic cyst in a panoramic radiograph, *Oral Surg Oral Med Oral Pathol Oral Radiol Endod* 101:638–642, 2006.

Metastatic Tumors

Ciola B: Oral radiographic manifestations of a metastatic prostatic carcinoma, *Oral Surg* 52:105–108, 1981.

D'Silva NJ, Summerlin DJ, Cordell KG, et al: Metastatic tumors in the jaws: a retrospective study of 114 cases, *J Am Dent Assoc* 137:1667–1672, 2006.

Hirshberg A, Leibovich P, Buchner A, et al: Metastatic tumors to the jawbones: analysis of 390 cases, *J Oral Pathol Med* 23:337–341, 1994.

Nevins A, Ruden S, Pruden P, et al: Metastatic carcinoma of the mandible mimicking periapical lesion of endodontic origin, *Endod Dent Traumatol* 4:238–239, 1988.

Van der Waal RI, Buter J, Van der Waal I, et al: Oral metastases: report of 24 cases, *Br J Oral Maxillofac Surg* 41:3–6, 2003.

Osteogenic Sarcoma

Bainchi SD, Boccardi A: Radiological aspects of osteosarcoma of the jaws, *Dentomaxillofac Radiol* 28:42–47, 1999.

Chindia ML: Osteosarcoma of the jaw bones, *Oral Oncol* 37:545–547, 2001.

Clark JL, Unni KK, Dahlin DC, et al: Osteosarcoma of the jaw, *Cancer* 51:2311–2316, 1983.

Gardner DG, Mills DM: The widened periodontal ligament of osteosarcoma of the jaws, *Oral Surg* 41:652–656, 1976.

Givol N, Buchner A, Taicher S, et al: Radiological features of osteogenic sarcoma of the jaws: a comparative study of different radiographic modalities, *Dentomaxillofac Radiol* 27:313–320, 1998.

Seeger LL, Gold RH, Chandnani VP: Diagnostic imaging of osteosarcoma, *Clin Orthop Relat Res* 270:254–263, 1991.

Chondrosarcoma

Garrington GE, Collett WK: Chondrosarcoma. I. A selected literature review, *J Oral Pathol* 17:1–11, 1988.

Garrington GE, Collett WK: Chondrosarcoma. II. Chondrosarcoma of the jaws: analysis of 37 cases, *J Oral Pathol* 17:12–20, 1988.

Gorsky M, Epstein JB: Craniofacial osseous and chondromatous sarcomas in British Columbia—a review of 34 cases, *Oral Oncol* 36:27–31, 2000.

Hayt MW, Becker L, Katz DS: Chondrosarcoma of the maxilla: panoramic radiographic and computed tomographic with multiplanar reconstruction findings, *Dentomaxillofac Radiol* 27:113–116, 1998.

Hertzanu Y, Mendelsohn DB, Davidge-Pitts K, et al: Chondrosarcoma of the head and neck—the value of computed tomography, *J Surg Oncol* 28:97–102, 1985.

Vener J, Rice D, Newman AN: Osteosarcoma and chondrosarcoma of the head and neck, *Laryngoscope* 94:240–242, 1984.

Ewing's Sarcoma

Karimi A, Shirinbak I, Beshkar M, et al: Ewing sarcoma of the jaws, *J Craniofac Surg* 22:1657–1660, 2011.

Wood RE, Nortje CJ, Hesseling P, et al: Ewing's sarcoma, *Oral Surg Oral Med Oral Pathol* 69:120–127, 1990.

Iwamoto Y: Diagnosis and treatment of Ewing's sarcoma, *Jpn J Clin Oncol* 37:79–89, 2007.

Fibrosarcoma

Slootweg PJ, Müller H: Fibrosarcoma of the jaws: a study of 7 cases, *J Maxillofac Surg* 12:157–162, 1984.

Taconis WK, van Rijssel TG: Fibrosarcoma of the jaws, *Skeletal Radiol* 15:10–13, 1986.

van Blarcom CW, Masson JMK, Dahlin DC: Fibrosarcoma of the mandible, *Oral Surg* 32:428–439, 1971.

Multiple Myeloma

Furutani M, Ohnishi M, Tanaka Y: Mandibular involvement in patients with multiple myeloma, *J Oral Maxillofac Surg* 52:23–25, 1994.

Huvos AG: *Bone tumors*, Philadelphia, 1979, Saunders.

Kaffe I, Ramon Y, Hertz M: Radiographic manifestations of multiple myeloma in the mandible, *Dentomaxillofac Radiol* 15:31–35, 1986.

Witt C: Radiographic manifestations of multiple myeloma in the mandible: a retrospective study of 77 patients, *J Oral Maxillofac Surg* 55:450–453, 1997.

Non-Hodgkin's Lymphoma

Maxymiw WG, Goldstein M, Wood RE: Extranodal non-Hodgkin's lymphoma of the maxillofacial region: analysis of 88 consecutive cases, *SADJ* 56:524–527, 2001.

Pazoki A, Jansisyanont P, Ord RA: Primary non-Hodgkin's lymphoma of the jaws: report of four cases and review of the literature, *J Oral Maxillofac Surg* 61:112–117, 2003.

Yamada T, Kitagawa Y, Ogasawara T, et al: Enlargement of the mandibular canal without hypesthesia caused by extranodal non-Hodgkin's lymphoma, *Oral Surg Oral Med Oral Pathol Oral Radiol Endod* 89:388–392, 2000.

Burkitt's Lymphoma

Adatia AK: Significance of jaw lesions in Burkitt's lymphoma, *Br Dent J* 145:263–266, 1978.

Burkitt DA: Sarcoma involving the jaws in African children, *Br J Surg* 46:218–223, 1958.

Jan A, Vora K, Sandor GKB: Sporadic Burkitt's lymphoma of the jaws: the essentials of prompt life-saving referral and management, *J Can Dent Assoc* 71:165–168, 2005.

Levine PH, Kamaraju LS, Connelly RR, et al: The American Burkitt's lymphoma registry: eight years' experience, *Cancer* 49:1016–1022, 1982.

Sariban E, Donahue A, Magrath IT: Jaw involvement in American Burkitt's lymphoma, *Cancer* 53:1777–1782, 1984.

Leukemia

Curtis AB: Childhood leukemias: initial oral manifestations, *J Am Dent Assoc* 83:159–164, 1971.

Greer RO, Mierau GW, Favara BE: *Tumors of the head and neck in children*, New York, 1983, Praeger Scientific.

Morgan L: Infiltrate of chronic lymphocytic leukemia appearing as a periapical radiolucent lesion, *J Endod* 21:475–478, 1995.

Sugihara Y, Wakasa T, Kameyama T, et al: Pediatric acute lymphocytic leukemia with osseous changes in jaws: literature review and report of a case, *Oral Radiol* 5:25–31, 1989.

25 Systemic Diseases

Fatima Jadu

DISEASE MECHANISM

This chapter addresses diseases that alter the normal form and function of bone and normal formation of teeth. These diseases produce abnormalities through a disturbance in the balanced serum concentrations of calcium and phosphate and/or through abnormal functioning osteoblasts, osteocytes, and osteoclasts (Fig. 25-1). These factors are essential for the normal development of the initial skeleton and for the continued bone remodeling that occurs thereafter—approximately 5% to 10% of total bone volume in an adult skeleton is replaced per year. For instance, a disease that causes a decrease in serum calcium alters the calcium and phosphate balanced levels, resulting in abnormal bone and tooth formation. A low serum calcium concentration can also result in the mobilization of calcium from bone, depleting the calcium content of bone. The reduced calcium level in bone results in bone with low density in the diagnostic image. Bone remodeling is also altered by the mobilization of calcium from bone resulting in an abnormal trabecular pattern in the diagnostic image. Dental anomalies such as enamel or dentin hypoplasia or hypocalcification are other possible consequences of a reduced serum calcium level. Other diseases can affect changes to bone and teeth through altered serum levels of phosphate or through abnormal numbers and function of osteoblasts, osteocytes, and osteoclasts.

DIAGNOSTIC IMAGING FEATURES

Because systemic disorders affect the entire body, the changes manifested in the appearance of the jaws in diagnostic images are usually generalized and often nonspecific, making it difficult to identify the diseases based on imaging characteristics alone (Table 25-1). The general changes that can be seen in the jaws include the following:

1. Change in size and shape of the bone
2. Change in the number, size, and orientation of trabeculae
3. Altered thickness and density of cortical structures
4. Increase or decrease in overall bone density

Changes in the first three elements can result in a decrease or increase in bone density.

Because many parameters in the production of a diagnostic image influence the density of the image, it may be difficult to detect genuine changes in the density of bone. Systemic conditions that result in a decrease in bone density do not affect mature teeth; the image of the teeth may stand out with normal density against a generally radiolucent jaw. In severe cases, the teeth may appear to lack any bony support. Also, cortical structures appear thin, are less defined, and occasionally disappear. A true increase in bone density may be detected by a loss of contrast of the inferior cortex of the mandible as the radiopacity of the cancellous bone approaches that of cortical bone. Often the radiolucent outline of the inferior alveolar nerve canal appears more distinct in contrast to the surrounding radiopaque dense bone.

Some systemic diseases that occur during tooth formation may result in dental alterations. Lamina dura is part of the bone structure of the alveolar process, but because it is usually examined in conjunction with the periodontal membrane space and roots of teeth, it is included with the description of the dental structures (Table 25-2). Changes to teeth and associated structures include the following:

1. Accelerated or delayed eruption
2. Hypoplasia
3. Hypocalcification
4. Loss of a distinct lamina dura

The teeth and their supporting structures often exhibit no detectable changes associated with systemic diseases. However, the first symptoms of a disease occasionally may manifest as a dental problem.

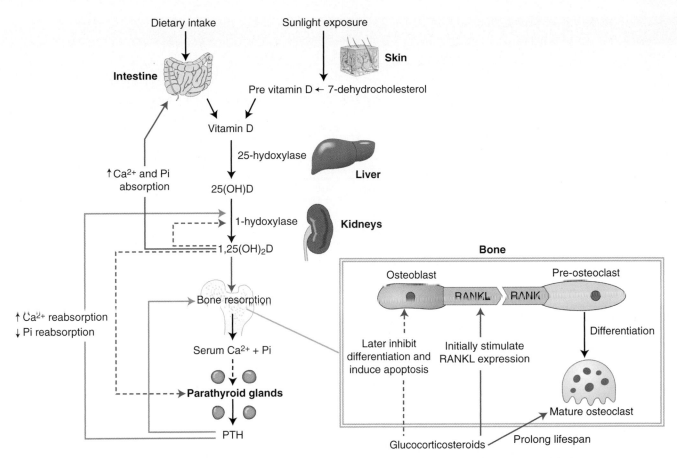

FIGURE 25-1 This figure shows the activity of vitamin D, parathyroid hormone (PTH), and glucocorticosteroids in bone and other tissues and outlines their roles in maintaining normal serum levels of calcium (Ca^{2+}) and phosphate (Pi) and bone metabolism. Bone metabolism entails the balanced process of osteoblastic bone formation and osteoclastic bone resorption. *Solid arrows* indicate a promotion effect, and *dashed arrows* indicate an inhibitory effect. Vitamin D, either ingested or produced in the skin, undergoes a series of hydroxylations, first in the liver and then in the kidneys, to the active form of $1,25(OH)_2D$ *(black arrows)*. $1,25(OH)_2D$ can increase serum Ca^{2+} and Pi by promoting their absorption in the intestine and tipping the balance of bone metabolism in favor of resorption, releasing Ca^{2+} and Pi from the bone to the serum *(solid blue arrows)*. This promotion of bone resorption is accomplished through the expression of receptor activator of nuclear factor kappa B ligand (RANKL) by osteoblasts, which interacts with a receptor activator of nuclear factor-kappa B (RANK) receptor on preosteoclasts differentiating these cells into active osteoclasts that resorb the bone *(lower right inset box)*. $1,25(OH)_2D$ can also inhibit the last hydroxylation of its precursor $25(OH)D$ within the kidneys and can inhibit the parathyroid glands from producing PTH *(dashed blue arrows)*. PTH can increase serum Ca^{2+} by directly increasing bone resorption through promoting the expression of RANKL and the differentiation of osteoclasts. PTH also increases serum Ca^{2+} by increasing reabsorption of Ca^{2+} in the kidneys and promoting the hydroxylation of vitamin D to its active form in the kidneys *(orange arrows)*. However, elevated serum Ca^{2+} can reduce production of PTH by the parathyroid glands *(dashed black arrow)*. Glucocorticosteroids initially increase bone resorption through increased osteoblastic expression of RANKL, increasing osteoclast differentiation, and can prolong the life span of the osteoclast. Later, glucocorticosteroids reduce bone formation by limiting differentiation and inducing apoptosis of osteoblasts.

ENDOCRINE DISORDERS

HYPERPARATHYROIDISM

Disease Mechanism

Hyperparathyroidism is an endocrine abnormality in which there is an excess of circulating parathyroid hormone (PTH). An excess of serum PTH increases bone remodeling but tips the balance of osteoblastic and osteoclastic activity in favor of osteoclastic resorption, which mobilizes calcium from the skeleton. This activity can alter the normal morphology of bone trabeculae into irregularly shaped, small trabeculae, which can result in a granular bone pattern in the diagnostic images. In addition, PTH increases renal tubular reabsorption of calcium and renal production of the active

vitamin D metabolite $1,25(OH)_2D$. The net result of these functions is an increase in serum calcium levels (see Fig. 25-1).

Primary hyperparathyroidism usually results from a benign tumor (adenoma) of one of the four parathyroid glands (80% to 85%), resulting in the production of excess PTH. The condition is often sporadic, but it may be part of a hereditary syndrome, such as hyperparathyroidism–jaw tumor syndrome, which involves tumors of parathyroid glands, jaws, and kidneys. Less frequently, individuals may have hyperplastic parathyroid glands that secrete excess PTH (10% to 15%). The incidence of primary hyperparathyroidism is about 0.1%.

Secondary hyperparathyroidism results from a compensatory increase in the output of PTH in response to hypocalcemia. The underlying hypocalcemia may result from inadequate dietary

TABLE 25-1 Changes in Bone Observed in Systemic Disease*

| Systemic Disease | Density | Size of Jaws | BONES | TRABECULAE | |
			Increase	Decrease	Granular
Hyperparathyroidism	Decrease	No	Yes	Yes	Yes
Hypoparathyroidism	Rare increase	No	No	No	No
Hyperpituitarism	No	Large	No	No	No
Hypopituitarism	No	Small	No	No	No
Hyperthyroidism	Decrease	No	No	No	No
Hypothyroidism	No	Small	No	No	No
Cushing's syndrome	Decrease	No	No	Yes	Yes
Osteoporosis	Decrease	No	No	Yes	No
Rickets	Decrease	No	No	Yes	No
Osteomalacia	Rare decrease	No	No	Rare decrease	No
Hypophosphatasia	Decrease	No	No	Yes	No
Renal osteodystrophy	Decrease; rare increase	Large	Rare	Yes	Yes
Hypophosphatemia	Decrease	No	No	Yes	Yes
Osteopetrosis	Increase	Large			
Sickle cell anemia	Decrease	Large maxilla			
Thalassemia	Decrease	Large maxilla			

*This table summarizes the major imaging changes to bone with endocrine and metabolic bone diseases. It does not include all the possible variable appearances.

TABLE 25-2 Effects on Teeth and Associated Structures*

Systemic Disease	Hypocalcification	Hypoplasia	Large Pulp Chamber	Loss of Lamina Dura	Loss of Teeth	Eruption
Hyperparathyroidism	No	No	No	Yes	Rare	No
Hypoparathyroidism	No	Yes	No	No	No	Delayed
Hyperpituitarism	No	No	No	No	No	Supereruption
Hypopituitarism	No	No	No	No	No	Delayed
Hypothyroidism	No	No	No	No	Yes	Early
Hyperthyroidism	No	No	No	Thin	Yes	Delayed
Cushing's syndrome	No	No	No	Partial	No	Premature
Osteoporosis	No	No	No	Thin	No	No
Rickets	Yes, enamel	Yes, enamel	No	Thin	No	Delayed
Osteomalacia	No	No	No	Thin	No	No
Hypophosphatasia	Yes	Yes	Yes	Yes	Yes	Delayed
Renal osteodystrophy	Yes	Yes	No	Yes	No	No
Hypophosphatemia	Yes	Yes	Yes	Yes	Yes	No
Osteopetrosis	Yes	Rare	No	Thick	Yes	Delayed

*This table summarizes the major imaging changes that can occur to teeth and associated structures with endocrine and metabolic bone diseases. It does not include all the possible variable appearances.

intake or poor intestinal absorption of vitamin D or from deficient metabolism of vitamin D in the liver or kidneys. This condition produces clinical and imaging features similar to primary hyperparathyroidism.

Clinical Features

Primary hyperparathyroidism affects females two to three times more commonly than males. The condition occurs mainly in adults 30 to 60 years old. Clinical manifestations of the disease cover a broad range, but most patients have renal calculi, peptic ulcers, cognitive impairment, or bone and joint pain. These clinical symptoms are mainly related to hypercalcemia. Gradual loosening, drifting, and loss of teeth may occur. The combination of hypercalcemia and an elevated serum level of PTH is diagnostic of primary hyperparathyroidism. Because of daily fluctuations, the serum calcium level should be tested at different intervals. The serum alkaline phosphatase level, a reliable indicator of bone turnover, may also be elevated in hyperparathyroidism.

Imaging Features

Only about one in five patients with hyperparathyroidism has observable bone changes.

General Features.
The major manifestations of hyperparathyroidism are as follows:
1. The earliest and most reliable changes of hyperparathyroidism are subtle erosions of bone from the subperiosteal surfaces of the phalanges of the hands.
2. Demineralization of the skeleton results in an unusual radiolucent appearance (generalized osteopenia).
3. Osteitis fibrosa cystica is seen in advanced cases as localized regions of bone loss produced by osteoclastic activity resulting in a loss of all apparent bone structure.

4. In about 10% of cases, brown tumors occur late in the disease. These lesions are called brown tumors because the gross specimen has a brown or reddish brown color. In diagnostic images, these tumors appear radiolucent.
5. The increased levels of serum calcium result in precipitation of the mineral in the soft tissues forming punctate or nodular calcifications in the joints and kidneys.
6. In prominent hyperparathyroidism, the entire calvaria has a granular appearance classically known as the "salt and pepper" skull. This appearance is caused by loss of the central (diploic) trabeculae and thinning of the cortical tables (Fig. 25-2).

Jaws.
Demineralization and thinning of cortical boundaries often occur in the jaws, including the inferior border of the mandible, the cortical boundaries of the mandibular canal, and the cortical outlines of the maxillary sinuses. The density of the jaws is decreased, resulting in a radiolucent appearance that contrasts with the normal density of the teeth (Fig. 25-3). The elevated rate of bone remodeling can cause an abnormal bone pattern secondary to replacement of normal trabeculae by numerous, small, randomly oriented trabeculae, resulting in a ground-glass appearance in the diagnostic image.

Brown tumors of hyperparathyroidism may appear in any bone but are frequently found in the facial bones and jaws, particularly in cases of long-standing disease. These lesions may be multiple within a single bone. They have variably defined margins and may produce cortical expansion. If solitary, the tumor may resemble a central giant cell granuloma or an aneurysmal bone cyst (Fig. 25-4). The histologic appearance of a brown tumor is identical to giant cell granuloma. If a giant cell granuloma occurs later than the second decade, the patient should be screened for an increase in serum calcium, PTH, and alkaline phosphatase levels.

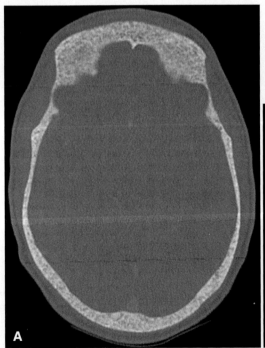
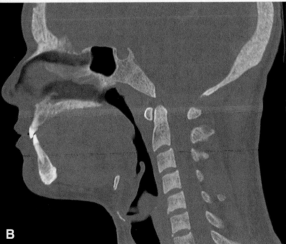

FIGURE 25-2 Axial **(A)** and sagittal **(B)** MDCT images with bone algorithm of a case of secondary hyperparathyroidism. Note the lack of normal cortical bone at the inner and outer tables of the skull, internal granular bone pattern, and generalized lack of defined outer cortical boundary of the osseous structures.

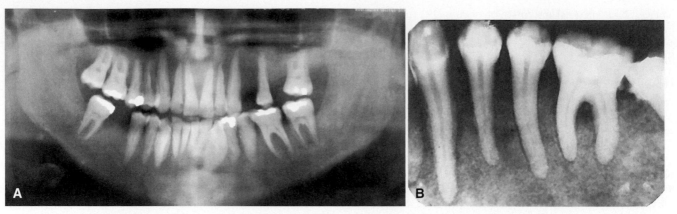

FIGURE 25-3 **A,** Panoramic image. The loss of bone in hyperparathyroidism results in the radiopaque teeth standing out in contrast to the radiolucent jaws. **B,** Periapical film of a different case demonstrates the loss of a distinct lamina dura and the granular texture of the bone pattern. (**B,** Courtesy H. G. Poyton, DDS, Toronto, Ontario, Canada.)

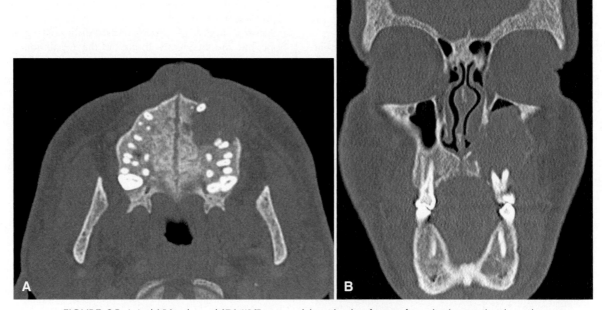

FIGURE 25-4 Axial (**A**) and coronal (**B**) MDCT images with bone algorithm of a case of secondary hyperparathyroidism with a brown tumor involving the maxilla. This tumor has features of a central giant cell granuloma with a granular expanded cortex of the maxilla and very subtle and ill-defined internal septa.

Teeth and Associated Structures. Occasionally, periapical images reveal loss of the lamina dura in patients (about 10%) with hyperparathyroidism. Depending on the duration and severity of the disease, loss of the lamina dura may occur around one tooth or all the remaining teeth (Fig. 25-5). The loss may be either complete or partial around a particular tooth. The result of lamina dura loss may give the root a tapered appearance because of loss of image contrast. Although PTH mobilizes minerals from the skeleton, mature teeth are immune to this systemic demineralizing process.

Management

After successful surgical removal of the causative parathyroid adenoma, almost all changes revert to normal. The only exception may be the site of a brown tumor, which often heals with bone that is more sclerotic than normal. Many people with this disease are being diagnosed earlier, resulting in fewer severe cases.

HYPOPARATHYROIDISM AND PSEUDOHYPOPARATHYROIDISM

Disease Mechanism

Hypoparathyroidism is an uncommon condition in which insufficient secretion of PTH occurs. Several causes exist, but the most common is damage or removal of the parathyroid glands during thyroid surgery. In pseudohypoparathyroidism, there is a defect in the response of the target tissue cells to normal levels of PTH. In both cases, the result is low serum levels of calcium.

Clinical Features

There are a variety of clinical manifestations. Most often, manifestations include sharp flexion (tetany) of the wrist and ankle joints (carpopedal spasm). Some patients have sensory abnormalities

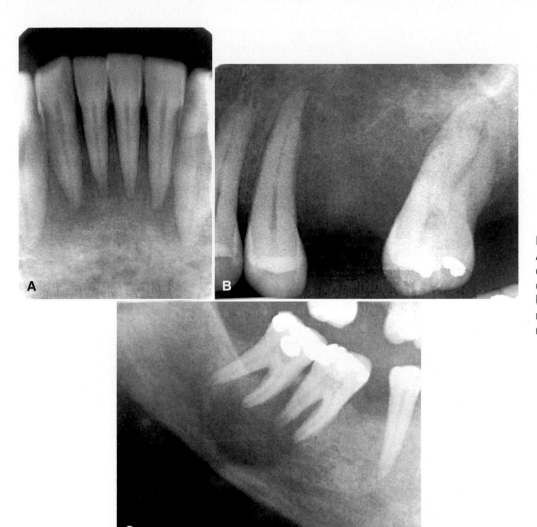

FIGURE   25-5 Hyperparathyroidism. **A** and **B,** Granular bone pattern that was characteristic in all intraoral films. Note the loss of a distinct lamina dura and floor of the maxillary antrum. **C,** This view of the same case reveals a brown tumor related to the apical region of the second and third molars.

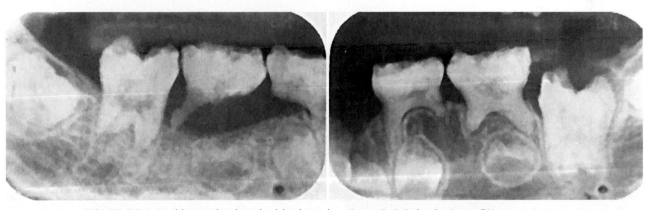

FIGURE 25-6 Pseudohypoparathyroidism-induced dental anomalies. *(Courtesy Dr. S. Bricker, San Antonio, TX.)*

consisting of paresthesia of the hands, feet, or the area around the mouth. Neurologic changes may include anxiety and depression, epilepsy, parkinsonism, and chorea. Chronic forms may produce a reduction in intellectual capacity. Some patients show no changes. Patients with pseudohypoparathyroidism often have early closure of certain bony epiphyses and manifest short stature or extremity disproportions.

Imaging Features

The principal change is calcification of the basal ganglia. On skull images, this calcification appears flocculent and paired within the cerebral hemispheres on the posteroanterior view. Imaging of the jaws may reveal dental enamel hypoplasia, external root resorption, delayed eruption, or root dilaceration (Fig. 25-6).

Management

These conditions are managed with orally administered supplemental calcium and vitamin D.

HYPERPITUITARISM

Synonyms

Synonyms for hyperpituitarism include acromegaly and gigantism.

Disease Mechanism

Hyperpituitarism results from hyperfunction of the anterior lobe of the pituitary gland, which increases the production of growth hormone. An excess of growth hormone causes overgrowth of all tissues in the body still capable of growth. The usual cause of this problem is a benign functioning tumor of the somatotrophs (growth hormone–secreting cells) in the anterior lobe of the pituitary gland.

Clinical Features

Hyperpituitarism in children involves generalized overgrowth of most hard and soft tissues, a condition termed gigantism. Active growth occurs in bones in which the epiphyses have not united with the bone shafts. Throughout adolescence, generalized skeletal growth is excessive and may be prolonged. Affected individuals ultimately may attain heights of 7 to 8 feet or more, but they exhibit remarkably normal proportions. The eyes and other parts of the central nervous system do not enlarge except in rare cases in which the condition manifests in infancy.

Adult hyperpituitarism, called acromegaly, has an insidious clinical course, quite different from the clinical profile seen in the childhood disease. In adults, the clinical effects of a pituitary adenoma develop quite slowly because many types of tissues have lost the capacity for growth. This is true of much of the skeleton; however, an excess of growth hormone can stimulate the mandible and the phalanges of the hand. Mandibular condylar growth may be very prominent. Also, the supraorbital ridges and the underlying frontal sinus may be enlarged. Excess growth hormone in adults may also produce hypertrophy of some soft tissues. The lips, tongue, nose, and soft tissues of the hands and feet typically overgrow in adults with acromegaly, sometimes to a striking degree.

Imaging Features

General Features. The pituitary tumor responsible for hyperpituitarism often produces enlargement ("ballooning") of the sella turcica (see Fig. 25-7, *B*). In some examples, the sella may not expand at all. Skull images characteristically reveal enlargement of the paranasal sinuses (especially the frontal sinus). These air sinuses are more prominent in acromegaly than in pituitary gigantism because sinus growth in gigantism tends to be more in step with the generalized enlargement of the facial bones. Hyperpituitarism in adults also produces diffuse thickening of the outer table of the skull.

Jaws. Hyperpituitarism causes enlargement of the jaws, most notably the mandible (Fig. 25-7, *A*). The increase in the length of the dental arches results in spacing of the teeth. In acromegaly, the angle between the ramus and body of the mandible may increase. This increase, in combination with the flaring of the anterior teeth caused by enlargement of the tongue (macroglossia), may result in development of an anterior open bite. The sign of incisor flaring is a helpful point of differentiation between acromegalic prognathism and inherited prognathism. In acromegaly, the most profound growth occurs in the condyle and ramus, often resulting in a class III skeletal relationship between the jaws. The thickness and height of the alveolar processes may also increase.

Teeth and Associated Structures. The tooth crowns are usually normal in size, although the roots of posterior teeth often enlarge as a result of hypercementosis. This hypercementosis may be the result of functional and structural demands on teeth instead of a secondary hormonal effect. Supereruption of the posterior teeth may occur in an attempt to compensate for the growth of the mandible.

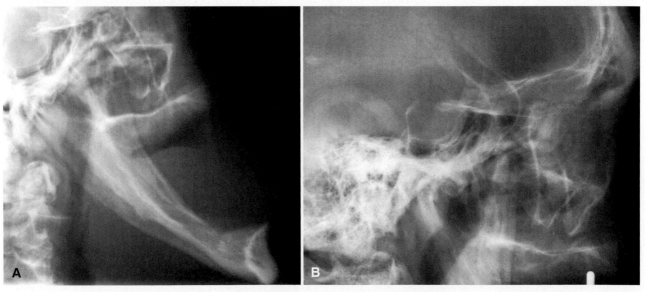

FIGURE 25-7 **A,** Example of acromegaly manifesting as excessive growth of the mandible, resulting in a class III skeletal relationship of the jaws. **B,** Portion of a lateral skull view of the same patient demonstrates enlargement of the sella turcica.

Management

Surgical removal of the pituitary gland is the first line of treatment. If surgery fails or is not possible, medications are given to reduce growth hormone levels. Radiation therapy may also be considered, but this usually takes several years to show an effect.

HYPOPITUITARISM

Definition

Hypopituitarism results from reduced secretion of pituitary hormones, the most common of which is growth hormone deficiency.

Clinical Features

Individuals with this condition exhibit dwarfism but have relatively well-proportioned bodies. One study reported a marked failure of development of the maxilla and the mandible. The dimensions of these bones in adults with this disorder were approximately the same as normal children 5 to 7 years old.

Imaging Features

Eruption of the primary dentition occurs at the normal time, but exfoliation is delayed by several years. The crowns of the permanent teeth form normally, but their eruption is delayed several years. The third molar buds may be completely absent. In hypopituitarism, the jaws, especially the mandible, are small, which results in crowding and malocclusion.

Management

Treatment is usually directed toward removal of the cause or replacement of the pituitary hormones or hormones of its target gland. The response of the dentition to treatment with growth hormone is variable but seems to parallel the skeletal response.

HYPERTHYROIDISM

Synonym

A synonym for hyperthyroidism is thyrotoxicosis.

Disease Mechanism

Hyperthyroidism is a syndrome that involves excessive production of thyroxine in the thyroid gland. The most common forms of hyperthyroidism are diffuse toxic goiter (Graves' disease); toxic nodular goiter (Plummer's disease); and toxic adenoma, a benign tumor of the thyroid gland. Each of these conditions results in increased levels of circulating thyroxine.

Clinical Features

Excessive thyroxine causes a generalized increase in the metabolic rate of all body tissues, resulting in tachycardia, increased blood pressure, sensitivity to heat, and irritability. Hyperthyroidism is more common in females.

Imaging Features

Hyperthyroidism results in an advanced rate of dental development and early eruption, with premature loss of the primary teeth. It also results in an increased rate of bone turnover that is imbalanced in favor of excessive bone resorption. This resorption is manifested in adults as a generalized decrease in bone density or loss of some areas of edentulous alveolar bone.

Management

Radioactive iodine is the most common treatment for hyperthyroidism followed by antithyroid medications and surgical removal of the thyroid gland.

HYPOTHYROIDISM

Synonyms

Synonyms for hypothyroidism are myxedema and cretinism.

Definition

Hypothyroidism usually results from insufficient secretion of thyroxine by the thyroid glands despite the presence of thyroid-stimulating hormone.

Clinical Features

In children, hypothyroidism may result in retarded mental and physical development. The base of the skull shows delayed ossification, and the paranasal sinuses show only partial pneumatization. Dental development is delayed, and the primary teeth are slow to exfoliate.

Hypothyroidism in an adult results in myxedematous swelling but not the dental or skeletal changes seen in children. Adult symptoms may range from lethargy, poor memory, inability to concentrate, constipation, and cold intolerance to the more florid clinical picture of dull and expressionless face, periorbital edema, large tongue, sparse hair, and skin that feels "doughy" to the touch.

Imaging Features

Features in children include delayed closing of the epiphyses and skull sutures with the production of numerous wormian bones (accessory bones in the sutures). Effects on the teeth include delayed eruption, short roots, and thinning of the lamina dura. The maxilla and mandible are relatively small. Patients with adult hypothyroidism may show periodontal disease, loss of teeth, separation of teeth as a result of enlargement of the tongue, and external root resorption.

Management

Patients with hypothyroidism are managed with hormone replacement and careful monitoring to prevent development of iatrogenic hyperthyroidism.

DIABETES MELLITUS

Disease Mechanism

Diabetes mellitus is a metabolic disorder that has two primary forms. Type 1, insulin-dependent diabetes mellitus (previously known as juvenile-onset diabetes), results from an absence or insufficiency of insulin, a hormone normally produced by the β cells of the islets of Langerhans in the pancreas. Type 2, non–insulin-dependent diabetes mellitus, results from insulin resistance. Patients with type 1 diabetes have virtually no β cells (in the islets), whereas patients with type 2 diabetes have approximately half the normal number. A shortage of insulin adversely affects carbohydrate metabolism. The principal clinical laboratory signs of the disease are hyperglycemia and glycosuria, both reflecting a complex biochemical imbalance between tissue demand for glucose and the release of this nutrient by the liver.

Clinical Features

Patients with untreated diabetes may present with classic symptoms and signs, such as polydipsia (excessive intake of fluids), polyuria (excessive urination), and, in more severe cases, acetone present in the urine and on the breath. This metabolic disorder, if not adequately treated, lowers the resistance of the body to infection. Diabetes may demonstrate numerous adverse effects in the oral cavity. Most prominently, uncontrolled diabetes acts as a continuing factor that predisposes to, aggravates, and accelerates periodontal disease. Patients with controlled diabetes do not appear to have more periodontal problems than persons without diabetes. Another occasional oral complication of diabetes mellitus is xerostomia resulting from a reduced salivary flow (about one third of normal). More recently, diabetes has been documented as a risk factor in the development of bisphosphonate-related osteonecrosis.

Imaging Features

Diabetes mellitus exhibits no characteristic imaging features of the jaws or teeth. Periodontal disease associated with diabetes is indistinguishable from periodontal disease in patients without diabetes.

Management

Type 1 diabetes is managed with lifelong insulin therapy. Type 2 diabetes is managed with dietary modifications, exercise, medications, and self-monitoring of blood glucose levels.

CUSHING'S SYNDROME

Disease Mechanism

Cushing's syndrome arises from prolonged exposure to elevated levels of either exogenous or endogenous glucocorticoids. Endogenous glucocorticoids are secreted by the adrenal glands and may be secreted in excess as a result of any of the following:

1. An adrenal adenoma
2. An adrenal carcinoma
3. Adrenal hyperplasia (usually bilateral)
4. A basophilic adenoma of the anterior lobe of the pituitary gland (Cushing's disease), producing excess adrenocorticotropic hormone

The increased level of glucocorticoid results in a loss of bone mass from reduced osteoblastic function and either directly or indirectly increased osteoclastic function (see Fig. 25-1).

Clinical Features

Patients with Cushing's syndrome often exhibit obesity that spares the extremities and is more pronounced in the face ("moon face") and upper back ("buffalo hump"). These patients also demonstrate violaceous striae and muscle weakness and may have hypertension and concurrent diabetes. This condition affects females three to five times as frequently as males. Onset may occur at any age but is usually seen in the third or fourth decade.

Imaging Features

The primary feature of Cushing's syndrome is generalized osteoporosis secondary to reduced osteoblastic and increased osteoclastic activity. This skeletal demineralization may result in pathologic fractures. The skeleton may also exhibit a granular pattern as a result of the abnormal formation of numerous, short, and randomly oriented bone trabeculae. The altered osteoblastic and osteoclastic activity also results in thinning of the skull, which may be accompanied by a mottled appearance. The teeth may erupt prematurely, and partial loss of the lamina dura may occur (Fig. 25-8).

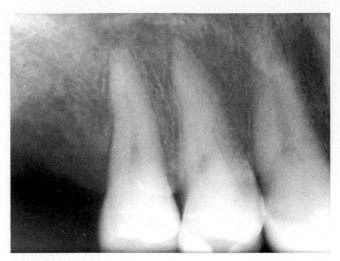

FIGURE 25-8 Cushing's syndrome manifested in the jaws as thinning of the lamina dura. (Courtesy H. G. Poyton, DDS, Toronto, Ontario, Canada.)

METABOLIC BONE DISEASES

OSTEOPOROSIS

Disease Mechanism

Osteoporosis is a generalized decrease in bone mass in which the histologic appearance of bone is normal. An imbalance occurs in the coupled bone resorption and formation process resulting in a decrease in bone formation and leading to changes in the volume of trabecular bone, trabecular architecture, and size and thickness of individual trabeculae.

Osteoporosis occurs with the aging process of bone and can be considered a variation of normal (primary osteoporosis). Bone mass normally increases from infancy to about 30 years of age. At this time, a gradual and progressive decline begins, occurring at a rate of about 8% per decade in females and 3% per decade in males. The loss of bone mass with age is so gradual that it is virtually imperceptible until it reaches significant proportions. Secondary osteoporosis may result from nutritional deficiencies, hormonal imbalance, inactivity, or corticosteroid or heparin therapy.

Clinical Features

The most important clinical manifestation of osteoporosis is fracture. The most common locations are the distal radius, proximal femur, ribs, and vertebrae. Patients may have bone pain. Postmenopausal women are most at risk.

Imaging Features

Osteoporosis results in an overall reduction in the density of bone. This reduction may be observed in the jaws by using the unaltered density of teeth as a comparison. There may be evidence of a reduced density and thinning of cortical boundaries, such as the inferior mandibular cortex (Fig. 25-9). Reduction in the volume of cancellous bone is more difficult to assess, although new techniques to analyze the trabecular pattern in intraoral films are being developed. Reduction in the number of trabeculae is least evident in the alveolar process, possibly because of the constant stress applied to this region of bone by the teeth. Occasionally, the lamina dura may appear thinner than normal. In other regions of the mandible, a reduction in the number of trabeculae may be evident. Accurate assessment of bone mineral density is difficult

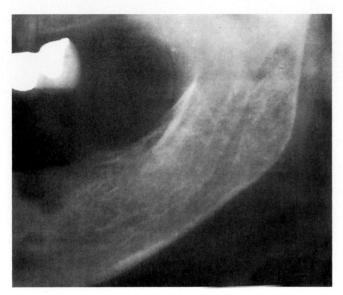

FIGURE 25-9 Osteoporosis evident as a loss of the normal thickness and density of the inferior cortex of the mandible.

but may be done with sophisticated techniques such as dual-energy photon absorption or quantitative computed tomographic (MDCT) protocols. Attempts have been made to use the commonly acquired periapical and panoramic radiographs to determine the risk of osteoporosis. Combined with clinical risk factors, it was found that a reduced width of the inferior cortex of the mandible may assist in identifying individuals with low bone mineral density.

Management

The administration of estrogens and calcium and vitamin D supplements after menopause helps to reduce the rate of cortical and trabecular bone loss. More recently, oral bisphosphonate medications have also been used to slow down bone loss. Weight-bearing exercise programs are an effective adjunct to the above-mentioned medications.

RICKETS AND OSTEOMALACIA

Synonym

A synonym for rickets and osteomalacia is calcipenic rickets.

Disease Mechanism

Rickets and osteomalacia result from inadequate serum and extracellular levels of calcium and phosphate, minerals required for the normal calcification of bone and teeth; this is seen as inadequately calcified osteoid in forming bone and hypocalcification of enamel and dentin in forming teeth. Both abnormalities result from a defect in the normal activity of the metabolites of vitamin D, especially $1,25(OH)_2D$, required for absorption of calcium in the intestine. The term rickets is usually applied when the disease affects the growing skeleton in infants and children. The term osteomalacia is used when this disease affects the mature skeleton in adults.

Failure of normal activity of vitamin D may occur as a result of:
1. Lack of vitamin D in the diet.
2. Lack of absorption of vitamin D resulting from various gastrointestinal malabsorption problems.
3. Lack of formation of the active metabolite $1,25(OH)_2D$, which is required for intestinal absorption of calcium. Interference in

the production of $1,25(OH)_2D$ may occur anywhere along its metabolic pathway (see Fig. 25-1).
4. Lack of exposure to ultraviolet light required for conversion of 7-dehydrocholesterol to provitamin D and then to active vitamin D.
5. Lack of conversion of vitamin D to $25(OH)D$ in the liver because of liver disease.
6. Lack of metabolism of $25(OH)D$ to $1,25(OH)_2D$ by the kidney because of kidney disease.
7. A defect in the intestinal target cell response to $1,25(OH)_2D$ or inadequate calcium supply.

Clinical Features

Rickets. In the first 6 months of life, tetany or convulsions are the most common clinical problems resulting from the hypocalcemia of rickets. Later in infancy, the skeletal effects of the disease may be more clinically prominent. Craniotabes, a softening of the posterior of the parietal bones, may be the initial sign of the disease. The wrists and ankles typically swell. Children with rickets usually have short stature and deformity of the extremities. Development of the dentition is delayed, and the eruption rate of the teeth is retarded.

Osteomalacia. Most patients with osteomalacia have some degree of bone pain and muscle weakness of varying severity. Other clinical features include a peculiar waddling or "penguin" gait, tetany, and greenstick bone fractures.

Imaging Features

General Features. The earliest and most prominent feature of rickets is widening of the epiphyses of the long bones. This is a manifestation of the wide uncalcified osteoid seams that are seen histologically. The resultant abnormal biomechanics lead to cupping and fraying of the metaphases of the long bones. The soft weight-bearing bones such as the femur and tibia undergo a characteristic bowing. Greenstick fractures (an incomplete fracture) occur in many patients with rickets.

In osteomalacia, the cortex of bone may be thin. Pseudofractures, which are poorly calcified, ribbon-like zones extending into bone at approximate right angles to the margin of the bone, may also be present. Pseudofractures occur most commonly in the ribs, pelvis, and weight-bearing bones and rarely in the mandible.

Jaws. In rickets, changes in the jaws generally occur after changes in the ribs and long bones. Jaw cortical structures, such as the inferior mandibular border or the walls of the mandibular canal, may be thin. Within the cancellous portion of the jaws, the trabeculae become reduced in density, number, and thickness. This imparts a generalized radiolucency to the jaws; in severe cases, the jaws appear so radiolucent that the teeth appear to lack bony support.

Most cases of osteomalacia produce no manifestations in the jaws. However, when manifestations are present in diagnostic images, there may be an overall radiolucent appearance and sparse trabeculae.

Teeth and Associated Structures. Rickets in infancy or early childhood may result in hypoplasia of developing dental enamel (Fig. 25-10). If the disease occurs before the age of 3 years, such enamel hypoplasia is fairly common. This early manifestation of rickets is demonstrated in diagnostic images to involve both unerupted and erupted teeth. Diagnostic images may also document retarded tooth eruption in early rickets. The lamina dura and the cortical boundary of tooth follicles may be thin or missing.

Osteomalacia does not alter the teeth because they are fully developed before the onset of the disease. The lamina dura may be especially thin in individuals with long-standing or severe osteomalacia.

Management

Because the cause of rickets and osteomalacia is vitamin D deficiency, the treatment of choice is vitamin D supplementation. Cholecalciferol is a vitamin D supplement that is stored in the

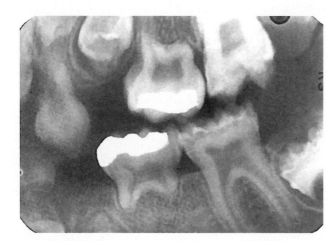

FIGURE 25-10 Rickets may cause thinning (hypoplasia) or decreased mineralization (hypocalcification) of the enamel as seen in this bitewing view. *(Courtesy H. G. Poyton, DDS, Toronto, Ontario, Canada.)*

body and released over several weeks. Signs of healing are seen 6 to 7 days after treatment.

RENAL OSTEODYSTROPHY

Synonym

A synonym for renal osteodystrophy is renal rickets.

Disease Mechanism

Chronic renal failure produces bone changes by interfering with the hydroxylation of 25(OH)D to 1,25(OH)$_2$D, which takes place in the kidneys. The various biologic functions of 1,25(OH)$_2$D outlined in Figure 25-1 are hindered, especially the absorption of calcium from the intestines. The result is a state of hypocalcemia and hyperphosphatemia. The imbalanced serum concentrations of calcium and phosphate inhibit the normal calcification of bone and teeth. Chronic low serum levels of calcium, in addition to affecting normal bone and teeth formation, also stimulate the parathyroid glands to secrete PTH, resulting in secondary hyperparathyroidism.

Clinical Features

The clinical features of renal osteodystrophy are the same as chronic renal failure. In children, growth retardation and frequent bone fractures may occur. Adults may have a gradual softening and bowing of the bones.

Imaging Features

General Features. The features of renal osteodystrophy are quite variable. Some changes of the skeleton resemble changes seen in rickets, and other changes are consistent with hyperparathyroidism, including generalized loss of bone density and thinning of bony cortices. An increase in bone density (Fig. 25-11) is an occasional

FIGURE 25-11 Two cases of renal osteodystrophy. **A,** Panoramic image reveals areas of radiolucency corresponding to loss of bone mass, loss of distinct lamina dura, and a sclerotic bone pattern around the roots of the teeth. **B,** Panoramic image reveals a diffuse sclerotic (radiopaque) bone pattern throughout the jaws. Note the loss of a distinct inferior cortex of the mandible resulting from an increase in the radiopacity of the internal aspect of the bone.

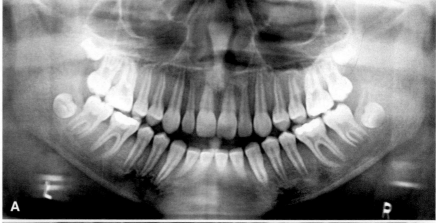

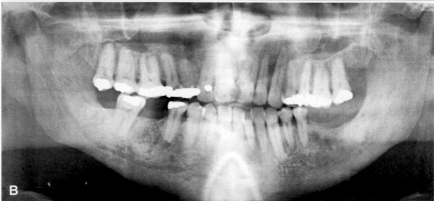

finding. There may be brown tumors, similar to lesions seen in primary hyperthyroidism, but these are less frequent.

Jaws. In renal osteodystrophy, the density of the mandible and maxilla is often less than normal with thin cortical boundaries. The density of the jaws occasionally may be greater than normal. The increased bone density is related to an increase in the bone turnover rate, which leads to an increase in the number and thickness of bone trabeculae. The altered bone trabeculae may also result in a granular bone pattern. Jaw enlargement has been reported in patients with renal disease. The size increase is due to enlargement of the cancellous bone component.

Teeth and Associated Structures. Hypoplasia and hypocalcification of the teeth are possible, sometimes resulting in loss of any evidence of enamel in diagnostic images. The lamina dura may be absent or less apparent in instances of bone sclerosis.

Management

In addition to treating the underlying renal disease, often with renal transplant, patients with renal osteodystrophy are given vitamin D supplements and phosphate binders. The imaging features of secondary hyperparathyroidism may persist even after a successful renal transplant because of hyperplasia of the parathyroid glands secondary to the previous chronic low serum levels of calcium.

HYPOPHOSPHATEMIC RICKETS

Synonyms

Vitamin D–resistant rickets and phosphopenic rickets are synonyms for hypophosphatemic rickets.

Disease Mechanism

Hypophosphatemic rickets represents a group of inherited conditions that produce renal tubular disorders resulting in excessive loss of phosphorus. There is a failure to reabsorb phosphorus in the distal renal tubules, resulting in a decrease in serum phosphorus (hypophosphatemia). Multiple myeloma may induce hypophosphatemia as a result of secondary damage to the kidneys. Normal calcification of the osseous structures requires the correct amount and ratio of serum calcium and phosphorus. Hypophosphatemia can result in low-density bone because of low calcium content and result in abnormal formation of trabeculae, which are sometimes short and irregular resulting in a granular-appearing bone pattern. Also, the hypophosphatemic state interferes with the normal calcification of dentin, resulting in larger than normal pulp chambers and canals.

Clinical Features

Children with hypophosphatemia show reduced growth and bony changes similar to rickets, including bowing of the legs, enlarged epiphyses, and skull changes. Adults have bone pain, muscle weakness, and vertebral fractures.

Imaging Features

General Features. In children with hypophosphatemia, findings are indistinguishable from rickets. In adults, the long bones may show persistent deformity, fractures, or pseudofractures.

Jaws. The jaws are usually osteoporotic and in extreme cases are remarkably radiolucent. Cortical boundaries may be unusually thin or not apparent at all (Fig. 25-12). Other manifestations include fewer visible trabeculae and a granular bone pattern.

Teeth and Associated Structures. The teeth may be poorly formed, with thin enamel caps and large pulp chambers and root canals (see Fig. 25-12, *B* and *C*). In addition, periapical and periodontal abscesses occur frequently. The occurrence of periapical rarefying osteitis without an etiology may be a result of large pulp chambers and defects in the formation of dentin. This may allow for the ingress of oral microorganisms and subsequent pulp necrosis. If the disease is severe, the patient has premature loss of the teeth. The lamina dura may become sparse, and cortical boundaries around tooth crypts may be thin or entirely absent.

Management

Treatment consists of administering vitamin D supplements, phosphates, and anticalciurics. Serum calcium concentrations must be closely monitored to prevent hypercalcemia and its complications. Nephrocalcinosis is a long-term complication that may arise from treatment.

HYPOPHOSPHATASIA

Disease Mechanism

Hypophosphatasia is a rare inherited disorder that is caused by a reduced activity of alkaline phosphatase, an enzyme that is produced by osteoblasts and odontoblasts and is required for the normal mineralization of osteoid and teeth. When deficient, the enzyme fails to cleave phosphate-containing substances, such as inorganic pyrophosphate, resulting in extracellular accumulation of inorganic pyrophosphate, a known inhibitor of hydroxyapatite formation. This condition is reflected in bone as abnormally low density and in teeth as inhibited dentin calcification and larger appearing pulp chambers and canals. The severe forms of the condition have an autosomal recessive mode of disease transmission, whereas the milder forms have a variable pattern of inheritance.

Clinical Features

Six clinical forms of the disease are recognized depending on the age at diagnosis: (1) perinatal (lethal), (2) perinatal (benign), (3) infantile, (4) childhood, (5) adult, and (6) odontohypophosphatasia. The disease in individuals with homozygous involvement is usually severe, has an early onset (in utero), and leads to death within the first year. These infants demonstrate bowed limb bones and a marked deficiency of skull ossification. Individuals with the milder forms of the disease show poor growth and deformities similar to rickets. A history may exist of fractures, delayed walking, or bone pain. About 85% of these children show premature loss of the primary teeth, particularly the incisors, and delayed eruption of the permanent dentition. Dental findings are often the first clinical sign of hypophosphatasia and the only sign of odontohypophosphatasia.

Imaging Features

General Features. In young children with hypophosphatasia, the long bones show irregular defects in the epiphysis, and the skull is poorly calcified. In older children, the premature closure of the skull sutures results in gyral impressions on the inner table of the skull. These are called convolutional markings and appear as multiple lucent areas that resemble hammered copper. The skull may assume a brachycephalic shape. A generalized reduction in bone density may occur in adults.

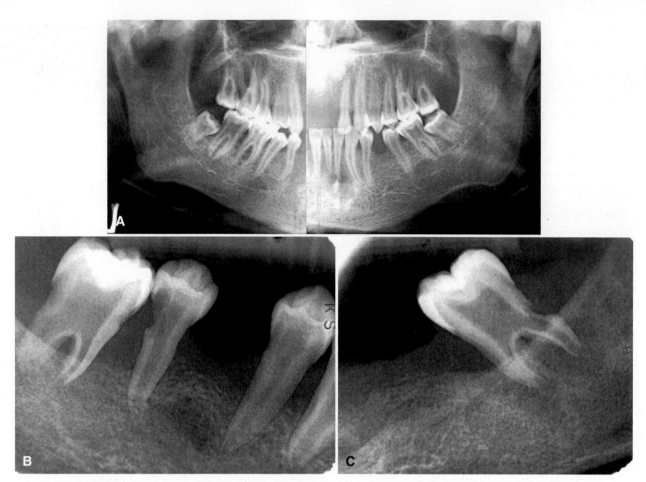

FIGURE 25-12 **A,** Panoramic image of hypophosphatemia. Note the radiolucent appearance of the jaws and the lack of bone density and large pulp chambers. **B** and **C,** These periapical films of a different case of hypophosphatemia demonstrate apparent bone loss around the teeth, a granular bone pattern, large pulp chambers, and external root resorption.

Jaws. A generalized radiolucency of the mandible and maxilla is evident. The cortical bone and lamina dura are thin, and the alveolar bone is poorly calcified and may appear deficient.

Teeth and Associated Structures. Both primary and permanent teeth have a thin enamel layer and large pulp chambers and root canals (Fig. 25-13). The teeth may also be hypoplastic and may be lost prematurely.

Management

There is no curative treatment for hypophosphatasia. However, enzyme replacement therapy is currently being investigated and has demonstrated improvement in children with life-threatening hypophosphatasia.

OSTEOPETROSIS

Synonyms

Albers-Schönberg disease and marble bone disease are synonyms for osteopetrosis.

Disease Mechanism

Osteopetrosis is a disorder of bone that results from a defect in the differentiation and function of osteoclasts. The lack of normally functioning osteoclasts results in abnormal formation of the primary skeleton and abnormal bone turnover thereafter. The failure of bone to remodel causes the bones to be dense, fragile, and susceptible to fracture and infection. The bone mass may also increase, leading to compression of the cranial nerves as they pass through the narrowed skull foramina and giving rise to numerous neuropathies. Obliteration of the marrow compromises hematopoiesis. This disorder is inherited as an autosomal recessive type (osteopetrosis congenita) and autosomal dominant type (osteopetrosis tarda).

Clinical Features

The more severe, recessive form of osteopetrosis is seen in infants and young children, and the more benign, dominant form appears later. The severe form is invariably fatal early in life. The patient has progressive loss of the bone marrow and its cellular products and a severe increase in bone density. The narrowing of bony canals results in hydrocephalus, blindness, deafness, vestibular nerve dysfunction, and facial nerve paralysis. The benign dominant form is milder and may be entirely asymptomatic. It may be discovered any time from childhood into adulthood. The disease may be discovered as an incidental finding or manifest as a pathologic fracture of a bone. In some more chronic cases, bone pain and cranial nerve palsies caused by neural compression may be clinical problems. Osteomyelitis may complicate this disease because of the relative lack of vascularity of the dense bone. This problem is more common

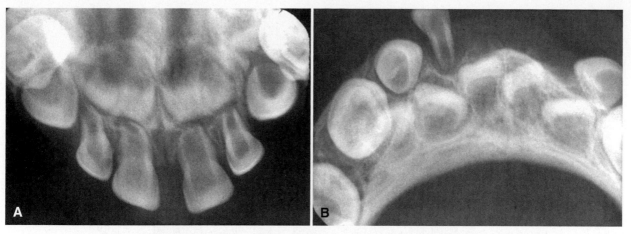

FIGURE 25-13 **A** and **B,** Example of hypophosphatasia. Note the large pulp chambers in the deciduous dentition and the premature loss of the mandibular incisors. *(Courtesy H. G. Poyton, DDS, Toronto, Ontario, Canada.)*

in the mandible, where periapical and periodontal infections are common.

Imaging Features

General Features. In the classic presentation of osteopetrosis, all bones show greatly increased density, which is bilaterally symmetric. The increased density throughout the skeleton is homogeneous and diffused (Fig. 25-14). The internal aspect of the involved bone may be so dense or radiopaque that the trabecular patterns of the medullary cavity may not be visible. The internal radiopacity also reduces the contrast between the outer cortical border and the cancellous portion of the bone. The entire bone may be mildly enlarged.

Jaws. The increased radiopacity of the jaws may be so great that the diagnostic image may fail to reveal any internal structure, and even the roots of the teeth may not be apparent. The increased bone density and relatively poor vascularity result in a susceptibility of the mandible to osteomyelitis, usually from odontogenic inflammatory lesions (Fig. 25-15).

Teeth and Associated Structures. Effects on teeth may include early tooth loss, missing teeth, malformed roots and crowns, and teeth that are poorly calcified and prone to caries. The normal eruption pattern of the primary and secondary dentition may be delayed as a result of bone density or ankylosis. The lamina dura and cortical borders may appear thicker than normal.

Management

Treatment of osteopetrosis consists of bone marrow transplants to attempt to stimulate the formation of functional osteoclasts. The hematologic complications are managed with systemic steroids. The osteomyelitis is difficult to treat, and a combination of antibiotics and hyperbaric oxygen therapy is used. It is imperative that affected patients avoid odontogenic inflammatory disease.

OTHER SYSTEMIC DISEASES
PROGRESSIVE SYSTEMIC SCLEROSIS
Synonym

A synonym for progressive systemic sclerosis (PSS) is scleroderma.

Disease Mechanism

PSS is a generalized connective tissue disease that causes excessive collagen deposition resulting in hardening (sclerosis) of the skin and other tissues. The involvement of the gastrointestinal tract, heart, lungs, and kidneys usually results in more serious complications. The cause of the disease is unknown.

Clinical Features

PSS is a disease of middle age, with the greatest incidence between the ages of 30 and 50 years. It is rarely seen in adolescents and elderly adults. Females are affected about three times as often as males.

In most patients with moderate to severe PSS, the involved skin has a thickened, leathery quality. The skin is not mobile over the underlying soft tissues, and involvement of the facial region may inhibit normal mandibular opening. Patients with diffuse disease are also likely to have xerostomia and increased numbers of decayed, missing, or filled teeth. Patients with this systemic disease are more likely to have deeper periodontal pockets and higher gingivitis scores. Patients with cardiac and pulmonary involvement may have varying degrees of heart failure and respiratory insufficiencies. Renal involvement usually leads to some degree of uremia, with or without hypertension.

Imaging Features

Jaws. A characteristic feature in some cases of PSS is an unusual pattern of mandibular erosions at regions of muscle attachment, such as the angles, coronoid process, digastric region, or condyles (Fig. 25-16). This type of resorption is typically bilateral and fairly symmetric. Most of these erosive borders are smooth and sharply defined. This resorption may progress with the disease.

Teeth and Associated Structures. The most common manifestation of PSS in images of the jaws is an increase in the width of the periodontal ligament (PDL) spaces around the teeth (Fig. 25-17). Approximately two thirds of patients with PSS exhibit this change. The PDL spaces affected by PSS usually are at least twice as thick as normal, and both anterior and posterior teeth are affected, although it is more pronounced around the posterior teeth. The lamina dura remains normal. Despite the widening of the PDL spaces, the clinician finds that involved teeth are often not mobile,

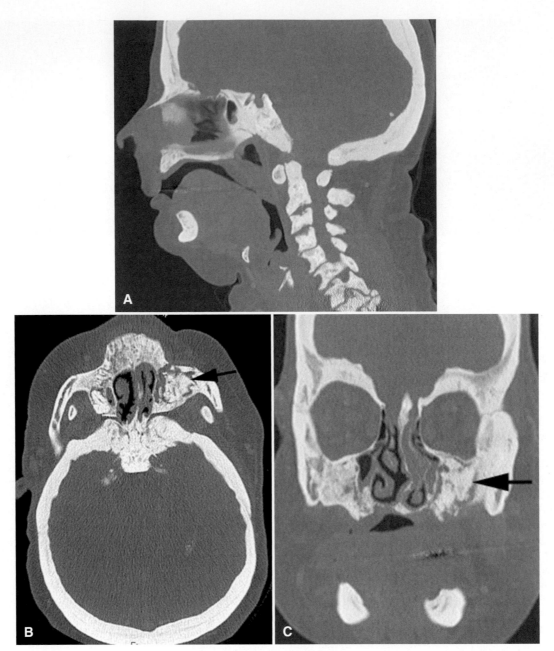

FIGURE 25-14 Osteopetrosis. Sagittal **(A)**, axial **(B)**, and coronal **(C)** MDCT images with bone algorithm show dense calcification of the bones. The case is complicated by osteomyelitis of the left maxilla with development of sequesta *(arrows in B and C)*.

FIGURE 25-15 Panoramic film of a patient with osteopetrosis. Note the increased density of the jaws, lack of eruption of the mandibular second bicuspids, narrow inferior alveolar nerve canal, and development of osteomyelitis in the body of the left mandible with periostitis *(arrow)*.

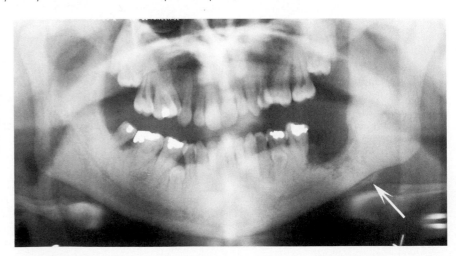

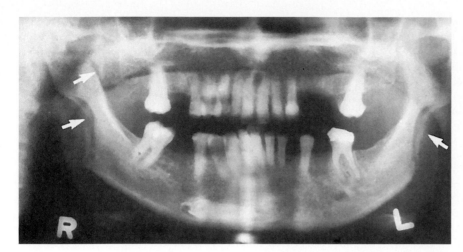

FIGURE 25-16 PSS demonstrating a loss of bone in the region of the angle of the mandible *(left arrows)* and at the right coronoid process *(right arrow)*, which are locations of muscle attachments.

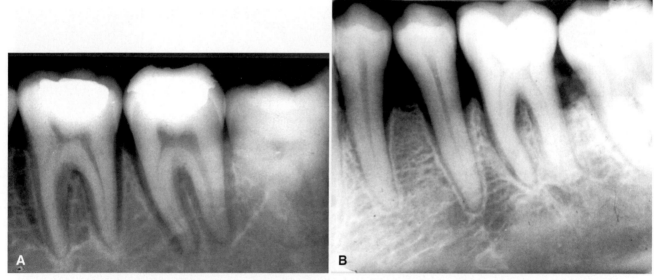

FIGURE 25-17 **A** and **B,** Two periapical films of two different patients with PSS. Note the widening of the periodontal membrane space around some of the teeth.

and their gingival attachments are usually intact. Almost half of patients with PDL space thickening also have some mandibular erosive bone changes.

Differential Diagnosis

Other causes of widening of the periodontal membrane space include tooth mobility, orthodontic tooth movement, intermaxillary fixation with arch bars, and invasion of the PDL by malignant neoplasms. Widening of the PDL space with malignant neoplasia differs in that it is irregular and accompanied by destruction of the lamina dura.

Management

The aforementioned thickening of PDL spaces does not seem to present any clinical difficulties. However, the progressive loss of bone in the region of the mandibular angle is more serious because of potential fracture. It is reasonable to obtain initial and periodic panoramic images in all patients with PSS to assess mandibular integrity.

SICKLE CELL ANEMIA

Disease Mechanism

Sickle cell anemia is an autosomal recessive, chronic hemolytic blood disorder. Patients with this disorder have abnormal hemoglobin (deoxygenated hemoglobin), which under low oxygen tension results in sickling of the red blood cells. These blood cells have a reduced capacity to carry oxygen to the tissues and adhere to vascular endothelium and obstruct capillaries because of damage to their membrane lipids and proteins. The spleen traps and readily destroys these abnormal red blood cells, resulting in anemia. The hematopoietic system responds to the resultant anemia by increasing the production of red blood cells, which requires compensatory hyperplasia of the bone marrow.

Clinical Features

The homozygous form of sickle cell anemia occurs in approximately 1 in every 400 African Americans. Although the gene is present in the heterozygous state in about 6% to 8% of African Americans, these individuals do not show related clinical findings.

Although symptoms and signs vary considerably, most patients with the disease normally manifest mild, chronic features. Long quiet spells of hemolytic latency occur, occasionally punctuated by exacerbations known as sickle cell crises. During the crisis state, patients often have severe abdominal, muscle, and joint pain and a high temperature and may experience circulatory collapse. During milder periods, the patient may complain of fatigability, weakness, shortness of breath, and muscle and joint pain. As in other chronic anemias, the heart is usually enlarged, and a murmur may be present. The disease occurs mostly in children and adolescents. It is compatible with a normal life span, although many patients die of complications of the disease before the age of 40 years.

Imaging Features

The hyperplasia of the bone marrow at the expense of cancellous bone is the primary reason for the abnormal manifestations of sickle cell anemia seen in diagnostic images. The extent of bone changes in sickle cell anemia relates to the degree of this hyperplasia.

General Features. The thinning of individual cancellous trabeculae and cortices is most common in the vertebral bodies, long bones, skull, and jaws. The skull may have widening of the diploic space and thinning of the inner and outer tables (Fig. 25-18). In extreme cases (5%), the outer table of the skull is not apparent, and a "hair-on-end" appearance may occur. Small areas of infarction may be present within bones after blockage of the microvasculature; these are seen as areas of localized bone sclerosis.

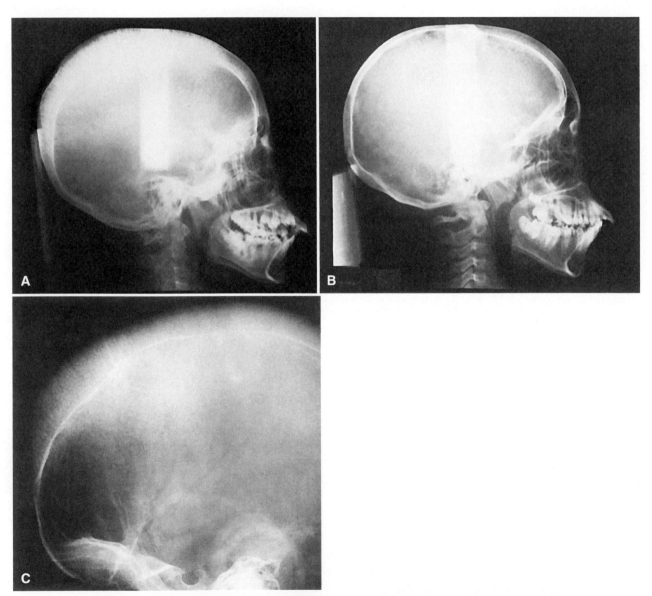

FIGURE 25-18 **A,** Image of a patient with sickle cell anemia shows a thickened diploic space and thinning of the skull cortex.
B, Normal skull for comparison. **C,** Skull showing the "hair-on-end" bone pattern. (**B,** Courtesy Dr. B. Sarnat, Los Angeles, CA;
C, courtesy H. G. Poyton, DDS, Toronto, Ontario, Canada.)

Osteomyelitis may complicate sickle cell anemia if infection begins in an area of pronounced hypovascularity. There also may be retardation of generalized bone growth.

Jaws. The manifestations of sickle cell anemia in the jaws include general osteoporosis. Osteoporosis occurs because of a decrease in the volume of trabecular bone and, to a lesser extent, thinning of the cortical plates. In most cases, the change is mild or moderate; extreme manifestations are unusual. Images of the jaws of children with sickle cell anemia have been reported to show a high frequency of severe osteoporosis. The bone pattern may be altered to one with fewer but coarser trabeculae. Rarely, bone marrow hyperplasia may cause enlargement and protrusion of the maxillary alveolar ridge.

Management

Management of patients with sickle cell anemia is supportive and aims to control the symptoms and prevent the complications of this multisystem disease. Bone marrow transplantation is a curative option, but its applicability is limited because of the associated risks.

THALASSEMIA

Synonyms

Synonyms for thalassemia include Cooley's anemia, Mediterranean anemia, and erythroblastic anemia.

Disease Mechanism

Thalassemia is a hereditary disorder that results in a defect in hemoglobin synthesis. This defect may involve either the α-globulin or β-globulin genes. The resultant red blood cells have reduced hemoglobin content, are thin, and have a shortened life span. The heterozygous form of the disease (thalassemia minor) is mild. The homozygous form (thalassemia major) may be severe. A less severe form, thalassemia intermedia, also occurs. As in sickle cell anemia, the result is hyperplasia of the bone marrow component of bone, which results in fewer trabeculae per unit area and can change the overall shape of the bone.

Clinical Features

In the severe form of the disease, the onset is in infancy, and the survival time may be short. The face develops prominent cheekbones and a protrusive premaxilla, resulting in a "rodent-like" face. The milder form of the disease occurs in adults.

Imaging Features

General Features. Similar to sickle cell anemia, the features of thalassemia generally result from hyperplasia of the ineffective bone marrow and its subsequent failure to produce normal red blood cells. However, these changes are usually more severe than with other anemias. There is a generalized radiolucency of the long bones with cortical thinning. In the skull, the diploic space exhibits marked thickening, especially in the frontal region. The skull also shows a generalized granular appearance (Fig. 25-19), and occasionally a "hair-on-end" effect may develop.

Jaws. Severe bone marrow hyperplasia prevents pneumatization of the paranasal sinuses, especially the maxillary sinus, and causes an expansion of the maxilla that results in malocclusion (Fig. 25-20, *A*). The jaws appear radiolucent, with thinning of the cortical borders and enlargement of the marrow spaces. The trabeculae are large and coarse (Fig. 25-20, *B*). The lamina dura is thin, and the roots of the teeth may be short.

Management

Patients with thalassemia minor require no treatment except for iron supplementation when iron deficiency is confirmed. Patients with thalassemia major require regular hypertransfusion to maintain their hemoglobin levels and iron chelation to prevent iron overload complications, such as cardiomyopathy and liver cirrhosis.

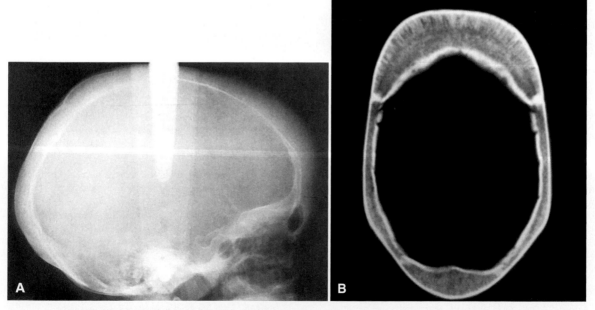

FIGURE 25-19 **A,** Skull image of a patient with thalassemia shows a granular appearance of the skull and thickening of the diploic space. **B,** Axial CT image of the skull of a patient with thalassemia. The diploic space is thickened, and there is a hint of linear orientation of the trabeculae, especially in the frontal bone. (**A,** *Courtesy H. G. Poyton, DDS, Toronto, Ontario, Canada.*)

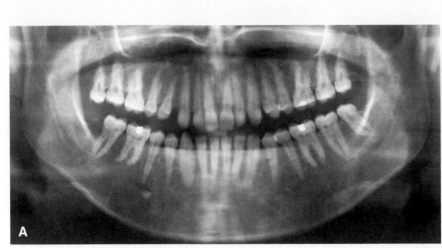
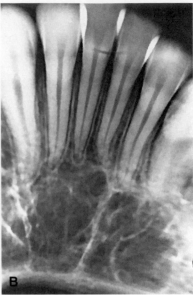

FIGURE 25-20 **A,** Panoramic film of a patient with thalassemia. Note the thickened body of the mandible and the sparse trabeculae and lack of maxillary antra. **B,** Image of a different patient with thalassemia with thick trabeculae and large bone marrow spaces. *(Courtesy H. G. Poyton, DDS, Toronto, Ontario, Canada.)*

BIBLIOGRAPHY

Adler C: *Bone diseases: macroscopic, histological and radiological diagnosis of structural changes in the skeleton,* Berlin, 2000, Springer-Verlag.

Paterson CR: *Metabolic disorders of bone,* Oxford, 1974, Blackwell Scientific.

Trapnell DH, Boweman JE: *Dental manifestation of systemic disease,* London, 1973, Butterworth.

Cushing's Syndrome

Kaltsas G, Makras P: Skeletal diseases in Cushing's syndrome: osteoporosis versus arthropathy, *Neuroendocrinology* 92(Suppl 1): 60–64, 2010.

Diabetes Mellitus

Collin HL, Niskanen L, Uusitupa M, et al: Oral symptoms and signs in elderly patients with type 2 diabetes mellitus: a focus on diabetic neuropathy, *Oral Surg Oral Med Oral Pathol Oral Radiol Endod* 90:299–305, 2000.

Lamey PJ, Darwazeh AM, Frier BM: Oral disorders associated with diabetes mellitus, *Diabetes Med* 9:410–416, 1992.

Murrah VA: Diabetes mellitus and associated oral manifestations: a review, *J Oral Pathol* 14:271–281, 1985.

Hyperparathyroidism

Aldred MJ, Talacko AA, Savarirayan R, et al: Dental findings in a family with hyperparathyroidism-jaw tumor syndrome and a novel HRPT2 gene mutation, *Oral Surg Oral Med Oral Pathol Oral Radiol Endod* 101:212–218, 2006.

Bilezikian JP: Hyper- and hypoparathyroidism. In Rakel R, editor: *Conn's current therapy,* Philadelphia, 1985, Saunders.

Daniels JM: Primary hyperparathyroidism presenting as a palatal brown tumor, *Oral Surg Oral Med Oral Pathol Oral Radiol Endod* 98:409–413, 2004.

Marcocci C, Cetani F: Clinical practice. Primary hyperparathyroidism, *N Engl J Med* 365:2389–2397, 2011.

Rosenberg EH, Guralnick W: Hyperparathyroidism: a review of 220 proved cases with special emphasis on findings in the jaws, *Oral Surg Oral Med Oral Pathol* 15(2 Suppl):84–94, 1962.

Hyperthyroidism

Little JW: Thyroid disorders. Part I: hyperthyroidism, *Oral Surg Oral Med Oral Pathol Oral Radiol Endod* 101:276–284, 2006.

Hypoparathyroidism

Frensilli J, Stoner R, Hinrichs E: Dental changes of idiopathic-hypoparathyroidism: report of three cases, *J Oral Surg* 29:727–731, 1971.

Glynne A, Hunter I, Thomson J: Pseudohypoparathyroidism with paradoxical increase in hypocalcemic seizures due to long-term anticonvulsant therapy, *Postgrad Med J* 48:632, 1972.

Hypophosphatasia

Eastman JR, Bixler D: Clinical, laboratory, and genetic investigations of hypophosphatasia: support for autosomal dominant inheritance with homozygous lethality, *J Craniofac Genet Dev Biol* 3:213–234, 1983.

Jedrychowski JR, Duperon D: Childhood hypophosphatasia with oral manifestations, *J Oral Med* 34:18–22, 1979.

Macfarlane JD, Swart JGN: Dental aspects of hypophosphatasia: a case report, family study, and literature review, *Oral Surg Oral Med Oral Pathol* 67:521–526, 1989.

Hypopituitarism

Conley H, Steflik DE, Singh B, et al: Clinical and histologic findings of the dentition in a hypopituitary patient: report of case, *ASDC J Dent Child* 57:376–379, 1990.

Edler RJ: Dental and skeletal ages in hypopituitary patients, *J Dent Res* 56:1145–1153, 1977.

Kosowicz J, Rzymski K: Abnormalities of tooth development in pituitary dwarfism, *Oral Surg Oral Med Oral Pathol* 44:853–863, 1977.

Myllarniemi S, Lenko HL, Perheentupa J: Dental maturity in hypopituitarism, and dental response to substitution treatment, *Scand J Dent Res* 86:307–312, 1978.

Whyte MP, Greenberg CR, Salman NJ, et al: Enzyme-replacement therapy in life-threatening hypophosphatasia, *N Engl J Med* 366:904–913, 2012.

Osteoporosis

Lee BD, White SC: Age and trabecular features of alveolar bone associated with osteoporosis, *Oral Surg Oral Med Oral Pathol Oral Radiol Endod* 100:92–98, 2005.

Mohammad AR, Alder M, McNally MA: A pilot study of panoramic film density at selected sites in the mandible to predict osteoporosis, *Int J Prosthodont* 9:290–294, 1996.

Taguchi A, Suei Y, Ohtsuka M, et al: Usefulness of panoramic radiography in the diagnosis of postmenopausal osteoporosis in women: width and morphology of inferior cortex of the mandible, *Dentomaxillofac Radiol* 25:263–267, 1996.

White SC: Oral radiographic predictors of osteoporosis, *Dentomaxillofac Radiol* 31:84–92, 2002.

Osteopetrosis

Barry CP, Ryan CD, Stassen LF: Osteomyelitis of the maxilla secondary to osteopetrosis: a report of two cases in sisters, *J Oral Maxillofac Surg* 65:144–147, 2007.

Ruprecht A, Wagner H, Engel H: Osteopetrosis: report of a case and discussion of the differential diagnosis, *Oral Surg Oral Med Oral Pathol* 66:674–679, 1988.

Waguespack SG, Hui SL, Dimeglio LA, et al: Autosomal dominant osteopetrosis: clinical severity and natural history of 94 subjects with a chloride channel 7 gene mutation, *J Clin Endocrinol Metab* 92:771–778, 2007.

Younai F, Eisenbud L, Sciubba JJ: Osteopetrosis: a case report including gross and microscopic findings in the mandible at autopsy, *Oral Surg Oral Med Oral Pathol* 65:214–221, 1988.

Progressive Systemic Sclerosis

Alexandridis C, White SC: Periodontal ligament changes in patients with progressive systemic sclerosis, *Oral Surg Oral Med Oral Pathol* 58:113–118, 1984.

Auluck A, Pai KM, Shetty C, et al: Mandibular resorption in progressive systemic sclerosis: a report of three cases, *Dentomaxillofac Radiol* 34:384–386, 2005.

Rout PG, Hamburger J, Potts AJ: Orofacial radiological manifestations of systemic sclerosis, *Dentomaxillofac Radiol* 25:193–196, 1996.

Wood RE, Lee P: Analysis of the oral manifestations of systemic sclerosis (scleroderma), *Oral Surg Oral Med Oral Pathol* 65:172–178, 1988.

Renal Osteodystrophy

Damm DD, Neville BW, McKenna S, et al: Macrognathia of renal osteodystrophy in dialysis patients, *Oral Surg Oral Med Oral Pathol Oral Radiol Endod* 83:489–495, 1997.

Hata T, Irei I, Tanaka K, et al: Macrognathia secondary to dialysis-related renal osteodystrophy treated successfully by parathyroidectomy, *Int J Oral Maxillofac Surg* 35:378–382, 2006.

Proctor R, Kumar N, Stein A, et al: Oral and dental aspects of chronic renal failure, *J Dent Res* 84:199–208, 2005.

Scutellari PN, Orzincolo C, Bedani PL, et al: Radiographic manifestations in teeth and jaws in chronic kidney insufficiency, *Radiol Med (Torino)* 92:415–420, 1996.

Rickets

Harris R, Sullivan HR: Dental sequelae in deciduous dentition in vitamin-D resistant rickets: case report, *Aust Dent J* 5:200–203, 1960.

Marks SC, Lindahl RL, Bawden JW: Dental and cephalometric findings in vitamin D resistant rickets, *J Dent Child* 32:259, 1965.

Sickle Cell Anemia

Brown DL, Sebes JI: Sickle cell gnathopathy: radiologic assessment, *Oral Surg Oral Med Oral Pathol* 61:653–656, 1986.

Ejindu VC, Hine AL, Mashayeckhi M, et al: Musculoskeletal manifestations of sickle cell disease, *Radiographics* 27:1005–1021, 2007.

Lawrenz DR: Sickle cell disease: a review and update of current therapy, *J Oral Maxillofac Surg* 57:171–178, 1999.

Sears RS, Nazif MM, Zullo T: The effects of sickle-cell disease on dental and skeletal maturation, *ASDC J Dent Child* 48:275–277, 1981.

White SC, Cohen JM, Mourshed FA: Digital analysis of trabecular pattern in jaws of patients with sickle cell anemia, *Dentomaxillofac Radiol* 29:119–124, 2000.

Thalassemia

Hazza'a AM, Al-Jamal G: Radiographic features of the jaws and teeth in thalassaemia major, *Dentomaxillofac Radiol* 35:283–288, 2006.

Poyton HG, Davey KW: Thalassemia: changes visible in radiographs used in dentistry, *Oral Surg Oral Med Oral Pathol* 25:564–576, 1968.

OUTLINE

The paranasal sinuses are the four paired sets of air-filled cavities of the maxillofacial complex, and they consist of the maxillary, frontal, and sphenoid sinuses and the ethmoid air cells. The maxillary sinuses are of particular importance to the dentist because of their proximity to the teeth and their associated structures. Abnormalities arising from within the maxillary sinuses can cause symptoms that may mimic diseases of odontogenic origin; conversely, abnormalities that arise in and around the teeth may affect the sinuses or mimic the symptoms of sinus disease. Because the paranasal sinuses may appear on many diagnostic images used in the practice of dentistry, the dentist should be familiar with variations in the normal appearances of the sinuses and the more common diseases that may affect them.

NORMAL DEVELOPMENT AND VARIATIONS

The paranasal sinuses develop as invaginations from the nasal fossae into their respective bones (maxillary, frontal, sphenoid, and ethmoid) and continue to enlarge until skeletal maturity. Consequently, the mucosal lining of the paranasal sinuses is similar to the lining found in the nasal cavity but with slightly fewer mucous glands. The epithelial cilia move these sinus secretions toward their respective communications, the ostia, with the nasal fossae.

The maxillary sinuses or antra are the first to develop in the second month of intrauterine life. An invagination develops in the lateral wall of the nasal fossa in the middle meatus, and the sinus cavity enlarges laterally into the body of the maxilla. At birth, each sinus is a thin, small slit, no more than 8 mm in length in its anteroposterior dimension. With time, the maxilla becomes progressively more pneumatized as the air cavity expands further into the bone both laterally under the orbits toward the zygomatic process and inferiorly into the alveolar process. Enlargement of the air space, or pneumatization, into the alveolar process superimposes the maxillary sinus and floor over the roots of the premolar or molar teeth to varying degrees on plain images.

The radiographic appearance of the floor of the maxillary sinus is a thin, radiopaque line. Where the alveolar process of the maxilla is not well pneumatized, the floor of the sinus may not be visible on periapical images (Fig. 26-1, *A*), or it may be seen superior to the roots of the maxillary premolar or molar teeth (Fig. 26-1, *B*). With greater pneumatization of the alveolar process, the floor of the sinus may appear to undulate or drape over or around the roots of the teeth or be superimposed over the roots of the adjacent teeth, giving the false impression that the tooth roots have penetrated the sinus floor (Fig. 26-1, *C* and *D*). Closer examination of the periapical areas of the teeth in such instances reveals intact laminae durae and periodontal ligament spaces. In patients with considerable pneumatization of the alveolar process of the maxilla, the lamina dura of a premolar or molar tooth may form a portion of the sinus floor. Maxillary pneumatization may also extend into the palatal, zygomatic, and frontal processes of the maxilla, and this can be appreciated on plain images and advanced imaging examinations such as cone-beam computed tomographic (CBCT), computed tomographic (CT), or magnetic resonance (MR) imaging (Fig. 26-2). In some instances, the appearance of the normally pneumatized maxilla may be mistakenly confused with a benign space-occupying lesion, particularly on plain images (Fig. 26-3).

Hypoplasia of the maxillary sinuses occurs unilaterally in about 1.7% of patients and bilaterally in 7.2%. In these patients, the images of the affected sinus may appear more radiopaque than normal because of the relatively large amount of surrounding maxillary bone. The configuration of the maxillary sinus walls frequently helps to distinguish between a hypoplastic sinus and a sinus that is pathologically radiopaque. An occipitomental (Waters) view shows an inward bowing of the sinus wall resulting in a smaller than normal air cavity. In contrast, extensive enlargement of the maxillary and other paranasal sinuses is a well-known feature of acromegaly.

The development of the frontal sinus does not usually begin until the fifth or sixth year of life. This sinus either develops directly as extensions from the nasal fossae or develops from the anterior ethmoid air cells (see Fig. 26-4, *B*). In about 4% of the population, the frontal sinuses fail to develop. As with the other paranasal sinuses, the right and left frontal sinus cavities develop separately, and as they expand, they approach each other in the midline. In such instances, a thin bony septum may partially

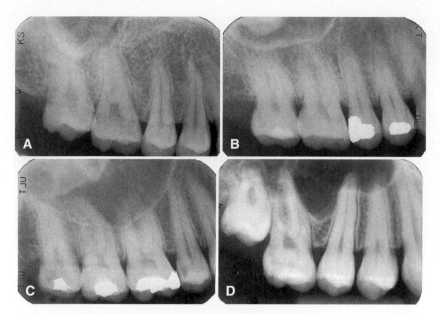

FIGURE 26-1 **A-D,** The range of normal of the position of the maxillary sinus relative to the premolar and molar teeth is shown in periapical images. There is no apparent floor in **A**, with progressively more pneumatization of the alveolar process in **B** and **C**; draping of the maxillary sinus border over the apices of the teeth is particularly evident in **D**.

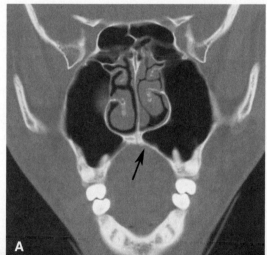

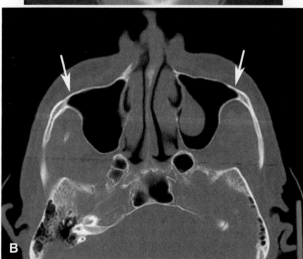

FIGURE 26-2 **A,** Example of pneumatization of the maxillary sinus into the palatal process of the maxilla *(arrow)* in coronal MDCT image. **B,** Examples of pneumatization of the zygomatic process of the maxilla *(arrows)* in axial MDCT image; also note the retention pseudocyst in the left maxillary sinus.

or completely separate the two asymmetric cavities. In adults, frontal sinus pneumatization may also extend posteriorly into the orbital roofs.

The sphenoid sinus begins growing in the fourth fetal month as invaginations from the sphenoethmoidal recesses of the nasal fossae. Located in the body of the sphenoid bone, the sinuses may be separated by a partial or complete bony septum that may result in sinus cavities that are asymmetric in size and shape. Similar to the other sinuses, the sphenoid sinuses may extend beyond the body of the bone into the dorsum sella, the clinoid processes, the greater or lesser wings, and the pterygoid processes. The ostium of the sphenoid sinus is a relatively large-diameter opening, which may explain why blockages of the sphenoid sinus ostium are uncommon (see the section on mucoceles later in this chapter).

The ethmoid air cells extend into the developing ethmoid bones during the fifth fetal month. They consist of multiple separate or interconnected air-filled chambers that border the medial and sometimes inferior aspects of the orbital cavities (Fig. 26-4, *A* and *B*). The number of air cells varies considerably, with each ethmoid bone containing 8 to 15 cells. In some cases, the ethmoid air cells may encroach into the neighboring maxillary, lacrimal, frontal, sphenoid, and palatine bones.

The function of the paranasal sinuses has been controversial. However, many authorities now believe the role of the paranasal sinuses is to insulate or protect deeper vital structures from external trauma.

DISEASES ASSOCIATED WITH THE PARANASAL SINUSES

The maxillary sinuses are of greatest concern to the dentist because of their proximities to the teeth and supporting structures. Therefore, the emphasis in this chapter is on diseases related to the maxillary sinus.

DEFINITION

Diseases associated with the maxillary sinuses include diseases that originate primarily from tissues within the sinus (intrinsic diseases) and diseases that originate outside the sinus (most commonly

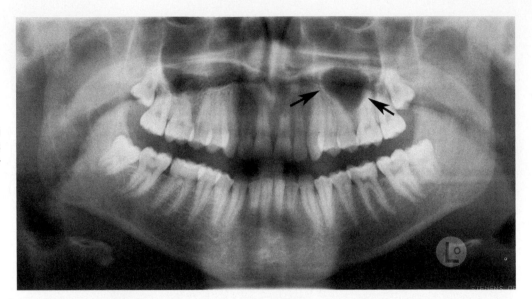

FIGURE 26-3 Panoramic image of a loculus *(arrows)* of the left maxillary sinus draping over the roots mimicking a benign space-occupying lesion.

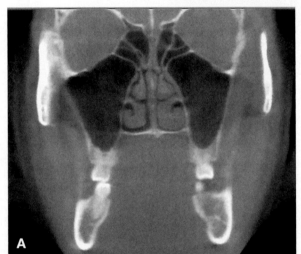

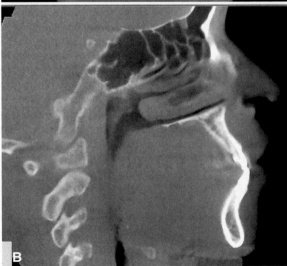

FIGURE 26-4 **A,** Coronal CBCT image of normal maxillary sinuses and ethmoid air cells. **B,** Sagittal CBCT image of normal frontal and sphenoid sinuses and ethmoid air cells.

diseases arising from odontogenic tissues) that either impinge on or infiltrate the sinus (extrinsic diseases). These types of diseases include inflammatory odontogenic disease, odontogenic cysts, benign and malignant odontogenic neoplasms, bone dysplasias, and trauma.

CLINICAL FEATURES

The clinical signs and symptoms of maxillary sinus disease include a sensation of pressure, altered voice characteristics, pain on head movement, percussion sensitivity of the teeth, regional dysesthesia, paresthesia or anesthesia, and swelling and tenderness of the facial structures adjacent to the maxilla.

APPLIED DIAGNOSTIC IMAGING

When maxillary sinus disease is suspected, it may be reasonable for the dentist to proceed with the initial radiologic investigation. A periapical image provides a detailed view of the periapical structures of the teeth and their relationships to the alveolar recess and floor of the maxillary antrum. Although this examination is limited, if the dentist suspects an abnormality, a maxillary lateral occlusal or panoramic image may be useful to obtain views of a greater region of the sinus as well as parts of the inferior, posterior, and anteromedial walls. In some cases, it may be difficult to compare the interior aspects of the right and left sinuses on the panoramic image because of overlapping of adjacent anatomic structures or ghost images.

If there are positive findings on these images, the patient should be referred to an oral and maxillofacial radiologist for a more comprehensive imaging examination. The occipitomental (Waters) skull projection is optimal for visualization of the maxillary sinuses, especially to compare internal radiopacities, and the frontal sinuses and ethmoid air cells. If the Waters view is made with the mouth open, parts of the sphenoid sinus may also be visualized.

Advanced imaging has become increasingly important for the evaluation of sinus disease and has virtually replaced plain images and conventional tomography for investigations of the paranasal sinuses. Because advanced imaging can produce multiplanar images through the sinuses, MDCT or CBCT examinations may contribute significantly to delineating the extent of disease, particularly in patients who have chronic or recurrent sinusitis. Coronal MDCT and CBCT imaging provide superior visualization of the ostiomeatal complex (the region of the ostia of the maxillary sinus and ethmoid air cells) and nasal cavities and for demonstrating any reaction in the surrounding bone to sinus disease. MRI provides superior visualization of the soft tissues, especially the extension of neoplasms developing or infiltrating into the sinuses or surrounding soft tissues, or the differentiation of retained fluid secretions from soft tissue masses in the sinuses.

INTRINSIC DISEASES OF THE PARANASAL SINUSES

This section describes abnormalities that originate from tissues within the sinuses.

INFLAMMATORY DISEASE

Inflammation may result from various causes, such as infection, chemical irritation, allergy, introduction of a foreign body, or facial trauma. The imaging changes associated with inflammation include thickened sinus mucosa, air-fluid levels, polyps, empyema, and retention pseudocysts. However, viral infections may not cause any imaging change in a sinus.

Mucositis

Synonym. A synonym for mucositis is localized thickened sinus mucosa.

Disease Mechanism. The mucosal lining of the paranasal sinuses is composed of respiratory epithelium and is normally about 1 mm thick. Normal sinus mucosa is not visualized on images; however, inflamed mucosa may increase in thickness 10 to 15 times, and this may be visualized with imaging. Localized inflammatory change is referred to as mucositis.

Clinical Features. Many patients may be unaware of a change to their sinus mucosa, and these changes are often discovered as incidental findings on images made for other purposes. Consequently, the discovery of thickened mucosa in an individual who is otherwise asymptomatic does not imply that further investigations are warranted or that treatment is required.

Imaging Features. Thickened mucosa is readily detectable in the image as a well-defined, noncorticated radiopaque band of increased radiopacity paralleling the bony wall of the sinus (Fig. 26-5).

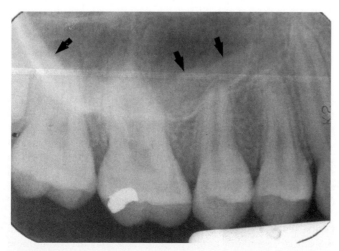

FIGURE 26-5 Thickened sinus mucosa *(arrows)* is portrayed as a radiopaque band paralleling the contour of the maxillary antral floor.

Sinusitis

Disease Mechanism. Sinusitis is a generalized inflammatory condition of the sinus mucosa caused by an allergen, bacteria, or a virus. Inflammatory changes may lead to ciliary dysfunction and retention of sinus secretions and sometimes blockage of the ostiomeatal complex. The term pansinusitis describes sinusitis affecting all the paranasal sinuses. In children with pansinusitis, the possibility of cystic fibrosis should be considered. Sinusitis is often categorized as acute or chronic based on the length of time that the disease is present. If the disease is present for 4 weeks or less, it is termed acute sinusitis; if it is present for more than 12 consecutive weeks, it is considered chronic. For sinusitis lasting from more than 4 weeks up to 12 weeks, the term subacute may be used.

Clinical Features. Acute sinusitis is the most common of the sinus conditions that cause pain and is often a complication of the common cold. After a few days, nasal congestion accompanied by a clear discharge can increase, and the patient may complain of pain and tenderness to pressure or swelling over the involved sinus. The pain may also be referred to the premolar and molar teeth on the affected side and these teeth may develop sensitivity to percussion. In the case of a bacterial sinusitis, a green or greenish yellow discharge may accompany the other aforementioned signs and symptoms. In such circumstances, it is important that the teeth be ruled out as a possible source of the pain or infection.

Chronic maxillary sinusitis is a sequela of an acute infection that fails to resolve by 3 months. Generally, no external signs occur except during periods of acute exacerbations when increased pain and discomfort are apparent. Chronic sinusitis may develop with anatomic derangements, including deviation of the nasal septum and the presence of concha bullosa (pneumatization of the middle concha) that inhibit the outflow of mucus, or with allergic rhinitis, asthma, cystic fibrosis, and dental infections.

Imaging Features. Thickening of sinus mucosa and the accumulation of secretions that accompany sinusitis reduce the air space of the sinus and cause it to become increasingly radiopaque. The most common radiopaque patterns that occur in the Waters view are localized mucosal thickening along the sinus floor, generalized thickening of the mucosal lining around the entire wall of the sinus, and near-complete or complete radiopacification of the sinus (Figs. 26-6 and 26-7). Such changes are best seen in the maxillary sinuses, but the frontal and sphenoid sinuses may be similarly affected. Scrutinizing the area around the maxillary ostium on plain images or CT images may reveal the presence of thickened mucosal tissue, which may cause blockage of the ostium. Mucosal thickening in just the base of the sinus may not represent sinusitis. Rather, it may represent the more localized thickening or mucositis that can occur in association with rarefying osteitis from a tooth with a nonvital pulp. However, this condition may progress to involve the entire sinus.

The image of thickened sinus mucosa may be uniform or polypoid. In the case of an allergic reaction, the mucosa tends to be more lobulated. In contrast, in cases of infection, the thickened mucosal outline tends to be smoother, with its contour following that of the sinus wall. The inability to perceive the delicate walls of the ethmoid air cells is a particularly sensitive sign of ethmoid sinusitis.

An air-fluid level resulting from the accumulation of secretions also may be present. Because the radiopacities of transudates, exudates, blood, and pathologically altered mucosa are similar, the

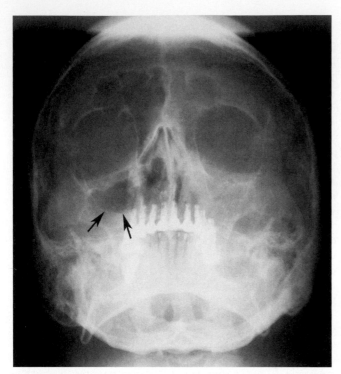

FIGURE 26-6 Waters view demonstrating complete radiopacification of the left maxillary and frontal sinuses and ethmoid air cells. An air-fluid level is visible in the right maxillary sinus (*arrows*).

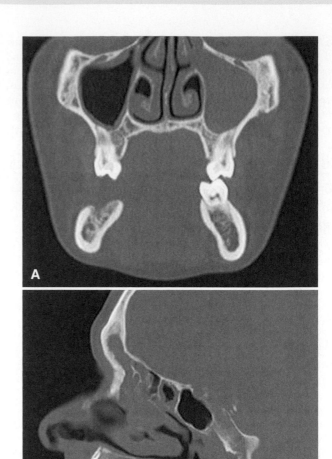

FIGURE 26-7 **A,** Coronal view of the maxillary sinuses showing complete radiopacification of the left sinus and circumferential mucosal thickening of the right sinus. **B,** Sagittal MDCT image of mucositis of the ethmoid air cells.

differentiation among them relies on their shape and distribution. When present, fluid appears radiopaque and occupies the inferior or so-called dependent aspect of the sinus. The border between the radiopaque fluid and the relatively radiolucent air in the antrum is horizontal and straight, and a meniscus may be seen at the periphery where the fluid meets a sinus wall (see Fig. 26-6). Chronic sinusitis may result in persistent radiopacification of the sinus with sclerosis and thickening of the bony walls as the sinus periosteum is stimulated (Fig. 26-8).

The resolution of acute sinusitis becomes apparent on the image as a gradual increase in the radiolucency of the sinus. This can first be recognized when a small clear area appears in the interior of the sinus; the thickened mucous membrane gradually shrinks so that it begins to follow the outline of the bony wall. In time, the image of the mucous membrane is not visible, and the sinus appears normal. In chronic sinusitis, the changes to the sinus wall may persist.

Management. The goals of treatment of sinusitis are to control the infection, promote drainage, and relieve pain. Acute sinusitis is usually treated medically with decongestants to reduce mucosal swelling and with antibiotics in the case of a bacterial sinusitis. Chronic sinusitis is primarily a disease of obstruction of the ostia; the goal is ventilation and drainage. Endoscopic surgery is often performed to enlarge obstructed ostia, or an alternative path of drainage is established.

Retention Pseudocyst

Synonyms. Synonyms for retention pseudocyst include antral pseudocyst, benign mucous cyst, mucus retention cyst, mucus retention pseudocyst, mesothelial cyst, pseudocyst, interstitial cyst, lymphangiectatic cyst, false cyst, retention cyst of the maxillary

sinus, benign cyst of the antrum, benign mucosal cyst of the sinus, serous nonsecretory retention pseudocyst, and mucosal antral cyst.

Disease Mechanism. The term retention pseudocyst is used to describe several related conditions that result in the development of cystlike lesions that are not lined by epithelium. The pathogenesis of these lesions is controversial, but because their clinical and imaging features are similar, no attempt is made to distinguish between them. One etiology suggests that blockage of the secretory ducts of seromucous glands in the sinus mucosa may result in a pathologic submucosal accumulation of secretions, resulting in swelling of the tissue. A second theory suggests that the serous nonsecretory retention pseudocyst arises as a result of cystic degeneration within an inflamed, thickened sinus lining.

Clinical Features. Retention pseudocysts may be found in any of the sinuses at any time of the year, although they may occur more often in the early spring or fall. This occurrence suggests that retention pseudocysts might be related to changes in seasonal allergies,

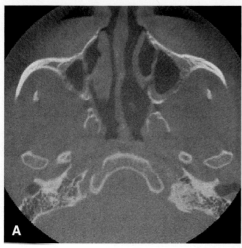

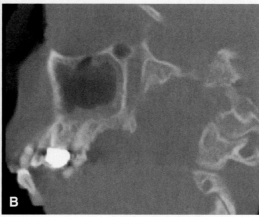

FIGURE 26-8 Axial (**A**) and sagittal (**B**) CBCT images show peripheral bony thickening of the left maxillary sinus from chronic sinusitis.

colds, humidity, or temperature changes. Most studies have found that retention pseudocysts are more common in males.

A retention pseudocyst rarely causes any signs or symptoms, and the patient is usually unaware of the lesion. It often is noticed as an incidental finding on images obtained for other purposes. Retention pseudocysts may range widely in size—from the size of a fingertip to a size large enough to fill the sinus completely and make it radiopaque. However, when a pseudocyst completely fills the maxillary sinus cavity, it may prolapse (extrude) through the ostium and cause nasal obstruction or rupture as a result of abrupt pressure changes caused by sneezing or blowing of the nose, producing postnasal discharge; this may be the only clinical evidence of the presence of the pseudocyst. The pseudocyst may be present on an imaging examination of the maxillary sinus and be absent only a few days later, only to reappear on subsequent examinations.

The maxillary sinus is the most common site of retention pseudocysts. Pseudocysts occasionally are found in the sphenoid sinus and less often are found in the frontal sinuses and ethmoid air cells. Antral retention pseudocysts are not related to dental extractions or associated with periapical disease.

Imaging Features

Location. Partial images of retention pseudocysts of the maxillary antrum may appear on maxillary posterior periapical images (Fig. 26-9, *A*), but they are best demonstrated on extraoral images (Fig. 26-9, *B*). One or more pseudocysts may occur within the same or different sinus cavities. These pseudocysts usually form on the floor of the sinus (Fig. 26-9, *D*), although they may form on any wall or the roof (Fig. 26-9, *C*).

Periphery and Shape. Retention pseudocysts usually appear as well-defined, noncorticated, smooth, dome-shaped, mostly sessile radiopaque masses. Because the lesion originates from within the sinus, it does not have a radiopaque, corticated border.

Internal Structure. The internal aspect is homogeneous and more radiopaque than the surrounding air of the sinus cavity (see Fig. 26-9, *B*). The radiopacity of the lesion is caused by the accumulation of fluid in the soft tissue lining of the sinus, which is relatively more radiopaque than air.

Effects on Surrounding Structures. There are no effects on the surrounding structures. The adjacent sinus floor is always intact. When a retention pseudocyst occurs adjacent to the root of a tooth, the lamina dura surrounding the root is intact, and the width of the periodontal ligament space is unaffected.

Differential Diagnosis. It is important to distinguish retention pseudocysts from antral polyps, odontogenic cysts, or neoplasms arising in the maxilla adjacent to the sinus; this can usually be done through imaging characteristics and by the patient's history. The floor of the maxillary sinus may be displaced by a developing odontogenic cyst or neoplasm as the border of the lesion becomes coincident with the bony sinus floor. In some instances, periodic fenestrations can be seen through the bony sinus floor depending on the growth rate or aggressiveness of the cyst or neoplasm. The retention pseudocyst is dome-shaped but lacks the thin marginal radiopaque line representing the corticated border characteristic of the odontogenic cyst or neoplasm. For example, in the case of a radicular cyst, the lamina dura of the involved tooth or teeth is not intact in the apical area.

Antral polyps of infectious or allergic origin may be difficult to distinguish from retention pseudocysts, but when there is concurrent mucositis and multiple soft tissue masses, the possibility of polyps should be considered. Benign neoplasms may also mimic retention pseudocysts. If benign neoplasms originate from outside the sinus, they are separated from the cavity of the sinus by a radiopaque border, similar to odontogenic cysts. Malignant neoplasms may destroy the osseous border of the sinus, whether they arise from within the sinus or from the alveolar process. However, a malignant neoplasm is less likely to appear as dome-shaped as a retention pseudocyst.

Management. Retention pseudocysts in the maxillary sinus usually require no treatment because they customarily resolve spontaneously without any residual effect on the antral mucosa.

Polyps

Disease Mechanism. The thickened mucous membrane of a chronically inflamed sinus frequently forms into irregular folds called polyps. Polyposis of the sinus mucosa may develop in an isolated area or in many areas throughout the sinus.

Clinical Features. Polyps may cause displacement or destruction of bone. In the ethmoid air cells, polyps may cause destruction of the medial wall of the orbit (lamina papyracea of the ethmoid bone) and an ipsilateral proptosis.

Imaging Features. A polyp may be differentiated from a retention pseudocyst on an image by noting that a polyp usually occurs with

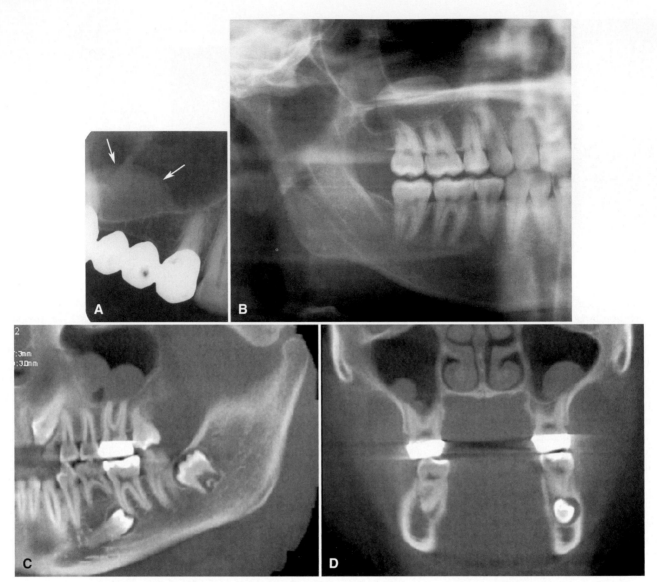

FIGURE 26-9 Noncorticated, dome-shaped retention pseudocyst *(arrows)* imaged on periapical **(A)**, panoramic **(B)**, reconstructed panoramic **(C)**, and coronal **(D)** CBCT images. Retention pseudocysts have noncorticated borders, indicating that they arise from within the sinus.

a thickened mucous membrane lining because the polypoid mass is no more than an accentuation of the mucosal thickening. In the case of a retention pseudocyst, the adjacent mucous membrane lining is not usually apparent. If multiple retention pseudocysts are seen within a sinus, the possibility of sinus polyposis should be considered.

The image of the bone displacement or destruction associated with polyps may mimic a benign or malignant neoplasm. Because many sinus neoplasms are asymptomatic, examination of a paranasal sinus that reveals bone destruction associated with increased radiopacity is an indication for additional imaging and biopsy; management should not be delayed by initial conservative treatment.

Antrolith

Disease Mechanism. Antroliths occur within the maxillary sinuses and are the result of deposition of mineral salts, such as calcium phosphate, calcium carbonate, and magnesium, around a nidus, which may be introduced into the sinus (extrinsic) or could be intrinsic such as masses of stagnant or inspissated mucus or cellular debris in sites of previous inflammation.

Clinical Features. Smaller antroliths are usually asymptomatic and discovered as incidental findings on imaging examination. If they continue to grow, the patient may have associated sinusitis, blood-stained nasal discharge, nasal obstruction, or facial pain.

Imaging Features

Location. Antroliths occur within the maxillary sinus and are positioned above the floor of the maxillary antrum in either periapical or panoramic images (Fig. 26-10).

Periphery and Shape. Antroliths have a well-defined periphery and may have a smooth or irregular shape.

Internal Structure. The internal aspect may vary from a barely perceptible radiopacity to an extremely radiopaque structure. The internal radiopacity may be homogeneous or heterogeneous. In some instances, alternating layers of radiolucency and radiopacity in the form of laminations may be seen.

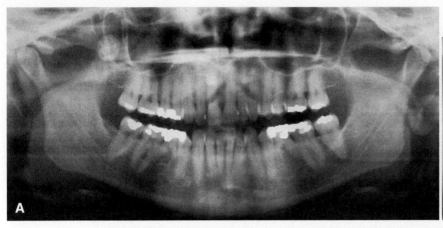
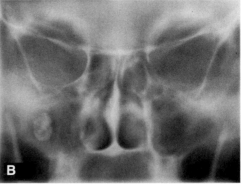

FIGURE 26-10 **A,** Alternating circular radiopaque and radiolucent pattern of an antrolith is seen on a panoramic image superimposed over the posterior wall of the right maxillary sinus. **B,** Coronal multidirectional tomographic image confirms the location of the antrolith within the sinus and shows the antrolith not to be attached to the adjacent sinus wall.

Differential Diagnosis. Antroliths may be distinguished from root fragments in the sinus by inspection of the mass for the usual root anatomy such as the presence of a root canal. A displaced root fragment in the sinus may move when imaging is performed with the head in different positions, unless it is lodged between the bone and the sinus lining. Rhinoliths are similar calcifications but are found within the nasal fossae. Posteroanterior and lateral skull views or advanced imaging can help identify the location of a rhinolith.

Management. An otolaryngologist may need to remove symptomatic antroliths.

Mucocele

Synonyms. Empyema, pyocele, and mucopyocele are synonyms for mucocele.

Disease Mechanism. A mucocele is an expanding, destructive lesion that results from a blocked sinus ostium. The blockage may result from intra-antral or intranasal inflammation, polyp, or neoplasm. The entire sinus becomes the pathologic cavity. As mucus secretions accumulate and the sinus cavity fills, the increase in pressure within the cavity results in thinning, displacement, and destruction of the sinus walls in some cases. When the cavity is filled with pus, it is termed an empyema, pyocele, or mucopyocele.

Clinical Features. A mucocele in the maxillary sinus may exert pressure on the superior alveolar nerves and cause radiating pain. The patient may first complain of a sensation of fullness in the cheek, and the area may swell. This swelling may first become apparent over the anteroinferior aspect of the antrum, the area where the wall is thin or destroyed. If the lesion expands inferiorly, it may cause loosening of the posterior teeth in the area. If the medial wall of the sinus is expanded, the lateral wall of the nasal cavity deforms, and the nasal airway may become obstructed. If the lesion expands into the orbit, it may cause diplopia (double vision) or proptosis (protrusion of the globe of the eye).

Imaging Features

Location. About 90% of mucoceles occur in the ethmoid air cells and frontal sinuses and rarely in the maxillary and sphenoid sinuses.

Periphery and Shape. The normal shape of the sinus is changed into a more circular, "hydraulic" shape as the mucocele enlarges.

Internal Structure. The internal aspect of the sinus cavity is uniformly radiopaque (Fig. 26-11, *A*).

Effects on Surrounding Structures. The shape of the sinus changes as its margins are displaced outward and the bone expands. Septa and the bony walls may be severely thinned. When the mucocele is associated with the maxillary antrum, teeth may be displaced or roots resorbed. In the frontal sinus, the usually scalloped border is smoothed by expansion, and any septum may be displaced (Fig. 26-11, *B*). The superomedial border of the orbit may be displaced or destroyed. In the ethmoid air cells, displacement of the lamina papyracea may occur, displacing the contents of the orbit. In the sphenoid sinus, the expansion may be in a superior direction, suggesting a pituitary neoplasm.

Differential Diagnosis. Although it may be impossible to distinguish between a mucocele in the maxillary antrum and a cyst or neoplasm, any suggestion that the lesion is associated with an occluded ostium should strengthen the likelihood of a mucocele. Blockage of the ostium is usually the result of a previous surgical procedure, although a deviated nasal septum or polyps may be a factor. A large odontogenic cyst displacing the maxillary antral floor may mimic a mucocele. One should look for any remnants of the internal aspect of the antrum between the wall of the cyst and the wall of the antrum. MDCT or CBCT imaging is the imaging method of choice for making these distinctions.

Management. Treatment of the mucocele is usually surgical, with a Caldwell-Luc operation to allow excision of the lesion. The prognosis is excellent.

NEOPLASMS

Benign neoplasms of the paranasal sinuses other than inflammatory polyps are rare. The imaging features of such benign neoplasms are nonspecific. Usually the involved portion of the sinus cavity appears radiopaque because of the presence of a mass, and there may be displacement of adjacent sinus borders.

The most common malignant neoplasms of the paranasal sinuses are squamous cell carcinomas and, to a lesser extent, malignant salivary gland neoplasms. Of carcinomas of the paranasal sinuses, 74% originate in the maxillary sinus. Although radiopacification is a

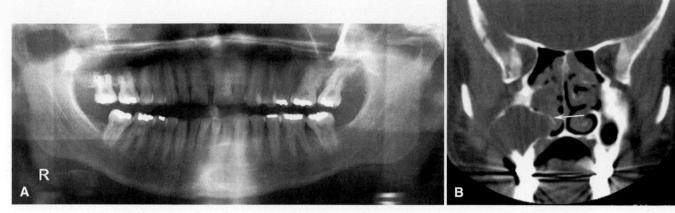

FIGURE 26-11 A mucocele has caused the radiopacification of the right maxillary sinus. **A,** Note the lack of a distinct border to the sinus on the panoramic image. **B,** Coronal MDCT image through the mucocele shows expansion into the nasal fossa *(arrow)* and the infratemporal fossa.

feature of both inflammatory conditions and neoplasms, bone destruction is more common with malignant neoplasms.

BENIGN NEOPLASMS OF THE PARANASAL SINUSES

Papilloma
Disease Mechanism. Epithelial papilloma is a rare neoplasm of respiratory epithelium that occurs in the nasal cavity and paranasal sinuses. It occurs predominantly in men.

Clinical Features. Unilateral nasal obstruction, nasal discharge, pain, and epistaxis may occur. The patient may have complained of recurring sinusitis for years and a subsequent nasal obstruction on the same side as the sinusitis. The epithelial papilloma, although benign, has a 10% incidence of associated carcinoma.

Imaging Features. Imaging features are nonspecific, and the diagnosis can be made only by histopathologic examination of the tissue.
    Location. The epithelial papilloma is usually in the ethmoidal or maxillary sinus. It may also appear as an isolated polyp in the nose or sinus.
    Internal Structure. This neoplasm appears as a homogeneous radiopaque mass of soft tissue density.
    Effects on Surrounding Structures. If bone destruction is apparent, it is the result of pressure erosion.

Osteoma
Disease Mechanism. The osteoma is the most common mesenchymal neoplasm in the paranasal sinuses. For a detailed description, see Chapter 22.

Clinical Features. Osteomas are almost twice as common in males compared with females and are most common in the second, third, and fourth decades. Most are usually slow growing and asymptomatic and are usually detected as an incidental finding in an examination performed for another purpose. When symptoms do occur, they are the result of obstruction of the sinus ostium or infundibulum or are the result of erosion or deformity, orbital involvement, or intracranial extension. Osteomas growing in the maxillary sinus may extend into the nose and cause nasal obstruction or a swelling of the side of the nose. They may expand the sinus and produce swelling of the cheek or hard palate. In cases extending to the orbit,

the patient may have proptosis. In some cases, external fistulas have developed. Osteomas of the maxillary sinus have been described after Caldwell-Luc operations.

Imaging Features
    Location. Although osteomas occasionally develop in the maxillary sinus, they more often occur in the frontal and ethmoidal sinuses. The incidence in the maxillary antrum ranges from 3.9% to 28.5% of the incidence in all paranasal sinuses.
    Periphery and Shape. An osteoma is usually lobulated or rounded and has a sharply defined margin (Fig. 26-12).
    Internal Structure. The internal aspect is homogeneous and extremely radiopaque.

Differential Diagnosis. The differential diagnosis includes antrolith, mycolith, teeth, odontomas, or odontogenic neoplasms, although these lesions are usually not as homogeneous in appearance as osteomas.

MALIGNANT NEOPLASMS OF THE PARANASAL SINUSES

Malignant neoplasms of the paranasal sinuses are exceptionally rare, accounting for less than 1% of all malignancies in the body. Squamous cell carcinoma accounts for 80% to 90% of the cancers in this site and is the most common primary malignant neoplasm of the paranasal sinuses. Other primary neoplasms include adenocarcinoma, carcinomas of salivary gland origin, soft and hard tissue sarcomas, melanoma, and malignant lymphoma. Factors that contribute to a poor prognosis for cancer of the paranasal sinuses include the advanced stage of the disease when it is finally diagnosed and the close proximity of vital anatomic structures. The clinical signs and symptoms may masquerade as an inflammatory sinusitis. The early primary lesions may appear only as a soft tissue mass in the sinus before they cause bone destruction. The lesion may become extensive, involving the entire sinus, with evidence of bone destruction before symptoms become apparent. Therefore, any unexplained radiopacity in the maxillary sinus of an individual older than 40 years should be investigated thoroughly.

Squamous Cell Carcinoma
Disease Mechanism. Squamous cell carcinoma likely originates from metaplastic epithelium of the sinus mucosal lining.

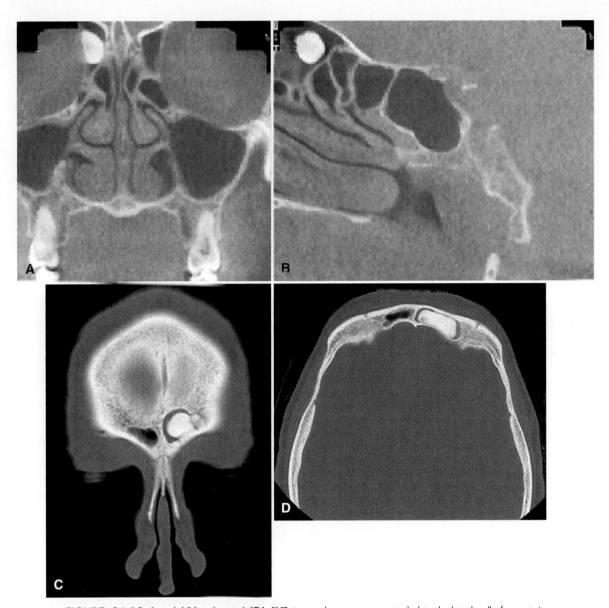

FIGURE 26-12 Coronal **(A)** and sagittal **(B)** CBCT images show an osteoma attached to the lateral wall of an anterior ethmoid air cell. Coronal **(C)** and axial **(D)** CT images of an osteoma in the frontal sinus. *(Courtesy Dr. Eugene Yu, Princess Margaret Hospital.)*

Clinical Features. The most common symptoms of cancer in the maxillary sinus are facial swelling, epistaxis, dysesthesia, paresthesia, nasal obstruction, and the presence of a lesion in the oral cavity. The mean patient age is 60 years (range, 25 to 89 years). Twice as many men as women are affected. Lymph nodes are involved in about 10% of cases, and symptoms are present for about 5 months before diagnosis.

The symptoms produced by malignant neoplasms in the maxillary sinus depend on which walls of the sinus are involved. The medial wall is usually the first to become eroded, leading to nasal signs and symptoms such as obstruction, discharge, bleeding, and pain. These symptoms may appear trivial, and their significance may be unappreciated. Lesions that arise on the floor of the sinus may first produce dental signs and symptoms, including enlargement of the alveolar process, unexplained pain and altered sensation of the teeth, loose teeth, swelling of the palate or alveolar ridge, and ill-fitting dentures. The neoplasm may erode the sinus floor and penetrate into the oral cavity. Such oral manifestations appear in 25% to 35% of patients with cancer in the maxillary sinus. When the lesion penetrates the lateral wall, facial and vestibular swelling becomes apparent, and the patient may complain of pain and hyperesthesia of the maxillary teeth. Involvement of the sinus roof and the floor of the orbit causes signs and symptoms related to the eye, including diplopia, proptosis, pain, and hyperesthesia or anesthesia and pain over the cheek and upper teeth. Invasion and penetration of the posterior wall lead to invasion of the muscles of mastication, causing painful trismus, obstruction of the eustachian tube causing a stuffy ear, and referred pain and hyperesthesia over the distribution of the second and third divisions of the fifth nerve.

Imaging Features. Sometimes the imaging findings, especially in early malignant disease of the paranasal sinuses, are nonspecific. It may be impossible to differentiate the early manifestations in

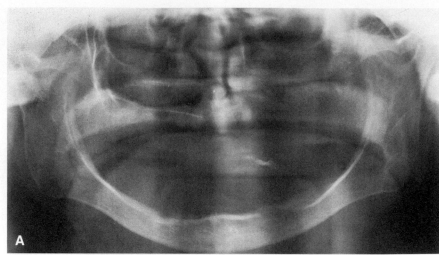

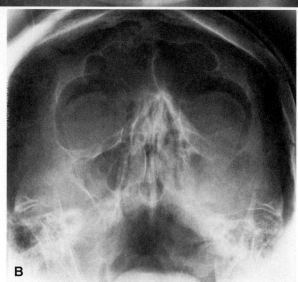

FIGURE 26-13 **A,** Panoramic image of a squamous cell carcinoma shows loss of definition of the cortex of the left maxillary sinus, nasal floor, and alveolar crest. **B,** Waters view of the same patient shows a similar loss of cortical integrity to the lateral wall of the left maxilla and radiopacification of the left maxillary sinus. *(Courtesy Dr. K. Dolan.)*

images of the maxillary sinus from the radiopacity of the sinus that develops in sinusitis and polyp formation. Evidence relies on changes seen in the surrounding bone, the sinus walls, and the maxillary alveolar process.

Location. Most carcinomas occur in the maxillary sinuses, but involvement of the frontal and sphenoid sinuses is also comparatively common.

Internal Structure. The internal aspect of the maxillary sinus has a soft tissue radiopaque appearance.

Effects on Surrounding Structures. As the lesion enlarges, it may destroy sinus walls and in general cause irregular radiolucent areas in the surrounding bone. A detailed examination of the adjacent alveolar process may reveal bone destruction around the teeth or irregular widening of the periodontal ligament space. Frequently, the medial wall of the maxillary sinus is thinned or destroyed, although there may also be destruction of the floor and anterior or posterior walls that may be detected in the panoramic film. The medial wall of the maxillary sinus is best seen on the Caldwell and Waters projections. In addition to loss of the medial wall, it may extend into the nasal cavity.

Additional Imaging. If a conventional image of any radiopacified sinus reveals the slightest suggestion of bone destruction, advanced

imaging, MDCT or MR imaging, is imperative; CBCT imaging is not the imaging modality of choice (Fig. 26-13). On MDCT imaging, the most characteristic sign of malignancy is invasion into the soft tissue facial planes beyond the sinus walls (Fig. 26-14). Consequently, MDCT imaging is useful in revealing the extent of paranasal sinus neoplasms, especially when extension into the orbit, infratemporal fossa, or cranial cavity has occurred. MRI examinations are excellent for revealing the extent of soft tissue penetration into adjacent structures and in differentiating mucus accumulation from the soft tissue mass of the neoplasm.

Differential Diagnosis. The differential diagnosis includes all the conditions that may cause radiopacity of the antrum, such as sinusitis, large retention pseudocysts, and odontogenic cysts. Bone destruction may also occur in infectious conditions and some benign conditions. Neoplasms should be suspected in any older patient in whom chronic sinusitis develops for the first time without an obvious cause.

Management. Treatment of squamous cell carcinoma in the paranasal sinuses may include radiation therapy, surgery, or a combination of the two. Malignant neoplasms in the paranasal sinuses usually have a poor prognosis because they are usually well

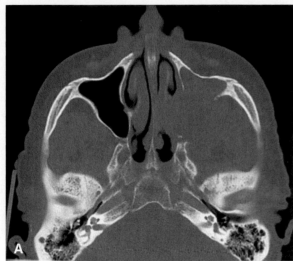

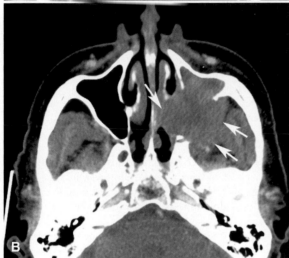

FIGURE 26-14 A, Axial bone algorithm CT image of a squamous cell carcinoma of the left maxillary sinus shows destruction of the posterolateral wall and the medial wall of the sinus. **B,** Same axial image slice with soft tissue algorithm demonstrates extension of the malignant neoplasm into the surrounding soft tissues *(arrows).*

advanced by the time of diagnosis. Other factors contributing to the poor prognosis include frequently inaccurate preoperative staging and the complex anatomy of the region.

Pseudotumor

Synonyms. Synonyms for pseudotumor include invasive fungal sinusitis, inflammatory pseudotumor, fibroinflammatory pseudotumor, plasma cell granuloma, sinonasal fungal disease, mucormycosis, aspergillosis, zygomycosis of the paranasal sinuses, and *Rhizopus* sinusitis.

Disease Mechanism. Pseudotumor is a descriptive name for a group of apparently related diseases of fungal origin that occur in the paranasal sinuses and in other parts of the head and neck.

Clinical Features. Pseudotumor often occurs after a series of recurrent infections. The symptoms may not be very specific. There may be recurring pain and a mass simulating a neoplasm. The latter may cause erosion of the walls of the involved sinus and proptosis if the orbit is involved. Altered nerve function resulting from

involvement of the nerve or occlusion of blood vessels by the mass has also been reported. Although cases have been reported in otherwise healthy individuals, many cases appear in patients who are immunocompromised or who have systemic diseases, such as diabetes mellitus, von Willebrand's disease, or myelodysplasia.

Imaging Features. The imaging findings in pseudotumor include masses simulating malignant neoplasms that cause erosion of bony walls of the involved sinuses.

Differential Diagnosis. The differential diagnosis includes benign and malignant neoplasms.

Management. The treatment of pseudotumor, which can include débridement of the sinuses by a Caldwell-Luc surgical approach, administration of antifungal medication, or other medicines, reflects the differences in the specific lesions included under the term pseudotumor of the sinuses, the exact location of the disease, the organism involved, and the medical status of the patient.

EXTRINSIC DISEASES INVOLVING THE PARANASAL SINUSES

INFLAMMATORY DISEASES

Perhaps 10% of inflammatory episodes of the maxillary sinuses are extensions of dental infections. Dental inflammatory lesions, such as periodontal disease or rarefying or sclerosing osteitis, may cause a localized mucositis in the adjacent floor of the maxillary antrum. This mucositis is a result of the diffusion of inflammatory exudate (mediators) beyond the cortical floor of the antrum and into the periosteum and the mucosal lining of the sinus. The localized type of mucositis related to dental inflammatory disease usually resolves in days or weeks after successful treatment of the underlying cause. This mucositis manifests as a homogeneous radiopaque, ribbon-shaped soft tissue that follows the contour of the maxillary sinus (see Fig. 26-5). The thickened mucosa is usually centered directly above the inflammatory lesion.

Periostitis and Periosteal New Bone Formation

Disease Mechanism. As previously described, the exudate from dental inflammatory lesions can diffuse through the cortical boundary of the antral floor. These products can strip and elevate the periosteal lining of the cortical bone of the floor of the maxillary antrum, stimulating the differentiation of pluripotential stem cells found within the cambium layer of the periosteum to produce an elevated thin layer of new bone adjacent to the root apex of the involved tooth (Fig. 26-15). The presence of one or more halo-like layers of new bone is a characteristic feature of inflammation of the periosteum.

Imaging Features. Although the periosteal tissue is not visible on the image per se, this process is referred to as periosteal new bone formation. This new bone may take the form of one or more thin radiopaque lines, or the line may be thick. This new bone should be centered directly above the inflammatory lesion.

BENIGN ODONTOGENIC CYSTS AND NEOPLASMS

The appearances and effects of benign odontogenic cysts and neoplasms on the maxillary sinuses may be similar. Odontogenic cysts are the most common group of extrinsic lesions that encroach

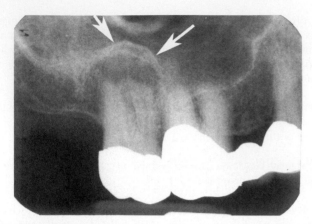

FIGURE 26-15 The halo-like appearance of bone surrounding the roots of a maxillary second molar is the result of periosteal new bone formation and displacement of the adjacent maxillary sinus floor *(arrows)*.

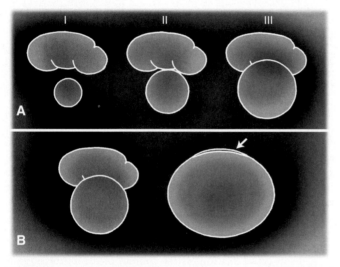

FIGURE 26-16 **A,** An odontogenic cyst or neoplasm develops adjacent to the floor of a sinus *(I)*. As the lesion enlarges, it abuts the maxillary sinus floor *(II)* and ultimately displaces the floor superiorly as it enlarges *(III)*. The border of the cyst and the border of the sinus are now the same line of bone. **B,** As it continues to enlarge, the lesion may encroach on almost all the space of the sinus, leaving a small saddle-like sinus over it *(arrow)*. The appearance may mimic sinusitis.

on the maxillary sinuses. The most common are radicular cysts and dentigerous cysts. Large cysts and neoplasms both can cause facial deformity, nasal obstruction, and displacement or loosening of teeth. For detailed descriptions of specific odontogenic cysts and neoplasms, see Chapters 21 and 22, respectively. Some odontogenic neoplasms, particularly ameloblastoma and myxoma, purportedly show a more aggressive pattern of growth in the maxilla because of the richer blood supply in the maxilla compared with the mandible and their closer proximities to vital structures in the skull base. Management of such neoplasms in the maxilla is often more aggressive than in cases involving the mandible.

As the cyst or neoplasm grows, its border becomes indistinguishable from the sinus border. With continued growth, the lesion encroaches on the space of the sinus and displaces its borders, and the air-filled space decreases in volume (Fig. 26-16). A thin radiopaque line divides the contents of the cyst from the sinus cavity. This appearance is in contrast to a retention

pseudocyst, which, being inside the sinus, does not have a cortex around its periphery.

Imaging Features

Periphery and Shape. The enlarging cyst or neoplasm can have a curved, oval, or "hydraulic" shape with cysts and with a corticated border. Both groups of lesions may have well-defined, thin cortical borders, although more aggressively growing lesions may lack areas of corticated.

Internal Structure. The internal structure of the cyst is homogeneous and radiopaque relative to the air-filled sinus cavity. Some neoplasms may also develop fine or coarse internal septation and appear multilocular or have regions of dystrophic calcification, depending on the histopathologic nature of the neoplasm. In some instances, the degree of radiopacity may mimic bone because of the extreme contrast to the radiolucent air within the sinus. Advanced imaging may be particularly useful in such situations to differentiate the area of increased radiopacity from bone.

Effects on Surrounding Structures. Both odontogenic cysts and neoplasms may displace the floor of the maxillary antrum and cause thinning of the peripheral cortex. These lesions may enlarge to the point where they almost completely encroach on the sinus air space. This residual air space may appear as a thin saddle over the cyst or neoplasm (see Fig. 26-16).

Differential Diagnosis

An antral loculation occasionally may have a round shape and sometimes appear to have a cortex. However, because the loculation contains air, which is more radiolucent than the fluid within a cyst, the loculation appears as, or more, radiolucent as the surrounding sinus.

Odontogenic cysts, in particular, must be differentiated from the common retention pseudocyst. Although odontogenic cysts may have a shape that is similar to that of a retention pseudocyst, only an odontogenic cyst demonstrates a peripheral cortex (Fig. 26-17). If the odontogenic cyst were to become infected, the cortex may be thickened, developing a sclerotic periphery or may be lost. Should the cortex become lost, it may be difficult to determine whether the lesion has arisen from outside or from within the sinus. However, in most cases, careful scrutiny of the lesion reveals some remaining cyst cortex, and the relationship to neighboring teeth may help to make this decision (Fig. 26-18). It may be difficult to differentiate a dentigerous cyst from a keratocystic odontogenic tumor if the latter develops in a pericoronal relationship to a tooth. Locating the association of the lesion with a tooth's cementoenamel junction on an advanced imaging examination may aid in the differentiation.

Very large cysts or neoplasms may completely efface the sinus cavity. When this occurs, little or no imaging evidence may exist of the air space left, and it may appear as if the cyst has developed within the sinus. In this case, because of the radiopacity of the cyst, the appearance may resemble sinusitis with radiopacification of the sinus. Evaluation of such a situation is aided by locating a region where both the displaced sinus floor and the unaffected sinus wall meet—the so-called double cortex (see Fig. 26-17, *C*). Additionally, noting that the wall of the cyst often has a more "hydraulic" shape than the wall of the sinus or the presence of normal vascular markings on the wall of the maxillary sinus that are not present on the walls of a cyst may be useful. A cyst that occupies the entire sinus usually causes expansion of the

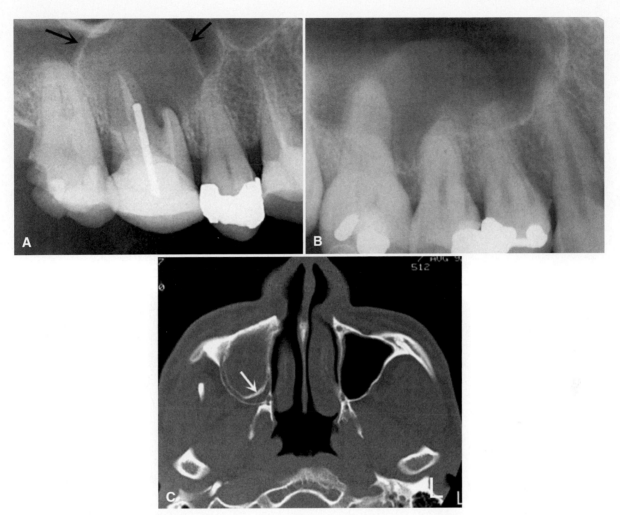

FIGURE 26-17 A, Periapical image of a small radicular cyst; note the peripheral cortex *(arrows)*. **B,** Periapical image of a pseudocyst; note the lack of a peripheral cortex. **C,** Axial CT image of a large radicular cyst; note the peripheral cortex *(arrow)* inside the outer cortex of the sinus.

medial wall (middle meatus) of the sinus and alters the sigmoid contour of the posterolateral wall of the sinus as viewed in axial CT images.

With or sometimes without treatment, an odontogenic cyst involving the sinus may "collapse" and heal. The end result is the appearance of an irregularly shaped bone formation with a radiolucent center projecting from the floor of the sinus (see Chapter 21). This bone formation should be differentiated from a bone-forming neoplasm, such as an osteoma or ossifying fibroma.

BONE DYSPLASIAS

Periapical and florid osseous dysplasias, when developing near the root apices of the maxillary premolar and molar teeth, behave in much the same way radiographically as benign cysts or neoplasms (Fig. 26-19). Fibrous dysplasia may arise adjacent to any of the paranasal sinuses, cause expansion of the bone, and cause displacement of sinus borders, which can result in a smaller sinus on the affected side. For a detailed description of bone dysplasias, see Chapter 23.

Clinical Features

The involvement of the facial skeleton with fibrous dysplasia can result in facial asymmetry, nasal obstruction, proptosis, pituitary gland compression, impingement on cranial nerves, or sinus obliteration. Sinus obliteration results when the expanding dysplastic bone encroaches on it. The lesion may displace the roots of teeth and cause teeth to separate or migrate, but it usually does not cause root resorption. Fibrous dysplasia is more common in children and young adults, and growth of the dysplastic bone usually ceases at the age of skeletal maturity.

Imaging Features

Location. The posterior maxilla is the most common location for fibrous dysplasia.

Periphery. The lesion itself is usually not well defined, tending to blend into the surrounding bone. The external cortex of the bone and the sinus border are intact but displaced.

Internal Structure. The normal radiolucent maxillary sinus may be partially or totally replaced by the increased radiopacity of this lesion. The degree of radiopacity depends on its stage of development and the relative amounts of bone and fibrous tissue present. Usually the radiopaque areas have a uniform characteristic ground-glass appearance on extraoral images or an orange-peel appearance on intraoral views (Fig. 26-20).

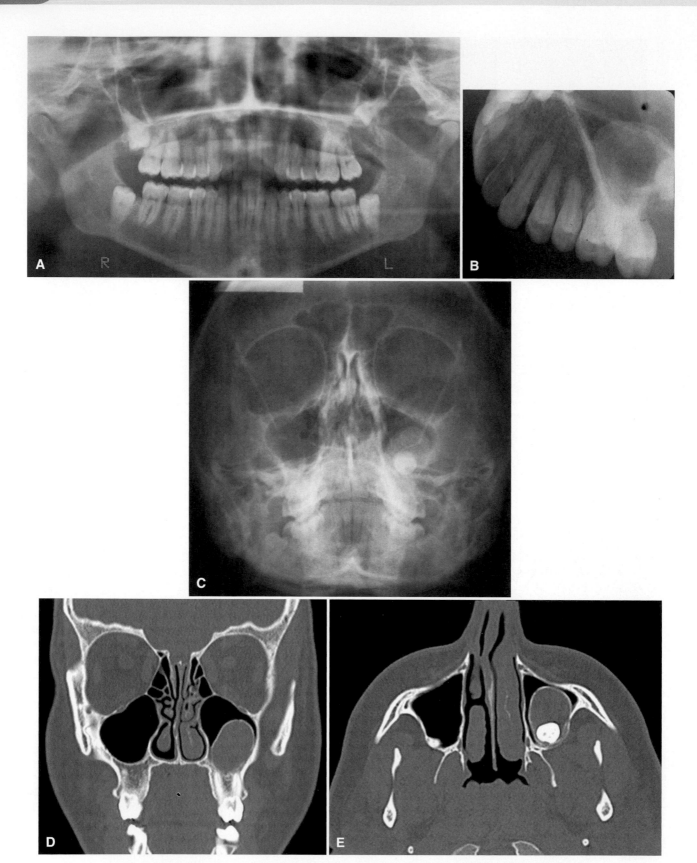

FIGURE 26-18 Series of images showing displacement of the left maxillary sinus floor as a result of a developing dentigerous cyst associated with the maxillary left third molar. **A-C,** The corticated periphery of the cyst is well seen in the panoramic **(A)**, occlusal **(B)**, and Waters **(C)** images. **D,** Coronal CT image shows the displaced floor of the left maxillary sinus. **E,** Axial image shows the bowing of the posterior sinus wall and the impacted tooth adjacent to it.

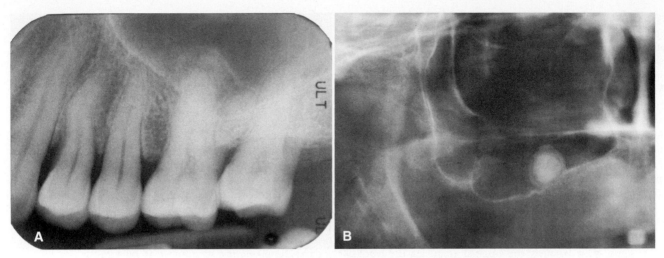

FIGURE 26-19 **A,** Periapical radiograph demonstrates elevation of the maxillary sinus floor by a focus of periapical osseous dysplasia located at the apices of the maxillary left first molar. **B,** Cropped panoramic image reveals a small region of osseous dysplasia invaginating into the inferior aspect of the sinus. Note the thin soft tissue capsule and cortex at the periphery.

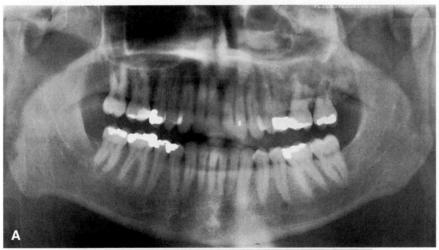

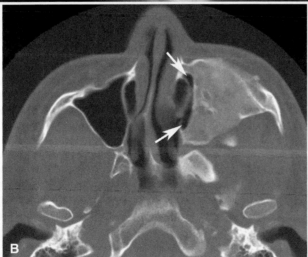

FIGURE 26-20 **A,** Panoramic image of involvement of the left maxillary sinus with fibrous dysplasia; note the radiopacification of the left maxillary sinus compared with the right sinus. **B,** Axial CT image of the same case reveals almost complete encroachment on the sinus; a small medial segment remains *(arrows)*. Note the very fine homogeneous bone pattern of fibrous dysplasia.

Effects on Surrounding Structures. Fibrous dysplasia may expand the alveolar process superiorly, elevating the orbital floor inferiorly and causing asymmetry of the alveolar process medially, facially, or posterolaterally. The new bone also may encroach on the dimensions of the air cavity causing it appear smaller in size but maintaining a resemblance of a normal shape.

Differential Diagnosis

The diagnosis of fibrous dysplasia in a relatively young person is usually not difficult. In contrast, Paget's disease of bone does not usually obliterate the sinus. Ossifying fibroma, which may have an appearance that is similar to fibrous dysplasia, may have a soft tissue capsule and may be more expansile. In some cases, however, the differential diagnosis of ossifying fibroma involving the antrum and fibrous dysplasia can be difficult. In fibrous dysplasia, the shape of the dysplastic bone encroaching on the internal aspect of the sinus often parallels the original shape of the external walls resulting in a smaller sinus but maintaining a similar shape (Fig. 26-21).

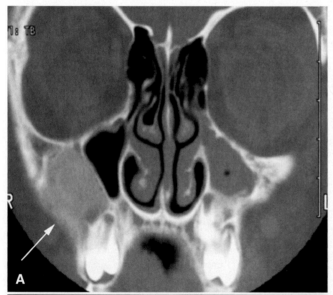

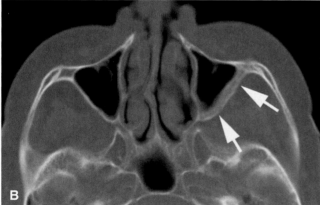

FIGURE 26-21 **A,** Coronal CT image using bone algorithm of fibrous dysplasia involving the right lateral wall of the maxilla *(arrow)* and causing parallel thickening into the sinus but leaving a relatively normal miniature shape of a sinus. **B,** Axial CT image using bone algorithm of the superior extent of a fibrous dysplasia lesion involving the posterior lateral wall of the sinus *(arrows)*. The fibrous dysplasia caused parallel thickening of the wall compared with the left side.

DENTAL STRUCTURES DISPLACED INTO THE SINUSES
Mechanism

Tooth roots may be fractured from various forms of trauma, including iatrogenic causes. They may be displaced into the sinus during extraction or subsequent attempts to retrieve them.

Clinical Features

No specific features may be visible if the root was displaced into the sinus recently. However, the dentist may note the absence of the root fragment on examining the extracted tooth and may be unable to locate it anywhere else. Sometimes asking the patient to hold his or her nose while attempting to breathe out through it, similar to a Valsalva maneuver, causes bubbles to appear within the blood contained within the fresh extraction socket. If the patient has had the root or tooth in the sinus for a number of days, the presenting symptom may be sinusitis (see the previous discussion on sinusitis).

Imaging Features

Location. Premolar or molar teeth or root fragments may be displaced into the sinus because of their proximity. These may be found anywhere within the sinus, but more often they are located near the floor of the sinus because of gravity (Fig. 26-22, *A*). Sometimes they may be submucosal, between the osseous wall of the sinus and the mucoperiosteum. Lateral maxillary occlusal views are useful for examining the maxillary sinus for displaced teeth or root fragments. Other images made along a different projection axis, such as a Waters view, may help in the three-dimensional localization.

Periphery and Shape. No immediate evidence of change may be appreciated in the sinus, even when an oroantral fistula has been created. The disruption of the sinus wall may be difficult or impossible to see on images if it is not in the mesial, distal, or superior (apical) part of the alveolar process.

Internal Structure. In the early stages, no internal structural changes are present except that the dental fragment may appear as a radiopaque mass of a size corresponding to the missing tooth or tooth root fragment.

Effects on Surrounding Structures. The dental fragment usually has no effect on surrounding structures; however, a sinusitis may result (see changes described earlier in this chapter under sinusitis). A break in the floor of the maxillary sinus caused by the displacement of the tooth or fragment into the sinus may be present but difficult to appreciate.

Differential Diagnosis

Bony masses that represent hyperostosis of the sinus wall or floor or septa within the sinus may mimic dental root fragments or even whole teeth (Fig. 26-22, *C*). Antroliths may also have a similar appearance. The shape of the radiopacity or the presence of a pulp canal or layer of enamel may help in the differential diagnosis. It may also be possible to displace the tooth fragment by having the patient move the head abruptly between views. If the root tip remains in its socket, it may be superimposed over the maxillary sinus, but the presence of a lamina dura and periodontal ligament space indicates a position within the alveolar process (Fig. 26-22, *B*).

The displaced tooth or root fragment may be subperiosteal and interior to the osseous wall of the sinus but not within the antral

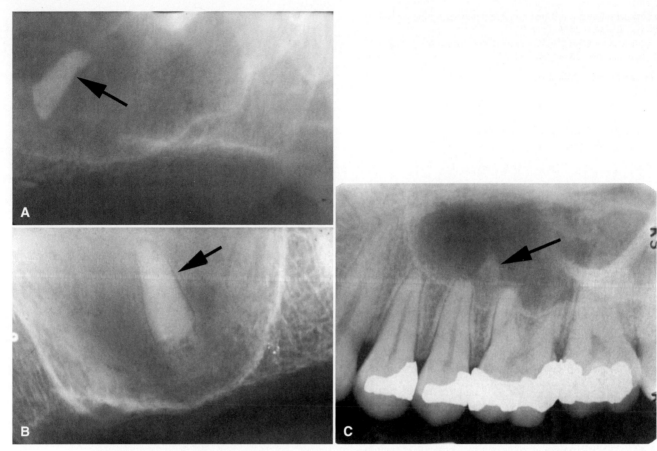

FIGURE 26-22 **A,** Periapical image revealing the presence of a portion of tooth root *(arrow)* within the maxillary sinus. **B,** Another periapical image of a retained root tip outside the sinus, but its image is superimposed over the sinus *(arrow)*. The presence of a periodontal membrane space indicates that it is in the alveolar process and not in the sinus. **C,** Periapical image of a region of hyperostosis *(arrow)* emanating from the floor of the maxillary sinus and mimicking the shape of a root tip.

lumen. Alternatively, the root may have been forced out of the socket into the surrounding bone, into the submucosal space, or into surrounding anatomic space such as the infratemporal space. Another possibility is for the fragment to be displaced into a cyst that was preoperatively mistaken for a loculus of the sinus cavity. Use of images at different angles should help localize the dental structure.

Management

Management ranges from follow-up with the patient to see whether a small root tip will be removed from the sinus through the ostium by ciliary action to entering the sinus surgically by a Caldwell-Luc procedure to remove the dental structure. Sinusitis may develop and should be managed with the appropriate treatment.

For other trauma involving the paranasal sinuses, see Chapter 30.

BIBLIOGRAPHY

Normal Development and Variations

Dodd GD, Jing BS: *Radiology of the nose, paranasal sinus and nasopharynx*, Baltimore, 1977, Williams & Wilkins.
DuBrul EL: *Sicher's oral anatomy*, ed 7, St Louis, 1980, Mosby.
Grant JCB: *A method of anatomy*, Baltimore, 1958, Williams & Wilkins.
Hengerer AS: Embryonic development of the sinuses, *Ear Nose Throat J* 63:134–136, 1984.

Karmody CS, Carter B, Vincent ME: Developmental anomalies of the maxillary sinus, *Trans Sect Otolaryngol Am Acad Ophthalmol Otolaryngol* 84:723–728, 1977.
Lusted LB, Keats TE: *Atlas of roentgenographic measurement*, ed 3, Chicago, 1972, Year Book Medical Publishers.
Ritter FN: *The paranasal sinuses: anatomy and surgical technique*, St Louis, 1973, Mosby.
Scuderi AJ, Harnsberger HR, Boyer RS: Pneumatization of the paranasal sinuses: normal features of importance to the accurate interpretation of CT scans and MR images, *AJR Am J Roentgenol* 160:1101–1104, 1993.
Shapiro R: *Radiology of the normal skull*, Chicago, 1981, Year Book Medical Publishers.
Som PM: The paranasal sinuses. In Bergeron RT, Osborn AG, Som PM, editors: *Head and neck imaging: excluding the brain*, St Louis, 1984, Mosby.
Takahashi R: The formation of the human paranasal sinuses, *Acta Otolaryngol Suppl (Stockh)* 408:1–28, 1984.

Applied Diagnostic Imaging

Lloyd GA: Diagnostic imaging of the nose and paranasal sinuses, *J Laryngol Otol* 103:453–460, 1989.
Zinreich SJ: Imaging of chronic sinusitis in adults: x-ray, computed tomography, and magnetic resonance imaging, *J Allergy Clin Immunol* 90:445–451, 1992.

Inflammatory Changes

Nurbakhsh B, Friedman S, Kulkarni GV, et al: Resolution of maxillary sinus mucositis after endodontic treatment of maxillary teeth with apical periodontitis: a cone-beam computerized tomography pilot study, *J Endod* 37:1504–1511, 2011.

Robinson K: Roentgenographic manifestations of benign paranasal disease, *Ear Nose Throat J* 63:144, 1984.

Thickened Mucous Membrane
Mucositis

Dolan K, Smoker W: Paranasal sinus radiology. Part 4A: maxillary sinuses, *Head Neck Surg* 5:345–362, 1983.

Killey HC, Kay LA: *The maxillary sinus and its dental implications*, Bristol, 1975, John Wright.

Periostitis
Sinusitis

Druce HM: Diagnosis and medical management of recurrent and chronic sinusitis in adults. In Gershwin ME, Incaudo GA, editors: *Diseases of the sinuses*, Ottawa, Canada, 1996, Humana Press.

Fireman P: Diagnosis of sinusitis in children: emphasis on the history and physical examination, *J Allergy Clin Immunol* 90:433–436, 1992.

Incaudo G, Gershwin ME, Nagy SM: The pathophysiology and treatment of sinusitis, *Allergol Immunopathol (Madr)* 14:423–434, 1986.

Kennedy DW: First-line management of sinusitis: a national problem? Surgical update, *Otolaryngol Head Neck Surg* 103:884–886, 1990.

Killey HC, Kay LA: *The maxillary sinus and its dental implications*, Bristol, 1975, John Wright.

Palacios E, Valvassori G: Computed axial tomography in otorhinolaryngology, *Adv Otorhinolaryngol* 24:1–8, 1978.

Paparella MM: Mucosal cyst of the maxillary sinus, *Arch Otolaryngol* 77:650–670, 1963.

Poyton HG: Maxillary sinuses and the oral radiologist, *Dent Radiogr Photogr* 45:43–50, 1972.

Reilly JS: The sinusitis cycle, *Otolaryngol Head Neck Surg* 103:856–861, 1990.

Shapiro GG, Rachelefsky GS: Introduction and definition of sinusitis, *J Allergy Clin Immunol* 90:417–418, 1992.

Zinreich SJ: Imaging of chronic sinusitis in adults: x-ray, computed tomography, and magnetic resonance imaging, *J Allergy Clin Immunol* 90:445–451, 1992.

Empyema

Ash JE, Raum M: *An atlas of otolaryngic pathology*, New York, 1956, American Registry of Pathology.

Groves J, Gray RF: *A synopsis of otolaryngology*, Bristol, 1985, John Wright.

Polyps

Potter GD: Inflammatory disease of the paranasal sinuses. In Valvassori GE, Potter GD, Hanefee WN, editors: *Radiology of the ear, nose and throat*, Philadelphia, 1982, Saunders.

Retention Pseudocysts

Allard RH, van der Kwast WA, van der Waal JI: Mucosal antral cysts: review of the literature and report of a radiographic survey, *Oral Surg Oral Med Oral Pathol* 51:2–9, 1981.

Dolan K, Smoker W: Paranasal sinus radiology. Part 4A: maxillary sinuses, *Head Neck Surg* 5:345–362, 1983.

Gothberg K, Little JW, King DR, et al: A clinical study of cysts arising from mucosa of the maxillary sinus, *Oral Surg* 41:52–58, 1976.

Hardy G: Benign cysts of the antrum, *Ann Otol Rhinol Laryngol* 48:649, 1939.

Kadymova MI: Lymphangiectatic (false) cysts of the maxillary sinuses and their relation with allergy, *Vestib Otorhinolaringol* 28:58, 1966.

Kaffe I, Littner MM, Moskona D: Mucosal-antral cysts: radiographic appearance and differential diagnosis, *Clin Prev Dent* 10:3–6, 1988.

McGregor GW: Formation and histologic structure of cysts of the maxillary sinus, *Arch Otolaryngol* 8:505, 1928.

Mills CP: Secretory cysts of the maxillary antrum and their relationship to the development of antrochoanal polypi, *J Laryngol Otol* 73:324–334, 1959.

Poyton HG: *Oral radiology*, Baltimore, 1982, Williams & Wilkins.

Ruprecht A, Batniji S, el-Neweihi E: Mucous retention cyst of the maxillary sinus, *Oral Surg Oral Med Oral Pathol* 62:728–731, 1986.

Shafer WG, Hine MK, Levy BM: *A textbook of oral pathology*, ed 4, Philadelphia, 1983, Saunders.

van Norstrand AWP, Goodman WS: Pathologic aspects of mucosal lesions of the maxillary sinus, *Otolaryngol Clin North Am* 9:21–34, 1976.

Mucocele

Atherino C, Atherino T: Maxillary sinus mucopyoceles, *Arch Otolaryngol* 110:200, 1984.

Jones JL, Kaufman PW: Mucopyocele of the maxillary sinus, *J Oral Surg* 39:948, 1981.

Zizmor JK, Noyek AM: The radiologic diagnosis of maxillary sinus disease, *Otolaryngol Clin North Am* 9:93, 1976.

Odontogenic Cysts

Killey HC, Kay LA: *The maxillary sinus and its dental implications*, Bristol, 1975, John Wright.

Poyton H: Maxillary sinuses and the oral radiologist, *Dent Radiogr Photogr* 45:43–50, 1972.

Van Alyea OE: *Nasal sinuses*, Baltimore, 1951, Williams & Wilkins.

Odontogenic Keratocysts

MacDonald-Jankowski DS: The involvement of the maxillary antrum by odontogenic keratocysts, *Clin Radiol* 45:31–33, 1992.

Neoplasms

Goepfert H, Luna MA, Lindberg RD, et al: Malignant salivary gland tumors of the paranasal sinuses and nasal cavity, *Arch Otolaryngol* 109:662–668, 1983.

St-Pierre S, Baker SR: Squamous cell carcinoma of the maxillary sinus: analysis of 66 cases, *Head Neck Surg* 5:508–513, 1983.

Epithelial Papilloma

Rogers JH, Fredrickson JM, Noyek AM: Management of cysts, benign tumors, and bony dysplasia of the maxillary sinus, *Otolaryngol Clin North Am* 9:233–247, 1976.

Osteoma

Dolan K, Smoker W: Paranasal sinus radiology. Part 4B: maxillary sinuses, *Head Neck Surg* 5:428–446, 1983.

Goodnight J, Dulguerov P, Abemayor E: Calcified mucor fungus ball of the maxillary sinus, *Am J Otolaryngol* 14:209–210, 1993.

Reuben BM: Odontoma of the maxillary sinus: a case report, *Quintessence Int Dent Dig* 14:287–290, 1983.

Samy LL, Mostofa H: Osteoma of the nose and paranasal sinuses with a report of twenty-one cases, *J Laryngol Otol* 85:449–469, 1971.

Ameloblastoma

Hames RS, Rakoff SJ: Diseases of the maxillary sinus, *J Oral Med* 27:90–95, 1972.

Reaume C, Wesley RK, Jung B, et al: Ameloblastoma of the maxillary sinus, *J Oral Surg* 38:520–521, 1980.

Malignant Neoplasms of the Paranasal Sinuses

Batsakis JG: *Tumors of the head and neck*, ed 2, Baltimore, 1979, Williams & Wilkins.

St-Pierre S, Baker S: Squamous cell carcinoma of the maxillary sinus: analysis of 66 cases, *Head Neck Surg* 5:508–513, 1983.

Zizmor J, Noyek AM: Cysts, benign tumors and malignant tumors of the paranasal sinuses, *Otolaryngol Clin North Am* 6:487–508, 1973.

Squamous Cell Carcinoma

Batsakis JG, Rice DH, Solomon AR: The pathology of head and neck tumors: squamous and mucous-gland carcinomas of the nasal cavity, paranasal sinuses and larynx. Part 6, *Head Neck Surg* 2:497–508, 1980.

Bridger M, Beale F, Bryce D: Carcinoma of the paranasal sinuses: a review of 158 cases, *J Otolaryngol* 7:379–388, 1978.

Eddleston B, Johnson R: A comparison of conventional radiographic imaging and computed tomography in malignant disease of the paranasal sinuses and the post-nasal space, *Clin Radiol* 34:161–172, 1983.

Hasso AN: CT of tumors and tumor-like conditions of the paranasal sinuses, *Radiol Clin North Am* 22:119–130, 1984.

Larheim TA, Kolbenstvedt A, Lien H: Carcinoma of maxillary sinus, palate and maxillary gingiva, occurrence of jaw destruction, *Scand J Dent Res* 92:235–240, 1984.

Lund VJ, Howard DJ, Lloyd GA: CT evaluation of paranasal sinus tumors for cranio-facial resection, *Br J Radiol* 56:439–446, 1983.

Mancuso A, Hanafee WN, Winter J, et al: Extensions of paranasal sinus tumors and inflammatory disease: an evaluation by CT and pluridirectional tomography, *Neuroradiology* 16:449–453, 1978.

St-Pierre S, Baker SR: Squamous cell carcinoma of the maxillary sinus: analysis of 66 cases, *Head Neck Surg* 5:508–513, 1983.

Thomas GK, Kasper KA: Ossifying fibroma of the frontal bone, *Arch Otolaryngol* 83:43–46, 1966.

Tsaknis PJ, Nelson JF: The maxillary ameloblastoma: an analysis of 24 cases, *J Oral Surg* 38:336–342, 1980.

Weber A, Tadmore R, Davis R, et al: Malignant tumors of the sinuses: radiologic evaluation, including CT scanning, with clinical and pathologic correlation, *Neuroradiology* 16:113–118, 1978.

Pseudotumor

Butugan O, Sanchez TG, Gonçalez F, et al: Rhinocerebral mucormycosis: predisposing factors, diagnosis, therapy, complications and survival, *Rev Laryngol Otol Rhinol (Bord)* 117:53, 1996.

Del Valle Zapico A, Rubio Suárez A, Mellado Encinas A, et al: Mucormycosis of the sphenoid sinus in an otherwise healthy patient: case report and literature review, *J Laryngol Otol* 110:471–473, 1996.

Ishida M, Taya N, Noiri T, et al: Five cases of mucormycosis in paranasal sinuses, *Acta Otolaryngol* 501(Suppl):92–96, 1993.

Lee BL, Holland GN, Glasgow BJ: Chiasmal infarction and sudden blindness caused by mucormycosis in AIDS and diabetes mellitus, *Am J Ophthalmol* 122:895–896, 1996.

Muzaffar M, Hussain SI, Chughtai A: Plasma cell granuloma: maxillary sinuses, *J Laryngol Otol* 108:357–358, 1994.

Ng TT, Campbell CK, Rothera M, et al: Successful treatment of sinusitis caused by Cunninghamella bertholetiae, *Clin Infect Dis* 19:313–316, 1994.

Ozhan S, Araç M, Isik S, et al: Pseudotumor of the maxillary sinus in a patient with von Willebrand's disease, *AJR Am J Roentgenol* 166:950–951, 1996.

Perolada Valmana JM, Morera Perez C, Blanes Julia M, et al: Mucormycosis of the paranasal sinuses, *Rev Laryngol Otol Rhinol (Bord)* 117:51–52, 1996.

Som PM, Brandwein MS, Maldjian C, et al: Inflammatory pseudotumor of the maxillary sinus: CT and MR findings in six cases, *AJR Am J Roentgenol* 163:689–692, 1994.

Tkatch LS, Kusne S, Eibling D: Successful treatment of zygomycosis of the paranasal sinuses with surgical debridement and amphotericin B colloidal dispersion, *Am J Otolaryngol* 14:249–253, 1993.

Utas C, Unlühizarci K, Okten T, et al: Acute renal failure associated with rhinosinuso-orbital mucormycosis infection in a patient with diabetic nephropathy [letter], *Nephron* 71:235, 1995.

Zapater E, Armengot M, Campos A, et al: Invasive fungal sinusitis in immunosuppressed patients: report of three cases, *Acta Otorhinolaryngol Belg* 50:137–142, 1996.

Fibrous Dysplasia

Malcolmson KG: Ossifying fibroma of the sphenoid, *J Laryngol Otol* 81:87–92, 1967.

Thomas GK, Kasper KA: Ossifying fibroma of the frontal bone, *Arch Otolaryngol* 83:43–46, 1966.

Wong A, Vaughan CW, Strong MS: Fibrous dysplasia of temporal bone, *Arch Otolaryngol* 81:131–133, 1965.

OUTLINE

DISEASE MECHANISM

Disorders of the temporomandibular joint (TMJ) include all abnormalities that interfere with the normal form or function of the TMJ. These disorders include developmental abnormalities that can result in an abnormal form of the osseous or soft tissue structures of the joint. Other disorders are acquired, such as dysfunction of the articular disc and associated ligaments and muscles, joint arthritides, inflammatory lesions, trauma, and neoplasms.

CLINICAL FEATURES

A wide variety of conditions can cause TMJ disorders that manifest with an extensive assortment of clinical features. Dysfunction of the joint is the most common disorder and is most likely to manifest with pain in the TMJ or ear or both, headache, muscle tenderness, joint stiffness, clicking or other joint noises, reduced range of motion, locking, and subluxation. Careful clinical assessment can help identify which structures are likely contributing to the joint dysfunction. For instance, pain to palpation of the muscles of mastication and headaches suggest a myofascial pain disorder, clicking or popping sounds in the joint and locking or reduced range of motion are often associated with disc abnormalities, and crepitus and pain over the joint itself commonly indicate arthritic involvement. A higher incidence of joint dysfunction has been reported in females, especially in their reproductive years, although the reason for this preponderance is unclear. In most cases, the clinical signs and symptoms are transitory, and often treatment is not indicated beyond patient reassurance and education. However, a small percentage (5%) of patients has severe dysfunction (e.g., severe pain, marked functional impairment, or both), which

requires a thorough diagnostic workup, including diagnostic imaging, before treatment.

Other disorders of the TMJ are less common. A neoplasm may manifest with swelling of the joint region, whereas redness and heat over the joint may indicate an inflammatory lesion. Developmental abnormalities are most likely to be unilateral and manifest with facial asymmetry. Changes in occlusion may also be a sign of an abnormality in one or both of the TMJs.

IMAGING ANATOMY OF THE TEMPOROMANDIBULAR JOINT

A thorough understanding of the anatomy and morphology of the TMJ is essential so that a normal variant is not mistaken for an abnormality. Each joint is formed by articulating components of the mandible and temporal bones. The TMJs are unique because although they constitute two separate joints anatomically, they function together as a single unit as the mandibular components are part of one bone. An articular disc composed of fibrocartilage is interposed between the osseous structures of each joint. Retrodiscal tissues help maintain the normal position of the disc. A fibrous capsule lined with synovial membrane surrounds and encloses the joint. The synovial tissue is present on non–force-bearing surfaces and secretes synovial fluid, which lubricates the joint. The muscles of mastication allow movement of the condyle, whereas ligaments limit the extent of movement.

MANDIBULAR COMPONENT

The mandibular condyle forms the mandibular component of the TMJ. The condyle is a bony ellipsoid structure connected to the mandibular ramus by a narrow neck (Fig. 27-1). The condyle is approximately 20 mm long mediolaterally and 8 to 10 mm thick anteroposteriorly. The shape of the condyle varies considerably; the superior aspect may be flattened, rounded, or markedly convex, whereas the mediolateral contour usually is slightly convex. These variations in shape may cause difficulty with radiographic interpretation; this underlines the importance of understanding the range of normal appearance (Fig. 27-2). The extreme ends of the condyle are called the medial and lateral poles. The long axis of the condyle

is formed between these poles and is slightly rotated on the condylar neck so that the medial pole is angled posteriorly, forming an angle of 15 to 33 degrees with the sagittal plane. The two condylar axes typically intersect near the anterior border of the foramen magnum in the axial or horizontal plane of the skull.

Most condyles have a pronounced ridge oriented mediolaterally on the anterior surface, marking the anteroinferior limit of the articulating area. This ridge is the upper limit of the pterygoid fovea, a small depression on the anterior surface at the junction of the condyle and condylar neck, which is the attachment site of the superior head of the lateral pterygoid muscle. The ridge should not be mistaken for an osteophyte (spur), which is a sign of degenerative joint disease (DJD).

Although the mandibular and temporal components of the TMJ are calcified by 6 months of age, complete calcification of cortical borders may not be completed until 20 years of age. As a result, radiographs of condyles in children may show little or no evidence of a cortical border. In the absence of disease, the cortical borders in adults are visible in the diagnostic image. However, a layer of fibrocartilage covering the condyle is not visible.

TEMPORAL COMPONENT

The articular component of the temporal bone is formed by the inferior aspect of the squamous process. It is composed of the glenoid or mandibular fossa posteriorly and the articular eminence and tubercle anteriorly (Fig. 27-3). Similar to the condyle, the mandibular fossa is covered with a thin layer of fibrocartilage. The posterior surface of the articular eminence is convex in shape, and its most inferior aspect is called the summit or apex. In a normal TMJ, the roof of the fossa, the posterior slope of the articular

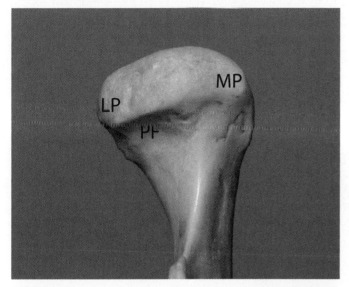

FIGURE 27-1 Anterior view of the mandibular condyle. *LP,* Lateral pole; *MP,* medial pole; *PF,* pterygoid fovea.

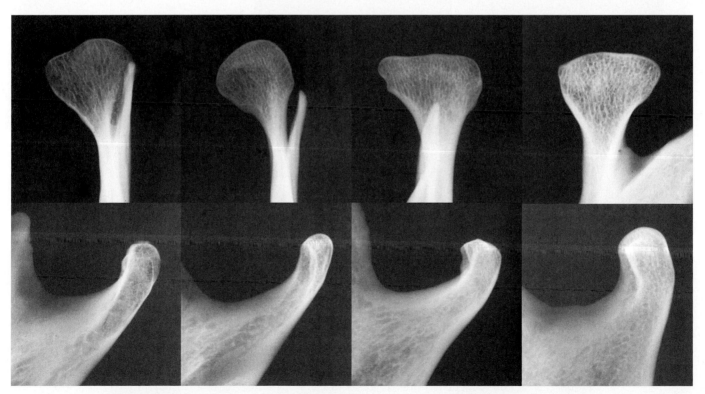

FIGURE 27-2 Composite of images of the mandibular condyle demonstrates the extensive variability in condylar shape from heart-shaped, round, flat, and large medial and lateral poles. The upper row comprises coronal views with corresponding lateral views immediately below.

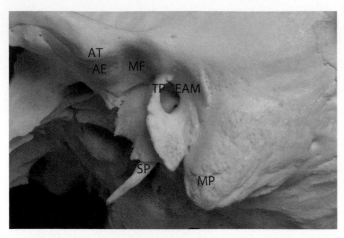

FIGURE 27-3 Lateral and inferior view of the skull showing the temporal component. *AE*, Articular eminence; *AT*, articular tubercle; *EAM*, external auditory meatus; *MF*, mandibular fossa; *MP*, mastoid process; *SP*, styloid process; *TP*, tympanic plate.

eminence, and the summit of the eminence form an "S" shape when viewed in the sagittal plane. The squamotympanic fissure and its medial extension, the petrotympanic fissure, form the posterior limit of the fossa. The middle portion of the roof of the fossa forms a small portion of the floor of the middle cranial fossa, and only a thin layer of cortical bone separates the joint cavity from the intracranial subdural space. The spine of the sphenoid forms the medial limit of the fossa. Fossa depth varies, and the development of the articular eminence relies on functional stimulus from the condyle. For example, the mandibular fossa is very flat and underdeveloped in patients with micrognathia or condylar agenesis. Young infants also lack a definite fossa and articular eminence; the fossa and articular eminence develop during the first 3 years and reach a mature shape by age 4 years, although the cortices may remain indistinct until adulthood (Fig. 27-4, *C* and *D*).

All aspects of the temporal component may be pneumatized with small air cells derived from the mastoid air cell complex

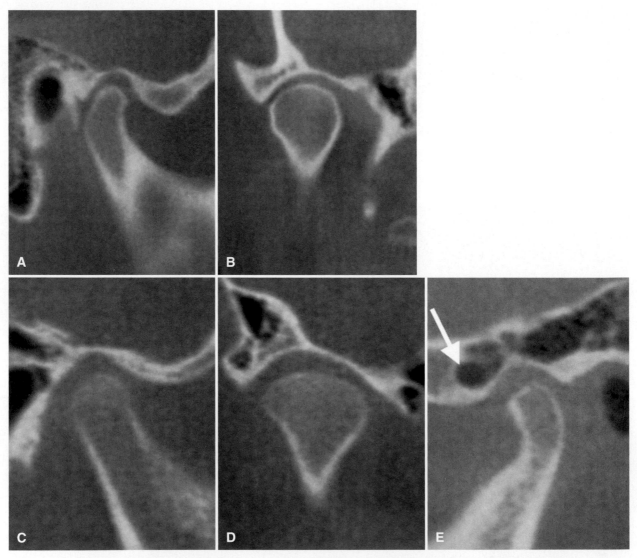

FIGURE 27-4 Sagittal reformat **(A)** and coronal reformat **(B)** CBCT images of the right TMJ in an adult. Note the thick regular cortication of all articulating surfaces and development of the glenoid fossa and articular eminence. Sagittal reformat **(C)** and coronal reformat **(D)** CBCT images of the right TMJ in a 7-year-old child. Note the thin cortication of the articulating surfaces, shallow glenoid fossa, and short articular eminence. Sagittal reformat **(E)** CBCT image of the left TMJ in an adult shows pneumatization of the temporal component including the articular eminence *(arrow)* with mastoid air cells.

(Fig. 27-4, *E*). Pneumatization of the articular eminence is seen radiographically in approximately 2% of patients.

INTERARTICULAR DISC

The interarticular disc (meniscus) is composed of avascular fibrous connective tissue and is positioned between the condylar and temporal components. The disc divides the joint cavity into two compartments, called the inferior (lower) and superior (upper) joint spaces, which are located below and above the disc, respectively (Fig. 27-5). A normal disc has a biconcave shape with a thick anterior band, thicker posterior band, and a thin middle part. The disc is also thicker medially than laterally. In a normal joint, the thin central portion serves as the articulating portion of the disc, acting as a cushion between the convex articulating surfaces of the condyle and articular eminence. The posterior band sits at the superior aspect of the condyle, or slightly anterior to it, in the 11 o'clock position. The periphery of the disc attaches to the inner surface of the joint capsule. The anterior band is also thought to be attached to some fibers of the superior head of the lateral pterygoid muscle. The posterior band attaches to the retrodiscal tissues. The disc and retrodiscal tissues are collectively called the soft tissue components of the TMJ.

During mandibular opening, as the condyle rotates and translates downward and forward, the disc also moves forward and rotates so that its thin central portion remains between the articulating convexities of the condylar head and articular eminence. The disc attaches to the condylar poles laterally and medially, helping to ensure passive movement of the disc with the condyle. On mandibular closing, this process reverses, with the disc moving back with the condyle into the mandibular fossa.

RETRODISCAL TISSUES (POSTERIOR DISC ATTACHMENT)

The retrodiscal tissues consist of superior and inferior lamellae enclosing a region of loose vascular tissue, which is often referred to as the bilaminar zone. The superior lamina, which is rich in elastin, inserts into the posterior wall of the mandibular fossa. The superior lamina stretches and allows the disc to move forward with condylar translation and then allows for the smooth recoil of the disc posteriorly as the mandible closes. The inferior lamina attaches more tightly to the posterior surface of the condyle. As the condyle moves forward, the retrodiscal tissues expand in volume, primarily as a result of venous distention, to fill the space created behind the condyle. The retrodiscal tissues are well innervated and may be the source of pain when the posterior attachment becomes trapped between the condyle and articular eminence in cases of anterior disc displacement.

TEMPOROMANDIBULAR JOINT BONY RELATIONSHIPS

Joint space is a general term used to describe the radiolucent area between the condyle and temporal component seen in diagnostic images. This term should not be confused with the terms superior joint space and inferior joint space described earlier, which refer to soft tissue spaces above and below the disc. The radiographic joint space contains the soft tissue components of the joint. The

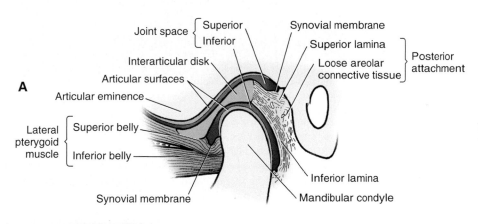

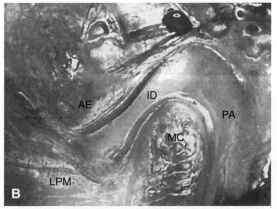

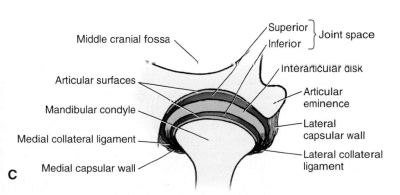

FIGURE 27-5 TMJ anatomy. **A,** Lateral view. **B,** Sectioned cadaver specimen in the same orientation. *AE,* Articular eminence; *ID,* interarticular disc; *LPM,* lateral pterygoid muscle; *MC,* mandibular condyle; *PA,* posterior attachment. **C,** Coronal view. *(Courtesy Dr. W. K. Solberg, Los Angeles, CA.)*

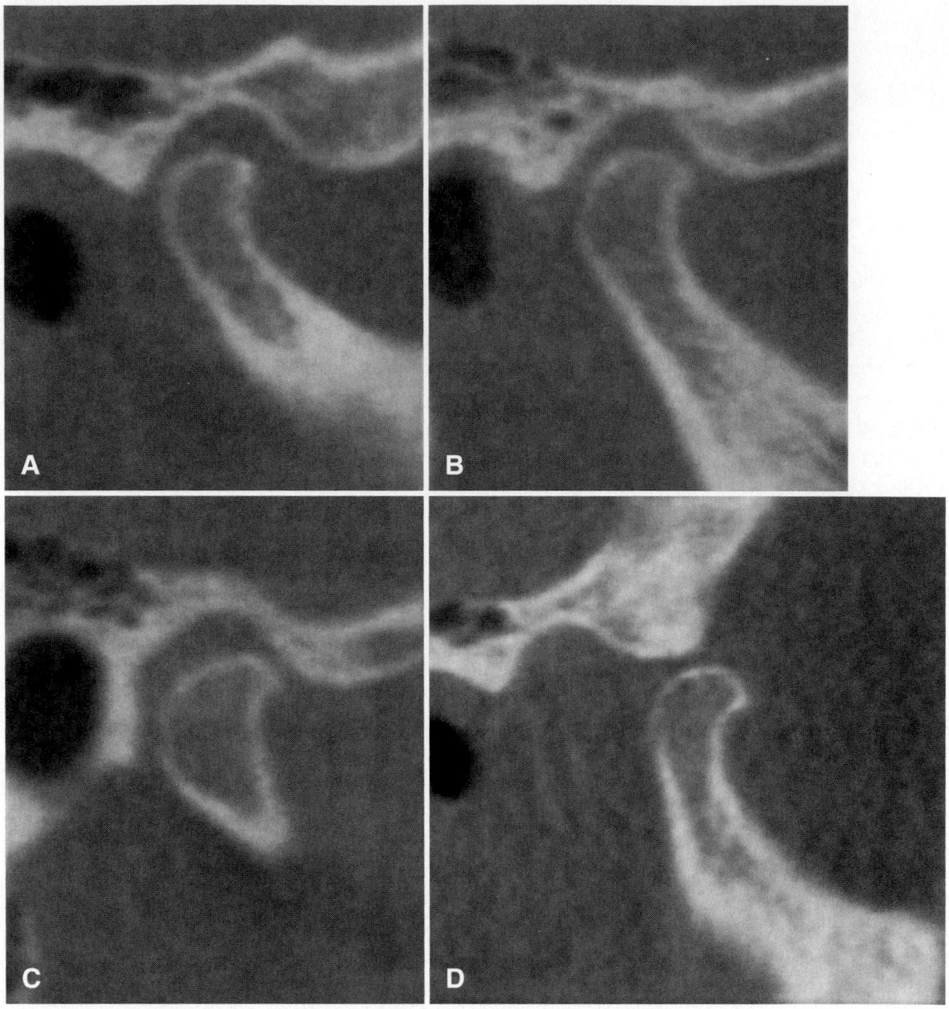

FIGURE 27-6 Sagittal reformat CBCT image. **A-C,** Closed position. Lateral image slice **(A)**, central image slice **(B)**, and medial image slice **(C)** of the same joint. The condyle appears retruded in the lateral slice, centered in the central slice, and anteriorly positioned in the medial slice. **D,** Open view shows the degree of condyle translation during mandibular opening.

condylar position within the fossa can be determined by examining the dimensions of the radiographic joint space viewed on corrected lateral images. A condyle is positioned concentrically when the anterior and posterior aspects of the radiolucent joint space are uniform in width; the condyle is retruded when the posterior joint space width is less than the anterior; and it is protruded when the posterior joint space is wider than the anterior. However, because the radiographic outline of the glenoid fossa and the condyle do not match similar to a smooth ball-and-socket joint, the dimensions of the joint space often vary from medial to lateral aspects of the normal joint (Fig. 27-6).

The diagnostic significance of mild or moderate condylar eccentricity is unclear; condylar eccentricity is seen in one third to one half of asymptomatic individuals and is not a reliable indicator of the soft tissue status of the joint, particularly because the shape of the condylar head is not concentric to the shape of the fossa. Markedly eccentric condylar positioning usually represents an abnormality. For example, inferior condylar positioning (widened joint space) may be seen in cases involving fluid or blood within the joint, and superior condylar positioning (decreased joint space or no joint space, with contact of osseous components) may indicate loss, displacement, or perforation of the disc or its attachments. Marked posterior condylar positioning is seen in some cases of anterior disc displacement, and pronounced anterior condylar positioning may be seen when there has been destruction of the articular eminence, such as in juvenile idiopathic arthritis (JIA).

CONDYLAR MOVEMENT

The condyle undergoes complex movement during mandibular opening. Downward and forward translation (sliding) of the condyle occurs where the superior surface of the disc slides against the articular eminence; at the same time, a hingelike, rotatory movement occurs with the superior surface of the condyle against the inferior surface of the disc. The extent of normal condylar translation varies considerably. In most individuals, at maximal opening, the condyle moves down and forward to the summit of the articular eminence or slightly anterior to it (see Fig. 27-6). The condyle typically is found within a range of 2 to 5 mm posterior and 5 to 8 mm anterior to the crest of the eminence. Reduced condylar translation, in which the condyle has little or no downward and forward movement and does not leave the mandibular fossa, is seen in patients who clinically have a reduced degree of mouth opening. Hypermobility of the joint may be suspected if the condyle translates more than 5 mm anterior to the eminence. If a superior movement also occurs anterior to the articular eminence, anterior locking or dislocation of the condyle may occur.

APPLICATION OF DIAGNOSTIC IMAGING

Imaging of the TMJ may be necessary to supplement information obtained from the clinical examination, particularly when an osseous abnormality or infection is suspected, conservative treatment has failed, or symptoms are worsening. Diagnostic imaging also should be considered for patients with a history of trauma, significant dysfunction, alteration in range of motion, sensory or motor abnormalities, or significant changes in occlusion. TMJ imaging is not indicated for joint sounds if other signs or symptoms are absent or for asymptomatic children and adolescents before orthodontic treatment. The purposes of TMJ imaging are to evaluate the integrity and relationships of the hard and soft tissues, confirm the extent or stage of progression of known disease, and evaluate the effects of treatment. There is often poor correlation between the severity of findings on TMJ imaging and the severity of the patient's symptoms or dysfunction. For instance, severe degenerative changes may be noted on an imaging study, but the patient has only mild discomfort, or vice versa. The clinician must correlate the imaging information with the patient's history and clinical findings to arrive at a final diagnosis and plan the management of the underlying disease process.

TEMPOROMANDIBULAR JOINT IMAGING MODALITIES

Several variables must be considered when selecting the type of imaging technique to use, including the specific clinical problem to be addressed, whether imaging of hard or soft tissues is desired, the strengths and limitations of the modalities being considered, the cost of the examination, and the radiation dose. Both joints should be imaged during the examination for comparison. Images of the osseous structures of the joints may be obtained using panoramic radiography, cone-beam computed tomographic (CBCT) imaging, or multidetector computed tomographic (MDCT) imaging. The soft tissues of the joints are best imaged with magnetic resonance imaging (MRI). The application of these techniques to TMJ diagnosis is discussed further in the following sections.

OSSEOUS STRUCTURES

Panoramic Projection

The panoramic image is a useful tool for providing a broad overview of the TMJ and surrounding structures. It serves the purpose of allowing the clinician to rule out gross disease, and for some patients, it is the only imaging required before conservative therapy is initiated. Gross osseous changes in the condyles may be identified, such as asymmetries, extensive erosions, large osteophytes, tumors, or fractures (Fig. 27-7). The panoramic projection also provides a means of comparing left and right sides of the mandible and can reveal odontogenic diseases and other disorders that may be the source of TMJ symptoms. However, no information about condylar position or function is provided because the mandible is partly opened and protruded when this image is exposed. Also, mild osseous changes may be obscured, and only marked changes in articular eminence morphology can be seen as a result of superimposition by the skull base and zygomatic arch. For these reasons, when a detailed assessment of the joint structures is desired, the panoramic view should be supplemented. The TMJ programs available on some panoramic machines do not provide the views required because of thick image layers and oblique, distorted views, and more advanced modalities are indicated.

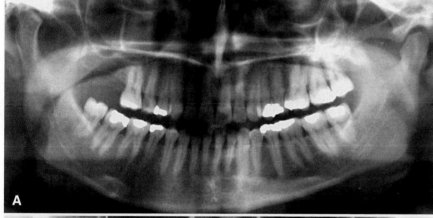

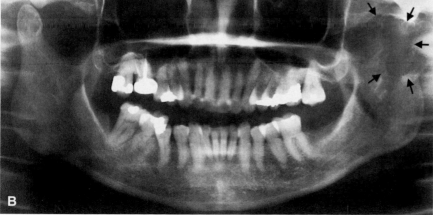

FIGURE 27-7 Panoramic images reveal right condylar hyperplasia **(A)** and destruction of the condyle by a malignant tumor **(B)** (arrows).

Cone-Beam Computed Tomographic Imaging

CBCT imaging produces volumetric imaging that allows reconstruction of thin section views in multiple, customizable planes. Thin sections allow the structures of the joints to be assessed without superimposition of surrounding anatomy. Classically, the joints are viewed in coronal and sagittal planes, corrected along the long axes of the condylar heads (Fig. 27-8). These views provide the least distorted representation of the condylar and temporal components and their relationship to each other. Panoramic and three-dimensional reformats also can be created, which are useful for assessing skeletal asymmetries or other osseous deformities. A CBCT scan is usually acquired with the patient's mouth in the closed position. Some machines allow low-resolution scans to be done in open mouth or other positions (see Chapter 12) to evaluate range of motion. CBCT imaging has the advantage of reduced radiation dose to the patient compared with MDCT. This reduced dose makes CBCT imaging ideal for imaging of osseous changes associated with DJD. CBCT imaging is also useful for determining the presence and extent of ankylosis and neoplasms, imaging fractures, evaluating complications from the use of polytetrafluoroethylene or silicon sheet implants, and examining for heterotopic bone growth. Soft tissue components including the discs cannot be adequately visualized with CBCT imaging. Metallic implants in or around the joints may create streak artifacts, which can obscure the joint structures.

Multidetector Computed Tomographic Imaging

MDCT imaging (see Chapter 14) is capable of providing the same information as CBCT imaging but additionally allows some visualization of the soft tissues. This additional visualization is required only in a few situations, such as when a neoplasm is suspected to extend beyond the osseous structures. The articular disc is not adequately visualized with this modality. Also, MDCT imaging exposes the patient to higher radiation doses than CBCT imaging.

SOFT TISSUE STRUCTURES

The most common indication for soft tissue imaging is when clinical findings suggest disc displacement with symptoms such as TMJ pain and dysfunction and when symptoms do not respond to conservative therapy. Soft tissue imaging may also be required to supplement osseous imaging in rare cases where infection or a neoplasm is suspected. As with any other modality, imaging should be prescribed only when the anticipated results are expected to influence the treatment plan. MR imaging is the modality of choice for visualizing the disc and other soft tissues of the TMJ.

Magnetic Resonance Imaging

MRI uses a magnetic field and radiofrequency pulses rather than ionizing radiation to produce multiple digital image slices (see Chapter 14). This imaging modality does not subject the patient to any ionizing radiation dose. Because MRI can provide a contrast between different soft tissues, this technique can be used for imaging the articular disc and other soft tissue components of the joint. Joint effusions can also be detected with MRI. MRI imaging displays the osseous structures of the TMJ but not in detail comparable to CBCT or MDCT imaging.

MRI allows construction of images in the sagittal and coronal planes without repositioning the patient (Fig. 27-9). These images usually are acquired in open and closed mandibular positions with use of surface coils to improve image resolution. Sagittal slices should be oriented perpendicular to the condylar long axis. The examinations usually are performed with use of T1-weighted, proton density–weighted, or T2-weighted pulse sequences. Proton density–weighted images are slightly superior to T1-weighted images in demonstrating osseous and discal tissues, whereas

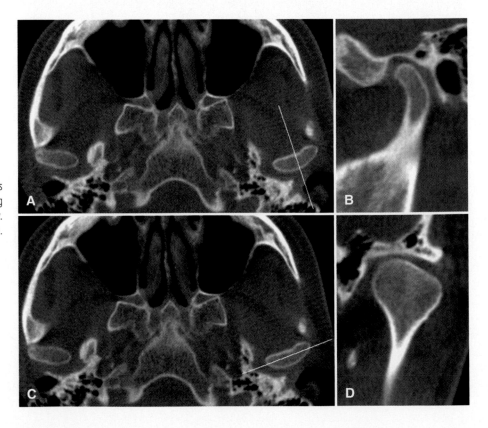

FIGURE 27-8 CBCT images show reconstruction planes for evaluating the TMJs. **A,** Axial view with line indicating corrected sagittal plane. **B,** Resultant corrected sagittal view. **C,** Axial view with line indicating corrected coronal plane. **D,** Resultant corrected coronal view.

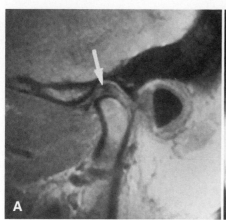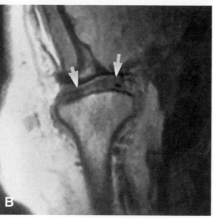

FIGURE 27-9   MRI of a normal TMJ. **A,** Closed sagittal view shows the condyle and temporal component. The biconcave disc is located with its posterior band *(arrow)* over the condyle. **B,** Closed coronal view shows the osseous components and disc *(arrows)* superior to the condyle. *(Courtesy Dr. Per-Lennart Westesson, Rochester, NY.)*

T2 weighted images demonstrate inflammation and joint effusion. Motion MRI studies during opening and closing can be obtained by having the patient open the jaw in a series of incremental distances and using rapid image acquisition ("fast scan") techniques.

MRI is contraindicated in patients who have pacemakers or some other implanted devices, intracranial vascular clips, or metal particles in vital structures. Orthodontic hardware may create artifacts over the dental region but are not a contraindication to imaging the joints. Some patients may be unable to tolerate the procedure because of claustrophobia or an inability to remain motionless.

ABNORMALITIES OF THE TEMPOROMANDIBULAR JOINT

DEVELOPMENTAL ABNORMALITIES

Disease Mechanism
Developmental abnormalities are the result of disturbance in the normal growth and development of the TMJ. The end result is abnormalities in the form or size of the joint components, most commonly the mandibular condyle. Because the condylar articular cartilage is considered the growth center for the mandible, disturbances involving this cartilage can result in altered growth of the mandibular condyle, ramus, body, and alveolar process on the affected side.

Condylar Hyperplasia
Disease Mechanism. Condylar hyperplasia is a developmental abnormality that results in enlargement and occasionally deformity of the condylar head; this may have a secondary effect on the mandibular fossa as it remodels to accommodate the abnormal condyle. Proposed etiologic factors include hormonal influences, trauma, infection, heredity, intrauterine factors, and hypervascularity. The mechanism may be overactive cartilage or persistent cartilaginous rests; the thickness of the entire cartilaginous and precartilaginous layers is increased. This condition usually is unilateral and may be accompanied by varying degrees of hyperplasia of the ipsilateral mandible.

Clinical Features. Condylar hyperplasia is more common in females and is most frequently discovered before age 20 years. The condition is self-limiting and tends to arrest with termination of skeletal growth, although a few cases continue to grow, and adult

onset has been reported. The condition may progress slowly or rapidly. Patients have a mandibular asymmetry that varies in severity, depending on the degree of condylar enlargement. The chin may be deviated to the unaffected side, or it may remain unchanged but with an increase in the vertical dimension of the ramus, mandibular body, or alveolar process of the affected side. As a result of this growth pattern, patients may have a posterior open bite on the affected side or a crossbite on the contralateral side with resultant problems with mastication or speech. Patients may also have symptoms related to TMJ dysfunction and may complain of limited or deviated mandibular opening, caused by restricted mobility of the enlarged condyle.

Imaging Features. The hyperplastic condyle may have a relatively normal shape but be enlarged, or its form could be altered (e.g., conical, spherical, elongated, lobulated) or irregular. It may appear to be more radiopaque in plain images because of the additional bone volume present. However, the cortical thickness and trabecular pattern of the enlarged condyle usually are normal, which helps to distinguish this condition from a condylar neoplasm. The glenoid fossa may be enlarged to compensate for the larger condylar head, usually as a result of remodeling of the posterior slope of the articular eminence. Secondary degenerative changes may be present because of the altered forces on the joint. The condylar neck may also be longer and thickened. Forward bending of the elongated condylar head and neck, to compensate for the increased bone volume, may result in an inverted "L" shape to these structures. The condylar neck may also bend laterally when viewed in the coronal (anteroposterior) plane (Fig. 27-10). Secondary enlargement of the ramus and mandibular body also may result in a characteristic downward bowing of the inferior mandibular border on the affected side. The ramus may have increased vertical and anteroposterior dimensions.

Differential Diagnosis. A condylar tumor, most notably an osteochondroma, is included in the differential diagnosis. An osteochondroma usually results in a condyle with a more irregular shape compared with a hyperplastic condyle because this tumor creates a more localized protruding growth. Surface irregularities and continued growth after cessation of skeletal growth should increase suspicion of this tumor. Occasionally, a condylar osteoma or large osteophyte that occurs in chronic DJD may simulate condylar hyperplasia. Associated ipsilateral hyperplasia of the mandible would not be seen in these other conditions.

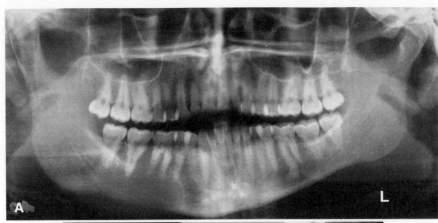

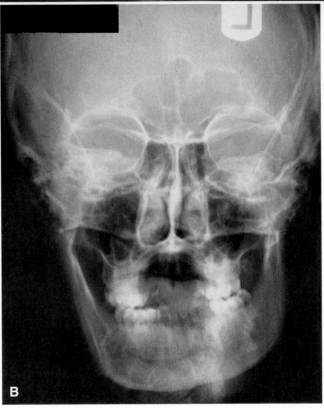

FIGURE 27-10 **A,** Panoramic image of condylar hyperplasia involving the right condyle. **B,** The resulting asymmetry of the mandible is apparent in the posteroanterior skull view.

Treatment. Treatment consists of a combination of condylectomy, orthognathic surgery, and orthodontics. Condylectomy removes the source of abnormal growth, whereas orthognathic surgery and orthodontics aim to correct any resultant functional and esthetic deficits. Initiation of treatment before condylar growth is complete helps limit the severity of mandibular deformation and compensatory changes in the maxilla and dentoalveolar structures. Treatment may also be delayed until growth is completed to avoid relapse and the need for additional interventions. A technetium bone scan may be helpful in determining if condylar growth is still active or not but may be misleading if there is increased activity secondary to concurrent remodeling or degenerative changes.

Condylar Hypoplasia

Disease Mechanism. Condylar hypoplasia is an undersized mandibular condyle, which may be the result of congenital, developmental, or acquired diseases that affect condylar growth. Severe congenital malformations may result in complete lack of formation of the condyle (aplasia). Rare congenital conditions causing hypoplasia of the condyle often also present with abnormalities of other structures of the face, such as the ear, eye, and zygomatic arch (see Chapter 32). Trauma, infection, and therapeutic radiation exposure to the condyle during growth are potential acquired causes of hypoplasia.

Clinical Features. Condylar hypoplasia is more commonly unilateral, unless it is a feature of a syndrome (e.g., Treacher Collins syndrome, Pierre Robin sequence). The condyle is a mandibular growth center; therefore, condylar hypoplasia is usually associated with some degree of unilateral mandibular hypoplasia and facial asymmetry. Deviation of the mandibular midline to the affected side and accentuation of this deviation on mandibular opening and malocclusion may develop. The amount of growth disturbance of the mandible is related to how early the onset of the disturbance to condylar growth occurs; earlier onset results in more severe underdevelopment of the ramus and mandibular body. Patients with condylar hypoplasia may develop symptoms of TMJ dysfunction.

Imaging Features.   The condyle may be normal in shape and structure but is diminished in size, and the mandibular fossa is proportionally small. The condylar neck is thinner and may appear short or elongated. The coronoid process is usually slender. The posterior border of the ramus and condylar neck may have a dorsal (posterior) inclination, creating a concavity in the outline of the posterior surface of the mandible in the panoramic image. If there is an associated mandibular hypoplasia, it manifests with a deepened antegonial notch and decreased vertical height of the mandibular body (Fig. 27-11). Occasional dental crowding may also result. Degenerative changes in the affected joint may be detected (Fig. 27-12).

Differential Diagnosis.   JIA may cause damage to the condyle, resulting in hypoplasia. However, other signs of joint destruction would also be seen. A survey of other joints or testing for rheumatoid factor may be helpful if there is uncertainty. Changes in condylar morphology in severe DJD or other arthritic conditions may also mimic a hypoplastic condyle, but other signs of arthritis are usually visible in the affected joint. Additionally, arthritis does not cause mandibular hypoplasia of the affected side unless it occurs during growth. Occasionally, it is difficult to determine if there is condylar hypoplasia or if the contralateral side is enlarged. Careful examination of the inferior border for a pronounced antegonial notch (hypoplasia) versus downward bowing (hyperplasia) is helpful.

Treatment.   Orthognathic surgery, bone grafts, and orthodontic therapy may be required.

Juvenile Arthrosis

Synonyms.   Synonyms for juvenile arthrosis include condylysis, Boering's arthrosis, and arthrosis deformans.

Disease Mechanism.   Juvenile arthrosis is a condylar growth disturbance first described by Boering, usually occurring in females during the second decade. During the first decade of growth, the mandibular condyle appears normal, but there is significant resorption of the condylar head during the second decade. The etiology is unknown, although theories involving a growth disturbance owing to an exuberant form of DJD, avascular necrosis, or hormonal abnormalities have been put forth. In cases where MRI was performed, all cases had severe anterior displacement of the articular disc. This finding supports the DJD theory. There is usually a secondary hypoplasia of the same side of the mandible. Juvenile arthrosis may be unilateral or bilateral.

Clinical Features.   Juvenile arthrosis affects mainly females during the second decade of growth. It usually is an incidental finding in a panoramic projection, or the patient may have mandibular asymmetry, signs and symptoms of TMJ dysfunction, or both. As the condylar changes progress, the patient often develops an anterior open bite.

Imaging Features.   The classic description is that the condylar head develops a characteristic "toadstool" appearance, with marked flattening and apparent elongation of the articulating condylar surface and dorsal (posterior) inclination of the condyle and neck. The condylar neck is shortened or absent in some cases, with the condyle resting on the upper margin of the ramus (Fig. 27-13). However, this description of the condylar changes was based on panoramic or transpharyngeal images with considerable image distortion of the condyle. CBCT images often reveal marked resorption of the superior aspect of the condylar head without a dorsal inclination. The articulating surface of the temporal component often is flattened. Progressive shortening of the ramus occurs on the affected side, and the antegonial notch may be deepened, indicating mandibular hypoplasia. Signs of DJD are always present.

Differential Diagnosis.   Resorption of the condylar head from JIA and severe DJD or severe condylar degeneration after orthognathic surgery or joint surgery may simulate juvenile arthrosis.

Treatment.   Orthognathic surgery and orthodontic therapy may be required to correct the mandibular asymmetry. Caution should be exercised in undertaking orthodontic therapy because stress on the joint may result in further degeneration and orthodontic relapse.

Coronoid Hyperplasia

Disease Mechanism.   Coronoid hyperplasia results in elongation of the coronoid process of the mandible. The etiology may be acquired or developmental. The coronoid processes may impinge

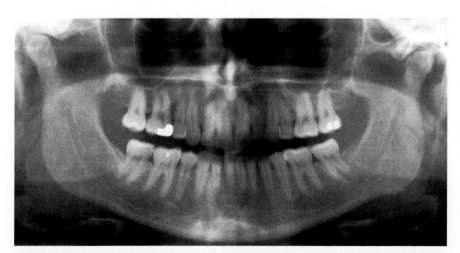

FIGURE 27-11 Panoramic image reveals hypoplasia of the left condyle. In this case, hypoplasia is restricted to the condylar head and neck with minimal involvement of the mandibular ramus and body.

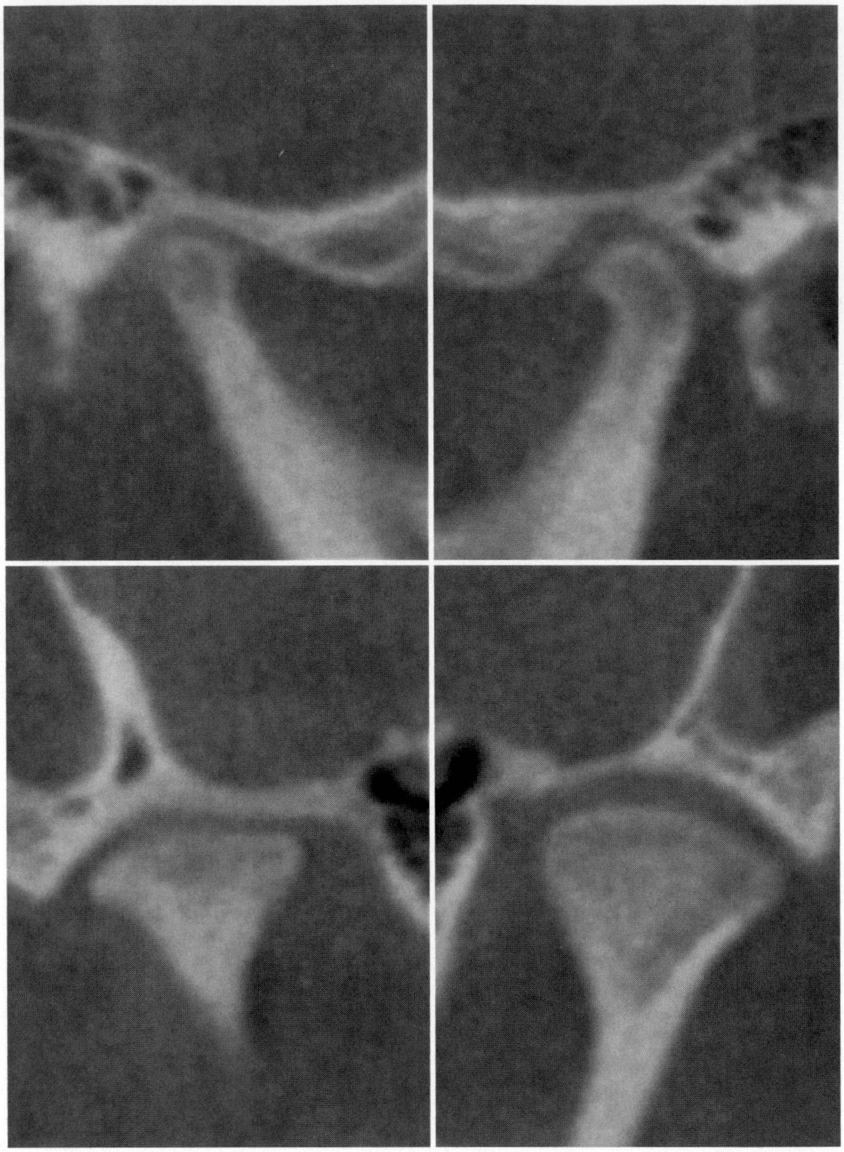

FIGURE 27-12 CBCT images of unilateral condylar hypoplasia. Sagittal (**A** and **B**) and coronal (**C** and **D**) reformatted images. **A** and **C,** The right condyle is hypoplastic, and there is secondary remodeling. The articular surfaces of the condyle and anterior aspect of the glenoid fossa are flattened, and the superior joint space is thinner compared with the left. **B** and **D,** Left side of same patient showing normal condyle.

on the posterior surface of the zygomatic arch during opening, restricting condylar translation. Sometimes a pseudojoint develops between the hyperplastic coronoid and the posterior surface of the zygoma, a condition called Jacob's disease.

Clinical Features.   The developmental variant of coronoid hyperplasia is more commonly bilateral. This form is most often diagnosed in young men who have a long history of progressive limitation of mouth opening. The resulting restricted opening may simulate the features of an apparent closed lock owing to disc displacement. Acquired coronoid hyperplasia usually develops secondary to restricted movement of the condyle, such as in ankylosis. The condition is painless.

Imaging Features.   Coronoid hyperplasia is best seen in panoramic images, Waters' images, and CBCT scans. The coronoid processes are elongated, and the tips extend at least 1 cm above the inferior rim of the zygomatic arch (Fig. 27-14). The coronoid processes may have a large but normal shape or may curve

anteriorly and may appear very radiopaque. Impingement of the coronoid against the zygomatic arch can be confirmed by performing CT imaging with the patient's mouth opened maximally (Fig. 27-15). Remodeling of the posterior surface of the zygomatic process of the maxilla, to accommodate the enlarged coronoid process during function, may also be seen. Because this condition is often bilateral, both sides should be examined for abnormality. The radiographic appearance of the TMJs usually is normal.

Differential Diagnosis.   Unilateral elongation of the coronoid process should be differentiated from a neoplasm, such as an osteochondroma or osteoma. In contrast to coronoid hyperplasia, tumors usually have an irregular shape. Clinical presentation of limited opening most often prompts examination of the TMJs for abnormalities that may restrict joint movement, such as internal derangement, neoplasm, or ankylosis. However, inclusion of the coronoid processes during TMJ imaging helps ensure that coronoid hyperplasia is not missed.

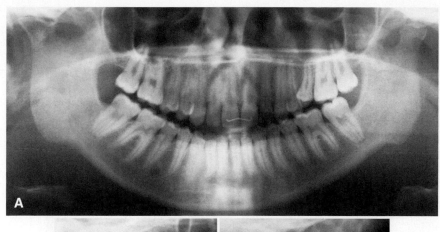

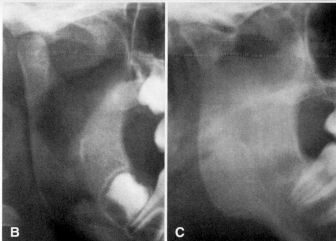

FIGURE 27-13 **A,** Panoramic image of juvenile arthrosis with the right condyle affected to a greater degree and displaying the traditional toadstool appearance and mild involvement of the left condyle. There is secondary mandibular hypoplasia. **B** and **C,** Cropped panoramic image **(B)** of the same case shows a normal-appearing right condyle 6 years before image **C** ot the same condyle.

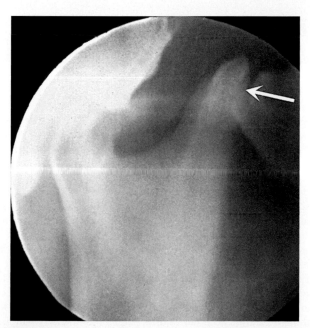

FIGURE 27-14 Sagittal tomogram of coronoid hyperplasia. The coronoid process is elongated and extends above the inferior rim of the zygomatic arch *(arrow)* but otherwise is shaped normally.

Treatment. Treatment consists of surgical removal of the coronoid process and postoperative physiotherapy. Regrowth of the coronoid process after surgery has been reported.

Bifid Condyle

Disease Mechanism. A bifid condyle has a vertical depression, notch, or deep cleft in the center of the condylar head, seen in the frontal or sagittal plane, resulting in the appearance of a "double" condylar head. There may be actual duplication of the condyle. This condition is rare and is more often unilateral, although it may be bilateral. It may result from an obstructed blood supply during development or other embryopathy, although a traumatic cause has been postulated with the divided condyle resulting from a longitudinal fracture.

Clinical Features. Bifid condyle usually is an incidental finding in panoramic views or anteroposterior projections. Some patients have signs and symptoms of TMJ dysfunction, including joint noises and pain.

Imaging Features. The orientation of the bifid condyle may be anteroposterior or mediolateral. Commonly, a depression or notch is present on the superior condylar surface, giving a heart-shaped outline when viewed in the frontal plane. The depth of the

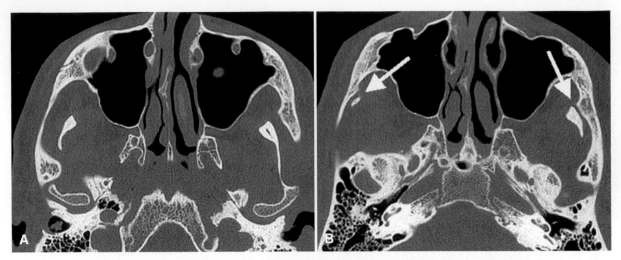

FIGURE 27-15 Two axial MDCT images taken in the closed mouth **(A)** and open mouth **(B)** positions showing impingement of hyperplastic coronoid processes with the medial aspect of the zygomatic arch *(arrows).* Note the hyperostosis on the medial surface of the zygomatic process at the point of impingement.

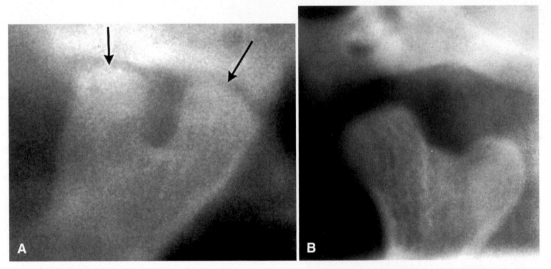

FIGURE 27-16 Bifid condyle. **A,** Sagittal tomogram shows a deep central notch with duplication of the condylar head *(arrows).* The glenoid fossa has remodeled (enlarged) to accommodate the abnormal condyle. **B,** Coronal tomogram shows a depression in the center of the condylar head.

depression is variable. A more remarkable presentation is complete duplication of the condylar head in the sagittal plane (Fig. 27-16). The mandibular fossa may remodel to accommodate the altered condylar morphology.

Differential Diagnosis. A slight medial depression on the superior condylar surface may be considered a normal variation; the point at which the depth of the depression signifies a bifid condyle is unclear. The differential diagnosis also includes a vertical fracture through the condylar head.

Treatment. Treatment is not indicated unless pain or functional impairment is present.

SOFT TISSUE ABNORMALITIES

Disc Displacement

Disease Mechanism. The articular disc may become abnormally positioned or displaced relative to the condylar and temporal components of the TMJ. The disc most often is displaced in an anterior direction, but it may be displaced anteromedially, medially, or anterolaterally. Lateral and posterior displacements are extremely rare. A displaced disc may interfere with normal function of the joint or cause pain, although it is a common finding in asymptomatic patients, leading to the hypothesis that disc displacements may be considered a normal variation. A disc that is displaced in the closed position may resume a normal relationship with the condyle when the mandible is opened, or it may remain displaced; the terms reducing and nonreducing are used to describe these situations, respectively (Fig. 27-17). A displaced disc may become deformed or be associated with other signs of TMJ dysfunction, including DJD, adhesion, effusion, and perforation. The cause of disc displacement is unknown, although parafunction, jaw injuries (e.g., direct trauma), whiplash injury, and forced opening beyond the normal range have been implicated. The term internal derangement is a nonspecific designation for an abnormality in the soft tissue components of

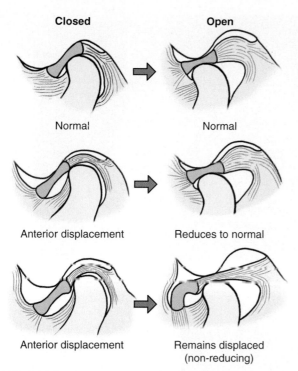

Closed   **Open**

Normal   Normal

Anterior displacement   Reduces to normal

Anterior displacement   Remains displaced
(non-reducing)

FIGURE 27-17 Position and movement of the disc during jaw opening. **A,** Normal position. **B,** Mildly displaced anteriorly (with reduction). **C,** Severely displaced anteriorly (without reduction). *(Courtesy Dr. W. K. Solberg, Los Angeles, CA.)*

the joint resulting in altered function, which may include disc displacement.

Clinical Features. Disc displacement has been found both in symptomatic and asymptomatic patients, and it is unknown why some individuals progress to more severe dysfunction, whereas others do not. Joint noises, such as popping or clicking, are a common sign of disc displacement but are most often nonpainful. Crepitus, a crunching or grinding sound, is suggestive of osseous degeneration associated with a long-term, nonreducing disc. Symptoms associated with a displaced disc include pain in the preauricular region, headaches, and closed or open locking of the joint. A decreased range of motion may be present, and when the displacement is unilateral, this may manifest as deviation of the mandible to the affected side on opening.

Imaging Features

Normal Disc Position. The articular disc cannot be visualized with conventional radiography or CBCT or MDCT imaging; MRI is the technique of choice. On MRI, the normal disc has a low signal intensity (i.e., is dark, between bone and muscle), and the signal intensity of the posterior attachment is usually higher (i.e., lighter). In a sagittal image slice, the normal biconcave disc appears as a "bow tie" shape. In the closed mouth position, the normal disc is positioned with the posterior band either directly superior to or slightly anterior to the condylar head (around the 11 o'clock position). The thin intermediate part of the disc sits between the anterosuperior surface of the condyle and the posterior surface of the articular eminence (see Fig. 27-9). In all positions of mouth opening, the thin intermediate part should remain the articulating surface of the disc between the condyle and articular eminence.

Disc Displacement. MR imaging is required for identification of a displaced disc. Although a retruded condylar position, seen in CBCT or MDCT imaging, has been associated with an anteriorly displaced disc, condylar position in maximal intercuspation is an unreliable indicator of disc displacement. Anterior displacement is the most common disc displacement. A disc is considered anteriorly displaced when its posterior band sits anterior to its normal position and the thin intermediate zone is no longer positioned between the condyle and articular eminence. This displacement may range from partial to full displacement with the posterior band sitting between the condyle and articular eminence in a mild partial displacement to sitting well anterior to the condylar head in a severe, full dislocation (Fig. 27-18). When the disc is severely anteriorly displaced, partial folding of the disc within the anterior joint space may be seen. Sometimes identification of the posterior band is difficult because of deformation of this part of the disc. Also, when the disc is chronically anteriorly positioned, the posterior attachment is pulled between the articulating surfaces of the condyle and temporal bone, and owing to resulting fibrosis, its tissue signal may become lower and approximate that of the posterior band. It is helpful to identify the position of the thin intermediate part of the disc to determine if it is anteriorly displaced from its normal position between the articulating surfaces of the condyle and articular eminence. Anteromedial displacement is indicated in sagittal image slices when the disc is in a normal position in the medial images of the joint but anteriorly positioned in the lateral images of the same joint. Medial or lateral displacement is indicated on coronal MRI when the body of the disc is positioned at the medial or lateral aspect of the condyle, respectively (see Fig. 27-18, *C*). Posterior disc displacement is rare.

Disc Reduction and Nonreduction. During mouth opening, an anteriorly displaced disc may reduce to a normal relationship with the condylar head during any part of the opening movement. In motion studies, this is usually a rapid posterior movement of the disc, and it is often accompanied by an audible click. This condition is referred to as disc reduction and can be diagnosed on MRI if the disc is anteriorly displaced in closed mouth views but is in a normal position in open mouth views (see Fig. 27-18). If the disc remains anteriorly displaced on opening, it is diagnosed as nonreducing. It may appear bent or deformed as the condyle pushes forward against it (Fig. 27-19). Fibrotic changes of the posterior attachment of a displaced disc may alter its tissue signal to approximate the signal of the disc and make identification of the disc itself difficult or impossible. In such cases, the disc may be erroneously interpreted as occupying a normal position at maximal opening. Identification of excessive tissue with low signal intensity anterior to the condylar head, representing the true disc tissue, should help confirm the nonreducing state of the disc.

Deformities and Perforation. If the disc remains chronically displaced, it undergoes permanent deformation, losing its biconcave shape. MRI can indicate alteration in the normal biconcave outline of the disc, which may vary from enlargement of the posterior band to a bilinear or biconvex disc outline. In cases of gross deformation or atrophy, identification of the disc may be difficult or impossible. Disc deformities may be accompanied by changes in its signal intensity, including an increase in signal. Changes to the condyle and temporal component of the joint consistent with DJD often accompany cases with long-standing displaced discs (Fig. 27-20). Perforations between the superior and inferior joint spaces most commonly occur in the retrodiscal tissue, just behind the posterior band of the disc (Fig. 27-21, *C*), and can be detected in arthrographic investigations but are not reliably detected with

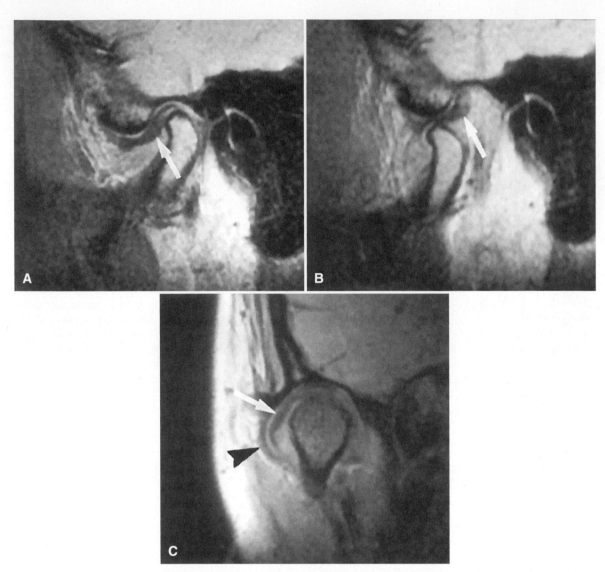

FIGURE 27-18 MRI of anterior disc displacement with reduction. **A,** Closed sagittal view shows the disc with its posterior band *(arrow)* anterior to the condyle; note the anterior position of the thin intermediate section of the disc. **B,** Open view shows the normal relationship of the disc and condyle and the posterior band of the disc *(arrow)*. **C,** Coronal view shows the disc *(arrow)* laterally displaced. The joint capsule *(arrowhead)* bulges laterally. (**B,** *Courtesy Dr. Per-Lennart Westesson, Rochester, NY.*)

MRI. Loss of the joint space, resulting in bone-to-bone contact between the osseous components, is suggestive of perforation of the disc or its attachment.

Fibrous Adhesions and Effusion.   Fibrous adhesions are masses of fibrous tissue or scar tissue that form in the joint space, particularly after TMJ surgery. Adhesions may restrict normal movement of the disc during mandibular opening, resulting in a "stuck disc" and possible closed lock. Adhesions are best identified with arthrography by resistance to injection of contrast agent, or they may be detected on MRI studies as tissue with low signal intensity. Adhesions may also be suspected when there is no movement of the disc relative to the articular eminence in mandibular open position in MRI. Joint effusion (fluid in the joint) is considered to be an early change that may precede DJD. MRI can detect joint effusion, which appears as an area of high signal intensity in the joint spaces on T2-weighted images (see Fig. 27-19, *B*).

Treatment.   Treatment of an asymptomatic displaced disc is not indicated. In symptomatic patients, conservative, noninvasive therapy should be initiated first. Most patients' symptoms resolve with time. Arthroscopy or arthrocentesis may be helpful in releasing adhesions and improving joint mobility. Open joint surgery is reserved for refractory cases.

REMODELING AND ARTHRITIC CONDITIONS
Remodeling
Disease Mechanism.   Remodeling is an adaptive response of cartilage and osseous tissue to forces applied to the joint that may be excessive, resulting in alteration of the shape of the condyle and articular eminence. This adaptive response may result in flattening of curved joint surfaces, which effectively distributes forces over a greater surface area. The number of trabeculae also increases, increasing the density of subchondral cancellous bone to resist applied forces better. No destruction or degeneration of fibrous

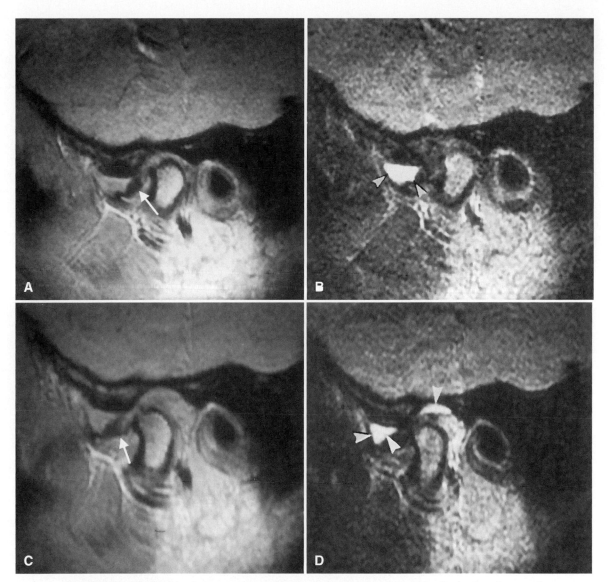

FIGURE 27-19 MRI of disc displacement without reduction in the presence of joint effusion. **A,** The disc *(arrow)* is anteriorly displaced in closed T1-weighted image. **B,** T2-weighted image of the same section shows the collection of joint effusion *(arrowheads)* in the anterior recess of the upper joint space. **C,** Open T1-weighted image shows the disc remains anterior to the condyle. The posterior band of the disc is indicated with an *arrow.* **D,** T2-weighted image is at the same level as image in **C**. Note the joint effusion *(arrowheads)* in the anterior and posterior recesses of the upper joint space. *(Courtesy Dr. Per-Lennart Westesson, Rochester, NY.)*

articular tissue covering the bony components occurs. TMJ remodeling occurs throughout adult life and is considered abnormal only if it is accompanied by clinical signs and symptoms of pain or dysfunction or if the degree of remodeling seen radiographically is judged to be severe. Remodeling may be unilateral and does not invariably serve as a precursor to DJD.

Clinical Features.   Remodeling may be asymptomatic, or patients may have signs and symptoms of TMJ dysfunction that may be related to the soft tissue components, associated muscles, or ligaments. Accompanying disc displacement may be a factor.

Imaging Features.   Changes noted in the diagnostic images may affect the condyle, temporal component, or both; they first occur on the anterosuperior surface of the condyle and the posterior slope of the articular eminence. The lateral aspect of the joint is affected in early stages, and the central and medial aspects become involved as remodeling progresses. These changes may include one or a combination of the following: flattening, thickening of the cortex of the articulating surfaces, and subchondral sclerosis (see Fig. 27-21).

Differential Diagnosis.   Severe joint flattening and subchondral sclerosis may be difficult to differentiate from early DJD. The microscopic changes of degeneration occur before they can be detected in the diagnostic image. The appearance of bone erosions, osteophytes, and loss of joint space in the diagnostic image are signs signifying DJD. Joints affected by degenerative changes may also remodel to have flattened surfaces during nondestructive phases; significant loss of bone volume of the condyle or eminence suggests previous erosion as opposed to adaptive remodeling.

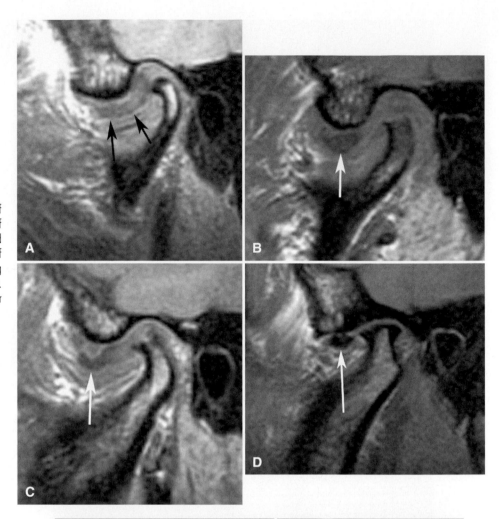

FIGURE 27-20 Sagittal MRI of several cases of anteriorly displaced discs *(arrows)* with various stages of DJD. **A,** Example of severe deformation of the disc and an increase in the tissue signal. **B,** Severe erosions of the superior aspect of the condyle. **C,** Erosions involving the condyle and a small osteophyte on the anterior aspect. **D,** Example of osteophytes forming on both the anterior and the posterior surfaces of the condyle.

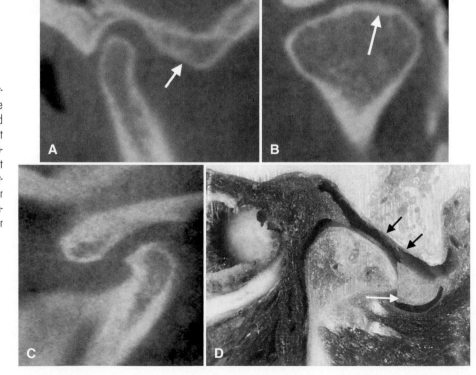

FIGURE 27-21 Sagittal **(A)** and coronal **(B)** reformat CBCT images of the right TMJ show remodeling. **A,** The right temporal component shows subchondral sclerosis and flattening of the articular eminence *(arrow).* **B,** The right condyle shows mild flattening of the lateral aspect and subchondral sclerosis of the medial aspect *(arrow).* The right temporal component is also flattened *(arrowhead).* **C,** Sagittal CBCT image shows significant flattening of the condylar head. **D,** Cadaver specimen. Note the flattening of the temporal component *(black arrows)* and large perforation posterior to a residual deformed disc *(white arrow).*

Treatment.   When no clinical signs or symptoms are present, treatment is not indicated. Otherwise, treatment directed to relieve stress on the joint, such as splint therapy, may be considered. This treatment should be preceded by an attempt to discover the cause of the joint stress.

Degenerative Joint Disease

Synonym.   Osteoarthritis is a synonym for DJD.

Disease Mechanism.   DJD is the breakdown of the articulating fibrocartilage covering the bony components of the joint leading to eventual deterioration of the osseous structures. DJD is thought to occur when the ability of the joint to adapt to excessive forces, through remodeling, is exceeded. Numerous etiologic factors may be important, including acute trauma, hypermobility, and loading of the joint such as occurs in parafunction. Disc displacement may also be a contributing element, and loss of normal lubrication within the joint has been suggested to play a part on the molecular level. DJD is a noninflammatory disorder characterized by both joint deterioration and bony proliferation. Joint deterioration is characterized by bone erosion, whereas new bone formation at the periphery of articular surfaces (osteophyte) and in the subchondral region (sclerosis) represents the proliferative component. Usually a variable combination of deterioration and proliferation occurs, but occasionally one aspect predominates; deterioration is more common in acute disease, and proliferation predominates in chronic disease. It has been reported that joints with long-term nonreducing disc displacement have a higher incidence of progressive radiographic changes of DJD than joints with no disc displacement or reducing discs.

Clinical Features.   DJD can occur at any age, although the incidence increases with age. DJD has a female preponderance. The disease may be asymptomatic, or patients may complain of signs and symptoms of TMJ dysfunction, including pain on palpation and movement, joint noises (crepitus), limited range of motion, and muscle spasm. The onset of symptoms may be sudden or gradual, and symptoms may disappear spontaneously, only to return in recurring cycles. Some studies report that the disease eventually "burns out," and symptoms disappear or decrease markedly in severity in long-standing cases.

Imaging Features.   Osseous changes in DJD are more accurately depicted on CT images, although osseous changes may also be detected on MRI, particularly T1-weighted images. Erosions are a sign of the deteriorating component of DJD. They manifest as small to large bites or scoops out of the articulating surfaces of the joint, resulting in loss of the continuity of the cortices and eventual loss of bone volume (Fig. 27-22). In severe DJD, the glenoid fossa may appear grossly enlarged because of erosion of the posterior slope of the articular eminence. This erosion may allow the condylar head to move forward and superiorly into an abnormal anterior position that may result in an anterior open bite. The condyle may also be markedly diminished in size and altered in shape because of severe erosions. In some cases, small, round, radiolucent areas with irregular margins surrounded by a varying area of increased density are visible deep to the articulating surfaces. These lesions are called Ely cysts or subchondral bone cysts, but they are not true cysts; they are areas of degeneration that contain fibrous tissue, granulation tissue, and osteoid (see Fig. 27-22, A and B). When the patient is in maximal intercuspation, the joint space may be narrow or absent. This finding often correlates with a displaced disc and frequently with a perforation of the disc or posterior attachment, resulting in bone-to-bone contact of the joint components.

In the proliferative phase of the disease, bone formation occurs at the periphery of the articulating surfaces. These projections of new bone are called osteophytes, and although they may form on any part of the joint, they are usually seen on the anterosuperior surface of the condyle, the lateral aspect of the temporal component, or both (Fig. 27-23). Osteophytes create broader, flatter articulating surfaces and serve to distribute the load on the joint over a greater area. In severe cases, osteophyte formation may extend from the articular eminence almost to encase the condylar head. Osteophytes may also break off and lie free within the joint space. These fragments are known as "joint mice," and they must be differentiated from other conditions that cause joint space radiopacities (Fig. 27-24). Variable degrees of sclerosis of the subchondral bone may accompany any of the changes described.

Differential Diagnosis.   DJD can have a spectrum of appearances ranging from extensive erosions (degenerative component) to substantial subchondral sclerosis and osteophyte formation (proliferative component). A more erosive appearance may simulate inflammatory arthritides, such as rheumatoid arthritis (RA), whereas a more proliferative appearance with extensive osteophyte formation may simulate a benign tumor, such as an osteoma or osteochondroma.

Treatment.   The changes to the joint produced by DJD cannot be reversed by any known treatment. Treatment is directed toward relieving joint stress (e.g., splint therapy), relieving secondary inflammation with antiinflammatory drugs, and increasing joint mobility and function (e.g., physiotherapy).

Rheumatoid Arthritis

Disease Mechanism.   RA is a heterogeneous group of systemic disorders that manifests mainly as synovial membrane inflammation in several joints. The TMJ becomes involved in approximately half of affected patients. The characteristic imaging findings are a result of villous synovitis, which leads to formation of synovial granulomatous tissue (pannus) that grows into fibrocartilage and bone, releasing enzymes that destroy the articular surfaces and underlying bone.

Clinical Features.   RA is more common in females and can occur at any age but increases in incidence with increasing age. A juvenile variant is discussed separately. Usually the small joints of the hands, wrists, knees, and feet are affected in a bilateral, symmetric fashion. TMJ involvement is variable; when the TMJ is affected, involvement is often bilateral and often occurs later than in other joints. Patients with TMJ involvement complain of swelling, pain, tenderness, stiffness on opening, limited range of motion, and crepitus. The chin appears receded, and an anterior open bite is a common finding because the condyles settle in an anterosuperior position as the articulating components are progressively destroyed.

Imaging Features.   CT imaging allows detailed assessment of the osseous changes associated with RA. MRI may demonstrate pannus, joint effusions, marrow edema, and disc abnormalities. The use of gadolinium as an MRI contrast agent has been shown to permit early detection of the inflammatory changes in joints with RA. The initial changes of RA may be generalized osteopenia (decreased density) of the condyle and temporal component and

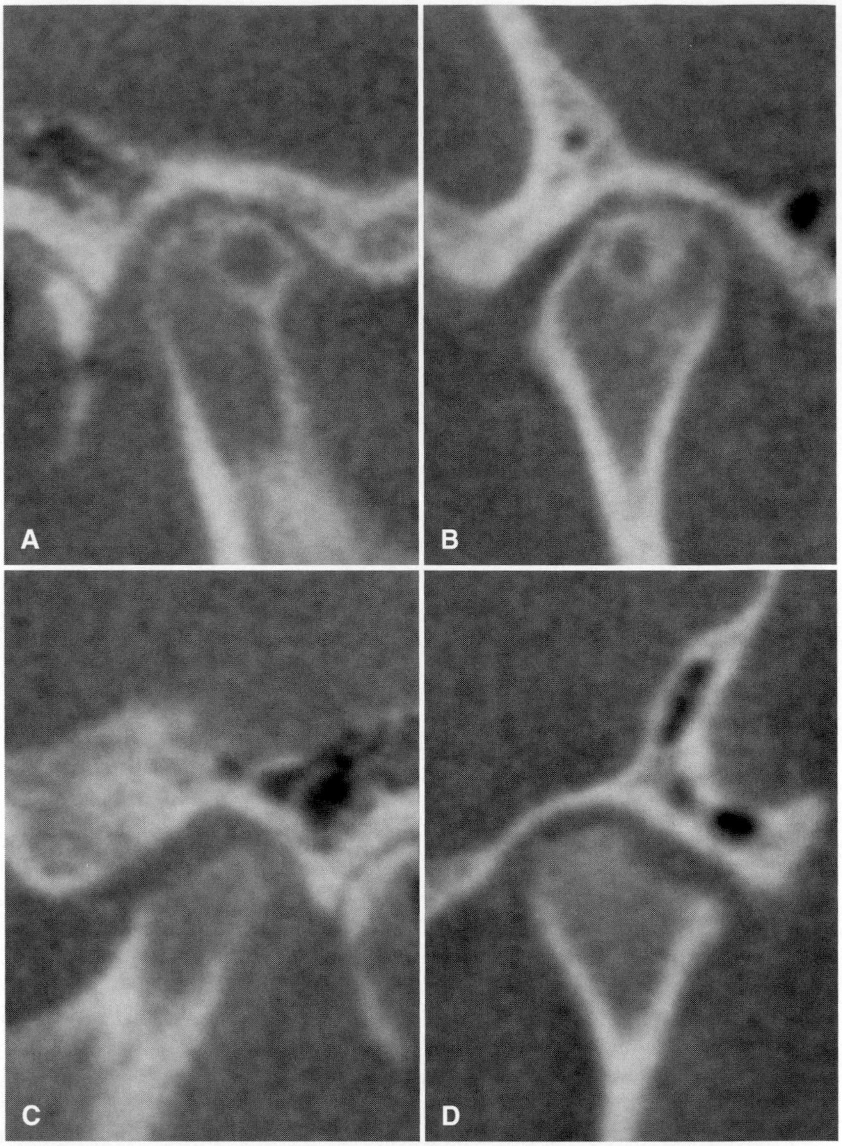

FIGURE 27-22 CBCT image, closed position depicting various erosions in DJD. **A** and **B,** Same patient, right side. Large subchondral cystlike erosion (Ely cyst) of the condyle surrounded by a broad zone of sclerosis. Note also the thin joint space. **C** and **D,** Same patient, left side. Broad erosion of the anterolateral condylar surface. Note also the lack of cortication of the remaining condylar surface and flattening of the temporal component.

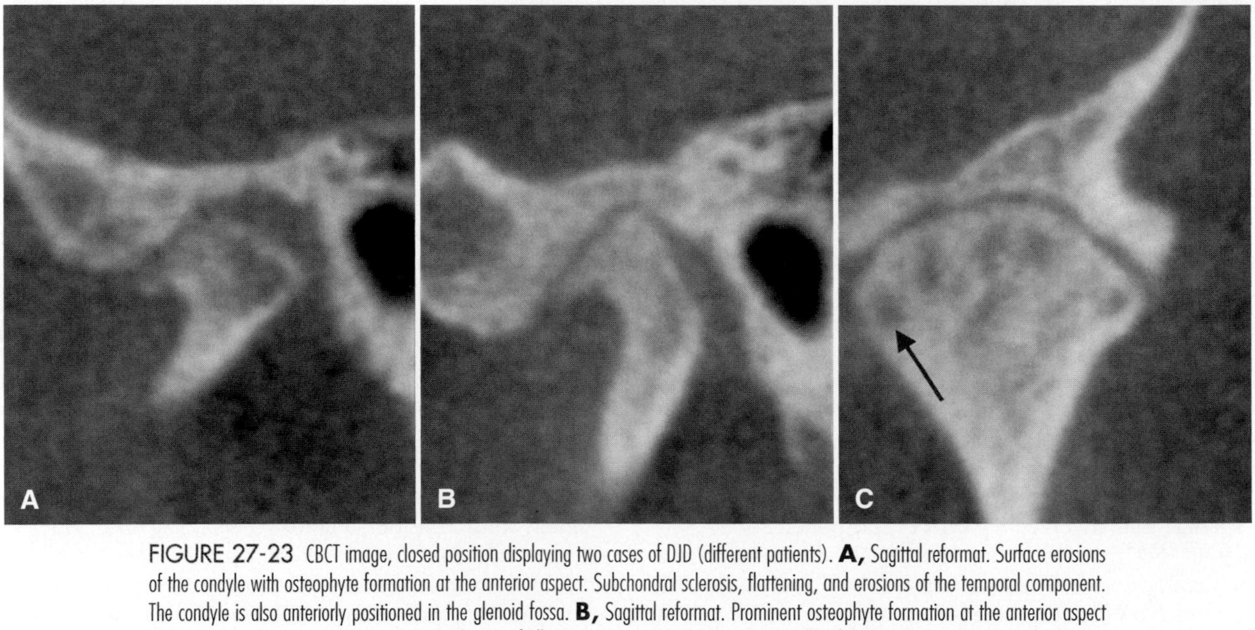

FIGURE 27-23 CBCT image, closed position displaying two cases of DJD (different patients). **A,** Sagittal reformat. Surface erosions of the condyle with osteophyte formation at the anterior aspect. Subchondral sclerosis, flattening, and erosions of the temporal component. The condyle is also anteriorly positioned in the glenoid fossa. **B,** Sagittal reformat. Prominent osteophyte formation at the anterior aspect of the condyle, flattening, and subchondral sclerosis of all joint components, with decreased width of the joint space. **C,** Coronal reformat, same patient as **B**. Multiple subchondral erosions are not visible in the sagittal reformat (one example indicated by *arrow*).

synovial inflammation. The pannus that develops may destroy the disc, resulting in diminished width of the joint space. Bone erosions by the pannus most often involve the articular eminence and the anterior aspect of the condylar head. Erosion of the anterior and posterior condylar surfaces at the attachment of the synovial lining may result in a "sharpened pencil" appearance of the condyle. Erosive changes may be so severe that the entire condylar head is destroyed, with only the neck remaining as the articulating

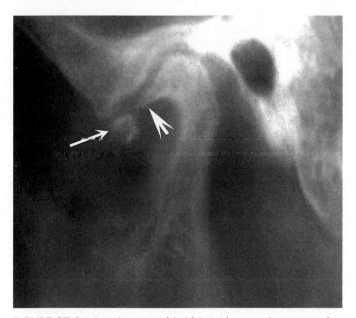

FIGURE 27-24 Sagittal tomogram of the left TMJ. A large osteophyte emanating from the anterior aspect of the condyle *(short arrow)* and a joint mouse *(long arrow)* positioned anterior to the condyle in the joint space.

surface. Similarly, the articular eminence may be destroyed to the extent that a concavity replaces the normally convex eminence. Such erosions permit anterosuperior positioning of the condyle when the teeth are in maximal intercuspation resulting in an anterior open bite (Fig. 27-25). Joint destruction eventually leads to secondary DJD. Subchondral sclerosis and flattening of articulating surfaces as well as subchondral "cyst" and osteophyte formation may occur. Fibrous ankylosis or, in rare cases, osseous ankylosis may occur (Fig. 27-26); reduced mobility is related to the duration and severity of the disease.

Differential Diagnosis. The differential diagnosis includes severe DJD and psoriatic arthritis. Osteopenia and severe erosions, particularly of the articular eminence, are more characteristic of RA. Involvement of other joints may increase suspicion of RA; a medical workup may be required when doubt exists. Psoriatic arthritis may be ruled out by the patient's history of skin lesions.

Treatment. Treatment is directed toward pain relief (analgesics), reduction or suppression of inflammation (nonsteroidal antiinflammatory drugs [NSAIDs], antirheumatic drugs, corticosteroids), and preservation of muscle and joint function (physiotherapy). Joint replacement surgery may be necessary in patients with severe joint destruction.

Juvenile Idiopathic Arthritis
Synonyms. Synonyms for JIA include juvenile RA, juvenile chronic arthritis, and Still's disease.

Disease Mechanism. JIA, formerly called juvenile RA and juvenile chronic arthritis, is a chronic rheumatologic inflammatory disease that manifests before age 16 years (mean age, 5 years). JIA is characterized by chronic, intermittent synovial inflammation that

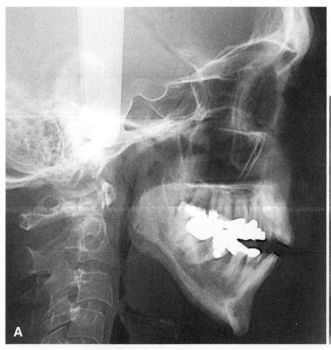
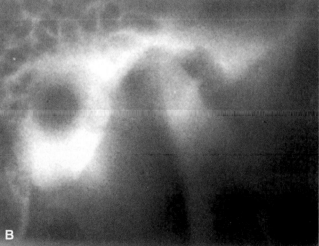

FIGURE 27-25 RA. **A,** Lateral cephalometric view illustrates a steep mandibular plane and anterior open bite. **B,** Lateral tomogram (closed position) illustrates a large erosion of the anterosuperior condylar head accompanied by severe erosions of the temporal component, including the articular eminence.

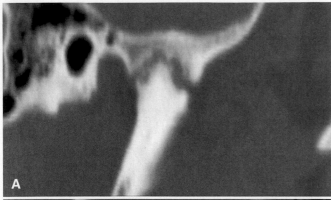

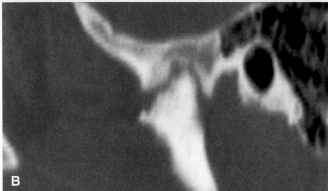

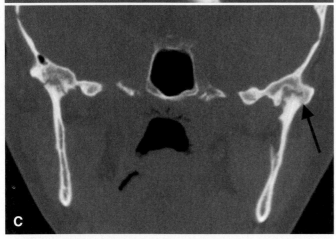

FIGURE 27-26 **A** and **B,** Sagittal reformat MDCT images with bone algorithm of the right and left joints of a case of RA. Note the irregular surface of the condyle and articular eminence and that the shapes are similar to opposing pieces of a puzzle, suggesting the possibility of fibrous ankylosis. Because of erosion of the articular eminence, the condyles have an abnormal anterior position near the residual articular eminence. **C,** Coronal MDCT image of the same case. Note osseous ankylosis on the lateral aspect of the left joint *(arrow).*

results in synovial hypertrophy, joint effusion, and swollen, painful joints. As the disease progresses, cartilage and bone are destroyed. Rheumatoid factor may be absent—hence the preferred terminology of JIA rather than juvenile RA. JIA differs from adult RA in that it has an earlier onset, and systemic involvement usually is more severe. TMJ involvement occurs in approximately 40% of patients and may be unilateral or bilateral.

Clinical Features.   JIA more commonly affects females. Children with JIA may have systemic symptoms including lethargy and pain. The TMJs in patients with JIA are often asymptomatic, even

when active disease affects these joints. When symptoms are present, they include pain in the muscles of mastication, pain and swelling over the joints, and limitations in mandibular movement. Unilateral onset is common, but contralateral involvement may occur as the disease progresses. Severe TMJ involvement results in inhibition of mandibular growth. Affected patients may have micrognathia and posteroinferior chin rotation, resulting in a facial appearance known as "bird face," which may also be accompanied by an anterior open bite. The degree of micrognathia is proportional to the severity of joint involvement and worse with earlier onset of the disease. Additionally, when only one TMJ is involved or if one side is more severely affected, the patient may have a mandibular asymmetry with the chin deviated to the affected side.

Imaging Features.   MRI with contrast agent is the modality of choice for assessing patients with JIA because it can demonstrate early synovial inflammation, even in asymptomatic patients or before bone destruction occurs. CT imaging can be performed for detailed assessment of osseous changes, whereas panoramic and cephalometric images are useful for evaluation of growth disturbances. Osteopenia (decreased density) of the affected TMJ components may be the only initial radiographic finding. Erosion of the articular eminence may result in the appearance of a large glenoid fossa. The condyle may be pointed (pencil-shaped) or concave or completely destroyed. As a result of bone destruction, the condylar head typically is positioned anterosuperiorly in the mandibular fossa (Fig. 27-27). Because the inflammation is intermittent, the cortex of the joint surfaces may reappear during quiescent periods, and the surfaces appear flattened. Secondary degenerative changes manifesting as sclerosis and osteophyte formation may be superimposed on the rheumatoid changes. Hypomobility at maximal opening is common, and fibrous ankylosis may occur in some cases. An abnormal disc shape is often observed in patients with long-term TMJ involvement. Manifestations of inhibited mandibular growth, such as deepening of the antegonial notch, diminished height of the ramus, and dorsal bending of the ramus and condylar neck, also may occur unilaterally or bilaterally, resulting in an obtuse angle between the mandibular body and the ascending ramus.

Treatment.   Early, aggressive treatment of JIA has resulted in improved outcomes. Medical treatments include NSAIDs, methotrexate, and biologic agents. Orthodontics and orthognathic surgery are often required to improve dentofacial form and function.

Psoriatic Arthritis and Ankylosing Spondylitis

Psoriatic arthritis and ankylosing spondylitis are seronegative, systemic arthritides that may affect the TMJs. Psoriatic arthritis occurs in patients with psoriasis of the skin, with inflammatory joint disease occurring in 7% of patients. Ankylosing spondylitis occurs predominantly in males and progresses to spinal fusion. TMJ imaging changes seen in these disorders may be indistinguishable from changes caused by RA, although occasionally a profound sclerotic change is seen in psoriatic arthritis.

Septic Arthritis

Synonym.   Infectious arthritis is a synonym for septic arthritis.

Disease Mechanism.   Septic arthritis is infection and inflammation of a joint that can result in joint destruction. Compared with the incidence of DJD and RA in the TMJ, septic arthritis is rare. Septic

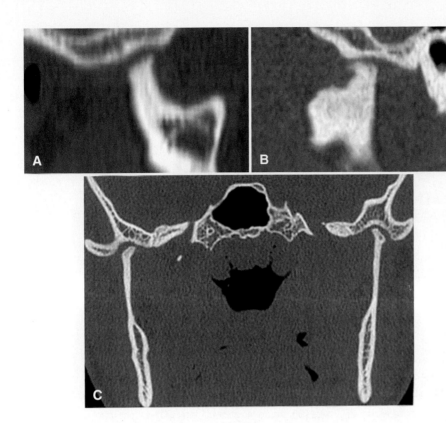

FIGURE 27-27 **A** and **B,** Sagittal MDCT reformat images of JIA. Note the severe erosion of the articular eminence and the condyles and the abnormal anterior positioning of both condyles. **C,** Coronal CT image of the same case shows small remnants of the condylar heads after severe erosion.

arthritis of the TMJ may be caused by direct spread of organisms from an adjacent cellulitis or from parotid, otic, or mastoid infections. It also may occur by direct extension of osteomyelitis of the mandibular body and ramus. Hematogenous spread from a distant, often occult, nidus has also been reported. Trauma and immunosuppression are also potential etiologic factors.

Clinical Features.   Individuals can be affected at any age, and the condition shows no sex predilection. It usually occurs unilaterally. The patient may have redness and swelling over the joint; trismus; severe pain on opening; inability to occlude the teeth; large, tender cervical lymph nodes; and fever and malaise. The mandible may be deviated to the unaffected side as a result of joint effusion.

Imaging Features.   CBCT imaging, MDCT imaging, and MRI are most useful for examining cases of suspected septic arthritis. No imaging signs may be present in acute stages of the disease, although the space between the condyle and the roof of the mandibular fossa may be widened because of inflammatory exudate in the joint spaces. Osteopenic (radiolucent) changes of the joint components and mandibular ramus may be evident. More obvious bony changes are seen approximately 7 to 10 days after the onset of clinical symptoms. As a result of the osteolytic effects of inflammation, the condylar articular cortex may become slightly radiolucent, erosions of the surface of the condyle and articular eminence may be seen, sequestra may become apparent, and there may be periosteal new bone formation (Fig. 27-28). Inflammatory changes that may accompany septic arthritis may be seen in MDCT images, such as opacification of mastoid air cells, osteomyelitis of the mandible, and cellulitis of surrounding soft tissue. MRI, with T2-weighted images, may show muscle enlargement and edema, joint effusion, or abscess. Nuclear medicine may have

a role in the diagnosis because technetium bone scan shows increased bone metabolism within the involved osseous components, especially the condyle, and a positive gallium scan confirms the presence of infection. As the disease progresses, the condyle and articular eminence, including the disc, may be destroyed. DJD is a common long-term sequela, and fibrous or osseous ankylosis may occur after the infection subsides. If the disease occurs during the period of mandibular growth, manifestations of inhibited mandibular growth may be evident in the diagnostic images.

Differential Diagnosis.   The diagnosis of septic arthritis is ideally made by identification of organisms in joint aspirate, although cultures occasionally remain negative. The imaging changes caused by septic arthritis may mimic the changes of severe DJD or RA, although septic arthritis usually occurs unilaterally. Also, the patient often has clinical signs and symptoms of infection.

Treatment.   Treatment includes antimicrobial therapy, drainage of effusion, arthrocentesis, and joint rest. Physiotherapy to reestablish joint mobility is initiated after the acute phase of infection has passed.

ARTICULAR LOOSE BODIES

Disease Mechanism

Articular loose bodies are radiopacities of varying origin that may be located in the synovium, inside the capsule in the joint spaces, or outside the capsule in soft tissue. They appear on images as calcifications seen around or superimposed over the condylar head. The loose bodies may represent bone that has separated from joint components, as in DJD (joint mice), hyaline cartilage metaplasia (calcification) that occurs in synovial chondromatosis, crystals deposited in the joint space in crystal-associated arthropathy (pseudogout), or tumoral calcinosis associated with renal disease.

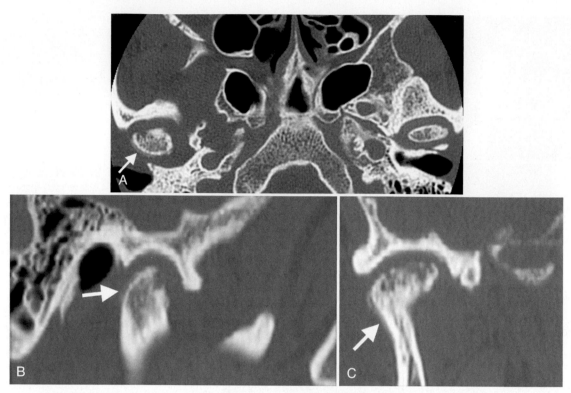

FIGURE 27-28 Axial MDCT image **(A)**, sagittal reformat MDCT image **(B)**, and coronal reformat CT image **(C)** of a case of septic arthritis involving the right joint. Note the erosions, sclerosis, and periosteal reaction that extends along the back of the condyle and lateral neck of the condyle *(arrows)*.

In rare cases, chondrosarcoma also may mimic the appearance of articular loose bodies.

Synovial Chondromatosis

Synonyms. Synonyms for synovial osteochondromatosis are synovial chondrometaplasia and osteochondromatosis.

Disease Mechanism. Synovial chondromatosis is an uncommon benign disorder characterized by metaplastic formation of multiple cartilaginous and osteocartilaginous nodules within the synovial membrane of joints. Some of these nodules may detach and form loose bodies in the joint space, where they persist and may increase in size, being nourished by synovial fluid. This condition is more common in the axial skeleton than in the TMJ. When the cartilaginous nodules ossify, the term synovial osteochondromatosis is appropriate.

Clinical Features. Females are more commonly affected in the TMJ than males. Patients may be asymptomatic or may complain of preauricular swelling, pain, change in occlusion, and decreased range of motion. Some patients have crepitus or other joint noises. The condition usually occurs unilaterally.

Imaging Features. The osseous components may appear normal or may exhibit osseous changes similar to changes in DJD. The joint space may be widened, and if ossification of the cartilaginous nodules has occurred, a radiopaque mass or several radiopaque loose bodies may be seen surrounding the condylar head (Fig. 27-29). There is considerable variation in the size of these

ossified loose bodies. CT imaging can indicate the location of these calcifications and confirm that they represent ossifications. Reactive sclerosis of the glenoid fossa and condyle may be seen. Occasionally, erosion through the glenoid fossa into the middle cranial fossa may occur, which is best detected with CT imaging. MRI can detect joint space effusion and enlargement and may be useful in defining the tissue planes between the synovial chondromatosis mass and surrounding soft tissue.

Differential Diagnosis. The appearance of synovial osteochondromatosis cannot always be differentiated from chondrocalcinosis; however, the ossified bodies in osteochondromatosis often are larger and may have a peripheral cortex that identifies their bony nature. Conditions that appear similar include DJD with joint mice (detached osteophytes) or chondrosarcoma or osteosarcoma. Sarcomas may be accompanied by severe bone destruction, which would help in differentiating the condition from synovial chondromatosis.

Treatment. Treatment consists of removal of the loose bodies and resection of abnormal synovial tissue in the joint by arthroscopic or open joint surgery.

Chondrocalcinosis

Synonyms. Pseudogout and calcium pyrophosphate dihydrate deposition disease are synonyms for chondrocalcinosis.

Disease Mechanism. Chondrocalcinosis is characterized by acute or chronic synovitis and precipitation of calcium pyrophosphate

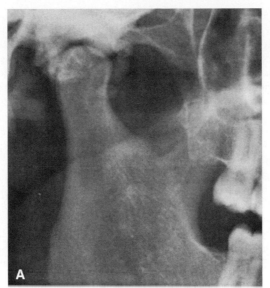

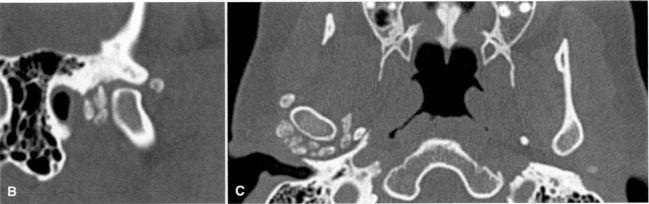

FIGURE 27-29 **A,** Cropped panoramic image of a right joint involved with osteochondromatosis. **B,** Sagittal CT reformat image. **C,** Axial MDCT image revealing multiple ossified bodies surrounding the condyle and within the joint capsule.

dihydrate crystals in the joint space. It differs from gout, in which urate crystals are precipitated—hence the term pseudogout.

Clinical Features.   More commonly affected joints are the knee, wrist, hip, shoulder, and elbow; TMJ involvement is uncommon. The condition occurs unilaterally. Patients most often complain of pain and swelling over the joint. Some patients are asymptomatic.

Imaging Features.   The appearance of chondrocalcinosis may simulate synovial chondromatosis, described previously. Often the radiopacities within the joint space are finer and have a more even distribution than in osteochondromatosis (Fig. 27-30). Crystal deposition may also extend to tissues surrounding the joint. Bone erosions and profound sclerosis of the osseous components have been described. Erosions of the glenoid fossa may be present, which require CT imaging for detection. Soft tissue swelling and edema of the surrounding muscles may be seen with MRI.

Differential Diagnosis.   The differential diagnosis is the same as for synovial chondromatosis.

Treatment.   Treatment consists of surgical removal of the large crystalline masses. Steroids, aspirin, and NSAIDs may provide relief. Colchicine may be used to alleviate acute symptoms and for prophylaxis.

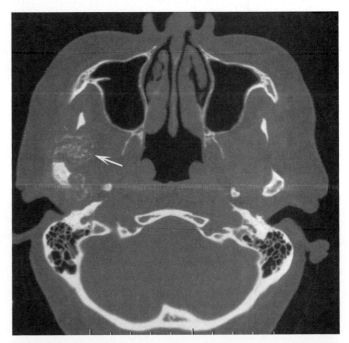

FIGURE 27-30   Axial bone algorithm MDCT image of chondrocalcinosis. Note the calcifications anterior to the right condyle *(arrow)* and the large erosion involving the medial pole of the condyle. Also, there is profound sclerosis of the lateral pole.

TRAUMA

Effusion

Disease Mechanism. Effusion is an influx of fluid into the joint and may be associated with trauma; soft tissue abnormalities, such as disc displacement; or arthritic conditions. Effusions within the joint after trauma most often represent hemorrhage into the joint spaces (hemarthrosis).

Clinical Features. The patient may have swelling over the affected joint; pain in the TMJ, preauricular region, or ear; and limited range of motion. Patients may also complain of the sensation of fluid in the ear, tinnitus, hearing difficulties, and difficulty occluding the posterior teeth.

Imaging Features. Joint effusions are best seen on T2-weighted MRI as bright signal (white) areas around the condyle. The involved joint spaces would be widened (see Fig. 27-19).

Differential Diagnosis. Effusion secondary to trauma must be differentiated from other conditions manifesting with effusion, including disc displacement and arthritis. Evidence of condylar fracture may be detected in cases of trauma. Patient history and clinical examination should be helpful.

Treatment. Treatment may include antiinflammatory drugs, although surgical drainage of the effusion occasionally is necessary.

Condylar Dislocation

Disease Mechanism. Condylar dislocation is abnormal positioning of the condyle out of the mandibular fossa but within the joint capsule. It usually occurs bilaterally and most commonly in an anterior direction. Dislocation may be caused by trauma and is often associated with a condylar fracture. Forced mouth opening, such as in an intubation procedure or failure of muscular coordination, may also lead to dislocation. Loose ligaments and joint capsule may predispose to chronic TMJ dislocation. Dislocation may also rarely occur superiorly through the roof of the glenoid fossa, into the middle cranial fossa, as a result of trauma.

Clinical Features. In anterior dislocation, patients are unable to close the mandible to maximal intercuspation. Some patients cannot reduce the dislocation, whereas others may be able to reduce the mandible by manipulation. Associated pain and muscle spasm often are present.

Imaging Features. CBCT imaging and MDCT imaging are most useful for evaluating the involved structures. Images show the condyle positioned outside the glenoid fossa, most commonly anterior and superior to the summit of the articular eminence. Signs of an associated condylar fracture may be present.

Differential Diagnosis. In patients with mandibular hypermobility, the condyles may translate anterior and superior to the articular eminence on opening. Clinical correlation to confirm that the patient cannot close the jaw normally is important to make the diagnosis of dislocation.

Treatment. Treatment consists of manual manipulation of the mandible to reduce the dislocation. Surgery occasionally is necessary to achieve reduction, especially in protracted cases.

Fracture

Disease Mechanism. Fractures of the TMJ may occur within the condylar head (intracapsular) or in the condylar neck (extracapsular). Condylar neck fractures are most common and are often accompanied by dislocation of the condylar head. Condylar head fractures may be horizontal, vertical, or compression fractures. Rarely, the fracture may involve the temporal component. Unilateral fractures, which are more common than bilateral fractures, may be accompanied by a parasymphyseal or mandibular body fracture on the contralateral side.

Clinical Features. The patient may have swelling over the TMJ, pain, limited range of motion, deviation to the affected side, and malocclusion or an anterior open bite. Some TMJ fractures are relatively asymptomatic and may not be discovered at the time of trauma; instead, these come to light as incidental findings at a later time when images are obtained for other reasons. Condylar fractures should be ruled out if the patient has a history of a blow to the mandible, especially to the mental region.

If a condylar fracture occurs during the period of mandibular growth, growth may be inhibited because of damage to the condylar growth center. The degree of subsequent hypoplasia is related to the severity of the injury and the stage of mandibular development at the time of injury (younger patients have more profound hypoplasia). Patients younger than 10 years old have a higher remodeling potential and may have less deformity compared with older patients, although injuries in patients younger than 3 years old tend to produce severe asymmetries. Injury to the joint may result in hemorrhage or effusion into the joint spaces that eventually may form bone during the healing process, which may result in ankylosis and limited joint function.

Imaging Features. In relatively recent condylar neck fractures, a radiolucent line limited to the outline of the neck may be visible. This line may vary in width, depending on whether the bone fragments are still aligned (narrow line) or displacement or dislocation has occurred (wider line). If the bone fragments overlap, an area of apparent increase in radiopacity may be seen instead of a radiolucent line (Fig. 27-31). Also, careful examination of the outer cortical boundary of the condyle and neck may reveal an irregular outline or a step defect. Approximately 60% of condylar fractures show evidence of fragment angulation and a variable degree of displacement (dislocation) of the fracture ends. Displacement of the condylar head most commonly occurs in an anterior and medial direction because of pull from the lateral pterygoid muscle. Fractures of the condylar head are less common and may be horizontal, vertical (responsible for the traumatic type of bifid condyle), or compressive types (Fig. 27-32). CBCT imaging is the preferred imaging modality to evaluate condylar fractures, because there is no superimposition of adjacent structures and TMJ reformats provide images in customizable planes. Two-dimensional and three-dimensional reformatted images are useful to localize a fractured fragment accurately. Alternatively, if CBCT imaging is unavailable, multiple right-angle plain film skull projections from the lateral, frontal, and basilar aspects may be used to detect a fracture.

The amount of remodeling seen in the TMJ after a condylar fracture with medial displacement varies considerably. In some cases, the bony fragments remodel to a form that is essentially normal, whereas in other cases the mandibular fossa may become shallow to compensate for a new condylar position. The condylar fragment may fuse to the condylar neck or ramus in a new,

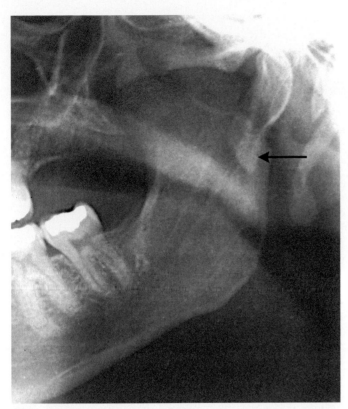

FIGURE 27-31 Panoramic image of condylar neck fracture. *Arrow* points to overlapped fragments, as evidenced by increased radiopacity.

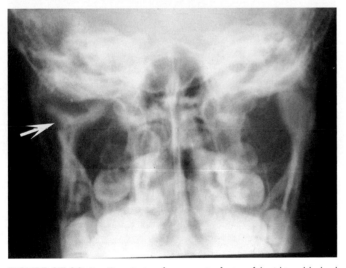

FIGURE 27-32 Open Towne's view of a compression fracture of the right condylar head (arrow).

abnormal position. The condyle eventually may show degenerative changes, including flattening, erosion, osteophyte formation, and ankylosis. These changes are more severe if the condyle is displaced. Condylar fractures can also be associated with damage of the intracapsular soft tissues, including the disc, joint capsule, and retrodiscal tissues, and with hemarthrosis and joint effusion.

Differential Diagnosis. Occasionally, old fractures that have remodeled may be difficult to differentiate from developmental abnormalities of the condyle. The most common difficulty is in determining whether a fracture is present. Panoramic views taken as an initial examination may not disclose a fracture, especially greenstick fractures of the condylar neck because changes in the mediolateral plane cannot be appreciated. Supplementation with a plain film at right angles (open Towne's view) or CBCT imaging is often necessary to visualize displacements.

Treatment. Treatment may not be indicated if mandibular function is adequate; otherwise, the fracture is reduced surgically. Physiotherapy may be important to maintain mobility and prevent the development of ankylosis.

Neonatal Fractures

Disease Mechanism. The use of forceps during delivery of neonates may result in fracture and displacement of the rudimentary condyle, which later manifests as severe mandibular hypoplasia and lack of development of the glenoid fossa and articular eminence. Such cases have a characteristic radiographic appearance in the panoramic image, having the appearance of a partly opened pair of scissors in place of a normal condyle (Fig. 27-33). This presentation results from the overlapping images of the medially displaced carrot-shaped rudimentary condyle and remnants of the condylar neck.

Differential Diagnosis. This condition often is not diagnosed until later in life, at which time a diagnosis of fracture may be made without a history that the fracture occurred at the time of birth. The condition must be differentiated from developmental hypoplasia of the mandible, which is unrelated to birth injury.

Treatment. The fracture usually is not treated, but the mandibular asymmetry may be corrected with a combination of orthodontics and orthognathic surgery.

ANKYLOSIS

Disease Mechanism

Ankylosis is a condition in which condylar movement is restricted because of fusion of the intraarticular joint components ("true" ankylosis) or a physical impediment caused by structures outside the joint. Intraarticular ankylosis may be bony or fibrous. In bony ankylosis, the condyle or ramus is attached to the temporal or zygomatic bone by an osseous bridge. In fibrous ankylosis, a soft tissue (fibrous) union of joint components occurs. Most unilateral cases are caused by mandibular trauma or infection. Severe arthritis, particularly related to rheumatic conditions, and therapeutic radiation exposure to the joint (cancer treatment) may also give rise to ankylosis. Extraarticular ankylosis may result from conditions that inhibit condylar movement, such as muscle spasm or fibrosis, myositis ossificans, or coronoid process hyperplasia.

Clinical Features

Patients have a history of progressively restricted jaw opening, or they may have a long-standing history of limited opening. Some degree of mandibular opening usually is possible through flexing of the mandible, although opening may be restricted to only a few millimeters, particularly in the case of bony ankylosis. Patients who develop ankylosis in childhood may have an associated facial asymmetry because of altered growth of the mandible. Pain is not commonly associated with ankylosis.

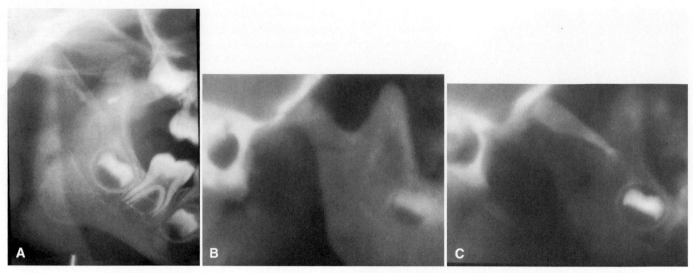

FIGURE 27-33 A, Cropped panoramic image of a neonatal fracture of the right condyle. Note the unusual shape of the coronoid notch, similar to a partially opened pair of scissors. **B,** Tomographic image slice of the lateral aspect of the same joint. Note the normal-appearing coronoid notch but lack of formation of the glenoid fossa and eminence and the abnormal anterior position of the condyle. **C,** Medial tomographic slice of the same case disclosing the fractured segment.

Imaging Features

In fibrous ankylosis, the articulating surfaces are usually irregular because of erosions. The joint space is usually very narrow, and although the bones are not fused, the two irregular surfaces may appear to fit one another like a jigsaw puzzle (see Fig. 27-26). Little or no condylar movement is seen. Radiographic signs of remodeling occasionally are visible as the joint components adapt to repeated attempts at mandibular opening. In bony ankylosis, the joint space may be partly or completely obliterated by the osseous bridge, which can vary from a slender segment of bone to a large bony mass (Fig. 27-34). Degenerative changes of the joint components are common. Morphologic changes often occur, such as compensatory progressive elongation of the coronoid processes and deepening of the antegonial notch in the mandibular ramus on the affected side, as a result of muscle function during attempted mandibular opening. If ankylosis occurs before mandibular growth is complete, growth of the affected side of the mandible is inhibited. Coronal CT images are the best diagnostic imaging method to evaluate ankylosis.

Differential Diagnosis

The major differential diagnosis is a condylar tumor. However, a history of trauma, infection, or other joint diseases should help rule out neoplastic disease. Differentiation of fibrous ankylosis from other causes of limited condylar movement is difficult because fibrous tissue is not visible in the diagnostic image.

Treatment

TMJ ankylosis requires surgical intervention. Gap arthroplasty involves removal of the osseous bridge or creation of a pseudarthrosis below the original joint space. Costochondral grafts are also used. Recurrence of ankylosis after surgery may develop.

TUMORS

Disease Mechanism

Benign and malignant tumors originating in or involving the TMJ are rare. Tumors affecting the TMJ may be intrinsic to the joint,

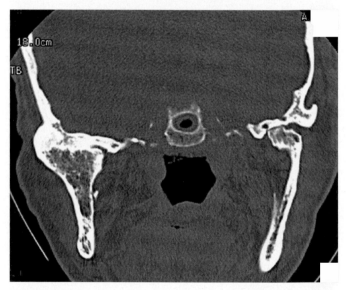

FIGURE 27-34 Coronal bone algorithm MDCT image slice of bony ankylosis. The right condyle and ramus are markedly enlarged. The articulating surface is irregular, and the central and lateral aspects are fused to the roof of the glenoid fossa, as evidenced by a lack of joint space. The left condylar articulating surface is eroded, and the joint space is decreased on the medial aspect; these changes are consistent with DJD.

developing in the condyle or temporal bone or soft tissue components of the joint, or they may be extrinsic, developing in the adjacent structures, such as the coronoid process or adjacent soft tissues. In either case, a tumor has the potential to affect joint morphology or function directly or indirectly. In extrinsic tumors, this effect on joint morphology or function may occur as a result of pressure exerted on the joint by the nearby tumor, or indirect effects on growth of the joint components as is sometimes seen with adjacent vascular lesions, or the tumor influencing mandibular positioning and range of motion during mandibular opening.

Benign Tumors

The most common benign intrinsic tumors involving the TMJ are osteochondromas; other tumors include osteomas, Langerhans' histiocytosis osteoblastomas, chondroblastomas, fibromyxomas, giant cell granulomas, and aneurysmal bone cysts. Benign tumors and cysts of the mandible (e.g., ameloblastomas, keratocystic odontogenic tumors, simple bone cysts) may involve the entire ramus and in rare cases extend into the condyle. In cases of extraarticular ankylosis, in which mandibular movement is restricted but the TMJs appear normal, hyperplasia or a tumor of the coronoid process must be ruled out.

Clinical Features.   Condylar tumors grow slowly and may attain considerable size before becoming clinically noticeable. Patients may complain of TMJ swelling, which may be accompanied by pain and decreased range of motion; the symptoms often mimic TMJ dysfunction. The clinical examination may reveal facial asymmetry, malocclusion, and deviation of the mandible to the unaffected side. Tumors of the coronoid process typically are painless, but patients may complain of progressive limitation of mandibular motion.

Imaging Features.   A benign tumor of the mandibular condyle usually manifests as an irregularly shaped enlargement of the condylar head. There may be decreased trabecular density owing to bony destruction or increased density owing to new, abnormal bone formed by the tumor. An osteoma or osteochondroma appears as an irregular, often pedunculated radiopaque mass attached to, or growing from, the condyle. Osteochondromas are benign tumors that most often extend from the anterior surface of the condyle near the attachment of the lateral pterygoid muscle. These bony growths usually have a cartilaginous cap. To differentiate these from osteomas, it is important to note that the internal

cancellous bone of the condyle is continuous with the internal structure of the osteochondroma (Fig. 27-35). Langerhans' histiocytosis creates well-defined radiolucent defects within the bone, and a laminated periosteal reaction may be seen along the adjacent cortices. Osteoblastomas manifest with mixed radiolucent and radiopaque patterns (see Chapter 22). Because benign tumors may interfere with normal joint function, secondary bone remodeling or degenerative changes may be seen in the affected joint. Tumors of the coronoid process may also affect TMJ function, which emphasizes the need to image and evaluate the coronoid process when evaluating joint abnormalities.

Differential Diagnosis.   Condylar tumors may simulate unilateral condylar hyperplasia because of condylar enlargement. Osteomas and osteochondromas generally create a more irregular appearance, with a bulbous or pedunculated growth pattern, whereas the characteristic condylar shape and proportions are better preserved in condylar hyperplasia. Coronoid tumors must be differentiated from coronoid hyperplasia, which differs from a tumor in that the coronoid process remains regular in shape.

Treatment.   Treatment consists of surgical excision of the tumor and occasionally excision of the condylar head or coronoid process.

Malignant Tumors

Disease Mechanism.   Malignant tumors of the TMJs may be primary or, more commonly, metastatic. Primary intrinsic malignant tumors of the condyle are extremely rare and include chondrosarcoma, osteogenic sarcoma, synovial sarcoma, and fibrosarcoma of the joint capsule. Extrinsic malignant tumors may represent direct extension of adjacent parotid salivary gland malignancies; rhabdomyosarcoma (particularly in children); or other regional carcinomas from the skin, ear, and nasopharynx. The most

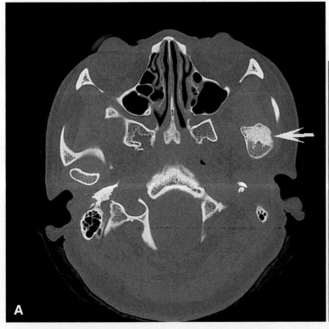
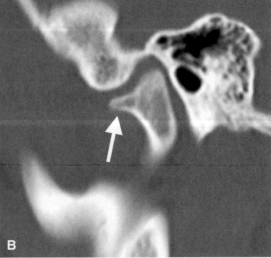

FIGURE 27-35 A, Axial bone algorithm MDCT image of an osteochondroma extending from the anterior surface of the left condylar head *(arrow)*. **B,** Sagittal reformat CT image of a different case; the internal aspect of the osteochondroma *(arrow)* is continuous with the cancellous portion of the condylar head.

common metastatic lesions include neoplasms originating in the breast, kidney, lung, colon, prostate, thyroid gland, and multiple myeloma.

Clinical Features.   Malignant tumors (primary or metastatic) may be asymptomatic, or patients may have symptoms of TMJ dysfunction, such as pain, limited mandibular opening, mandibular deviation, and swelling. A patient occasionally is treated for TMJ dysfunction without recognition that the underlying condition is a malignancy.

Imaging Features.   Malignant primary and metastatic TMJ tumors manifest with a variable degree of bone destruction with ill-defined, irregular margins. Most lack tumor bone formation, with the exception of osteogenic sarcoma, which often has a radiopaque component. Chondrosarcoma may appear as an indistinct, essentially radiolucent destructive lesion of the condyle with surrounding discrete soft tissue calcifications that may simulate the appearance of the articular loose bodies seen in chondrocalcinosis or pseudogout (Fig. 27-36). In the case of metastatic tumors, the radiographic appearance usually is nonspecific condylar destruction (with a few exceptions, such as metastatic prostate carcinoma, which may have osteoblastic reaction) and does not indicate the site of origin (Fig. 27-37). Pathologic fracture of the condyle may be seen as a sequela of destruction of the bony structure of the joint (Fig. 27-38). CT imaging is the imaging modality of choice to view bone involvement. MRI is useful for displaying the extent of involvement into the surrounding soft tissues.

Differential Diagnosis.   Joint destruction caused by a malignant tumor must be differentiated from the osseous destruction seen in severe DJD. Malignant tumors cause profound central bone

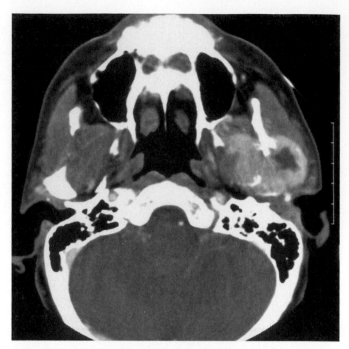

FIGURE 27-37 Axial soft tissue algorithm CT image of a metastatic lesion from a carcinoma of the thyroid gland that has destroyed all of the left mandibular condyle.

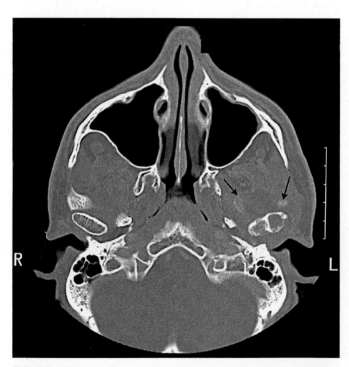

FIGURE 27-36 Axial bone algorithm MDCT image of chondrosarcoma. A radiolucent destructive lesion is present in the left condylar head, and faint radiopacities (soft tissue calcifications) are visible anterior to the condylar head *(arrows)*.

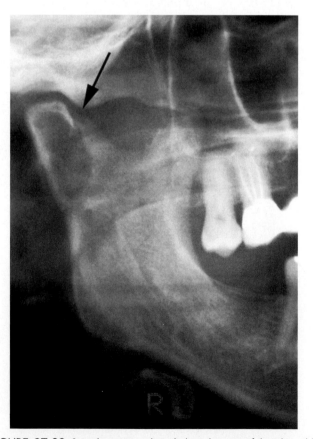

FIGURE 27-38 Cropped panoramic radiograph shows destruction of the right condyle owing to a metastatic lung carcinoma with a secondary pathologic fracture *(arrow)*.

destruction, whereas the bone resorption seen in DJD is more peripheral. Also, no soft tissue mass is seen in association with DJD but would be expected when a malignant tumor is present. Chondrosarcoma may simulate joint space calcifications (discussed earlier) but is also associated with severe bone destruction, in contrast to other conditions forming loose joint bodies.

Treatment. In the case of primary malignant tumors, treatment consists of wide surgical removal of the tumor. Tumor extension to vital anatomic structures may compromise survival. Metastatic tumors of the TMJ rarely are treated surgically; treatment mainly is palliative and may include radiotherapy and chemotherapy.

BIBLIOGRAPHY

Disorders of the Temporomandibular Joint

Brooks SL, Brand JW, Gibbs SJ, et al: Imaging of the temporomandibular joint, position paper of the American Academy of Oral and Maxillofacial Radiology, *Oral Surg Oral Med Oral Pathol Oral Radiol Endod* 83:609–618, 1997.

Helkimo M: Studies on function and dysfunction of the masticatory system, II: index for anamnestic and clinical dysfunction and occlusal state, *Sven Tandlak Tidskr* 67:101–121, 1974.

McNeill C, Mohl ND, Rugh JD, et al: Temporomandibular disorders: diagnosis, management, education, and research, *J Am Dent Assoc* 120:253, 255, 257, 1990.

Petrikowski CG, Grace MG: Temporomandibular joint radiographic findings in adolescents, *Cranio* 14:30–36, 1996.

Rugh JD, Solberg WK: Oral health status in the United States: temporomandibular disorders, *J Dent Educ* 49:398–406, 1985.

Wänman A, Agerberg G: Mandibular dysfunction in adolescents, I: prevalence of symptoms, *Acta Odontol Scand* 44:47–54, 1986.

Anatomy of the Temporomandibular Joint

Blaschke DD, Blaschke TJ: A method for quantitatively determining temporomandibular joint bony relationships, *J Dent Res* 60:35–43, 1981.

Drace JE, Enzmann DR: Defining the normal temporomandibular joint: closed, partially open, and open mouth MR imaging of asymptomatic subjects, *Radiology* 177:67–76, 1990.

Hansson LG, Hansson T, Petersson A: A comparison between clinical and radiologic findings in 259 temporomandibular joint patients, *J Prosthet Dent* 50:89–94, 1983.

Ingervall B, Carlsson GE, Thilander B: Postnatal development of the human temporomandibular joint. II. A microradiographic study, *Acta Odont Scand* 34:133–139, 1976.

Larheim TA: Radiographic appearance of the normal temporomandibular joint in newborns and small children, *Acta Radiol Diagn (Stockh)* 22:593–599, 1981.

Pullinger AG, Hohender L, Solberg WK, et al: A tomographic study of mandibular condyle position in an asymptomatic population, *J Prosthet Dent* 53:706–713, 1985.

Taylor RC, Ware WH, Fowler D, et al: A study of temporomandibular joint morphology and its relationship to the dentition, *Oral Surg* 33:1002–1013, 1972.

Ten Cate AR: Gross and micro anatomy. In Zarb GA, Carlsson BJ, Mohl ND, editors: *Temporomandibular joint and masticatory muscle disorders*, ed 2, Copenhagen, 1994, Munksgaard.

Westesson P-L, Kurita K, Eriksson L, et al: Cryosectional observations of functional anatomy of the temporomandibular joint, *Oral Surg Oral Med Oral Pathol* 68:247–251, 1989.

Yale SH, Allison BD, Hauptfuehrer JD: An epidemiological assessment of mandibular condyle morphology, *Oral Surg* 21:169–177, 1966.

Diagnostic Imaging of the Temporomandibular Joint

Brooks SL, Brand AW, Gibbs SJ, et al: Imaging of the temporomandibular joint: position paper of the American Academy of Oral and Maxillofacial Radiology, *Oral Surg Oral Med Oral Pathol Oral Radiol Endod* 83:609–618, 1997.

Helms CA, Kaplan P: Diagnostic imaging of the temporomandibular joint: recommendations for use of the various techniques, *AJR Am J Roentgenol* 154:319–322, 1990.

Katzberg RW: Temporomandibular joint imaging, *Radiology* 170:297–307, 1989.

Hard Tissue Imaging

Christiansen EL, Chan TT, Thompson JR, et al: Computed tomography of the normal temporomandibular joint, *Scand J Dent Res* 95:499–509, 1987.

Coin CG: Tomography of the temporomandibular joint, *Med Radiogr Photogr* 50:26–39, 1974.

Tsiklakis K, Syriopoulos K, Stamatakis HC: Radiographic examination of the temporomandibular joint using cone beam computed tomography, *Dentomaxillofac Radiol* 33:196–201, 2004.

Soft Tissue Imaging

Conway WF, Hayes CW, Campbell RL: Dynamic magnetic resonance imaging of the temporomandibular joint using FLASH sequences, *J Oral Maxillofac Surg* 46:930–938, 1988.

Hansson LG, Westesson PL, Eriksson L: Comparison of tomography and midfield magnetic resonance imaging for osseous changes of the temporomandibular joint, *Oral Surg Oral Med Oral Pathol Oral Radiol Endod* 82:698–703, 1996.

Moses JJ, Salinas E, Goergen T, et al: Magnetic resonance imaging or arthrographic diagnosis of internal derangement of the temporomandibular joint, *Oral Surg Oral Med Oral Pathol* 75:268–272, 1993.

Tomas X, Pomes J, Berenquer J, et al: MR imaging of temporomandibular joint dysfunction: a pictorial review, *Radiographics* 26:765–781, 2006.

Radiographic Abnormalities of the Temporomandibular Joint
Condylar Hyperplasia

Gray RJM, Sloan P, Quayle AA, et al: Histopathological and scintigraphic features of condylar hyperplasia, *Int J Oral Maxillofac Surg* 19:65–71, 1990.

Rubenstein LK, Campbell RL: Acquired unilateral condylar hyperplasia and facial asymmetry: report of a case, *ASDC J Dent Child* 52:114–120, 1985.

Shira RB: Facial asymmetry and condylar hyperplasia, *Oral Surg* 40:567, 1975.

Wolford LM, Mehra P, Reiche-Fischel O, et al: Efficacy of high condylectomy for management of condylar hyperplasia, *Am J Orthod Dentofac Orthop* 121:136–151, 2002.

Condylar Hypoplasia

Jerell RG, Fuselier B, Mahan P: Acquired condylar hypoplasia: report of a case, *ASDC J Dent Child* 58:147–153, 1991.

Worth HM: Radiology of the temporomandibular joint. In Zarb GA, Carlsson BJ, Mohl ND, editors: *Temporomandibular joint function and dysfunction*, Copenhagen, 1979, Munksgaard.

Juvenile Arthrosis

Boering G: Temporomandibular joint arthrosis and facial deformity, *Trans Int Conf Oral Surg* 258–260, 1967.

Worth HM: Radiology of the temporomandibular joint. In Zarb GA, Carlsson BJ, Mohl ND, editors: *Temporomandibular joint function and dysfunction*, Copenhagen, 1979, Munksgaard.

Coronoid Hyperplasia

Daniels JSM, Ali I: Post-traumatic bifid condyle associated with temporomandibular joint ankylosis: report of a case and review of the literature, *Oral Surg Oral Med Oral Pathol Oral Radiol Endod* 99:682–688, 2005.

Loh FC, Yeo JF: Bifid mandibular condyle, *Oral Surg Oral Med Oral Pathol* 69:24–27, 1990.

McLoughlin PM, Hopper C, Bowley NB: Hyperplasia of the mandibular coronoid process: an analysis of 31 cases and a review of the literature, *J Oral Maxillofac Surg* 53:250–255, 1995.

Satoh K, Ohno S, Aizawa T, et al: Bilateral coronoid hyperplasia in an adolescent: report of a case and review of the literature, *J Oral Maxillofac Surg* 64:334–338, 2006.

Soft Tissue Abnormalities

Dolwick MF, Sanders B: TMJ internal derangement and arthrosis. In *Surgical atlas,* St. Louis, 1985, Mosby.

Helms CA, Kaban LB, McNeill C, et al: Temporomandibular joint: morphology and signal intensity characteristics of the disc at MR imaging, *Radiology* 172:817–820, 1989.

Katzberg RW: Temporomandibular joint imaging, *Radiology* 170:297, 1989.

Katzberg RW, Tallents RH, Hayakawa K, et al: Internal derangements of the temporomandibular joint: findings in the pediatric age group, *Radiology* 154:125–127, 1985.

Larheim TA: Current trends in temporomandibular joint imaging, *Oral Surg Oral Med Oral Pathol Oral Radiol Endod* 80:555–576, 1995.

Larheim TA: Role of magnetic resonance imaging in the clinical diagnosis of the temporomandibular joint, *Cells Tissues Organs* 180:6–21, 2005.

Nuelle DG, Alpern MC, Ufema JW: Arthroscopic surgery of the temporomandibular joint, *Angle Orthod* 56:118–142, 1986.

Rammelsberg P, Pospiech PR, Jäger L, et al: Variability of disc position in asymptomatic volunteers and patients with internal derangements of the TMJ, *Oral Surg Oral Med Oral Pathol Oral Radiol Endod* 83:393–399, 1997.

Sano T, Westesson PL: Magnetic resonance imaging of the temporomandibular joint: increased T2 signal in the retro-discal tissue of painful joints, *Oral Surg Oral Med Oral Pathol Oral Radiol Endod* 79:511–516, 1995.

Wilkes CH: Internal derangements of the temporomandibular joint: pathological variations, *Arch Otolaryngol Head Neck Surg* 115:469–477, 1989.

Remodeling and Arthritic Conditions

Remodeling

Brooks SL, Westesson PL, Eriksson L, et al: Prevalence of osseous changes in the temporomandibular joint of asymptomatic persons without internal derangement, *Oral Surg Oral Med Oral Pathol* 73:118–122, 1992.

Moffett BC, Johnson LC, McCabe JB, et al: Articular remodeling in the adult human temporomandibular joint, *Am J Anat* 115:119–141, 1964.

Degenerative Joint Disease

de Leeuw R, Boering G, Stegenga B, et al: Temporomandibular joint osteoarthrosis: clinical and radiographic characteristics 30 years after nonsurgical treatment–a preliminary report, *Cranio* 11:15–24, 1993.

Helenius LMJ, Tervahartiala P, Helenius I, et al: Clinical, radiographic and MRI findings of the temporomandibular joint in patients with different rheumatic diseases, *Int J Oral Maxillofac Surg* 35:983–989, 2006.

Kurita H, Uehara S, Yokochi M, et al: A long-term follow-up study of radiographically evident degenerative changes in the temporomandibular joint with different conditions of disc displacement, *Int J Oral Maxillofac Surg* 35:49–54, 2006.

Mayne JG, Hatch GS: Arthritis of the temporomandibular joint, *J Am Dent Assoc* 79:125–130, 1969.

Radin EL, Paul IL, Rose RM: Role of mechanical factors in pathogenesis of primary osteoarthritis, *Lancet* 1:519–522, 1972.

Sato H, Fujii T, Yamada N, et al: Temporomandibular joint osteoarthritis: a comparative clinical and tomographic study pre- and post-treatment, *J Oral Rehabil* 21:383–395, 1994.

Rheumatoid Arthritis

Gynther GW, Tronje G, Holmlund AB: Radiographic changes in the temporomandibular joint in patients with generalized osteoarthritis and rheumatoid arthritis, *Oral Surg Oral Med Oral Pathol Oral Radiol Endod* 81:613–618, 1996.

Larheim TA, Smith HJ, Aspestrand F: Rheumatic disease of the temporomandibular joint: MR imaging and tomographic manifestations, *Radiology* 175:527–531, 1990.

Syrjänen SM: The temporomandibular joint in rheumatoid arthritis, *Acta Radiol Diagn (Stockh)* 26:235–243, 1985.

Juvenile Idiopathic Arthritis

Ganik R, Williams FA: Diagnosis and management of juvenile rheumatoid arthritis with TMJ involvement, *Cranio* 4:254–262, 1986.

Hu Y-S, Schneiderman ED: The temporomandibular joint in juvenile rheumatoid arthritis. I: computed tomographic findings, *Pediatr Dent* 17:46–53, 1995.

Hu Y-S, Schneiderman ED, Harper RP: The temporomandibular joint in juvenile rheumatoid arthritis. II: relationship between computed tomographic and clinical findings, *Pediatr Dent* 18:312–319, 1996.

Karhulahti T, Ylijoki H, Rönning O: Mandibular condyle lesions related to age at onset and subtypes of juvenile rheumatoid arthritis in 15-year-old children, *Scand J Dent Res* 101:332–338, 1993.

Stoll ML, Sharpe T, Beukelman T, et al: Risk factors for temporomandibular joint arthritis in children with juvenile idiopathic arthritis, *J Rheumatol* 39:1880–1887, 2012.

Psoriatic Arthritis

Koorbusch GF, Zeitler DL, Fotos PG, et al: Psoriatic arthritis of the temporomandibular joints with ankylosis, *Oral Surg Oral Med Oral Pathol* 71:267–274, 1991.

Wilson AW, Brown JS, Ord RA: Psoriatic arthropathy of the temporomandibular joint, *Oral Surg Oral Med Oral Pathol* 70:555–558, 1990.

Ankylosing Spondylitis

Locher MC, Felder M, Sailer HF: Involvement of the temporomandibular joints in ankylosing spondylitis (Bechterew's disease), *J Craniomaxillofac Surg* 24:205–213, 1996.

Ramos-Remus C, Major P, Gomez-Vargas A, et al: Temporomandibular joint osseous morphology in a consecutive sample of ankylosing spondylitis patients, *Ann Rheum Dis* 56:103–107, 1997.

Septic Arthritis

Leighty SM, Spach DH, Myall RW, et al: Septic arthritis of the temporomandibular joint: review of the literature and report of two cases in children, *Int J Oral Maxillofac Surg* 22:292–297, 1993.

Sembronio S, Albiero AM, Robiony M, et al: Septic arthritis of the temporomandibular joint successfully treated with arthroscopic lysis and lavage: case report and review of the literature, *Oral Surg Oral Med Oral Pathol Oral Radiol Endod* 103:e1–e6, 2007.

Articular Loose Bodies

Ardekian L, Faquin W, Troulis MJ, et al: Synovial chondromatosis of the temporomandibular joint: report and analysis of eleven cases, *J Oral Maxillofac Surg* 63:941–947, 2005.

Carls FR, von Hochstetter A, Engelke W, et al: Loose bodies in the temporomandibular joint, *J Craniomaxillofac Surg* 23:215–221, 1995.

Chuong R, Piper MA: Bilateral pseudogout of the temporomandibular joint: report of a case and review of the literature, *J Oral Maxillofac Surg* 53:691–694, 1995.

Dijkgraaf LC, Liem RS, de Bont LG, et al: Calcium pyrophosphate dihydrate crystal deposition disease: a review of the literature and a light and electron microscopic study of a case of the temporomandibular joint with numerous intracellular crystals in the chondrocytes, *Osteoarthritis Cartilage* 3:35–45, 1995.

Lustmann J, Zeltser R: Synovial chondromatosis of the temporomandibular joint: review of the literature and case report, *Int J Oral Maxillofac Surg* 18:90–94, 1989.

Orden A, Laskin DM, Lew D: Chronic preauricular swelling, *J Oral Maxillofac Surg* 47:390–397, 1989.

Pynn BR, Weinberg S, Irish J: Calcium pyrophosphate dihydrate deposition disease of the temporomandibular joint: a case report and review of the literature, *Oral Surg Oral Med Oral Pathol Oral Radiol Endod* 79:278–284, 1995.

Yu Q, Yang J, Wang P, et al: CT features of synovial chondromatosis in the temporomandibular joint, *Oral Surg Oral Med Oral Pathol Oral Radiol Endod* 97:524–528, 2007.

Trauma
Effusion
Emshoff R, Brandimaier I, Bertram S, et al: Magnetic resonance imaging findings of osteoarthrosis and effusion in patients with unilateral temporomandibular joint pain, *Int J Oral Maxillofac Surg* 31:598–602, 2002.

Schellhas KP, Wilkes CH: Temporomandibular joint inflammation: comparison of MR fast scanning with T1- and T2-weighted imaging techniques, *AJR Am J Roentgenol* 153:93–98, 1989.

Schellhas KP, Wilkes CH, Baker CC: Facial pain, headache, and temporomandibular joint inflammation, *Headache* 29:229–232, 1989.

Westesson P-L, Brooks SL: Temporomandibular joint: relationship between MR evidence of effusion and the presence of pain and disc displacement, *AJR Am J Roentgenol* 159:559, 1992.

Dislocation
Kai S, Kai H, Nakayama E, et al: Clinical symptoms of open lock position of the condyle: relation to anterior dislocation of the temporomandibular joint, *Oral Surg Oral Med Oral Pathol* 74:143–148, 1992.

Ohura N, Ichioka S, Sudo T, et al: Dislocation of the bilateral mandibular condyle into the middle cranial fossa: review of the literature and clinical experience, *J Oral Maxillofac Surg* 64:1165–1172, 2006.

Wijmenga JP, Boering G, Blankestijn J: Protracted dislocation of the temporomandibular joint, *Int J Oral Maxillofac Surg* 15:380–388, 1986.

Fracture
Choi J, Oh I-K: A follow-up study of condyle fracture in children, *Int J Oral Maxillofac Surg* 34:851–858, 2005.

Dahlström L, Kahnberg KE, Lindahl L: Fifteen years follow-up on condylar fractures, *Int J Oral Maxillofac Surg* 18:18–23, 1989.

Gerhard S, Ennemoser T, Rudisch A, et al: Condylar injury: magnetic resonance imaging findings of the temporomandibular joint soft tissue changes, *Int J Oral Maxillofac Surg* 36:214–218, 2007.

Horowitz I, Abrahami E, Mintz SS: Demonstration of condylar fractures of the mandible by computed tomography, *Oral Surg* 54:263–268, 1982.

Lindahl L, Hollender L: Condylar fractures of the mandible, II: a radiographic study of remodeling processes in the temporomandibular joint, *Int J Oral Surg* 6:153–165, 1977.

Pharoah MJ: Radiology of the temporomandibular joint. In Zarb GA, Carlsson BJ, Mohl ND, editors: *Temporomandibular joint and masticatory muscle disorders*, ed 2, Copenhagen, 1994, Munksgaard.

Raustia AM, Pyhtinen J, Oikarinen KS, et al: Conventional radiographic and computed tomographic findings in cases of fracture of the mandibular condylar process, *J Oral Maxillofac Surg* 48:1258–1264, 1990.

Schellhas KP: Temporomandibular joint injuries, *Radiology* 173:211–216, 1989.

Zachariades N, Mezitis M, Mourouzis C, et al: Fractures of the mandibular condyle: a review of 466 cases. Literature review, reflections on treatment and proposals, *J Craniomaxillofac Surg* 34:421–432, 2006.

Neonatal Fractures
Pharoah MJ: Radiology of the temporomandibular joint. In Zarb GA, Carlsson BJ, Mohl ND, editors: *Temporomandibular joint and masticatory muscle disorders*, ed 2, Copenhagen, 1994, Munksgaard.

Worth HM: Radiology of the temporomandibular joint. In Zarb GA, Carlsson GE, editors: *Temporomandibular joint function and dysfunction*, Copenhagen, 1979, Munksgaard.

Ankylosis
Ferretti C, Bryant R, Becker P, et al: Temporomandibular joint morphology following post-traumatic ankylosis in 26 patients, *Int J Oral Maxillofac Surg* 34:376–381, 2005.

Rowe NL: Ankylosis of the temporomandibular joint, *J R Coll Surg Edinb* 27:67–79, 1982.

Wood RE, Harris AM, Nortjé CJ, et al: The radiologic features of true ankylosis of the temporomandibular joint: an analysis of 25 cases, *Dentomaxillofac Radiol* 17:121–127, 1988.

Tumors
Benign Tumors
James RB, Alexander RW, Traver JG Jr: Osteochondroma of the mandibular coronoid process: report of a case, *Oral Surg* 37:189–195, 1974.

Nwoku AL, Koch H: The temporomandibular joint: a rare localisation for bone tumors, *J Maxillofac Surg* 2:113–119, 1974.

Pharoah MJ: Radiology of the temporomandibular joint. In Zarb GA, Carlsson BJ, Mohl ND, editors: *Temporomandibular joint and masticatory muscle disorders*, ed 2, Copenhagen, 1994, Munksgaard.

Svensson B, Isacsson G: Benign osteoblastoma associated with an aneurysmal bone cyst of the mandibular ramus and condyle, *Oral Surg Oral Med Oral Pathol* 76:433–436, 1993.

Thoma KH: Tumors of the mandibular joint, *J Oral Surg Anesth Hosp Dent Serv* 22:157–167, 1964.

Worth HM: Radiology of the temporomandibular joint. In Zarb GA, Carlsson GE, editors: *Temporomandibular joint function and dysfunction*, Copenhagen, 1979, Munksgaard.

Malignant Tumors
Morris MR, Clark SK, Porter BA, et al: Chondrosarcoma of the temporomandibular joint: case report, *Head Neck Surg* 10:113–117, 1987.

Rubin MM, Jui V, Cozzi GM: Metastatic carcinoma of the mandibular condyle presenting as temporomandibular joint syndrome, *J Oral Maxillofac Surg* 47:507–510, 1989.

Takehana dos Santos D, Cavalcanti MGP: Osteosarcoma of the temporomandibular joint: report of 2 cases, *Oral Surg Oral Med Oral Pathol Oral Radiol Endod* 94:641–647, 2002.

DISEASE MECHANISMS

The deposition of calcium salts, primarily calcium phosphate, usually occurs in the skeleton. When it occurs in an unorganized fashion in soft tissue, it is referred to as heterotopic calcification. This soft tissue mineralization may develop in a wide variety of unrelated disorders and degenerative processes. Heterotopic calcifications may be divided into three categories, as follows:

- Dystrophic calcification
- Idiopathic calcification
- Metastatic calcification

Dystrophic calcification refers to calcification that forms in degenerating, diseased, and dead tissue despite normal serum calcium and phosphate levels. The soft tissue may be damaged by blunt trauma, inflammation, injections, the presence of parasites, soft tissue changes arising from disease, and many other causes. This calcification usually is localized to the site of injury. Idiopathic calcification (or calcinosis) results from deposition of calcium in normal tissue despite normal serum calcium and phosphate levels. Examples include chondrocalcinosis and phleboliths. Metastatic calcification results when minerals precipitate into normal tissue as a result of higher than normal serum levels of calcium (e.g., hyperparathyroidism, hypercalcemia of malignancy) or phosphate (e.g., chronic renal failure). Metastatic calcification usually occurs bilaterally and symmetrically.

When the mineral is deposited in soft tissue as organized, well-formed bone, the process is known as heterotopic ossification. The term heterotopic indicates that bone has formed in an abnormal (extraskeletal) location. The heterotopic bone may be all compact bone, or it may exhibit some trabeculae and fatty marrow. The deposits may range from 1 mm to several centimeters in diameter, and one or more may be present. Causes range from posttraumatic ossification, bone produced by tumors, and ossification caused by diseases such as progressive myositis ossificans and ankylosing spondylitis.

CLINICAL FEATURES

Sites of heterotopic calcification or ossification may not cause significant signs or symptoms; they most often are detected as incidental findings during radiographic examination.

IMAGING FEATURES

Soft tissue opacities are common, present on about 4% of panoramic radiographs (Fig. 28-1). In most cases, the goal is to identify the calcification correctly to determine whether treatment or further investigation is required. Some soft tissue calcifications require no intervention or long-term surveillance, whereas others may be life-threatening and the underlying cause requires treatment. When the soft tissue calcification is adjacent to bone, it sometimes is difficult to determine whether the calcification is within bone or soft tissue. Another radiographic view at right angles is useful. The important criteria to consider in arriving at the correct interpretation are the anatomic location, number, distribution, and shape of the calcifications. Analysis of the location requires knowledge of soft tissue anatomy, such as the position of lymph nodes, stylohyoid ligaments, blood vessels, laryngeal cartilages, and the major ducts of the salivary glands.

HETEROTOPIC CALCIFICATIONS

Heterotopic calcifications are calcifications that occur in an unorganized fashion in soft tissue.

DYSTROPHIC CALCIFICATION

Disease Mechanism

Dystrophic calcification is the precipitation of calcium salts into primary sites of chronic inflammation or dead and dying tissue. This process is usually associated with a high local concentration of phosphatase, as in normal bone calcification; an increase in local alkalinity; and anoxic conditions within the inactive or devitalized tissue. A long-standing chronically inflamed cyst is a common location of dystrophic calcification.

Clinical Features

Common soft tissue sites include the gingiva, tongue, lymph nodes, and cheek. Dystrophic calcifications may produce no signs or symptoms, although occasionally enlargement and ulceration of overlying soft tissues may occur, and a solid mass of calcium salts sometimes can be palpated.

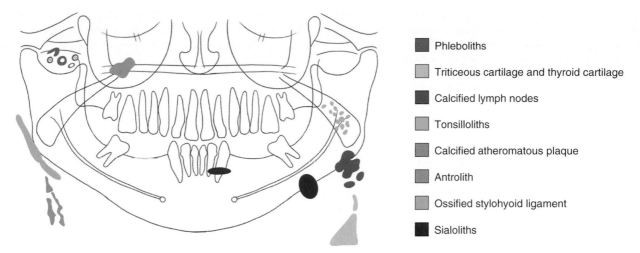

Phleboliths

Triticeous cartilage and thyroid cartilage

Calcified lymph nodes

Tonsilloliths

Calcified atheromatous plaque

Antrolith

Ossified stylohyoid ligament

Sialoliths

FIGURE 28-1 Schematic of panoramic radiograph demonstrating the typical geometry and location of selected soft tissue calcifications and ossifications.

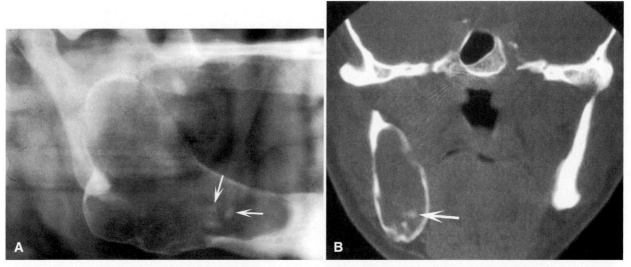

FIGURE 28-2 **A,** Large residual cyst with ill-defined calcifications seen in a panoramic image *(arrows).* **B,** Coronal MDCT image with bone algorithm of the same case, which demonstrates the dystrophic calcification within the cyst *(arrow).*

Imaging Features

The radiographic appearance of dystrophic calcification varies from barely perceptible, fine grains of radiopacities to larger, irregular radiopaque particles that rarely exceed 0.5 cm in diameter. One or more of these radiopacities may be seen, and the calcification may be homogeneous or may contain punctate areas. The outline of the calcified area usually is irregular or indistinct. Common sites are long-standing chronically inflamed cysts (Fig. 28-2) and polyps (Fig. 28-3).

Calcified Lymph Nodes

Disease Mechanism. Dystrophic calcification occurs in lymph nodes that have been chronically inflamed because of various diseases, frequently granulomatous disorders. The lymphoid tissue becomes replaced by hydroxyapatite-like calcium salts, nearly effacing all nodal architecture. The presence of calcifications in lymph nodes implies disease, either active or the result of previously treated pathosis. In the past, tuberculosis was the most

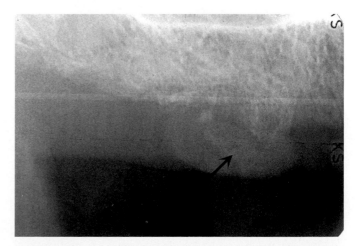

FIGURE 28-3 Periapical film shows the soft tissue mass, inflammatory fibrous hyperplasia, emanating from the edentulous ridge. This soft tissue mass contains a dystrophic calcification *(arrow).*

common disease causing calcified lymph nodes (scrofula or cervical tuberculous adenitis). Other well-known causes of lymph node calcification include bacille Calmette-Guérin vaccination, sarcoidosis, cat-scratch disease, rheumatoid arthritis and systemic sclerosis, lymphoma previously treated with radiation therapy, fungal infections, and malignancy (treated Hodgkin's lymphoma and metastases from distant calcifying neoplasms, most notably metastatic thyroid carcinoma).

Clinical Features. Calcified lymph nodes are generally asymptomatic, and the nodes are first discovered as an incidental finding on a panoramic radiograph. The most commonly involved nodes are the submandibular and superficial and deep cervical nodes. Less commonly, the preauricular and submental nodes are involved. When these nodes can be palpated, they are hard, lumpy, round to oblong masses.

Imaging Features

Location. The most common location is the submandibular region, either at or below the inferior border of the mandible near the angle or between the posterior border of the ramus and cervical spine. The image of the calcified node sometimes overlaps the inferior aspect of the ramus. Lymph node calcifications may affect a single node or a linear series of nodes in a phenomenon known as lymph node "chaining" (Fig. 28-4).

Periphery. The periphery is well defined and usually irregular, occasionally having a lobulated appearance similar to the outer shape of cauliflower. This irregularity of shape is of great significance in distinguishing node calcifications from other potential soft tissue calcifications in the area.

Internal Structure. The internal aspect is without pattern but may vary in the degree of radiopacity, giving the impression of a collection of spherical or irregular masses. Occasionally, the lesion has a laminated appearance, or the radiopacity may appear only on the surface of the node (eggshell calcification). The pattern of nodal calcification does not reliably distinguish between benign and malignant disease.

Differential Diagnosis. Differentiation between a single calcified lymph node and a sialolith in the hilar region of the submandibular gland may be difficult because both may appear near or adjacent to the inferior cortex of the mandible just anterior to the angle. Usually a sialolith has a smooth outline, whereas a calcified lymph node is usually irregular and sometimes lobulated. The differentiation can be made if the patient has symptoms related to the submandibular salivary gland (see Chapter 29). Occasionally, sialography may be necessary to make the differentiation. Another calcification that may have a similar appearance in this region is a phlebolith; however, phleboliths are usually smaller and multiple, with concentric radiopaque and

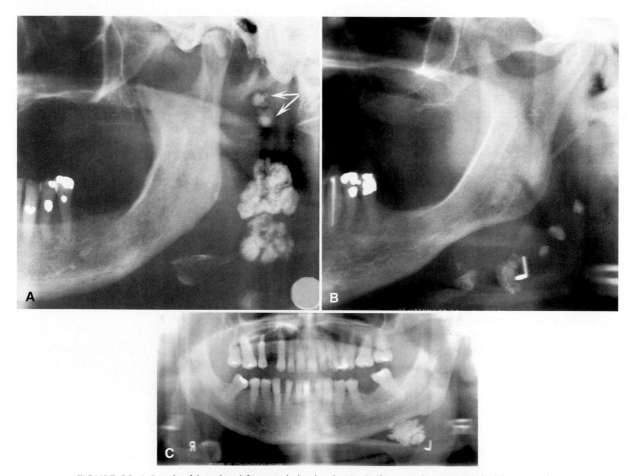

FIGURE 28-4 Examples of dystrophic calcification in the lymph nodes. **A,** Two large examples positioned behind the ramus with a cauliflower-like shape and two smaller examples in a more superior position (arrows). **B,** Several smaller examples positioned below the lower border of the mandible. **C,** Larger example.

radiolucent rings, and their shape may mimic a portion of a blood vessel.

Management. Calcified lymph nodes usually do not require treatment; however, the underlying cause should be established in case treatment is required, such as in the case of active disease.

Dystrophic Calcification in the Tonsils

Synonyms. Synonyms for dystrophic calcification in the tonsils include tonsillar calculi, tonsil concretions, and tonsilloliths.

Disease Mechanism. Tonsillar calculi are formed when repeated bouts of inflammation enlarge the tonsillar crypts. Incomplete resolution of organic debris (dead bacteria and pus, epithelial cells, and food) can serve as the nidus for dystrophic calcification.

Clinical Features. Tonsilloliths usually manifest as hard, round, white or yellow objects projecting from the tonsillar crypts, usually of the palatine tonsil. Small calcifications usually produce no clinical signs or symptoms. However, pain, swelling, fetor oris, dysphagia, or a foreign body sensation on swallowing has been reported with larger calcifications. Giant tonsilloliths stretching lymphoid tissue and resulting in ulceration and extrusion are much less common. These calcifications have been reported to occur in individuals between 20 and 68 years old; they are found more often in older age groups.

Imaging Features
Location. In a panoramic image, tonsilloliths appear as single or multiple radiopacities that overlap the midportion of the mandibular ramus in the region where the image of the dorsal surface of the tongue crosses the ramus in the oropharyngeal air spaces. Tonsilloliths frequently appear immediately inferior to the mandibular canal in the panoramic image (Fig. 28-5). On axial computed tomographic (CT) images, they appear in the soft tissue medial to the mandibular ramus and next to the lateral wall of the oropharyngeal air space.
  Periphery. The most common appearance of tonsilloliths is a cluster of multiple small, ill defined radiopacities. Rarely, this calcification may attain a large size.
  Internal Structure. These calcifications appear slightly more radiopaque than cancellous bone and approximately the same as cortical bone.

Differential Diagnosis. The clinical differential diagnosis includes calcified granulomatous disease, syphilis, mycosis, or lymphoma, which may produce a firm tonsillar mass. The essential radiographic differential diagnosis is a radiopaque lesion within the mandibular ramus, such as a dense bone island. When in doubt, a right-angle view such as a posteroanterior skull view or an open Towne's view may show that the calcification lies to the medial aspect of the ramus. Three-dimensional imaging such as MDCT or cone-beam computed tomographic (CBCT) imaging may be necessary for precise localization.

Management. No treatment is required for most tonsillar calcifications. In symptomatic patients, tonsilloliths may be expressed manually, possibly with the patient under sedation to suppress the gag reflex. Large calcifications with associated symptoms are removed surgically. Treatment of asymptomatic tonsilloliths may be considered in elderly patients with mechanical deglutition

disorders and immunocompromised patients because of the risk for aspiration pneumonia.

Cysticercosis
Disease Mechanism. When humans ingest eggs or gravid proglottids from the parasite *Taenia solium* (pork tapeworm), the covering of the eggs is digested in the stomach, and the larval form (*Cysticercus cellulosae*) of the parasite is hatched. The larvae penetrate the mucosa, enter the blood vessels and lymphatics, and are distributed as cysticerci in the tissues all over the body, but they preferentially locate to brain, muscle, skin, liver, lungs, subcutaneous tissues, and heart. They are also found in oral and perioral tissues, especially the muscles of mastication. The glycoprotein-rich cyst wall is greater than 100 μm thick and rarely elicits any host response when intact. In tissues other than the intestinal mucosa, the larvae eventually die years after infection and are treated as foreign bodies, eliciting a strong inflammatory reaction causing granuloma formation, scarring, and calcification. There is currently an increased incidence of cysticercosis in the American Southwest and urban Northeast, especially among Koreans and Hispanics. The problem is endemic in developing countries of Central and South America, Asia, and Africa, where there is fecal contamination of agricultural soil and pork is a valued food.

Clinical Features. Mild cases of cysticercosis are completely asymptomatic. More severe cases have symptoms that range from mild to severe gastrointestinal upset with epigastric pain and severe nausea and vomiting. Invasion of the brain may result in seizures, headache, visual disturbances, acute obstructive hydrocephalus, irritability, loss of consciousness, and death. Examination of the oral mucosa may disclose palpable, well-circumscribed soft fluctuant swellings, which resemble a mucocele or benign mesenchymal neoplasm. Multiple small nodules may be felt in the region of the masseter and suprahyoid muscles and in the tongue, buccal mucosa, or lip.

Imaging Features. While alive, larvae are not visible radiographically. Death of the parasites and development of calcifications in subcutaneous and muscular sites occurs years after the initial infection.
  Location. The oral locations of calcified cysticerci include the muscles of mastication and facial expression, the suprahyoid muscle, and the postcervical musculature as well as the tongue, buccal mucosa, and lip.
  Periphery and Shape. Multiple well-defined elliptic radiopacities that resemble grains of rice are viewed.
  Internal Structure. The internal aspect is homogeneous and radiopaque.

Differential Diagnosis. Cysticercus may appear similar to a sialolith. However, the small size of the calcified nodules of cysticerci and their widespread dissemination, particularly in brain and muscles, are highly suggestive of the diagnosis.

Management. Although basic sanitation (proper preparation of pork and avoiding fecal contamination of water supplies and vegetables) is needed to extinguish this source of infection, the symptoms that accompany the initial infestation are best treated by a physician using an anthelmintic such as albendazole or praziquantel. Adjunctive corticosteroids help stem the inflammatory reaction, and anticonvulsants may prevent epileptic seizures. After the larvae have settled and calcified in the oral tissues, they are

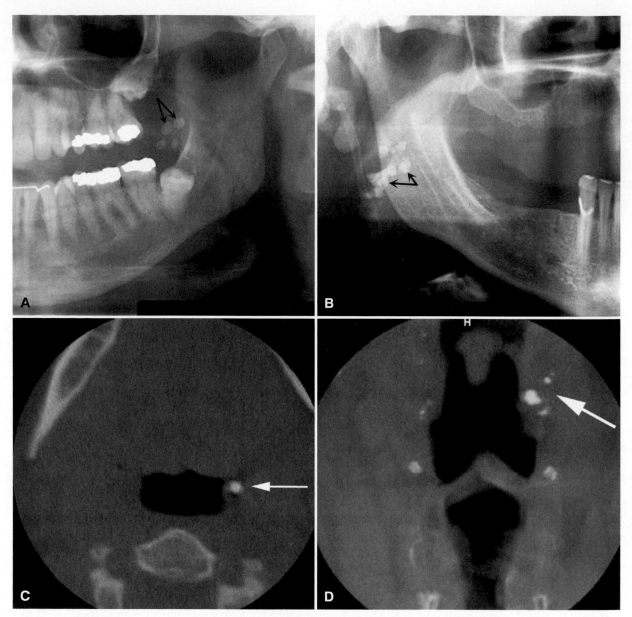

FIGURE 28-5 Dystrophic calcification of the tonsils. **A** and **B,** These two examples show positions anterior to the ramus **(A)** and overlapping the posterior aspect of the ramus **(B)** *(arrows)*. Note the calcified stylohyoid ligament. **C,** Axial CBCT image of a calcification within the tonsils *(arrow)*. **D,** Coronal CBCT image of the same case with several calcifications within the tonsils *(arrow)*.

harmless. However, it is important to carry out a detailed investigation in each patient to rule out the presence of the parasite in other locations and to perform serologic testing on close contacts to identify a possible source of infection.

Mönckeberg's Medial Calcinosis (Arteriosclerosis)

Two distinct patterns of arterial calcification can be identified radiographically and histologically: Mönckeberg's medial calcinosis and calcified atherosclerotic plaque.

Disease Mechanism. The hallmark of arteriosclerosis is the fragmentation, degeneration, and eventual loss of elastic fibers followed by the deposition of calcium within the medial coat of the vessel.

Clinical Features. Most patients are asymptomatic initially, although late in the course of the disease clinical pathosis such as cutaneous gangrene, peripheral vascular disease, and myositis as a result of vascular insufficiency may occur. Patients with Sturge-Weber syndrome also develop intracranial arterial calcifications.

Imaging Features

Location. Medial calcinosis involving the facial artery or, less commonly, the carotid artery may be viewed on panoramic radiographs.

Periphery and Shape. The calcific deposits in the wall of the artery outline an image of the artery. From the side, the calcified vessel appears as a parallel pair of thin, radiopaque lines (Fig. 28-6)

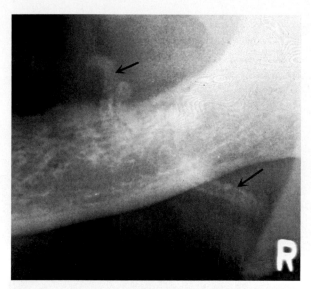

FIGURE 28-6 Section of a panoramic image shows calcification of a blood vessel, probably the facial vein *(arrows)*.

that may have a straight course or a tortuous path and is described as a "pipe stem" or "tram-track" appearance. In cross section, involved vessels display a circular or ringlike pattern.

Internal Structure.   There is no internal structure because the diffuse, finely divided calcium deposits occur solely in the medial wall of the vessels.

Differential Diagnosis.   The radiographic appearance of arteriosclerosis is so distinctive as to be pathognomonic of the condition.

Management.   Evaluation of the patient for occlusive arterial disease and peripheral vascular disease may be appropriate. In addition, hyperparathyroidism may be considered because medial calcinosis frequently develops as a metastatic calcification in patients with this condition.

Calcified Atherosclerotic Plaque

Disease Mechanism.   Stenotic atheromatous plaque in the extracranial carotid vasculature is the major contributing source of cerebrovascular embolic and occlusive disease. Dystrophic calcification can occur in the evolution of plaque within the intima of the involved vessel.

Imaging Findings

Location.   Atherosclerosis first develops at arterial bifurcations as a result of increased endothelial damage from shear forces at these sites. When calcification has occurred, these lesions may be visible in the panoramic radiograph in the soft tissues of the neck either superior or inferior to the greater cornu of the hyoid bone (where the common carotid artery splits into the external and internal carotid arteries) and adjacent to the cervical vertebrae C3, C4, or the intervertebral space between them (Fig. 28-7).

Periphery and Shape.   These soft tissue calcifications are usually multiple, irregular in shape, and sharply defined from the surrounding soft tissues, and they have a vertical linear distribution.

Internal Structure.   The internal aspect is composed of a heterogeneous radiopacity with radiolucent voids.

Differential Diagnosis.   Calcified triticeous cartilage may be mistaken for atheromatous plaque, although the uniform size, shape, and location of calcified triticeous cartilage in the laryngeal cartilage skeleton identify this innocuous condition.

Management.   Many published case reports and case series report individual instances of patients with calcified carotid atheromas on panoramic radiographs who were found to have clinically significant stenoses with a heightened risk for a cerebrovascular accident. However, further research needs to be conducted with case-control or cohort studies with a control group to determine whether calcified carotid atheromas represent an independent risk factor for stroke. In the meantime, patients with calcified carotid atheromas, especially patients with established risk factors for cerebrovascular and cardiovascular disease, should be referred to their physicians for further investigation.

IDIOPATHIC CALCIFICATION

Idiopathic calcification (or calcinosis) results from deposition of calcium in normal tissue despite normal serum calcium and phosphate levels. They are fairly common in the head and neck.

Sialolith

Disease Mechanism.   Sialoliths are stones found within the ducts of salivary glands (see Chapter 29). Mechanical conditions leading to a slow flow rate and physiochemical characteristics of the gland secretion both contribute to the formation of a nidus and subsequent precipitation of calcium and phosphate salts. Mid-infrared spectroscopic analysis has determined that sialoliths consist of hydroxyapatite, amorphous carbonated calcium phosphate, carbonated apatite, and whitlockite in combination with fibrous proteins such as mucins.

Clinical Features.   Sialoliths are most common in the submandibular glands of middle-aged and older men. They usually occur singly (70% to 80%) but may be multiple, especially in the parotid gland. Patients with salivary stones may be asymptomatic, but they usually have a history of pain and swelling in the floor of the mouth and in the involved submandibular gland or in the cheek in the case of parotid sialoliths. This discomfort may intensify at mealtimes, when salivary flow is stimulated. Because the stone usually does not block the flow of saliva completely, the pain and swelling gradually subside. Recurrent sialolithiasis occurs in 9% of patients, and about 10% of patients with sialolithiasis also have nephrolithiasis.

Imaging Features

Location.   The submandibular gland is involved more often (83% to 94% of cases) than the parotid gland (4% to 10%) or the sublingual gland (1% to 7%), probably because the submandibular gland has a longer and more tortuous duct, an uphill flow in the proximal portion, and more viscous saliva with a higher mineral content. About 50% of submandibular stones lie in the distal portion of Wharton's duct, 20% in the proximal portion, and 30% in the gland itself.

Periphery and Shape.   Sialoliths located in the duct of the submandibular gland usually are cylindric and very smooth in their outlines (Fig. 28-8). Stones that form in the hilus of a

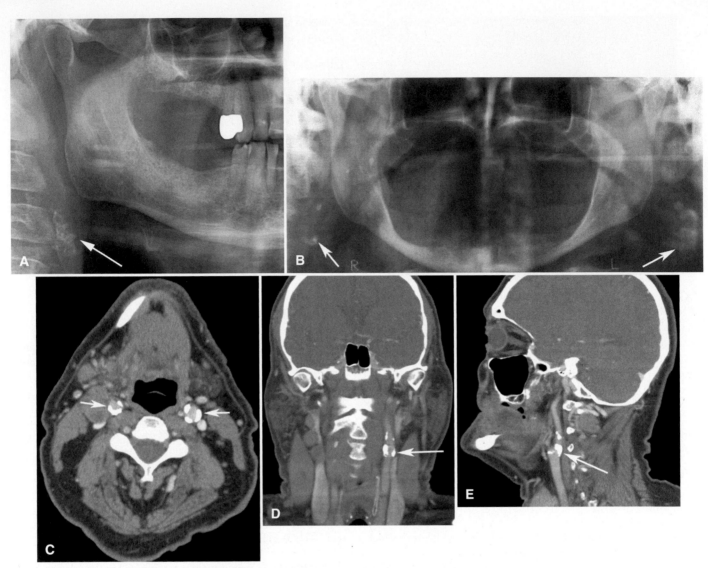

FIGURE 28-7 **A,** Cropped panoramic image shows calcifications related to the carotid artery. **B,** Panoramic image with bilateral examples of calcifications associated with the carotid arteries *(arrows)*. **C,** Axial MDCT image with soft tissue algorithm of the same case shown in **B** demonstrates bilateral calcification within the walls of the carotid arteries *(arrows)*. **D** and **E,** Coronal **(D)** and sagittal **(E)** MDCT images of the same case demonstrate the carotid calcifications *(arrows)*.

submandibular gland tend to be larger and more irregularly shaped (Fig. 28-9, *A*).

Internal Structure.   Some stones are homogeneously radiopaque, and others show evidence of multiple layers of calcification (see Fig. 28-9, *A*). Less than 20% of submandibular gland sialoliths and 40% of sialoliths in the parotid gland are radiolucent because of the low mineral content of the parotid secretions.

Radiologic Investigation.   Salivary stones occasionally are seen on periapical views superimposed over the mandibular premolar and molar apices (see Fig. 28-9, *C*). The best view for visualizing stones in the distal portion of Wharton's duct is a standard mandibular occlusal view using half the usual exposure time, which displays the floor of the mouth without overlap from the mandible. Stones in a more posterior location are best visualized on lateral oblique views of the mandible or on a panoramic film. To demonstrate stones in the parotid gland duct, the clinician places a periapical film in the buccal vestibule, reduces the exposure time, and orients

the x-ray beam through the cheek. Also, stones in the parotid duct can be seen if the patient "blows out" the cheek as an anteroposterior skull view is exposed. An open mouth lateral skull projection can be used, or sometimes sialoliths are visible in a panoramic view (Fig. 28-9, *B*). When radiographs to detect sialoliths are produced, the exposure time should be reduced to about half of normal; this helps in detecting stones that are lightly calcified. If a noncalcified stone is suspected, sialography is used (see Chapter 29).

Differential Diagnosis.   Sialoliths can be distinguished from other soft tissue calcifications because they usually are associated with pain or swelling of the involved salivary gland. Other calcifications (e.g., lymph node calcifications) are asymptomatic. If the diagnosis is unclear, the clinician can prescribe a sialogram.

Management.   Small stones often may be "milked out" through the duct orifice by bimanual palpation. If the stone is too large or located in the proximal duct, nonsurgical or minimally invasive

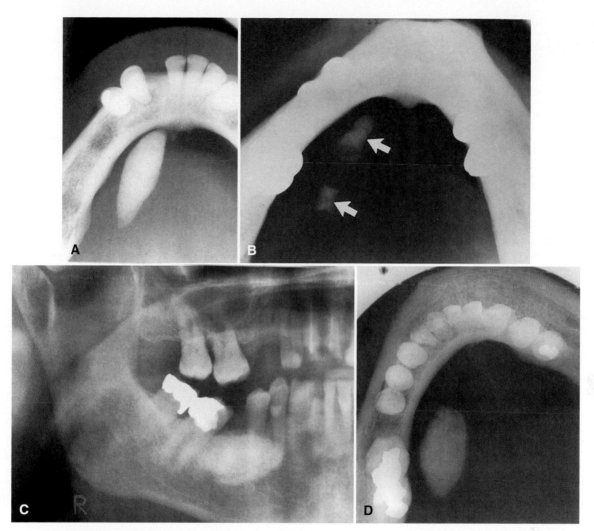

FIGURE 28-8 **A** and **B,** Standard occlusal projections of single and multiple examples of calcified sialoliths *(arrows)* in the duct of a submandibular gland. Exposure times have been reduced to demonstrate these calcifications better, which are less calcified than the mandible. **C,** In another example, the image of the sialolith is superimposed over the mandibular alveolar process in this cropped panoramic image. **D,** Occlusal view of the same case shown in **C**.

sialolithotomy using intracorporeal lithotriptors has become a popular treatment modality in Europe. The U.S. Food and Drug Administration has not approved extracorporeal shock wave lithotripsy for treatment of sialoliths in the United States. Sialendoscopes with various grasping forceps and baskets have been developed for extraction of stones from salivary gland ducts using ductoplasty and in some cases preventing the removal of the submandibular gland. In cases of exceedingly large or intraparenchymal sialoliths, surgical removal of the stone or gland may be required.

Phleboliths

Disease Mechanism.
Intravascular thrombi, which arise from venous stagnation, sometimes become organized or even mineralized. Mineralization begins in the core of the thrombus and consists of crystals of calcium carbonate–fluorohydroxyapatite. Phleboliths are calcified thrombi found in veins, venulae, or the sinusoidal vessels of hemangiomas (especially the cavernous type).

Clinical Features.
In the head and neck, phleboliths nearly always signal the presence of a hemangioma. In an adult, phleboliths may be the sole residua of a childhood hemangioma that has long since regressed. The involved soft tissue may be swollen, throbbing, or discolored by the presence of veins or a soft tissue hemangioma. Hemangiomas often fluctuate in size, associated with changes in body position or during a Valsalva maneuver. Applying pressure to the involved tissue should cause a blanching or change in color if the lesion is vascular in nature. Auscultation may reveal a bruit in cases of cavernous hemangioma but not in the capillary type.

Imaging Features
Location. Phleboliths most commonly are found in hemangiomas (see Chapter 22).

Periphery and Shape. In cross section, the shape is round or oval, up to 6 mm in diameter with a smooth periphery. If the involved blood vessel is viewed from the side, the phlebolith may resemble a straight or slightly curved sausage.

Internal Structure. The internal aspect may be homogeneously radiopaque but more commonly has the appearance of laminations, giving phleboliths a bull's-eye or targetoid appearance. Radiolucent flow voids may be seen, which may represent the remaining patent portions of the vessel (Fig. 28-10).

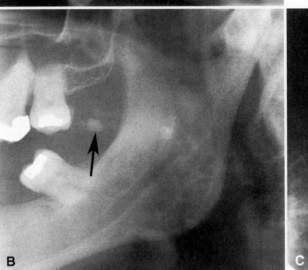

FIGURE 28-9 **A,** Cropped panoramic image of a submandibular gland sialolith. Note the position and the hint at a laminated internal pattern. **B,** Cropped panoramic image of a sialolith *(arrow)* involving the parotid gland. **C,** Intraoral periapical image of a superimposed submandibular sialolith that could be difficult to differentiate from a dense bone island without an occlusal film. *(***B,** *Courtesy Drs. John Lovas and Nick Hogg, Dalhousie University.)*

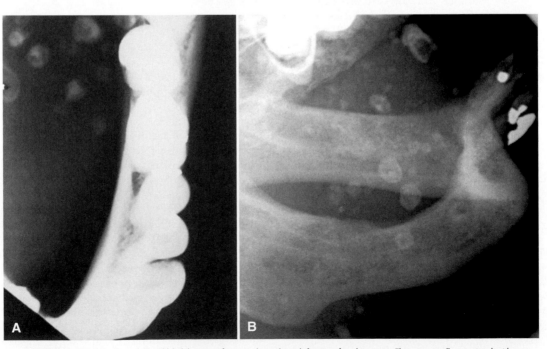

FIGURE 28-10 **A** and **B,** Phleboliths are soft tissue dystrophic calcifications found in veins. They are usually associated with hemangiomas.

Differential Diagnosis.   A phlebolith may have a shape similar to that of a sialolith. Submandibular sialoliths usually occur singly; if more than one is present, they usually are oriented in a single line, whereas phleboliths are usually multiple and have a more random, clustered distribution. The importance of correctly identifying phleboliths lies in the identification of a possible vascular lesion, such as a hemangioma. This is critical if surgical procedures are contemplated.

Laryngeal Cartilage Calcifications

Disease Mechanism.   The epiglottis and vocal processes of the arytenoid cartilages are fibroelastic cartilages, whereas all the remaining laryngeal cartilages are made of hyaline cartilage. Enchondral calcification and ossification of the hyaline laryngeal cartilages begins on attainment of skeletal maturity and progresses thereafter as a physiologic process. Calcified triticeous and thyroid cartilages are the laryngeal cartilages that are most frequently demonstrated on panoramic radiographs.

Clinical Features.   Calcification of laryngeal cartilages is an incidental radiographic finding with no clinical features.

Imaging Features
   Location.   The small, paired triticeous cartilages are found within the lateral thyrohyoid ligaments. The calcified triticeous cartilage is located on a lateral skull or panoramic image within the soft tissues of the pharynx inferior to the greater cornu of the hyoid bone and adjacent to the superior border of C4. The superior cornu of a calcified thyroid cartilage appears medial to C4 and is superimposed on the prevertebral soft tissue (Fig. 28-11).
   Periphery and Shape.   The word triticeous means "grain of wheat," and the cartilage measures 7 to 9 mm in length and 2 to 4 mm in width. The periphery of the calcified triticeous cartilage is well defined and smooth, and the geometry is exceedingly regular. Usually only the top 2 to 3 mm of a calcified thyroid cartilage is visible at the lower edge of a panoramic radiograph with 6-inch systems.
   Internal Structure.   Calcified tracheal cartilages generally demonstrate a homogeneous radiopacity but may occasionally demonstrate an outer cortex.

Differential Diagnosis.   Calcified triticeous cartilage may be confused with calcified atheromatous plaque in the carotid bifurcation, but the solitary nature and extremely uniform size and shape of the former should be discriminatory.

Management.   No treatment is needed for calcified tracheal cartilages, but careful attention to the differences in morphology and location enable the clinician to distinguish between calcified triticeous cartilage and calcified carotid atheromas.

Rhinoliths and Antroliths

Disease Mechanism.   Calcareous concretions that occur in the nose (rhinoliths) or the antrum of the maxillary sinus (antroliths) arise from the deposition of nasal, lacrimal, and inflammatory mineral salts, such as calcium phosphate, calcium carbonate, and magnesium, by accretion around a nidus. Rarely, concretions form in the frontal or ethmoid sinus. In cases of rhinolith, the nidus is usually an exogenous foreign body (e.g., coins, beads, seeds and fruit pits), especially in pediatric patients. Adult drug smugglers who carry the contraband in packets in the nose sometimes forget to remove one, and a rhinolith develops around it over time. The route of entry is usually anterior, but some may enter the choana posteriorly during sneezing, coughing, or emesis. The nidus for an antrolith is usually endogenous (e.g., root tip, bone fragment, blood clot, inspissated mucus, ectopic tooth), especially in adults. Dystrophic calcification may occur within chronically inflamed mucosa of the maxillary sinus in long-standing sinusitis. The appearance is usually of small scattered and faint calcifications in the thickened mucosal lining. Occasionally, a noninvasive aspergillosis mycetoma may develop in the antrum, especially in patients with chronic sinus disease. This mycetoma may manifest as a muddy, necrotic fungus ball, or calcareous deposits may transform it into a hard mycolith.

Clinical Features.   The patient may be asymptomatic for extended periods, but the expanding mass may impinge on the mucosa, producing pain, congestion, and ulceration. The patient may have nasal obstruction, unilateral purulent or blood-stained rhinorrhea, sinusitis, headache, epistaxis, anosmia, fetor, and fever.

Imaging Features
   Location.   Rhinoliths develop in the nose (Fig. 28-12, *A*), whereas antroliths develop in the antrum of the maxillary sinus (see Fig. 28-12, *C*).
   Periphery and Shape.   These stones have various shapes and sizes, depending on the nature of the nidus.
   Internal Structure.   Rhinoliths and antroliths may manifest as homogeneous or heterogeneous radiopacities, depending on the nature of the nidus, and sometimes may have laminations. Occasionally, the density exceeds the surrounding bone.

Differential Diagnosis.   The differential diagnosis includes osteoma, odontoma, calcified polyp, and surgical ciliated cyst.

Management.   Patients should be referred to an otorhinolaryngologist for endonasal or sinus endoscopic surgical removal of the mass. In some cases, lithotripsy has been used to debulk large rhinoliths.

METASTATIC CALCIFICATION

Metastatic calcification of the soft tissues in the oral region is caused by conditions involving elevated serum calcium and phosphate levels, such as hyperparathyroidism (see Chapter 25) or hypercalcemia of malignancy. These calcifications are extremely rare.

HETEROTOPIC OSSIFICATIONS
OSSIFICATION OF THE STYLOHYOID LIGAMENT

Disease Mechanism
Embryologically, the styloid process arises from the second branchial arch (Reichert's cartilage), which consists of four sections that give rise to the stylohyoid complex. Ossification of the stylohyoid ligament usually extends downward from the base of the skull and commonly occurs bilaterally. However, in rare cases, the ossification begins at the lesser horn of the hyoid and in fewer still in a central area of the ligament.

Clinical Features
The ossified ligament usually can be detected by palpation over the tonsil as a hard, pointed structure. Only a few patients have symptoms, and there is very little correlation between the extent

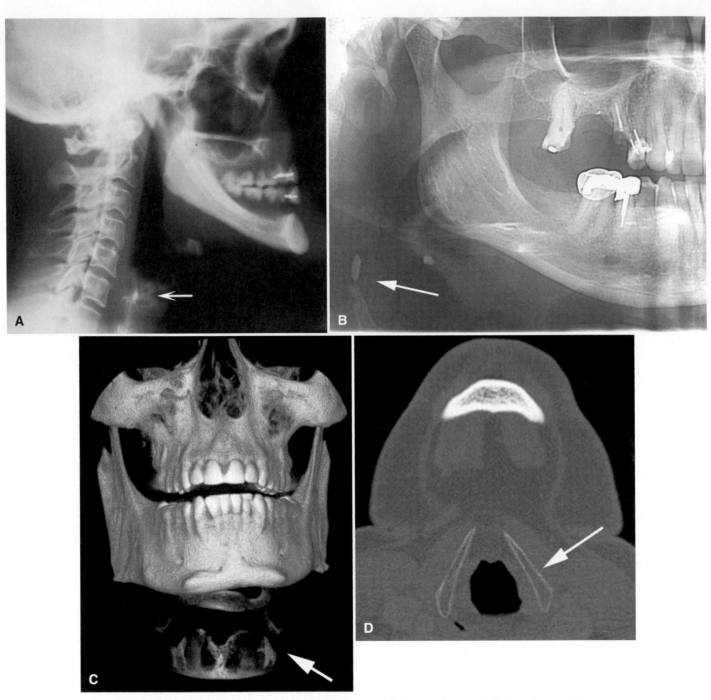

FIGURE 28-11 A, Lateral cephalometric film reveals calcification of the thyroid cartilage *(arrow)*. **B,** Cropped panoramic image reveals calcification of the triticeous cartilage and greater cornu of the thyroid cartilage *(arrow)*. **C,** Three-dimensional reconstruction of a CBCT study shows extensive calcification of the thyroid cartilage *(arrow)*. **D,** Axial CT image of calcification of the thyroid cartilage *(arrow)*. *(**C,** Courtesy Dr. Susanne Perschbacher.)*

of ossification and the intensity of the accompanying symptoms. Symptoms related to this ossified ligament are termed Eagle's syndrome, which is expressed as one of two subtypes: (1) classic Eagle's syndrome, resulting from cranial nerve impingement, and (2) the carotid artery syndrome, resulting from impingement on the carotid vessels. When this entity is associated with discomfort and the patient has a recent history of neck trauma (typically tonsillectomy), the condition is called classic Eagle's syndrome. The ossified stylohyoid complex and local scar tissue are thought to

cause symptoms by impinging on cranial nerves V, VII, IX, X, or XII, all of which pass in close proximity to the styloid process. Symptoms may include vague, nagging to intense pain in the pharynx on speaking, chewing, swallowing, turning the head, or opening the mouth widely, especially on singing or yawning; a foreign body sensation in the throat on swallowing; and tinnitus or otalgia. Clinical findings without a history of neck trauma constitute carotid artery syndrome. The patient may describe referred pain along the distribution of the external carotid artery or internal

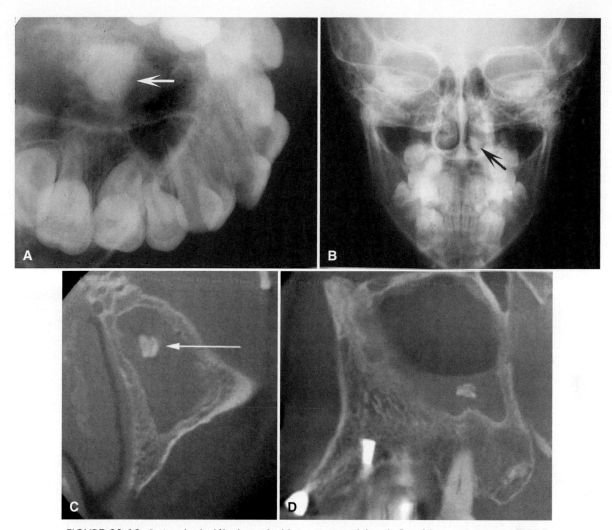

FIGURE 28-12 **A,** Lateral occlusal film shows a rhinolith *(arrow)* positioned above the floor of the nose. **B,** Posteroanterior skull film of the same case shown in **A** demonstrates that the rhinolith is positioned within the nasal fossa *(arrow).* **C,** Axial CBCT image reveals the presence of an antrolith *(arrow).* **D,** Coronal CBCT of the same case shown in **C** demonstrates the antrolith above the floor of the maxillary sinus.

carotid artery. This pain is the result of mechanical impingement of the involved artery and stimulation of its sympathetic nerve plexus. When the external carotid artery is impinged and stimulated, the patient may feel suborbital facial pain. Symptoms when the internal carotid artery is affected may include eye pain, temporal or parietal headache, migraines, aphasia, visual symptoms, weakness, and transient hemispheric ischemia with vertigo or syncope, notably on turning the head to the ipsilateral side. Pain is produced in these patients by mechanical irritation of the periarterial sympathetic nerve plexus overlying the artery, producing regional carotidynia; this may occur even in the absence of ossification of the stylohyoid complex. Only deviation of the styloid process, usually medially, is required for the tip of the process to impinge an artery. These individuals usually are older than 40 years. This condition is more prevalent than classic Eagle's syndrome.

Imaging Features

Ossification of the stylohyoid ligament is detected commonly as an incidental feature on panoramic images. In one study,

approximately 18% of a population examined showed ossification of more than 30 mm of the stylohyoid ligament. The ligament may have at least some calcification in individuals of any age.

Location.   In a panoramic image, the linear ossification extends forward from the region of the mastoid process and crosses the posteroinferior aspect of the ramus toward the hyoid bone. The hyoid bone is positioned roughly parallel to or superimposed on the posterior aspect of the inferior cortex of the mandible.

Shape.   The styloid process appears as a long, tapering, thin, radiopaque process that is thicker at its base and projects downward and forward (Fig. 28-13). It normally ranges from about 0.5 to 2.5 cm in length. The ossified ligament has roughly a straight outline, but in some cases some irregularity may be seen in the outer surface. The farther the radiopaque ossified ligament extends toward the hyoid bone, the more likely it is that it will be interrupted by radiolucent, jointlike junctions (pseudoarticulations).

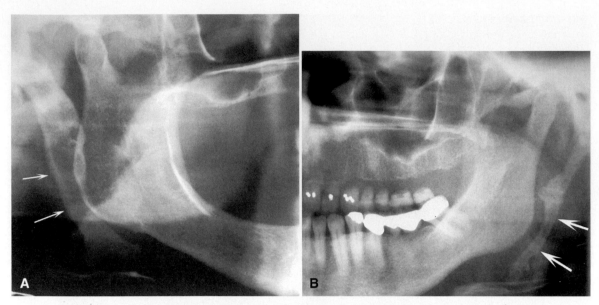

FIGURE 28-13 **A** and **B,** Examples of prominent ossification of the stylohyoid ligament *(arrows)*. These individuals did not have any symptoms.

Internal Structure. Small ossifications of the stylohyoid ligament appear homogeneously radiopaque. As the ossification increases in length and girth, the outer cortex of this bone becomes evident as a radiopaque band at the periphery.

Differential Diagnosis

The symptoms accompanying stylohyoid ligament ossification and Eagle's syndrome or stylohyoid syndrome generally are vague; however, when they occur with the distinctive evidence of ligament ossification in the diagnostic images, little chance exists that the complaint will be confused with another entity. Occasionally, the symptoms may be similar to symptoms seen in temporomandibular joint dysfunction. With topical anesthesia to suppress the gag reflex, palpation of the tonsillar fossa to reproduce the symptoms and detect the hard submucosal mass may serve as a diagnostic confirmation.

Management

Most patients with ossification of the stylohyoid ligament are asymptomatic, and no treatment is required. For patients with vague symptoms, a conservative approach of reassurance and steroid or lidocaine injections into the tonsillar fossa would be recommended initially. However, for patients with persistent or intense symptoms, the recommended treatment is amputation of the stylohyoid process (stylohyoidectomy).

OSTEOMA CUTIS

Disease Mechanism

Osteoma cutis is a rare soft tissue ossification in the skin or subcutaneous tissues that manifests as focal development of bone within the dermis physically removed from any original osseous tissue. Osteoma cutis may be primary, occurring in normal tissue without any preexisting condition, or secondary, developing in damaged or disrupted skin. Approximately 85% of cases are secondary and occur as a result of acne of long duration, developing in a scar or chronic inflammatory dermatosis. They occasionally

are found in diffuse scleroderma, replacing the altered collagen in the dermis and subcutaneous septa.

Clinical Features

Osteoma cutis can occur anywhere, but the face is the most common site. The tongue is the most common intraoral site (osteoma mucosae or osseous choristoma). Osteoma cutis does not cause any visible change in the overlying skin other than an occasional color change that may appear yellowish white. If the lesion is large, the individual osteoma may be palpated. A needle inserted into one of the papules is met with stonelike resistance. Some patients have numerous (dozens to hundreds) of lesions, usually on the face in female patients and on the scalp or chest in male patients. This form is known as multiple miliary osteoma cutis.

Imaging Features

Location. Radiographically, osteoma cutis most commonly appears in the cheek and lip regions (Fig. 28-14). In this location, the image can be superimposed over a tooth root or alveolar process, giving the appearance of an area of dense bone. Accurate localization can be achieved by placing an intraoral film between the cheek and alveolar process to image the cheek alone. Alternatively, a posteroanterior skull view with the cheek blown outward by use of a soft tissue technique of 60 kVp helps localize osteomas in the skin.

Periphery and Shape. Osteoma cutis appears as smoothly outlined, radiopaque, washer-shaped images. These single or multiple radiopacities usually are very small, although the size can range from 0.1 to 5 cm.

Internal Structure. The internal aspect may be homogeneously radiopaque but usually has a radiolucent center that represents normal fatty marrow, giving the lesion a donut appearance radiographically. Trabeculae occasionally develop in the marrow cavity of larger osteomas. Individual lesions of calcified cystic acne

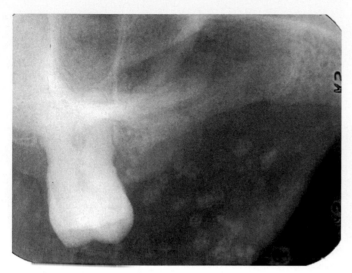

FIGURE 28-14 Osteoma cutis is seen as faint radiopaque calcifications in the cheek.

resemble a snowflake-like radiopacity, which corresponds to the clinical location of the scar.

Differential Diagnosis

The differential diagnosis should include myositis ossificans, calcinosis cutis, and osteoma mucosae. If the blown-out cheek technique is used, the lesions of osteoma cutis appear much more superficial than mucosal lesions. Myositis ossificans is of greater proportions, in some cases causing noticeable deformity of the facial contour.

Management

No treatment is required, but primary osteoma cutis is occasionally removed for cosmetic reasons. Resurfacing of the skin with the erbium:yttrium-aluminum-garnet laser with tretinoin cream or curettage and the carbon dioxide continuous wave laser has been successful in treating multiple miliary osteoma cutis. More recently, good cosmetic results have been reported with a needle microincision-extirpation technique in patients with multiple miliary osteoma cutis.

MYOSITIS OSSIFICANS

In myositis ossificans, fibrous tissue and heterotopic bone form within the interstitial tissue of muscle and associated tendons and ligaments. Secondary destruction and atrophy of the muscle occur as this fibrous tissue and bone interdigitate and separate the muscle fibers. There are two principal forms: (1) localized and (2) progressive.

Localized (Traumatic) Myositis Ossificans

Synonyms.   Synonyms for localized myositis ossificans include posttraumatic myositis ossificans and solitary myositis.

Disease Mechanism.   Localized myositis ossificans results from acute or chronic trauma or from heavy muscular strain caused by certain occupations and sports. Muscle injury from multiple injections (occasionally from dental anesthetic) also may be a cause. Skeletal muscle has limited capacity for regeneration after significant physical trauma. The injury leads to considerable hemorrhage into the muscle or associated tendons and fascia. It has been proposed that exuberant proliferation of vascular granulation tissue subsequently undergoes metaplasia to cartilage and bone during the healing process. The term myositis is misleading because no inflammation is involved. The fibrous tissue and bone form within the interstitial tissue of the muscle; no actual ossification of the muscle fibers occurs.

Clinical Features.   Localized myositis ossificans can develop at any age in either sex, but it occurs most often in young men who engage in vigorous activity. The site of the precipitating trauma remains swollen, tender, and painful much longer than expected. The overlying skin may be red and inflamed, and when the lesion involves a muscle of mastication, opening the jaws may be difficult. After about 2 or 3 weeks, the area of ossification becomes apparent in the tissues; a firm intramuscular mass can be palpated. The localized lesion may enlarge slowly, but eventually it stops growing. The lesion may appear fixed, or it may be freely movable on palpation.

Imaging Features

Location.   The most commonly involved muscles of the head and neck are the masseter and sternocleidomastoid. However, other muscles of mastication may be involved, such as the medial and lateral pterygoid, buccinator, and temporalis muscles. The anterior attachments of the temporalis and the medial pterygoid muscles are at risk of injury on administration of mandibular block anesthesia. A radiolucent band usually can be seen between the area of ossification and adjacent bone, and the heterotopic bone may lie along the long axis of the muscle (Fig. 28-15). Masses generally measure less than 6 cm in greatest dimension.

Periphery and Shape.   The periphery commonly is more radiopaque than the internal structure. There is a variation in shape from irregular oval to linear streaks (pseudotrabeculae) running in the same direction as the normal muscle fibers. These pseudotrabeculae are characteristic of myositis ossificans and strongly imply a diagnosis.

Internal Structure.   The internal structure varies with time. By 3 to 4 weeks after injury, the radiographic appearance is a faintly homogeneous radiopacity. This radiopacity organizes further, and by 2 months a delicate lacy or feathery radiopaque internal structure develops. These changes indicate the formation of bone; however, this bone does not have a normal-appearing trabecular pattern. Gradually, the image of this entity becomes denser, more homogeneous, and better defined, maturing fully in about 5 to 6 months, although some lesions progress more slowly and do not reach maturation until 12 months. After this period, the lesion may shrink.

Differential Diagnosis.   The differential diagnosis of localized myositis ossificans includes ossification of the stylohyoid ligament and other soft tissue calcifications. However, the form and the location of myositis ossificans often are enough to make the differential diagnosis. Other lesions to consider are bone-forming tumors. Although tumors such as osteogenic sarcoma can form a linear bone pattern (see Chapter 24), the tumor is contiguous with the adjacent bone, and signs of bone destruction often are present.

Management.   Microinjury and subsequent muscle necrosis attract macrophages, which elaborate osteogenic growth factors. One strategy during the evolution of the lesion is bone morphogenetic protein type I receptor inhibition to reduce the heterotopic ossification. Rest and limitation of use are recommended to diminish the extent of the calcific deposit. For lesions that cause a functional restriction or neurologic impairment, surgical excision of

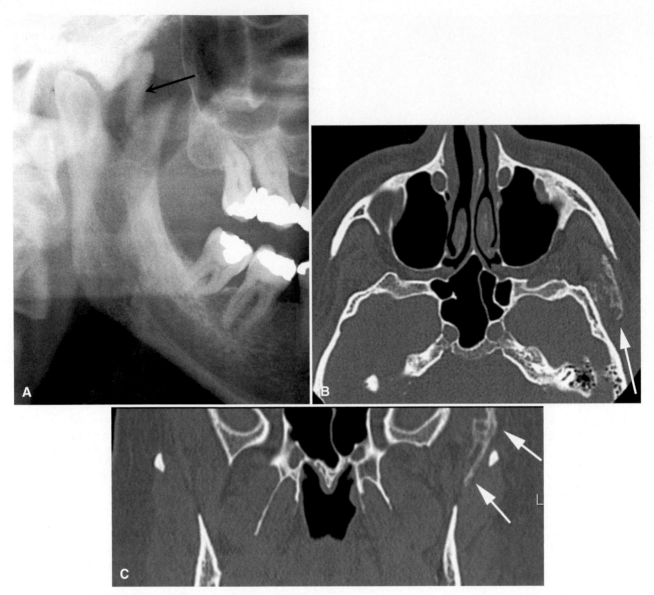

FIGURE 28-15 A, Soft tissue ossification extending from the coronoid process in a superior direction, following the anatomy of the temporalis muscle *(arrow)*. This condition arose after several attempts were made to provide a submandibular nerve block, leaving the patient unable to open the mandible. **B,** Axial MDCT image of ossification along the temporalis muscle *(arrow)* after a surgical procedure. **C,** Coronal MDCT image of the same case shown in **B** reveals the calcifications *(arrows)*.

the entire calcified mass with intensive physiotherapy to minimize postsurgical scarring is the recommended treatment. Complete maturation of myositis ossificans occurs between 6 and 12 months. Incomplete excision or excision at an immature stage can result in recurrence.

Progressive Myositis Ossificans

Synonym.   A synonym for progressive myositis ossificans is fibrodysplasia ossificans progressiva.

Disease Mechanism.   Progressive myositis ossificans is a rare hereditary disease with autosomal dominant transmission; less commonly, it arises as a result of spontaneous mutation. It is more common in males and causes symptoms from early infancy. Progressive formation of heterotopic bone occurs within the

interstitial tissue of muscles, tendons, ligaments, and fascia, and the involved muscles atrophy.

Clinical Features.   In most cases, heterotopic ossification starts in the muscles of the neck and upper back and moves to the extremities. The disease commences with soft tissue swelling that is tender and painful and may show redness and heat, indicating the presence of inflammation. The acute symptoms subside, and a firm mass remains in the tissues. This condition may affect any of the striated muscles, including the heart and diaphragm. In some cases, the spread of ossification is limited; in others, ossification becomes extensive, affecting almost all of the large muscles of the body. Stiffness and limitation of motion of the neck, chest, back, and extremities (especially the shoulders) gradually increase. Functional deficits are progressive and handicapping. Advanced stages of the

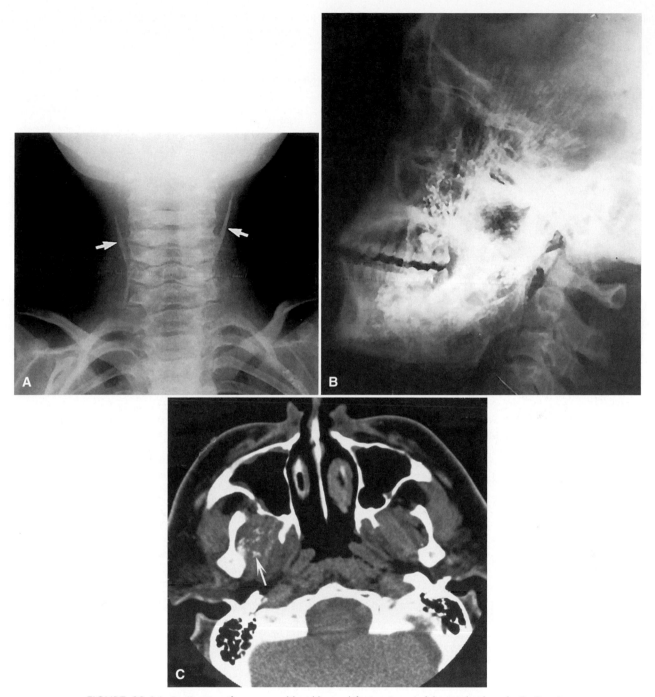

FIGURE 28-16 **A,** Myositis ossificans, seen as bilateral linear calcifications *(arrows)* of the sternohyoid muscle. **B,** Extensive ossification of the masseter and temporalis muscles. **C,** Axial CT scan with soft tissue algorithm demonstrates calcifications in the lateral pterygoid muscle *(arrow)*. (**A,** *Courtesy Dr. H. Worth, Vancouver, British Columbia.*)

disease result in the "petrified man" condition. During the third decade, the process may spontaneously arrest; however, most patients die during the third or fourth decades. Premature death usually results from respiratory embarrassment or from inanition through the involvement of the muscles of mastication.

Imaging Features. The radiographic appearance of progressive myositis ossificans is similar to appearance of the limited form. The heterotopic bone more commonly is oriented along the long axis of the involved muscle (Fig. 28-16). Osseous malformation of

the regions of muscle attachment, such as the mandibular condyles, also may be seen.

Differential Diagnosis. In the initial stages of the disease, distinguishing between progressive myositis ossificans and rheumatoid arthritis may be difficult. However, the presence of specific anomalies suggests the diagnosis. In the case of calcinosis, the deposits of amorphous calcium salts frequently resorb, but in progressive myositis ossificans, the bone never disappears.

Management.   No effective treatment exists for progressive myositis ossificans. Nodules that are traumatized and that ulcerate frequently should be excised. If interference with respiration or respiratory infection occurs in the later stages of the disease, supportive therapy may be required.

BIBLIOGRAPHY

Banks K, Bui-Mansfield L, Chew F, et al: A compartmental approach to the radiographic evaluation of soft-tissue calcifications, *Semin Roentgenol* 40:391–407, 2005.

Carter L: Lumps and bumps—what is that stone? *Alpha Omegan* 103:151–156, 2010.

Keberle M, Robinson S: Physiologic and pathologic calcifications and ossifications in the face and neck, *Eur Radiol* 17:2103–2111, 2007.

Monsour PA, Romaniuk K, Hutchings RD: Soft tissue calcifications in the differential diagnosis of opacities superimposed over the mandible by dental panoramic radiography, *Aust Dent J* 36:94–101, 1991.

Worth HM: *Principles and practice of oral radiologic interpretation*, St. Louis, 1963, Mosby.

Calcified Lymph Nodes

Carter L: Decoding cervical soft tissue calcifications on panoramic dental radiographs, *Va Dent J* 83:18–19, 2006.

Eisenkraft B, Som P: The spectrum of benign and malignant etiologies of cervical node calcification, *AJR Am J Roentgenol* 172:1433–1437, 1999.

Paquette M, Terezhalmy G, Moore W: Calcified lymph nodes, *Quintessence Int* 34:562–563, 2003.

Shin L, Fischbein N, Kaplan M, et al: Metastatic squamous cell carcinoma presenting as diffuse and punctate cervical lymph node calcifications: sonographic features and utility of sonographically guided fine-needle aspiration biopsy, *J Ultrasound Med* 28:1703–1707, 2009.

Dystrophic Calcification in the Tonsils

Guevara C, Mandel L: Panoramic radiographic demonstration of bilateral tonsilloliths, *N Y State Dent J* 77:28–30, 2011.

Lo R-H, Chang K-P, Chu S-T: Upper airway obstruction caused by bilateral giant tonsilloliths, *J Chinese Med Assoc* 74:329–331, 2011.

Siber S, Hat J, Brakus I, et al: Tonsillolithiasis and orofacial pain, *Gerodontology* 29:e1157–e1160, 2012.

Cysticercosis

Delgado-Azañero WA, Mosqueda-Taylor A, Carlos-Bregni R, et al: Oral cysticercosis: a collaborative study of 16 cases, *Oral Surg Oral Med Oral Pathol Oral Radiol Endod* 103:528–533, 2007.

Kimura-Hayama E, Higuera J, Corona-Cedillo R, et al: Neurocysticercosis: radiologic-pathologic correlation, *Radiographics* 30:1705–1719, 2010.

Sathe N, Acharya R, Patil M, et al: An unusual case of labial cysticercosis with a natural history, *Nat J Maxillofac Surg* 1:100–102, 2011.

Sorvillo F, Wilkins P, Shafir S, et al: Public health implications of cysticercosis acquired in the United States, *Emerg Infect Dis* 17:1–6, 2011.

Calcified Blood Vessel

Almog DM, Horev T, Illig K, et al: Correlating carotid artery stenosis detected by panoramic radiography with clinically relevant carotid artery stenosis determined by duplex ultrasound, *Oral Surg Oral Med Oral Pathol Oral Radiol Endod* 94:768–773, 2002.

Beckstrom B, Horsley S, Scheetz J, et al: Correlation between carotid area calcifications and periodontitis: a retrospective study of digital panoramic radiographic findings in pretreatment cancer patients, *Oral Surg Oral Med Oral Pathol Oral Radiol Endod* 103:359–366, 2007.

Henriques J, Kreich M, Baldani M, et al: Panoramic radiography in the diagnosis of carotid artery atheromas and the associated risk factors, *Open Dent J* 5:79–83, 2011.

Johansson E, Ahlqvist J, Garoff M, et al: Ultrasound screening for asymptomatic carotid stenosis in subjects with calcifications in the area of the carotid arteries on panoramic radiographs: a cross-sectional study, *BMC Cardiovasc Disord* 11:44, 2011.

Rhinoliths and Antroliths

Güneri P, Kaya A, Caliskan M: Antroliths: survey of the literature and report of a case, *Oral Surg Oral Med Oral Pathol Oral Radiol Endod* 99:517–521, 2005.

Henriques J, Kreich E, Rosa R, et al: Noninvasive aspergillosis as a maxillary antrolith: report of a rare case, *Quintessence Int* 43:143–146, 2012.

Nass Duce M, Talas DU, Ozer C, et al: Antrolithiasis: a retrospective study, *J Laryngol Otol* 117:637–640, 2003.

Orhan K, Kocyigit D, Kisnisci R, et al: Rhinolithiasis: an uncommon entity of the nasal cavity, *Oral Surg Oral Med Oral Pathol Oral Radiol Endod* 101:e28–e32, 2007.

Pinto LS, Campagnoli EB, de Souza Azevedo R, et al: Rhinoliths causing palatal perforation: case report and literature review, *Oral Surg Oral Med Oral Pathol Oral Radiol Endod* 104:e42–e46, 2007.

Sümbüllü M, Tozoğlu U, Yörük O, et al: Rhinolithiasis: the importance of flat panel detector-based cone beam computed tomography in diagnosis and treatment, *Oral Surg Oral Med Oral Pathol* 107:e65–e67, 2009.

Sialolith

McGurk M, Escudier M, Thomas B, et al: A revolution in the management of obstructive salivary gland disease, *Dent Update* 33:28–30, 2006; erratum: *Dent Update* 33:83, 2006.

Nahlieli O, Nakar L, Nazarian Y, et al: Sialoendoscopy: a new approach to salivary gland obstructive pathology, *J Am Dent Assoc* 137:1394–1400, 2006.

Nakayama E, Okamura K, Mitsuyasu T, et al: A newly developed interventional sialendoscope for a completely nonsurgical sialolithectomy using intracorporeal electrohydraulic lithotripsy, *J Oral Maxillofac Surg* 65:1402–1405, 2007.

Sabot J-F, Gustin M-P, Delahougue K, et al: Analytical investigation of salivary calculi, by mid-infrared spectroscopy, *Analyst* 137:2095–2100, 2012.

Witt R, Iro H, Koch M, et al: Minimally invasive options for salivary calculi, *Laryngoscope* 122:1306–1311, 2012.

Phleboliths

Altug H, Büyüksoy V, Okçu K, et al: Hemangiomas of the head and neck with phleboliths: clinical features, diagnostic imaging, and treatment of 3 cases, *Oral Surg Oral Med Oral Pathol Oral Radiol Endod* 103:e60–e64, 2007.

Eivazi B, Fasunla A, Güldner C, et al: Phleboliths from vascular malformations of the head and neck, *Phlebology* 2012 [Epub ahead of print].

Mandel L, Perrino M: Phleboliths and the vascular maxillofacial lesion, *J Oral Maxillofac Surg* 68:1973–1976, 2010.

Calcified Laryngeal Cartilages

Carter L: Discrimination between calcified triticeous cartilage and calcified carotid atheroma on panoramic radiography, *Oral Surg Oral Med Oral Pathol Oral Radiol Endod* 90:108–110, 2000.

Kamikawa R, Pereira M, Fernandes Â, et al: Study of the localization of radiopacities similar to calcified carotid atheroma by means of panoramic radiography, *Oral Surg Oral Med Oral Pathol Oral Radiol Endod* 101:374–378, 2006.

Mupparrapu M, Vuppalapati A: Ossification of laryngeal cartilages on lateral cephalometric radiographs, *Angle Orthod* 75:196–201, 2005.

Zan E, Yousem D, Aygun N: Asymmetric mineralization of the arytenoid cartilages in patients without laryngeal cancer, *AJNR Am J Neuroradiol* 32:1113–1118, 2011.

Ossified Stylohyoid Ligament

Bafaqeeh SA: Eagle syndrome: classic and carotid artery types, *J Otolaryngol* 29:88–94, 2000.

Chuang WC, Short JH, McKinney AM, et al: Reversible left hemispheric ischemia secondary to carotid compression in Eagle syndrome: surgical and CT angiographic correlation, *AJNR Am J Neuroradiol* 28:143–145, 2007.

Colby C, Del Gaudio J: Stylohyoid complex syndrome, *Arch Otolaryngol Head Neck Surg* 137:248–252, 2011.

Eagle WW: Elongated styloid process, symptoms and treatment, *AMA Arch Otolaryngol* 67:172–176, 1958.

Farhat H, Elhammady MS, Ziayee H, et al: Eagle syndrome as a cause of transient ischemic attacks: case report, *J Neurosurg* 110:90–93, 2009.

Klécha A, Hafian H, Devauchelle B, et al: A report of post-traumatic Eagle's syndrome, *Int J Oral Maxillofac Surg* 37:970–972, 2008.

Osteoma Cutis

Baskan EB, Turan H, Tunali S, et al: Miliary osteoma cutis of the face: treatment with the needle microincision-extirpation method, *J Dermatol Treat* 18:252–254, 2007.

Davis M, Pittelkow M, Lindor N, et al: Progressive extensive osteoma cutis associated with dysmorphic features: a new syndrome? Case report and review of the literature, *Br J Dermatol* 146:1075–1080, 2002.

Johann A, Garcia B, Nacif T, et al: Submandibular osseous choristoma, *J Craniomaxillofac Surg* 34:57–59, 2006.

Shigehara H, Honda Y, Kishi K, et al: Radiographic and morphologic studies of multiple miliary osteomas of cadaver skin, *Oral Surg Oral Med Oral Pathol Oral Radiol Endod* 86:121–125, 1998.

Talsania N, Jolliffe V, O'Toole E, et al: Platelike osteoma cutis, *J Am Acad Dermatol* 64:613–615, 2011.

Thielen AM, Stucki L, Braun RP, et al: Multiple cutaneous osteomas of the face associated with chronic inflammatory acne, *J Eur Acad Dermatol Venereol* 20:321–326, 2006.

Myositis Ossificans

Findlay I, Lakkireddi P, Gangone R, et al: A case of myositis ossificans in the upper cervical spine of a young child, *Spine (Phila Pa 1976)* 35:E1525–E1528, 2010.

Kaplan F, Le Merrer M, Glaser D, et al: Fibrodysplasia ossificans progressive, *Best Pract Res Clin Rheumatol* 22:191–205, 2008.

Kruse A, Danneman C, Grätz KW: Bilateral myositis ossificans of the masseter muscle after chemoradiotherapy and critical illness neuropathy—case report of a rare entity and review of the literature, *Head Neck Oncol* 1:30, 2009.

Lin T-Y, Wu C-C, Chiang F-Y, et al: Noninfectious painful neck mass mimicking malignancy in a child, *Head Neck* 33:753–755, 2011.

St-Hilaire H, Weber W, Ramer M, et al: Clinicopatholgic conference: trismus following dental treatment, *Oral Surg Oral Med Oral Pathol Oral Radiol Endod* 98:261–266, 2004.

SALIVARY GLAND DISEASE

DISEASE MECHANISM

Dental diagnosticians have professional responsibility for detecting disorders of the salivary glands. A familiarity with salivary gland disorders and applicable current imaging technology is an essential element of the clinician's armamentarium. Both major and minor salivary glands may be involved pathologically; however, this chapter deals only with the major glands. Salivary gland disease processes may be divided into the following clinical categories: inflammatory disorders, noninflammatory disorders, and space-occupying masses. Inflammatory disorders are acute or chronic and may be secondary to ductal obstruction by sialoliths, trauma, infection, or space-occupying lesions such as neoplasia. Noninflammatory disorders are metabolic and secretory abnormalities associated with diseases of nearly all the endocrine glands, malnutrition, and neurologic disorders. Space-occupying masses are cystic or neoplastic; the neoplasms are benign or malignant.

CLINICAL SIGNS AND SYMPTOMS

Diseases of the major salivary glands may have single or multiple clinical features. Swelling in the areas of the parotid and submandibular glands should create a clinical suspicion of salivary gland disease until ruled out. Pain and altered salivary flow may be present. Because the periodicity and longevity of these symptoms are important in the differential diagnosis, a review of the medical history and physical condition of the patient may provide important information. A history of skin, endocrine, or swallowing abnormalities may suggest a systemic collagen disease or metabolic disorder.

DIFFERENTIAL DIAGNOSIS OF SALIVARY ENLARGEMENTS

Enlargements of the Parotid Area

Unilateral enlargements of the parotid area are categorized by the presence of a discrete, palpable mass or a diffuse swelling. If no mass is apparent, sialadenitis should be considered. Sialadenitis may be primary or secondary to ductal obstruction (retrograde). A mass superficial to the gland may represent lymphadenitis, infected preauricular cyst, infected sebaceous cyst, benign lymphoid hyperplasia, or extraparotid tumor. A mass intrinsic to the gland suggests a neoplasm (benign or malignant), intraglandular lymph node, or hamartoma. Rapid growth, facial nerve paralysis, rock-hard texture, pain, and older age of occurrence are clinical features of malignant neoplasms.

The differential diagnosis of asymptomatic bilateral enlargements of the parotid area may include benign lymphoepithelial lesion, Sjögren's syndrome, alcoholism, medication (iodine and certain heavy metals), and Warthin's tumor. Painful bilateral enlargement may occur after radiation treatment or as a result of bacterial or viral sialadenitis (including mumps) when accompanied by systemic symptoms.

The differential diagnosis of diffuse facial swelling in the parotid region, not related to abnormalities of the gland, includes hypertrophy of the masseter muscle, accessory parotid gland, lesions related to the temporomandibular joint, and osteomyelitis of the ramus of the mandible. A palpable mass superficial to the gland suggests lymphadenitis, an infected preauricular or sebaceous cyst, benign lymphoid hyperplasia, or extraparotid tumor (Box 29-1).

Enlargements of the Submandibular Area

Unilateral enlargement of the submandibular area associated with tender lymph nodes is suggestive of sialadenitis, which may be primary or secondary to ductal obstruction or decreased salivary flow (retrograde). Unilateral enlargement without tender lymph nodes suggests a neoplasm, cyst, lymphoepithelial lesion, or fibrosis. An intraglandular mass may be neoplastic or cystic. Neoplasms of the submandibular gland have a greater chance of being malignant than neoplasms of the parotid gland. Sublingual gland neoplasms have a still greater chance of being malignant than neoplasms of the submandibular glands. Rapid growth, rock-hard texture, pain, and older age of occurrence are clinically suggestive of malignancy. Masses superficial or adjacent to the submandibular gland may be lymph nodes or extraglandular neoplasms.

Bilateral enlargement of the submandibular gland area suggests bacterial or viral sialadenitis. Although mumps is primarily a viral infection of the parotid glands, it may also occur in the submandibular glands. Other causes of swelling in the submandibular region include Sjögren's syndrome, enlarged lymph nodes, submandibular space infection, and branchial cleft cyst (see Box 29-1).

APPLIED DIAGNOSTIC IMAGING

Diagnostic imaging of salivary gland disease may be undertaken to differentiate inflammatory processes from neoplastic disease, distinguish diffuse disease from focal suppurative disease, identify and localize sialoliths, and demonstrate ductal morphology. In addition, diagnostic imaging attempts to determine the anatomic location of a tumor, differentiate benign from malignant disease, demonstrate the relationship between a mass and adjacent anatomic structures, and aid in the selection of biopsy sites.

STRATEGIES FOR DIAGNOSTIC IMAGING

Projection (plain film) radiographs are two-dimensional images acquired without special effects. They are an appropriate starting point for imaging the major salivary glands from a cost-benefit point of view. These images can demonstrate moderately calcified sialoliths and the possible involvement of adjacent osseous structures. Because obstructive and associated inflammatory conditions are the most common disorders and primarily involve the ductal system, conventional sialography is typically the most appropriate next imaging modality. If the patient is allergic to the iodine contrast agent used in sialography, magnetic resonance imaging (MRI), multidetector computed tomographic (MDCT) imaging, or ultrasonography (US) may be selected as alternative imaging modalities. More recent studies comparing the diagnostic yield of MRI with sialography suggest that MRI might replace sialography in the future as the imaging modality of choice for ductal pathosis. Sialography, cone beam computed tomographic (CBCT) imaging, and MDCT imaging are the best imaging modalities for the detection of sialoliths (sialolithiasis) if they are calcified enough to be radiopaque. If sialography eliminates inflammatory disorders or suggests the presence of a space-occupying mass (either cystic or solid), contrast-enhanced MDCT imaging or MRI is appropriate for evaluation. US is an alternative technique to differentiate cystic lesions from solid masses and to identify advanced autoimmune lesions. Functional disorders such as xerostomia are appropriately imaged with sialography or scintigraphy (nuclear medicine scan). Scintigraphy can provide important physiologic information that may be helpful in forming the differential diagnosis.

PROJECTION RADIOGRAPHY

Projection or plain radiography is a fundamental part of the examination of the salivary glands and may provide sufficient information to preclude the use of more sophisticated and expensive imaging techniques. Both intraoral and extraoral techniques are appropriate, depending on the patient's clinical presentation and history. These images have the potential to identify unrelated pathoses in the areas of the salivary glands that may be mistakenly identified as salivary gland disease, such as resorptive or osteoblastic changes in adjacent bone causing periauricular swelling mimicking a parotid tumor. Panoramic and posteroanterior skull radiographs may demonstrate bony lesions, eliminating salivary pathosis from the differential diagnosis. Unilateral or bilateral functional or congenital hypertrophy of the masseter muscle may clinically mimic a salivary tumor. An extraoral image may demonstrate a deep antegonial notch, overdeveloped mandibular angle, and exostosis on the outer surface of the angle in cases of masseter hypertrophy.

Projection images are useful when the clinical impression, supported by a compatible history, suggests the presence of sialoliths (stones or calculi). The examination should include both intraoral and extraoral images to demonstrate the entire region of the gland. Sialoliths may be multiple at different locations. It is expedient to decrease the usual exposure by about half to avoid overexposure of the sialoliths. However, this technique is limited by the fact that 20% of the sialoliths of the submandibular gland and 40% of the sialoliths of the parotid gland are not well calcified, rendering them radiolucent and not visible on projection images. When acquired digitally, the images can be enhanced to assist in visualizing anatomic structures and pathologic abnormalities. Radiolucent sialoliths are rarely found in the sublingual glands.

Intraoral Radiography

Sialoliths in the anterior two thirds of the submandibular duct are typically imaged with a cross-sectional mandibular occlusal projection as described in Chapter 7 (Fig. 29-1). The posterior portion of the duct may be demonstrated with an over-the-shoulder occlusal projection view, where the directing cone is placed on the shoulder and the central ray is directed in an anterior direction through the angle of the mandible, with the patient's head rotated back and tilted to the unaffected side (Fig. 29-2).

Parotid sialoliths are more difficult to demonstrate than the submandibular variety owing to the tortuous course of Stensen's duct around the anterior border of the masseter and through the buccinator muscle. As a rule, only sialoliths anterior to the masseter muscle can be imaged on an intraoral image. To demonstrate sialoliths in the anterior part of the duct, an intraoral image receptor is stabilized with a holder inside the cheek, as high as possible in the buccal sulcus and over the parotid papilla. The central ray is directed perpendicular to the center of the receptor.

Extraoral Radiography

A panoramic projection frequently demonstrates sialoliths in the posterior duct or reveals intraglandular sialoliths in the submandibular gland if they are within the image layer (Fig. 29-3). The image of most parotid sialoliths is superimposed over the ramus and body of the mandible at the level of or just superior to the occlusal plane, making oblique lateral radiographs of the mandible of limited value. To demonstrate sialoliths in the submandibular gland, the lateral projection is modified by opening the mouth, extending the chin, and depressing the tongue with the index finger; this improves the image of the sialolith by moving it inferior to the mandibular border.

Sialoliths in the distal portion of Stensen's duct or in the parotid gland are difficult to demonstrate by intraoral or lateral extraoral views. However, a posteroanterior skull projection with the cheeks puffed out may move the image of the sialolith free of the adjacent bone, rendering it visible on the projected image (see Fig. 29-2). This technique may also demonstrate interglandular sialoliths that may be obscured during sialography.

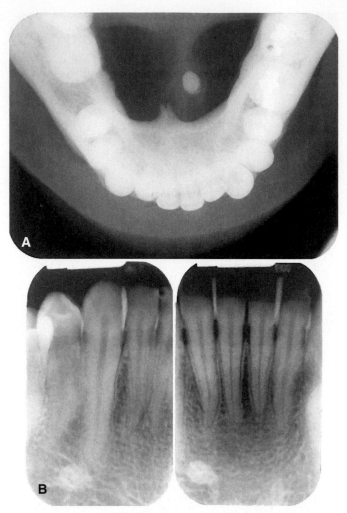

FIGURE 29-1 Intraoral radiographic projections. **A,** Underexposed mandibular occlusal radiograph demonstrates a radiopaque sialolith in Wharton's duct. Note the classic laminated appearance. **B,** Periapical radiographs of the same case. The radiopaque calculus can be localized lingual to the teeth by applying appropriate object localization rules.

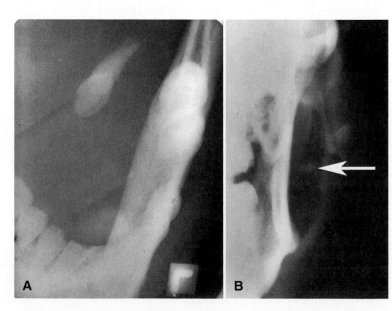

FIGURE 29-2 Extraoral radiographic projections. **A,** Over-the-shoulder occlusal projection reveals a sialolith. **B,** Anteroposterior skull view with cheek blown out to provide air contrast to reveal a parotid sialolith *(arrow)*.

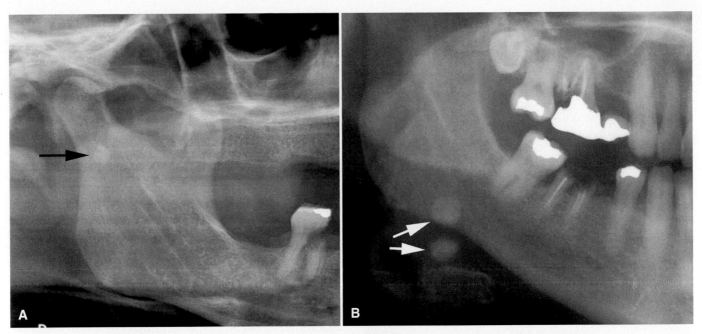

FIGURE 29-3 Cropped panoramic radiographs. **A,** Parotid sialolith superimposed over condylar neck *(arrow)* is superior to the plane of occlusion, which differentiated it from a palatine tonsillolith. **B,** Submandibular sialoliths *(arrows)* near the antegonial notch of the mandible and superior to the hyoid bone.

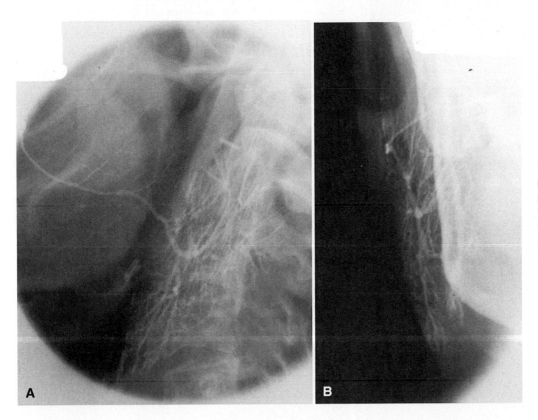

FIGURE 29-4 Sialography of normal parotid gland. **A,** Lateral projection of the parotid demonstrates opacification all the way to the terminal ducts and acini. **B,** Anteroposterior projection of the same gland demonstrates "parenchymal blushing" from acinar opacification.

CONVENTIONAL SIALOGRAPHY

First performed in 1902, sialography is a radiographic technique where a radiopaque contrast agent is infused into the ductal system of a salivary gland before imaging with plain films/digital image receptors, fluoroscopy, panoramic radiography, CBCT imaging, or MDCT imaging. Sialography is the most detailed way to image the ductal system (Figs. 29-4 to 29-6). CBCT imaging has been developed more recently as an imaging modality for conventional sialography. Its advantages are multiplanar and three-dimensional visualization of the ductal structures and the ability to remove overlapping anatomic structures from the image for better visualization of the gland.

The ductal systems of the parotid and submandibular glands are most readily studied with this technique. Although the sublingual gland is difficult to infuse intentionally, it may be fortuitously opacified while Wharton's duct is infused to image the submandibular gland. A survey or "scout" image is usually acquired before infusion of the contrast solution into the ductal system as an aid in verifying the optimal exposure factors and patient positioning parameters as well as detection of radiopaque sialoliths or extraglandular pathosis.

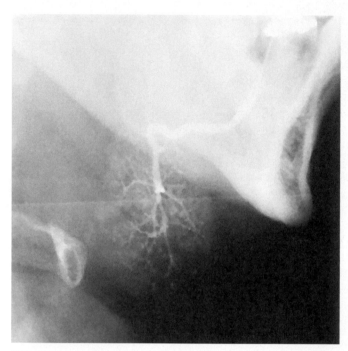

FIGURE 29-5 Sialography of normal submandibular gland. Lateral view demonstrates parenchymal blushing. Normal fine branching is visible. Lack of parenchymal blushing at the anteroinferior margin is caused by radiographic burnout.

With this technique, a lacrimal or periodontal probe is used to dilate the sphincter at the ductal orifice before the passage of a cannula (blunt needle or catheter) connected by extension tubing to a syringe containing contrast agent. Lipid-soluble (e.g., Ethiodol) or non–lipid-soluble (e.g., Sinografin) contrast solution is slowly infused until the patient feels discomfort (usually between 0.2 and 1.5 mL, depending on the gland being studied). These iodine-containing agents render the ductal system radiopaque. The filling phase can be monitored by fluoroscopy or with static projection images. The intent is to opacify the ductal system proximally to the acini. The image of the ductal system appears as "tree limbs," with no area of the gland devoid of ducts. With acinar filling, the "tree" comes into "bloom," which is the typical appearance of the parenchymal opacification phase (see Figs. 29-4 to 29-6). The gland is allowed to empty for 5 minutes without stimulation. If postevacuation images suggest retention of contrast agent, a sialagogue, such as lemon juice or 2% citric acid, may be administered to augment evacuation by stimulating secretion. Non–lipid-soluble contrast agents are preferred because of reports of inflammatory reactions subsequent to inadvertent extravasation of lipid-soluble agents. In addition to static projection radiographic images, the opacified gland can be imaged with CBCT, MDCT, or panoramic imaging techniques. CBCT imaging and MDCT imaging have the advantage of providing three-dimensional visualization.

Sialography is indicated for the evaluation of chronic inflammatory diseases and ductal pathoses. Contraindications include acute infection, known sensitivity to iodine-containing compounds, and immediately anticipated thyroid function tests.

CONE-BEAM COMPUTED TOMOGRAPHIC IMAGING

CBCT imaging is useful in evaluating structures in and adjacent to salivary glands but cannot resolve differences in soft tissue densities. Minimally calcified sialolithiasis is well depicted on CBCT imaging, and it is useful as a recording modality for conventional sialography, providing three-dimensional visualization of the ductal structure (Fig. 29-7).

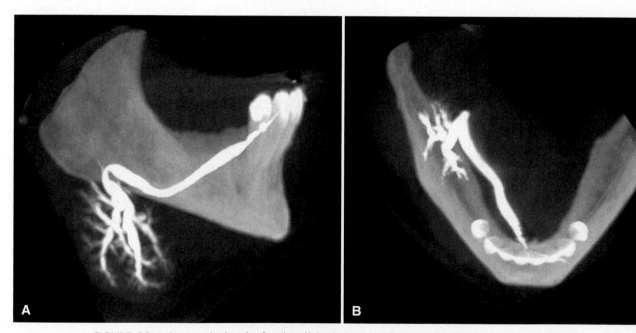

FIGURE 29-6 Conventional sialography of a submandibular gland imaged with CBCT imaging. The images are rendered in lateral **(A)** and axial **(B)** views. (Courtesy Dr. Fatima Jadu.)

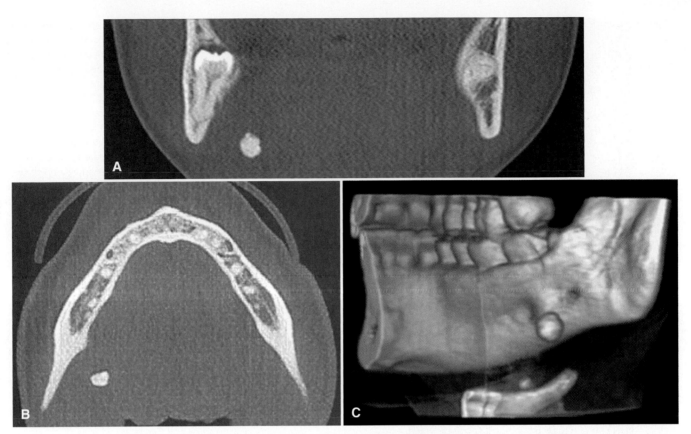

FIGURE 29-7 CBCT imaging of a submandibular sialolith. Coronal **(A)**, axial **(B)**, and three-dimensional renditions **(C)**.

MULTIDETECTOR COMPUTED TOMOGRAPHIC IMAGING

MDCT imaging is useful in evaluating structures in and adjacent to salivary glands; it displays both soft and hard tissues and minute differences in soft tissue densities. Thin axial and coronal images with a soft tissue algorithm are commonly acquired after intravenous administration of a contrast agent (Fig. 29-8). (See Chapter 14 for a description of the MDCT imaging process.) The imaging study is typically assessed in both hard and soft tissue windows. Glandular tissues are usually easily discernible from surrounding fat and muscle. The parotid glands are more radiopaque than the surrounding fat but less opaque than adjacent muscles. Although the submandibular and sublingual glands are similar in density to adjacent muscles, they are readily identified on the basis of shape and location. The submandibular and sublingual glands are most easily identified on directly acquired contrast-enhanced coronal MDCT scans. MDCT imaging is useful in assessing acute inflammatory processes and abscesses, cysts, mucoceles, and neoplasia. Calcifications such as sialoliths are also well depicted with MDCT imaging (Fig. 29-9). However, MDCT is not recognized as a sensitive study for salivary tumors per se.

MAGNETIC RESONANCE IMAGING

MRI typically provides a different and superior soft tissue contrast resolution than MDCT imaging; it also results in fewer problems with streak artifacts from metallic dental restorative materials (Fig. 29-10). (See Chapter 14 for a description of the basic concepts and principles of MRI.)

MRI can be an alternative to conventional sialography in evaluating ductal pathosis, especially when ductal catheterization is either problematic or contraindicated. Before imaging, the patient is given lemon juice or a similar sialagogue to stimulate salivation. The MRI study is performed using rapid acquisition with relaxation enhancement sequence and a three-dimensional constructive interference in steady state sequence. The images may be reformatted using a multiplanar reconstruction software algorithm.

Although indications for MDCT imaging and MRI occasionally overlap, MRI is usually the imaging method of choice in evaluating parenchymal masses or cystic lesions because of superior display of salivary gland masses, internal structures, and regional extension of the lesions into adjacent tissues or spaces, especially in examining the submandibular glands. The use of intravenous contrast agent (most commonly gadolinium) is helpful in distinguishing between cystic and solid masses and in evaluating perineural spread of malignant tumors. Sublingual masses should always be studied by MRI because of their high incidence of malignancy. Studies have shown MRI with evoked salivation, sometimes termed "MR sialography," as a natural contrast medium to reveal ductal morphology accurately and to identify sialoliths. Axial views are acquired for all sequences, with coronal and sagittal views as needed. Noncontrast T1-weighted and T2-weighted sequences are obtained, followed by T1-weighted postcontrast, fat-suppressed images. Fast spin echo T2-weighted images may also require fat suppression.

SCINTIGRAPHY (NUCLEAR MEDICINE, POSITRON EMISSION TOMOGRAPHY)

Nuclear medicine, or scintigraphy, provides a functional study of the salivary glands, taking advantage of the selective concentration

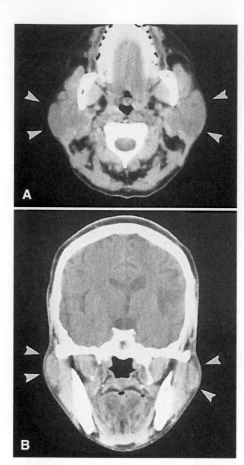

FIGURE 29-8 CT images with soft tissue algorithm. **A,** Axial view demonstrates bilateral enlargement of the parotid glands (arrowheads). **B,** Coronal view of the same patient. The clinical and histopathologic diagnosis was autoimmune parotitis. (*Courtesy Department of Radiology, Baylor University Medical Center, Dallas, TX.*)

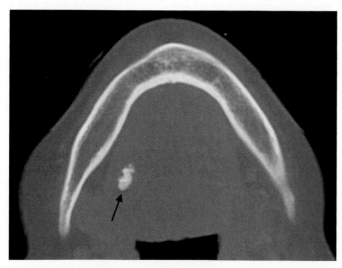

FIGURE 29-9 Axial bone algorithm MDCT image shows a sialolith in the submandibular (Wharton's) duct.

of specific radiopharmaceuticals in the glands. (See Chapter 14 for a description of the nuclear medicine procedures used to acquire images.) When technetium 99m (^{99m}Tc)-pertechnetate is injected intravenously, it is concentrated in and excreted by glandular structures, including the salivary, thyroid, and mammary glands. The

radionuclide appears in the ducts of the salivary glands within minutes and reaches maximal concentration within 30 to 45 minutes. A sialagogue is then administered to evaluate secretory capacity. All major salivary glands can be studied at once.

Although this technique has high diagnostic sensitivity, it lacks specificity and demonstrates minimal morphology. Pathosis may be demonstrated by an increased, decreased, or absent radionuclide uptake (Fig. 29-11). Lesions that concentrate ^{99m}Tc-pertechnetate are Warthin's tumors and oncocytomas. The diagnosis of salivary gland tumors from nuclear medicine scans is not completely reliable. Because of relatively low image resolution, MDCT imaging and MRI are preferred for the evaluation of salivary masses. A specialized form of nuclear medicine is positron emission tomography (PET). Despite a much greater resolution than scintigraphy, PET has not been useful for classifying salivary tumors as benign or malignant.

ULTRASONOGRAPHY

Compared with MDCT imaging and MRI, US has the following advantages: relatively inexpensive, widely available, painless, easy to perform, no ionizing radiation risk, and noninvasive. (For a full description of US, see Chapter 14.) The primary applications of US are the differentiation of solid masses from cystic ones (Fig. 29-12) and guided fine-needle aspiration biopsies. More recent studies suggest that this technique may also be helpful in detecting sialoliths and diagnosing advanced autoimmune lesions (Sjögren's syndrome). However, US does not reliably demonstrate the extent of tumors in the deep lobe of the parotid.

IMAGE INTERPRETATION OF SALIVARY GLAND DISORDERS

OBSTRUCTIVE AND INFLAMMATORY DISORDERS

Sialolithiasis

Synonyms. Synonyms for sialolithiasis are calculus and salivary stones.

Disease Mechanism. Sialolithiasis is the formation of a calcified obstruction within the salivary duct. Sialoliths may form in any of the major or minor salivary glands or their ducts, but usually only one gland is involved. The submandibular gland and Wharton's duct are the most frequently involved (83% of cases). If one stone is found, at least a one in four chance exists that others are present. Sialoliths can obstruct the secretory ducts, resulting in chronic retrograde infections because of a decrease in salivary flow.

Clinical Features. Clinical symptoms include intermittent swelling and pain with eating and signs of infection.

Imaging Features. Depending on their degree of calcification, sialoliths may appear either radiopaque or radiolucent on radiographic examinations (20% to 40% of cases may not be calcified enough to be radiopaque and are sometimes referred to as "mucous plugs") (Fig. 29-13; see Fig. 29-1). Sialoliths vary in shape from long cigar shapes to oval or round shapes. When visible, they usually have a homogeneous radiopaque internal structure. Sialography is helpful in locating obstructions that are undetectable with plain radiography, especially if the sialoliths are radiolucent. The contrast agent usually flows around the sialolith, filling the duct

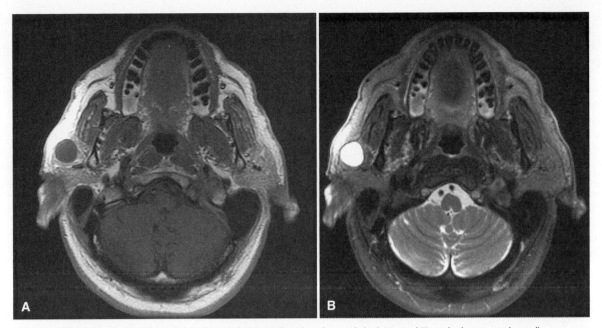

FIGURE 29-10 MRI reveal a lymphoepithelial cyst involving the right parotid gland. **A,** Axial T1-weighted image reveals a well-defined circular lesion involving the right parotid gland with an internal signal isointense to muscle. **B,** Matching T2-weighted image reveals that the lesion has a high internal signal because of the fluid content.

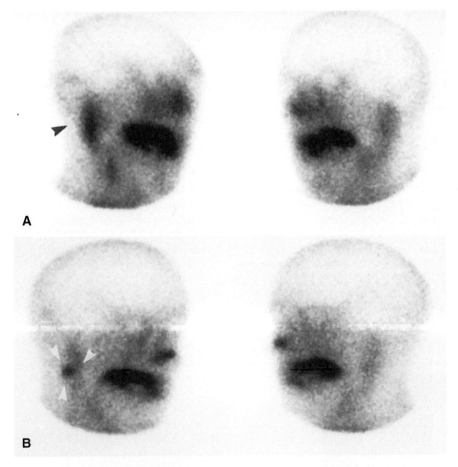

FIGURE 29-11 Scintigraphy **A,** ^{99m}Tc-pertechnetate scan of the salivary glands (right and left anterior oblique views) demonstrates increased uptake of radioisotope in the right parotid gland *(black arrowhead).* **B,** Scintigram obtained after administration of a sialagogue (lemon juice) demonstrates retention of isotope in the right parotid gland *(white arrowheads).* This is a typical presentation of salivary stasis, Warthin's tumor, or oncocytoma.

proximal to the obstruction (Fig. 29-14; see Fig. 29-13). The ductal system is frequently dilated proximal to the obstruction and implies the presence of an obstruction even when it is not visible. The contrast agent that flows around the sialolith is more radiopaque and may obscure small sialoliths. Radiolucent sialoliths appear as ductal filling voids (Fig. 29-15; see Fig. 29-13). Sialography should not be performed if a radiopaque stone has been shown on projection radiography to be in the distal portion of the duct because the procedure may displace it proximally into the ductal system, complicating subsequent removal. MDCT imaging may also detect minimally calcified sialoliths not visible on projection or plain images. Size measurements of radiopaque sialoliths have been reported to differ little from measurement made with US and histomorphometry.

US is of limited value in the diagnosis of inflammatory and obstructive diseases, but more recent studies indicate it is fairly reliable in demonstrating sialoliths. More than 90% of stones larger than 2 mm are detected as echo-dense spots with a characteristic acoustic shadow.

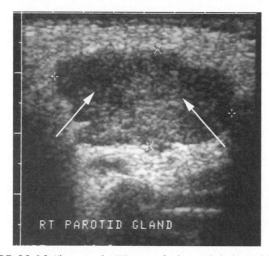

FIGURE 29-12 Ultrasonography (US) image of right parotid gland. A well-delineated solid mass is suggested by echo returns within the lesion *(arrows)*. US appearance is typical of a benign salivary tumor. *(Courtesy Department of Radiology, Baylor University Medical Center, Dallas, TX.)*

Sialoliths must be differentiated from phleboliths and dystrophic calcification of lymph nodes. Phleboliths typically have a radiolucent center. Calcified lymph nodes usually appear to be "cauliflower" shaped. In the panoramic image, palatine tonsilliths have a similar location as parotid sialoliths, superimposed over the ramus, but can be differentiated in that they are typically multiple, punctate, and imaged inferior to the occlusal plane.

Treatment. Treatment of sialolithiasis may consist of encouragement of spontaneous discharge through the use of sialagogues to stimulate secretion. Sialography may also stimulate discharge, especially if an oil-based contrast agent is used. If discharge does not occur, the sialolith may be removed by surgery, by more conservative "basket" retrieval methods, and as a last resort by total excision of the involved salivary gland.

Bacterial Sialadenitis

Synonyms. Synonyms for bacterial sialadenitis are parotitis and submandibulitis.

Disease Mechanism. Bacterial sialadenitis is an acute or chronic bacterial infection of the terminal acini or parenchyma of the salivary glands. Acute bacterial infections most commonly affect the parotid gland, but the submandibular gland may also be involved. These infections are the result of reduced salivary secretion and retrograde infection by the oral flora (usually *Staphylococcus aureus* and *Streptococcus viridans*). Reduced salivary secretion may also be drug related or the result of occlusion of a major duct.

Chronic inflammation may affect any of the major salivary glands, causing extensive swelling and culminating in fibrosis. Chronic inflammation may be a consequence of an untreated acute sialadenitis or associated with some type of obstruction resulting from sialolithiasis, noncalcified organic debris, or stricture (scar or fibrosis) formation in the excretory ducts. Bacteria or viruses may not be detected in the gland or saliva. The parotid is most often involved.

Clinical Features. Most cases are unilateral and may occur at any age. In acute cases, the typical clinical presentation is swelling, redness, tenderness, and malaise. Enlarged regional lymph nodes and suppuration may also be noted. Elderly patients, postoperative patients, and debilitated patients who have poor hygiene and low

FIGURE 29-13 A, Partial image of a standard mandibular occlusal film reveals the presence of a sialolith *(arrow)*. **B,** Sialogram of the same patient demonstrates flow of contrast material past the stone *(short arrows)* and a negative filling defect *(long arrow)* from a smaller radiolucent sialolith. The proximal secondary ducts within the gland show abnormal irregular widening, indicating sialodochitis.

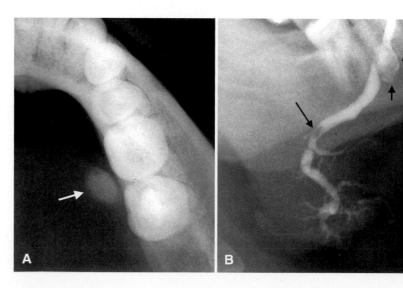

sialectasia. An even distribution throughout the gland is seen in recurrent parotitis and autoimmune disorders. If connected to the ductal system, abscess cavities may fill with contrast media during sialography. Abscess cavities appear on MDCT images as walled-off areas of lower attenuation within an enlarged gland. US may distinguish between diffuse inflammation (echo-free, high signal, light image) and suppuration (less echo-free, low signal, darker image) and detect sialoliths greater than 2 mm in diameter. Examination by US may also demonstrate abscess cavities, if present, and may be the study of choice for recurrent parotitis, especially in children. Contrast-enhanced MDCT imaging may demonstrate glandular enlargement (Fig. 29-16). However, MRI is an appropriate alternative examination in cases in which sialography is contraindicated or not technically possible. On MRI, inflamed glands are usually enlarged and demonstrate a lower tissue signal on T1-weighted images and a higher signal on T2-weighted images compared with the surrounding muscle. Advanced sialadenitis may occur in combination with sialolithiasis, sialodochitis, abscess formation, and fistulas.

Treatment.   Treatment of bacterial sialadenitis typically begins conservatively with attention to oral hygiene, local massage, increased fluid intake, and the use of oral sialagogues (sour citrus fruit wedges or salivary stimulants). An appropriate antibiotic regimen may also be indicated. If symptoms continue, surgical remedies ranging from partial to total excision of the gland may be considered.

Sialodochitis

Synonym.   A synonym for sialodochitis is ductal sialadenitis.

Disease Mechanism.   Sialodochitis is an inflammation of the ductal system of the salivary glands. The result is dilation of the involved ductal system; in chronic cases, interstitial fibrosis may also develop causing constriction of a small segment of the dilated duct. It is common in both the submandibular and the parotid glands.

Imaging Features.   Sialectasia or dilation of the ductal system is a prominent manifestation of sialodochitis on sialography (see Fig. 29-15). If interstitial fibrosis develops, it is apparent on sialography as a "sausage-string" appearance of the main duct and its major branches produced by alternating strictures and dilations. More recently, these changes have been seen with the use of thin section MRI. Scintigraphy and MDCT imaging are not typically indicated in the diagnosis of inflammatory ductal diseases of the salivary glands. They are costly and nonspecific and typically do not provide any more useful information than sialography does.

Treatment.   The management of sialodochitis is similar to that described for sialadenitis.

Autoimmune Sialadenitis

Synonyms.   Synonyms for autoimmune sialadenitis include myoepithelial sialadenitis, Sjögren's syndrome, benign lymphoepithelial lesion, Mikulicz's disease, sicca syndrome, dacryosialoadenopathia atrophicans, and autoimmune sialosis.

Disease Mechanism.   Autoimmune sialadenitis represents a group of disorders that affect the salivary glands and share an autosensitivity. The range of clinical and histopathologic manifestations suggests that these disorders represent different developmental stages of the same immunologic mechanisms, differing only in the

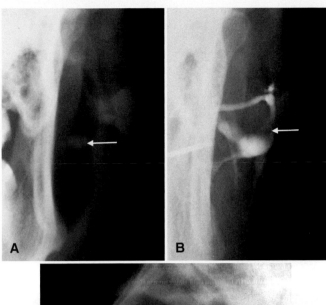
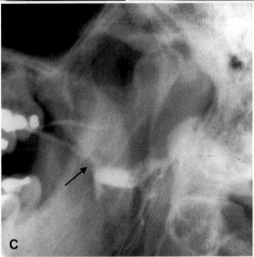

FIGURE 29-14 **A,** Cropped view of a posteroanterior skull view as part of a parotid investigation; the cheek has been puffed out, providing air contrast and revealing a poorly calcified sialolith (arrow). **B,** Cropped view of a posteroanterior skull view of the sialogram of the same patient with the negative filling defect representing the sialolith (arrow) seen in **A. C,** Lateral view of the same patient revealing the filling defect (arrow) and abnormal dilation of the proximal ducts.

salivary secretion are most commonly affected. Untreated acute suppurative infections typically form abscesses. The diagnosis is based on clinical observation, systemic symptoms, and the expression of pus from the duct.

In chronic cases, pus may be expressed from the ductal orifice and salivary stimulation may cause pain during periods of painful swelling. This condition is episodic in nature, and signs of generalized sepsis are seldom present. The obstruction may be congenital or caused by sialolithiasis, trauma, infection, or neoplasia. Typical clinical symptoms include intermittent swelling, pain when eating, and superimposed infection resulting from salivary stasis.

Imaging Features.   Sialography is contraindicated in acute infections because disrupted ductal epithelium may allow extravasation of contrast agent, resulting in a foreign body reaction and severe pain. However, this technique is appropriate for use in cases of suspected chronic infections. Epithelial flattening may lead to mildly dilated terminal ducts and saclike acini, which is demonstrable with sialography. The saclike acinar areas are referred to as

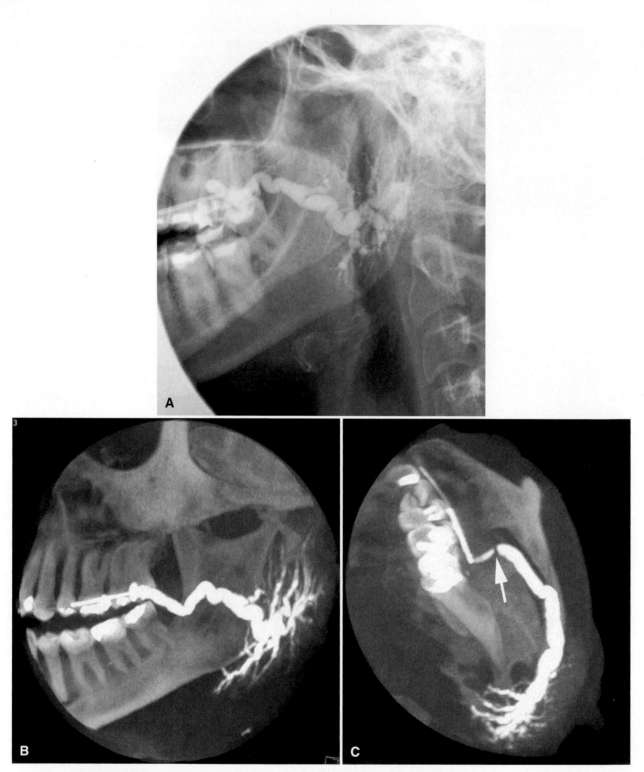

FIGURE 29-15 Conventional sialography of the parotid recorded as a plain lateral projection **(A)** and on CBCT imaging as lateral **(B)** and axial **(C)** renditions. A negative (radiolucent) filling defect *(arrow)* in the proximal portion of Stensen's duct **(C)** is not depicted in the lateral plain projection; the defect suggests a minimally calcified sialolith. Prominent intermittent strictures and dilation of the main and secondary ducts are typical of advanced sialodochitis. *(Courtesy Dr. Fatima Jadu.)*

extent and intensity of tissue reaction. Different forms may share a common etiology.

Clinical Features. Clinical manifestations range from recurrent painless swelling of the salivary glands (usually the parotid gland) to a stage that includes enlargement of the lacrimal glands. Glandular swelling may be accompanied by xerostomia and exophthalmia (primary Sjögren's syndrome) and subsequently by connective tissue disease, such as rheumatoid arthritis, progressive systemic sclerosis, systemic lupus erythematosus, or polymyositis (secondary Sjögren's syndrome). The process may progress to benign lymphoepithelial lesions that can assume the proportions of a tumor. A presumptive diagnosis can be made on the basis of any two of the following three features: (1) dry mouth, (2) dry eyes, and (3) rheumatoid disease. The disease is most common in adults primarily in the 40 to 60 year age range, and there is a 90% to 95%

female prevalence. The childhood form is only one tenth as common as the adult form, and there is much less chance of advanced parotid disease. Studies have shown a 44 times greater risk for development of non-Hodgkin's lymphoma compared with control subjects. Mikulicz's disease has been included within the diagnosis of primary Sjögren's syndrome but represents a unique condition consisting of enlargement of the lacrimal and salivary glands and characterized by few autoimmune reactions.

Imaging Features.   Sialography is helpful in the diagnosis and staging of autoimmune disorders. In the early stages of disease, sialography demonstrates the initiation of punctate (<1 mm) and globular (1 to 2 mm) spherical collections of contrast agent evenly distributed throughout the glands. These collections are referred to as sialectases (Fig. 29-17). At this stage, the main duct may appear normal, but the intraglandular ducts may be narrowed or not evident. Sialectasia typically remains after the administration of a sialagogue, which is an indication that contrast agent is pooled extraductally.

As the disease progresses, the collections of contrast agent increase in size (>2 mm in diameter) and are irregular in shape. These pools of contrast agent are termed *cavitary sialectases*. These larger sialectases are fewer in number and less uniformly distributed throughout the glands than punctate or globular sialectases (Fig. 29-18). Progressively larger cavities of contrast agent and dilation of the main ductal system may also be present. At the end stage of this disorder, complete destruction of the gland occurs. Cavitation and glandular fibrosis are the result of recurrent inflammation. The differential diagnosis for this appearance includes chronic bacterial or granulomatous infections and multiple parotid cysts associated with human immunodeficiency virus (HIV) infection. However, diffuse cervical lymphadenopathy is common in HIV disease and uncommon in Sjögren's syndrome. Thin section MRI has been shown to be reliable in depicting sialodochitis and sialectasia, especially when globular changes are present (Fig. 29-19).

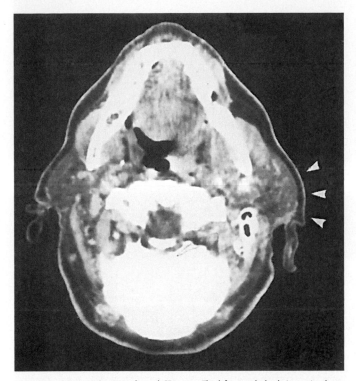

FIGURE 29-16 Contrast-enhanced CT image. The left parotid gland *(arrows)* is larger than the right, with no suggestion of abscess formation. This appearance is consistent with diffuse parotitis and cellulitis. *(Courtesy Department of Radiology, Baylor University Medical Center, Dallas, TX.)*

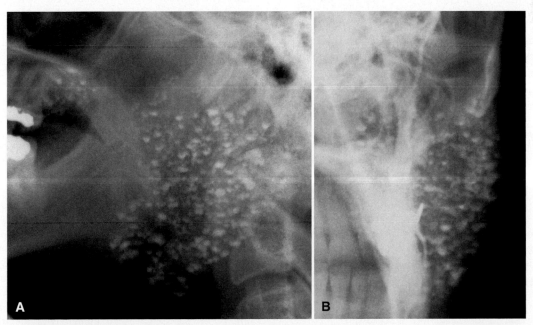

FIGURE 29-17 Conventional sialography of left parotid. **A,** Lateral projection demonstrates punctate sialectases distributed throughout the gland, which is suggestive of autoimmune sialadenitis. Clinical and histopathologic diagnosis was Sjögren's syndrome. **B,** Anteroposterior projection of the same gland.

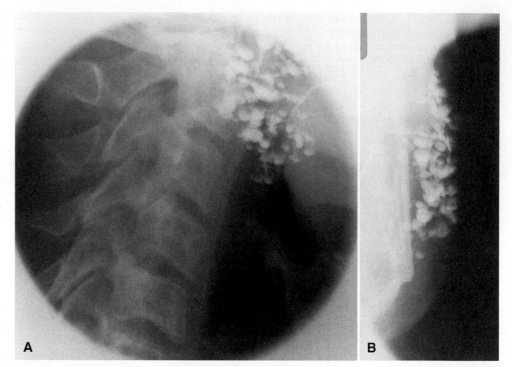

FIGURE 29-18 Sialography of the left parotid. Punctate (small spherical), globular (larger spherical), and cavitary (larger, irregular) sialectases with some dilation of the main duct are suggestive of advanced autoimmune disease with parenchymal destruction with retrograde infection in lateral **(A)** and anteroposterior **(B)** projections. Clinical and histopathologic diagnosis was Sjögren's syndrome.

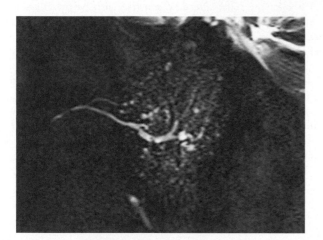

FIGURE 29-19 T2-weighted MRI enhances structures high in water content. Note the multiple punctate sialectases of the parotid gland in this case of Sjögren's syndrome. *(Courtesy Dr. Alan G. Lurie, Farmington, CT.)*

Treatment. The management of autoimmune disorders of the salivary glands is directed toward relief of symptoms. Underlying systemic rheumatoid conditions are typically treated with antiinflammatory agents, corticosteroids, and immunosuppressive therapeutic agents. Salivary stimulants, increased fluid intake, and artificial saliva and tears are symptomatic treatment regimens for the eyes and mouth. More advanced inflammatory changes may be treated surgically by local incision or total excision of the symptomatic gland.

NONINFLAMMATORY DISORDERS

Sialadenosis

Synonym. A synonym for sialadenosis is sialosis.

Disease Mechanism. Sialadenosis is a nonneoplastic, noninflammatory enlargement of primarily the parotid salivary glands. It is usually related to metabolic and secretory disorders of the parenchyma associated with diseases of nearly all the endocrine glands (hormonal sialadenoses), protein deficiencies, malnutrition in alcoholics (dystrophic-metabolic sialadenoses), vitamin deficiencies, and neurologic disorders (neurogenic sialadenoses).

Clinical Features. Affected glands are typically enlarged.

Imaging Features. Sialography may demonstrate enlargement of the affected glands or a normal appearance. In enlarged glands, the ducts are splayed. MDCT imaging and MRI provide a more straightforward depiction of the glands but are nonspecific and require correlation with the clinical findings and history.

Treatment. The management of sialadenosis hinges on identifying the cause of the metabolic or secretory disorder. Conservative treatment, including local massage, increased fluid intake, and the use of oral sialagogues (sour citrus fruit wedges or salivary stimulants), is appropriate.

Cystic Lesions

Disease Mechanism. Cysts of the salivary glands are rare (<5% of all salivary gland masses) and most commonly occur unilaterally in the parotid gland (see Fig. 29-10). They may be congenital (branchial), lymphoepithelial, dermoid, or acquired, including mucous retention cysts (obstructions from any etiology). Cystic salivary lesions may be intraglandular or extraglandular in nature and may progress to such proportions that they are clinically palpable and must be distinguished from neoplasia. Cystic neoplasms are discussed separately in this chapter. Mucous extravasation pseudocysts lack an epithelial lining and result from ductal rupture. Ranulas are retention cysts that usually occur as a result of obstruction of the sublingual duct. Benign lymphoepithelial cysts are thought to be sequelae of cystic degeneration of salivary inclusions within lymph nodes. Multicentric parotid cysts associated with HIV have been reported and are termed benign lymphoepithelial lesions of human immunodeficiency syndrome. These lesions are accompanied by cervical lymphadenopathy, occur bilaterally, and are usually in the superficial portion of the parotid gland (Fig. 29-20). Secondary parotitis may develop.

Imaging Features.   Cystic masses may be indirectly visualized on sialography only by the displacement of the ducts arching around them. Cystic lesions typically appear as well-circumscribed, non-enhancing (when imaged with contrast agent administration), low-density areas on MDCT imaging. Cysts appear as well-circumscribed, high signal areas on T2-weighted MRI, but they do not enhance after administration of gadolinium contrast agent, as do benign mixed tumors. When imaged with US, cysts are sharply marginated and echo-free (represented as a dark area) (Fig. 29-21).

Treatment.   Management of cystic lesions is typically surgical, involving local or total excision of the gland.

Benign Tumors

Disease Mechanism.   Salivary gland tumors are uncommon, occurring in less than 0.003% of the population. They account for about 3% of all tumors. Approximately 80% of salivary tumors arise in the parotid gland, 5% arise in the submandibular gland, 1% arise in the sublingual gland, and 10% to 15% arise in the minor salivary glands. Most (70% to 80%) of these tumors occur in the superficial lobe of the parotid gland. Most are benign or low-grade malignancies. High-grade malignancies are uncommon. The chance of neoplasms of major salivary glands being benign varies directly with the size of the gland.

Imaging Features.   Benign tumors and low-grade malignancies may have a similar appearance, with well-defined margins, which are most apparent on MDCT or MRI examinations. Because of the greater density of the submandibular gland, which can equal that of the neoplasm and obscure the tumor, intravenous contrast enhancement is required during the MDCT examination. Contrast enhancement causes the tumor to appear more radiopaque because

the vascularity of the tumor is greater than that of the adjacent salivary gland tissue. MRI is a preferential modality for salivary gland neoplasia, especially for the submandibular gland, because of its superior soft tissue contrast resolution. On US, benign masses are typically less echogenic than parenchyma, sharply defined, and of essentially homogeneous echo strength and density. Benign tumors may present as low-intensity (dark) or high-intensity (light) tissue signals on MRI, although the relative intensity of the signal may indicate the presence of lipid, vascular, or fibrous tissues. Sialography may suggest a space-occupying mass when the ducts are compressed or smoothly displaced around the lesion (the "ball-in-hand" appearance) (Fig. 29-22).

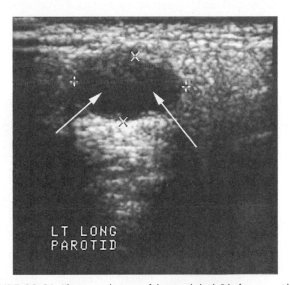

FIGURE 29-21 Ultrasonography image of the parotid gland. Echo-free mass with well-defined margins presents a typical cystic appearance *(arrows)*. *(Courtesy Department of Radiology, Baylor University Medical Center, Dallas, TX.)*

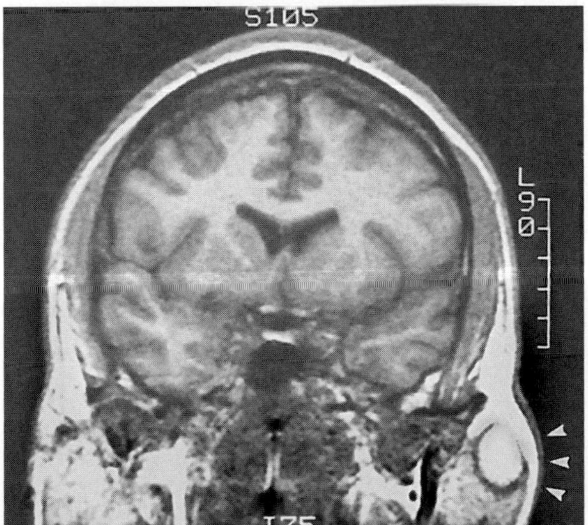

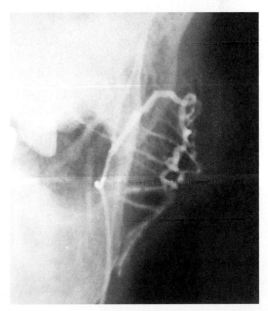

FIGURE 29-20 Coronal section MRI. The high signal mass *(arrows)* in the left parotid gland was diagnosed as a cyst. This patient was found to be HIV positive. *(Courtesy Department of Radiology, Baylor University Medical Center, Dallas, TX.)*

FIGURE 29-22 Sialogram of left parotid (anteroposterior view). A mass within the gland is inferred by the appearance of the ducts displaced around the lesion. This is referred to as the "ball-in-hand" appearance, which is suggestive of a space-occupying mass. *(Courtesy Department of Radiology, Baylor University Medical Center, Dallas, TX.)*

Treatment.   The management of benign tumors of the major salivary glands is typically surgical. Benign tumors of the parotid gland may be either partially incised or totally excised. Submandibular and sublingual glands are invariably totally excised.

Pleomorphic Adenoma

Synonym.   A synonym for pleomorphic adenoma is benign mixed tumor.

Disease Mechanism.   A pleomorphic adenoma is a neoplasm arising from the ductal epithelium of major and minor salivary glands exhibiting epithelial and mesenchymal components.

Clinical Features.   Pleomorphic adenoma accounts for 75% of all salivary gland tumors; 80% are found in the parotid gland, 4% are found in the submandibular gland, 1% are found in the sublingual gland, and 10% are found in the minor salivary glands. This tumor typically occurs in the fifth decade of life as a slow-growing, unilateral, encapsulated, asymptomatic mass. A slight female predilection exists. Recurrence occurs in 50% of cases after excision. Malignant transformation is reported in 15% of untreated cases.

Imaging Features.   On MDCT imaging, benign mixed tumor is a sharply circumscribed, infrequently lobulated, and essentially round homogeneous lesion that has a higher density than the adjacent glandular tissue (Fig. 29-23, *A*). Calcifications within the tumor are commonly seen and are well depicted on MDCT. This tumor has various tissue signals in different MRI techniques, such as relatively low (dark) in T1-weighted images, intermediate on proton density–weighted images, and homogeneous high intensity (bright) on T2-weighted images (see Fig. 29-23, *C*). Foci of low signal intensity (dark areas) usually represent areas of fibrosis or dystrophic calcifications. If a calcification is present (signal void),

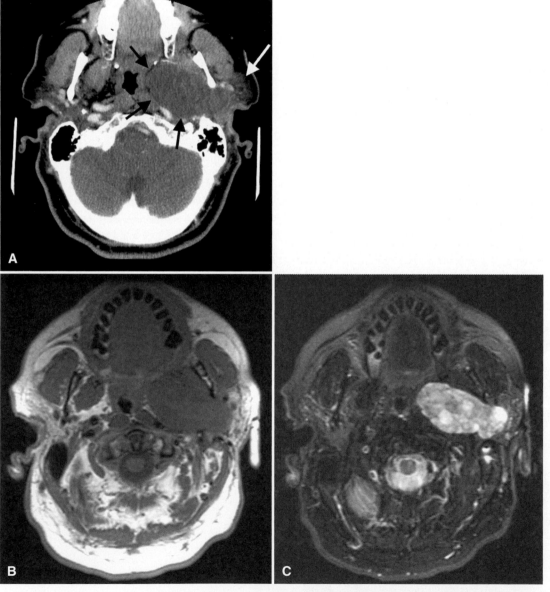

FIGURE 29-23 CT and MRI of a pleomorphic adenoma. **A,** Axial CT soft tissue algorithm image. Note the well-defined periphery *(black arrows)* and the internal density that is less than surrounding muscles. The remaining parotid gland *(white arrow)* is displaced laterally. **B,** T1-weighted MR image. The tissue signal of the tumor is isointense with muscle. **C,** T2-weighted image. Note the increased signal of the tumor, which is now hyperintense to muscle.

the diagnosis favors a benign mixed tumor; otherwise, it is difficult to differentiate this tumor from other parotid masses.

Benign mixed tumor does not usually concentrate ^{99m}Tc-pertechnetate, and the tumor appears as a cold spot when examined by scintigraphy. Solid tumors larger than 5 mm are usually well visualized. There is a rare malignant form of this tumor, called malignant mixed tumor or carcinoma ex pleomorphic adenoma.

Warthin's Tumor

Synonyms.   Synonyms for Warthin's tumor include papillary cystadenoma lymphomatosum, adenolymphoma, and lymphomatous adenoma.

Disease Mechanism.   Warthin's tumor is a benign tumor arising from proliferating salivary ducts trapped in lymph nodes during embryogenesis of the salivary glands.

Clinical Features.   Warthin's tumor is the second most common benign neoplasm of the salivary glands, accounting for 2% to 6% of parotid tumors. In the parotid, it is usually found in the inferior lobe of the gland. This unusual type of tumor is a slow-growing, painless, round-to-ovoid mass. The tumors are multiple in 20% of cases. Warthin's tumor typically affects men older than 40 years and may be unilateral or bilateral (Fig. 29-24).

Imaging Features.   MDCT imaging and MR imaging are the preferred techniques for imaging Warthin's tumor. The imaging appearance of this tumor is not specific and is typical of benign salivary tumors as described for benign mixed tumor. On MDCT imaging, this tumor may be of either soft tissue or cystic density. On MR imaging, it is heterogeneous and may demonstrate hemorrhagic foci. Warthin's tumor is characteristically intensely hot (high signal) on ^{99m}Tc-pertechnetate scans. Oncocytoma (oxyphilic adenoma) may also accumulate ^{99m}Tc-pertechnetate, but this tumor is uncommon and more likely to be bilateral (see Fig. 29-11). However, oncocytoma has been reported to be present in essentially everyone older than 70 years. US shows Warthin's tumor as a solid mass (anechoic), unless the mass is cystic, as some are (see Fig. 29-12).

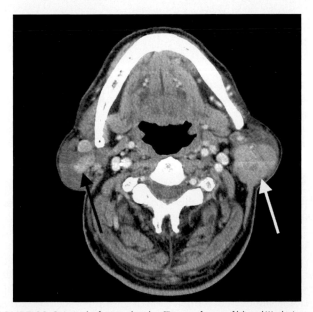

FIGURE 29-24 Axial soft tissue algorithm CT image of a case of bilateral Warthin's tumor, a large tumor involving the left parotid *(white arrow)* and a much smaller tumor on the right side *(black arrow)*.

Hemangioma

Synonym.   A synonym for hemangioma is vascular nevus.

Disease Mechanism.   Hemangioma is a benign neoplasm of proliferating endothelial cells (congenital hemangioma) and vascular malformations, including lesions resulting from abnormal vessel morphogenesis.

Clinical Features.   Hemangioma is the most frequently occurring nonepithelial salivary neoplasm, accounting for 50% of the cases. Of hemangiomas, 85% arise in the parotid gland. It is the most common salivary gland tumor during infancy and childhood. The average age at diagnosis is 10 years, with 65% occurring in the first 2 decades of life. They are frequently unilateral and asymptomatic. A 2:1 female-to-male predilection exists. Treatment is by local excision for patients who do not undergo spontaneous remission.

Imaging Features.   Phleboliths, discrete soft tissue calcifications associated with vascular lesions, are a common feature of this tumor (see Chapter 28) and are best identified on projection or plain images and MDCT images. When this tumor occurs in association with a salivary gland, the ducts of the gland may be displaced curving about the mass, which may be apparent on sialography. MDCT imaging shows hemangioma as a soft tissue mass that is well distinguished from surrounding tissue, especially when intravenous contrast enhancement is used. On MRI, the tumor has a signal similar to that of adjacent muscle on T1-weighted images and a very high signal on T2-weighted images. Although US usually demonstrates well-defined margins in hemangioma, ill-defined margins may also be noted. Strongly hypoechoic hemangioma may have a complex appearance on US resulting from the multiple interfaces in the lesion. Phleboliths are seen on imaging as multiple hyperechoic areas within the body of the gland itself.

Malignant Tumors

Disease Mechanisms.   About 20% of tumors in the parotid are malignant compared with 50% to 60% of submandibular tumors, 90% of sublingual tumors, and 60% to 75% of minor salivary gland tumors.

Imaging Features.   The imaging presentation of malignant tumors is variable and is related to the grade, aggressiveness, location, and type of tumor. In many cases, it is impossible to determine whether a tumor is malignant or benign (Fig. 29-25). However, features such as ill-defined margins (Fig. 29-26), invasion of adjacent soft tissues (e.g., fat spaces), and destruction of adjacent osseous structures are considered to be typical indicators of malignancy.

Treatment.   Management of malignant tumors of the major salivary glands is typically surgical. Low-grade malignant tumors of the parotid gland may be either partially incised or totally excised. Submandibular and sublingual glands are invariably totally excised. High-grade tumors may require radical neck dissection. Combinations of surgery, therapeutic radiation, and chemotherapy may also be used.

Mucoepidermoid Carcinoma

Disease Mechanism.   Mucoepidermoid carcinoma is a malignant tumor composed of a variable admixture of epidermoid and mucous cells arising from the ductal epithelium of the salivary glands.

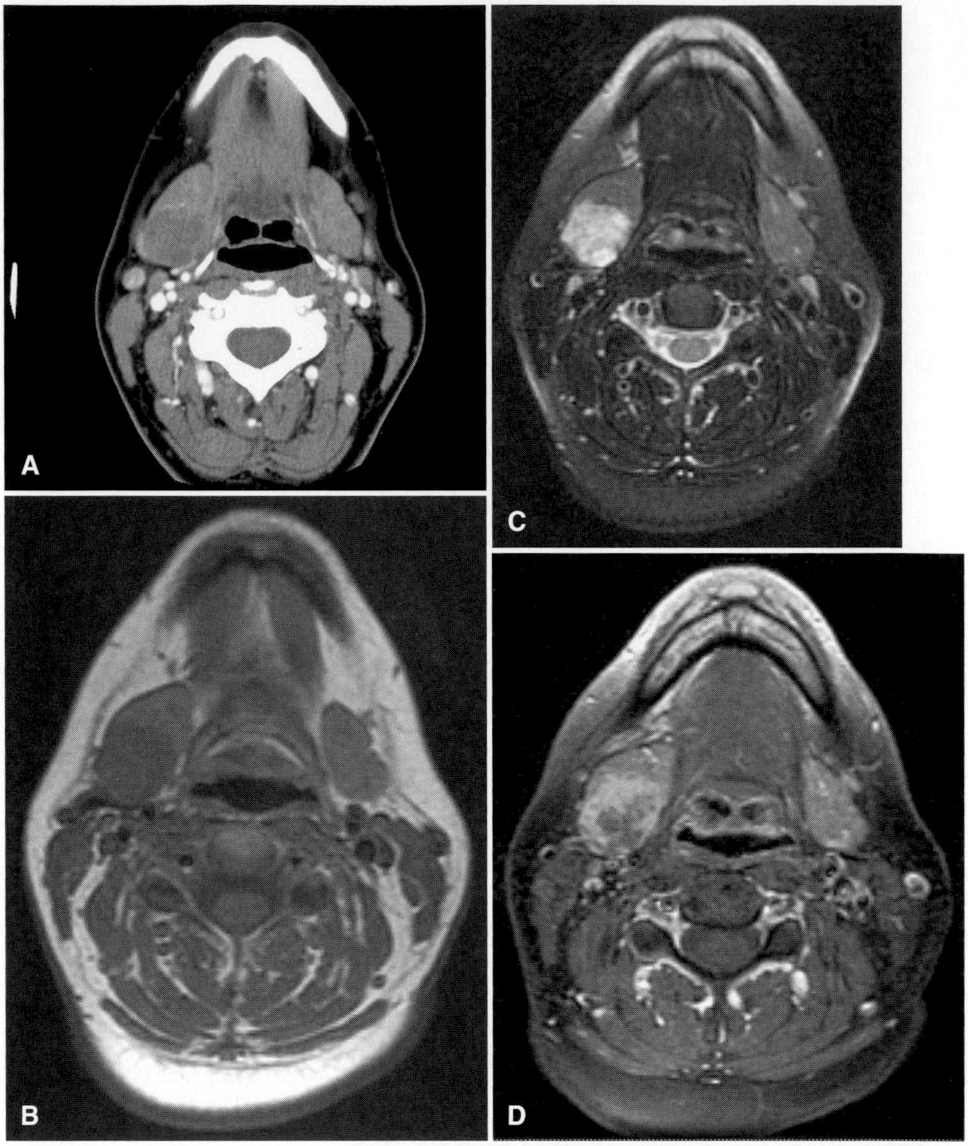

FIGURE 29-25 Four axial CT and MRI depict an adenoid cystic carcinoma of the right submandibular gland. Note the well-defined periphery, making it difficult to differentiate from a benign tumor. **A,** The internal density of the tumor in this soft tissue algorithm CT image is almost equal to the remaining gland. **B,** The tissue signal in this T1-weighted MR image is slightly less than the remaining gland. **C,** In a T2-weighted MR image, the high signal of the tumor contrasts with the remaining gland. **D,** In a T1-weighted postgadolinium, fat saturation image, the tumor has a higher signal than in the remaining gland.

Clinical Features. Mucoepidermoid carcinoma is the most common malignant salivary gland tumor (35%). Slightly more than half occur in the major salivary glands, most commonly the parotid gland; the rest are found in the minor glands, with the palate being the most frequent location. The aggressiveness of the lesion varies with its histologic grade. A wide age range exists, with the highest prevalence in the fifth decade of life. A slight predilection for females exists. The low-grade variety rarely metastasizes. Clinically, this tumor appears as a movable, slowly growing, painless nodule similar to a benign mixed tumor. It is usually only 1 to 4 cm in diameter. The prognosis is good; the 5-year survival rate is greater than 95%.

In contrast to low-grade mucoepidermoid carcinomas, high-grade tumors often cause facial pain and paralysis, have ill-defined margins, and are relatively immobile. Metastasis by blood and lymph are common, with recurrence in half of patients after excision. The prognosis is poor and varies with the histologic grade; the 5-year survival rate may be 25% in some cases.

Imaging Features. Low-grade mucoepidermoid carcinomas are typically not apparent on projection or plain images unless destructive changes to adjacent osseous structures have occurred. Presentations of this tumor on sialography, MDCT imaging, MR imaging, US, and scintigraphy are similar to presentations previously described for benign salivary tumors. However, low-grade mucoepidermoid carcinoma may have a lobulated or irregularly sharply circumscribed appearance on contrast-enhanced MDCT imaging or MRI (Fig. 29-27). Cystic areas may present, and calcifications rarely may be seen.

The imaging diagnosis of high-grade mucoepidermoid carcinoma typically relies on the appearance of irregular margins and ill-defined form when the mass is examined with MDCT imaging or MRI. On MDCT images, the tumor manifests as an irregular homogeneous mass, slightly more dense than the glandular parenchyma. If intravenous contrast agent is added to the MDCT study, the result is a sharply defined homogeneous mass that is considerably more opaque. MDCT imaging and CBCT imaging are also reliable techniques for the detection of invasion of adjacent osseous structures.

In contrast to low-grade malignancies and benign neoplasms, high-grade mucoepidermoid carcinoma, similar to most high-grade

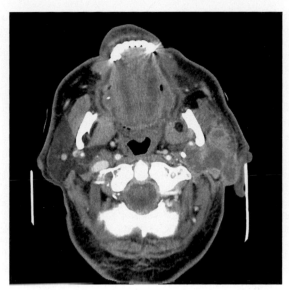

FIGURE 29-26 Axial soft tissue algorithm CT image reveals an adenocarcinoma of the left parotid gland. Almost all of the gland has been replaced by this ill-defined tumor that has some peripheral enhancement and lower density internal structure, likely representing necrotic regions.

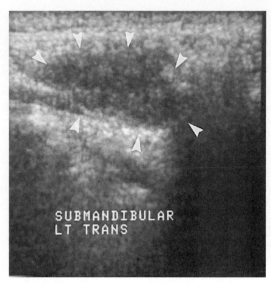

FIGURE 29-28 Ultrasonography demonstrates a mass in the submandibular gland *(arrowheads)* that has a heterogeneous hypoechoic pattern compared with the adjacent tissue. The histopathologic diagnosis was adenoid cystic carcinoma. *(Courtesy Department of Radiology, Baylor University Medical Center, Dallas, TX.)*

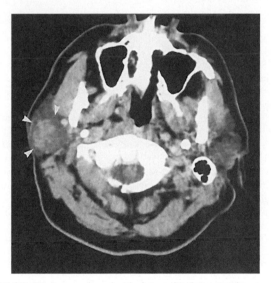

FIGURE 29-27 Contrast-enhanced axial soft tissue algorithm computed tomographic (CT) image demonstrates a mass in the right parotid gland with a poorly marginated, heterogeneous, slightly lobulated appearance *(white arrowheads)*. Poorly defined margins suggest a low-grade malignancy rather than a benign tumor, although the CT appearance of both is similar. The histopathologic diagnosis was low-grade mucoepidermoid carcinoma. *(Courtesy Department of Radiology, Baylor University Medical Center, Dallas, TX.)*

malignancies, has homogeneous low signal intensity (dark) on T1-weighted images, but T2-weighted images are more heterogeneous and intense (brighter) than T1-weighted images, although still slightly darker (low signal) relative to the surrounding tissues in MRI. Regardless of clinical presentation and margins, low signal intensity is suggestive of a high-grade malignancy. Cavitary sialectasia and ductal displacement may be noted on sialography of this tumor.

Other Malignant and Metastatic Tumors.   Although the incidence of other malignant tumors of the major salivary glands is low,

a significant variety exists in their histogenesis. Of all malignant salivary gland tumors, 23% are adenoid cystic carcinomas; however, most of these neoplasms develop in the minor salivary glands.

Adenocarcinoma accounts for only 6.4% of all salivary gland malignancies, with acinic cell carcinoma, primary lymphoma, and squamous cell carcinoma occurring with even less frequency. Pain, paresthesia, and paralysis may be present, especially in high-grade tumors. The pain associated with acinic cell carcinoma is not considered to be as grave a sign as in other malignant salivary tumors. Tumor spread may be by direct invasion or metastasis. Adenoid cystic carcinoma also spreads along nerve sheaths and is best demonstrated on postcontrast MRI where nerve enhancement and enlargement are present. Metastasis of tumors of the salivary glands is not unusual. Metastatic lesions in the parotid gland are more common than in the other salivary glands because of the extensive lymphatic and circulatory components of the parotid gland. Most metastatic lesions of the parotid gland occur through the lymphatic system and include squamous cell carcinoma, lymphoma, and melanoma. Although considerably fewer lesions are the result of hematogenous dissemination, metastasis from the lung, breast, kidney, and gastrointestinal tract has been reported.

Imaging Features.   The presentation of these tumors is nonspecific and similar to high-grade mucoepidermoid carcinoma previously described. US may demonstrate echo-free cystic areas in adenoid cystic carcinomas (Fig. 29-28).

BIBLIOGRAPHY

Del Balso AM, Ellis GE, Hartman KS, et al: Diagnostic imaging of the salivary glands and periglandular regions. In Del Balso AM, editor: *Maxillofacial imaging*, Philadelphia, 1990, Saunders.

Freling NJM: Imaging of salivary gland disease, *Semin Roentgenol* 35:12–20, 2000.

Harnsberger HR, Hudgins PA, Wiggins RW III, et al: *Pocket radiologist, head and neck 100 top diagnoses*, Salt Lake City, 2002, Amirsys.

Harnsberger HR, Hudgins R, Wiggins P, et al: *Diagnostic imaging head and neck*, Salt Lake City, 2004, Amirsys.

Koenig LJ, Tamimi D, Harnsberger HR, et al: *Diagnostic imaging—oral and maxillofacial*, Salt Lake City, 2012, Amirsys.

Lufkin RB, Hanafee WN: *MRI of the head and neck*, New York, 1992, Raven Press.

Rabinov K, Weber AL: *Radiology of the salivary glands*, Boston, 1985, GK Hall Medical Publishers.

Rice DH, Becker TS: The salivary glands. In Hanafee WN, Ward PH, editors: *Clinical correlations in the head and neck*, vol 2, New York, 1994, Thieme Medical Publishers.

Seifert G, Miehlke A, Hanbrich J, et al: *Diseases of the salivary glands*, Stuttgart, Germany, 1986, George Thieme Verlag.

Van den Akker HP: Diagnostic imaging in salivary gland disease, *Oral Surg* 66:625–637, 1988.

Watson MG: Investigation of salivary gland disease, *Ear Nose Throat J* 68:84, 87–93, 1989.

Projection Radiography

Ollerenshaw R, Ross SS: Radiological diagnosis of salivary gland disease, *Br J Radiol* 24:538–548, 1951.

Silvers AR, Som PM: Salivary glands, *Radiol Clin North Am* 36:941–966, 1998.

Weissmari JL: Imaging of the salivary glands, *Semin Ultrasound CT MR* 16:546–568, 1995.

Yousem DM, Kraut MA, Chalian AA: Major salivary gland imaging, *Radiology* 216:19–29, 2000.

Conventional Sialography

Eisenbud L, Cranin N: The role of sialography in the diagnosis and therapy of chronic obstructive sialadenitis, *Oral Surg Oral Med Oral Pathol* 16:1181–1199, 1963.

Jadu FM, Yaffe MJ, Lam EW: A comparative study of the effective doses from cone beam computed tomography and plain radiography for sialography, *Dentomaxillofac Radiol* 39:257–263, 2010.

Kalinowski M, Heverhagen T, Rehberg E, et al: Comparative study of MR sialography and digital subtraction sialography for benign salivary gland disorders. *AJNR Am J Neuroradiol* 23:1485–1492, 2002.

Kalk WW, Vissink A, Spijkervet HK, et al: Parotid sialography for diagnosing Sjögren syndrome, *Oral Surg Oral Med Oral Pathol Oral Radiol Endod* 94:131–137, 2002.

Li B, Long X, Cheng Y, et al: Cone beam CT sialography of Stafne bone cavity. *Dentomaxillofac Radiol* 40:519–523, 2011.

Manashil GB: *Clinical sialography*, Springfield, 1978, Charles C Thomas.

Ozdemir D, Polat NT, Polat S: Lipiodol UF retention in dental sialography, *Br J Radiol* 77:1040–1041, 2004.

Varghese JC, Thornton F, Lucey BC, et al: A prospective comparative study of MR sialography and conventional sialography of salivary duct disease, *AJR Am J Roentgenol* 173:1497–1503, 1999.

Whaley K, Blair S, Low PS, et al: Sialographic abnormalities in Sjögren's syndrome, rheumatoid arthritis, and other arthritides and connective tissue diseases: a clinical and radiological investigation using hydrostatic sialography, *Clin Radiol* 23:474–482, 1972.

Cone-Beam Computed Tomographic Imaging of the Major Salivary Glands

Dreiseidler T, Ritter L, Rothamel D, et al: Salivary calculus diagnosis with 3-dimensional cone-beam computed tomography, *Oral Surg Oral Med Oral Pathol Oral Radiol Endod* 110:94–100, 2010.

Multidetector Computed Tomographic Imaging of the Major Salivary Glands

Bryan RN, Miller RH, Ferreyro RI, et al: Computed tomography of the major salivary glands, *AJR Am J Roentgenol* 139:547–554, 1982.

Casselman JW, Mancuso AA: Major salivary gland masses: comparison of MR imaging and CT, *Radiology* 165:183–189, 1987.

Choi DS, Na DG, Byn HS, et al: Salivary gland tumors: evaluation with two-phase helical CT. *Radiology* 214:231–236, 2000.

Kosaka M, Kamiishi H: New strategy for the diagnosis of parotid gland lesions utilizing three-dimensional sialography, *Comput Aided Surg* 5:42–45, 2000.

Lloyd RE, Ho KH: Combined CT scanning and sialography in the management of parotid tumors, *Oral Surg Oral Med Oral Pathol* 65:142–144, 1988.

Magnetic Resonance Imaging of the Major Salivary Glands

Browne RFJ, Golding SJ, Watt-Smith SR: The role of MRI in facial swelling due to presumed salivary gland disease, *Br J Radiol* 74:127–133, 2001.

Jäger L, Menauer F, Holzknecht N, et al: MR sialography of the submandibular duct—an alternative to conventional sialography and US? *Radiology* 216:665–671, 2000.

Jungehulsing M, Fischbach R, Schroder U, et al: Magnetic resonance sialography, *Otolaryngol Head Neck Surg* 121:488–494, 1999.

Kaneda T, Minami M, Ozawa K, et al: MR of the submandibular gland: normal and pathologic states, *AJNR Am J Neuroradiol* 17:1575–1581, 1996.

Mandelblatt S, Braun IF, Davis PC, et al: Parotid masses: MR imaging, *Radiology* 163:411–414, 1987.

Som PM, Biller HF: High-grade malignancies of the parotid gland: identification with MR imaging, *Radiology* 173:823–826, 1989.

Swartz JD, Rothman MI, Marlowe FI, et al: MR imaging of parotid mass lesions: attempts at histopathologic differentiation, *J Comput Assist Tomogr* 13:789–796, 1989.

Scintigraphy (Nuclear Medicine) of the Major Salivary Glands

Chaudhuri TK, Stadalnik RC: Salivary gland imaging, *Semin Nucl Med* 10:400–401, 1980.

Garcia RR: Differential diagnosis of tumors of the salivary glands with radioactive isotopes, *Int J Oral Surg* 3:330–334, 1974.

Greyson ND, Noyek AM: Radionuclide salivary scanning, *J Otolaryngol Suppl* 10:1–47, 1982.

Keyes JW Jr, Harkness BA, Greven KM, et al: Salivary gland tumors: pretherapy evaluation with PET, *Radiology* 192:99–102, 1994.

Mishkin FS: Radionuclide salivary gland imaging, *Semin Nucl Med* 11:258–265, 1981.

Tonami H, Higashi K, Matoba M, et al: A comparative study between MR sialography and salivary gland scintigraphy in the diagnosis of Sjögren syndrome. *J Comput Assist Tomogr* 25:262–268, 2001.

Van den Akker HP, Busemann-Sokole E: Absolute indications for salivary gland scintigraphy with ^{99m}Tc-pertechnetate, *Oral Surg* 60:440–447, 1985.

Ultrasonography of the Major Salivary Glands

El-Khateeb SM, Abou-Khalaf AE, Farid MM, et al: A prospective study of three diagnostic sonographic methods in differentiation between benign and malignant salivary gland tumours, *Dentomaxillofac Radiol* 40:476–485, 2011.

Gritzmann G: Sonography of the salivary glands, *AJR Am J Roentgenol* 153:161–166, 1989.

Howlett DC: High resolution ultrasound assessment of the parotid gland, *Br J Radiol* 76:271–277, 2003.

Mandel LK: Ultrasound findings in HIV-positive patients with parotid swellings, *J Oral Maxillofac Surg* 59:283–286, 2001.

Martinoli C, Derchi LE, Solbiati L, et al: Color Doppler sonography of salivary glands, *AJR Am J Roentgenol* 163:933–941, 1994.

Shimizu M, Ussmüller J, Donath K, et al: Sonographic analysis of recurrent parotitis in children: a comparative study with sialographic findings, *Oral Surg Oral Med Oral Pathol Oral Radiol Endod* 86:606–615, 1998.

Obstructive and Inflammatory Disorders

Aung W, Yamada I, Umehara I, et al: Sjögren's syndrome: comparison of assessments with quantitative salivary gland scintigraphy and contrast sialography, *J Nucl Med* 41:257–262, 2000.

Brook I: Acute bacterial suppurative parotitis: microbiology and management, *J Craniofac Surg* 14:37–40, 2003.

Hughes M, Carson K, Hill J: Scintigraphic evaluation of sialadenitis, *Br J Radiol* 67:328–331, 1994.

Kassan SS, Moutsopoulos HM: Clinical manifestations and early diagnosis of Sjögren syndrome, *Arch Intern Med* 164:1275–1284, 2004.

Lemon SI, Imbesi SG, Shikhman AR: Salivary gland imaging in Sjögren syndrome, *Future Rheumatol* 2:83–92, 2007.

Sobrino-Guijarro B, Cascarini L, Lingam RK: Advances in imaging obstructed salivary glands can improve diagnostic outcomes, *Oral Maxillofac Surg* 17:11–19, 2013.

Som PM, Shugar JM, Train JS, et al: Manifestations of parotid gland enlargement: radiographic, pathologic, and clinical correlation–part 1, the autoimmune pseudosialectasias, *Radiology* 141:415–419, 1981.

Tomita M, Ueda T, Nagata H, et al: Usefulness of magnetic resonance sialography in patients with juvenile Sjogren syndrome, *Clin Exp Rheumatol* 23:540–544, 2005.

Yamamoto Y, Harada S, Ohara M, et al: Clinical and pathological differences between Mikulicz's disease and Sjögren's syndrome, *Rheumatology (Oxford)* 44:227–234, 2005.

Noninflammatory Disorders

Chilla R: Sialadenosis of the salivary glands of the head: studies on the physiology and pathophysiology of parotid secretion, *Adv Otorhinolaryngol* 26:1–38, 1981.

Cysts and Neoplasms

Boahene DKO, Olsen KD, Lewis JE, et al: Mucoepidermoid carcinoma of the parotid gland–the Mayo Clinic experience, *Arch Otolaryngol Head Neck Surg* 130:849–856, 2004.

Boles R, Raines J, Lebovits M, et al: Malignant tumors of salivary glands: a university experience, *Laryngoscope* 90:729–736, 1980.

Byrne MN, Spector JG, Garvin CF, et al: Preoperative assessment of parotid masses: a comparative evaluation of radiographic techniques to histologic diagnosis, *Laryngoscope* 99:284–292, 1989.

Day TA, Deveikis J, Gillespie MB, et al: Salivary gland neoplasms, *Curr Treat Options Oncol* 5:11–26, 2004.

Del Balso AM, Williams E, Tane TT: Parotid masses: current modes of diagnostic imaging, *Oral Surg* 54:360–364, 1982.

Gottesman RI, Som PM, Mester J, et al: Observations on two cases of apparent submandibular gland cysts in HIV positive patients: MR and CT findings, *J Comput Assist Tomogr* 20:444–447, 1996.

Lee YYP, Wong KT, King AD, et al: Imaging of salivary gland tumours, *Eur J Radiol* 66:419–436, 2008.

Madani G, Beale T: Tumors of the salivary glands, *Semin Ultrasound CT MRI* 27:452–464, 2006.

Mirich DR, McArdle CB, Kulkarni MV: Benign pleomorphic adenomas of the salivary glands: surface coil MR imaging versus CT, *J Comput Assist Tomogr* 11:620–623, 1987.

Thawley SE, Panbje WR: *Comprehensive management of head and neck tumors*, Philadelphia, 1987, Saunders.

Thoeny HC: Imaging of salivary gland tumours, *Cancer Imaging* 7:52–62, 2007.

Tsai SC, Hsu HT: Parotid neoplasms: diagnosis, treatment, and intraparotid facial nerve anatomy, *J Laryngol Otol* 116:359–362, 2002.

Trauma

Ernest W. N. Lam

OUTLINE

Radiologic examination is essential for evaluating trauma to the teeth and jaws. The presence, location, and orientation of fracture planes and fragments can be determined, and the involvement of nearby vital anatomic structures can be assessed. Foreign objects that have become embedded within the soft tissues as a result of trauma can be detected. Follow-up images are useful in evaluating the extent of healing after an injury and long-term changes resulting from the trauma.

APPLIED RADIOLOGY

The ideal imaging study may be difficult to perform after trauma because of the nature of the injury and patient discomfort. Although the prescription of the appropriate images should be ordered only after a careful clinical examination, in some cases this is not always possible.

DENTOALVEOLAR FRACTURES

Although a panoramic image may be useful for localizing injuries to the teeth and supporting structures, it may not have the image resolution to reveal injuries involving the anterior mandible or maxillae or the teeth. Dentoalveolar trauma always requires intraoral images to obtain adequate anatomic detail. A minimum of two intraoral periapical images should be made at different horizontal x-ray beam angulations to identify tooth fractures. Additionally, it is important to image the teeth of the opposing arch. Occlusal views may also be particularly useful depending on the severity of the trauma and the ability of the patient to open the mouth. More recently, small field of view cone-beam computed tomographic (CBCT) imaging has been used to identify tooth fractures, although the results have been variable. The high resolution of the small field systems may be beneficial to imaging such fractures.

If a tooth or a large fragment of a tooth is missing, a chest or abdominal image may be considered to locate the tooth. If there are lacerations in the lips or cheek, a soft tissue image of the area may be obtained by placing an intraoral film or receptor in the mouth adjacent to the traumatized soft tissue and then exposing it. If the laceration is in the tongue, a standard mandibular occlusal image may be exposed, or the tongue can be protruded and then imaged.

MANDIBULAR FRACTURES

Panoramic imaging may be useful as an initial investigation for assessing mandibular fractures. Should a fracture be suspected to involve the body or alveolar process of the mandible, the addition of an intraoral cross-sectional occlusal view of the mandible may be useful, if this is possible. The open mouth Towne view may be useful in cases of suspected trauma to the mandibular condylar head and neck areas. This view may supplement panoramic imaging, especially in cases of nondisplaced greenstick fractures of the condylar neck. For suspected multiple and complex fractures of the mandible, either CBCT or multidetector computed tomographic imaging (MDCT) is the modality of choice for imaging mandibular trauma, although magnetic resonance imaging (MRI) may be useful to assess soft tissue injury to the temporomandibular joint capsule or articular disk.

MAXILLOFACIAL FRACTURES

Computed tomographic (CT) imaging is the method of choice for imaging fractures of the maxillofacial skeleton, particularly fractures that involve multiple bones.

RADIOLOGIC SIGNS OF FRACTURE

Fractures are often erroneously referred to as "lines" despite their three-dimensional nature. Fractures represent planes of cleavage through a tooth or bone, and these planes extend deep into the tissues. A fracture may be missed if the plane of the fracture is not aligned with the direction of the incident x-ray beam on a single plane image.

The following are general signs that may indicate the presence of a fracture of a tooth or bone:
1. The presence of one or two usually sharply defined radiolucent lines within the anatomic boundaries of a structure. If the line

or lines extend beyond the boundaries of the mandible, more than likely they represent an overlapping structure. If a line extends beyond the boundaries of a tooth root, the line may represent a superimposed neurovascular canal.

2. A change in the normal anatomic outline or shape of the structure. A mandible that is noticeably asymmetric between the left and right sides may be fractured. A fracture of the mandible may also manifest as a change in the contour of the occlusal plane at the location of the fracture site.

3. A loss of continuity of an outer border. This may appear as a gap in the continuity of the otherwise smooth tooth or cortical border. Such a gap may also produce a step-type defect where the two fragments have become displaced relative to one another.

4. An increase in the radiopacity of a structure. This can be caused by the overlapping of two fragments of tooth or bone such that a particular area appears "doubly" radiopaque.

TRAUMATIC INJURIES OF THE TEETH

CONCUSSION

Definition

The term concussion refers to a crush injury to the vascular structures at the tooth apex and the periodontal ligament resulting in inflammatory edema. There is no displacement, and only minimal loosening of the tooth occurs. The injury may result in mild avulsion of the tooth from its socket, causing its occlusal surface to make premature contact with an opposing tooth during mandibular closing.

Clinical Features

The patient usually complains that the traumatized tooth is tender to touch, which can be confirmed by gentle horizontal or vertical percussion of the tooth. The tooth may also be sensitive to biting forces, although patients usually try to modify their occlusion to avoid contacting the traumatized tooth.

Imaging Features

The imaging appearance of a dental concussion may be subtle. No changes may be visible, or there may be localized widening of the apical periodontal ligament space (Fig. 30-1). Changes to the size of the pulp chamber and root canals may develop in the months and years after traumatic injury to the teeth, and this may be particularly evident in teeth that are still developing. Should pulpal necrosis occur after trauma, there may be no further deposition of (secondary) dentin as the odontoblasts and the pulpal and pulpal stem cell populations die.

Teeth that have undergone trauma before apical closure may develop a morphologically abnormal apex, the osteodentin cap. As the pulpal necrosis process begins incisally and progresses apically, vital odontoblasts may remain at the developing root apex, and tertiary dentin (osteodentin) may be deposited ahead of the advancing front of pulpal necrosis. The disorganized and sparse matrix of mineralized material that does develop may resemble bone in structure and a root apex morphologically; as such, it "caps" the end of the root. The osteodentin cap in some instances may appear to be contiguous with the developing root apex or appear separate from it. In contrast to internal resorption where the root canal is focally widened (Fig. 30-2), the root canal seen in association with an osteodentin cap appears uniformly widened from pulp chamber to apex (Fig. 30-3). The development of the canal and deposition of dentin is "frozen in time" at the developmental stage at which pulpal necrosis occurred. When the cap is covered or "hidden" from view, the apex of the root resembles that of a developing tooth (see Fig. 30-3, C).

Management

Because significant displacement of the tooth or teeth does not occur, the appropriate treatment is conservative and may include slight adjustment of the opposing teeth (if necessary) or the application of a flexible splint. Periodic monitoring in the first year with repeated vitality testing and radiographs are indicated. Should rarefying osteitis develop, endodontic treatment is appropriate.

LUXATION

Definition

Luxation is a dislocation of the tooth from its socket after severing of the periodontal attachment. Such teeth are abnormally mobile

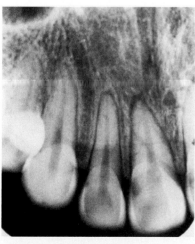

FIGURE 30-1 Widening of the periodontal ligament spaces of the incisors after dental concussion.

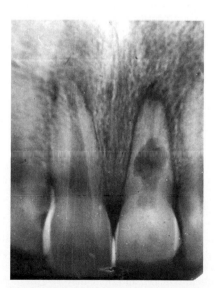

FIGURE 30-2 Obliteration of the pulp chamber but not the root canal, internal root resorption, and an incisal fracture of the maxillary left central incisor after dental concussion. Also note the area of rarefying osteitis involving the maxillary right central incisor and the widened pulp chamber and canal.

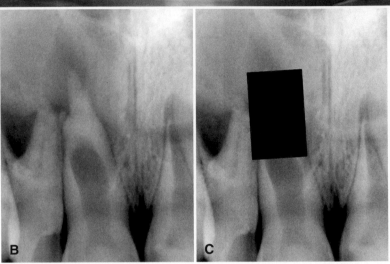

FIGURE 30-3 Panoramic **(A)** and periapical **(B)** images showing an osteodentin cap associated with the maxillary right central incisor. There is a large area of rarefying osteitis extending from the maxillary midline to the mesial surface of the maxillary right canine. Note the uniformly wide root canal of the incisor. When the osteodentin cap is "obscured," the apex of the root is reminiscent of a developing root apex **(C)**.

and displaced. Subluxation of the tooth denotes an injury to the supporting structures of the tooth that results in abnormal loosening of the tooth without frank dislocation.

Depending on their magnitude and direction, traumatic forces can cause intrusive luxation (displacement of a tooth into the alveolar process), extrusive luxation (partial displacement of a tooth out of its socket), or lateral luxation (movement of a tooth in a direction other than intrusive or extrusive displacement). In intrusive and lateral luxation, comminution or crushing of the alveolar process may accompany tooth dislocation.

The movement of the apex and disruption of the circulation to the traumatized tooth that accompanies luxation can produce either temporary or permanent changes to the dental pulp, and these changes may result in pulpal necrosis. If the pulp survives the traumatic incident, the rate of dentin formation may accelerate and continue until it obliterates the pulp chamber and root canal. This process may occur in permanent and deciduous teeth.

Clinical Features

An adequate clinical history is helpful in identifying luxation and ordering the appropriate radiographs. Subluxated teeth are in their normal location but are abnormally mobile. There may be extravasated blood emanating from the gingival crevice, indicating periodontal ligament damage, and there may be extreme sensitivity to percussion and masticatory forces.

The clinical crowns of intruded teeth may appear reduced in height. Maxillary incisors may be intruded so deeply into the alveolar process that they appear to be completely avulsed or lost.

The displaced tooth may cause some damage to adjacent teeth, particularly if any developing permanent teeth are present in the underlying bone.

Depending on the orientation and magnitude of the force and the shape of the root, it may be pushed through the buccal or, less commonly, the lingual cortex of the alveolar process where it may be seen and palpated. On repeated vitality testing, the sensitivity of a luxated tooth may be temporarily decreased or undetectable, especially shortly after the injury. Vitality may return weeks or several months later.

Usually two or more teeth are involved in luxation injuries, and the teeth most frequently affected are the deciduous and permanent maxillary incisors. The mandibular teeth are seldom affected. The type of luxation appears to vary with age, and this may reflect changes to the nature of maturing bone. Intrusions and extrusions are often found in the deciduous dentition. In the permanent dentition, the intrusive type of luxation is seen less frequently.

Imaging Features

Radiographic examinations of luxated teeth may demonstrate the extent of injury to the root, periodontal ligament, and alveolar process. An image made at the time of injury serves as a valuable reference point for comparison with subsequent radiographs. As with dental concussion, the minor damage associated with subluxation may be subtle and limited to elevation of the tooth from its socket. The sole radiographic finding may be a widening of the apical portion of the periodontal ligament space. Elevation of the tooth may not be apparent on the image.

The depressed position of the crown of an intruded tooth is often apparent on an image (Fig. 30-4), although a minimally intruded tooth may be difficult to demonstrate. Intrusion may result in partial or total obliteration of the apical periodontal ligament space. Multiple radiologic projections, including occlusal views, may be necessary to show the direction of tooth displacement and the relationship of the displaced tooth to adjacent teeth and the outer cortex of bone.

A tooth that has been extruded may demonstrate varying degrees of apical widening of the periodontal ligament space, depending on the magnitude of the extrusive force (Fig. 30-5). A laterally luxated tooth with some degree of extrusion may show a widened periodontal ligament space, with greater width on the side of impact.

Management

A subluxated permanent tooth may be restored to its normal position by digital pressure shortly after the accident. If inflammation precludes repositioning, minimal reduction of opposing teeth may be necessary to minimize any discomfort. The use of a flexible splint may provide additional stability and prevent further damage to the pulp and periodontal ligament. A subluxed deciduous tooth may potentially damage its underlying successor. Consequently, extraction may be considered. If the alveolar bone over the root of a luxated tooth has been fragmented and displaced, the fragments should be repositioned by digital pressure. A subluxated primary tooth should be periodically examined after the injury. If it causes discomfort because of extrusion, it can be removed without undue concern for occlusal problems. Subluxed permanent teeth should be monitored in the same manner as teeth that have been concussed.

AVULSION

Definition

The term avulsion is used to describe the complete displacement of a tooth from the alveolar process. Teeth may be avulsed by direct trauma when the force is applied directly to the tooth or by indirect trauma (i.e., when indirect force is applied to teeth as a result of the jaws striking together). Avulsion occurs in about 15% of traumatic injuries to the teeth, with fights being responsible for the avulsion of most permanent teeth and accidental falls accounting for the traumatic loss of most deciduous teeth.

Clinical Features

Maxillary central incisors are the most commonly avulsed teeth from both dentitions. Most often only a single tooth is lost. This injury typically occurs in a relatively young age group when the permanent central incisors are just erupting. Fractures of the alveolar process and lip lacerations may be seen with an avulsed tooth.

Imaging Features

In a recent avulsion, the lamina dura of the empty socket is apparent and usually persists for several months. The missing tooth may be displaced into the adjacent soft tissue, and its image may project over the image of the alveolar process, giving the false impression that it lies within the bone. To differentiate between an intruded tooth and an avulsed tooth lying within the adjacent soft tissues, a soft tissue image of the lacerated lip or tongue should be made. In some instances, new bone within the healing socket may be very dense and simulate a retained root tip (Fig. 30-6).

Management

If the avulsed tooth is not found by clinical or radiologic examination, a chest or abdominal image may be considered to locate it within the airway or gastrointestinal tract. Reimplanting permanent teeth after avulsion is possible; however, the prognosis of the reimplantation depends on the condition of the tooth while it is outside the mouth, the time it is out of its socket, and the viability of the residual periodontal ligament fibers. Endodontic therapy may be necessary after reimplantation, and there may be external root resorption in the months and years after reimplantation. Reimplanting an avulsed deciduous tooth carries the danger of interfering with the underlying developing permanent tooth.

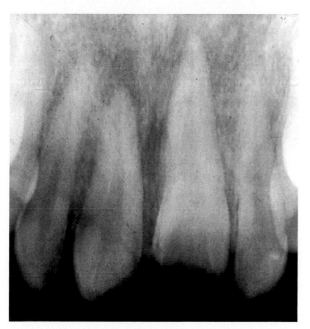

FIGURE 30-4 Intruded maxillary central incisor after trauma. Note the fractured incisal edges of both central incisors.

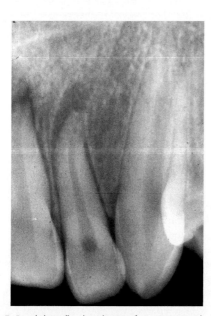

FIGURE 30-5 Extruded maxillary lateral incisor after trauma. Note the localized increase to the width of the apical periodontal ligament space.

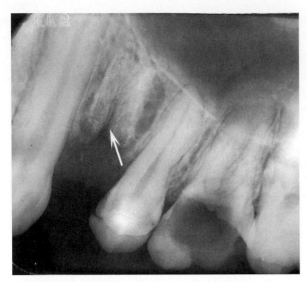

FIGURE 30-6 Bone formation during healing of a first premolar tooth socket. Note how the bone is developing from the lateral walls of the socket. The central radiolucent line *(arrow)* may have a similar appearance to that of a pulp canal, falsely giving the impression of a retained tooth fragment.

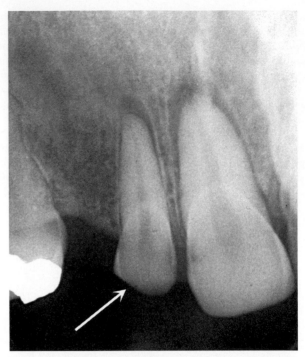

FIGURE 30-7 Incisal edge fracture involving the right maxillary lateral incisor *(arrow)* and subluxation of both the central and the lateral incisors. Note the increases to the widths of the apical periodontal ligament spaces.

FRACTURES OF THE TEETH
DENTAL CROWN FRACTURES

Definition

Fractures of the dental crown account for about 25% of traumatic injuries to the permanent teeth and 40% of injuries to the deciduous teeth. The most common event responsible for the fracture of permanent teeth is a fall, followed by accidents involving vehicles (e.g., bicycles, automobiles) and blows from foreign objects striking the teeth. Fractures involving only the crown normally fall into three categories:

1. Fractures that involve only the enamel without the loss of enamel substance (infraction of the crown or crack)
2. Fractures that involve enamel or enamel and dentin with loss of tooth substance but without pulpal involvement (uncomplicated fracture)
3. Fractures that pass through enamel, dentin, and pulp with loss of tooth substance and exposure of the pulp (complicated fracture)

Clinical Features

Fractures of the dental crowns most frequently involve anterior teeth. Infractions or cracks in the enamel are common, although frequently they may not be readily detectable unless by illumination. Histologic studies show that such cracks pass through the enamel but not into the dentin.

Uncomplicated fractures that involve both the enamel and the dentin of permanent teeth are more common than complicated fractures that include the pulp. In contrast, complicated and uncomplicated fractures occur with near-equal proportions in the deciduous teeth. Uncomplicated crown fractures that involve dentin can be recognized by the contrast in color between dentin and the peripheral layer of enamel. The exposed dentin is usually sensitive to chemical, thermal, and mechanical stimulation. In deep fractures, the pink blush of the pulp may be appreciated through the thin remaining dentin wall. Complicated crown fractures are distinguishable by bleeding from the exposed pulp or by droplets of blood forming from pinpoint exposures. The pulp is visible and may extrude from the open pulp chamber if the fracture is old. The exposed pulp is sensitive to most forms of stimulation.

Imaging Features

Imaging provides information regarding the location and extent of the fracture and the relationship of the fracture plane and fragment to the pulp chamber. The stage of root development of the involved tooth also can be assessed (Fig. 30-7). This initial image also provides a means of comparison for follow-up examinations of the involved teeth.

Management

Although crown infractions do not require treatment, the vitality of the tooth should be evaluated. The sharp edges of enamel that result from an uncomplicated fracture should be smoothed and may require restoration for cosmetic reasons. It is reasonable to delay this procedure for a number of weeks until the pulp has recovered and secondary dentin is laid down. The prognosis for teeth with fractures limited to the enamel is quite good, and pulpal necrosis develops in less than 2% of such cases. If a fracture involves both dentin and enamel, the frequency of pulpal necrosis is about 3%. Oblique fractures have a worse prognosis than horizontal fractures because potentially a greater amount of dentin is exposed. The frequency of pulpal necrosis increases greatly with concussion and mobility of the tooth.

Treatment of complicated crown fractures of permanent teeth may involve pulp capping, pulpotomy, or pulpectomy, depending on the stage of root formation. If a coronal fracture of a deciduous tooth involves the pulp, it is usually best treated by extraction.

DENTAL ROOT FRACTURES

Definition

For horizontal root fractures, the plane of cleavage may extend across the long axis of the root either perpendicularly or obliquely. In contrast, vertical root fractures represent fracture planes that run lengthwise from the crown toward the apex of the tooth, usually through the facial and lingual root surfaces.

Clinical Features

Horizontal root fractures occur more commonly in maxillary central incisors and result from the direct application of traumatic force to the face, alveolar processes, or teeth. In contrast, vertical fractures usually involve the molar teeth in adults. Vertical fractures may be iatrogenic, following the insertion of retention screws or pins into teeth, or the result of high occlusal forces, particularly in restored teeth. Endodontically treated posterior teeth that have not been restored with a full coverage restoration are also at risk.

The mobility of the fractured tooth crown relates to the level of the fracture. That is, the closer the fracture plane is located to the apex, the more stable the tooth is. When testing the mobility of a traumatized tooth, the clinician places a finger over the alveolar process. If movement of only the crown is detected, a root fracture is likely. Fractures of the root may occur with fractures of the alveolar process and are often not detected. This situation is most commonly observed in the anterior region of the mandible where root fractures are infrequent. Although root fracture is usually associated with temporary loss of sensitivity (by all usual criteria), the sensitivity of most teeth returns to normal within about 6 months.

Imaging Features

Horizontal fractures of the dental root may occur at any level and involve one (Fig. 30-8) or all of the roots of multirooted teeth. Most of the fractures confined to the root occur in the middle third of the root. The ability of an image to reveal the presence of a root fracture depends on the relative angulation of the incident x-ray beam to the fracture plane and the degree of separation of the fragments. If the x-ray beam is aligned along the fracture plane, a single sharply defined radiolucent line confined to the anatomic limits of the root may be seen. However, if the orientation of the x-ray beam meets the fracture plane in a more oblique manner, the fracture plane may appear as a more poorly defined single line or as two lines that converge at the mesial and distal surfaces of the root. The appearance of a comminuted root fracture may also be less well defined. Most nondisplaced root fractures are usually difficult to detect, and several views at differing angles may be necessary. In some instances when the fracture line is not visible, the only evidence of a fracture may be a localized increase in the width of the periodontal ligament space adjacent to the fracture site (Fig. 30-9).

Longitudinal or vertical root fractures are uncommon but are most likely in teeth with posts that have been subjected to trauma. The width of the fracture plane tends to increase with time, probably because of resorption of the fractured surfaces (Fig. 30-10). Over time, calcification and obliteration of the pulp chamber and canal may be seen.

More recently, high-resolution, small field of view CBCT imaging has been used to examine root fractures, although with varying sensitivity and specificity. Several small field of view CBCT systems can resolve 150 μm or less and may be of great value in the identification of tooth fractures (Fig. 30-11). Small field of view CBCT also enables the user to visualize the fracture in multiple planes of view. Many teeth that are investigated for root fractures have been endodontically treated and root canal filling materials or metal posts are in place. These high-density, highly attenuated materials can create substantial image artifacts that can degrade image quality making fracture identification very difficult, if not impossible (Fig. 30-12). Although x-ray orientation no longer is a limitation for CBCT imaging, image artifact from root canal filling material and metal posts and lack of separation of fracture

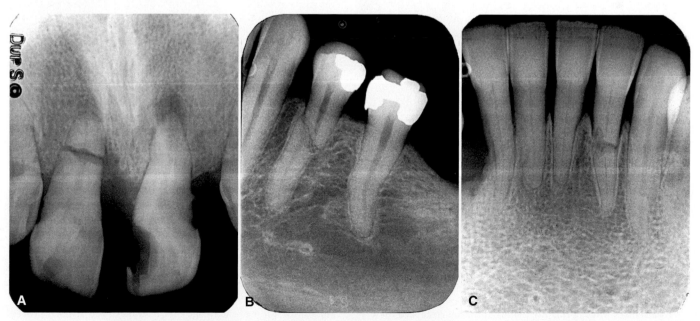

FIGURE 30-8   **A,** Recent horizontal fracture of the right maxillary central incisor and apical rarefying osteitis involving the adjacent left central incisor. **B,** Healed fracture with slight displacement of the fragments. **C,** Healed fracture with an increase in the distance between the fracture segments as a result of root resorption.

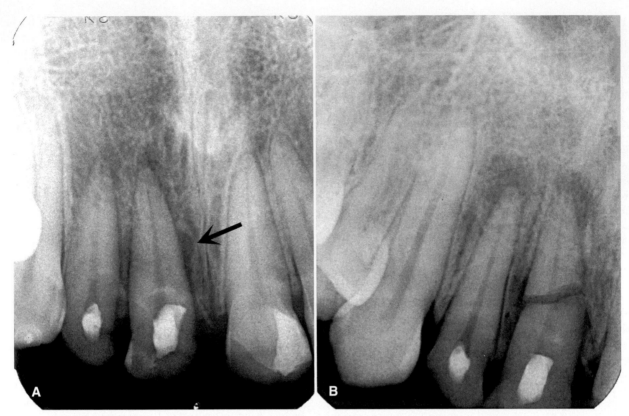

FIGURE 30-9 **A,** Subtle evidence of a root fracture involving the root of the maxillary right central incisor. Although a fracture plane is not apparent on the mesial aspect of the root because of malalignment of the x-ray beam, there is widening of the periodontal membrane space on the mesial surface *(arrow)* at the site of the fracture. **B,** Later dislocation of the root fragments.

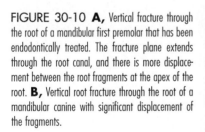

FIGURE 30-10 **A,** Vertical fracture through the root of a mandibular first premolar that has been endodontically treated. The fracture plane extends through the root canal, and there is more displacement between the root fragments at the apex of the root. **B,** Vertical root fracture through the root of a mandibular canine with significant displacement of the fragments.

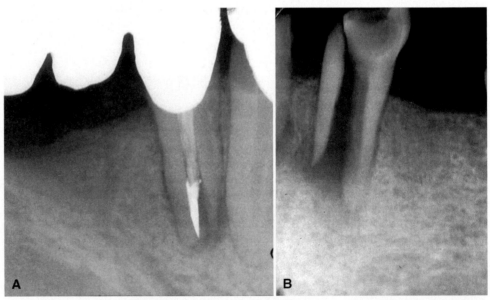

fragments continue to make identification of radiologic root fracture a challenge.

In instances where a fracture plane cannot be visualized on any imaging modality, focal widening of the periodontal ligament space along the tooth root surface can be used as an indirect sign of root fracture.

Differential Diagnosis

Superimposition of the image of a fracture of the alveolar process or small neurovascular canals or soft tissue structures such as the lip, ala of the nose, or nasolabial fold over the image of a root may mimic a root fracture.

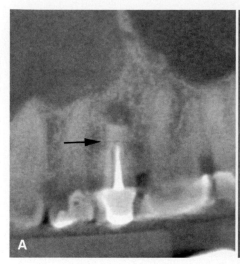
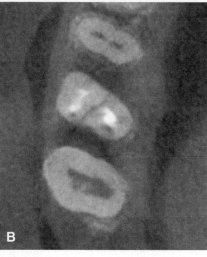

FIGURE 30-11 **A,** Panoramic-type reconstruction from small field of view CBCT volume showing a horizontal fracture through the apical one third of the tooth root of a maxillary left second premolar *(arrow)*. **B,** Axial CBCT image of a vertical fracture involving a maxillary first molar and extending from the crown into the furcation region.

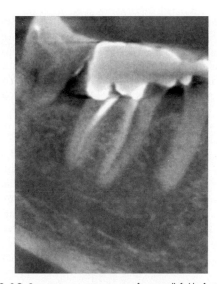

FIGURE 30-12 Panoramic-type reconstruction from small field of view CBCT volume showing a dark line running parallel to the root canal filling material in the mesial root of the mandibular molar. This "cupping" or "beam hardening" artifact could be misinterpreted as a vertical root fracture.

Management

Horizontal fractures in the middle or apical third of the root of permanent teeth can be manually reduced to the proper position and immobilized. The prognosis is generally favorable because of the relatively low incidence of pulpal necrosis. The more apical the fracture is, the better the prognosis. Endodontic therapy is performed when evidence of pulpal necrosis exists. It is common for bone resorption to occur at the site of the fracture rather than at the apex. When the fracture occurs in the coronal third of the root, the prognosis is poor, and extraction is indicated unless the apical portion of the root fragment can be extruded orthodontically and restored. The roots of fractured deciduous teeth that are not badly dislocated may be retained with the expectation that they will be normally resorbed. Attempts at removal may result in damage to the developing succedaneous tooth.

Single-rooted teeth with vertical root fractures must be extracted. Multirooted teeth may be hemisected, and the intact remaining half of the tooth may be restored with endodontic therapy and a crown.

COMBINATION CROWN AND ROOT FRACTURES

Definition

Crown-root fractures involve both the crown and roots. Although uncomplicated fractures may occur, crown-root fractures usually involve the pulp. The permanent teeth are affected about twice as much as the deciduous teeth. Most crown and root fractures of the anterior teeth are the result of direct trauma. Many posterior teeth are predisposed to such fractures by large restorations or extensive caries.

Clinical Features

The fracture plane of a typical crown-root fracture of an anterior tooth extends obliquely from the labial surface near the gingival third of the crown to a position apical to the gingival attachment on the lingual surface. Displacement of the fragments is usually minimal. Crown-root fractures occasionally manifest with bleeding from the pulp. Because these teeth are sensitive to occlusal forces that may cause separation of the fragments, a patient with a crown and root fracture usually complains of pain during mastication.

Imaging Features

The identification of crown-root fractures is fraught with the same problems as identifying standalone root fractures due to the amount of fragment distraction, primary x-ray beam angulation, and artifacts derived from intracanal restorative materials.

Management

Removal of the coronal fragment permits the evaluation of the extent of the fracture. If the coronal fragment includes 3 to 4 mm of clinical root, successful restoration of the tooth is doubtful, and removal of the residual root is recommended. If the crown-root fracture is vertically oriented, prognosis is poor regardless of treatment.

If the pulp is not exposed and the fracture does not extend more than 3 to 4 mm below the epithelial attachment, conservative treatment is likely to be successful. Uncomplicated crown and root fractures are frequently encountered in posterior teeth, and the tooth is likely to be restorable with crown lengthening procedures. If only a small amount of root is lost with the coronal fragment but the pulp has been compromised, it is likely that the tooth can be restored after endodontic treatment.

TRAUMATIC INJURIES TO THE FACIAL BONES

Facial fractures most frequently affect the mandible and the midface and, to a lesser extent, the maxillae. Radiologic examinations play a crucial role in the diagnosis and management of traumatic injuries to these and the other facial bones. Superficial signs of injury, such as soft tissue swelling, hematoma formation, or hemorrhage from a laceration or abrasion, may focus the radiologic examination. Localized injuries may be investigated with plain imaging. Maxillofacial fracture imaging is conducted primarily in hospitals using medical CT systems.

MANDIBULAR FRACTURES

The most common mandibular fracture sites are the condyle, body, and angle, followed less frequently by the parasymphyseal region, ramus, coronoid process, and alveolar process. Trauma to the mandible is often associated with other injuries, most commonly concussion (loss of consciousness) and other fractures, usually of the maxillae, zygomatic bones, and cranial vault.

The most common causes of mandibular fractures are assault, falls, and sports injuries. About half of all mandibular fractures occur in individuals 16 to 35 years old, and injuries in males are reportedly three times more common than in females. Fractures are more likely to occur on weekend days than on other days of the week.

Mandibular Body Fractures

Definition.   The mandible is the most commonly fractured facial bone. A fracture of the mandibular body on one side can be accompanied by a fracture of the condylar neck on the opposite side. Trauma to the anterior mandible may also result in unilateral or bilateral fractures of the condylar necks. When a localized heavy force is directed posteriorly to the mandible, there may be fractures of the angle, ramus, or coronoid process. In children, fractures of the mandibular body usually occur in the anterior region.

Mandibular fractures are classified as being either favorable or unfavorable, depending on the orientation of the fracture plane. Unfavorable fractures are fractures in which the action of muscles attached to the mandibular fragments displaces the fragments away from one another. For example, if a fracture plane in the body of the mandible slants obliquely posteriorly and inferiorly from the base of the anterior border of the ramus, the masseter and medial pterygoid muscles may displace the ramal fragment superiorly and

away from the body of the mandible. In favorable fractures, the muscle action tends to reduce the fracture.

Clinical Features.   A history of injury is typical, substantiated by some evidence of the trauma that caused the fracture, such as injury to the overlying skin. The patient frequently has swelling and a deformity that is accentuated when the patient opens the mouth. A discrepancy is often present in the occlusal plane, and manipulation may produce crepitus or abnormal mobility. Intraoral examination may reveal ecchymosis in the floor of the mouth. In the case of bilateral fractures to the mandible, a risk exists that the digastric, mylohyoid, and omohyoid muscles will displace the anterior mandibular fragment posteriorly and inferiorly, causing impingement on the airway.

Imaging Features.   The examination of a suspected mandibular fracture may include panoramic imaging or CT imaging. In some cases if the patient is cooperative and conscious, intraoral periapical and occlusal images may be beneficial given their higher resolution.

The margins of fracture planes usually appear as sharply defined radiolucent lines of separation that are confined to the structure of the mandible (Fig. 30-13). Displacement of the fragments results in a cortical discontinuity or "step" or an irregularity in the occlusal plane. Occasionally, the margins of the fracture overlap each other, resulting in an area of increased radiopacity at the fracture site.

Nondisplaced mandibular fractures may involve one or both buccal and lingual cortical plates (Fig. 30-14). An incomplete fracture involving only one cortical plate is often called a greenstick fracture, and these usually occur in children. An oblique fracture that involves both cortical plates may cause some diagnostic difficulties if the fracture lines in the buccal and lingual plates are not superimposed (Fig. 30-15). In this case, two lines are seen that converge at the periphery, suggesting two distinct fractures when in reality only one exists. CT imaging would preferable in this case, but if this imaging is not available, an occlusal view would be helpful.

Differential Diagnosis.   The superimposition of soft tissue images on a panoramic image of the mandible may simulate a fracture. A narrow air space between the dorsal surface of the tongue and the soft palate superimposed across the angle of the mandible in a panoramic image may simulate a fracture. The air space between the dorsal surface of the tongue and the posterior pharyngeal wall can appear similar to a fracture on lateral views of the mandible.

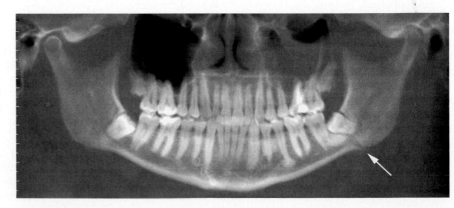

FIGURE 30-13 Reconstructed panoramic image from large field of view CBCT volume shows an oblique fracture through the left posterior mandible.

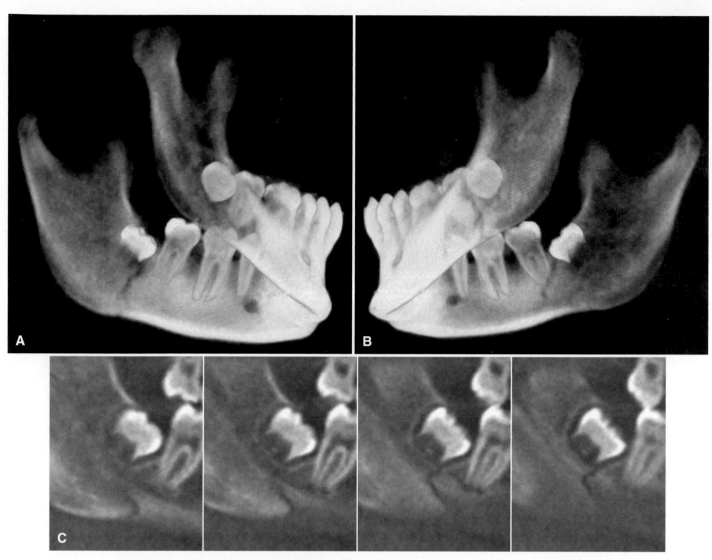

FIGURE 30-14 Three-dimensional surface renderings of oblique fractures through the posterior mandibular bodies and rami (**A** and **B**) and sagittal CBCT images through the fracture on the right side (**C**).

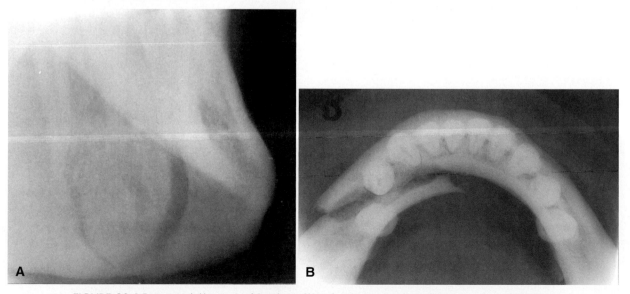

FIGURE 30-15 **A,** Lateral oblique image of the right mandible in the premolar region shows what appears to be two fracture lines that converge at the inferior cortex. **B,** True occlusal image of the mandible of the same case demonstrates only a single fracture plane. The two lines seen in **A** reflect the obliquity of the fracture plane relative to the x-ray beam.

Similar appearances can occur in the region of the soft palate where it superimposes over the ramus.

Management.
The management of a fracture of the mandible presents a variety of surgical problems that involve the proper reduction, fixation, and immobilization of the fractured bone fragments. Minimally displaced fractures are managed by closed reduction and intermaxillary fixation, whereas fractures with more severely displaced fragments may require open reduction. Treatment for fractures of the body often includes antibiotic therapy because a tooth root may be in the line of the fracture. When the fracture line involves third molars, severely mobile teeth, or teeth with at least half their roots exposed in the fracture line, the involved teeth are often extracted to reduce the risk of infection and problems with fixation.

Mandibular Condyle Fractures

Definition.
Fractures involving the mandibular condyle can be divided into condylar neck fractures and condylar head fractures. Of the two, condylar neck fractures are more common, and when they occur, the condylar head is usually displaced medially, inferiorly, and anteriorly as a result of lateral pterygoid muscle contraction (Fig. 30-16). Fractures of the condylar head may result in a vertical cleft dividing the condylar head fragments or may produce multiple fragments in a compression-like injury (Fig. 30-17). Almost half of patients with condylar fractures also have fractures in the mandibular body.

Clinical Features.
The clinical symptoms of a fractured mandibular condylar head are not always apparent, so the preauricular area must be carefully examined and palpated. The patient may have pain on opening or closing the mouth or trismus from local swelling. An anterior open bite may be present with only distal molar contacts, and there may be deviation of the mandible on opening. A significant feature may be the inability of the patient to protrude the mandible because the lateral pterygoid muscle is attached to the condyle.

Imaging Features.
Nondisplaced fractures of the mandibular condylar head may be difficult, if not impossible, to detect on a panoramic image. CT imaging is the modality of choice because it enables the clinician to visualize the three-dimensional relationship of the displaced condylar head to the glenoid fossa and to adjacent anatomic structures in the skull base and infratemporal fossa.

Studies of remodeled previously fractured condyles show that children and adolescents have much greater remodeling potential than adults. In children younger than 12 years, most fractured condyles show a return to normal morphology after healing, whereas the remodeling is less complete in teenagers. In adults, only minor remodeling is observed. The extent of remodeling is also greater with fractures of the condylar head than with condylar neck fractures with displacement of the condylar head. The most common deformities are medial inclination of the condyle, abnormal shape of the condyle, shortening of the neck, erosion, and flattening. Early condylar fractures commonly result in hypoplasia of the ipsilateral side of the mandible.

Management.
The technical details of treating mandibular condylar fractures vary according to whether one or both condyles are involved, the extent of displacement, and the occurrence and severity of concomitant fractures. The treatment is directed to

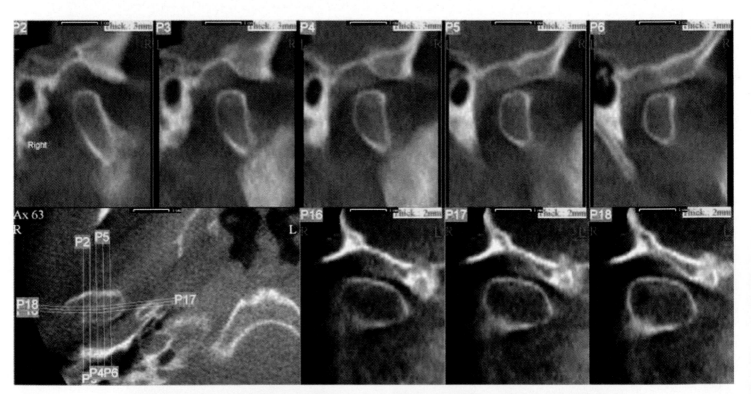

FIGURE 30-16 Corrected sagittal and coronal CBCT images through the right temporomandibular joint shows a condylar neck fracture. The corrected sagittal images *(top row)* show anterior and inferior displacement of the condylar head. The corrected coronal images *(bottom row)* show medial rotation of the condylar head.

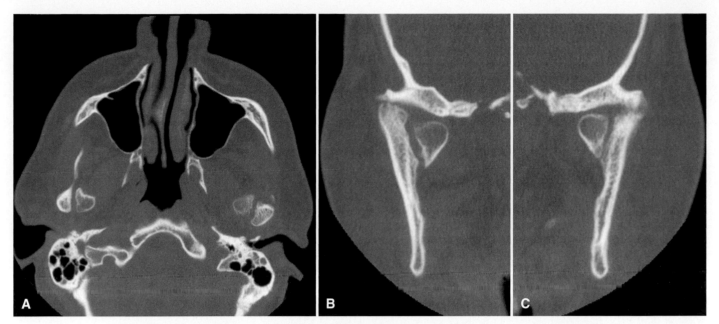

FIGURE 30-17 Example of CT images of bilateral condylar neck fractures showing medial displacement of the condylar heads in line with the lateral pterygoid muscles in the axial image **(A)** and medial displacement in the coronal images **(B** and **C)**; also, in **C** there is osseous ankylosis between the residual condylar neck and the temporal bone.

relieve acute symptoms, restore proper anatomic relationships, and prevent bony ankylosis. If a malocclusion develops, intermaxillary fixation may be provided in an attempt to restore proper occlusion. Often condylar head and neck fractures are not reduced because of the morbidity of the procedure and the size and position of the fracture fragments.

Fractures of the Alveolar Processes

Definition. Simple fractures of the alveolar process may involve the buccal or lingual cortical plates of the alveolar processes of the maxillae or mandible. These fractures commonly are associated with traumatic injuries to teeth that are luxated with or without dislocation. Several teeth are usually affected, and the fracture plane is most often horizontally oriented. Some fractures extend through the entire alveolar process (in contrast to the simple fracture that involves only one cortical plate), and the fracture plane may be located apical to the teeth or involve the tooth socket. These are also commonly associated with dental injuries and extrusive luxations with or without root fractures.

Clinical Features. A common location of alveolar fractures is the anterior maxilla. Simple alveolar fractures are relatively rare in the posterior segments of the arches. In this location, fracture of the buccal plate usually occurs during removal of a maxillary posterior tooth. Fractures of the entire alveolar process occur in the anterior and premolar regions and in an older age group.

A characteristic feature of an alveolar process fracture is marked malocclusion with displacement and mobility of the fragment, and when the practitioner tests the mobility of a single tooth, the entire fragment of bone moves. The teeth in the fragment have a recognizable dull sound when percussed, and the attached gingiva may have lacerations. The detached bone may include the floor of the maxillary sinus, in which case bleeding from the nose on the involved side may occur as well as ecchymosis of the buccal vestibule.

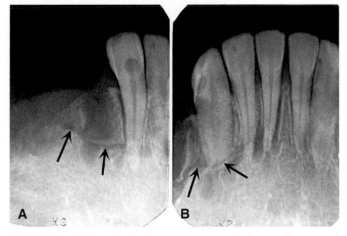

FIGURE 30-18 **A** and **B,** Two images demonstrate an alveolar process fracture extending from the distal aspect of the mandibular right cuspid in an anterior direction *(arrows)* and through the tooth socket of the right central incisor.

Imaging Features. Periapical images, if they can be made, often do not reveal fractures of a single cortical wall of the alveolar process, although evidence exists that the teeth have been luxated. However, a fracture of the anterior labial cortical plate may be apparent on an occlusal image or on a lateral extraoral image of the mandible if bone displacement has occurred and the x-ray beam is oriented at near right angles to the direction of bone displacement. Fractures of both cortical plates of the alveolar process are usually apparent (Fig. 30-18).

The closer the fracture is to the alveolar crest, the greater the possibility that root fractures are present. It may be difficult to differentiate a root fracture from an overlapping fracture line of the alveolar bone. Several images produced with different projection angles may help with this differentiation. If the fracture plane is truly associated with the tooth, the line should not shift relative to the tooth. Fractures of the posterior alveolar process may involve the floor of the maxillary sinus and result in abnormal thickening of the sinus mucosa or the accumulation of blood and sinus secretions, in which case an air-fluid level may be appreciated.

Management.   Fractures of the alveolar process are treated by repositioning the displaced teeth and associated bone fragments with digital pressure. Gingival lacerations are sutured. If the luxated permanent teeth are splinted and stable, intermaxillary fixation may be unnecessary. Teeth that have lost their vascular supply may eventually require endodontic treatment.

A soft diet for 10 to 14 days is recommended. Antibiotic coverage is provided because of communication with tooth sockets.

MIDFACIAL FRACTURES INCLUDING MAXILLARY FRACTURES

Fractures of the midfacial region involving one or multiple bones are discussed in this section.

Orbital Wall Blow-Out Fractures

Definition.   Blow-out fractures of the orbital walls result from a direct blow to the orbit by an object that is too large to enter the orbital cavity, such as a fist or a baseball. The force of the impact travels through the bone and is transferred to one or more of the very thin walls of the orbit. By definition, the orbital rim in blow-out fractures remains intact. The most common fractures involve the medial wall of the orbit formed by the lamina papyracea of the ethmoid bone and the floor of the orbit that separates this space from the maxillary sinus.

Clinical Features.   Periorbital edema is a common feature of the orbital blow-out fracture, as is enophthalmos. Eye movements may be restricted if one or more of the periorbital muscles becomes entrapped in the bony defect created by the fracture. If the ethmoid air cells are involved, there may be epistaxis.

Imaging Features.   Coronal CT imaging reconstructions best demonstrate a discontinuity of the lamina papyracea in a medial wall blow-out fracture or the accumulation of soft tissue in the roof of the maxillary sinus in an orbital floor blow-out fracture. Coronal CT imaging may show the classic "trapdoor" appearance of the displaced orbital floor (Fig. 30-19, *A*). CT imaging also may show soft tissue densities or air-fluid levels in the adjacent ethmoid air cells or maxillary sinus (Fig. 30-19, *B*) or herniation of periorbital fat and entrapment of periorbital muscle through the bony defect in the orbital floor (Fig. 30-19, *C*).

Management.   Surgical repair may be attempted for patients who have severely affected eye movements as a result of muscle entrapment or unacceptable enophthalmos.

Zygomatic Fractures

Definition.   Fractures involving the zygomatic bone may include tripod fractures, in which the zygomatic bone and adjacent areas of the maxillary, frontal, sphenoid, and temporal bones may be involved; zygomatic arch fractures, in which the zygomatic process of the temporal bone is fractured; and Le Fort type II and III fractures (described in the following section).

Injuries to the zygomatic bone or arch usually result from a forceful blow to the cheek or side of the face. Although a zygomatic bone fracture may rotate or displace the fragments medially, support by the adjacent temporalis and masseter muscles may limit displacement.

Clinical Features.   Flattening of the upper cheek with tenderness and dimpling of the skin over the side of the face may occur, although some of the clinical characteristics of zygomatic fractures may not be apparent much longer than an hour after trauma because they may be masked by edema. In most cases, periorbital ecchymosis and hemorrhage into the sclera (near the outer canthus) occur. Additional symptoms may include unilateral epistaxis (for a short time after the accident), anesthesia or paresthesia of the cheek, and compromised eye movements. The presence of diplopia suggests a significant injury to the floor of the orbit. Mandibular movement may be limited if the displaced zygomatic bone impinges on the coronoid process.

Imaging Features.   Because of edema obscuring the clinical features, the imaging examination may provide the only means of determining the presence and extent of the injury (Fig. 30-20). CT imaging is the modality of choice for imaging these fractures (Fig. 30-21).

The zygomatic arch may fracture at its weakest point, about 1 cm posterior to the zygomaticotemporal suture. Separation or fracture of the frontozygomatic suture may also occur. Fractures do not usually occur through the zygomaticomaxillary suture; however, in some cases, a fracture plane may extend obliquely, involving the inferior rim of the orbit and the lateral wall of the maxilla. If the fracture plane involves the maxillary sinus, the sinus may exhibit increased radiopacity as a result of the accumulation of blood and mucus secretions, an air-fluid level.

Panoramic images of the zygomatic arch often reveal the zygomaticotemporal suture as a radiolucent line that may have the appearance of a discontinuity in the inferior border. This is a variation of normal anatomy and should not be misinterpreted as a fracture.

Management.   When symptoms include minimal displacement of the zygomatic arch and no cosmetic deformity or impairment of eye movement, no treatment may be required. Otherwise, reduction is usually indicated. Fractures of the zygomatic bone and arch maybe reduced through an intraoral or extraoral approach.

Le Fort Fractures

Complex fractures involving multiple facial bones may be quite variable but often follow general patterns classified by the French surgeon Le Fort. By definition, all Le Fort fractures include fractures of one or more of the pterygoid plates of the sphenoid bone. Although Le Fort fractures may be bilateral, they are most often unilateral.

The detection of fractures of the midface in images is difficult because of the complex anatomy in this region and the multiple superimpositions of structures. CT imaging is the diagnostic imaging method of choice for complex facial fractures because it provides multiple image slices in orthogonal planes through the face allowing for the display of osseous structures without the complication of overlapping anatomy that is problematic with plain imaging. CT also provides suitable image detail to detect secondary changes associated with trauma, including herniation of orbital fat and extraocular muscle, soft tissue swelling or emphysema, and blood or fluid accumulation. As an aid in determining the spatial orientation of fractures or bone fragments, CT images

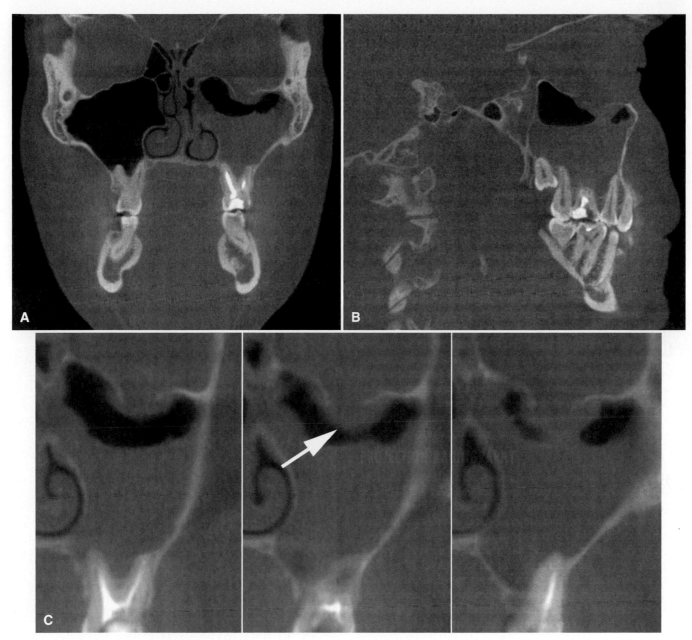

FIGURE 30-19 CBCT images show orbital blow-out fractures involving the lamina papyracea of the left ethmoid bone and the orbital floor in the coronal **(A)** and sagittal **(B)** planes. Note the fluid/soft tissue densities in the adjacent ethmoid air cells and the air-fluid level in the left maxillary sinus. **C,** These CBCT reconstructions, made perpendicular to the track of the optic nerve, show an intact orbital rim and the "trapdoor" appearance of the orbital floor blow-out fracture with herniation of soft tissue into the maxillary sinus *(arrow)*.

may be reformatted so that three-dimensional images may be evaluated.

Le Fort I (Horizontal Fracture)

Definition. A Le Fort I fracture is a relatively horizontal fracture in the body of the maxilla that results in detachment of the alveolar process and adjacent bone of the maxilla from the middle face. This fracture is the result of a horizontally directed traumatic force directed posteriorly at the base of the nose. The fracture plane passes superior to the roots of the teeth and nasal floor and posteriorly through the base of the maxillary sinus and the tuberosity to the pterygoid processes (Fig. 30-22). In the unilateral fracture,

an auxiliary fracture exists in the midline of the palate. The unilateral fracture must be distinguished from a fracture within the alveolar process (discussed previously) that does not extend to the midline or involve the pterygoid plates posteriorly. Fractures of the mandible (54%) and zygomatic bone (23%) may also be found in these patients.

Clinical Features. If the fragment is not distally impacted, it can be manipulated by holding onto the teeth. If the fracture line is at a high level, the fragment may include the pterygoid muscle attachments, which pull the fragment posteriorly and inferiorly. As a result, the posterior maxillary teeth contact the mandibular teeth first, resulting in an anterior open bite, retruded chin, and long

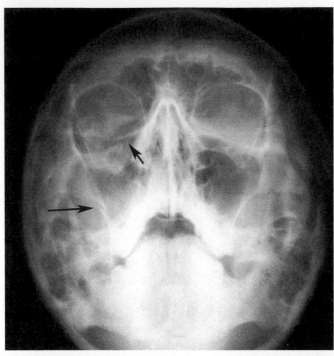

FIGURE 30-20 Waters view shows a tripod fracture involving the right zygomatic bone. Note the fracture through the right orbital rim *(short arrow)* and lateral wall of the maxillary sinus *(long arrow)*. Also, there is radiopacification of the right maxillary sinus.

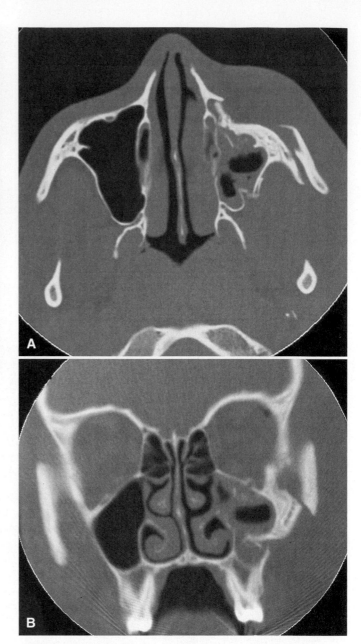

FIGURE 30-21 Axial **(A)** and coronal **(B)** CT images show depression and rotation of a left tripod fracture. An air-fluid level is also visible in the left maxillary sinus.

face. If the fracture is at a low level, no displacement may occur. Other symptoms may include associated swelling and bruising about the eyes, pain over the nose and face, deformity of the nose, and flattening of the middle of the face. Epistaxis is inevitable, and occasionally double vision and varying degrees of paresthesia over the distribution of the infraorbital nerve may occur. Manipulation may reveal a mobile maxilla and crepitation.

Imaging Features.   CT imaging reveals an air-fluid level or radiopacification in the maxillary sinus (Fig. 30-23, *A*). Coronal images may reveal the plane of the fracture extending posteriorly through the maxilla, whereas coronal or axial images together may reveal involvement of the pterygoid plates posteriorly. Three-dimensional reconstructions of the CT data set may show the plane of the fracture to greatest advantage (Fig. 30-23, *B*).

Management.   If the fracture is not displaced and is at a relatively low level in the maxilla, it can be treated by intermaxillary fixation. Fractures that are high, with the fragment displaced posteriorly or with pronounced separation, require craniomaxillary fixation in addition to intermaxillary fixation.

Le Fort II (Pyramidal Fracture)

Definition.   A Le Fort II fracture has a pyramidal shape on posteroanterior skull images—hence the name. It results from a violent force applied posteriorly and superiorly through the base of the nose. This force separates the maxilla from the base of the skull. The fracture plane extends from the bridge of the nose inferiorly, laterally, and posteriorly through the nasal and lacrimal bones, the orbital floor and inferior rim obliquely, inferiorly across the maxilla, and posteriorly to the pterygoid processes (Figs. 30-24 and 30-25). The frontal and ethmoid sinuses are involved in about 10% of cases, especially in severe comminuted fractures.

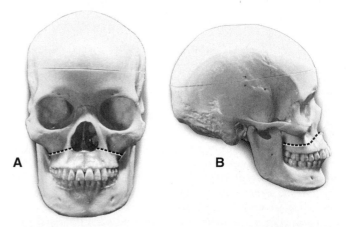

FIGURE 30-22 Usual position of a Le Fort I fracture on frontal **(A)** and lateral **(B)** views.

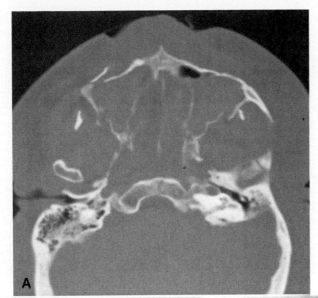

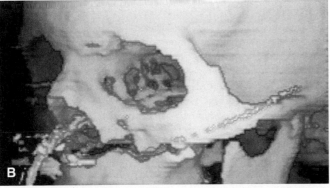

Clinical Features.   In contrast to Le Fort I fracture, which may be characterized by only slight swelling about the upper lips, a Le Fort II fracture results in massive edema and marked swelling of the middle third of the face. Typically, ecchymosis develops around the eyes within minutes of the injury. The edema is likely to be so severe that it is impossible to see the globes. The conjunctivae over the inner quadrants of the eyes are bloodshot, and if the zygomatic bones are involved, this ecchymosis extends to the outer quadrant.

The broken nose is displaced because the face has fallen, and the nose and face are lengthened. An anterior open bite occurs. Epistaxis is inevitable, and cerebrospinal fluid rhinorrhea may occur. Palpation reveals the discontinuity of the lower borders of the orbits. By applying pressure between the bridge of the nose and the palate, the "pyramid" of bone can be moved. Other common symptoms include double vision and variable degrees of paresthesia over the distribution of the infraorbital nerve.

FIGURE 30-23 **A,** Axial image of Le Fort I fractures involving the anterior and postero-lateral walls of the right and left maxilla and the pterygoid plates. Opacification of the maxillary sinuses is also seen with a small retained collection of air in the left maxillary sinus. **B,** Three-dimensional reconstruction of the image data shows extension of the fracture plane from above the base of the nose posteriorly through the maxillary tuberosity.

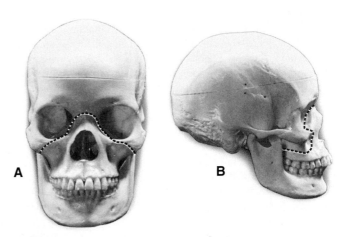

FIGURE 30-24 Usual position of the Le Fort II fracture on frontal **(A)** and lateral **(B)** views.

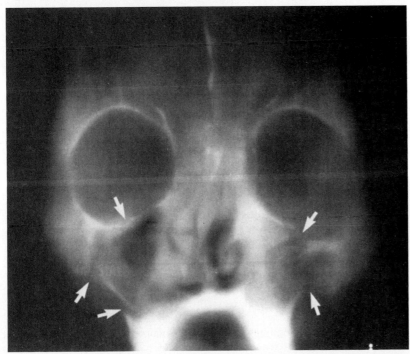

FIGURE 30-25 Coronal tomographic view of a Le Fort II fracture. Note the fractures through the orbital rims bilaterally. Also, there are fractures through the ethmoid bones and the lateral walls of the maxillae *(arrows)*. *(Courtesy Dr. C. Schow, Galveston, TX.)*

Imaging Features.   The radiologic examination reveals fractures of the nasal bone, frontal process of the maxilla, infraorbital rim, and orbital floor. More inferiorly and posteriorly, there would be involvement of the zygomatic bone or zygomatic process of the maxilla, separation of the zygomaticomaxillary suture, and fracture of the lateral wall of the maxillary sinus and the pterygoid plates. Involvement of the ethmoid air cells and frontal and maxillary sinuses would result in thickening of the sinus mucosa or the accumulation of blood-fluid levels in the air spaces. CT imaging is the modality of choice for imaging such complex fractures.

Management.   The treatment of this fracture is accomplished by reduction of the displaced maxilla by intermaxillary fixation, open reduction, and interosseous wiring of the infraorbital rims and plating of the accompanying fractures of the nose, nasal septum, and orbital floor. Repair of the detached medial canthal ligaments may also be required. Leakage of cerebrospinal fluid requires the attention of a neurosurgeon if the posterior or superior walls of the frontal sinuses are involved.

Le Fort III (Craniofacial Disjunction)

Definition.   A Le Fort III midface fracture results when the traumatic force is of sufficient magnitude to separate the middle third of the facial skeleton completely from the cranium. The fracture plane usually extends from the nasal bone and frontal process of the maxilla or nasofrontal and maxillofrontal sutures, across the orbital floor, through the ethmoid air cells and sphenoid sinus to the zygomaticofrontal sutures (Fig. 30-26). More posteriorly and inferiorly, the fracture plane passes across the pterygomaxillary fissure and separates the bases of the pterygoid plates from the sphenoid bone. If the maxilla is displaced and freely movable, a fracture must also have occurred in the area of the zygomaticotemporal suture. Because the zygomatic bone or zygomatic arch is involved, these injuries are associated with multiple other maxillary fractures. Mandibular fractures are also observed in half the cases.

Clinical Features.   Craniofacial disjunction produces a clinical appearance similar to that of a pyramidal fracture. However, this injury is considerably more extensive. The soft tissue injuries are severe, with massive edema. The nose may be blocked with blood or blood clot, or cerebrospinal fluid rhinorrhea may be present. Bleeding may occur into the periorbital tissues and the conjunctiva, and numerous eye signs of neurologic importance

are likely to be present. A "dished-in" or concave deformity of the face is characteristic of this fracture pattern, as is an anterior open bite because of the retroclined positions of the maxillary incisors with only the posterior teeth in occlusion. Even on mandibular opening, the patient is unable to separate the molars. Intraoral and extraoral palpation reveals irregular contours and step deformities, and crepitation is apparent when the fragments are moved.

Imaging Features.   It is virtually impossible to document these multiple fractures with plain films, and CT images in concert with the clinical information are required. The main radiologic findings are distractions of the frontonasal, frontomaxillary, zygomaticofrontal, and zygomaticotemporal sutures and fractures through the nasal bone, frontal process of the maxilla, orbital floor, and pterygoid plates (Fig. 30-27). Associated fractures involving the walls of all the paranasal sinuses result in radiopaque air-fluid levels with mucosal thickening. Three-dimensional reconstructions show the fracture planes and the large bone fragments (see Fig. 30-27, *D* and *E*).

Management.   The associated severe soft tissue injury necessitates airway management, initial hemorrhage control, and repair of lacerations. Surgery may be delayed until the edema has sufficiently resolved. The treatment of transverse fractures is complicated because fixation of the loose middle third of the facial skeleton is difficult owing to the fact that fractures of the zygomatic arch occur. The only possibilities are external immobilization or immobilization within the tissues. In the former, the loose maxilla is suspended by wires through the cheeks from a metal head frame (halo) or fixed by external pins anchored in bone. The other possibility is immobilization within the tissues by using internal wiring to the closest solid bone superior to the fracture. Many complications may develop during or after this treatment.

MONITORING THE HEALING OF FRACTURES

Imaging examination of the facial bones after trauma is usually necessary to measure the degree of reduction from treatment and to monitor the continued immobilization of the fracture site during repair. Typically, monitoring of this type is accomplished by use of plain imaging. The monitoring of fracture repair should include examination of both the alignment of the cortical plates of the involved bone and remodeling and remineralization of the fracture site. During normal healing, the fracture line increases in width about 2 weeks after reduction of the fracture. This increase in width results from the resorption of the fractured ends and small sequestered fragments of bone. Evidence of remineralization usually occurs 5 to 6 weeks after treatment. In contrast to the long bones of the skeleton, rarely is a callus formed in healing jaw fractures. The complete remodeling of the fracture site with obliteration of the fracture line may take several months. Fracture lines may persist for years on rare occasions, even when the patient has made a clinically complete recovery. Possible complications of healing include malalignment of the fracture segments and inflammatory lesions related to nonvital teeth near or in the line of the fracture. Other complications include nonunion of the fractured segments seen as increased width of fracture line, cortication of the fractured surfaces, and rounding of the sharp edges of the segments. The development of osteomyelitis of the fracture site appears as an increase in sclerosis of the surrounding bone, inflammatory periosteal new bone, and development of sequestra.

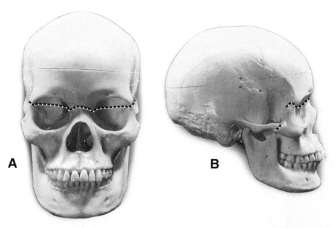

FIGURE 30-26 *Usual position of a Le Fort III fracture on frontal* (**A**) *and lateral* (**B**) *views.*

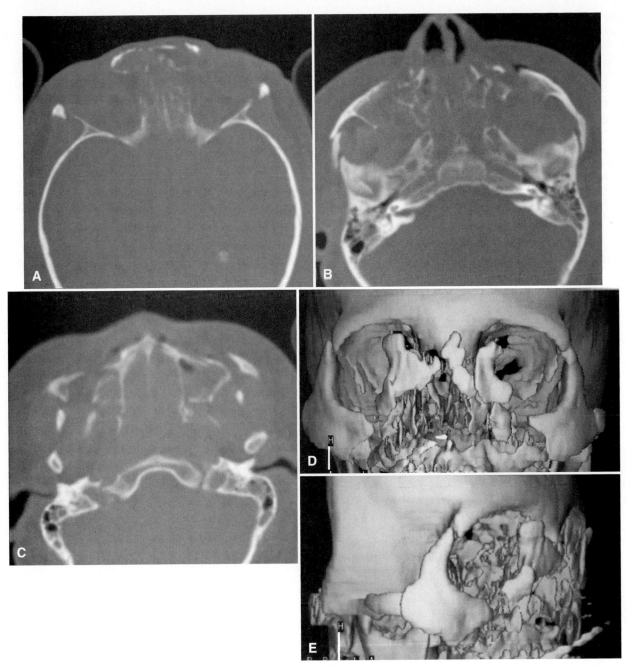

FIGURE 30-27 Axial CT images show a bilateral Le Fort III fracture with distractions of the frontonasal **(A)**, frontomaxillary, zygomaticofrontal, and zygomaticotemporal sutures **(B)** and fractures of the nasal bone, frontal process of the maxilla, orbital floor, and pterygoid plates **(C)**. Note the near-total radiopacification of the maxillary sinuses. Three-dimensional reconstructions, frontal view **(D)** and lateral view **(E)**, of the axial CT images reveal substantial fragmentation of the periorbital bones, zygomatic bone, and arch, posteriorly.

BIBLIOGRAPHY

Brook IW, Wood N: Aetiology and incidence of facial fractures in adults, *Int J Oral Surg* 12:293–298, 1983.

Daffner RH: Imaging of facial trauma, *Curr Probl Diagn Radiol* 26:153–184, 1997.

Dingman TM, Natvig AC: *Surgery of facial fractures*, Philadelphia, 1967, Saunders.

Gerlock AJ Jr, Sinn DP, McBride KL: *Clinical and radiographic interpretation of facial fractures*, Boston, 1981, Little, Brown.

Hunter JG: Pediatric maxillofacial trauma, *Pediatr Clin North Am* 39:1127–1143, 1992.

Kaban LB: Diagnosis and treatment of fractures of the facial bones in children 1943–1993, *J Oral Maxillofac Surg* 51:722–729, 1993.

Koltai PJ, Rabkin D: Management of facial trauma in children, *Pediatr Clin North Am* 43:1253–1275, 1996.

Laine FJ, Conway WF, Laskin DM: Radiology of maxillofacial trauma, *Curr Probl Diagn Radiol* 22:145–188, 1993.

Matteson SR, Deahl ST, Alder ME, et al: Advanced imaging methods, *Crit Rev Oral Biol Med* 7:346–395, 1996.

Matteson SR, Tyndall DA: Pantomographic radiology. Part II. Pantomography of trauma and inflammation of the jaws, *Dent Radiogr Photogr* 56:21–48, 1983.

Newman J: Medical imaging of facial and mandibular fractures, *Radiol Technol* 69:417–435, 1998.

Shumrick KA: Recent advances and trends in the management of maxillofacial and frontal trauma, *Facial Plast Surg* 9:16–28, 1993.

Trauma to Teeth

Andreasen JO: *Traumatic injuries of the teeth*, Philadelphia, 1981, Saunders.

Andreasen JO, Andreasen FM, Skeie A, et al: Effect of treatment delay upon pulp and periodontal healing of traumatic dental injuries—a review article, *Dent Traumatol* 18:116–128, 2002.

Josell SD, Abrams RG: Traumatic injuries to the dentition and its supporting structures, *Pediatr Clin North Am* 29:717–741, 1982.

Luxation

Andreasen JO: Luxation of permanent teeth due to trauma: a clinical and radiographic follow-up study of 189 injured teeth, *Scand J Dent Res* 78:273–286, 1970.

Avulsion

Donaldson M, Kinirons MJ: Factors affecting the time of onset of resorption in avulsed and replanted incisor teeth in children, *Dent Traumatol* 17:205–209, 2001.

Tooth Crown Fracture

Ravn JJ: Follow-up study of permanent incisors with enamel fractures as a result of acute trauma, *Scand J Dent Res* 89:213–217, 1981.

Ravn JJ: Follow-up study of permanent incisors with enamel-dentin fracture after acute trauma, *Scand J Dent Res* 89:355–365, 1981.

Stockton LW, Suzuki M: Management of accidental and iatrogenic injuries to the dentition, *J Can Dent Assoc* 64:378–382, 1998.

Cracked Tooth Syndrome

Fox K, Youngson CC: Diagnosis and treatment of the cracked tooth, *Prim Dent Care* 4:109–113, 1997.

Turp JC, Gobetti JP: The cracked tooth syndrome: an elusive diagnosis, *J Am Dent Assoc* 127:1502–1507, 1996.

Tooth Root Fracture

Cvek M, Mejare I, Andreason JO: Healing and prognosis of teeth with intra-alveolar fractures involving the cervical part of the root, *Dent Traumatol* 18:57–65, 2002.

Hovland EJ: Horizontal root fractures: treatment and repair, *Dent Clin North Am* 36:509–525, 1992.

Luebke RG: Vertical crown-root fractures in posterior teeth, *Dent Clin North Am* 28:883–894, 1984.

Majorana A, Pasini S, Bardellini E, et al: Clinical and epidemiological study of traumatic root fractures, *Dent Traumatol* 18:77–80, 2002.

Schetritt A, Steffensen B: Diagnosis and management of vertical root fractures, *J Can Dent Assoc* 61:607–613, 1995.

Schmidt BL, Stern M: Diagnosis and management of root fractures and periodontal ligament injury, *J Calif Dent Assoc* 24:51–55, 1996.

Walton RE, Michelich RJ, Smith GN: The histopathogenesis of vertical root fractures, *J Endodont* 10:48–56, 1984.

Wright EF: Diagnosis, treatment, and prevention of incomplete tooth fractures, *Gen Dent* 40:390–399, 1992.

Computed Tomographic Imaging of Jaw Fractures

Creasman CN, Markowitz BL, Kawamoto HK Jr, et al: Computed tomography versus standard radiography in the assessment of fractures of the mandible, *Ann Plast Surg* 29:109–113, 1992.

Johnson DH: CT of maxillofacial trauma, *Radiol Clin North Am* 22:131–144, 1984.

Kassel EE, Noyek AM, Cooper PW: CT in facial trauma, *J Otolaryngol* 12:2–15, 1983.

Marsh JL, Vannier MW, Gado M, et al: In vivo delineation of facial fractures: the application of advanced medical imaging technology, *Ann Plast Surg* 17:364–376, 1986.

Raustia AM, Pyhtinen J, Oikarinen KS, et al: Conventional radiographic and computed tomographic findings in cases of fracture of the mandibular condylar process, *J Oral Maxillofac Surg* 48:1258–1264, 1990.

Trauma to the Mandible

Bailey BJ, Clark WD: Management of mandibular fractures, *Ear Nose Throat J* 62:371–378, 1983.

Chayra GA, Meador LR, Laskin DM: Comparison of panoramic and standard radiographs for the diagnosis of mandibular fractures, *J Oral Maxillofac Surg* 44:677–679, 1986.

Clark WD: Management of mandibular fractures, *Am J Otolaryngol* 13:125–132, 1992.

Ellis E III, Moos KF, El-Attar A: Ten years of mandibular fractures: an analysis of 2,137 cases, *Oral Surg* 59:120–129, 1985.

Olson RA, Fonseca RJ, Zeitler DL, et al: Fractures of the mandible: a review of 580 cases, *J Oral Maxillofac Surg* 40:23–28, 1982.

Reiner SA, Schwartz DL, Clark KF, et al: Accurate radiographic evaluation of mandibular fractures, *Arch Otolaryngol Head Neck Surg* 115:1083–1085, 1989.

Winstanley RP: The management of fractures of the mandible, *Br J Oral Maxillofac Surg* 22:170–177, 1984.

Condylar Fractures

Consensus Conference on Open or Closed Management of Condylar Fractures, 12th ICOMS, Budapest, 1995, *Int J Oral Maxillofac Surg* 27:243–267, 1998.

Dahlström L, Kahnberg KE, Lindahl L: 15 years follow-up on condylar fractures, *Int J Oral Maxillofac Surg* 18:18–23, 1989.

Dimitroulis G: Condylar injuries in growing patients, *Aust Dent J* 42:367–371, 1997.

Hall MB: Condylar fractures: surgical management, *J Oral Maxillofac Surg* 52:1189–1192, 1994.

Hayward JR, Scott RF: Fractures of the mandibular condyle, *J Oral Maxillofac Surg* 51:57–61, 1993.

Sahm G, Witt E: Long-term results after childhood condylar fractures: a computer-tomographic study, *Eur J Orthod* 11:154–160, 1989.

Silvennoinen U, Iizuka T, Lindqvist C, et al: Different patterns of condylar fractures: an analysis of 382 patients in a 3-year period, *J Oral Maxillofac Surg* 50:1032–1037, 1992.

Walker RV: Condylar fractures: nonsurgical management, *J Oral Maxillofac Surg* 52:1185–1188, 1994.

Fractures of the Alveolar Process

Andreasen JO: Fractures of the alveolar process of the jaw: a clinical and radiographic follow-up study, *Scand J Dent Res* 78:263–272, 1970.

Giovannini UM, Goudot P: Radiologic evaluation of mandibular and dentoalveolar fractures, *Plast Reconstr Surg* 109:2165–2166, 2002.

Trauma to the Maxilla

Banks P: *Kiley's fractures of the middle third of the facial skeleton*, Bristol, UK, 1981, Wright.

Close LG: Fractures of the maxilla, *Ear Nose Throat J* 62:365–370, 1983.

Luce EA: Developing concepts and treatment of complex maxillary fractures, *Clin Plast Surg* 19:125–131, 1992.

Marciani RD: Management of midface fractures: fifty years later, *J Oral Maxillofac Surg* 51:960–968, 1993.

Teichgraeber JF, Rappaport NJ, Harris JH Jr: The radiology of upper airway obstruction in maxillofacial trauma, *Ann Plast Surg* 27:103–109, 1991.

Tung TC, Chen YR, Santamaria E, et al: Dislocation of anatomic structures into the maxillary sinus after craniofacial trauma, *Plast Reconstr Surg* 101:1904–1908, 1998.

Zygomatic Complex Fractures

Fujii N, Yamashiro M: Classification of malar complex fractures using computed tomography, *J Oral Maxillofac Surg* 41:562–567, 1983.

McLoughlin P, Gilhooly M, Wood G: The management of zygomatic complex fractures–results of a survey, *Br J Oral Maxillofac Surg* 32:284–288, 1994.

Prendergast ML, Wildes TO: Evaluation of the orbital floor in zygoma fractures, *Arch Otolaryngol Head Neck Surg* 114:446–450, 1988.

Sands T, Symington O, Katsikeris N, et al: Fractures of the zygomatic complex: a case report and review, *J Can Dent Assoc* 59:749–755, 1993.

Winstanley RP: The management of fractures of the zygoma, *Int J Oral Surg* 10(Suppl 1):235–240, 1981.

OUTLINE

Dental anomalies may be congenital, developmental, or acquired and may include variations in the normal number, size, morphology, or eruptive pattern of the teeth. Congenital abnormalities are typically genetically inherited anomalies, and developmental anomalies occur during the formation of a tooth or teeth. In contrast, acquired abnormalities result from changes to teeth after normal formation. Teeth that form abnormally short roots may represent congenital or developmental anomalies, whereas the shortening of normal tooth roots by external resorption represents an acquired change.

DEVELOPMENTAL ABNORMALITIES

NUMBER OF TEETH

Supernumerary Teeth

Synonyms. Synonyms for supernumerary teeth include hyperdontia, distodens, mesiodens, peridens, parateeth, and supplemental teeth.

Disease Mechanism. Supernumerary teeth are teeth that develop in addition to the normal complement as a result of excess dental lamina in the jaws. The tooth or teeth that develop may be morphologically normal or abnormal. When supernumerary teeth have normal morphologic features, the term supplemental is sometimes used. Supernumerary teeth that occur between the maxillary central incisors are termed mesiodens, those that occur in the premolar area are peridens, and those that occur in the molar area are distodens.

Clinical Features. Supernumerary teeth are easily identified by counting and identifying all the teeth in the jaws. They occur in 1% to 4% of the population, may have a greater incidence in Asians and Native American and indigenous populations, and occur twice as often in males. Although supernumerary teeth can arise in either the deciduous or the permanent dentitions, they are more common in the permanent dentition and can arise anywhere in either jaw. Single supernumerary teeth are most common in the anterior maxilla, where they are referred to as mesiodens (Figs. 31-1 to 31-3), and in the maxillary molar region (Fig. 31-4), whereas multiple supernumerary teeth occur most frequently in the premolar regions, usually in the mandible and usually positioned in the lingual aspect of the alveolar process (Figs. 31-5 and 31-6).

Supernumerary teeth are usually discovered on images because they may interfere with normal tooth eruption (Fig. 31-7). When a supernumerary tooth does erupt, it commonly does so outside the normal arch form because of space restrictions.

Imaging Features. The imaging features of supernumerary teeth are variable. They may appear entirely normal in both size and shape, but they may also be smaller in size compared with the adjacent normal dentition or have a conical shape with the appearance of a canine tooth. In extreme cases, the supernumerary teeth may appear grossly deformed.

Images may reveal supernumerary teeth in the deciduous dentition (Fig. 31-8) after 3 or 4 years of age when the deciduous teeth have formed or in the permanent dentition of children older than 9 to 12 years. In addition to periapical images, occlusal and cone-beam computed tomographic (CBCT) images may aid in determining the location and number of unerupted supernumerary teeth. Care should be taken to review panoramic images for supernumerary teeth because these may be obscured in the anterior maxillae by the image of the cervical spine, or they may appear distorted if they lie outside the focal trough.

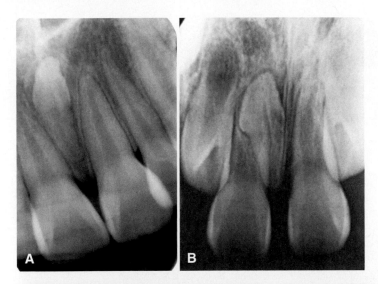

FIGURE 31-1 **A** and **B,** Periapical images of inverted mesiodens.

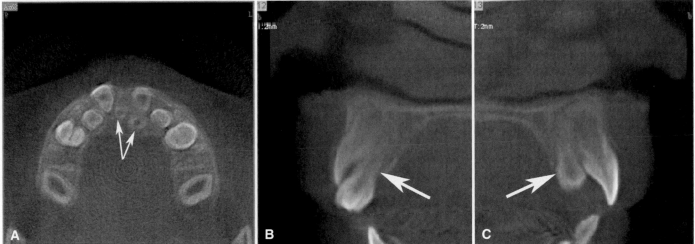

FIGURE 31-2 Axial **(A)** and cross-sectional **(B** and **C)** CBCT views of two mesiodens *(arrows)* erupting to the palatal aspect of the adjacent permanent central incisors.

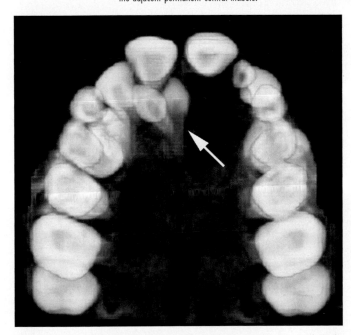

FIGURE 31-3 CBCT three-dimensional rendering of two supernumerary teeth in the anterior maxillae, palatal to the central incisors *(arrow).*

Differential Diagnosis. Multiple supernumerary teeth have been associated with numerous genetically inherited syndromes, including cleidocranial dysplasia (see Chapter 32), familial adenomatous polyposis (Gardner's syndrome) (see Chapter 22), and pyknodysostosis.

Management. The management of supernumerary teeth depends on many factors, including their potential effect on the developing normal dentition, their position and number, and the potential complications that may result from surgical intervention. If supernumerary teeth erupt, they can cause malalignment of the normal dentition. Supernumerary teeth that remain in the jaws may cause root resorption of adjacent teeth and their follicles may develop dentigerous cysts or interfere with the normal eruption sequence. All the preceding factors influence the decision either to remove a supernumerary tooth or to keep it under observation.

Missing Teeth

Synonyms. Synonyms for missing teeth are hypodontia, oligodontia, and anodontia.

Disease Mechanism. The expression of developmentally missing teeth includes the absence of one or a few teeth (hypodontia), the

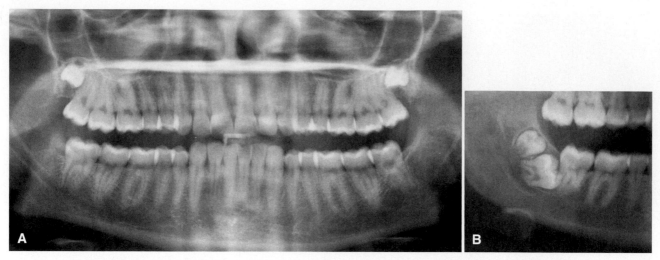

FIGURE 31-4 **A,** Example of two supplemental teeth in the maxillary third molar area (distodens). **B,** Example in the mandibular third molar region. (**A,** *Courtesy Dr. H. Grubisa, Oakville, Ontario, Canada.*)

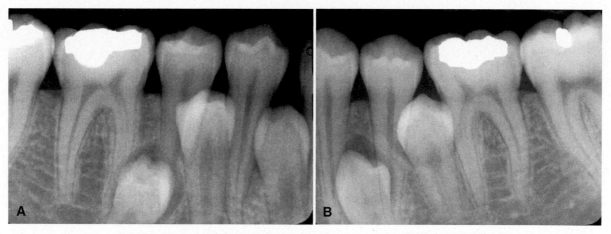

FIGURE 31-5 **A** and **B,** Periapical images show bilateral supplemental premolar teeth (peridens).

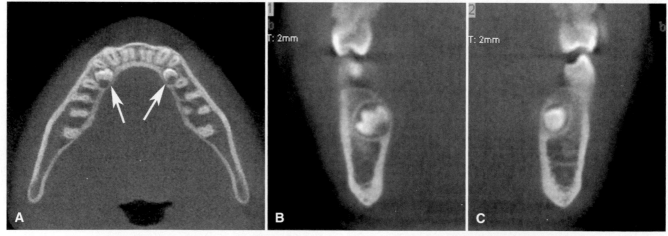

FIGURE 31-6 Axial **(A)**, right cross-sectional **(B)**, and left cross-sectional **(C)** CBCT views of peridens *(arrows)* developing to the lingual of the adjacent mandibular first premolars.

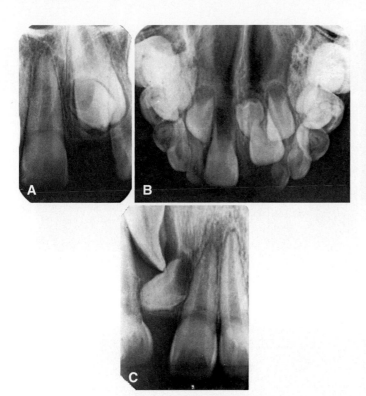

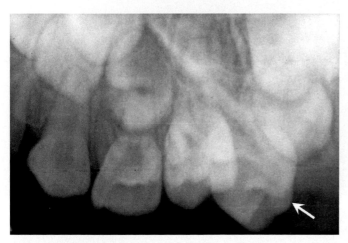

FIGURE 31-7 **A-C,** Examples of mesiodens interfering with eruption of adjacent permanent teeth.

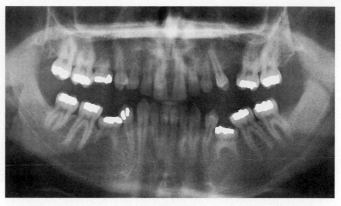

FIGURE 31-9 Developmental absence of maxillary and mandibular second premolars and maxillary canines. Note the apically positioned deciduous mandibular second molars. This appearance is suggestive of ankylosis of the teeth.

FIGURE 31-8 Supplemental deciduous molar *(arrow).*

absence of numerous teeth (oligodontia), and the failure of all teeth to develop (anodontia). Developmentally missing teeth may also be the result of numerous independent pathologic mechanisms that can affect the orderly formation of the dental lamina (e.g., orofaciodigital syndrome), failure of a tooth germ to develop at the optimal time, lack of necessary space imposed by a malformed jaw, or disproportion between tooth mass and jaw size.

Clinical Features.   Hypodontia in the permanent dentition, excluding third molars, is found in 3% to 10% of the population. Hypodontia is more frequently found in Asian and Native American and indigenous populations. Although missing primary teeth are relatively uncommon, when one tooth is missing, it is usually

a maxillary incisor. The most commonly missing teeth are third molars, followed by mandibular second premolars (Fig. 31-9) and maxillary lateral and mandibular central incisors. The absence may be either unilateral or bilateral. Children who have developmentally missing teeth tend to have more than one absent and more than one morphologic group (incisors, premolars, and molars) involved.

Imaging Features.   The development of teeth may vary markedly among individuals. Missing teeth may be recognized by identifying and counting the teeth present. For some individuals, the eruption of some teeth may be delayed by a number of years after the established time (especially mandibular second premolars), whereas others may erupt up to 1 year after the contralateral tooth.

Differential Diagnosis.   A tooth may be considered to be developmentally missing when it cannot be discerned clinically or through imaging, and no history exists of its extraction. Anodontia or oligodontia may occur in patients with ectodermal dysplasia (Fig. 31-10). This genetically diverse group of abnormalities includes 186 distinct diseases involving 64 gene mutations. In addition to missing teeth, phenotypically, these individuals may also lack sweat glands; have thin, fine hair; thin, delicate skin; and malformed nails. When the teeth are involved, the condition may manifest with multiple missing or malformed teeth that often have a conical or canine shape or a notable decrease in tooth size. The ectodermal dysplasias have been subdivided into two groups. Group A includes entities with abnormalities involving two or more of the classically involved structures previously identified, whereas group B includes abnormalities of one of these structures and another abnormality of ectodermal origin that may include the mammary glands, thyroid glands, thymus, anterior pituitary gland, cornea, conjunctiva, lacrimal gland, lacrimal duct, or meibomian glands.

Management.   Missing teeth, abnormal occlusion, or altered facial appearance may cause some patients psychological distress. If the extent of hypodontia is mild, the associated changes likewise may be slight and manageable by orthodontics. In more severe cases, restorative, implant, and prosthetic procedures can be undertaken.

SIZE OF TEETH

A positive correlation exists between tooth size (mesiodistal or buccolingual dimension) and body height. Males also have larger

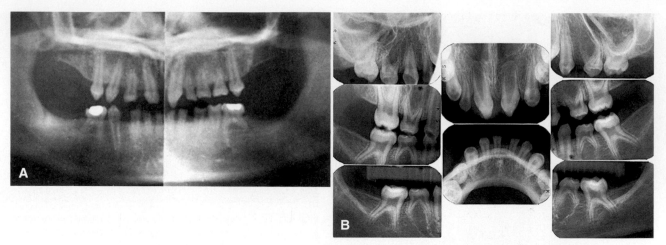

FIGURE 31-10 **A** and **B,** Two examples of multiple missing and malformed teeth in ectodermal dysplasia.

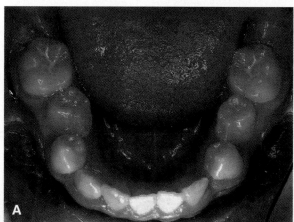

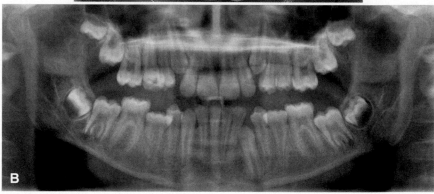

FIGURE 31-11 **A,** Clinical photograph of mandibular second premolar macrodontia. **B,** Panoramic image shows the greater mesial/distal widths of the tooth crowns compared with their respective first premolars. (**A,** *Courtesy Dr. H. Grubisa, Oakville, Ontario, Canada.*)

primary and permanent teeth than females. Beyond these normal variations, however, individuals may occasionally have unusually large or small teeth.

Macrodontia

Disease Mechanism. In macrodontia, the teeth are larger than normal. Macrodontia rarely affects the entire dentition. Often a single tooth, individual contralateral teeth, or a group of teeth may be involved (Fig. 31-11). Macrodontia may occur sporadically, and its cause is unknown. Vascular abnormalities such as a hemangioma (arising from within the bone or the soft tissues) can result in an increase in the size and accelerate the development of adjacent teeth. Macrodontia can also occur in hemihypertrophy of the face or in pituitary gigantism.

Clinical Features. Clinically, macrodont teeth appear large and may be associated with crowding, malocclusion, or impaction.

Imaging Features. Images reveal the increased size of both unerupted and erupted macrodont teeth. The shape of the tooth is usually normal, but some cases may exhibit mildly distorted morphology. Crowding may cause impaction of adjacent teeth.

Differential Diagnosis. The differential diagnosis of a sporadic macrodont tooth includes gemination and fusion. When fusion occurs, a count of the teeth present reveals a missing tooth. In gemination, all the teeth may be present, and often evidence exists of a division or cleft of the crown or root of the tooth. The differentiation between these three conditions may not influence the treatment provided.

Management.   In most cases, macrodontia does not require treatment. Orthodontic treatment may be necessary if a malocclusion is present.

Microdontia

Disease Mechanism.   In microdontia, the teeth are smaller than normal. As with macrodontia, microdontia may involve all the teeth or be limited to a single tooth or group of teeth. Often the lateral incisors and third molars may be small. Generalized microdontia is extremely rare, although it does occur in some patients with pituitary dwarfism. Supernumerary teeth may also be microdont teeth.

Clinical Features.   The involved teeth are noticeably small and may have altered morphology. Microdont molars may have an altered shape. For example, mandibular molars may have four cusps rather than five, and maxillary molars may have four cusps rather than three (Fig. 31-12). Microdont lateral incisors may be peg-shaped (Fig. 31-13).

Imaging Features.   These small teeth are frequently malformed.

Differential Diagnosis.   The recognition of small teeth indicates the diagnosis. The number and distribution of microdont teeth may also suggest consideration of syndromes (e.g., congenital heart disease, progeria).

Management.   Restorative or prosthetic treatment may be considered to create a more normal-appearing tooth, especially when considering esthetic concerns in the anterior dentition.

ERUPTION OF TEETH

Transposition

Disease Mechanism.   Transposition is the condition in which two typically adjacent teeth have exchanged positions in the dental arch.

Clinical Features.   The most frequently transposed teeth are the permanent canine and the first premolar. Second premolars infrequently lie between the first and second molars. The transposition of central and lateral incisors is rare. Transposition can occur with hypodontia, supernumerary teeth, or the persistence of a deciduous predecessor. Transposition in the primary dentition has not been reported.

Imaging Features.   Images reveal transposition when the teeth are not in their usual sequence in the dental arch (Fig. 31-14).

Differential Diagnosis.   Transposed teeth are usually easily recognized.

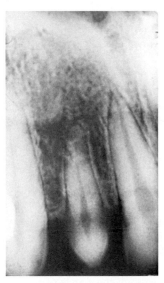

FIGURE 31-13 Peg-shaped deformity in microdontia of a maxillary lateral incisor.

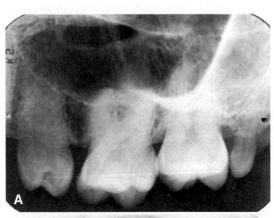

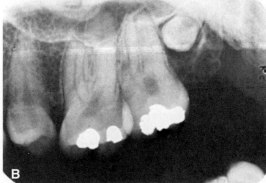

FIGURE 31-12 **A** and **B,** Periapical images show a reduction in both the size and the number of cusps in microdontia of the maxillary third molars.

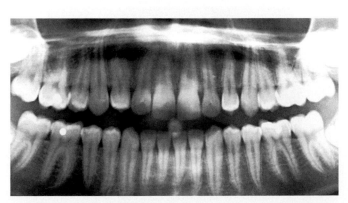

FIGURE 31-14 Cropped panoramic image demonstrating bilateral transposition of the maxillary canines and first premolars.

Management.   Transposed teeth are frequently altered prosthetically for function or esthetics or both.

ALTERED MORPHOLOGY OF TEETH

Fusion

Synonym.   A synonym for fusion is synodontia.

Disease Mechanism.   Fusion of teeth results from the union of adjacent tooth germs of developing teeth. Some authors think that fusion results when two tooth germs develop so close together that, as they grow, they contact and fuse before calcification. Other authors contend that a physical force or pressure produced during development causes contact of adjacent tooth buds. Males and females experience fusion in equal numbers; the incidence is higher in Asian and Native American and indigenous populations.

Clinical Features.   Fusion results in a reduced number of teeth in the arch. Although fusion is more common in the deciduous dentition, it may also occur in the permanent dentition. When a deciduous canine and lateral incisor fuse, the corresponding permanent lateral incisor may be absent. Fusion is more common in anterior teeth of both the permanent and the deciduous dentition (Fig. 31-15). Fusion may be total or partial, depending on the stage of odontogenesis and the proximity of the developing teeth. The result can vary from a single tooth of about normal size to a tooth of nearly twice the normal size. The crowns of fused teeth usually appear to be large and single, although incisal clefts of varying depth or a bifid crown can sometimes occur.

Imaging Features.   Images disclose the unusual shape or size of the fused teeth. The true nature and extent of the union are frequently more evident on the image than can be determined by clinical examination. Fused teeth may also show an unusual configuration of the pulp chamber or root canal.

Differential Diagnosis.   The differential diagnosis for fused teeth includes gemination and macrodontia. Fusion may be differentiated from gemination when the number of teeth is reduced by one except in the unusual case in which a normal tooth and a supernumerary tooth have fused. The differentiation is usually academic because little difference exists in the treatment provided.

Management.   The management of a case of fusion depends on which teeth are involved, the degree of fusion, and the morphologic result. If the affected teeth are deciduous, they may be retained as they are. If the clinician contemplates extraction, it is important first to determine whether the permanent teeth are present. In the case of fused permanent teeth, the fused crowns may be reshaped with a restoration that mimics two independent crowns. The morphology of fused teeth requires radiologic examination before the teeth are reshaped. Endodontic therapy may be necessary and perhaps may be difficult or impossible if the root canals are of unusual shape. In some cases, it is most prudent to leave the teeth as they are.

Concrescence

Disease Mechanism.   Concrescence occurs when the roots of two or more primary or permanent teeth are fused by cementum. Although the cause is unknown, many authorities suspect that space restriction during development, local trauma, excessive occlusal force, or local infection after development plays an important role. If the condition occurs during development, it is sometimes referred to as true concrescence. If the condition occurs later, it is referred to as acquired concrescence.

Clinical Features.   Maxillary molars are the teeth most frequently involved, especially a third molar and a supernumerary tooth. Involved teeth may fail to erupt or may erupt incompletely. The sexes are equally affected.

Imaging Features.   An imaging examination may not always distinguish between concrescence and teeth that are in close contact or that are simply superimposed (Fig. 31-16). When the condition is suspected on an image and extraction of one of the teeth is being considered, additional projections at different angles may be obtained to delineate the condition better.

Differential Diagnosis.   It is usually impossible to determine with certainty whether teeth whose root images are superimposed are actually joined. If the roots are joined, it may be impossible to tell whether the union is by cementum or by dentin (fusion). In this regard, the absence of a periodontal ligament (PDL) space between the roots may be helpful.

Management.   Concrescence affects treatment only when the decision is made to remove one or both of the involved teeth because this condition complicates the extraction. The clinician should warn the patient that an effort to remove one might result in the unintended and simultaneous removal of the other.

Gemination

Synonym.   A synonym for gemination is twinning.

Disease Mechanism.   Gemination is a rare anomaly that arises when a single tooth bud attempts to divide. The result may be an invagination of the crown with partial division or, in rare cases, complete division through the crown and root, producing identical structures. Complete twinning results in a normal tooth plus a supernumerary tooth in the arch. The cause of gemination is unknown, but some evidence suggests that it is familial.

Clinical Features.   Although gemination may occur in both the deciduous and the permanent dentitions, it more frequently affects the primary teeth, usually in the incisor region. It can be detected clinically after the anomalous tooth erupts. The occurrence in males and females is about equal. The enamel or dentin of geminated teeth may be hypoplastic or hypocalcified.

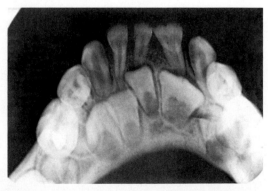

FIGURE 31-15 Fusion of the central and lateral incisors in both the primary and the permanent dentitions. Note the reduction in number of teeth and the increased width of the fused tooth mass.

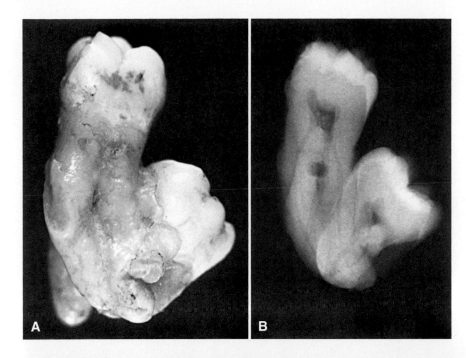

FIGURE 31-16 **A,** Concrescence occurs when two teeth are joined by cementum. **B,** Extraction of one tooth may result in the unintended removal of the second because the cementum bridge may not be well visualized. *(Courtesy Dr. R. Kienholz, Dallas, TX.)*

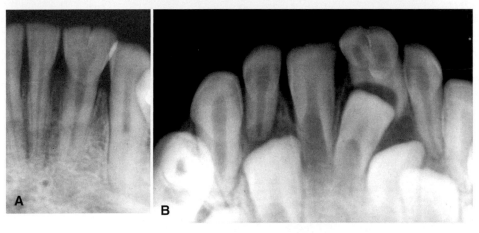

FIGURE 31-17 **A,** Gemination of a mandibular lateral incisor showing bifurcation of the crown and pulp chamber. **B,** Almost complete gemination of a deciduous lateral incisor.

Imaging Features.   Images reveal the altered shape of the hard tissue and pulp chamber of the geminated tooth. Radiopaque enamel outlines the clefts in the crowns and invaginations and accentuates them. The pulp chamber is usually single and enlarged and may be partially divided (Figs. 31-17 and 31-18). In the rare case of premolar gemination, the tooth image suggests a molar with an enlarged crown and two roots.

Differential Diagnosis.   The differential diagnosis of gemination includes fusion. If the malformed tooth is counted as one, individuals with gemination have a normal tooth count, whereas individuals with fusion are seen to be missing a tooth.

Management.   A geminated tooth in the anterior region may compromise arch esthetics and arch length. Areas of hypoplasia and invagination lines or areas of coronal separation represent caries-susceptible sites that may in time result in pulpal inflammation. Affected teeth can cause malocclusion and lead to periodontal disease. Consequently, the affected tooth may be removed (especially if it is deciduous), the crown may be restored or reshaped, or the tooth may be left untreated and periodically examined to preclude the development of complications. Before treatment is

initiated on a primary tooth, the status of the permanent tooth and configuration of its root canals should be determined by imaging.

Taurodontism
Disease Mechanism.   The bodies of taurodont teeth appear elongated, and the roots are short. The pulp chamber extends from a normal position in the crown throughout the length of the elongated body, leading to a more apically positioned pulpal floor.

Taurodontism may occur in any tooth in either the permanent or the primary dentition; however, it is usually fully expressed in the molars and less often in the premolars. Single or multiple teeth may show taurodont features.

Clinical Features.   Because the body and roots of taurodont teeth lie below the alveolar margin, the distinguishing features of these teeth are not recognizable clinically.

Imaging Features.   The distinctive morphology of taurodont teeth is quite apparent on images. The peculiar feature is the elongated pulp chamber and the more apically positioned furcation (Fig. 31-19). The shortened roots and root canals are a function of the

FIGURE 31-18 **A,** Gemination of a maxillary left second premolar on cross-sectional slices. **B,** Three-dimensional surface rendering demonstrating the geminating tooth and its association with the premolar. **C,** Coronal CBCT image of another case of gemination of a second premolar. Note the common root canal. (**A** and **B,** Courtesy Dr. B. Friedland, Cambridge, MA.)

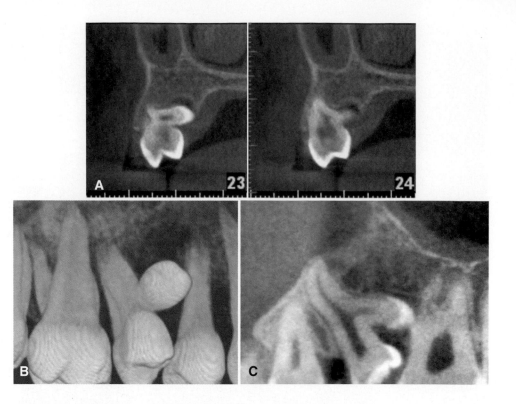

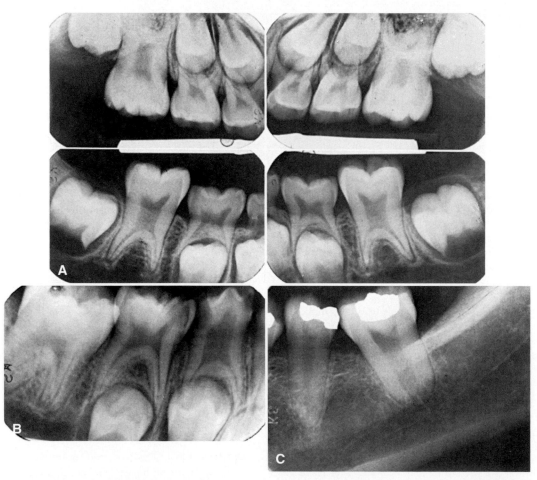

FIGURE 31-19 Periapical images reveal enlarged pulp chambers and apically positioned furcations in permanent first molars **(A)**, a primary first molar **(B)**, and a permanent molar **(C)**.

long body and normal length of the tooth. The dimensions of the crown are normal.

Differential Diagnosis.   The image of the taurodont tooth is characteristic and easily recognized on imaging. The developing molar may appear similar; however, identification of the wide apical foramina and incompletely formed roots aids in the differential diagnosis. Taurodontism has been reported with greater frequency in patients with trisomy 21 syndrome.

Management.   Taurodont teeth do not require treatment.

Dilaceration

Disease Mechanism.   Dilaceration is a disturbance in tooth formation that produces a sharp bend or curve in the tooth anywhere in the crown or the root. Although this anomaly is likely developmental in nature, one of the oldest concepts is that dilaceration is the result of mechanical trauma to the calcified portion of a partially formed tooth.

Clinical Features.   Most cases of radicular dilaceration are not recognized clinically. If the dilaceration is so pronounced that the tooth does not erupt, the only clinical indication of the defect is a missing tooth. If the defect is in the crown of an erupted tooth, it may be readily recognized as an angular distortion (Fig. 31-20).

Imaging Features.   Images provide the best means of detecting a radicular dilaceration. The condition occurs most often in maxillary premolars. One or more teeth may be affected. If the roots dilacerate mesially or distally, the condition is clearly apparent on a periapical image (Fig. 31-21). However, when the roots are dilacerated buccally (labially) or lingually, the central x ray passes approximately parallel with the deflected portion of the root, and the apical end of the root may have the appearance of a circular or oval radiopaque area with a central radiolucency (the apical foramen and root canal), giving the appearance of a "bull's eye." The PDL space around this dilacerated portion may be seen as a radiolucent halo encircling the radiopaque area (Fig. 31-22). In some cases, especially in the maxilla, the

geometry of the projections may preclude the recognition of a dilaceration.

Differential Diagnosis.   Occasionally, dilacerated roots may be difficult to differentiate from fused roots, sclerosing osteitis, or a dense bone island. However, these usually can be discerned by images made at different angles.

Management.   A dilacerated root generally does not require treatment because it provides adequate support. If the tooth is to be extracted for some other reason, the removal can be complicated, especially if the surgeon is not prepared with a preoperative image. In contrast, dilacerated crowns are frequently restored with a prosthetic crown to improve esthetics and function.

Dens Invaginatus, Dens in Dente, and Dilated Odontome

Synonyms.   Gestant odontome and "tooth within a tooth" are synonyms for dens invaginatus, dens in dente, and dilated odontome.

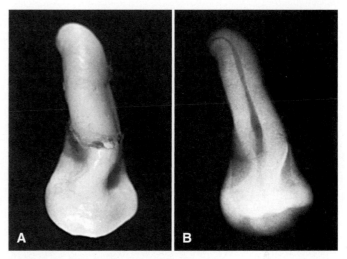

FIGURE 31-20 **A,** Dilaceration of the crown may be recognized clinically. **B,** Image of the specimen in **A**. *(Courtesy Dr. R. Kienholz, Dallas, TX.)*

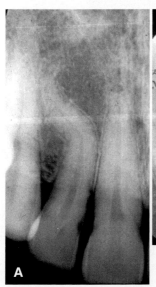

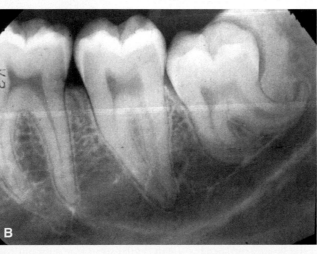

FIGURE 31-21 Dilaceration of the root of a maxillary lateral incisor **(A)** and mandibular third molar **(B)**.

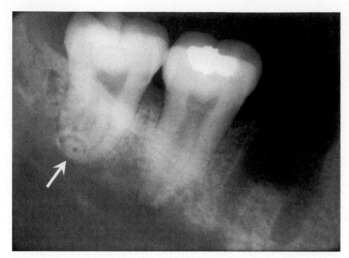

FIGURE 31-22 The most apical portion of this third molar root is dilacerated in the buccal-lingual direction so that its long axis lies along the path of the x-ray beam. Note the "bull's eye" appearance of the root apex produced by the root canal, tooth root, and PDL space (arrow).

Disease Mechanism.

The three entities dens invaginatus, dens in dente, and dilated odontome all result from varying degrees of invagination or infolding of the enamel surface into the interior of a tooth. The least severe form of this infolding is dens invaginatus, and the most severe form is dilated odontome. The invagination can occur in either the cingulum area (dens invaginatus) or the incisal edge (dens in dente) of the crown or in the root during tooth development. It may also involve the pulp chamber or root canal system; this may result in a deformity of either the crown or the root, although these anomalies are seen most often in tooth crowns. Coronal invaginations usually originate from an anomalous infolding of the enamel organ into the dental papilla. In a mature tooth, the result is a fold of hard tissue within the tooth characterized by enamel lining the fold (Fig. 31-23). When the abnormality involves the root, it may be the result of an invagination of Hertwig's epithelial root sheath and produce an accentuation of the normal longitudinal root groove.

In contrast to the coronal type, which is lined with enamel, the radicular type of defect is lined with cementum. If the invagination retracts and is cut off, it leaves a longitudinal structure of cementum, bone, and remnants of the PDL within the pulp canal. The structure often extends for most of the root length. In other cases, the root sheath may bud off a saclike invagination that produces a circumscribed cementum defect in the root. Mandibular first premolars and second molars are especially prone to develop the radicular variety of this invagination anomaly.

Among whites and Asians, there is little difference in frequency of occurrence. If all grades of expression of invagination—from mild to severe—are included, the condition is found in approximately 5% of these two ethnic groups. The condition appears to be rare in individuals of African descent. No sexual predilection exists. Although no specific mode of inheritance seems to fit all the data, a high degree of inheritability seems to exist.

Clinical Features.

Dens invaginatus may appear as nothing more than a small pit between the cingulum and the lingual surface of an incisor tooth (Fig. 31-24). In dens in dente, the pit is located at the incisal edge of the tooth, and crown morphology may appear

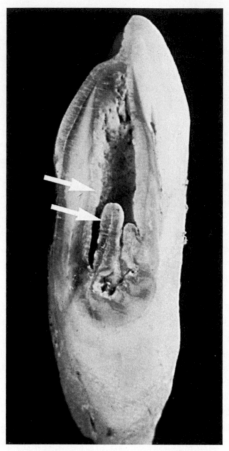

FIGURE 31-23 Dens in dente is characterized by an infolding of enamel into the tooth. This sectioned canine with a dens in dente shows enamel (arrows) folded into the tooth's interior.

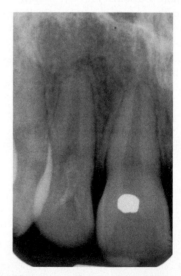

FIGURE 31-24 Radiopaque, inverted teardrop outline of dens invaginatus in a maxillary lateral incisor. Note the position of the invagination in the cingulum area of the tooth crown.

abnormal, having the appearance of a peg-shaped microdont tooth (Fig. 31-25). A dilated odontome can be thought of as the most extreme dens invaginatus and has roughly the shape of a doughnut with central soft tissue surrounded by dental hard tissue.

Dens invaginatus and dens in dente occur most frequently in the permanent maxillary lateral incisors, followed by (in decreasing

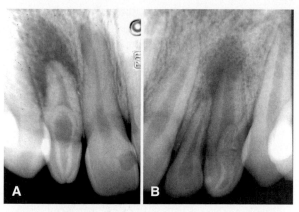

FIGURE 31-25 A and **B,** Infolding of enamel is more severe in dens in dente as seen in these two periapical images. The invagination begins near the incisal edge of these abnormally peg-shaped lateral incisors.

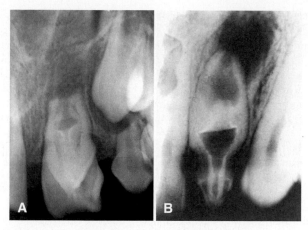

FIGURE 31-26 A and **B,** Severe forms of dens in dente usually result in necrosis of the pulp, open apices, and rarefying osteitis at the tooth apices.

frequency) the maxillary central incisors, premolars, and canines and less often the posterior teeth. Invagination is rare in the crowns of mandibular teeth and in deciduous teeth. The abnormality occurs symmetrically in about half the cases, and concomitant involvement of the central and lateral incisors may occur.

The clinical importance of dens invaginatus and dens in dente is the risk of pulpal inflammation. Although enamel lines the coronal defect, it is frequently thin, often of poor quality, and even missing in some areas. The cavity is usually separated from the pulp chamber by a relatively thin wall that opens into the oral environment through a narrow constriction. The pit is often difficult if not impossible to keep clean, and consequently it offers conditions favorable for the development of caries. Carious lesions are difficult to detect clinically and rapidly involve the pulp. In addition, sometimes fine canals extend between the invagination and the pulp chamber, resulting in pulpal disease even in the absence of caries.

Imaging Features. Most cases of dens invaginatus or dens in dente are discovered with imaging and can be identified in the image even before the tooth erupts. The infolding of the enamel lining is more radiopaque than the surrounding tooth structure and can be identified easily as an inverted teardrop-shaped radiolucency with a radiopaque border (see Figs. 31-24 and 31-25). Less frequently, the radicular invaginations appear as poorly defined, slightly radiolucent structures running longitudinally within the root. The defects, especially the coronal variety, may vary in size and shape from small and superficial to large and deep. If a coronal invagination is extensive, the crown is almost invariably malformed, and the apical foramen is usually wide (Fig. 31-26). A frequent cause of an open apical foramen is the cessation of root development that occurs as a result of death of the pulpal tissue. In the most severe form (dilated odontome), the tooth is severely deformed, having a circular or oval shape with a radiolucent interior (Fig. 31-27).

Differential Diagnosis. The appearance and usual occurrence in incisors are so characteristic that, once recognized, little probability exists that the anomaly will be confused with another condition.

Management. Although it is important to evaluate every case individually, the placement of a prophylactic restoration in the defect is typically the treatment of choice and should ensure a

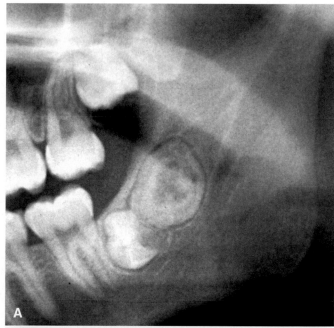

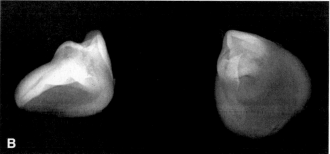

FIGURE 31-27 A, Dilated odontome, the most severe enamel invagination, is positioned just posterior to the developing mandibular third molar in this panoramic image. **B,** Images of the extracted dilated odontome from two different angulations.

normal life span for the tooth. Failure of early identification and treatment may result in premature tooth loss or the requirement for root canal therapy.

Dens Evaginatus

Synonym. A synonym for dens evaginatus is Leong's premolar.

Disease Mechanism. In contrast to dens invaginatus or dens in dente, dens evaginatus is the result of an outpouching of the enamel organ. The resultant enamel-covered tubercle usually occurs in or near the middle of the occlusal surface of a premolar or occasionally a molar (Fig. 31-28). Lateral incisors are most commonly involved, whereas canines are rarely affected. The frequency of occurrence of dens evaginatus is highest in Asian and Native American and indigenous populations.

Clinical Features. Clinically, dens evaginatus appears as a tubercle of enamel on the occlusal surface of the affected tooth. A hard, polyp-like protuberance predominantly exists in the central groove or lingual ridge of a buccal cusp of posterior teeth and in the cingulum fossa of anterior teeth. Dens evaginatus may occur bilaterally and usually in the mandible. The tubercle often has a dentin core, and a very slender pulp horn frequently extends into the evagination. After the tubercle is worn down by the opposing teeth, it appears as a small circular facet with a small black pit in the center (Fig. 31-29). Wear, fracture, or indiscriminate surgical removal of this tubercle may precipitate a pulpal infection because of the exposure of the pulp horn. In rare cases, a microscopic direct communication may occur between the pulp and the oral cavity through this tubercle. In these instances, the pulp may become infected shortly after eruption.

Imaging Features. Imaging shows an extension of a dentin tubercle on the occlusal surface unless the tubercle is already worn down. The dentin core is usually covered with opaque enamel. A fine pulp horn may extend into the tubercle, but this may not be visible in the image. If the tubercle has been worn to the point of pulpal exposure or has fractured, pulpal necrosis may result (see Fig. 31-29). Necrosis is indicated by an open apical foramen and periapical radiolucency. Multiple root formation is often associated with dens evaginatus, especially in mandibular premolars.

Differential Diagnosis. The clinical and imaging appearances may be characteristic or may be difficult to visualize if the tubercle has been worn down to the occlusal surface.

Management. If the tubercle causes any occlusal interference or shows evidence of marked abrasion, it probably should be removed under aseptic conditions, and the pulp should be capped, if necessary. Such a precaution may preclude pulpal exposure and infection as the result of accidental fracture or advanced abrasion.

Amelogenesis Imperfecta

Disease Mechanism. Amelogenesis imperfecta is a genetic anomaly arising from mutations that may have occurred in one or more of four candidate genes that play some role in enamel formation: (1) amelogenin (*AMELX*), (2) enamelin (*ENAM*), (3) enamelysin

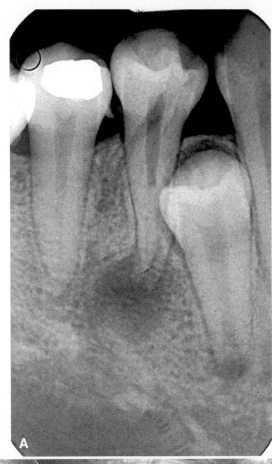

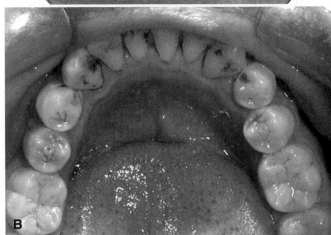

FIGURE 31-29 **A,** Periapical image of a mandibular first premolar with a dens evaginatus and apical rarefying osteitis. **B,** Clinical photograph of another case of dens evaginatus involving both mandibular second premolars. Note the worn tubercles located in the center of the occlusal surfaces, now seen as black pits representing communication with the pulp chamber.

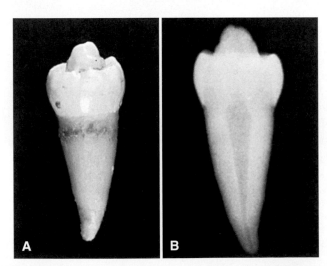

FIGURE 31-28 **A,** Occlusal tubercle of dens evaginatus as seen in a mandibular premolar. **B,** Periapical image of the specimen. *(Courtesy Dr. R. Kienholz, Dallas, Texas.)*

(*MMP20*), and (4) kallikrein 4 (*KLK4*). The mutation may be inherited in an autosomal dominant or recessive manner, or it may be inherited in an X-linked pattern. These mutations lead to marked changes in the enamel of all or nearly all the teeth in both dentitions and is not related to any time or period of enamel development or any clinically demonstrable alteration (disease or dietary abnormality) in other tissues. The enamel may lack the normal prismatic structure and be laminated throughout its thickness or at the periphery. As a result, these teeth are more resistant to decay. The dentin and root form are usually normal. Eruption of the affected teeth is often delayed, and a tendency for tooth impaction exists. Although at least 14 variants of the condition have been described, four general types have been delineated on the basis of their clinical or imaging appearances: (1) a hypoplastic type, (2) a hypomaturation type, (3) a hypocalcified type, and (4) a hypomaturation type associated with taurodontism.

Clinical Features

Hypoplastic Type. The enamel of the affected teeth fails to develop to its normal thickness. Consequently, the color of the underlying dentin imparts a yellowish brown color to the tooth. In addition, the enamel may be abnormal; it may be rough, pitted, smooth, or glossy. The crowns of the teeth may appear undersized with a roughly square shape. The reduced enamel thickness also causes a loss of contact between adjacent teeth (Fig. 31-30). The occlusal surfaces of the posterior teeth are relatively flat with low cusps. This is a result of the attrition of cusp tips that were initially low and not fully formed. Hypoplastic amelogenesis imperfecta type is the most easily identifiable on imaging.

Hypomaturation. In the hypomaturation form of amelogenesis imperfecta, the enamel has a mottled appearance but is of normal thickness. The enamel is softer than normal, its density comparable to dentin, and it may break away from the crown. Its color may range from clear to cloudy white, yellow, or brown. In one form of hypomaturation amelogenesis imperfecta, the teeth may be capped with white, opaque enamel. This appearance has been referred to as "snow-capped" teeth.

Hypocalcification. The hypocalcific form of amelogenesis imperfecta is more common than the hypoplastic variety. The crowns of the teeth are normal in size and shape when they erupt because the enamel is of regular thickness (Fig. 31-31). However, because the enamel is poorly mineralized (it is less dense than dentin), it starts to fracture away shortly after it comes into function, and this creates clinically recognizable defects. The soft enamel abrades rapidly, and the softer dentin also wears down rapidly, resulting in a grossly worn tooth, sometimes to the level of the gingiva. An explorer point under pressure can penetrate the soft enamel, yet caries in these worn teeth is unusual. The hypocalcified enamel has increased permeability and becomes stained and darkened. The teeth of a young person with generalized hypomineralization of the enamel are frequently dark brown from food stains.

Hypomaturation with Taurodontism. This classification indicates a combination of hypomaturation with taurodontism.

Imaging Features. Amelogenesis imperfecta is identified primarily by clinical examination, although the imaging features substantiate the clinical impression. The imaging signs of hypoplastic amelogenesis imperfecta include a square crown, a relatively thin radiopaque layer of enamel, low or absent cusps, and multiple open contacts between the teeth. The anterior teeth on images are said to have a "picket fence"–type appearance. The density of the enamel is normal. Pitted enamel appears as sharply localized areas

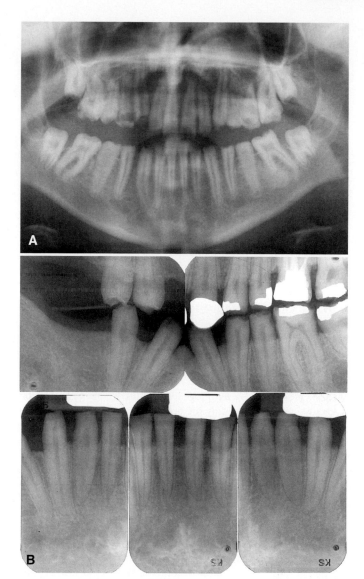

FIGURE 31-30 **A,** Cropped panoramic image of hypoplastic amelogenesis imperfecta. Note the absence of interproximal contacts and the "picket fence"–like appearance of the teeth. **B,** Intraoral images of another case of amelogenesis imperfecta. Note the very thin enamel layer. (**A,** *Courtesy Dr. S. Roth, Halifax, Nova Scotia, Canada.*)

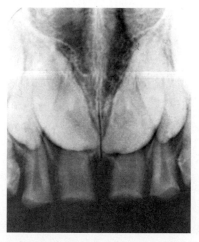

FIGURE 31-31 The reduced radiopacity of the enamel and the rapid abrasion of the crowns of the primary teeth are features of hypomineralized amelogenesis imperfecta.

of mottled density, quite different from the image cast by a tooth that is normal in shape and density. The hypomaturation form exhibits a normal thickness of the enamel, but its density is the same as that of dentin. In the hypocalcified forms, the enamel thickness is normal, but its density is even less (more radiolucent) than that of dentin. With advanced abrasion, obliteration of the pulp chambers may complicate recognition of the image.

Differential Diagnosis.   If advanced abrasion is present and secondary dentin obliterates the pulp chambers, the imaging picture of amelogenesis imperfecta appears similar to that of dentinogenesis imperfecta. However, the presence of bulbous crowns and narrow roots, the relatively normal density of any remaining enamel, and the obliteration of pulp chambers and root canals, in the absence of marked attrition, are characteristic of dentinogenesis imperfecta (see the following section) and should distinguish it from amelogenesis imperfecta.

Management.   Appropriate treatment for amelogenesis imperfecta is restoration of the esthetics and function of the affected teeth.

Dentinogenesis Imperfecta

Synonym.   A synonym for dentinogenesis imperfecta is hereditary opalescent dentin.

Disease Mechanism.   Dentinogenesis imperfecta is a genetic anomaly involving primarily the dentin, although the enamel may be thinner than normal in this condition. Three types of dentinogenesis imperfecta exist, and each has been associated with a particular genetic. Type I dentinogenesis imperfecta, which is associated with osteogenesis imperfecta (see the following section) is caused by mutations of one of two genes involved in collagen synthesis: (1) collagen type I, alpha 1 (*COL1A1*) or (2) collagen type I, alpha 2 (*COL1A2*) genes. Types II and III dentinogenesis imperfecta are caused by mutations of the dentin sialoprotein (*DSP*) and dentin sialophosphoprotein (*DSPP*) genes.

The tooth roots and pulp chambers of type I teeth are generally small and underdeveloped, and the primary dentition may be more severely affected than the permanent dentition. Type II dentinogenesis imperfecta is similar to type I but affects the dentin only without any skeletal defects. The expression of type II dentinogenesis imperfecta is variable, and occasionally individuals exhibit enlarged pulp chambers in the primary teeth. Type III dentinogenesis imperfecta, or the so-called Brandywine isolate, was described in a population of less than 200 persons in the Brandywine, Maryland, region. There is some controversy regarding the differentiation between types II and III; however, type III teeth are said to exhibit enlarged pulp chambers, making them more susceptible to pulp exposure.

Dentinogenesis imperfecta occurs with equal frequency in both sexes. Both the deciduous and the permanent dentition may have this defect.

Clinical Features.   The appearance of teeth with dentinogenesis imperfecta is characteristic. They exhibit a high degree of amber-like translucency and various colors from yellow to blue-gray. The colors change according to whether the teeth are observed by transmitted light or reflected light. The enamel easily fractures from the teeth, and the crowns wear readily. In adults, the teeth frequently may wear down to the gingiva. The exposed dentin becomes stained. The color of the abraded teeth may change to dark brown or black. Some patients demonstrate an anterior open bite.

Imaging Features.   The crowns in patients with dentinogenesis imperfecta are usually normal in size, but there is a constriction of the cervical portion of the tooth that gives the crown a bulbous appearance. Images may reveal slight to marked attrition of the occlusal surface. The roots are usually short and slender. There may be partial or complete obliteration of the pulp chambers. Early in development, the teeth may appear to have large pulp chambers, but these are quickly obliterated by the formation of dentin. Ultimately, the root canals may be absent or threadlike (Fig. 31-32). Occasionally, areas of rarefying osteitis may be seen in association with what appear to be sound teeth without evidence of pulpal involvement. These changes may occur as a result of microscopic communications between the residual pulp and the oral cavity. These lesions do not occur as frequently as in dentin dysplasia. The architecture of the bone in the maxilla and mandible is normal.

Differential Diagnosis.   Dentin dysplasia (see the following section) is in the differential diagnosis.

Management.   The placement of prosthetic crowns on the affected teeth is usually unsuccessful unless the teeth have good root support. The teeth should not be extracted from patients 5 to 15 years old. It is generally preferable to place full overdentures on the teeth to prevent alveolar resorption. In adults, extraction of the teeth and their replacement can be recommended.

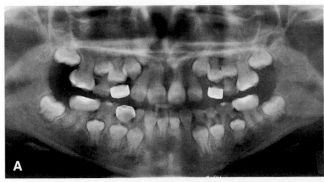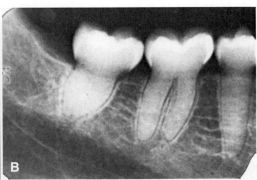

FIGURE 31-32 **A** and **B**, Dentinogenesis imperfecta characteristically shows bulbous crowns, constriction of tooth at the cementoenamel junction, short roots, and a reduced size of the pulp chamber and root canals.

Osteogenesis Imperfecta

Osteogenesis imperfecta is a hereditary disorder characterized by osseous fractures. The pathogenesis is thought to be an inborn error in the synthesis of type I collagen, which results in brittle bones. It is usually transmitted as an autosomal dominant trait. Patients may have blue sclerae, wormian bones (bones in skull sutures), skeletal deformities, and progressive osteopenia. Dentinogenesis imperfecta is found in approximately 25% of cases. Oral findings may also include class III malocclusions and an increased incidence of impacted first and second molars.

Dentin Dysplasia

Disease Mechanism.   Dentin dysplasia is a genetically inherited autosomal dominant abnormality that resembles dentinogenesis imperfecta. Two types have been described: (1) type I (radicular) and (2) type II (coronal). In type I, the most marked changes are found in the appearances of the roots. In type II, changes in the crown are most clearly seen in the altered shape of the pulp chambers. Mutations of the dentin sialophosphoprotein (*DSPP*) gene, the same gene that has been implicated in dentinogenesis imperfecta types II and III, have also been implicated in type II dentin dysplasia. Dentin dysplasia is less frequent than dentinogenesis imperfecta (1 : 100,000 compared with 1 : 8000).

Clinical Features.   Clinically, teeth with dentin dysplasia have characteristic features. Type I (radicular form) teeth have mostly normal color and shape in both dentitions. Occasionally, a slight bluish brown translucency is apparent. The teeth are often misaligned in the arch, and patients may describe drifting and spontaneous exfoliation with little or no trauma. In type II (coronal form), the crowns of the primary teeth appear to be of the same color, size, and contour as in dentinogenesis imperfecta; this is interesting in light of the purported close genetic linkage between the two dentin abnormalities. Although not universally accepted, reports exist that primary teeth rapidly abrade. The permanent teeth have clinically normal-appearing crowns.

Imaging Features.   In type I dentin dysplasia, the roots of both the primary and the permanent teeth are either short or abnormally shaped (Fig. 31-33). The molar roots have been described as having a shallow "W" shape. The roots of primary teeth may be only thin spicules. The pulp chambers and root canals completely fill in before eruption. The extent of obliteration of the pulp chambers and canals is variable. In addition, about 20% of teeth with type I dentin dysplasia are associated with rarefying osteitis; this is likely the result of microscopic communications between the residual pulp and the oral cavity. Association of these inflammatory lesions with noncarious teeth is an important feature for recognition of this particular entity. In type II dentin dysplasia, obliteration of the pulp chamber (Fig. 31-34) and reduction in the caliber of the root canals occurs after eruption (at least by 5 or 6 years). These changes are not seen before eruption. As the chambers of the molars are being filled with hypertrophic dentin, the pulp chambers may become flame-shaped or thistle-shaped and may have multiple pulp stones. Occasionally, the anterior teeth and premolars develop a pulp chamber that is thistle tube in shape because of its extension into the root. The roots of the coronal variety are normal in shape and proportions.

Differential Diagnosis.   The differential diagnosis for dentin dysplasia includes only one other entity, dentinogenesis imperfecta,

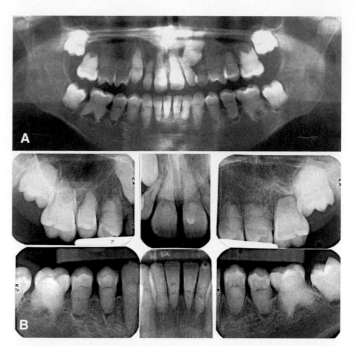

FIGURE 31-33 Panoramic **(A)** and periapical **(B)** images of the same case show the short, poorly developed roots; obliterated pulp chambers and root canals; and periapical rarefying osteitis associated with type 1 (radicular) dentin dysplasia. Note the half-moon or "demilune" shape of the pulp chambers.

because both abnormalities can appear clinically similar. Both entities can produce crowns with altered color and occluded pulp chambers. The finding of a thistle tube–shaped pulp chamber in a single-rooted tooth strengthens the probability of dentin dysplasia. However, in type II dentin dysplasia, the pulp chambers become obliterated after eruption. Sometimes, crown size can help distinguish between the two. The teeth in dentinogenesis imperfecta typically have bulbous-shaped crowns with a constriction in the cervical region, whereas the crowns in dentin dysplasia are usually of normal shape, size, and proportion. If the roots are short and narrow, the condition is likely to be dentinogenesis imperfecta. Normal-appearing roots or practically no roots at all should suggest dentin dysplasia. Periapical rarefying osteitis in association with noncarious teeth is more commonly seen in dentin dysplasia.

Management.   Teeth with type I dentin dysplasia have such poor root support that prosthetic replacement is about the only practical treatment. Teeth that are of normal shape, size, and support (type II) can be crowned if they seem to be rapidly abrading. The esthetics of discolored anterior teeth can be improved by prosthetic treatment.

Regional Odontodysplasia

Synonyms.   Synonyms for regional odontodysplasia include odontogenesis imperfecta and ghost teeth.

Disease Mechanism.   Regional odontodysplasia is a rare condition in which both enamel and dentin are hypoplastic and hypocalcified. This localized arrest in tooth development typically affects only a few adjacent teeth in a quadrant. These teeth may be either primary or permanent. If the primary teeth are affected, their successors are usually involved. Although many theories exist regarding the etiology of this condition, its cause is unknown.

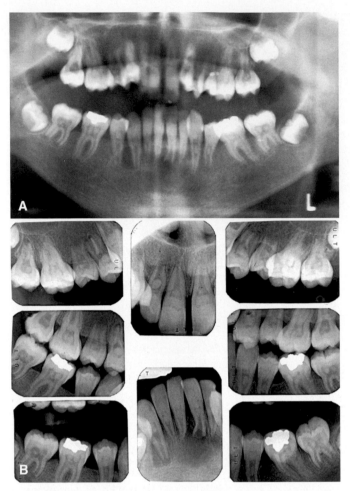

Clinical Features.

Teeth affected with regional odontodysplasia are small and mottled brown as a result of staining of the hypocalcified and hypoplastic enamel. They are especially susceptible to caries, are brittle, and are subject to fracture and pulpal infection. Central incisors are most often affected, with lateral incisors and canines also occasionally exhibiting the defect (most often in the maxilla). Eruption of the defective teeth is often delayed, and in severe cases they may not erupt.

Imaging Features.

Because these teeth are very poorly mineralized, the images of teeth with regional odontodysplasia have been described as having a "ghostlike" appearance. The pulp chambers are large and the root canals are wide because the hypoplastic dentin is thin, serving just to outline the image of the root (Fig. 31-35). Also, the poorly outlined roots are short. The enamel likewise is thin and less dense than usual, sometimes so thin and poorly mineralized that it may not be evident on the image. The tooth is little more than a thin shell of hypoplastic enamel and dentin. Teeth that do not erupt are so hypomineralized and hypoplastic that they appear to be resorbing.

Differential Diagnosis.

The malformed teeth occasionally seen in one of the expressions of dentinogenesis imperfecta occasionally may be confused with teeth in regional odontodysplasia. However, the fact that the dentinogenesis imperfecta trait usually carries a history of familial involvement, in contrast to odontodysplasia (which is not hereditary), is an important distinguishing feature. Also, the enamel in regional odontodysplasia is hypoplastic, which is not the case in dentinogenesis imperfecta. Finally, only a few teeth of either dentition in an isolated segment of the arch are affected in regional odontodysplasia, whereas the type of dentinogenesis imperfecta that resembles regional odontodysplasia involves all primary teeth.

Management.

With the advent of newer restorative materials, it is recommended to retain and restore the affected teeth as much

FIGURE 31-34 Panoramic **(A)** and periapical **(B)** images of the same case show obliteration of the pulp chamber, reduction in the caliber of root canals, and pulp stones obscuring the flame-shaped or thistle-shaped pulp chambers associated with type II (coronal) dentin dysplasia. Note the areas of rarefying osteitis associated with some of the mandibular anterior teeth.

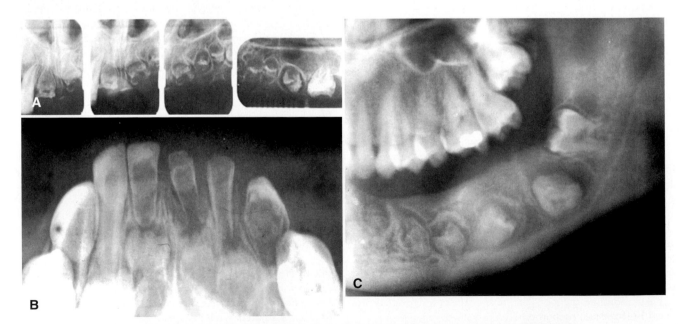

FIGURE 31-35 Periapical images reveal poor mineralization of all of the dental hard tissues in regional odontodysplasia. Note in the images how only one portion of the arch is involved. **A,** Involvement of the maxillary left dentition. **B,** Involvement of the primary incisors and canines. **C,** Involvement of the left mandibular premolars and first and second molars. Note the lack of eruption and hypoplasia of enamel and dentin expressed mainly as short roots.

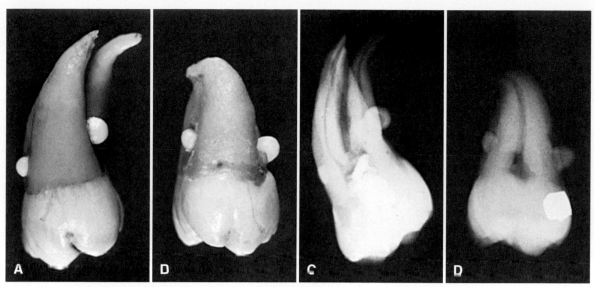

FIGURE 31-36 **A** and **B,** Enamel pearls are small outgrowths of enamel and dentin in the furcation areas of teeth. **C** and **D,** Images of the teeth in **A** and **B**. *(Courtesy Dr. R. Kienholz, Dallas, TX.)*

as possible. Unerupted teeth should be retained during the period of skeletal growth. Severely damaged permanent teeth with pulpal involvement may require removal and replacement.

Enamel Pearl

Synonyms.   Enamel drop, enamel nodule, and enameloma are synonyms for enamel pearl.

Disease Mechanism.   An enamel pearl is a small globule of enamel 1 to 3 mm in diameter that occurs on the roots of molars (Fig. 31-36). It is found in about 3% of the population, probably formed by Hertwig's epithelial root sheath before the epithelium loses its enamel-forming potential. Usually only one pearl develops, but occasionally more develop. Enamel pearls may have a core of dentin and rarely a pulp horn extending from the chamber of the host tooth.

Clinical Features.   Most enamel pearls form below the crest of the gingiva and are not detected during a clinical examination. They typically develop in the furcal areas of molar teeth, often lying at or just apical to the cementoenamel junction. Enamel pearls that form on the maxillary molars are usually in the mesial or distal furca, and pearls that develop in mandibular molars are more often in the buccal or lingual furca. Usually no clinical symptoms are associated with their presence, although they may predispose to formation of a periodontal pocket and subsequent periodontal disease.

Imaging Features.   The enamel pearl appears smooth, round, and comparable in degree of radiopacity to the enamel covering the crown (Fig. 31-37). Occasionally the dentine casts a small, round, radiolucent shadow in the center of the radiopaque sphere of enamel. If projected over the crown, it may be obscured.

Differential Diagnosis.   It is possible to mistake an enamel pearl for an isolated piece of calculus or a pulp stone. The differentiation between a pulp stone and an enamel pearl can be made by increasing the vertical angle of projection to move the image of the enamel pearl away from the pulp chamber. If the opacity is a

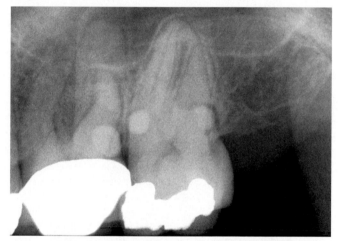

FIGURE 31-37 Three enamel pearls (one attached to the first molar and two on the second molar) are apparent in this periapical image.

calculus, it is usually clinically detectable. Occasionally, oblique views of maxillary or mandibular molars may cause superimposition of a portion of the roots in the region of the furcation, producing a density that appears similar to that of an enamel pearl. In this case, producing another image at a slightly different horizontal angle eliminates this radiopaque region.

Management.   As a rule, the recognition that a radiopaque mass superimposed on the tooth is an enamel pearl precludes the necessity for treatment. The clinician can remove the mass if its location at the cementoenamel junction predisposes to periodontal disease. The possibility must always be considered that it may contain a pulp horn.

Talon Cusp

Disease Mechanism.   The talon cusp is an anomalous hyperplasia of the cingulum of a maxillary or mandibular incisor. It results in the formation of a supernumerary cusp. Normal enamel covers the cusp and fuses with the lingual aspect of the tooth. Any developmental grooves that are present may become caries-susceptible areas. The cusp may or may not contain an extension (horn) of the pulp. No apparent ethnic predilection exists.

Clinical Features.   The talon cusp is infrequently encountered. It may be found in either sex and on both primary and permanent incisors. It varies in size from that of a prominent cingulum to a cusplike structure extending to the level of the incisal edge. When viewed from its incisal edge, an incisor bearing the cusp is T-shaped with the top of the "T" representing the incisal edge. Although it usually occurs as an isolated entity, its incidence has been reported to be increased in teeth related to cleft palate syndromes and in association with other anomalies.

Imaging Features.   The radiopaque image of a talon cusp is superimposed on that of the crown of the involved incisor (Fig. 31-38). Its outline is smooth, and a layer of normal-appearing enamel is generally distinguishable. The image may not reveal a pulp horn. The cusp is often apparent before eruption and may simulate the presence of a supernumerary tooth.

Differential Diagnosis.   The appearance of a talon cusp is quite distinctive. Although it may not be distinguishable from a

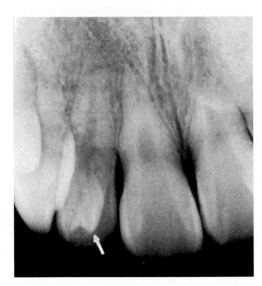

FIGURE 31-38 *Maxillary lateral incisor bearing a talon cusp (arrow). The tooth also has two enamel invaginations, one near the incisal edge and a second in the cingulum area. (Courtesy Dr. R. A. Cederberg, Dallas, TX.)*

supernumerary tooth with a single film, a second image with either the parallax or the buccal object technique can demonstrate a connection to the tooth.

Management.   If developmental grooves are present where the cusp fuses with the lingual surface of the incisor, treatment may be required to prevent the development of decay. If the cusp is large, it may pose an esthetic or occlusal problem. Slowly removing the cusp over a long period may stimulate the formation of secondary dentin and prevent exposure of a pulp horn.

Turner's Hypoplasia

Synonym.   A synonym for Turner's hypoplasia is Turner's tooth.

Disease Mechanism.   Turner's hypoplasia is a term used to describe a permanent tooth with a local hypoplastic defect in its crown. This defect may have been caused by the extension of a periapical infection from its deciduous predecessor or by mechanical trauma transmitted through the deciduous tooth. If the trauma (whether infectious or mechanical) occurs while the crown is forming, it may adversely affect the ameloblasts of the developing tooth and result in some degree of enamel hypoplasia or hypomineralization.

Clinical Features.   Turner's hypoplasia most often affects the mandibular premolars, generally because of the relative susceptibility of the deciduous molars to caries, their proximity to the developing premolars, and their relative time of mineralization. The severity of the defect depends on the severity of the infection or mechanical trauma and on the stage of development of the permanent tooth. It may disturb matrix formation or calcification, in which case the result varies from a hypoplastic defect to a hypomineralization spot in the enamel. The hypomineralized area may become stained, and the tooth usually shows a brownish spot on the crown. If the insult is severe enough to cause hypoplasia, the crown may show pitting or a more pronounced defect.

Imaging Features.   The enamel irregularities associated with Turner's hypoplasia alter the normal contours of the affected tooth and are often apparent on an image (Fig. 31-39). The involved region of the crown may appear as an ill-defined radiolucent region. A stained hypomineralized spot may not be apparent because of an insufficient difference in the degree of radiopacity between the spot and the crown of the tooth. Also, the hypomineralized areas may become remineralized by continued contact with saliva.

FIGURE 31-39 **A,** Turner's hypoplasia shown as an extensive malformation and hypomineralization of the crowns of both premolars. **B,** Band of hypoplasia extending across the crown of the mandibular left central incisor.

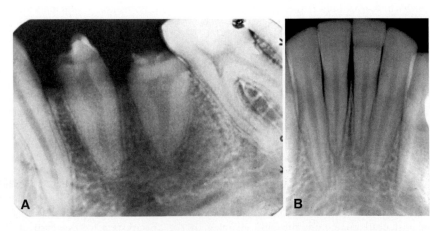

Differential Diagnosis.   Other conditions that result in deformation of the tooth crown, such as the delivery of high doses of therapeutic radiation, should be considered, although usually several adjacent teeth are involved. Small defects may simulate the appearance of carious lesions but can be easily differentiated by clinical inspection.

Management.   If an image of a tooth affected by Turner's hypoplasia shows that the tooth has good root support, the esthetics and function of the deformed crown can be restored.

Congenital Syphilis

Disease Mechanism.   About 30% of people with congenital syphilis have dental hypoplasia that involves the permanent incisors and first molars. Development of primary teeth is seldom disturbed. The affected incisors are called Hutchinson's incisors, and the molars are called "mulberry molars." The changes characteristic of the condition seem to result from a direct infection of the developing tooth because the syphilitic spirochete has been identified in the tooth germ.

Clinical Features.   The affected incisor has a characteristic screwdriver-shaped crown, with the mesial and distal surfaces tapering from the middle of the crown to the incisal edge (Fig. 31-40). The effect is that the edge may be no wider than the cervical area of the tooth. The incisal edge is also frequently notched. Although maxillary central incisors usually demonstrate these syphilitic changes, the maxillary lateral and mandibular central incisors may also be involved.

As with incisor crowns, the crowns of affected first molars are quite characteristic, usually smaller than normal and may be even smaller than second molar crowns. The most distinctive feature is the constricted occlusal third of the crown, with the occlusal surface no wider than the cervical portion of the tooth. The cusps of these molars are also reduced in size and poorly formed. The enamel over the occlusal surface is hypoplastic, unevenly formed in irregular globules, similar to the surface of a mulberry, a small berry having an appearance similar to a blackberry.

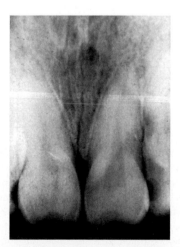

FIGURE 31-40 Congenital syphilis may induce a developmental malformation of the maxillary central incisors referred to as "Hutchinson's incisors." The abnormal morphology is characterized by tapering of the mesial and distal surfaces toward the incisal edge with notching of the incisal edge.

Imaging Features.   The characteristic shapes of the affected incisor and molar crowns can be identified in the image. Because the crowns of these teeth form at about 1 year of age, images may reveal the dental features of congenital syphilis 4 to 5 years before the teeth erupt.

Management.   Hutchinson's teeth and mulberry molars often do not require dental treatment. Esthetic restorations may be used to correct the hypoplastic defects as indicated clinically.

ACQUIRED ABNORMALITIES

Acquired changes of the dentition—changes that are initiated after development of the tooth—range in severity from changes that have no clinical significance to changes that cause tooth loss. In the latter case, early detection and treatment are required to preserve the tooth.

ATTRITION

Disease Mechanism

Attrition is physiologic wearing of the dentition resulting from occlusal contacts between the maxillary and mandibular teeth. It occurs on the incisal, occlusal, and interproximal surfaces. Interproximal wear causes the contact points to become broad and flattened. Attrition occurs in more than 90% of young adults and is generally more severe in men than women. The extent of attrition depends on the abrasiveness of the diet, salivary factors, mineralization of the teeth, and emotional tension. Physiologic attrition is a component of the aging process. When the loss of dental tissue becomes excessive such as from bruxism, the attrition becomes pathologic.

Clinical Features

The tooth wear patterns from attrition are characteristic. Wear facets first appear on cusps and marginal oblique and transverse ridges. The incisal edges of the maxillary and mandibular incisors show evidence of broadening. The wear facets on the occlusal surfaces of molars become more pronounced, with the lingual cusps of maxillary teeth and the buccal cusps of mandibular posteriors showing the most wear. When the dentin is exposed, it usually becomes stained, and the color contrast between stained dentin and enamel highlights the areas of attrition. The incisal edges of mandibular incisors tend to become pitted because the dentin wears more rapidly than its surrounding enamel. In the case of pathologic attrition, the patterns of wear are generally not as uniformly progressive as the patterns described for physiologic attrition. The wear facets develop at a faster rate. However, physiologic attrition is a relative term, and its clinical manifestations vary with the customs (dietary and otherwise) of the population in question.

Imaging Features

The imaging appearance of attrition results in a change in the normal outline of the tooth structure, altering the normal curved surfaces into flat planes. The crown is shortened and is bereft of the incisal or occlusal surface enamel (Fig. 31-41). Often many adjacent teeth in each arch show this wear pattern. Reduction in the size of the pulp chambers and canals may occur because attrition stimulates the deposition of secondary dentin. This secondary dentin may result in complete obliteration of the pulp chamber and canals. A simultaneous widening of the PDL space frequently occurs if the tooth is mobile. Occasionally, evidence of hypercementosis is present.

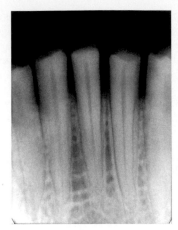

FIGURE 31-41 Physiologic wear or attrition is demonstrated on this periapical image of the mandibular incisors.

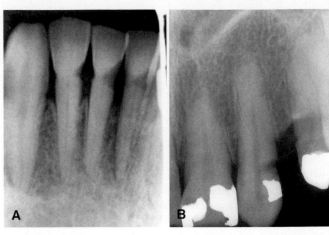

FIGURE 31-42 **A,** Abrasion of the cervical areas of these incisor teeth is evident from excessive (and improper) use of dental floss. Note the obliteration of the pulp chambers and reduction in size of the root canals. **B,** Abrasion on the distal aspect of the maxillary canine from a denture clasp.

Differential Diagnosis

Recognition of physiologic attrition is usually not difficult given the characteristic history, location, and extent of wear. The general pattern is predictable and familiar.

Management

Physiologic attrition does not generally require treatment unless the teeth become symptomatic or there is some cosmetic concern.

ABRASION

Abrasion is the nonphysiologic wearing of teeth in contact with foreign substances as a result of friction induced by factitious habits or occupational hazards. A history or clinical examination usually reveals the cause. Although many causes exist, two occur with moderate frequency and can usually be eliminated: (1) toothbrush injury and (2) dental floss injury. Other causes include pipe smoking, opening hairpins with the teeth, improper use of toothpicks, denture clasps, and cutting thread with the teeth.

Toothbrush Injury

Clinical Features. Toothbrush abrasion is probably the most frequently observed type of injury to the dental hard tissues. Improper "back-and-forth" movements of the toothbrush with heavy pressure cause the bristles to assume a wedge-shaped arrangement between the crowns and the gingiva. This improper brushing technique wears a V-shaped wedge or groove into the cervical area of the tooth, usually involving enamel and the softer root surface.

Abraded teeth may become sensitive as the dentin is exposed. The abraded areas are usually most severe at the cementoenamel junction on the labial and buccal surfaces of maxillary premolars, canines, and incisors, in approximately that order. The enamel generally limits the coronal extension of abrasion. The lesions are more common and more pronounced on the left side for a right-handed person, and vice versa. The deposition of secondary dentin opposite the abraded areas usually keeps pace with the destruction at the surface, so pulpal exposure is rarely a complication.

Imaging Features. The imaging appearance of toothbrush abrasion is radiolucent defects at the cervical level of teeth. These defects have well-defined semicircular or semilunar shapes with borders of increasing radiopacity. The pulp chambers of the more seriously involved teeth are frequently partially or completely

obliterated. The most common location of this injury is the premolar areas, usually in the upper arch.

Dental Floss Injury

Clinical Features. Excessive and improper use of dental floss, particularly in conjunction with toothpaste, may result in abrasion of the dentition (Fig. 31-42). The most frequent site is the cervical portion of the proximal surfaces just above the gingiva.

Imaging Features. The imaging appearance of dental floss abrasion is narrow semilunar radiolucency in the interproximal surfaces of the cervical area. Most often the radiolucent grooves on the distal surfaces of the teeth are deeper than the grooves on the mesial surfaces, probably because it is easier to exert more pressure in a forward direction by pulling than by pushing the floss backward into the mouth.

Differential Diagnosis. Dental floss abrasion is readily identified by its clinical and imaging appearances. Its location provides some evidence regarding the nature of the cause. This can be verified by the patient history. Occasionally, the radiolucencies simulate carious lesions located at the cervical region of the tooth. The differential diagnosis is accomplished with clinical inspection.

Management. The primary treatment recommended for abrasion is elimination of the causative agents or habits. Extensively abraded areas can be restored.

EROSION

Disease Mechanism

Erosion of teeth results from a chemical action not involving bacteria. Although in many cases the cause is not apparent, in others it is obviously the contact of acid with teeth. The source of the acid may be from chronic vomiting or acid reflux from gastrointestinal disorders or from a diet rich in acidic foods, citrus fruits, or carbonated beverages. Regurgitated acids attack lingual or palatal tooth surfaces, and dietary acids primarily demineralize labial surfaces. Some occupations involve contact with acids that can induce dental erosion. The location of the erosion, the pattern of eroded areas, and the appearance of the lesion usually provide clues regarding the origin of the decalcifying agent.

Clinical Features

Dental erosion is usually found on incisors, often involving multiple teeth. The lesions are generally smooth, glistening depressions in the enamel surface, frequently near the gingiva. Erosion may result in so much loss of enamel that a pink spot shows through the remaining enamel.

Imaging Features

Areas of erosion appear as radiolucent defects on the crown. Their margins may be either well defined or diffuse. A clinical examination usually resolves any questionable lesions.

Differential Diagnosis

The diagnosis of erosion is based on the recognition of dished-out or V-shaped defects in the buccal and labial enamel and the dentinal surfaces. The margins of a restoration may project above the remaining tooth surface. The edges of lesions caused by erosion are usually more rounded off compared with lesions caused by abrasion.

Management

As with abrasion, erosion is managed with identification and removal of the causative agent. If the cause is chronic vomiting from a psychological disorder, a daily fluoride rinse should be prescribed during counseling therapy. If the cause is unknown, management depends solely on restoration of the defect. Restoration prevents additional damage, possible pulp exposure, and objectionable esthetic appearance.

RESORPTION

Resorption is the removal of tooth structure by osteoclasts, referred to as odontoclasts when they are resorbing tooth structure. Resorption is classified as internal or external on the basis of the surface of the tooth being resorbed. External resorption affects the outer tooth surface, and internal resorption affects the inner surface of the pulp chamber and canal. These two types differ in their imaging appearance and treatment. The resorption discussed here is not that associated with the normal physiologic loss of deciduous teeth. Although the etiology of most resorptive lesions is unknown, at least presumptive evidence exists that some lesions are the sequelae of chronic infection (inflammation), excessive pressure and function, or factors associated with local tumors and cysts.

Internal Resorption

Disease Mechanism.   Internal resorption occurs within the pulp chamber or canal and involves resorption of the surrounding dentin. This resorption results in enlargement of the size of the pulp space at the expense of tooth structure. This condition may be transient and self-limiting or progressive. The etiology of the recruitment and activation of odontoclasts is unknown but may be related to inflammation of the pulpal tissues. Internal resorption has been reported to be initiated by acute trauma to the tooth, direct and indirect pulp capping, pulpotomy, and enamel invagination.

Clinical Features.   Internal resorption may affect any tooth in either the primary or the secondary dentition. It occurs most frequently in permanent teeth, usually in central incisors and first and second molars. The resorptive process most commonly begins during the fourth and fifth decades and is more common in men. When the lesion is in the pulp chamber of the crown, a radiolucent area may appear to envelope the crown. If the enlarging pulp perforates the dentin and the enamel becomes involved, the area may appear clinically as a pink spot. If the condition is not intercepted, it may perforate the crown, with hemorrhagic tissue projecting from the perforation, and lead to infectious pulpitis. When the lesion occurs in the root of a tooth, it is, for the most part, clinically silent. If resorption is extensive, it may weaken the tooth and result in fracture. It is also possible that the pulp may expand into the PDL and communicate with a deep periodontal pocket or the gingival sulcus, leading to pulpal infection.

Imaging Features.   Images can reveal symptomless early lesions of internal resorption. The lesions are localized; radiolucent; and round, oval, or elongated within the root or crown and are continuous with the image of the pulp chamber or root canal. These changes are now easily demonstrated using small field of view, high-resolution CBCT imaging. The outline is usually sharply defined and smooth or slightly scalloped. The result is an irregular widening of the pulp chamber or canal (Fig. 31-43). It is characteristically homogeneously radiolucent, without bony trabeculation or pulp stones. However, the internal structure may seem to be apparent if the surface of the resorbed tooth structure is very irregular and has a scalloped texture. In some cases, virtually the entire pulp may enlarge within a tooth, although more commonly the lesion remains localized.

Differential Diagnosis.   The most common lesions to be confused with internal root resorption are dental caries on the buccal or lingual surface of a tooth and external root resorption. Carious lesions have more diffuse margins than lesions caused by internal root resorption. Clinical inspection quickly reveals caries on the buccal or lingual surface of a tooth. Also, the mesial and distal surfaces of the pulp chamber and canal can usually be separated from the borders of the carious lesion. However, with internal root resorption, the image of the resorption cannot be separated from the pulp chamber or canal by altering the horizontal angulation of the x-ray beam.

Management.   The treatment for internal resorption depends on the condition of the tooth. If the process has not led to a serious weakening defect in the structure, endodontic treatment halts the resorption. If the expanding pulp has not structurally compromised the tooth but a perforation of the root has occurred, the perforated surface may be surgically exposed and retrofilled. If the tooth has been badly excavated and weakened by the resorption, extraction may be the only alternative.

External Resorption

Disease Mechanism.   In external resorption, odontoclasts resorb the outer surface of the tooth. This resorption most commonly involves the root surface but may also involve the crown of an unerupted tooth. The resorption may involve cementum and dentin and in some cases gradually extends to the pulp. Because the recruitment of odontoclasts requires an intact blood supply, only sections of the tooth with soft tissue coverage are susceptible to this resorption. This resorption may occur to a single tooth, multiple teeth, or, in rare cases, all of the dentition. In many cases, the etiology is unknown, but causes can be attributed in

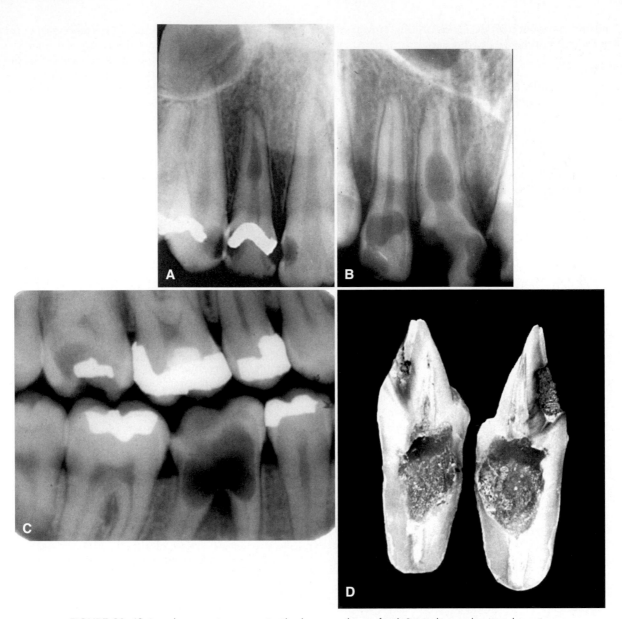

FIGURE 31-43 Internal root resorption may occur in either the crown or the root of teeth. Periapical images show internal resorption centered in the root canal system (**A** and **B**) and in both the crown and the roots (**C** and **D**) in a sectioned incisor (after crown reduction).

other cases to localized inflammatory lesions, reimplanted teeth, tumors and cysts, excessive mechanical and occlusal forces, and impacted teeth.

Clinical Features.
External resorption is usually not recognized because often no characteristic signs or symptoms exist. Even when considerable loss of tooth structure occurs, the tooth in question is frequently firm and immobile in the dental arch. In advanced resorption, some nonspecific pain or fracture of the resorbed root occurs.

External resorption may appear at the apex of the tooth or on the lateral root surface, although it most commonly occurs in the apical and cervical regions. It is slightly more prevalent in mandibular teeth than in maxillary teeth and involves primarily the central incisors, canines, and premolars. External root resorption is common. One study of men and women 18 to 25 years old found that all patients exhibited some degree of external root resorption in four or more teeth.

Imaging Features.
Common sites for external root resorption are the apical and cervical regions. When the lesion begins at the apex, it generally causes a smooth resorption of the tooth structure, resulting in blunting of the root apex (Fig. 31-44). Almost always the bone and lamina dura follow the resorbing root and exhibit a normal appearance around this shortened structure. When external root resorption occurs as the result of a periapical inflammatory lesion, the lamina dura is lost around the apex. After normal apexification (constriction of the walls of the pulp canal at the apex) of the pulp canal, it is very difficult or impossible to see the canal exit at the apex of the tooth. However, if resorption of the apical region has occurred, the pulp canal is visible and is abnormally wide at the apex (Fig. 31-45).

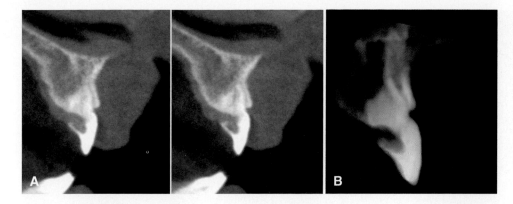

FIGURE 31-44 **A,** CBCT cross sections in the buccal and palatal plane demonstrate an area of external resorption affecting the palatal surface of the crown of a maxillary central incisor at the cementoenamel junction and proceeding internally into the tooth crown. **B,** Three-dimensional surface rendering of the maxillary central incisor shows the resorptive defect on the palatal aspect of the tooth.

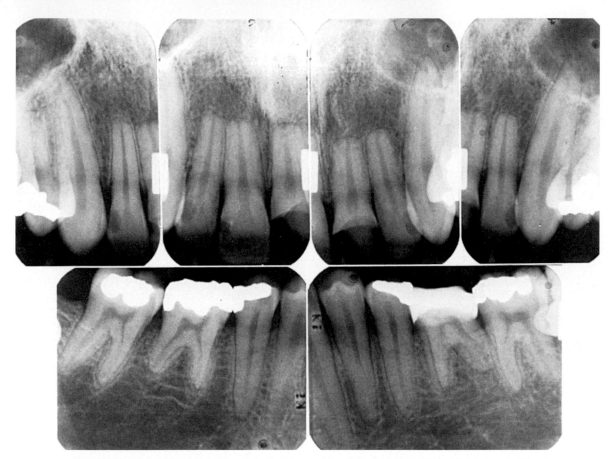

FIGURE 31-45 External root resorption results in a loss of tooth structure from the apex. Note the blunted root apices, the widened pulp root canals, and the intact lamina dura.

Occasionally, external root resorption involves the lateral aspects of roots (Fig. 31-46). Such lesions tend to be irregular, may involve one side more than the other, and occur in any tooth. A common cause of external resorption on the side of a root is the presence of an unerupted adjacent tooth. Examples of external root resorption include resorption of the distal aspect of the roots of an upper second molar by the crown of the adjacent third molar and resorption of the root of a permanent central or lateral incisor, or both, by an unerupted maxillary canine. External resorption of an entire tooth can occur when the tooth is unerupted and completely embedded in bone (Fig. 31-47), usually involving the maxillary canine or third molar. In such instances, the entire tooth, including the root and crown, may undergo resorption.

Differential Diagnosis. External root resorption on the apex or lateral surface of a root is easily visualized with imaging. When the lesion lies on the buccal or lingual surface of a root and above the level of the adjacent bone, the differential diagnosis includes caries and internal resorption. Internal resorption characteristically appears as an expansion of the pulp chamber or canal. In the case of external resorption, the image of the normal intact pulp chamber or canal may be traced through the radiolucent area of external resorption. Also, projections made at different angles can be compared. The location of the radiolucency caused by external root resorption moves with respect to the pulp canal, whereas the image of internal resorption remains fixed to the canal.

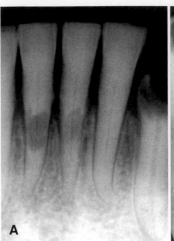
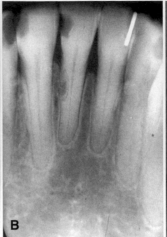
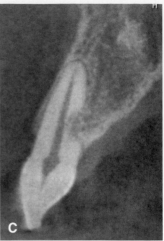

FIGURE 31-46 **A,** External root resorption of the lateral surface of the root of the mandibular central incisors. These are sharply defined radiolucencies confined to the root surfaces. **B,** The root has been replaced by an ingrowth of bone. This is sometimes referred to as inostosis. **C,** Sagittal CBCT image of external resorption of the palatal surface of the root of a central incisor with bone ingrowth into the defect.

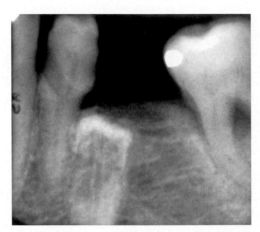

FIGURE 31-47 External resorption of an impacted second premolar. Although both enamel and dentin have been resorbed, the residual enamel of the crown can still be seen as well as a hint of a pulp chamber.

Management. When the cause of external root resorption is known, the treatment is usually to remove the etiologic factors. Treatment may involve cessation of excessive mechanical forces; removal of an adjacent impacted tooth; or eradication of a cyst, tumor, or source of inflammation. If the area of resorption is broad and on an accessible surface of the root (e.g., at the cervical location), curettage of the defect and the placement of a restoration usually stops the process.

SECONDARY DENTIN

Mechanism

Secondary dentin is dentin deposited in the pulp chamber after the formation of primary dentin has been completed. Secondary dentin deposition may be part of physiologic aging and may result from such innocuous stimuli as chewing or slight trauma. Secondary dentin also develops after long-term trauma from pathologic conditions such as moderately progressive caries, trauma, erosion, attrition, abrasion, or a dental restorative procedure. This specific stimulus promotes a more rapid and localized coronal response than that seen as a result of normal aging. The term tertiary dentin has been suggested to identify dentin specifically initiated by stimuli other than the normal aging response and normal biologic function.

Clinical Features

The response of odontoblasts in producing secondary dentin reduces the sensitivity of teeth to stimuli from the external environment. In elderly individuals with extensive secondary dentin formation, this reduced sensitivity may be especially pronounced. Similarly, the formation of an additional layer of dentin between the pulp and a region of insult reduces the sensitivity often felt by individuals with recent dental restorations or coronal fractures.

Imaging Features

Secondary dentin is indistinguishable from primary dentin on imaging. Its presence is manifested as a reduction in size of the normal pulp chamber and canals (Fig. 31-48). When secondary dentin formation results from the normal aging process, the result is a generalized reduction in pulp chamber and canal size, maintaining a relatively normal shape. Often there remains only a thin, narrow pulp chamber and canal. The pulp horns usually disappear relatively early, followed by a reduction in size of the pulp chamber and narrowing of the canals. When more specific stimuli initiate secondary dentin formation, it begins in the region adjacent to the source of stimuli and alters the normal shape of the pulp chamber. Although formation of secondary dentin may continue until the pulp appears to be completely obliterated, histologic studies show that even in these extreme cases a small thread of viable pulp tissue remains.

Differential Diagnosis

Secondary dentin is recognized indirectly by the reduction in size of the pulp chamber. This appearance differs from that of the pulp stone. The pulp stone (see the following description) simply occupies some pulp chamber or canal space, but it has a round-to-oval shape (conforming to the chamber).

Management

Secondary dentin per se does not require treatment. The precipitating cause is removed if possible, and the tooth is restored when appropriate.

PULP STONES

Mechanism

Pulp stones are foci of calcification in the dental pulp. They are probably apparent microscopically in more than half of teeth from

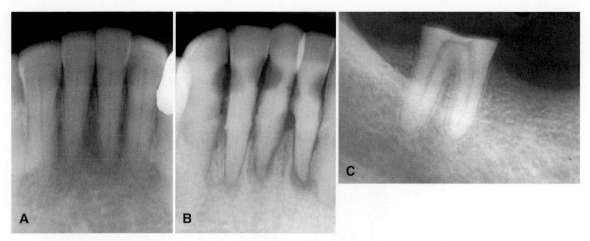

FIGURE 31-48 **A,** Normal formation of secondary dentin causes recession of the pulp chamber and narrowing of the root canals. **B,** Secondary dentin has obliterated the pulp chambers and narrowed the root canals. This is likely a result of the carious lesions. **C,** Secondary dentin formation has obliterated the pulp chamber stimulated by the severe attrition of the coronal aspect of this molar.

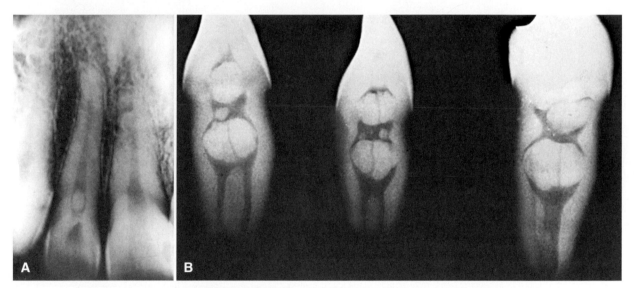

FIGURE 31-49 **A,** Pulp stones may be found as isolated calcifications in the pulp. **B,** When large, they may cause deformation of the pulp chamber and root canals.

young people and in almost all teeth from people older than 50 years. Although most are microscopic, they vary in size, with some 2 or 3 mm in diameter, almost filling the pulp chamber. Only these larger concretions can be visualized on imaging. Although the larger masses represent only 15% to 25% of pulpal calcification, they are a common imaging finding and may appear in a single tooth or several teeth. Their cause is unknown, and no firm evidence exists that they are associated with any systemic or pulpal disturbance.

Clinical Features

Pulp stones are not clinically discernible.

Imaging Features

The imaging appearance of pulp stones is quite variable. They may be seen as radiopaque structures within pulp chambers or root canals, or they may extend from the pulp chamber into the root canals (Fig. 31-49). No uniform shape or number exists. They may occur as a single dense mass or as several small radiopacities. They

may be round or oval, and some pulp stones that potentially occupy most of the pulp chamber conform to its shape. Their outline likewise varies from sharply defined to a more diffuse margin. They occur in all tooth types but most commonly in molars. In rare instances, the canal remodels and increases its girth to accommodate a large stone.

Differential Diagnosis

Although pulp stones are variable in size and form, their recognition is usually not difficult. However, in some cases, differentiation from pulpal sclerosis is difficult.

Management

Pulp stones do not require treatment.

PULPAL SCLEROSIS

Mechanism

Pulpal sclerosis is another form of calcification in the pulp chamber and canals of teeth. In contrast to pulp stones, pulpal

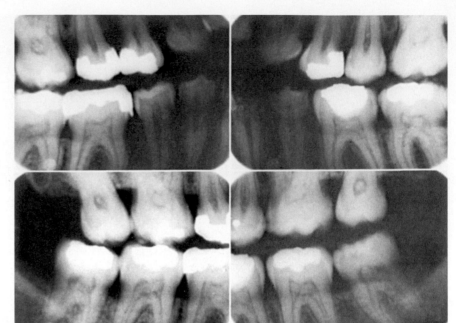

FIGURE 31-50 Pulpal sclerosis is seen as diffuse calcification of the pulp chamber and canals.

sclerosis is a diffuse process. Its specific cause is unknown, although its appearance correlates strongly with age. About 66% of all teeth in individuals 10 to 20 years old and 90% of all teeth in individuals 50 to 70 years old show histologic evidence of pulpal sclerosis. Histologically, the pattern of calcification is amorphous and unorganized, being evident as linear strands or columns of calcified material paralleling blood vessels and nerves in the pulp.

Clinical Features

Pulpal sclerosis is a clinically silent process without clinical manifestations.

Imaging Features

Early pulpal sclerosis, a degenerative process, is not demonstrable on imaging. Diffuse pulpal sclerosis produces a generalized, ill-defined collection of fine radiopacities throughout large areas of the pulp chamber and pulp canals (Fig. 31-50).

Differential Diagnosis

The differential diagnosis includes small pulp stones, but this differentiation is academic because neither pulpal sclerosis nor pulp stones require treatment.

Management

Pulpal sclerosis does not require treatment. As with pulp stones, its only importance may be that it can cause difficulty in the performance of endodontic therapy when such a procedure is indicated for other reasons.

HYPERCEMENTOSIS

Disease Mechanism

Hypercementosis is excessive deposition of cementum on the tooth roots. In most cases, its cause is unknown. Occasionally, it appears on a supraerupted tooth after the loss of an opposing tooth. Another cause of hypercementosis is inflammation, usually resulting from rarefying or sclerosing osteitis. In the context of

inflammation, cementum is deposited on the root surface adjacent to the apex. Hypercementosis occasionally has been associated with teeth that are in hyperocclusion or that have been fractured. Finally, hypercementosis occurs in patients with Paget's disease of bone (see Chapter 23) and with hyperpituitarism (gigantism and acromegaly).

Clinical Features

Hypercementosis does not cause any clinical signs or symptoms.

Imaging Features

Hypercementosis is evident on images as an excessive buildup of cementum around all or part of a root (Fig. 31-51). The outline is usually smooth but occasionally may be seen as an irregular but bulbous enlargement of the root. It is most evident at the apical end and is usually seen as a mildly irregular accumulation of cementum. This cementum is slightly more radiolucent than dentin. Of importance is the fact that the lamina dura and PDL space encompass the extra dentin. In the case of Paget's disease, the hypercementosis is usually very exuberant and irregular in outline.

Differential Diagnosis

The differential diagnosis may include any radiopaque structure that is seen within the vicinity of the root, such as a dense bone island or mature periapical osseous dysplasia. The differentiating characteristic is the presence of the periodontal membrane space around the hypercementosis. There may be a resemblance to a small cementoblastoma. Occasionally, a severely dilacerated root may have the appearance of hypercementosis.

Management

Hypercementosis requires no treatment. If a related condition, such as a periapical inflammatory lesion, exists, treatment may be necessary. The primary significance of hypercementosis may relate to the difficulty that the root configuration can pose if extraction is indicated.

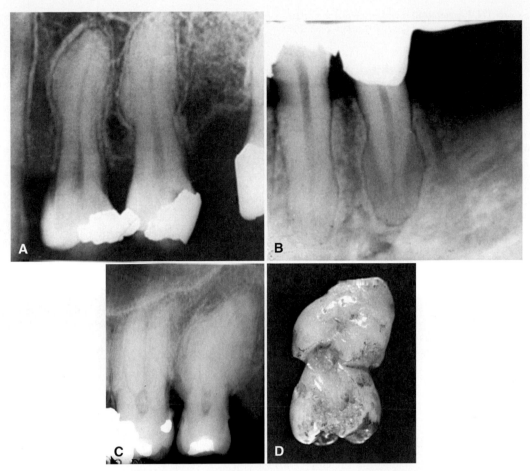

FIGURE 31-51 Hypercementosis of the roots. **A-C,** In all cases, note the continuity of the lamina dura and the PDL space that encompasses the extra cementum. **D,** An extracted molar exhibits extensive hypercementosis. *(Courtesy Dr. R. Kienholz, Dallas, TX.)*

BIBLIOGRAPHY

Developmental Abnormalities

Bergsma D, editor: *Birth defects compendium*, ed 2, New York, 1979, Alan R Liss.

Dixon GH, Stewart RE: Genetic aspects of anomalous tooth development. In Stewart RE, Prescott GH, editors: *Oral facial genetics*, St Louis, 1976, Mosby.

MacDougall M, Dong J, Acevedo AC: Molecular basis of human dentin diseases, *Am J Med Genet A* 140A:2536–2546, 2006.

Pindborg JJ: *Pathology of the dental hard tissues*, Copenhagen, 1970, Munksgaard.

Schulze C: Developmental abnormalities of the teeth and jaws. In Gorlin RJ, Goldman HM, editors: *Thoma's oral pathology*, ed 6, vol 1, St Louis, 1970, Mosby.

Witkop CJ Jr: Amelogenesis imperfecta, dentinogenesis imperfecta and dentin dysplasia revisited: problems with classification, *J Oral Pathol* 17:547–553, 1989.

Witkop CJ Jr, Rao S: Inherited defects in tooth structure. In Bergsma D, editor: *Birth defects, XI: orofacial structures*, vol 7, no 7, Baltimore, 1971, Williams & Wilkins.

Worth HM: *Principles and practice of oral radiologic interpretation*, Chicago, 1963, Year Book Medical.

Wright JT: The molecular etiologies and associated phenotypes of amelogenesis imperfecta, *Am J Med Genet A* 140A:2547–2555, 2006.

Supernumerary Teeth

Grahnen H, Lindahl B: Supernumerary teeth in the permanent dentition: a frequency study, *Odontol Rev* 12:290–294, 1961.

Grimanis GA, Kyriakides AT, Spyropoulos ND: A survey on supernumerary molars, *Quintessence Int* 22:989–995, 1991.

Niswander JD: Effects of heredity and environment on development of the dentition, *J Dent Res* 42:1288–1296, 1963.

Rao SR: Supernumerary teeth. In Bergsma D, editor: *Birth defects compendium*, ed 2, New York, 1979, Alan R Liss.

Yusof WZ: Non-syndrome multiple supernumerary teeth: literature review, *J Can Dent Assoc* 56:147–149, 1990.

Developmentally Missing Teeth

al-Emran S: Prevalence of hypodontia and developmental malformation of permanent teeth in Saudi Arabian school children, *Br J Orthod* 17:115–118, 1990.

Garn SM, Lewis AB: The relationship between third molar agenesis and reduction in tooth number, *Angle Orthod* 32:14–18, 1962.

Keene HJ: The relationship between third molar agenesis and the morphologic variability of the molar teeth, *Angle Orthod* 35:289–298, 1965.

Levin LS: Dental and oral abnormalities in selected ectodermal dysplasia syndromes, *Birth Defects Orig Artic Ser* 24:205–227, 1988.

O'Dowling IB, McNamara TG: Congenital absence of permanent teeth among Irish school-children, *J Ir Dent Assoc* 36:136–138, 1990.

Visioni AF, Lisboa-Costa TN, Pagnan NAB, et al: Ectodermal dysplasias: clinical and molecular review, *Am J Med Genet* 149A:1980–2002, 2009.

Macrodontia

Garn SM, Lewis AB, Kerewsky BS: The magnitude and implications of the relationship between tooth size and body size, *Arch Oral Biol* 13:129–131, 1968.

Transposition

Schacter H: A treated case of transposed upper canine, *Dent Rec (London)* 71:105–108, 1951.

Fusion

Hagman FT: Anomalies of form and number, fused primary teeth, a correlation of the dentitions, *ASDC J Dent Child* 55:359–361, 1988.

Sperber GH: Genetic mechanisms and anomalies in odontogenesis, *J Can Dent Assoc (Tor)* 33:433–442, 1967.

Gemination

Tannenbaum KA, Alling EE: Anomalous tooth development: case report of gemination and twinning, *Oral Surg Oral Med Oral Pathol* 16:883–887, 1963.

Taurodontism

Bixler D: Heritable disorders affecting dentin. In Steward RE, Prescott GA, editors: *Oral facial genetics*, St Louis, 1976, Mosby.

Dens in Dente

Oehlers FA: The radicular variety of dens invaginatus, *Oral Surg Oral Med Oral Pathol* 11:1251–1260, 1958.

Rushton MA: A collection of dilated composite odontomes, *Br Dent J* 63:65–86, 1937.

Soames JV, Kuyebi TA: A radicular dens invaginatus, *Br Dent J* 152:308–309, 1982.

Dens Invaginatus

Oehlers FA, Lee KW, Lee EC: Dens invaginatus (invaginated odontome): its structure and responses to external stimuli, *Dent Pract Dent Rec* 17:239–244, 1967.

Sykaras SN: Occlusal anomalous tubercle on premolars of a Greek girl, *Oral Surg Oral Med Oral Pathol* 38:88–91, 1974.

Yip WK: The prevalence of dens invaginatus, *Oral Surg Oral Med Oral Pathol* 38:80–87, 1974.

Amelogenesis Imperfecta

Bailleul-Forestier I, Molla M, Verloes A, et al: The genetic basis of inherited anomalies of the teeth. Part 1: clinical and molecular aspects of non-syndromic dental disorders, *Eur J Med Genet* 51:273–291, 2008.

Wright JT: The molecular etiologies and associated phenotypes of amelogenesis imperfecta, *Am J Med Genet A* 140:2547–2555, 2006.

Dentinogenesis Imperfecta and Dentin Dysplasia

Kim JW, Simmer JP: Hereditary dentin defects, *J Dent Res* 86:292–299, 2007.

MacDougall M, Dong J, Acevedo AC: Molecular basis of human dentin diseases, *Am J Med Genet A* 140:2536–2546, 2006.

O'Carroll MK, Duncan WK, Perkins TM: Dentin dysplasia: review of the literature and a proposed subclassification based on imaging findings, *Oral Surg Oral Med Oral Pathol* 72:119–125, 1991.

Regional Odontodysplasia

Crawford PJ, Aldred MJ: Regional odontodysplasia: a bibliography, *J Oral Pathol Med* 18:251–263, 1989.

Enamel Pearl

Moskow BS, Canut PM: Studies on root enamel, II: enamel pearls: a review of their morphology, localization, nomenclature, occurrence, classification, histogenesis, and incidence, *J Clin Periodontol* 17:275–281, 1990.

Talon Cusp

Meskin LH, Gorlin RJ: Agenesis and peg-shaped permanent lateral incisors, *J Dent Res* 42:1476–1479, 1963.

Natkin E, Pitts DL, Worthington P: A case of talon cusp associated with other odontogenic abnormalities, *J Endod* 9:491–495, 1983.

Turner's Hypoplasia

Via WF Jr: Enamel defects induced by trauma during tooth formation, *Oral Surg Oral Med Oral Pathol* 25:49–54, 1968.

Congenital Syphilis

Bradlaw RV: The dental stigmata of prenatal syphilis, *Oral Surg Oral Med Oral Pathol* 6:147–158, 1953.

Putkonen T: Dental changes in congenital syphilis: relationship to other syphilitic stigmata, *Acta Derm Venereol* 42:44–62, 1962.

Sarnat BG, Shaw NG: Dental development in congenital syphilis, *Am J Orthod* 29:270, 1943.

Acquired Abnormalities

Baden E: Environmental pathology of the teeth. In Gorlin RJ, Goodman HM, editors: *Thoma's oral pathology*, ed 6, vol 1, St Louis, 1970, Mosby.

Mitchell DF, Standish SM, Fast TB: *Oral diagnosis/oral medicine*, Philadelphia, 1978, Lea & Febiger.

Pindborg JJ: *Pathology of the dental hard tissues*, Philadelphia, 1970, Saunders.

Shafer WG, Hine MK, Levy BM: *Oral pathology*, ed 4, Philadelphia, 1983, Saunders.

Attrition

Johnson GK, Sivers JE: Attrition, abrasion, and erosion: diagnosis and therapy, *Clin Prev Dent* 9:12–16, 1987.

Murphy TR: Reduction of the dental arch by approximal attrition: quantitative assessment, *Br Dent J* 116:483–488, 1964.

Russell MD: The distinction between physiological and pathological attrition: a review, *J Ir Dent Assoc* 33:23–31, 1987.

Seligman DA, Pullinger AG, Solberg WK: The prevalence of dental attrition and its association with factors of age, gender, occlusion, and TMJ symptomatology, *J Dent Res* 67:1323–1333, 1988.

Abrasion

Bull WH, Callender RM, Pugh BR, et al: The abrasion and cleaning properties of dentifrices, *Br Dent J* 125:331, 1968.

Erwin JC, Buchner CM: Prevalence of tooth root exposure and abrasion among dental patients, *Dent Items Interest* 66:760, 1944.

Erosion

Stafne EC, Lovestedt SA: Dissolution of tooth substance by lemon juice, acid beverages, and acid from some other sources, *J Am Dent Assoc* 34:586–592, 1947.

ten Bruggen Cate HJ: Dental erosion in industry, *Br J Ind Med* 25:249, 1968.

Resorption

Bakland LK: Root resorption, *Dent Clin North Am* 36:491–507, 1992.

Bennett CG, Poleway SA: Internal resorption, postpulpotomy type, *Oral Surg* 17:228–234, 1964.

Goldman HM: Spontaneous intermittent resorption of teeth, *J Am Dent Assoc* 49:522–532, 1954.

Massler M, Perreault JG: Root resorption in the permanent teeth of young adults, *J Dent Child* 21:158–164, 1954.

Phillips JR: Apical root resorption under orthodontic therapy, *Angle Orthod* 20:1–22, 1955.

Simpson HE: Internal resorption, *J Can Dent Assoc* 30:355, 1964.

Solomon CS, Notaro PJ, Kellert M: External root resorption: fact or fancy, *J Endod* 15:219–223, 1989.

Stafne EC, Austin LT: Resorption of embedded teeth, *J Am Dent Assoc* 32:1003–1009, 1945.

Tronstad L: Root resorption: etiology, terminology, and clinical manifestations, *Endod Dent Traumatol* 4:241–252, 1988.

Secondary Dentin

Kuttler Y: Classification of dentine into primary, secondary and tertiary, *Oral Surg Oral Med Oral Pathol* 12:966–969, 1959.

Pulp Stones

Moss-Salentijn L, Hendricks-Klyvert M: Calcified structures in human dental pulps, *J Endod* 14:184–189, 1988.

32

Craniofacial Anomalies

Carol Anne Murdoch-Kinch

OUTLINE

Developmental disturbances can affect the normal growth and differentiation of craniofacial structures. As a consequence, they are usually first discovered in infancy or childhood. Many of the conditions discussed in this chapter have an unknown etiology. Some are caused by known and recently discovered genetic mutations, whereas others result from environmental factors. These conditions result in a variety of abnormalities of the face and jaws, including abnormalities of structure, shape, organization, and function of hard and soft tissues. A multitude of conditions affect the morphogenesis of the face and jaws, many of which are rare syndromes. This chapter briefly reviews more common developmental abnormalities that may be encountered in dental practice.

CLEFT LIP AND PALATE

DISEASE MECHANISM

A failure of fusion of the developmental processes of the face during fetal development may result in a variety of facial clefts. Cleft lip and cleft palate are the most common developmental craniofacial anomalies. Their incidence varies with geographic location, ethnicity, and socioeconomic status. In white populations, the incidence of cleft lip is 1:800 to 1:1000 live births, and the incidence of cleft palate is approximately 1:1000. Cleft lip with or without cleft palate (CL/P) and cleft palate are two different conditions with different etiologies. CL/P results from a failure of fusion of the medial nasal process with the maxillary process. This condition can range in severity from a unilateral cleft lip to bilateral complete clefting through the lip, alveolus, and hard and soft palate in the most severe cases. Cleft palate develops from a failure of fusion of the lateral palatal shelves. The minimal manifestation of cleft palate is a submucous cleft in which the palate appears to be intact except for notching of the uvula (bifid uvula) or notching in the posterior border of the hard palate detectable by palpation. The most severe presentation is complete clefting of the hard and soft palate. The precise etiology of orofacial clefting is not completely understood. However, most cases of CL/P and cleft palate are considered to be multifactorial with a strong genetic component. CL/P and cleft palate each can be associated with other abnormalities, as part of a genetic malformation syndrome, such as 22q.11 deletion syndrome (velocardiofacial syndrome—cleft palate and facial and cardiac abnormalities) or van der Woude syndrome (cleft lip or cleft palate or both and lip pits). Other factors that are implicated in the development of orofacial clefts include nutritional disturbances (prenatal folate deficiency); environmental teratogenic agents (maternal smoking, in utero exposure to anticonvulsants); stress, which results in increased secretion of hydrocortisone; defects of vascular supply to the involved region; and mechanical interference with the fusion of the embryonic processes (cleft palate in Pierre Robin sequence). Clefts involving the lower lip and mandible are extremely rare.

CLINICAL FEATURES

The frequency of CL/P and cleft palate varies with gender and race, but in general CL/P is more common in males, whereas cleft palate is more common in females. Both conditions are more common in Asians and Hispanics than African Americans or Caucasians. The severity of CL/P varies from a notch in the upper lip, to a cleft involving only the lip, to extension into the nostril resulting in deformity of the ala of the nose. As CL/P increases in severity, the cleft includes the alveolar process and palate. Bilateral cleft lip is more frequently associated with cleft palate. Cleft palate also varies in severity, ranging from involvement of only the uvula or soft palate to extension all the way through the palate to include the alveolar process in the region of the lateral incisor on one or both sides. With involvement of the alveolar process, there is an increase in frequency of dental anomalies in the region of the cleft, including missing, hypoplastic, and supernumerary teeth and enamel hypoplasia. Dental anomalies are also more prevalent in the mandible in these patients. In both CL/P and cleft palate, the palatal defects interfere with speech and swallowing. Affected individuals with palatal clefts are also at increased risk for recurrent middle ear infections because of the abnormal anatomy and function of the eustachian tube.

IMAGING FEATURES

The typical imaging appearance is a well-defined vertical radiolucent defect in the alveolar bone and numerous associated dental anomalies (Figs. 32-1 and 32-2). These anomalies may include the absence of the maxillary lateral incisor and the presence of supernumerary teeth in this region. The involved teeth often are malformed and poorly positioned. In patients with cleft lip and palate,

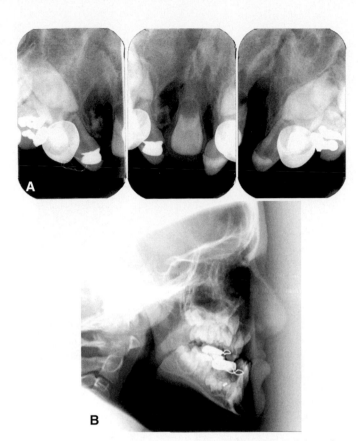

FIGURE 32-1 Cleft lip/palate results in defects in the alveolar ridge and abnormalities of the dentition. **A,** Bilateral clefts of the maxilla in the lateral incisor regions and defects of the dentition. **B,** Lateral cephalometric view shows underdevelopment of the maxilla.

DISEASE MECHANISM

Crouzon syndrome is an autosomal dominant skeletal dysplasia characterized by variable expressivity and almost complete penetrance. It is one of many diseases characterized by premature craniosynostosis (closure of cranial sutures). Its incidence is estimated at 1:25,000 births. Of these cases, 33% to 56% may arise as a consequence of spontaneous mutations, with the remaining being familial. Crouzon syndrome is caused by a mutation in fibroblast growth factor receptor II on chromosome 10. Mutations at this site are also responsible for other craniosynostosis syndromes with similar facial features but clinically visible limb abnormalities. In patients with Crouzon syndrome, the coronal suture usually closes first, and eventually all cranial sutures close early. There is also premature fusion of the synchondroses of the cranial base. The subsequent lack of bone growth perpendicular to the synchondroses and cranial coronal sutures produces the characteristic cranial shape and facial features.

CLINICAL FEATURES

Patients characteristically have brachycephaly (short skull front to back), hypertelorism (increased distance between eyes), and orbital proptosis (protruding eyes) (Fig. 32-3, *A* and *B*). In familial cases, the minimal criteria for diagnosis are hypertelorism and orbital proptosis. Patients may become blind as a result of early suture closure and increased intracranial pressure. The nose often appears prominent and pointed because the maxilla is narrow and short in a vertical and anteroposterior dimension. The anterior nasal spine is hypoplastic and retruded, failing to provide adequate support to the soft tissue of the nose. The palatal vault is high, and the maxillary arch is narrow and retruded, resulting in crowding of the dentition.

IMAGING FEATURES

The earliest radiographic signs of cranial suture synostosis are sclerosis and overlapping edges. Sutures that normally should look radiolucent on the skull film are not detectable or show sclerotic changes. Rarely, the facial features may manifest before evidence of sutural synostosis. Premature fusion of the cranial base leads to diminished facial growth. In some cases, prominent cranial markings are noted, which are also seen in normal growing patients, but are more prominent because of an increase in intracranial pressure from the growing brain. These markings may be seen as multiple radiolucencies appearing as depressions (so-called digital impressions) of the inner surface of the cranial vault, which results in a beaten metal appearance (Fig. 32-3, *C-E*).

In the jaws, the lack of growth in an anteroposterior direction at the cranial base results in maxillary hypoplasia, creating a class III malocclusion in some patients. The maxillary hypoplasia contributes to the characteristic orbital proptosis because the maxilla forms part of the inferior orbital rim and, if severely hypoplastic, fails to support the orbital contents adequately. The mandible is typically smaller than normal but appears prognathic in relation to the severely hypoplastic maxilla.

DIFFERENTIAL DIAGNOSIS

Premature craniosynostosis, either isolated or as part of a genetic syndrome, is a common disorder. The incidence of Crouzon syndrome is reported to range from 1:2100 to 1:2500 births. Other causes of craniosynostosis must be differentiated from Crouzon syndrome, including other syndromic forms of

there may be a mild delay in the development of maxillary and mandibular teeth and an increased incidence of hypodontia in both arches. The osseous defect may extend to include the floor of the nasal cavity. In patients with a repaired cleft, a well-defined osseous defect may not be apparent but only a vertically short alveolar process at the cleft site.

MANAGEMENT

Management of CL/P and cleft palate is complex, requiring the coordinated efforts of a multidisciplinary team known as a cleft palate/craniofacial anomalies team. This team usually includes a plastic and reconstructive surgeon; oral and maxillofacial surgeon; ear, nose, and throat surgeon; orthodontist; dentist; speech therapist; psychologist; nutritionist; and social worker. Clefts of the palate are usually surgically repaired within the first year of life, whereas clefts of the lip are usually repaired within the first 3 months to aid in feeding and maternal-infant bonding. The bone in the cleft site is often augmented with bone grafting before replacement of missing teeth with either fixed or removable prosthodontics or dental implants. Orthodontic treatment is usually necessary to recreate a normal arch form and functional occlusion.

CROUZON SYNDROME

SYNONYMS

Synonyms for Crouzon syndrome include craniofacial dysostosis, syndromic craniosynostosis, and premature craniosynostosis.

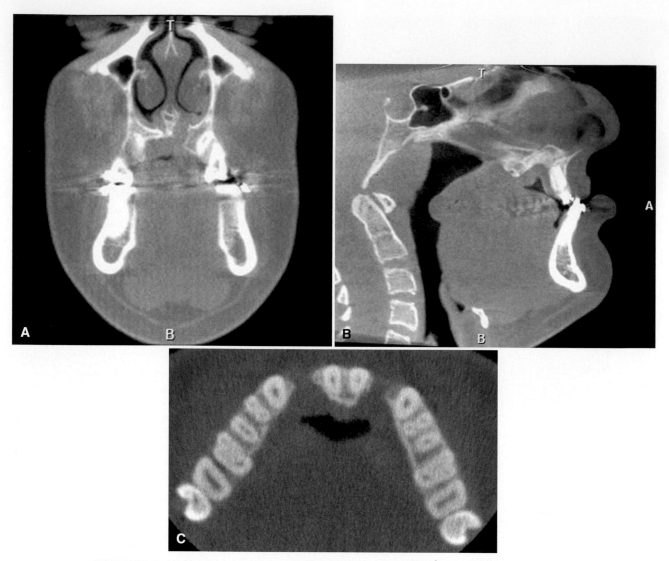

FIGURE 32-2 Cone-beam CT images of a patient with left unilateral cleft lip/palate. **A,** Coronal view. Note the discontinuity in the nasal floor visible on the patient's left side. **B,** Sagittal view of the same patient shows maxillary hypoplasia and deficient palatal anatomy. **C,** Axial cone-beam CT image of a different patient with bilateral clefts shows bilateral defects in the maxillary alveolar process. *(A and B, Courtesy Dr. Sean Edwards, Department of Oral and Maxillofacial Surgery, University of Michigan, Ann Arbor, MI.)*

craniosynostosis and nonsyndromic coronal craniosynostosis. The characteristic facial features must be present to suggest Crouzon syndrome.

MANAGEMENT

The craniofacial features of Crouzon syndrome worsen over time because of the abnormal craniofacial growth. Early diagnosis permits surgical and orthodontic treatment from infancy through adolescence, coordinated by a cleft palate/craniofacial anomalies team. The objectives of these treatments are to allow normal brain growth and development by preventing increased intracranial pressure, protect the eyes by providing adequate bony support, and improve facial esthetics and occlusal function. Because of early diagnosis and improvements in medical and dental care, most patients have normal intelligence and good functional outcomes and can expect a normal life span.

HEMIFACIAL MICROSOMIA

SYNONYMS

Synonyms for hemifacial microsomia include hemifacial hypoplasia, craniofacial microsomia, lateral facial dysplasia, Goldenhar syndrome, and oculoauriculovertebral dysplasia (OAV) spectrum.

DISEASE MECHANISM

Hemifacial microsomia is the second most common developmental craniofacial anomaly after cleft lip and palate and affects approximately 1:56,000 live births. Hemifacial microsomia is a feature of Goldenhar syndrome. This syndrome can also include a broader array of anomalies within the oculoauriculovertebral dysplasia (OAV) complex. Patients with hemifacial microsomia typically display reduced growth and development of half of the face owing to abnormal development of the first and second

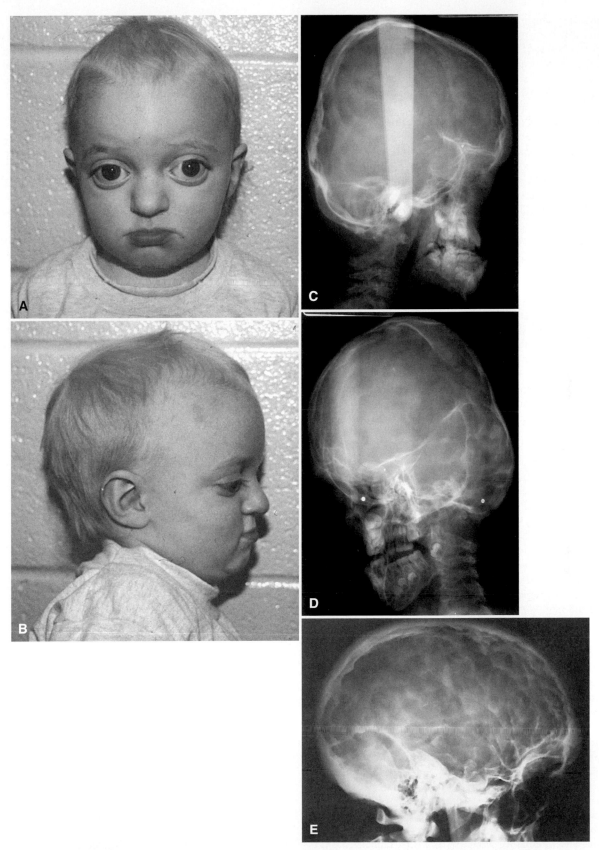

FIGURE 32-3 **A** and **B,** Characteristic facial features of Crouzon syndrome in this 2-year-old boy include orbital proptosis, hypertelorism, and midfacial hypoplasia. Rarely, these facial features may precede the radiographic features of sutural synostosis. **C,** Crouzon syndrome results in early closure of the cranial sutures and depressions (digital impressions) on the inner surface of the calvaria from growth of the brain. **D** and **E,** Closure of the cranial sutures in another patient. Note also the prominent digital markings. (**D** and **E,** Courtesy Department of Radiology, Baylor University Hospital, Dallas, TX.)

branchial arches. This malformation sequence is usually unilateral but occasionally may involve both sides (craniofacial microsomia). When the whole side of the face is involved, the mandible, maxilla, zygoma, external and middle ear, hyoid bone, parotid gland, vertebrae, fifth and seventh cranial nerves, musculature, and other soft tissues are diminished in size and sometimes fail to develop. Delayed dental eruption and hypodontia on the affected side also have been reported. Most cases occur spontaneously, but familial cases demonstrating autosomal dominant inheritance have been reported. There is a male predominance of 3:2 and a right-side predominance of 3:2. Cases have been reported with epibulbar dermoids, preauricular skin appendages, and preauricular fistulas; additional vertebral anomalies; and cardiac, cerebral, and renal malformations (Goldenhar syndrome and OAV complex). Genetic mutations at chromosome 14q32 and microdeletions at 22q11 have been associated with some cases of Goldenhar syndrome; however, in most cases, a clear genetic cause is not found.

CLINICAL FEATURES

Hemifacial microsomia is usually apparent at birth. Patients with this condition have a striking appearance caused by progressive failure of the affected side to grow, which gives the involved side of the face a reduced dimension. In addition, aplasia or hypoplasia of the external ear (microtia) is common, and the ear canal is often missing. In some patients, the skull is diminished in size. In about 90% of cases, there is malocclusion on the affected side. The midsagittal plane of the patient's face is curved toward the affected side. The occlusal plane often is canted up to the affected side.

IMAGING FEATURES

The primary radiographic finding is a reduction in the size of the bones on the affected side. This change is clearest in the mandible, which may show a reduction in the size of or, in severe cases, lack of any development of the condyle, coronoid process, or ramus. The body is reduced in size, and a portion of the distal aspect may be missing (Fig. 32-4). The dentition on the affected side may show a reduction in the number or size of the teeth. Multidetector computed tomographic (MDCT) examination shows a reduction in the size of the muscles of mastication and muscles of facial expression and hypoplasia or atresia of the auditory canal and ossicles of the middle ear. The course of the facial nerve is often shown to be abnormal on MDCT examination of the temporal bone. Magnetic resonance imaging (MRI) can also be useful in demonstrating the extent of inner ear abnormalities and involvement of the facial nerve and other soft tissues of the mouth and eyes. Thin section MDCT imaging of the temporal bone is often performed to assess the degrees of stenosis of the external auditory meatus and middle and inner ear malformations to plan treatment, including the use of cochlear implants, bone-anchored hearing aids, or implant-retained ear prostheses. This imaging is particularly important for patients with Goldenhar syndrome and the broader OAV complex. A multimodality approach to imaging can be optimal, including panoramic images to demonstrate dental development, cephalometric images and cone-beam CT (CBCT) imaging to assess the facial asymmetry and plan orthodontic treatment, two-dimensional CT imaging of the temporal bones to assess the external and internal ear anatomy, and three-dimensional CT imaging for surgical treatment planning.

DIFFERENTIAL DIAGNOSIS

The features of hemifacial microsomia are characteristic. Condylar hypoplasia, especially caused by a fracture at birth or by juvenile arthrosis (Boering's arthrosis), may be similar, but it does not produce the ear changes. Exposure of the face of a child to radiation therapy during growth also may result in underdevelopment of the irradiated tissues. In progressive hemifacial atrophy (Parry-Romberg syndrome), the changes become more severe over time but are generally not present at birth, and the ears are normal.

MANAGEMENT

The mandibular abnormalities may be corrected by conventional orthognathic surgery or distraction osteogenesis to lengthen the ramus on the affected side. Orthodontic intervention may correct or prevent malocclusion. The ear abnormalities may be repaired by plastic surgery or corrected with prosthetic ears, and the hearing loss may be partly corrected by hearing aids, such as bone-anchored hearing aids. In bilateral cases with profound hearing loss (Goldenhar syndrome and OAV complex), cochlear implants may be used to correct severe hearing loss.

TREACHER COLLINS SYNDROME

SYNONYM

Mandibulofacial dysostosis is a synonym for Treacher Collins syndrome.

DISEASE MECHANISM

Treacher Collins syndrome is an autosomal dominant disorder of craniofacial development. It is the most common type of mandibulofacial dysostosis, with an incidence of 1:50,000. Treacher Collins syndrome has variable expressivity and complete penetrance. Approximately half of cases arise as the result of sporadic mutation; the rest are familial. Treacher Collins syndrome is caused by a mutation in the *TCOF1* gene on chromosome 5.

CLINICAL FEATURES

Individuals with Treacher Collins syndrome have a wide range of anomalies, depending on the severity of the condition. The most common clinical findings are relative underdevelopment or absence of the zygomatic bones, resulting in a small narrow face; a downward inclination of the palpebral fissures; underdevelopment of the mandible, resulting in a down-turned, wide mouth; malformation of the external ears; absence of the external auditory canal; and occasional facial clefts (Fig. 32-5, *A* and *B*). The palate develops with a high arch or cleft in 30% of cases. Hypoplasia of the mandible and a steep mandibular angle results in an Angle class II anterior open bite malocclusion. Hypoplasia or atresia of the external ear, auditory canal, and ossicles of the middle ear may result in partial or complete deafness.

IMAGING FEATURES

A striking finding is the hypoplastic or missing zygomatic bones, and hypoplasia of the lateral aspects of the orbits. The auditory canal, mastoid air cells, and articular eminence often are smaller than normal or absent. The maxilla and especially the mandible are hypoplastic, showing accentuation of the antegonial notch and a steep mandibular angle, which gives the impression that the body of the mandible is bending in an inferior and posterior direction (Fig. 32-5, *C-F*). The ramus is especially short. The condyles are positioned posteriorly and inferiorly. The maxillary sinuses may be underdeveloped or absent. Cervical spine anomalies have also been reported in 18% of patients with Treacher Collins syndrome, including spina bifida occulta, dysmorphic C1,

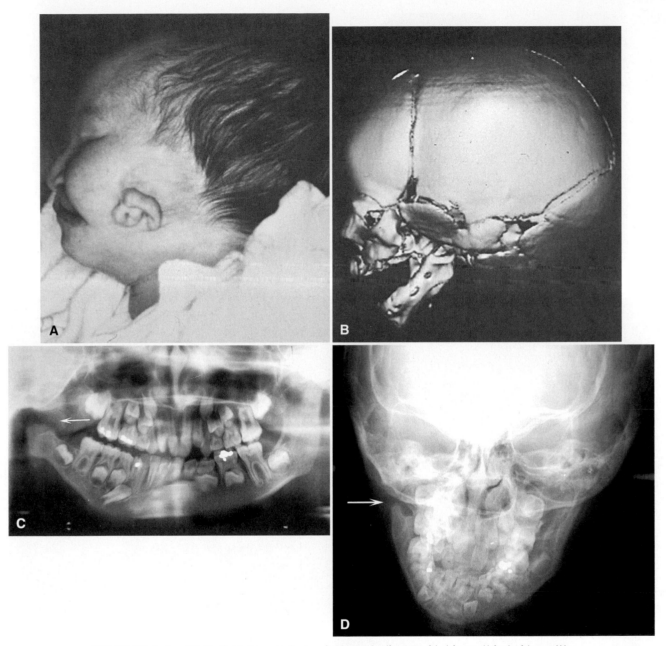

FIGURE 32-4 **A** and **B,** Hemifacial microsomia, showing reduced size and malformation of the left ear and left side of the mandible. **A,** Clinical photograph of an infant with hemifacial microsomia. **B,** Three-dimensional CT image of the affected side shows the extent of the bony malformation. Note the complete absence of the temporomandibular joint and coronoid process as well as auditory canal atresia. **C** and **D,** Panoramic image **(C)** and posteroanterior skull view **(D)** of other cases show lack of development of the ramus, coronoid process, and condyle *(arrows)*. (**A** and **B,** *Courtesy Dr. Arlene Rozzelle, Children's Hospital of Michigan, Detroit, MI.*)

and reduced C2-C3 space. In one case series, five of seven patients with cervical spine anomalies also had cleft palate. This finding suggests that patients with Treacher Collins syndrome and cleft palate may be at higher risk for cervical spine anomalies and should be targeted for assessment. A more recent study has also reported dysplasia or aplasia of major salivary glands, as detected by ultrasound imaging, in half of patients with Treacher Collins syndrome followed at a major craniofacial anomalies center. This finding is important because these salivary gland anomalies could significantly increase risk for dental caries in patients with Treacher Collins syndrome.

DIFFERENTIAL DIAGNOSIS

Other disorders that may result in severe hypoplasia of the entire mandible include condylar agenesis, Hallermann-Streiff syndrome, Nager syndrome, and Pierre Robin sequence, which can be a part of several other genetic syndromes or an isolated anomaly.

Management

Comprehensive treatment of patients with Treacher Collins syndrome is optimally provided by a multidisciplinary cleft palate/craniofacial anomalies team. Growth of the facial bones during

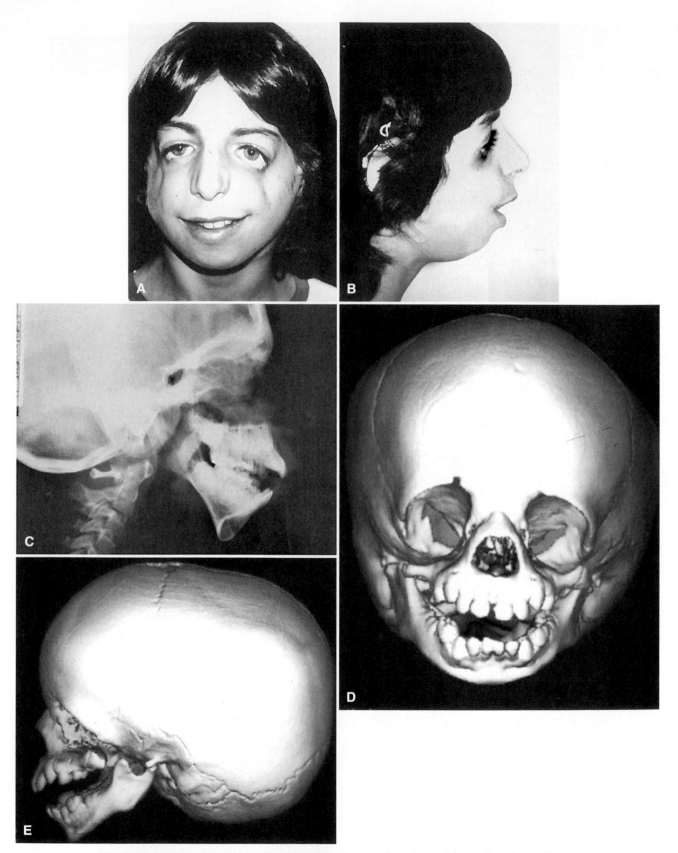

FIGURE 32-5 Treacher Collins syndrome. **A** and **B,** Note the characteristic facies: downward-sloping palpebral fissures, colobomas of the outer third of the lower lids, depressed cheekbones, receding chin, little if any nasofrontal angle, and a nose that appears relatively large. **C,** Correlation of radiographic features with clinical features: short mandibular rami, steep mandibular angle, and anterior open bite. The zygomas are poorly formed. **D** and **E,** Three-dimensional CT images of young child with Treacher Collins syndrome show the extent of the bony abnormalities, including bilateral auditory canal atresia, aplasia of the zygomatic arch, and hypoplasia of the mandibular ramus with characteristic "curved" shape of the mandibular body and pronounced antegonial notching.

adolescence may result in some cosmetic improvement. Surgical intervention, including bilateral distraction osteogenesis of the mandible, may improve the osseous defects. Treatment of the external ear defects may involve plastic and reconstructive surgery or prostheses or both. Hearing aids or cochlear implants may be used to treat the hearing loss, depending on the severity. Coordinated orthodontics and orthognathic surgery are often used to treat malocclusion and improve function and esthetics.

CLEIDOCRANIAL DYSPLASIA

SYNONYM

Cleidocranial dysostosis is a synonym for cleidocranial dysplasia.

DISEASE MECHANISM

Cleidocranial dysplasia is an autosomal dominant malformation syndrome affecting bones and teeth; it affects both sexes equally. The prevalence is estimated at 1.1 million. It can be inherited or arise as a result of sporadic mutation. Cleidocranial dysplasia is caused by a mutation in the *Runx2* gene on chromosome 6. This gene codes for an osteoblast-specific transcription factor. It has variable expressivity and almost complete penetrance.

CLINICAL FEATURES

Although the disease affects the entire skeleton, cleidocranial dysplasia primarily affects the skull, clavicles, and dentition. Affected individuals have been shown to be of shorter stature than unaffected relatives but not short enough for this to be considered a form of dwarfism. The face appears small in contrast to the cranium because of hypoplasia of the maxilla and a brachycephalic skull (reduced anteroposterior dimension with increased skull width) and the presence of frontal and parietal bossing. The paranasal sinuses may be underdeveloped. There is delayed closure of the cranial sutures, and the fontanels may remain patent years beyond the normal time of closure. The bridge of the nose may be broad and depressed, with hypertelorism (excessive distance between the eyes). The complete absence (aplasia) or reduced size (hypoplasia) of the clavicles allows excessive mobility of the shoulder girdle (Fig. 32-6, *A* and *B*).

The dental abnormalities produce most of the morbidity associated with cleidocranial dysplasia and are often the reason for diagnosis in mildly affected individuals. Characteristically, patients with this disease show prolonged retention of the primary dentition and delayed eruption of the permanent dentition. Extraction of primary teeth does not adequately stimulate eruption of underlying permanent teeth. A study of teeth from patients with cleidocranial dysplasia revealed a paucity or complete absence of cellular cementum on both erupted and unerupted teeth. Often unerupted supernumerary teeth are present, and considerable crowding and disorganization of the developing permanent dentition may occur. The number of supernumerary teeth has been correlated with a reduction in skeletal height in these patients.

IMAGING FEATURES

The characteristic skull findings are brachycephaly, delayed or failed closure of the fontanels, open skull sutures including a persistent metopic open suture, and multiple wormian bones (small, irregular bones in the sutures of the skull that are formed by secondary centers of ossification in the suture lines) (Figs. 32-6, *C-G*, and 32-7). In the most severe cases, very little formation of the parietal and frontal bones may occur. Typically, the clavicles are underdeveloped to varying degrees, and they are completely absent in approximately 10% of cases. Other bones also may be affected, including the long bones, vertebral column, pelvis, and bones of the hands and feet.

In the jaws, the maxilla and paranasal sinuses characteristically are underdeveloped, resulting in maxillary micrognathia. The mandible is usually normal in size. A patent (open) mandibular symphysis has been reported in 3% of adults and 64% of children. Several investigators have described the alveolar bone overlying unerupted teeth as being denser than usual, with a coarse trabecular pattern in the mandible. This finding correlates to the histologic findings of decreased resorption and multiple reversal lines, and it may account for the delayed eruption in teeth not mechanically obstructed by supernumerary and other unerupted teeth.

Characteristically, there is prolonged retention of the primary dentition and multiple unerupted permanent and supernumerary teeth (Fig. 32-8, *A* and *B*). The number of supernumerary teeth varies; 63 in one individual have been reported. The unerupted teeth develop most commonly in the anterior maxilla and premolar regions of the jaws. Many resemble premolars, and these unerupted teeth may develop dentigerous cysts. The supernumerary teeth develop, on average, 4 years later than the corresponding normal teeth. Because of this delayed development, it has been proposed that the supernumerary teeth represent a third dentition.

DIFFERENTIAL DIAGNOSIS

Cleidocranial dysplasia may be identified by the family history, excessive mobility of the shoulders, clinical examination of the skull, and pathognomonic radiographic findings of prolonged retention of the primary teeth with multiple unerupted supernumerary teeth. Other conditions associated with multiple unerupted and supernumerary teeth, such as Gardner's syndrome and pyknodysostosis, must be considered in the differential diagnosis.

MANAGEMENT

In cleidocranial dysplasia, dental care should include the removal of primary and supernumerary teeth to improve the possibility of spontaneous eruption of the permanent teeth. The bone overlying the normal permanent teeth should be removed to expose the crown when half of the root is formed to aid their eruption. Autotransplantation of teeth has been shown to be a successful strategy to treat older patients. Ideally, patients should be identified early, before age 5 years, to take advantage of combined orthodontic and surgical treatment. Prosthodontic rehabilitation with dental implants has been used in some cases. Patients should be monitored for development of distal molars and cysts until late adolescence. Surgical treatment of the bony defects of the skull is often performed to address esthetic concerns. In those cases, three-dimensional CT imaging is used to visualize the size and thickness of such defects and plan for harvesting of bone graft material from other parts of the skull (see Fig. 32-7, *A-C*).

HEMIFACIAL HYPERPLASIA

SYNONYMS

Hemifacial hypertrophy and hemihyperplasia are synonyms for hemifacial hyperplasia.

DISEASE MECHANISM

Hemifacial hyperplasia is a condition in which half of the face, including the maxilla alone or with the mandible or in concert with other parts of the body, grows to unusual proportions. The

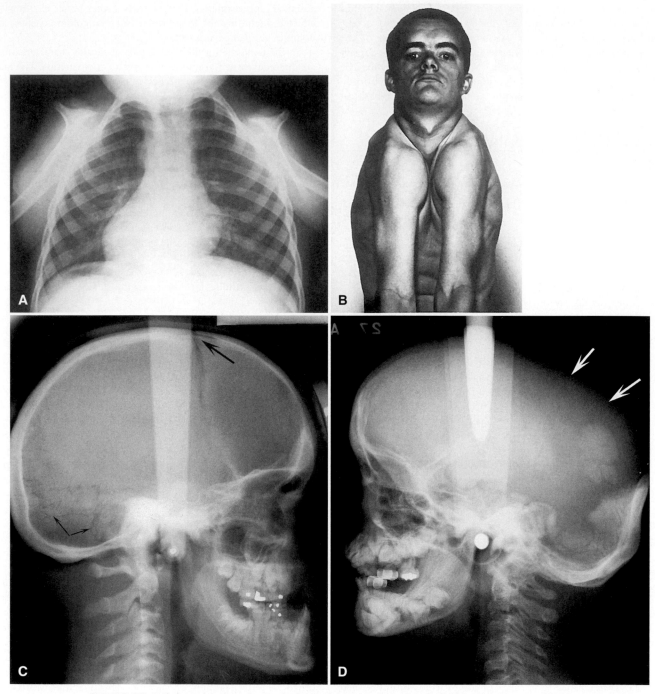

FIGURE 32-6 Cleidocranial dysplasia. **A,** Note the absence of clavicles on chest radiograph. **B,** The result is excessive mobility of the shoulders. Note also the frontal bossing and underdeveloped maxilla. **C,** Lateral radiograph shows the wormian (sutural) bones in the occipital region *(small arrows)* and the open fontanel *(large arrow).* **D,** Lateral skull film shows a lack of development of the parietal bones *(arrows).*

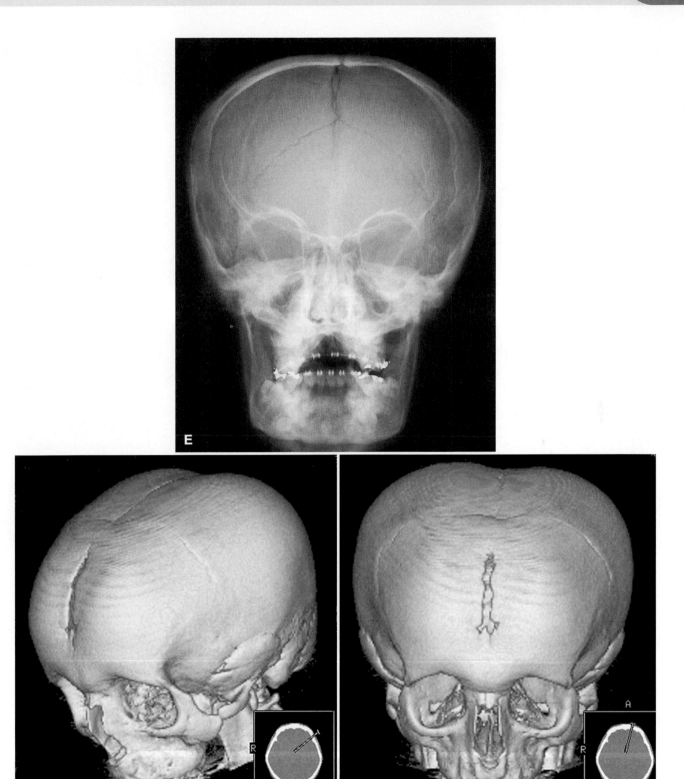

FIGURE 32-6, cont'd **E,** Posteroanterior skull film. Brachycephaly results in a light bulb–like shape to the silhouette of the skull and mandible. **F,** Three-dimensional reconstruction of a CT study with oblique orientation shows the typical skull shape seen in this condition. Note the parietal and frontal bossing and open metopic suture in this 18-year-old man. **G,** Direct frontal view of same three-dimensional reconstruction shows the light-bulb shape of the skull and the open metopic suture. (*A, Courtesy Department of Radiology, Baylor University Hospital, Dallas, TX.*)

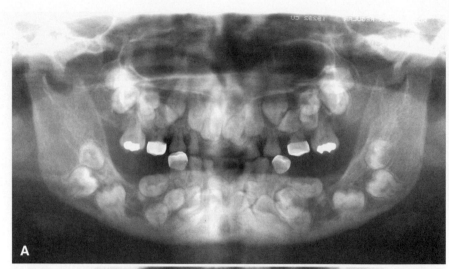

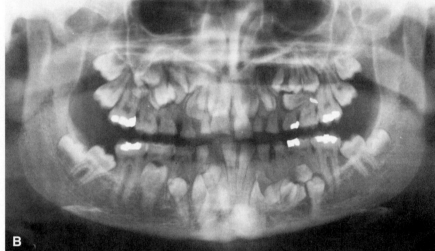

FIGURE 32-7 **A** and **B,** Panoramic images of cleidocranial dysplasia. Note the prolonged retention of the primary dentition and multiple unerupted supernumerary teeth and lack of normal coronoid notches. **C,** Axial CT image of the mandible demonstrates multiple unerupted teeth. This type of imaging can be used to localize the unerupted teeth to assist in treatment planning of extractions and orthodontic tooth movement. *(Courtesy Dr. Sean Edwards, Department of Oral and Maxillofacial Surgery, University of Michigan, Ann Arbor, MI.)*

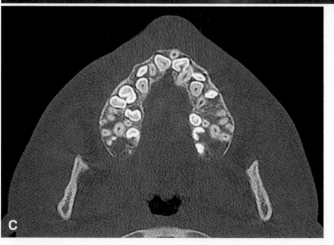

cause of this condition is unknown. Some cases are associated with genetic diseases, such as Beckwith-Wiedemann syndrome.

CLINICAL FEATURES

Hemifacial hyperplasia begins at birth and usually continues throughout the growing years. In some cases, it may not be recognized at birth but becomes more apparent with growth. It often occurs with other abnormalities, including mental deficiency, skin abnormalities, compensatory scoliosis, genitourinary tract anomalies, and various neoplasms, including Wilms' tumor of the kidney, adrenocortical tumor, and hepatoblastoma (Beckwith-Wiedemann syndrome). Females and males are affected with approximately equal frequency. The dentition of affected individuals may show unilateral enlargement, accelerated development, and premature loss of primary teeth. The tongue and alveolar bone enlarge on the involved side.

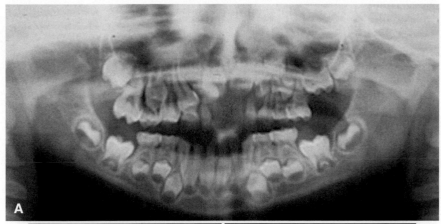

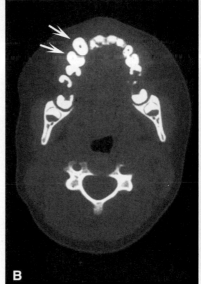

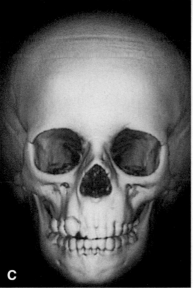

FIGURE 32-8 Hemifacial hyperplasia, revealing enlargement of the right maxilla only. **A,** Panoramic radiograph shows accelerated dental development limited to the right maxilla in a 5-year-old boy. **B,** CT axial image using bone algorithm of the same patient demonstrates enlargement of the maxillary cuspid and first bicuspid *(arrows)* compared with the contralateral side. **C,** three-dimensional CT scan shows subtle bony enlargement of the right maxilla and the right cuspid.

IMAGING FEATURES

Radiologic examination of the skulls of patients reveals enlargement of the bones on the affected side, including the mandible (see Fig. 32-8), maxilla, zygoma, and frontal and temporal bones. A few cases have been reported involving only one side of the maxilla or one side of the mandible.

DIFFERENTIAL DIAGNOSIS

The differential diagnosis should consider hemifacial hypoplasia of the opposite side, arteriovenous aneurysms, hemangioma, and congenital lymphedema. Also, severe condylar hyperplasia that may involve half of the mandible should be considered. The presence of enlarged teeth together with rapid eruption of the dentition suggests hemifacial hyperplasia. Cases limited to one side of the maxilla must be differentiated from monostotic fibrous dysplasia and segmental odontomaxillary dysplasia, both of which have characteristic changes in the radiographic appearance of the alveolar bone, not present in hemifacial hyperplasia.

MANAGEMENT

An insufficient number of cases of hemifacial hyperplasia with long-term follow-up have been reported to make definitive recommendations for treatment. Although most cases are isolated,

a child with suspected hemifacial hyperplasia should be referred to a medical geneticist for diagnosis and early detection of one of several genetic syndromes that can be associated with this condition.

SEGMENTAL ODONTOMAXILLARY DYSPLASIA

SYNONYM

A synonym for segmental odontomaxillary dysplasia is hemimaxillofacial dysplasia.

DISEASE MECHANISM

Segmental odontomaxillary dysplasia is a developmental abnormality of unknown etiology that affects the posterior alveolar process of one side of the maxilla, including the teeth and attached gingiva.

CLINICAL FEATURES

The abnormality is always unilateral and results in enlargement of the alveolar process, with or without enlargement of the gingiva, and dental anomalies. Teeth frequently are missing (most commonly the premolars), or hypoplastic, and some of the teeth that remain are unerupted. Ipsilateral hypertrichosis and other skin anomalies, including closely packed sebaceous glands in the upper lip, hyperpigmentation, hypopigmentation, Becker's nevus, and clefting, have also been reported in 23% of cases. Mild facial enlargement has also been reported in a few cases. Most cases are detected in childhood because a parent notices the lack of tooth eruption or mild facial asymmetry, or the dentist notices missing premolars on diagnostic images.

IMAGING FEATURES

The density of the maxillary alveolar process is increased, with a greater number of thick trabeculae that appear to be aligned in a vertical orientation (Fig. 32-9). There have been some reports of missing buccal cortical plate, but this is not a consistent feature.

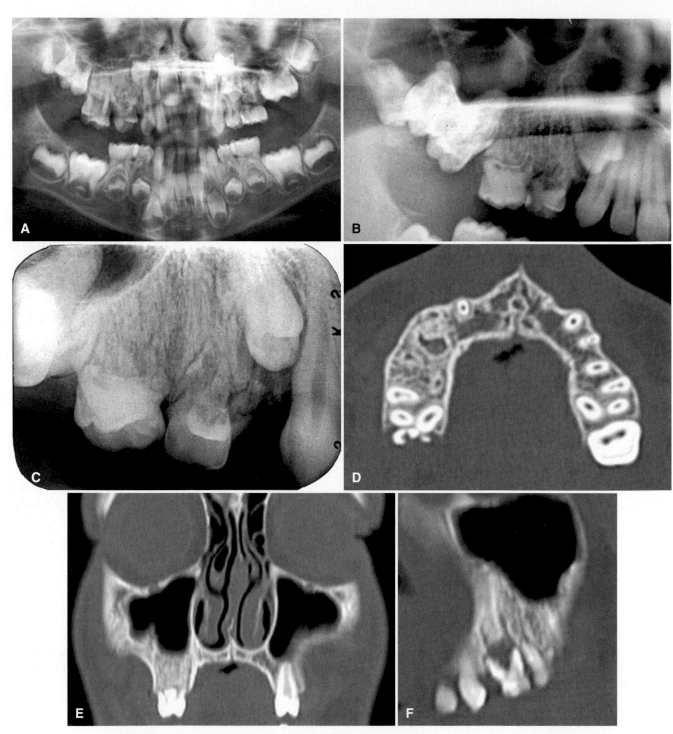

FIGURE 32-9 **A,** Panoramic view of segmental odontomaxillary dysplasia. Note the large left maxillary deciduous molars compared with the right side and the lack of formation of the bicuspids, delayed eruption of the first molar, and the dense bone pattern of the left maxillary alveolar process. **B** and **C,** A second case demonstrating the coarse trabecular pattern of the right maxillary alveolar process and delayed eruption of the maxillary right first bicuspid and molars. **D-F,** Cone-beam CT images of another case involving the right maxilla. **D,** Axial image shows an increase in internal bone density within the right maxilla. **E,** Coronal image shows increase in width of the alveolar process. **F,** Multiple vertical radiolucent linear structures, which likely represent nutrient canals.

The roots of the deciduous teeth are larger than on the unaffected side and usually are splayed in shape. The crowns of the deciduous teeth and sometimes the permanent teeth are enlarged. Enlargement of pulp chambers and irregular resorption of the roots of deciduous teeth also may be seen. The alveolar process is not pneumatized by the maxillary sinus and appears smaller than on the contralateral side. There is often delayed eruption of the first and second permanent molars.

DIFFERENTIAL DIAGNOSIS

Other conditions that must be differentiated from segmental odontomaxillary dysplasia include segmental hemifacial hyperplasia, monostotic fibrous dysplasia, and regional odontodysplasia. Hemifacial hyperplasia is not associated with coarse vertically oriented trabeculae in the bone; monostotic fibrous dysplasia is not typically associated with missing teeth and, in contrast to segmental odontomaxillary dysplasia, will continue to show disproportionate growth of the affected side, and regional odontodysplasia typically is associated with ghost teeth and is not associated with expansion and alteration in trabecular pattern in the alveolar bone.

LINGUAL SALIVARY GLAND DEPRESSION

SYNONYMS

Synonyms for lingual salivary gland depression include lingual mandibular bone depression, developmental salivary gland defect, Stafne defect, Stafne bone cyst, static bone cavity, and latent bone cyst.

DISEASE MECHANISM

Lingual mandibular bone depressions represent a group of concavities in the lingual surface of the mandible, where the depression is lined with an intact outer cortex. Historically, they were referred to as pseudocysts because they resemble cysts radiographically, but they are not true cysts because no epithelial lining is present. The most common location is within the submandibular gland fossa and often close to the inferior border of the mandible. This lingual posterior variant of these depressions was first described by Stafne in 1942. This well-defined deep depression is thought to result from or be associated with growth of the salivary gland adjacent to the lingual surface of the mandible. Similar defects have also been described in the anterior region near the apical region of the bicuspids, associated with the sublingual glands (lingual anterior variant) and very rarely on the medial surface of the ascending ramus, associated with the parotid gland (medial ramus variant). In lingual posterior variant developmental bone defects investigated surgically, an aberrant lobe of the submandibular gland has been described to extend into the bony depression; however, CT imaging of some of these defects reveals fat tissue and no evidence of gland. The etiology remains unknown, but the condition is a developmental anomaly that has been documented to develop in patients ranging in age from 11 to 30 years. These defects may continue to grow slowly in size.

CLINICAL FEATURES

Although lingual mandibular bone depressions appear to be rare, with an incidence of lingual posterior variant of about 0.10% to 0.48%, it is likely that many go unreported. The incidence of lingual anterior variant is even less at 0.009%. Lingual mandibular bone depressions are asymptomatic and next to impossible to palpate and generally discovered only incidentally during radiographic examination of the area. In a review of a large number of cases, males were affected more than females with a predominance of 6.1:1, and peak incidence was in the fifth and sixth decades.

IMAGING FEATURES

A lingual mandibular bone depression is a well-defined round, ovoid, or occasionally lobulated radiolucency that ranges in diameter from 1 to 3 cm (Fig. 32-10). The lingual posterior defect is located below the inferior alveolar nerve canal and anterior to the angle of mandible, in the region of the antegonial notch and submandibular gland fossa. Rare lingual anterior variant examples are located in the apical region of the mandibular premolars or cuspids and are related to the sublingual gland fossa, above the mylohyoid muscle. The margins of the radiolucent defect are well defined by a dense sclerotic radiopaque margin of variable width, which is usually thicker on the superior aspect. This appearance is the result of the x-rays passing tangentially through the relatively thick walls of the depression. This cortical outline is often less distinct in the lingual anterior variant. The lingual posterior defect may involve the inferior border of the mandible. MDCT images reportedly reveal tissue of fat density within the defect (Fig. 32-11), or in some cases there is continuity of the tissue within the defect with the adjacent salivary gland.

DIFFERENTIAL DIAGNOSIS

The appearance and location of the radiographic image of this developmental bone defect are characteristic and easily identified. Lingual mandibular bone depressions can be readily differentiated from odontogenic lesions such as cysts because the epicenter of odontogenic lesions is located above the inferior alveolar canal. However, when the defect is related to the sublingual gland and appears above the canal, odontogenic lesions should be considered in the differential diagnosis.

MANAGEMENT

Recognition of the lesion should preclude any treatment or surgical exploration or the need for advanced imaging such as CT imaging. The defect may increase in size with time. There are rare reports of salivary gland neoplasms developing in the soft tissue within the defect. Destruction of the well defined cortex of the defect may indicate the presence of a neoplasm.

FOCAL OSTEOPOROTIC BONE MARROW

SYNONYM

A synonym for focal osteoporotic bone marrow is marrow space.

DISEASE MECHANISM

Focal osteoporotic bone marrow is a radiologic term indicating the presence of radiolucent defects within the cancellous portion of the jaws. Histologic examination reveals normal areas of hematopoietic or fatty marrow. The etiology is unknown but has been postulated to be: (1) bone marrow hyperplasia; (2) persistent embryologic marrow remnants; or (3) sites of abnormal healing after extraction, trauma, or local inflammation. This entity is a variation of normal anatomy.

CLINICAL FEATURES

Focal osteoporotic bone marrow defects are usually clinically asymptomatic and are commonly an incidental radiographic finding. These marrow spaces are more common in middle-aged women.

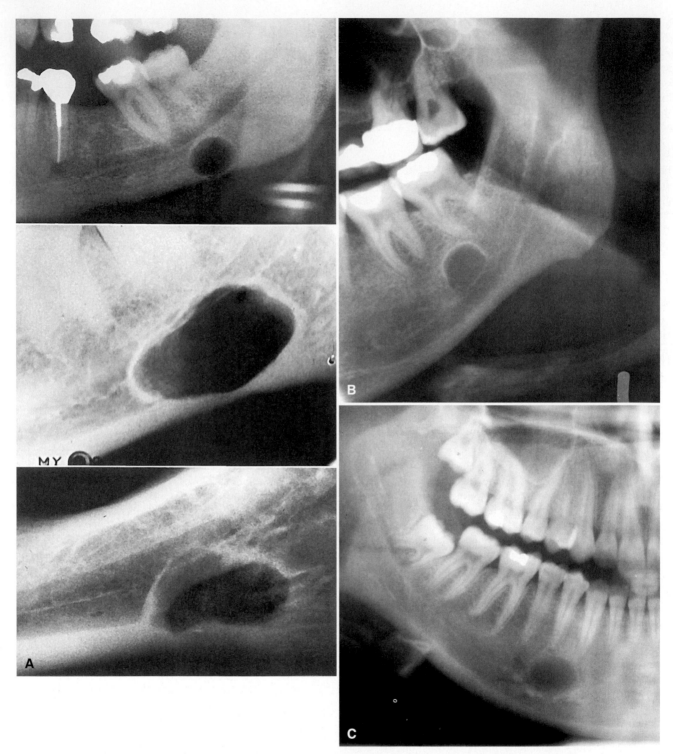

FIGURE 32-10 **A-C,** Lingual mandibular bone depressions of the posterior variant usually are seen as sharply defined radiolucencies beneath the mandibular canal in the region of the submandibular gland fossa. These defects can erode the inferior border of the mandible. Image in **B** is an unusual variant with a superior position above the inferior alveolar canal. Image in **C** represents an anterior variant within the sublingual gland fossa.

IMAGING FEATURES

A common site for focal osteoporotic bone marrow is the mandibular molar-premolar region. Other sites include the maxillary tuberosity region, mandibular retromolar area, edentulous locations, occasionally the furcation region of mandibular molars, and rarely near the apex of teeth. The radiographic appearance of focal osteoporotic bone marrow space is quite variable. The internal aspect is radiolucent because of the presence of fewer trabeculae compared with the surrounding bone. The periphery may be ill-defined and blending or may appear to be corticated. The immediate surrounding bone is normal without any sign of a bone reaction (Fig. 32-12).

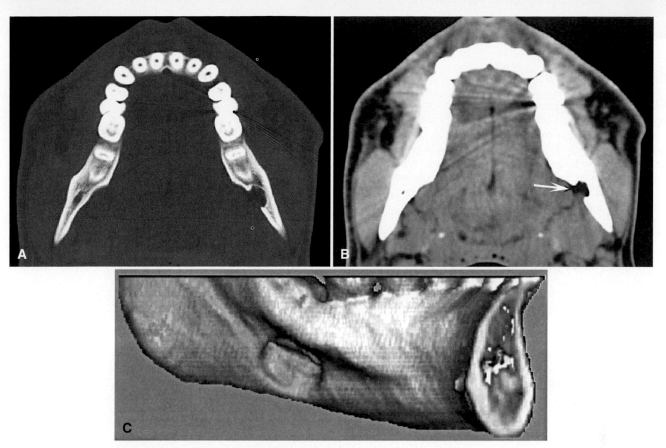

FIGURE 32-11 CT scans of lingual mandibular bone depressions, posterior variant. **A** and **B,** Axial bone and soft tissue windows of the same case. Note the well-defined defect extending from the medial surface of the mandible and the corresponding soft tissue image, which shows radiolucent tissue within the defect that has the density equivalent of fat tissue (*arrow* in **B**). **C,** Three-dimensional, reformatted CT image revealing a defect extending from the medial surface of the mandible.

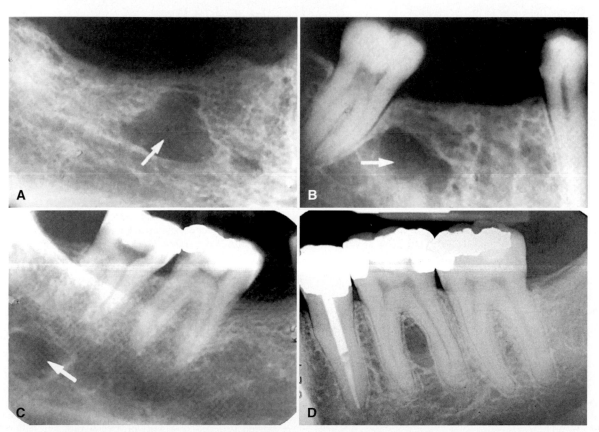

FIGURE 32-12 **A-C,** Focal osteoporotic bone marrow defect, seen as a radiolucency (*arrow*). A few internal trabeculae may be present, and the periphery varies from well defined to ill defined. **D,** Example located in the furcation of a mandibular first molar. The periodontal ligament space and lamina dura are intact.

DIFFERENTIAL DIAGNOSIS

A small simple bone cyst may have a similar appearance because there is usually no bone reaction at the periphery of a simple bone cyst. When the osteoporotic bone marrow occurs in the furcation region or at the apex of a tooth, the differential diagnosis includes the presence of an inflammatory lesion. If the area is normal bone marrow, the lamina dura should be intact. Very early inflammatory lesions that have not yet stimulated a visible osteoblastic response may appear similar.

MANAGEMENT

No treatment is required for osteoporotic bone marrow space. Prior radiographs of the region should always be obtained if available. When doubt exists about the true nature of the radiolucency, a longitudinal study with films at 3-month intervals may be prescribed. The marrow space should not increase in size.

BIBLIOGRAPHY

Cohen MM Jr, McLean RE: *Craniosynostosis: diagnosis, evaluation, and management*, ed 2, New York, 2000, Oxford University Press.

Gorlin RJ, Cohen MM Jr, Hennekam RCM: *Syndromes of the head and neck*, ed 4, New York, 2001, Oxford University Press.

Neville BW, Damm DD, Allen CM, et al: *Oral and maxillofacial pathology*, ed 2, Philadelphia, 2002, Saunders.

Worth HM: *Principles and practice of oral radiologic interpretation*, Chicago, 1963, Year Book Medical.

Cleft Lip and Cleft Palate

Habel A, Sell D, Mars M, et al: Management of cleft lip and palate, *Arch Dis Child* 74:360, 1996.

Harris EF, Hullings JG: Delayed dental development in children with isolated cleft lip and palate, *Arch Oral Biol* 35:469, 1990.

Hibbert SA, Field JK: Molecular basis of familial cleft lip and palate, *Oral Dis* 2:238, 1996.

Honein MA, Rasmussen SA, Reefhuis J, et al: Maternal and environmental tobacco smoke exposure and the risk of orofacial clefts, *Epidemiology* 18:226–233, 2007.

Shapira Y, Lubit E, Kuftinec MM: Hypodontia in children with various types of clefts, *Angle Orthod* 70:16–21, 2000.

Wyszynski DF, Beaty TH, Maestri NE, et al: Genetics of nonsyndromic oral clefts revisited, *Cleft Palate Craniofac J* 33:406, 1996.

Crouzon Syndrome

Murdoch-Kinch CA, Bixler D, Ward RE: Cephalometric analysis of families with dominantly inherited Crouzon syndrome: an aid to diagnosis in family studies, *Am J Med Genet* 77:405–411, 1998.

Tuite GF, Evanson J, Chong WK, et al: The beaten copper cranium: a correlation between intracranial pressure, cranial radiographs, and computed tomographic scans in children with craniosynostosis, *Neurosurgery* 39:691–699, 1996.

Hemifacial Microsomia

al-Haddidi A, Cevidanes LHS, Mol A, et al: Comparison of two methods for quantitative assessment of mandibular asymmetry using cone beam computed tomography image volumes, *Dentomaxillofac Radiol* 40:351–357, 2011.

Johnson JM, Moonis G, Green GE, et al: Syndromes of the first and second branchial arches, part 2: syndromes, *AJNR Am J Neuroradiol* 32:230–237, 2011.

Maruko E, Hayes C, Evans CA, et al: Hypodontia in hemifacial microsomia, *Cleft Palate Craniofac J* 38:15–19, 2001.

Monahan R, Seder K, Patel P, et al: Hemifacial microsomia: etiology, diagnosis and treatment, *J Am Dent Assoc* 132:1402–1408, 2001.

Senggen E, Laswed T, Meuwly J-Y, et al: First and second branchial arch syndromes: multimodality approach, *Pediatr Radiol* 41:549–561, 2011.

Treacher Collins Syndrome

Osterhus IN, Skogedal N, Akre H, et al: Salivary gland pathology as a new finding in Treacher Collins syndrome, *Am J Med Genet Part A* 158A:1320–1325, 2012.

Posnick JC: Treacher Collins syndrome: perspectives in evaluation and treatment, *J Oral Maxillofac Surg* 55:1120, 1997.

Pun AH-Y, Clark BE, David DJ, et al: Cervical spine in Treacher Collins syndrome, *J Craniofac Surg* 23:218–220, 2012.

Cleidocranial Dysplasia

Dalessandri D, Laffranchi L, Tonni I, et al: Advantages of cone beam computed tomography (CBCT) in the orthodontic treatment planning of cleidocranial dysplasia patients: a case report, *Head Face Med* 7:6, 2011.

Golan I, Baumert U, Hrala BP, et al: Dentomaxillofacial variability of cleidocranial dysplasia: clinicoradiological presentation and systematic review, *Dentomaxillofac Radiol* 32:347–354, 2003.

McGuire TP, Gomes PP, Lam DK, et al: Cranioplasty for midline metopic suture defects in adults with cleidocranial dysplasia, *Oral Surg Oral Med Oral Pathol Oral Radiol Endod* 103:175–179, 2007.

Seow WK, Hertzberg J: Dental development and molar root length in children with cleidocranial dysplasia, *Pediatr Dent* 17:101–105, 1995.

Yoshida T, Kanegane H, Osata M, et al: Functional analysis of RUNX2 mutations in Japanese patients with cleidocranial dysplasia demonstrates novel genotype-phenotype correlations, *Am J Hum Genet* 71:724–738, 2002.

Hemifacial Hyperplasia

Fraumeni JF, Geiser CF, Manning MD, et al: Wilms' tumor and congenital hemihypertrophy: report of five new cases and review of the literature, *Pediatrics* 40:886, 1967.

Hoyme HE, Seaver LH, Procopio F, et al: Isolated hemihyperplasia (hemihypertrophy): report of a prospective multicenter study of the incidence of neoplasia and review, *Am J Med Genet* 79:274–278, 1998.

Kogon SL, Jarvis AM, Daley TD, et al: Hemifacial hypertrophy affecting the maxillary dentition: report of a case, *Oral Surg Oral Med Oral Pathol* 58:549–553, 1984.

Segmental Odontomaxillary Dysplasia

Danforth RA, Melrose RJ, Abrams AM, et al: Segmental odontomaxillary dysplasia: report of eight cases and comparison with hemimaxillofacial dysplasia, *Oral Surg Oral Med Oral Pathol* 70:81, 1990.

Miles DA, Lovas JL, Clhen MM, et al: Hemimaxillofacial dysplasia: a newly recognized disorder of facial asymmetry, hypertrichosis of the facial skin, unilateral enlargement of the maxilla, and hypoplastic teeth in two patients, *Oral Surg Oral Med Oral Pathol* 64:445, 1987.

Minett CP, Daley TD: Hemimaxillofacial dysplasia segmental odontomaxillary dysplasia): case study with 11 years of follow-up from primary to adult dentition, *J Oral Maxillofac Surg* 70:1183–1191, 2012.

Packota GV Pharoah MJ, Petrikowski CG, et al: Radiographic features of segmental odontomaxillary dysplasia: a study of 12 cases, *Oral Surg Oral Med Oral Pathol Oral Radiol Endod* 82:577, 1996.

Whitt JC, Rokos JW, Dunlap CL, et al: Segmental odontomaxillary dysplasia: report of a series of 5 cases with long-term follow-up, *Oral Surg Oral Med Oral Pathol Oral Radiol Endod* 112:e29–e47, 2011.

Lingual Mandibular Bone Depression

Parvizi F, Rout PG: An ossifying fibroma presenting as Stafne's idiopathic bone cavity, *Dentomaxillofac Radiol* 26:361, 1997.

Philipsen HP, Takata T, Reichart PA, et al: Lingual and buccal mandibular bone depressions: a review based on 583 cases from a world-wide literature survey, including 69 new cases from Japan, *Dentomaxillofac Radiol* 31:281–290, 2002.

Focal Osteoporotic Bone Marrow

Schneider LC, Mesa ML, Fraenkel D, et al: Osteoporotic bone marrow defect: radiographic features and pathogenic factors, *Oral Surg* 65:127, 1988.

Standish S, Shafer W: Focal osteoporotic bone marrow defects of the jaws, *J Oral Surg* 20:123, 1997.

33 Implants

Byron W. Benson and Vivek Shetty

OUTLINE

Few advances in dentistry have been as remarkable as the use of dental implants (Fig. 33-1) to restore orofacial form and function. Implant technology has enabled the dentist to help patients regain the ability to chew normally and function without embarrassment. With the application of precise surgical and restorative techniques, implant-facilitated restorations provide a predictable and successful rehabilitation of patients with a broad spectrum of prosthodontic needs. The predictable results of contemporary implant systems derive in part from increasingly sophisticated imaging techniques and software programs used in all phases of implant treatment. These imaging modalities contribute information for every stage of the treatment, from presurgical diagnosis and treatment planning, through surgical placement and postoperative assessment of the implant, to the prosthetic restoration and long-term maintenance phase.

Acceptance of dental implantology as an integral part of conventional practice requires the general dentist to be knowledgeable of implant imaging techniques and their clinical application. With the exception of occasionally used subperiosteal, blade, and transosteal implant systems, dental implants used today are almost exclusively root-form devices (see Fig. 33-1) embedded within the jaw bone (endosseous implants). This chapter focuses on current imaging concepts and describes the applications and value of imaging techniques in the various stages of contemporary implant dentistry.

DIAGNOSTIC IMAGING

Commonly used two-dimensional imaging, such as panoramic and periapical images, is generally useful and cost-effective for patient selection and initial assessment. However, these modalities lack the cross-sectional visualization or interactive image analysis that can be obtained with the more sophisticated imaging techniques now available. Numerous imaging techniques can be applied to various phases of implant case management (Table 33-1). The selection of a specific imaging technique should be based on the examination best suited to provide the information required by the implant team—the restorative dentist, surgeon, and radiologist (Table 33-2).

IMAGING TECHNIQUES

The ideal imaging technique for dental implant care should have several essential characteristics, including the ability to visualize the implant site in the mesiodistal, faciolingual, and superoinferior dimensions; the ability to allow reliable, accurate measurements; a capacity to evaluate trabecular bone density and cortical thickness; a capacity to correlate the imaged site with the clinical site; reasonable access and cost to the patient; and minimal radiation risk. Usually a combination of imaging techniques is used. Available imaging techniques include intraoral (film and digital), cephalometric, and panoramic imaging; cone-beam computed tomographic (CBCT) imaging; and multidetector computed tomographic imaging (MDCT). A review of these imaging techniques as applied to dental implant case management is provided here.

INTRAORAL IMAGING

Intraoral images may be acquired on film or as digital images. Periapical and occlusal radiographs provide images with superior resolution and sharpness. Periapical radiographs commonly are used to evaluate the status of adjoining teeth and remaining alveolar bone in the mesiodistal dimension. They also have been used for determining vertical height, morphology, and bone quality (bone density, amount of cortical bone, and amount of trabecular bone). Although readily available and relatively inexpensive, periapical radiography has geometric and anatomic limitations. When teeth are present, images are typically made with the paralleling technique, creating an image with minimal foreshortening and elongation (Fig. 33-2). Because of variations in the morphology of the residual edentulous alveolar ridge (Fig. 33-3), the ridge may not have the same "long axis" as a tooth. The position of the image receptor may not result in an accurate display of the height of the alveolar ridge as a result of image foreshortening or elongation. Also, placing the image receptor either superior or inferior enough to capture an image of the entire maxillary or mandibular ridge can prove to be challenging. Reportedly, 25% of mandibular periapical radiographs do not demonstrate the mandibular canal. In cases in which the canal is identifiable, only 53% of measurements from the alveolar crest to the superior wall of the mandibular canal are accurate within 1 mm.

Because periapical images are unable to provide any cross-sectional information, occlusal radiographs may be used occasionally to determine the faciolingual dimensions of the mandibular alveolar ridge (Fig. 33-4). Although useful, the occlusal image

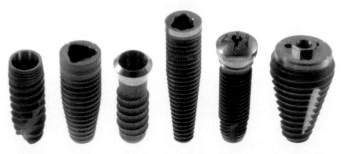

FIGURE 33-1 Six common root-form dental implants that represent the variety of morphologic designs and sizes available for different applications. Generally, it is desirable to place the largest implant possible for greatest support.

TABLE 33-1	Implant Imaging Strategies
Stage of Treatment	**Radiographic Procedures**
Initial examination	• Panoramic supplemented by intraoral periapical images • Cross-sectional imaging, including CBCT imaging, not appropriate for initial examination
Preoperative site specific	• Cross-sectional imaging orthogonal to site (CBCT imaging considered modality of choice) • CBCT imaging if osseous augmentation considered • CBCT imaging to assess previous bone reconstruction and augmentation procedures
Postoperative	• For asymptomatic implants, intraoral periapical or panoramic if case is extensive; CBCT imaging is not appropriate for periodic review of clinical asymptomatic implants • For implant mobility or altered sensation, cross-sectional imaging (CBCT imaging) • For anticipated implant retrieval, cross-sectional imaging (CBCT imaging)

CBCT, Cone-beam computed tomographic.
From Tyndall DA, Price JB, Tetradis S, et al: Position statement of the American Academy of Oral and Maxillofacial Radiology on selection criteria for the use of radiology in dental implantology with emphasis on cone beam computed tomography, *Oral Surg Oral Med Oral Pathol Oral Radiol* 113:817–826, 2012.

TABLE 33-2	Imaging Technique			
Imaging Technique	**Applications**	**Advantages**		**Disadvantages**
Periapical imaging	S, M, E, A	• Readily available • High image definition • Minimal distortion • Least cost and radiation exposure		• Limited imaging area • No faciolingual dimension • Limited reproducibility • Image elongation and foreshortening
Panoramic imaging	S, M, E, A	• Readily available • Large imaging area • Minimal cost and radiation exposure		• No faciolingual dimension • Image distortion • Technique errors common • Inconsistent magnification • Geometric distortion
Reformatted CBCT imaging	M, E, A	• Allows evaluation of all possible sites • No superimposition • Uniform magnification • Measurements accurate within about 1 mm • Estimates internal bone density • Simulates placement with software		• Limited availability • Sensitive to technique errors • Some metallic image artifacts • Special training for interpretation • Moderate cost and radiation risk • Volume averaging contributes to measurement error • Relative bone density measurements (HU) are not calibrated
Reformatted MDCT imaging	M, E, A	• Allows evaluation of all possible sites • No superimposition • Uniform magnification • Measurements accurate within about 1 mm • Estimates internal bone density in HU are calibrated • Simulates placement with software		• Limited availability • Sensitive to technique errors • Metallic image artifacts • Special training for interpretation • Higher cost and radiation risk • Volume averaging contributes to measurement error

A, Augmentation; *CBCT,* cone-beam computed tomographic; *E,* edentulous (6+); *HU,* Hounsfield units; *M,* multiple implants; *MDCT,* multidetector computed tomographic; *S,* single implant.

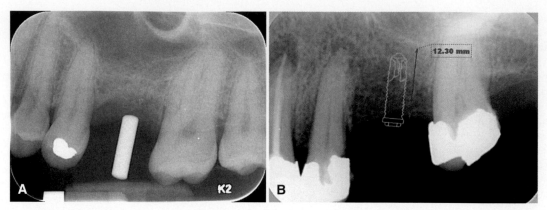

FIGURE 33-2 Intraoral periapical radiographs of a potential implant site. **A,** Imaging guide/stent may be used to indicate the desired axis of insertion. **B,** Digital overlay library allows simulated implant placement as well as measurements in the two-dimensional plane.

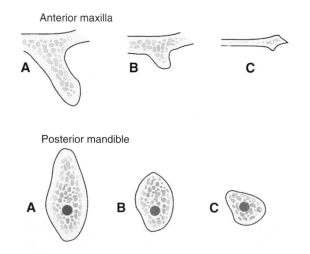

Anterior maxilla

Posterior mandible

FIGURE 33-3 Patterns of bone morphology in the anterior maxilla *(above)* and posterior mandible *(below)* in potential patients for implant therapy. Minimal resorption **(A)**, moderate resorption **(B)**, and severe resorption **(C)** of alveolar bone. *(Modified from Brånemark P-L, Zarb GA, Albrektsson T: Tissue-integrated prostheses: osseointegration in clinical dentistry, Chicago, 1985, Quintessence.)*

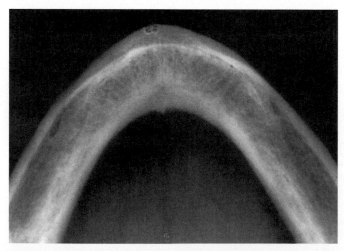

FIGURE 33-4 Intraoral mandibular cross-sectional occlusal radiograph depicts the maximal buccolingual dimension of the mandible but not the residual alveolar ridge.

records only the widest portion of the mandible, which typically is located inferior to the alveolar ridge. This image may give the clinician the impression that more bone is available in the cross-sectional (faciolingual) dimension than actually exists. The occlusal technique is not useful in imaging the maxillary arch because of anatomic limitations.

LATERAL AND LATERAL-OBLIQUE CEPHALOMETRIC IMAGING

Lateral cephalometric imaging provides an image of known magnification (usually 7% to 12% for midline structures) that documents axial tooth inclinations and the dentoalveolar ridge relationships in the midline of the jaws. The soft tissue profile also is apparent on this film and can be used to evaluate profile alterations after prosthodontics rehabilitation. However, this projection can provide a cross-sectional view of only the maxillary and mandibular midline. Images of nonmidline structures are superimposed on the contralateral side, complicating the evaluation of other implant sites. Occasionally, lateral-oblique cephalometric radiographs are used with one side of the mandibular body positioned parallel to the film cassette. Image magnification on these views is unpredictable because the body of the mandible is not the same distance from the film as is the rotation center of the cephalostat (used to calculate object-receptor distance for image magnification values). Thus, measurements made from these images are unreliable. In general, cephalometric images have significant limitations but may be useful in the placement of some implants near the midline for overdentures.

PANORAMIC IMAGING

Although the resolution and sharpness of panoramic radiographs are less than those of intraoral radiographs, panoramic projections provide a broader visualization of the jaws and adjoining anatomic structures. Panoramic units are widely available, making this imaging technique useful and popular as a screening and assessment instrument for preliminary estimations of crestal alveolar bone and cortical boundaries of the mandibular canal, maxillary sinus, and nasal fossa (Fig. 33-5).

Information acquired from panoramic images must be applied judiciously because this technique has significant limitations as a definitive presurgical planning tool. Angular measurements on panoramic radiographs tend to be accurate, but linear

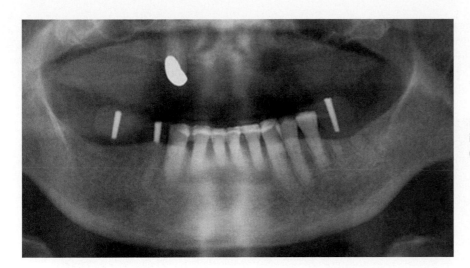

FIGURE 33-5 Cropped portion of panoramic radiograph with imaging guide/stent in place to indicate the desired axis of insertion at three mandibular sites.

measurements are not. Image size distortion (magnification) varies significantly between images acquired on different panoramic units and even within different areas of the same image. Vertical measurements are unreliable owing to foreshortening and elongation of the anatomic structures because the central ray of the x-ray beam is perpendicular neither to the long axis of the anatomic structures nor to the plane of the image receptor. The negative vertical angulation of the x-ray beam also causes lingually positioned objects, such as mandibular tori, to be projected superiorly on the film, resulting in an overestimation of vertical bone height. The anatomic vertical axis varies within the image, particularly in nonmidline areas. Compared with contact radiographs of dissected anatomic specimens, only 17% of panoramic measurements between the alveolar crest and superior wall of the mandibular canal were found to be accurate within 1 mm.

Similarly, dimensional accuracy in the horizontal plane of panoramic radiographs is highly dependent on the position of the structures of interest relative to the central plane of the image layer. The horizontal dimension of images of structures located facial or lingual to the central plane but still within the image layer tends to be minified or magnified, respectively. The degree of horizontal size distortion is difficult to ascertain on panoramic radiographs because the shape of the image layer is configured to a population average, and the anatomic morphology of only a few individuals conforms totally to that image layer. Horizontal image magnification with panoramic radiographs ranges from 0.70 to 2.2 times the actual size, which some manufacturers report as a 1.25 average magnification (at the central plane of the image layer). Errors in patient positioning can further exacerbate measurement error in the horizontal dimension. The deficient dimensional accuracy of the two-dimensional panoramic image is further limited by the lack of any cross-sectional information.

REFORMATTED CONE-BEAM AND MULTIDETECTOR COMPUTED TOMOGRAPHIC IMAGING

The three-dimensional visualizations of craniofacial structures initially led to the application of MDCT imaging in implant dentistry. However, concerns about excessive radiation risk and increased costs led to the replacement of MDCT imaging with more refined modalities such as CBCT imaging. Newer CBCT techniques provide high-resolution images of high diagnostic quality with significantly reduced acquisition times and radiation burden. Patients who are edentulous or who are being considered for multiple implants and augmentation procedures may be best imaged with either CBCT imaging or MDCT imaging to investigate potential implant sites. For MDCT imaging, a lateral scout image of the selected jaw with the necessary alignment corrections for the mandible or maxilla is typically an essential initial step. The jaws are aligned so that the acquired axial computed tomographic image slices are parallel to the occlusal plane. These axial images are thin (1 to 2 mm) and overlapping, resulting in approximately 30 axial image slices per jaw. The image information of these sequential axial images can be postprocessed to produce multiple two-dimensional images in various planes using a computer-based process called multiplanar reformatting.

CBCT images are acquired with an initial scout image followed by a single revolution imaging sequence. The vertical height of the imaging sequence can be adjusted to include only one jaw, both, or a larger area, especially if the temporomandibular joint needs to be included in the imaged area. Multiplanar reformatting processing is also accomplished with CBCT imaging data. Some investigators have suggested that the field of view include the entire maxillary sinus if a sinus-lift graft is planned. Several units are available with limited fields of view and smaller voxel sizes; these images include only several adjacent teeth. Regardless of the field of view size, a voxel size of less than 0.3 to 0.4 mm is rarely required for implant planning purposes.

The reformatted images of both types of volumetric data result in three basic image types: (1) axial images with a computer-generated superimposed curve of the alveolar process, (2) associated reformatted alveolar cross-sectional images, and (3) panoramic-like (pseudopanoramic or curved-linear) images. An axial image that includes the full contour of the mandible (or maxilla) at a level corresponding to the dental roots is typically selected as a reference for the reformatting process. With use of a computer program, a series of sequential dots on the selected axial scan are connected to develop a customized arch or curve unique for each jaw. The computer program then generates a series of lines perpendicular to the curve of the individual arch. These lines are made at constant intervals (usually 1 to 2 mm) and numbered sequentially on the axial and pseudopanoramic images to indicate the position at which each cross-sectional slice will be reconstructed (Figs. 33-6 and 33-7). Cross-sectional alveolar reconstructions are made perpendicular to the curve, and pseudopanoramic reconstructions are made parallel with the curve. Three-dimensional representations may also be constructed in various orientations.

Such reformatted images provide the clinician with accurate two-dimensional diagnostic information in all three dimensions. Typical MDCT studies provide information on the continuity of the cortical bone plates, residual bone in the mandible and maxilla, the relative location of adjoining vital structures, and the contour

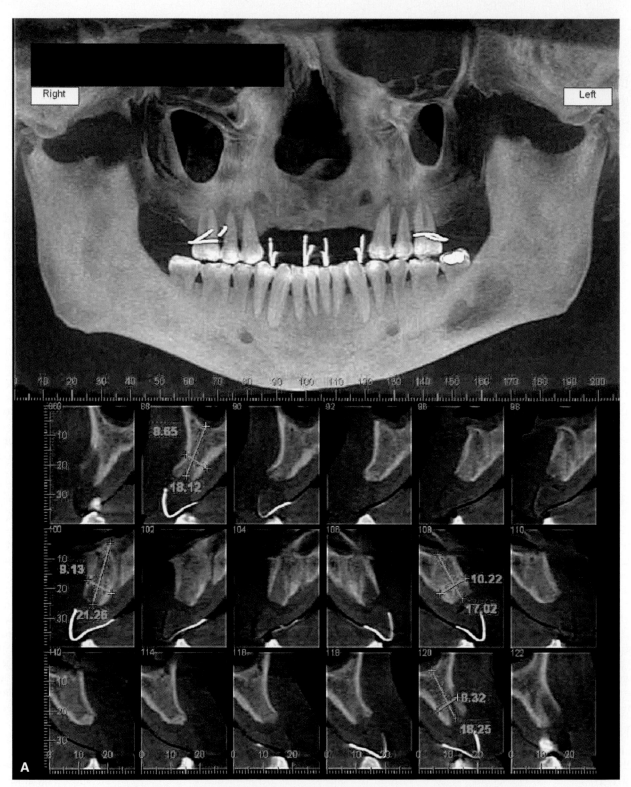

FIGURE 33-6 Reformatted CBCT study of the maxilla. **A,** Pseudopanoramic (maximum intensity projection) image *(above)* and alveolar cross-sectional reconstructed images using an imaging stent incorporating radiopaque strips to define the buccal and palatal contours of the planned prosthesis *(below)*. Note the measurements on the cross-sectional images.

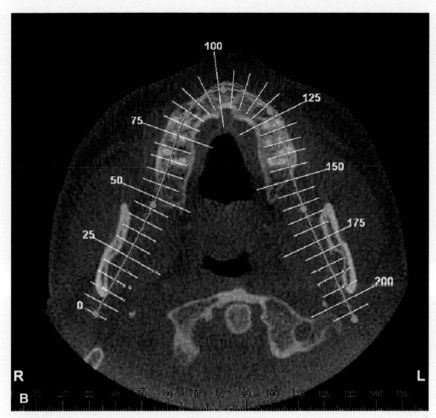

FIGURE 33-6, cont'd B, Axially reformatted image defines the central plane of the pseudopanoramic image and serves as a reference image for the alveolar cross-sectional images.

of soft tissues covering the osseous structures. Studies have reported that 94% of MDCT imaging measurements between the alveolar crest and wall of the mandibular canal were accurate within 1 mm. Reformatted images from CBCT imaging data have been shown to have measurement accuracy equivalent to MDCT imaging data. These reformations are also useful in the planning augmentation procedures such as a sinus lift and can provide an estimate of the internal density. A three-dimensional image can provide visualization of the overall morphology of the intended implant site. Bone density at the intended implant sites can be assessed from MDCT images by selecting the area of interest and assessing the mean density in Hounsfield units (HU). Several studies have correlated these data to predict implant stability (Table 33-3). Density values measured in HU are not calibrated for use with CBCT imaging data volumes.

Reformatted CBCT images and MDCT images may be printed as 1:1 images on high-grade photographic paper or plastic film. If the study is to be viewed electronically as individual static images on a monitor, a measurement scale is typically incorporated into the image for calibration. Alternatively, the reformatted study may be viewed with interactive software. The pseudopanoramic images are helpful in identifying mesiodistal relationships and minimally corticated mandibular canals. However, the quality of the reformatted imaging study depends on the ability of the patient to remain still during image acquisition because movement may produce geometric image distortion. Because of the shorter acquisition times, this is less of an issue with CBCT imaging compared with MDCT imaging. Metallic restorations typically cause streak image artifacts, but the impact of this streaking can be minimized by aligning the jaws so that the acquired axial scans are parallel to

the occlusal plane, which sometimes keeps the artifact from obscuring the alveolar crest. Metallic artifacts are less prominent on CBCT imaging because of the image acquisition physics. All the images in computed tomographic studies for dental implant studies should be adequately interpreted by an oral and maxillofacial radiologist or other appropriately trained dentist or physician; this is especially important because a large anatomic area outside the region of interest is included in the primary images and must be interpreted.

IMAGING ALTERNATIVES

Less commonly, magnetic resonance imaging has been suggested as an alternative modality for implant sites. The primary advantages are superior soft tissue visualization to localize the mandibular canal and the absence of risk from ionizing radiation. Disadvantages include acquisition cost, imaging artifacts from ferromagnetic metals, and difficulty in estimating bone quality and quantity because cortical bone margins are challenging to differentiate from adjacent air. Magnetic resonance imaging is contraindicated for patients with ferromagnetic metallic implants because there is a potential for the magnetic field to cause movement of the implants. Most implants that are currently available are made of titanium, a nonferromagnetic metal.

PREOPERATIVE PLANNING

Preoperative imaging allows a qualitative and quantitative evaluation of potential implant sites and is an important extension of clinical examination and assessment. Radiographs help the clinician visualize the alveolar ridges and adjacent structures in all three

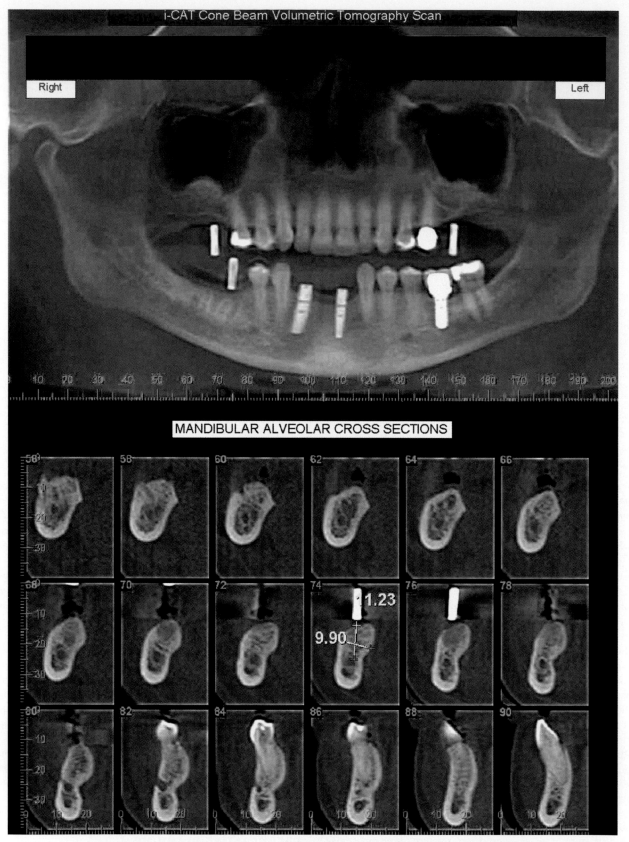

FIGURE 33-7 Reformatted CBCT study of the mandible. Pseudopanoramic and alveolar cross-sectional reconstructed images. The imaging stent incorporates metal rods indicating the intended path of insertion for the implants. The rods are subsequently removed, converting the imaging guide into a surgical stent when the implants are placed. *(Courtesy Dr. Hui Liang, Dallas, TX.)*

TABLE 33-3   Bone Density Correlation

Misch Bone Density Class	Bone Type	MDCT Imaging Density Range (HU)
D1	Dense cortical	>1250
D2	Porous cortical and coarse trabecular	850–1250
D3	Porous cortical (thin) and fine trabecular	350–850
D4	Fine trabecular	150–350
D5	Immature and nonmineralized	<150

HU, Hounsfield units, MDCT, multidetector computed tomographic.
Adapted from Misch CE: Contemporary implant dentistry, ed 3, St Louis, 2008, Mosby, pp 134–137.

dimensions and guide the choice of site, number, size, and axial orientation of the implants. Site selection includes consideration of the desired position of an implant and its relationship to adjacent anatomic structures, such as the incisive and mental foramina, inferior alveolar canal, existing teeth, nasal fossae, and maxillary sinuses. The incidence of implant-related injuries to the inferior alveolar nerve has been reported to be 0% to 33.2%, and inadequate preoperative imaging is a contributing factor. Conditions such as retained root fragments, impacted teeth, osteosclerosis, and any osseous pathoses that could compromise the outcome must be identified and localized relative to the proposed implant site.

Diagnostic images of potential implant sites can provide information about the quality and quantity of bone that would be adequate to support the implant fixture. The quality of bone includes assessment of the cortical bone because it is best suited to withstand the functional loading forces of dental implants. There is a greater likelihood of successful osseous integration when there is a thicker cortical bone. A greater number of internal trabeculae per unit area is also advantageous. Mean bone density assessments, measured in HU, can be assessed with MDCT studies. However, measurements in HU are not calibrated for CBCT imaging data volumes.

Bone quantity is assessed by documenting the height and width of available alveolar bone and the morphology of the ridge. The chances of a successful outcome increase with a greater amount of bone available for anchorage. A cross-sectional image to document the faciolingual width and height of the ridge, along with the inclination of the bone contours, is especially useful in the preoperative planning phase. Alveolar ridge width measurements aid in selecting the implant diameter and implant placement for maximal engagement of cortical bone. Ridge height measurements help select the largest appropriate fixture to maximize anchorage and distribution of masticatory forces. Morphologic features not immediately apparent on clinical examination, such as osseous undercuts and ridge concavities, become evident with cross-sectional imaging.

Accurate bone measurements are essential for determining the optimal size and length and orientation of the proposed implants. The shape and amount of residual bone tends to dictate the size and shape of the implants. Generally, the largest possible implant is chosen because it presents the greatest surface areas available for osseointegration. To maximize the chances for success, the implants are sized so that there is 1 to 1.5 mm of residual bone surrounding the implant and at least 1 to 2 mm of bone interposed between the implant and adjacent structures, such as the mandibular canal and nasal fossa. Consequently, precise measurements acquired from images are very important in the planning process, and it is important to correct for any magnification factor associated with a particular imaging technique. Except for specialized interactive reformatted MDCT imaging and CBCT imaging implant programs, all other projection-type radiographic images have a magnification factor, which must be taken into account when the dimensions of the bone are calculated. The measurements obtained from the images (usually in millimeters) are divided by the magnification factor for that particular imaging technique. As described earlier, the magnification factor of some techniques may be variable (periapical, panoramic), and a constant magnification factor cannot be applied. With dental implant MDCT imaging and CBCT imaging reformatting software, the image is reproduced in the actual size of the jaw without magnification. The magnification of digital projection-type images can also be calibrated with the measurement tool.

IMAGING GUIDES/STENTS

The clinical utility of presurgical imaging studies can be enhanced by the use of an imaging guide/stent that helps relate the radiographic image and its information to a precise anatomic location or a potential surgical site. In the case of MDCT imaging and CBCT imaging, an imaging stent also facilitates correlation of the individual image slices to an anatomic location in the scout films. The intended implant sites are identified by markers made of radiopaque spheres or rods (metal, composite resin, or gutta-percha) retained within an acrylic stent (Fig. 33-8; see Fig. 33-7), which the patient wears during the imaging procedure so that images of the markers are captured in the diagnostic images. The imaging stent subsequently may be used as a surgical guide to orient the insertion angle of the surgical drills and the angle of the implant. Diagnostic dentures coated with barium paste may be used during imaging for localization and can establish the spatial relationships between the anticipated prosthesis and the implant fixtures. Generally, nonmetallic radiopaque markers (gutta-percha, composite resin) are used in MDCT imaging and CBCT imaging studies to minimize the effect of image artifacts produced by metal markers. However, some metals scatter less than others, and metallic scatter artifact of some CBCT units appears to be less than that of MDCT units. Existing root-form implants do not produce a significant axial scatter artifact.

INTERACTIVE DIAGNOSTIC SOFTWARE

Several different interactive software packages are available to simulate implant orientation and placement on a computer screen before surgery. They are designed for use on personal computers, typically requiring a Windows (Microsoft, Redmond, WA) operating system. These programs provide an interactive analysis of potential implant sites for bone quantity, quality, and morphology and can simulate the surgical placement of the implant. Visualization of anatomic structures, volumetric analysis for bone grafts, and mechanical analysis of structural forces during restoration are also within the capability of the software packages (Fig. 33-9).

SELECTING DIAGNOSTIC IMAGING FOR PREOPERATIVE PLANNING

Panoramic images, supplemented by intraoral periapical images, provide a good starting point for initial assessment. Periapical radiographs provide the greatest image detail. These survey radiographs

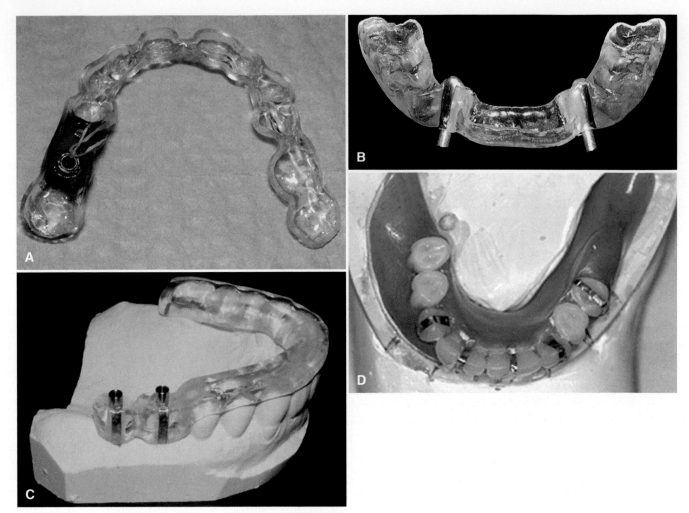

FIGURE 33-8 Four examples of imaging guides/stents. **A,** Vacuum-formed imaging stent with copper cylinders to indicate desired axes of insertion. The predicted contour of the completed implant restoration is filled with acrylic mixed with barium to depict the buccal and lingual emergence profile on the cross-sectional image. A piece of dental floss is tied through the guide to prevent swallowing or aspiration. **B,** Processed stent with metal cylinders marking the implant sites. This can also be used as a surgical stent by inserting the guide bur through the cylinders. **C,** Another processed stent with metal rod insertion axis markers, along with radiopaque strips outlining the buccal and lingual contours of the planned restoration. **D,** Existing denture is modified to become an imaging guide by adding radiopaque strips along the buccal and lingual contours of the denture teeth.

help determine whether the patient is a good candidate for implant procedures. For instance, the presence of a pathologic lesion or severe alveolar atrophy at the planned implant site would preclude the use of additional MDCT imaging and CBCT imaging studies with their attendant financial and radiation risk burdens. If the initial survey radiographs reveal reasonable conditions for placing implants, CBCT imaging is optimally appropriate to obtain cross-sectional images of these sites (Fig. 33-10 and see Table 33-2). Generally, comprehensive imaging of the maxilla and mandible is required to evaluate multiple implant sites and a medium to large field of view CBCT image would be a reasonable selection. If potential sites are restricted to a few selected regions, a small field of view CBCT image is preferred. Inadequate treatment planning may lead to failure of the implant and harm to the patient. Iatrogenic inferior alveolar nerve injuries related to implant placement have been reported to range from 0% to 33.2% and are a common cause of medicolegal litigation. In general, the ease of acquisition, isotropic voxel dimensions, and lower radiation burden make CBCT

imaging the cross-sectional imaging modality of choice compared with MDCT imaging.

INTRAOPERATIVE AND POSTOPERATIVE ASSESSMENTS

Periapical and panoramic imaging usually are adequate for both intraoperative and postoperative assessments (Figs. 33-11 through 33-13). Intraoperative imaging may be required to confirm correct placement of the implant or to locate a lost implant (Fig. 33-14). Frequently, intraoral images are used to ensure that the bodies of the healing abutments are fully seated on the implant before any dental impression is acquired. After surgery, the successful integration of the implant is assessed through a combination of alveolar bone height around the implant and the appearance of the peri-implant bone. Periapical images of the entire implant fixture are useful in assessing the bone-implant interface. If threaded

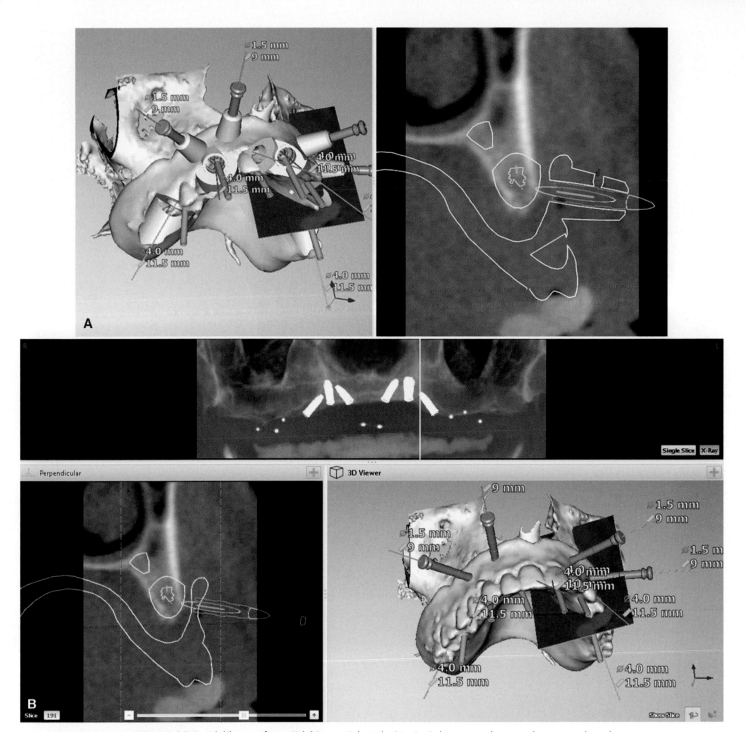

FIGURE 33-9 NobelClinician software (Nobel Biocare, Yorba Linda, CA). **A,** Evaluating an implant site with an imaging/surgical guide. **B,** Visualization of an implant site in three dimensions. In this case, the implant was angled to avoid the maxillary sinus. *(Courtesy Dr. Jorge Gonzalez, Dallas, TX.)*

root-form fixtures have been placed, the optimal radiographic image must separate the threads for best visualization; this may not always be a predictable procedure because the exact angulation of the implant is unknown. The angulation of the x-ray beam must be within 9 degrees of the long axis of the fixture to open the threads on the image on most threaded fixtures (Figs. 33-15 and 33-16). Angular deviations of 13 degrees or more result in complete overlap of the threads. For longitudinal assessments, an effort should be made to reproduce the vertical angulation of the central ray of the x-ray beam as closely as possible between radiographs to duplicate the image geometry closely. Mesial and distal marginal bone height is measured from a standard landmark at the collar of the implant or, in the case of threaded implants, by use of known interthread distances and compared with bone levels in previous periapical radiographs. The presence of relatively distinct bone margins with a constant height relative to the implant suggests successful osseous integration. Clinical symptoms suggestive of a failing implant should be corroborated by a radiographic

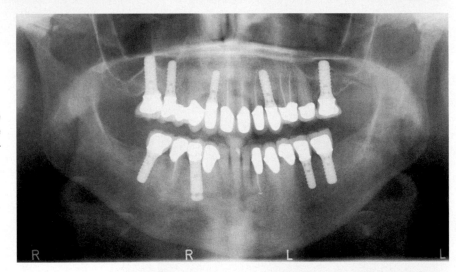

FIGURE 33-10 Reformatted coronal **(A)** and axial **(B)** cross-sectional regional CBCT images to assess the integrity of an osseous graft before implant placement.

FIGURE 33-11 Panoramic radiograph used for postoperative assessment of multiple successfully restored root-form implants. The threads are visualized on all of the implants except for the mandibular right premolar, which is a smooth cylinder.

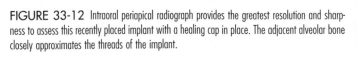

FIGURE 33-12 Intraoral periapical radiograph provides the greatest resolution and sharpness to assess this recently placed implant with a healing cap in place. The adjacent alveolar bone closely approximates the threads of the implant.

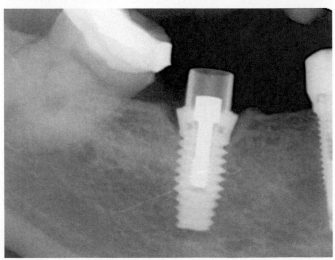

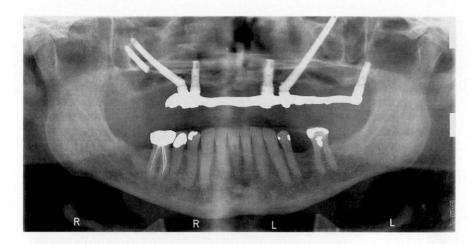

FIGURE 33-13 Panoramic radiograph used for postoperative assessment of a case that employed a combination of alveolar and zygomatic arch implants.

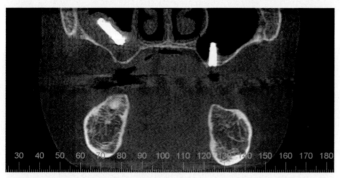

FIGURE 33-14 Reformatted CBCT study for postoperative assessment of an implant displaced into the right maxillary sinus and associated with mucositis in the right antrum. The implant on the left alveolus is not well supported by bone and extends well into the antrum.

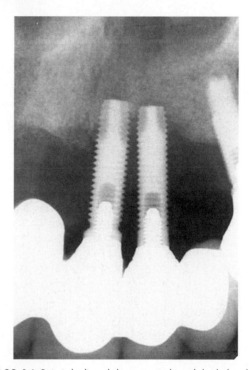

FIGURE 33-16 Periapical radiograph demonstrates advanced alveolar bone loss adjacent to failing dental implants.

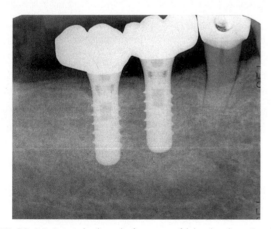

FIGURE 33-15 Periapical radiograph of two successful dental implants. Note the close apposition of the bone to the surface of each implant. A minor amount of saucerization is present at the alveolar crest adjacent to the distal fixture.

examination of the bone-implant interface. Radiographic signs of failure include a loss of crestal bone (saucerization) evidenced by apical migration of the alveolar bone or indistinct osseous margins. These adverse changes are progressive and should be differentiated from the initial circumscribed resorptive osseous changes around the cervical area of the fixture occurring during the first 6 months that are induced by the surgical procedure itself (Fig. 33-17). Studies suggest that the rate of marginal bone loss after successful implantation is approximately 1.2 mm in the first year, subsequently tapering off to about 0.1 mm in succeeding years. Subtle areas of bone resorption adjacent to the fixture may be made more evident with intraoral digital images by evaluating a density profile graph of radiographic density values, a feature available on most digital imaging units. If intraoral digital images are acquired at surgery, they may be compared with subsequent digital images either by subjective visualization or by digital subtraction (see Chapter 4). Occasionally, areas of marginal bone gain also may be noted.

The success of an implant also can be evaluated by the appearance of normal bone surrounding it and its apposition to the surface of the implant body. The development of a thin radiolucent area that closely follows the outline of the implant usually correlates to clinically detectable implant mobility; it is an important indicator of failed osseointegration (Figs. 33-18 and 33-19). Changes in the periodontal ligament space of associated teeth (natural abutment) are also useful in monitoring the functional

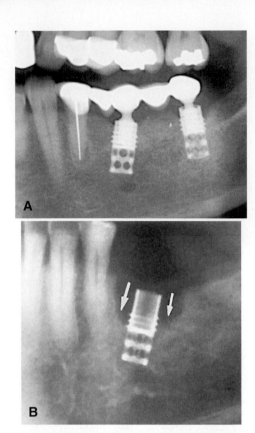

A

B

FIGURE 33-17 **A,** Marginal bone loss around the cervical region of a root-form dental implant (portion of a panoramic radiograph). **B,** Periapical radiograph of moderate bone loss (saucerization type) around the cervical region of a root-form dental implant *(arrows).*

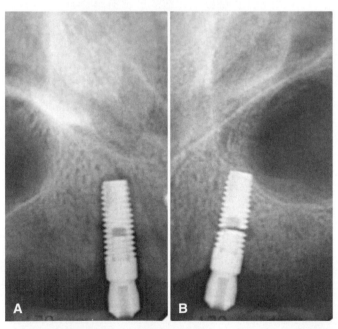

A   **B**

FIGURE 33-18 **A,** Periapical radiograph of bone loss around a root-form dental implant (thin radiolucent band surrounding the implant), indicating failure of osseous integration. **B,** Periapical view of fractured endosseous implant.

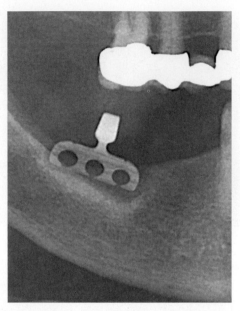

FIGURE 33-19 Cropped panoramic radiograph demonstrates severe bone loss adjacent to a failing blade-type dental implant.

TABLE 33-4   Radiographic Signs Associated with Failing Endosseous Implants

Imaging Appearance	Clinical Implications
Thin radiolucent area that closely follows the entire outline of implant	Failure of implant to integrate with adjoining bone
Crestal bone loss around the coronal portion of implant	Osteitis resulting from poor plaque control, adverse loading, or both
Apical migration of alveolar bone on one side of implant	Nonaxial loading resulting from improper angulation of implant
Widening of the periodontal ligament space of nearest natural (tooth) abutment	Poor stress distribution resulting from biomechanically inadequate prosthesis-implant system
Fracture of implant fixture	Unfavorable stress distribution during function

competence of the implant-prosthesis composite. Any widening of the periodontal ligament space compared with baseline radiographs indicates poor stress distribution and forecasts implant failure (Table 33-4). After successful implantation, radiographs may be made at regular intervals to assess the success or failure of the implant fixture. Cross-sectional imaging, ideally with CBCT imaging, may be necessary for adequate assessment in cases demonstrating implant mobility or altered sensation (Figs. 33-20 through 33-22). CBCT imaging is also appropriate if implant retrieval is being considered but is inappropriate for periodic review of clinically asymptomatic implants.

In summary, diagnostic imaging using a variety of imaging techniques is an integral part of dental implant therapy for presurgical planning, intraoperative assessment, and postoperative assessment. Cross-sectional imaging is considered essential for optimal implant placement, especially in the case of complex reconstructions.

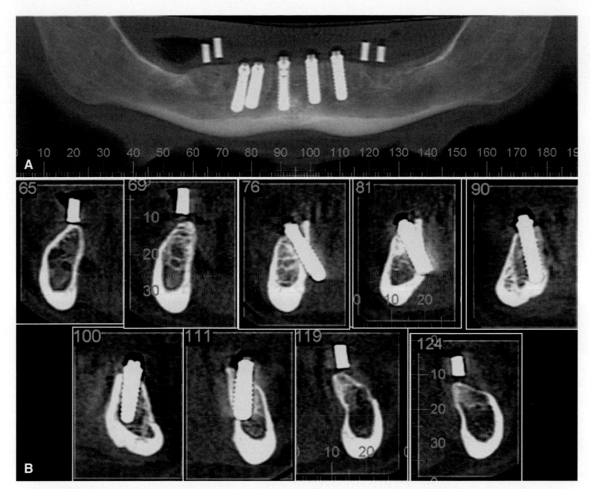

FIGURE 33-20 **A,** Pseudopanoramic reformatted CBCT image initially made to evaluate new implant sites as well as the existing implants. In this image, the existing implants appear reasonably normal in orientation. **B,** Cross-sectional reformatted CBCT images reveal nonrestorable ectopic placement of the existing implants with lingual cortical perforation and extension into the lingual tissues.

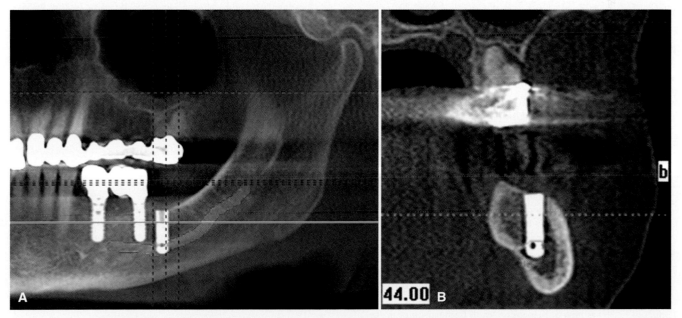

FIGURE 33-21 **A** and **B,** Reformatted CBCT images demonstrate embarrassment and compression of the mandibular canal by a dental implant. The mandibular canal is radiopaque in the pseudopanoramic rendition **(A)** because the canal was mapped to identify its anatomic course more easily. The same canal is radiolucent in the alveolar cross-sectional rendition **(B)** because mapping was not employed.

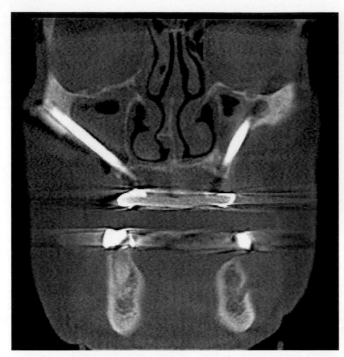

FIGURE 33-22 Coronal reformatted CBCT image depicts advanced maxillary sinusitis secondary to failing zygomatic arch implants. Note the axial scatter artifact from metallic materials in the maxillary hybrid denture and mandibular dental restorations.

BIBLIOGRAPHY

Comparative Dosimetry

Cohnen M, Kemper J, Möbes O, et al: Radiation dose in dental radiology, *Eur Radiol* 12:634–637, 2002.

Lecomber AR, Yoneyama Y, Lovelock DJ, et al: Comparison of patient dose from imaging protocols for dental implant planning using conventional radiography and computed tomography, *Dentomaxillofac Radiol* 30:255–259, 2001.

Loubele M, Bogaerts R, Van Dijck E, et al: Comparison between effective radiation dose of CBCT and MSCT scanners for dentomaxillofacial applications, *Eur J Radiol* 71:461–468, 2009.

Ludlow JB, Davies-Ludlow LE, Brooks SL, et al: Dosimetry of 3 CBCT devices for oral and maxillofacial radiology: CB Mercuray, NewTom 3G and i-CAT, *Dentomaxillofac Radiol* 35:219–226, 2006 [erratum *Dentomaxillofac Radiol* 35:392].

Pauwels R, Beinsberger J, Collaert B, et al; SEDENTEXCT Project Consortium: Effective dose range for dental cone beam computed tomography scanners, *Eur J Radiol* 81:267–271, 2012.

Pauwels R, Theodorakou C, Walker A, et al; SEDENTEXCT Project Consortium: Dose distribution for dental cone beam CT and its implication for defining a dose index, *Dentomaxillofac Radiol* 41:583–593, 2012.

Schulze D, Heiland M, Thurmann H, et al: Radiation exposure during midfacial imaging using 4- and 16-slice computed tomography, cone beam computed tomography systems and conventional tomography, *Dentomaxillofac Radiol* 33:83–86, 2004.

Computed Tomographic Imaging

Hashimoto K, Kawashima S, Araki M, et al: Comparison of image performance between cone-beam computed tomography for dental use and four-row multidetector helical CT, *J Oral Sci* 48:27–34, 2006.

Hashimoto K, Kawashima S, Kameoka S, et al: Comparison of image validity between cone beam computed tomography for dental use and multidetector row helical computed tomography, *Dentomaxillofac Radiol* 36:465–471, 2007.

Hiasa K, Abe Y, Okazaki Y, et al: Preoperative computed tomography-derived bone densities in Hounsfield units at implant sites acquired primary stability, *ISRN Dent* 2011:678729, 2011.

Lascala CA, Panella J, Marques MM: Analysis of the accuracy of linear measurements obtained by cone beam computed tomography (CBCT-NewTom), *Dentomaxillofac Radiol* 33:291–294, 2004.

Scarfe WC, Farman AG, Sukovic P: Clinical applications of cone-beam computed tomography in dental practice, *J Can Dent Assoc* 72:75–80, 2006.

Sukovic P: Cone beam computed tomography in craniofacial imaging, *Orthod Craniofac Res* 6(Suppl 1):31–36, 2003.

Worthington P, Rubenstein J, Hatcher DC: The role of cone-beam computed tomography in the planning and placement of implants, *J Am Dent Assoc* 141(Suppl 10):S19–S24, 2010.

Zhang L, Zhu XR, Lee AK, et al: Reducing metal artifacts in cone-beam CT images by preprocessing projection data, *Int J Radiat Oncol Biol Phys* 67:924–932, 2007.

General Imaging Techniques

Benson BW: Presurgical radiographic planning for dental implants, *Oral Maxillofac Surg Clin North Am* 13:751–761, 2001.

DeSmet E, Jacobs R, Gijbels F, et al: The accuracy and reliability of radiographic methods for the assessment of marginal bone level around oral implants, *Dentomaxillofac Radiol* 31:176–181, 2002.

Gray CF, Redpath TW, Smith FW: Magnetic resonance imaging: a useful tool for evaluation of bone prior to implant surgery, *Br Dent J* 184:603–607, 1996.

Holmes SM: iCAT scanning in the dental office, *Fortress Guardian* 9:2, 2007.

Sahiwal IG, Woody RD, Benson BW, et al: Radiographic identification of nonthreaded endosseous dental implants, *J Prosthet Dent* 87:552–562, 2002.

Sahiwal IG, Woody RD, Benson BW, et al: Radiographic identification of threaded endosseous dental implants, *J Prosthet Dent* 87:563–577, 2002.

Schropp L, Stavropoulos A, Spin-Neto R, et al: Evaluation of the RB-RB/LB-LB mnemonic rule for recording optimally projected intraoral images of dental implants: an in vitro study, *Dentomaxillofac Radiol* 41:298–304, 2012.

Sonick M, Abrahams J, Faiella RA: A comparison of the accuracy of periapical, panoramic, and computerized tomographic radiographs in locating the mandibular canal, *Int J Oral Maxillofac Implants* 9:455–460, 1994.

Tyndall DA, Brooks SL: Selection criteria for dental implant site imaging: a position paper of the American Academy of Oral and Maxillofacial Radiology, *Oral Surg Oral Med Oral Pathol Oral Radiol Endod* 89:630–637, 2000.

Tyndall DA, Price JB, Tetradis S, et al: Position statement of the American Academy of Oral and Maxillofacial Radiology on selection criteria for the use of radiology in dental implantology with emphasis on cone beam computed tomography, *Oral Surg Oral Med Oral Pathol Oral Radiol* 113:817–826, 2012.

General Implantology

Misch CE: *Contemporary Implant Dentistry*, ed 3, St Louis, 2008, Mosby.

Miyamoto I, Tsuboi Y, Suwa H, et al: Influence of cortical bone thickness and implant length on implant stability at the time of surgery—clinical, prospective, biomechanical, and imaging study, *Bone* 37:776–780, 2005.

Renton T, Dawood A, Shah A, et al: Post-implant neuropathy of the trigeminal nerve: a case series, *Br Dent J* 212:E17, 2012.

Sahiwal I, Woody RD, Benson BW, et al: Macro design morphology of endosseous dental implants, *J Prosthet Dent* 87:543–551, 2002.

Imaging Guides/Stents

Cehreli MC, Aslan Y, Sahin S: Bilaminar dual-purpose stent for placement of dental implants, *J Prosthet Dent* 84:55–58, 2000.

Kopp KC, Koslow AH, Abdo OS: Predictable implant placement with a diagnostic/surgical template and advanced radiographic imaging, *J Prosthet Dent* 89:611–615, 2003.

Ku YC, Shen YF: Fabrication of a radiographic and surgical stent for implants with a vacuum former, *J Prosthet Dent* 83:252–253, 2000.

Interactive Computer Software

Fortin T, Bosson JL, Coudert JL, et al: Reliability of preoperative planning of an image-guiding system for oral implant placement based on 3-dimensional images: an in vivo study, *Int J Oral Maxillofac Implants* 18:886–893, 2003.

Guerrero ME, Jacobs R, Loubele M, et al: State-of-the-art cone beam CT imaging for preoperative planning of implant placement, *Clin Oral Invest* 10:1, 2006.

Rosenfeld AL, Mandelaris GA, Tardieu PB: Prosthetically directed implant placement using computer software to ensure precise placement and predictable prosthetic outcomes, 1: diagnostics, imaging, and collaborative accountability, *Int J Periodont Restor Dent* 26:215–221, 2006.

Panoramic Radiography

Tal H, Moses O: A comparison of panoramic radiography with computed tomography in the planning of implant surgery, *Dentomaxillofac Radiol* 20:40–42, 1991.

Truhlar RS, Morris HF, Ochi S: A review of panoramic radiography and its potential use in implant dentistry, *Implant Dent* 2:122–130, 1993.

34 Forensics

R. E. Wood

SCOPE OF FORENSICS IN DENTISTRY

The scope of forensics in dentistry (also called forensics in odontology) includes both the identification of human remains and the associated legal responsibilities. Dental forensics may involve the identification of an individual or in some cases multiple individuals, such as from a mass disaster. In the latter case, the task would be preferably handled by a team that includes forensic odontologists, a forensic anthropologist, and a forensic pathologist for biologic profiling or population stratification.

Stratification is the sorting of multiple individuals based on age and, to a lesser extent, race and gender. When this process is applied to a group of unidentified human remains, it enhances the chance to make a positive match between one individual and the dental records of missing persons. If a match is impossible, at least the assessment of the developmental age of the dentition of individuals using diagnostic imaging allows the forensic dentist to determine the age. This determination involves a process where the developmental age of the dentition of an individual is compared with the mean developmental ages of a standard population to arrive at a chronologic age. This process also can be performed on living individuals, such as when identifying individuals with amnesia. There are other methods (not included in this chapter) besides the developmental age of teeth to determine chronologic age, such as determining the developmental age of the bones of the wrist and hand. Virtually all age determinations by any scientific process have an associated error rate. According to Saks in his publication, "The Coming Paradigm Shift in Forensic Identification Science," quantification of error rates in the comparative forensic sciences has been problematic. For this reason, it is imperative that the forensic dentist understands the inherent scientific errors and is cautious in selecting language used to state opinions in official reports.

Forensic dentists also contribute to cases involving bite-mark injuries including recognition, documentation, and analysis of injuries. Analysis involves comparison of a known dentition with a bite mark in a substance, including human skin. Such cases may involve civil litigation or providing aid to dental regulatory authorities. Radiology often provides objective data that are useful in supporting the opinions of a forensic dentist. This chapter focuses primarily on the role of the forensic dentist in identifying human remains.

NEED FOR IDENTIFICATION OF HUMAN REMAINS

Human remains are identified for personal, legal, and societal reasons. People place great importance on verification of the identity of the deceased from a personal perspective because doing so gives a measure of closure to loved ones, permits appropriate funerary rites, and allows appropriate religious ceremonies to be undertaken. In the absence of knowing for certain that a loved one has died, the grieving process may be delayed or interrupted.

From a legal perspective, certification of death is required before payment of life insurance; settling of wills and estates; dissolution of business partnerships, contracts, and marriage; and settling of debts. Just as important from a legal perspective is the commencement of suspicious death investigation. Knowing the identity of a person who died under suspicious circumstances may instigate the investigation. Also, fulfilling the legal requirements for the identification of an individual has importance for society as a whole. A competent forensic death investigation of human remains has four goals: determination of the means, manner, and cause of death and identification of the remains.

METHODS OF BODY IDENTIFICATION

The primary methods used in body identification are visual identification, fingerprint identification, DNA identification, identification by the presence of unique skeletal or medical devices, and dental identification. Visual identification, although the most common method, is unpleasant and may be unreliable. This method can be considered a form of comparative science practiced by someone without scientific training and at a time of high stress and in difficult circumstances. Errors in visual identification are well documented. Fingerprint identification is common but requires that the deceased individual has fingerprint records before death (e.g., criminal record, military or police service) and for the cadaveric fingerprints to remain intact after death. The fingerprints

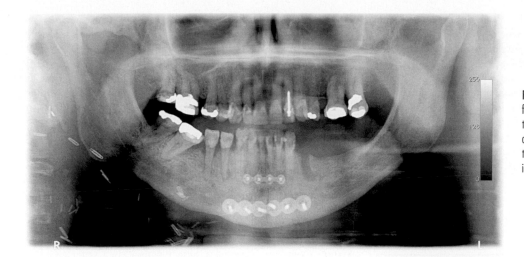

FIGURE 34-1 Panoramic image reveals two fixation plates with 10 intraosseous screws placed in the anterior mandible after a mandibulotomy procedure. The shape and position of the plates and orientation of individual fixation screws provide unique information that could be used for identification.

may not be intact in cases where the body has undergone decomposition, maceration, or incineration. Fingerprint identification is impossible with skeletonized remains.

DNA identification, accomplished by comparing an antemortem (before death) sample with an unknown set of human remains, provides confident identification except between identical twins who have the same DNA. In addition to comparative identification, DNA analysis can be used for racial stratification where a DNA trait may indicate the ethnocultural group of a deceased individual.

Identification by skeletal or medical devices can be made if these devices have serial numbers or if they are unusual in form (Fig. 34-1). Additionally, frontal sinus morphology is quite variable, and this region may be used to compare antemortem and postmortem (after death) diagnostic images for the purpose of identification.

Dental identification has many advantages over the other techniques. Empirical testing has proven that it is reliable, straightforward when antemortem images are available, and readily demonstrable in courts of law. It is also quick and inexpensive.

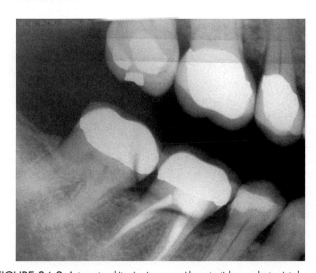

FIGURE 34-2 Antemortem bitewing image provides potential concordant points because of the presence and unique shape of the restorations and root canal filling material.

UTILITY OF DENTAL RADIOLOGY FOR BODY IDENTIFICATION

Diagnostic images are used in dental identification because they provide objective evidence of the antemortem and postmortem condition. Conventional radiographs and digital images are a permanent record of the antemortem condition at the time they were exposed and are difficult to misinterpret. In contrast, a dental charting by one dentist may not be directly comparable to a dental charting by a second dentist of the same patient. Despite the forensic utility of antemortem dental images, most dentists (appropriately) do not expose a full-mouth set of images at each appointment. As a consequence, antemortem images should be analyzed in conjunction with the antemortem dental chart. Antemortem dental images should never be exposed for the purpose of providing a record for later comparison, even in high-risk groups such as convicted criminals or sex-trade workers. Use of the chart and antemortem images of known date allows the forensic dentist to produce an antemortem odontogram, a record of the patient's dentition, which can be compared with the postmortem conditions for the purposes of identification.

IDENTIFICATION OF A SINGLE BODY

The process of body identification using dental criteria is relatively straightforward and is outlined in the American Society of Forensic Odontology manual. Using diagnostic images, the forensic dentist identifies points of agreement (concordance) between the antemortem and postmortem images and lists them numerically. There is no set number of points needed for an identification to be made. A decedent who was edentulous before death may not have any concordant points with any other edentulous candidate, but if there are teeth present with restorations, this may provide enough unique information to eliminate all other possible candidates and provide a match for only one putative decedent (Fig. 34-2). Useful concordant points may include the specific teeth present, with unique features such as shape of crown and roots, and the presence of restorations, including endodontic fillings, the materials used, and their unique shape.

In undertaking a dental identification, the concordant points are listed and incorporated into a report. Discordant points are also listed. Discordant points include explainable discrepancies; points that do not match up based on explainable circumstances, such as a restoration placed after the antemortem images were exposed; and unexplainable discrepancies, where the findings cannot be explained without further investigation. An example of an unexplainable discrepancy would be a tooth missing on an antemortem examination but present on a postmortem examination. Unexplainable discrepancies, if they remain unaccounted for, preclude a positive identification using dental means. All of these findings must be listed in detail in a formal report.

Figure 34-3 shows antemortem and postmortem bitewing images used in an identification of an individual. After comparing images for concordant points, determine whether this is a positive identification.

RADIOLOGIC TECHNIQUES IN BODY IDENTIFICATION

Either conventional radiographs or digital images may be used in single-person or multiple-fatality dental forensics. Using conventional radiographs in postmortem examinations requires the films to be developed on-site. The result is a slight delay compared with using digital imaging. However, conventional radiographic images provide the flexibility of using various image receptor sizes. For example, occlusal films can be used for bitewing radiographs (Fig. 34-4). Using larger image films (e.g., occlusal), a complete radiographic survey can be accomplished in six radiographs (Fig. 34-5). In cases where the remains are decomposed, conventional films or specimens can readily be wrapped in polyethylene stock bags to prevent contamination (Fig. 34-6). A further advantage of using conventional radiographs is that their latitude allows images of decent quality in cases ranging from extremely bloated remains with soft tissue thickness up to five times normal to skeletonized remains and burned and partly carbonized remains resulting from fire.

Most forensic dentists use digital systems. The advantages of digital systems include the ability make retakes to modify the imaging angle to replicate the antemortem images or to augment the examination instantly and improve the speed of identification. However, there are some limitations with the use of digital systems. Occasionally, the wider latitude of conventional film is superior for imaging small amounts of remaining material where there has been considerable loss of tooth structure or soft tissue coverage (Fig. 34-7). There are procedures that can be used with digital imaging to help mitigate these problems. Lucite sheets can be used to mimic soft tissue, x-ray generator exposure settings can be reduced, and the x-ray tube head can be moved away from the receptor. However, in some cases, there is so little tissue left that these measures may not result in more acceptable images (see Fig. 34-7). Also, digital systems can be expensive, and the image receptor and a significant amount of the attached cord must be thoroughly protected lest they become contaminated from the human remains.

Regardless of which image receptor is selected, it is imperative for the forensic dentist to operate safely by practicing body substance precautions and x-ray safety. With respect to precautions from the body being examined, it is prudent to wrap equipment in impermeable membranes to avoid contamination and to drape bodies with disposable covers so that all government-mandated laws on the handling of body substances are obeyed.

Handheld dental x-ray generators (Fig. 34-8) may be considered mandatory for dental forensics. These devices involve only minimal operator exposure, allow battery packs to be switched out in cases of heavy use, and are highly portable. They are compatible with either conventional film or digital systems.

Finally, with regard to forensics, it is better to take too many images than too few. There is no concern for radiation dose in the deceased, so the entire tooth-bearing parts of the jaws should be imaged. Equally importantly, the forensic dentist or forensic radiographer should keep in mind the goal of postmortem radiography, which is to provide images of high quality for forensic comparison with antemortem images. Diagnosis of disease is not the goal of forensic radiography. Postmortem images may be made in advance of receipt of any antemortem records, so with respect to radiologic imaging, the maxim "when in doubt—max out" is operative. Finally, in situations where the case is being entered into a "found-human-remains/missing persons" database such as National Missing and Unidentified Persons System (NamUs), National Crime Information Center (NCIC), INTERPOL, or others, the body may be buried or otherwise irretrievable by the time any antemortem-postmortem comparison is performed.

FORENSIC DENTAL IDENTIFICATION REPORT

After the examination is conducted, the forensic dentist writes a report for the coroner or medical examiner. The following are points that should appear in the report, regardless of the style of report employed.

- What *must* be in a report:
  - Title of the report
  - Name of the coroner or medical examiner
  - Name of the pathologist
  - Autopsy number or case agency number assigned to the deceased
  - Name of the putative deceased person whose records are compared with the records of the remains
  - Date of the postmortem examination
  - Date of your report
  - Brief description of the materials provided to you (e.g., radiographs, charts)
  - Brief description of how the postmortem examination was conducted
  - Points of concordance between the antemortem and postmortem materials
  - Points of discordance between the antemortem and postmortem materials
  - Results of your comparison
  - Your name and signature but without your address, phone number, or other contact information
- What *should* be in a report:
  - Where the examination took place
  - What the examination consisted of in detail (e.g., postmortem images exposed)
  - Who provided materials (e.g., radiographs, charts) not generated by yourself and how they came to be in your possession.
  - Means of your comparison
  - Points of identification listed and individually numbered
  - Points of discordance listed and individually numbered
  - Statement saying that your report is based only on the materials available to you such as: "This report is based on the materials provided to me at the time of the comparison. If new evidence is made available, the author

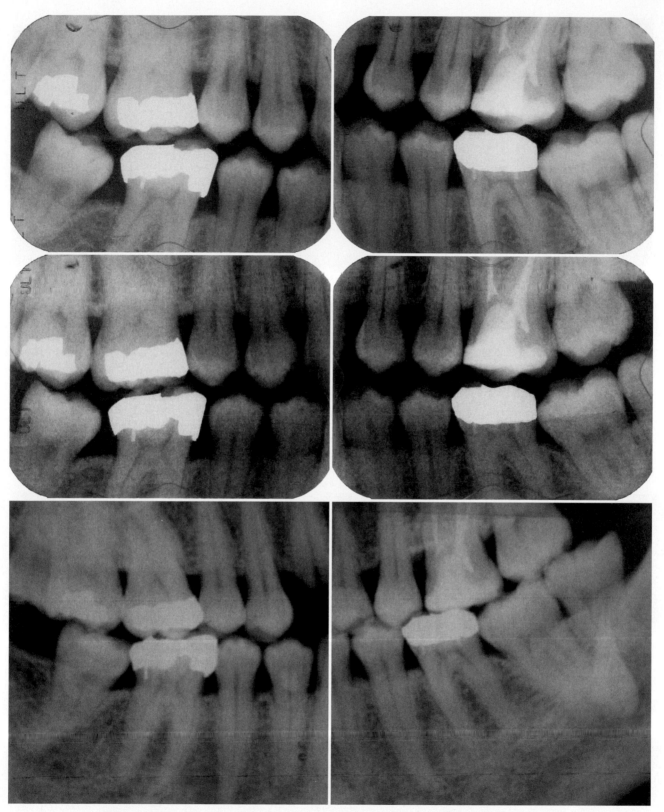

FIGURE 34-3 Four antemortem conventional bitewing images *(top)* and two postmortem bitewing images *(bottom)*. A positive match can be made using teeth present and the morphology of the teeth, such as root structure and pulp chambers, number and shape of metallic restorations, and endodontic filling material.

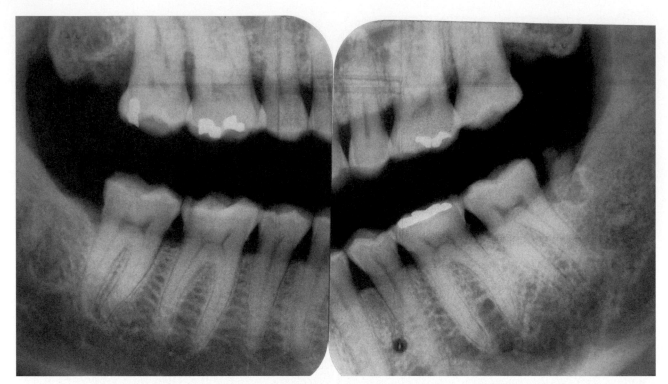

FIGURE 34-4 The use of two conventional occlusal films as bitewing images allows for a greater amount of tissue to be imaged than if No. 2 size film had been used.

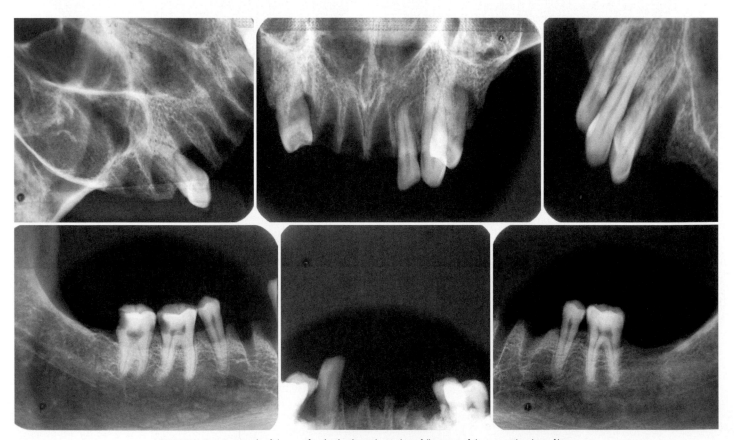

FIGURE 34-5 Example of the use of occlusal radiographs to obtain full imaging of the jaws with only six films.

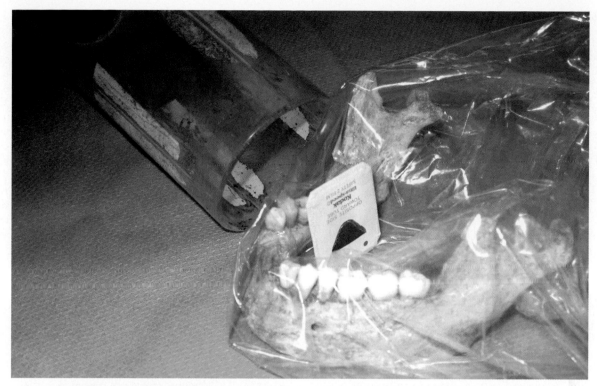

FIGURE 34-6 A polyethylene stock bag is used to wrap the specimen for conventional radiographic imaging to protect the forensic dentist and others handling the material.

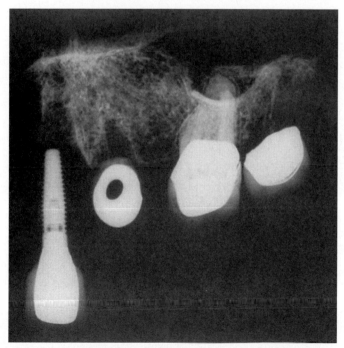

FIGURE 34-7 This dark image demonstrates the difficulty in obtaining images with acceptable density when dealing with very small amounts of tissue.

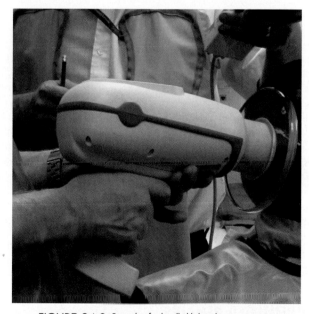

FIGURE 34-8 Example of a handheld dental x-ray generator.

of this report reserves the right to amend or change this report."
- Statement that your report was returned to the authorizing agency along with materials provided and the date this was done.

STYLE OF REPORTING CONCORDANT POINTS

It is recommended to spell out the name of each tooth described rather than using a tooth numbering system. This procedure reduces the chance of error in the event that the report is read by persons not accustomed to using either the FDI (World Dental Federation) tooth-numbering system or the Universal (U.S.) numbering system. For example, the report may include the following statement: "The maxillary right third molar is present and malformed with especially stunted roots on both antemortem and postmortem radiographic examinations."

MATERIALS USED IN A REPORT

The forensic dentist must keep materials used in the examination in a secure place while they are in use. After the examination is completed and the report submitted, however, it is recommended to retain a copy of the report but to return all materials to the coroner or medical examiner. This individual will return them to the dentist or retain them in his or her own file. This practice places the onus for safe, secure, and permanent storage of all materials on the coroner or medical examiner, and chain of custody is maintained.

APPLICATIONS OF RADIOLOGY IN MASS DISASTERS

Forensic dental identification is very useful in multiple-fatality incidents that result in a large number of human remains that may be commingled, macerated, burnt, or otherwise damaged. If the multiple-fatality event is small and can be managed by local providers, it may be simply a matter of undertaking multiple single identifications. However, if the incident is too large for local authorities to manage with confidence, it may be necessary to call on trained and experienced teams of forensic dentists from outside the local jurisdiction. Such situations are not the place for a well-meaning dentist lacking training or extensive case experience. Most people underestimate the stress involved with these situations, even on seasoned practitioners.

The process of identification of remains in multiple-fatality situations is the same as the individual identification except for the organization. Normally, three teams are formed: (1) an antemortem team that collects, organizes, and collates incoming data obtained by investigators; (2) a postmortem team that examines, radiographs, and charts the remains; and (3) a comparison team that makes identifications. In all cases, it is imperative to work with at least two members in each team so that errors can be caught.

In situations where the number of remains is large or fragmentation of the remains occurs, the comparisons become especially complex. Numerous computer software programs are available that can aid in the comparison, such as WinID3, Plass Data or DVI System (for websites see Resources section at the end of this chapter). These programs rank possible matches and mismatches using simple algorithms. However, all final identifications are made by experts.

APPLICATION OF RADIOLOGY TO LONG-TERM UNIDENTIFIED REMAINS

Methods of identification of long-term unidentified remains are limited to situations where there are antemortem records of acceptable quality for comparison with postmortem records. In the United States, there are 100,000 active missing persons cases and 40,000 sets of human remains contained in depositories at any given time. This situation has been termed a silent, slow, mass disaster. In many instances, radiologic evaluation of human remains can identify potential objective points of concordance and, with some degree of age stratification, can suggest a possible match of this set of human remains to a missing person. Many agencies attempt to provide this service, including the NamUs (National Missing and Unidentified Persons System), NCIC (National Crime Information Center), and INTERPOL. These agencies use methods of coding the features of the dentition that facilitate the comparison process. In most cases, this comparison process is ongoing and updated at regular intervals. Once the information for a set of remains is entered into one or more databases, it remains there until an identification is made. Similarly, antemortem records remain on the database until the person returns (in the case of a missing person) or until a match to postmortem remains is made. The information in some of these programs is available for public view on websites, whereas other programs keep the information exclusively for law enforcement. Generally, the wider the dissemination of this information, the greater is the benefit. Also, and perhaps counterintuitively, for best results the less dental minutiae entered into the coding system, the better. The presence of excessive detail increases the chance of false rejection of a match.

RESOURCES

Adams BJ: The diversity of adult dental patterns in the United States and the implications for personal identification, *J Forensic Sci* 48:497–503, 2003.

American Board of Forensic Odontology: http://www.abfo.org/.

Kirk NJ, Wood RE, Goldstein M: Skeletal identification using the frontal sinus region: a retrospective study of 39 cases, *J Forensic Sci* 47: 318–323, 2002.

National Research Council: Strengthening forensic science in the United States: a path forward (2009): http://www.nap.edu/catalog .php?record_id=12589.

Saks MJ, Koehler JJ: The coming paradigm shift in forensic identification science, *Science* 309:892–895, 2005.

Wood RE, Kirk NJ, Sweet DJ: Digital dental radiographic identification in the pediatric, mixed and permanent dentitions, *J Forensic Sci* 44:910–916, 1999.

Dental Identification Websites

DVI guide: www.interpol.int/Media/Files/INTERPOL-Expertise/DVI/ DVI-Guide.

WinID3: www.winid.com/.

Missing Persons Websites

British Columbia: Ministry of Public Safety and Solicitor General, Unidentified Human Remains in B.C.: http://www.missing-u.ca/ britishcolumbia.htm.

FBI: NCIC Missing Person and Unidentified Person Statistics for 2010: http://www.fbi.gov/about-us/cjis/ncic/ncic-missing-person-and -unidentified-person-statistics-for-2010.

National Institute of Justice (U.S.): Missing persons and unidentified remains: the nation's silent mass disaster: http://www.nij.gov/ journals/256/missing-persons.html.

National Missing and Unidentified Persons System (NamUs): http://www.namus.gov/.

OPP: Missing Persons and Unidentified Bodies Unit: http://www.missing-u.ca/.

Index

Page numbers followed by f indicate figures; t, tables; b, boxes.